W9-BCL-944

SECOND EDITION

BEST PRACTICES for
Occupational Therapy
in Schools

Edited by Gloria Frolek Clark, PhD, OTR/L, BCPP, SCSS, FAOTA;
Joyce E. Rioux, EdD, OTR/L, SCSS; and
Barbara E. Chandler, PhD, OTR/L, FAOTA

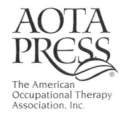
AOTA PRESS
The American
Occupational Therapy
Association, Inc.

AOTA Vision 2025
Occupational therapy maximizes health, well-being, and quality of life for all people, populations, and communities through effective solutions that facilitate participation in everyday living.

Mission Statement
The American Occupational Therapy Association advances occupational therapy practice, education, and research through standard-setting and advocacy on behalf of its members, the profession, and the public.

AOTA Staff
Sherry Keramidas, *Executive Director*
Christopher M. Bluhm, *Chief Operating Officer*

Chris Davis, *Associate Chief Officer for AOTA Press and Content Strategy*
Caroline Polk, *Digital Manager and* AJOT *Managing Editor*
Ashley Hofmann, *Development/Acquisitions Editor*
Barbara Dickson, *Production Editor*

Rebecca Rutberg, *Director, Marketing*
Amanda Goldman, *Marketing Manager*
Jennifer Folden, *Marketing Specialist*

American Occupational Therapy Association, Inc.
4720 Montgomery Lane
Bethesda, MD 20814
Phone: 301-652-AOTA (2682)
TDD: 800-377-8555
Fax: 301-652-7711
www.aota.org
To order: 1-877-404-AOTA or store.aota.org

© 2019 by the American Occupational Therapy Association, Inc. All rights reserved.
No part of this book may be reproduced in whole or in part by any means without permission. Printed in the United States of America.

Disclaimers
This publication is designed to provide accurate and authoritative information in regard to the subject matter covered. It is sold or distributed with the understanding that the publisher is not engaged in rendering legal, accounting, or other professional service. If legal advice or other expert assistance is required, the services of a competent professional person should be sought.
—*From the Declaration of Principles jointly adopted by the American Bar Association and a Committee of Publishers and Associations*

It is the objective of the American Occupational Therapy Association to be a forum for free expression and interchange of ideas. The opinions expressed by the contributors to this work are their own and not necessarily those of the American Occupational Therapy Association.

ISBN: 978-1-56900-411-1
Ebook ISBN: 978-1-56900-591-0
Library of Congress Control Number: 2019934181

Cover design by Debra Naylor, Naylor Design, Inc., Washington, DC
Composition by Manila Typesetting Company, Makati City, Philippines
Printed by Automated Graphic Systems, White Plains, MD

Dedication

To our families who supported us throughout this project; to our colleagues whose research has provided evidence-based interventions for children; and to school practitioners who implement best practices to enhance the engagement and participation of students throughout their daily occupations.

Contents

Section I. Foundations of Occupational Therapy in Schools — 1

Section II. Evidence-Guided Practices: System-Level Considerations to Support Participation — 69

Section III.   Evidence-Guided Practices: Population-Level Considerations to Support Participation — 209

Figures, Tables, Exhibits, and Case Examples

Exhibits

Case Examples

About the Editors

Gloria Frolek Clark, PhD, OTR/L, BCP, SCSS, FAOTA, received a bachelor's degree in occupational therapy from the University of North Dakota and a doctorate in human development and family studies (early childhood special education) from Iowa State University (ISU). She was part of ISU's early childhood special education leadership grant program, funded through the U.S. Office of Special Education Programs.

Dr. Frolek Clark has worked more than 40 years in early intervention and school practice in addition to 15 years as a state consultant at the Iowa Department of Education. She was cofounder and first chairperson of the American Occupational Therapy Association's (AOTA's) Early Intervention and School Special Interest Section, member of the Commission on Practice, member of the Pediatric Specialty Board, and liaison to the School System Specialty Certification Panel. Dr. Frolek Clark has coauthored multiple book chapters, AOTA official documents, and systematic reviews. She is coeditor of *Best Practices for Documenting Occupational Therapy Services in Schools.* Currently, Dr. Frolek Clark works with children and their families in a community-based program, presents nationally on a variety of topics, and consults with educational agencies to enhance effectiveness of services. She is an AOTA Board Director.

Joyce E. Rioux, EdD, OTR/L, SCSS, is the Assistant Director of Therapies at the Capitol Region Education Council in Connecticut. She received her bachelor's degree in occupational therapy from Quinnipiac College (now Quinnipiac University), her master's degree in educational technology from Central Connecticut State University, and her doctorate in educational leadership from the University of Hartford.

Dr. Rioux has more than 35 years' experience in school system practice. At the local level, she is an advocate for promoting and protecting the full scope of occupational therapy practice in schools. She has co-led and actively contributed to the writing, editing, and publication of the current occupational therapy guidelines for Connecticut's schools. She is an active member of ConnOTA and participates in a local school focus group along with a dedicated group of occupational therapy practitioners. At the national level, Dr. Rioux is a member of the AOTA Commission on Continuing Competence and Professional Development. She also serves as chair of the AOTA Board for Advanced and Specialty Certification and in this role actively monitors trends in occupational therapy practice. She was instrumental in leading 2 Ad Hoc Panels to determine the need for and then develop a School System Specialty Certification. Dr. Rioux presents at local, state, and national conferences on topics specific to school therapy practice and professional development.

Barbara E. Chandler, PhD, OTR/L, FAOTA, has been an occupational therapist for more than 40 years. She received a bachelor of arts in American studies and sociology from the University of Tennessee and a master's in occupational therapy from Western Michigan University. She has a doctorate in educational leadership (higher education administration).

Dr. Chandler worked in the schools and operated a private practice in western North Carolina for 12 years before serving as the first AOTA pediatric program manager from 1988 to 1993. She worked in academia and practice (e.g., home health, early intervention) and provided consultation services through her private practice, Therapeutic Services and Design. Dr. Chandler has lectured and written extensively on occupational therapy services under the Individuals With Disabilities Education Act, including editing *Early Childhood: Occupational Therapy Services for Children Birth to Five* (AOTA Press, 2010). She served as chairperson of the AOTA Early Intervention and School Special Interest Section from 1993 to 1996. She recently retired to her mountain home in beautiful Virginia.

About the Contributors

Rebecca E. Argabrite Grove, MS, OTR/L, FAOTA
Practice Manager, Governance, Leadership Development,
    and International
American Occupational Therapy Association
Bethesda, MD

Rachel Ashcraft, OTR/L, TBRI® Practitioner
Founder
Foster the Future Alabama
Clinical Supervisor
Child'sPlay Therapy Center
Birmingham

Sue Bainter, MA, OTR/L
Getting Ready Coach
University of Nebraska–Lincoln

Susan Bazyk, PhD, OTR/L, FAOTA
Director
Every Moment Counts, LLC
Professor Emerita, Master of Occupational Therapy
    Program
Cleveland State University
Cleveland

Christopher M. Bluhm, CAE, CPA, CMA
Chief Operating Officer
American Occupational Therapy Association
Bethesda, MD

Ellenmarie Brady, OTD, OTR/L, RN
Private Practice
Adjunct Faculty, Department of Occupational Therapy
New York University
Staten Island

Susan M. Cahill, PhD, OTR/L, FAOTA
Occupational Therapy Program Director and Associate
    Professor
Lewis University
Romeoville, IL

Catherine Candler, OTR, PhD, BCP
Professor
Abilene Christian University
Abilene, TX

Barbara E. Chandler, PhD, OTR/L, FAOTA
Therapeutic Services and Design
Winchester, VA

Gloria Frolek Clark, PhD, OTR/L, BCP, SCSS, FAOTA
Owner, Gloria Frolek Clark, LLC
Adel, IA
Adjunct Professor of Occupational Therapy
Drake University
Des Moines, IA

Sherrilene Classen, PhD, MPH, OTR/L, FAOTA, FGSA
Professor and Chair
Department of Occupational Therapy
College of Public Health and Health Professions
University of Florida
Gainesville

Cynthia Clough, PhD, OT/L
Assistant Professor
Mount Mary University
Milwaukee

Cheryl Colangelo, MS, OT/L
Instructor in Clinical Rehabilitation Medicine
Columbia University
New York

Shannon Corkrean, MOT/L
Heartland Area Education Agency
Johnston, IA

Lisa A. Crabtree, PhD, OTR/L, FAOTA
Department of Occupational Therapy
    and Occupational Science
Towson University
Towson, MD

Winnie Dunn, PhD, OTR, FAOTA
Distinguished Professor
University of Missouri
Columbia

Christina M. Edelbrock, MA, OTR/L, BCP, SCSS
Occupational Therapy Team Coordinator
Munroe–Meyer Institute, University of Nebraska
    Medical Center
Omaha

Charlotte E. Exner, PhD, OT/L, FAOTA
Department of Occupational Therapy
    and Occupational Science
Towson University
Towson, MD

Sarah E. Fabrizi, PhD, OTR/L
Occupational Therapy Program
Department of Rehabilitation Sciences
Marieb College of Health and Human Services
Florida Gulf Coast University
Fort Myers

Alyssa M. Fagan, OTD, OTR/L, LMT
Cooke School & Institute
New York
Private Practice
Brooklyn

Elizabeth A. Fain, EdD, OTR/L
Occupational Therapy Program Director/Associate Dean
    of Applied Health Sciences
Pfeiffer University
Misenheimer, NC

Jayna Fischbach, OTD, OTR/L, BCP
Assistant Professor, Occupational Therapy Department
Drake University
Des Moines
Senior Advisor of Occupational Therapy Services
DotCom Therapy
Des Moines

Janice Harman Flegle, MA, OTR/L, BCP
Director, Occupational Therapy, and Associate Professor
Munroe–Meyer Institute, University of Nebraska
    Medical Center
Omaha

Jane Galvin, MOT
Senior Occupational Therapist
Victorian Paediatric Rehabilitation Service
The Royal Children's Hospital
Melbourne, Victoria, Australia

Elizabeth Goodrich, OTR, ATP, PhD, FAOTA
Related Services Team Lead
Tomball Independent School District
Tomball, TX

Lenin C. Grajo, PhD, EdM, OTR/L
Director, Post-Professional Doctor of Occupational Therapy
    (OTD) Program
Assistant Professor, Programs in Occupational Therapy
Department of Rehabilitation and Regenerative Medicine
Vagelos College of Physicians and Surgeons
Columbia University
New York

Meredith P. Gronski, OTD, OTR/L, CLA
Director and Assistant Professor, OTD Program
Methodist University
Fayetteville, NC

Dottie Handley-More, MS, OTR/L, FAOTA
Highline Public Schools
Burien, WA
Assistant Clinical Professor, Division
    of Occupational Therapy
University of Washington
Seattle

Barbara Hanft, MA, OTR, FAOTA
Developmental Consultant
Kill Devil Hills, NC

Lauren Holahan, PhD, OT/L, FAOTA
Occupational Therapy and Medicaid Consultant,
    Exceptional Children Division
North Carolina Department of Public Instruction
Associate Professor, Division of Occupational Science/
    Occupational Therapy
University of North Carolina at Chapel Hill

Jan Hollenbeck, OTD, OTR
Medford Public Schools
Medford, MA
Partnership for Advancement of School Service-Providers,
    LLC
Watertown, MA

Elizabeth G. Hunter, PhD, OTR/L
Assistant Professor
Graduate Center for Gerontology
University of Kentucky
Lexington

Leslie L. Jackson, DrOT, MEd, OT/L, FAOTA
Assistant Professor and Program Coordinator, Occupational
    Therapy
Chicago State University
Chicago

Amanda C. Jozkowski, PhD, OTR/L
Assistant Professor, Graduate Faculty
Department of Occupational Therapy and Occupational
    Science
Towson University
Towson, MD

Heather Kuhaneck, PhD, OTR/L, FAOTA
Associate Professor
Sacred Heart University
Fairfield, CT

Jessica Lampert, OTR, PhD, COMS, CLVT
Occupational Therapist, Therapy 2000
Private Practice Orientation and Mobility Specialist
Dallas

Patricia Laverdure, OTD, OTR/L, BCP
Assistant Professor
Department of Occupational Therapy
Virginia Commonwealth University
Richmond

Deborah Lieberman, MHSA, OTR/L, FAOTA
Director, Evidence-Based Practice Project
Staff Liaison to the Commission on Practice
American Occupational Therapy Association
Bethesda, MD

Amy K. Lynch, PhD, TBRI® Educator, OTR/L, SCFES
Associate Professor, Program of Occupational Therapy
College of Public Health
Temple University
Philadelphia

Lucy Jane Miller, PhD, OTR
Associate Clinical Professor, Department of Pediatrics
University of Colorado Denver
Professor of Pediatrics
Rocky Mountain University of Health Profession
    Graduate Program
Provo, UT

Miriam Monahan, OTD, OTR/L, CDRS, CDI
Dominican University of California
San Rafael, CA

Elizabeth O. Morejon, OTD, OTR/L, C–SIPT
President, Best Onsite Therapy Services, Inc.
School Board of Broward County
Adjunct Professor, Occupational Therapy Program
Florida International University
Miami

Christine Teeters Myers, PhD, OTR/L
Clinical Associate Professor and Program Director
Department of Occupational Therapy
University of Florida
Gainesville

Rebecca Nicholson, OTD, OTR/L
University of Kansas Medical Center
Kansas City

Laurette Olson, PhD, OTR/L, FAOTA
Professor and Program Director
Graduate Occupational Therapy Program
Iona College
New Rochelle, NY

Meira L. Orentlicher, PhD, OTR/L, FAOTA
Professor and Associate Director of Research
    and Scholarship
Occupational Therapy Department
Touro College
New York City and Bay Shore, NY

Mara C. Podvey, PhD, OTR
Associate Professor, Department of Occupational Therapy
Seton Hall University
South Orange, NJ
Co-Owner, Maternal Insights, LLC
West Caldwell, NJ

Jean E. Polichino, OTR, MS, FAOTA
Jean Polichino Consulting, LLC
Fredricksburg, TX

Michelle Ponsolle-Mays, MS, OTR/L
OT and PT Team Lead
Related Services Facilitator
Community High School District 155
Crystal Lake, IL

Matthew Press, MHS, OTR/L, ATP
Assistive Technology Specialist–Peoria Unified School
    District
Coordinator of Graduate Certificate in AT
Northern Arizona University
Peoria

Jo Smith Read, PhD
Curriculum Director
Vance Charter School
Henderson, NC

Kathlyn L. Reed, PhD, MLIS, OTR, FAOTA
Self-Employed
Houston, TX

Elizabeth Richardson, MS, OTR/L
Academic Fieldwork Coordinator
Department of Health Professions
James Madison University
Harrisonburg, VA

Joyce E. Rioux, EdD, OTR/L, SCSS
Assistant Director of Therapies
Capitol Region Education Council
Windsor, CT

Sandra Schefkind, OTD, OTR/L, FAOTA
Pediatric Practice Manager
American Occupational Therapy Association
Bethesda, MD

Gretchen Scheibel, MS, OTR/L, BCBA
Gretchen Scheibel Consulting, LLC
Portland, ME

Colleen Schneck, ScD, OTR/L, FAOTA
Chair and Part-Time Associate Dean
Department of Occupational Science and Occupational
    Therapy
College of Health Sciences
Eastern Kentucky University
Richmond

Elizabeth Schneider, EdS, OTR/L, BCP
Boulder Valley School District
Boulder, CO

Judith Schoonover, MEd, OTR/L, ATP, FAOTA
Specialized Instructional Facilitator–Assistive Technology
Loudoun County Public Schools
Ashburn, VA

Winifred Schultz-Krohn, PhD, OTR/L, BCP, SWC, FAOTA
Professor and Chair of Occupational Therapy
San Jose State University
San Jose, CA

Deborah B. Schwind, DHSc, MEd, OTR/L
Loudoun County Public Schools
Ashburn, VA
Adjunct Professor, OTA Program
Northern Virginia Community College
Springfield

Jayne Shepherd, MS, OTR/L, FAOTA
Rural Infant Services Program
Middle Peninsula and Northern Neck Community Services Board
Urbanna, VA

Susan Englert Shutrump, OTR/L
Supervisor OT/PT Services
Trumbull County Educational Service Center
Niles, OH

Meghan E. Spielman, COTA/L
East Windsor Public Schools,
East Windsor, CT

Virginia Spielmann, MSOT
Executive Director
STAR Institute for Sensory Processing Disorder
Greenwood Village, CO

Pam Stephenson, OTD, OTR/L
Assistant Professor
Occupational Therapy Program
Murphy Deming College of Health Sciences
Fishersville, VA

Meghan Suman, OTD, OTR/L, BCP, SCSS
Assistant Professor
Lewis University
Romeoville, IL

Yvonne Swinth, PhD, OTR/L, FAOTA
Professor and Department Chair
University of Puget Sound
Editor, *Journal of Occupational Therapy: Schools and Early Intervention*
Co-chair, Washington Occupational Therapy Association OT in the Schools
Tacoma, WA

Steven D. Taff, PhD, OTR/L, FNAP, FAOTA
Director
Division of Professional Education
Washington University Program in Occupational Therapy
St. Louis

Lisa Tekell, OTD, OTR/L
Private Practice
Mediapolis, IA

Renee Watling, PhD, OTR/L, FAOTA
Visiting Assistant Professor
School of Occupational Therapy
University of Puget Sound
Tacoma, WA

Lorienne Watson, DrOT, MOT, OTR/L
Occupational Therapist
Miami-Dade County Public Schools
Adjunct Lecturer
Florida International University
Miami

Naomi Weintraub, PhD, OTR
Head, Neuro-Developmental Disabilities and Writing Research Laboratory
School of Occupational Therapy, Faculty of Medicine
Hadassah-Hebrew University of Jerusalem
Jerusalem, Israel

Amy Russell Yun, OTD, MS, OTR/L
Assistant Professor, Occupational Therapy Program
Department of Health Professions
James Madison University
Harrisonburg, VA

Foreword

When I was asked to write the foreword to this second edition of *Best Practices for Occupational Therapy in Schools,* I was surprised, delighted, and more than a little intimidated. I am not an occupational therapy practitioner. I wondered whether I had the grounding to convey the importance of this volume to the vast number of occupational therapy practitioners who work in schools today. To answer this question, I looked to the foreword written for the original edition. In that piece, Drs. Dunn and Rourk wrote from the perspective of changes across the time span of a career. They captured the essential changes that were once seen as unimaginable, and they chronicled the adaptive responses that the field of occupational therapy made in response to those changes. They recounted the foundational role for related services in the Education for All Handicapped Children Act of 1975 (Pub. L. 94–12) and expressed their faith in the ability of a new generation of occupational therapy practitioners to face the continuing challenges.

In reading the words of these occupational therapy icons, I realized that I follow them, not as an occupational therapy professional but as a witness to the ongoing changes and new roles that professionals must undertake together to improve the academic, social, emotional, and life outcomes for individuals with disabilities. In that role, I am confident.

I will forever be grateful to have assumed the directorship of a new national initiative at the National Association of State Directors of Special Education (NASDSE) following the landmark 1997 amendments to the Individuals With Disabilities Education Act (IDEA; Pub. L. 105–117). These amendments were a guide to a new kind of educational environment for individuals with disabilities. Like Drs. Dunn and Rourk, I found that practices we take for granted today were contentious just 20 years ago. The 1997 amendments placed access to the general curriculum in the national spotlight. A focus on placement-neutral funding formulas made it less advantageous to service students in a segregated environment and more fundable to serve them in an integrated setting. The introduction of positive behavioral interventions and supports helped us to understand the importance of proactive strategies and the connection between behavior and learning. The demand to act on what we know launched a national priority for evidence-based practice and data-based decision making. To benefit from these changes, we—policymakers, administrators, practitioners, and families—needed to learn together. Into this landscape, more than 50 national organizations entered as partners.

Through NASDSE's IDEA Partnership, we looked at issues across disciplines. We learned why we each cared about these issues, what we each knew, and what work was already underway. We identified messaging and action we could advance through our own networks. We worked on issues in which we had shared interests to make it safer to talk about areas in which we had little agreement. We kept our organizational identities while we acted as partners. Moreover, we modeled what it meant to be in this work together.

For the American Occupational Therapy Association (AOTA), this collaboration was natural. Soon occupational therapy practitioners at the national, state, and local levels were leading activities in the IDEA Partnership. Occupational therapy practitioners played a key role in translating response to intervention to practitioners and families who were steeped in medical models of disability. Practitioners brought new attention to their role in school-to-career or school-to-community transition when occupational therapy services were underused in secondary settings. They played lead roles in bridging education and mental health and helped to define the ways in which connectedness could advance wellness.

As an organization, AOTA built communities of practice among its members, creating a venue for practitioner wisdom to be acknowledged, connected to, and active in national work on issues. With its openness to learning from and with the field, AOTA became an exemplar of organizational ability to influence practice change.

Given this history of leading and implementing change, it is no surprise that AOTA is on the forefront of the newest changes. With the passage of the Every Student Succeeds Act (ESSA; 2015; Pub. L. 114–95), related service providers were recognized for their important role in advancing school success. Under ESSA, these practitioners are identified as specialized instructional support personnel. This change foreshadows some important new work ahead in ESSA as it is implemented and in IDEA as it is reauthorized. In this edition, occupational therapy leaders from across the nation show the profession's preparation to assume those roles.

Many thanks to the editors for the invitation to write this foreword and for all the work on this critical update of the original volume; to Sandy Schefkind for her unwavering support for working across groups; and to the many occupational therapy leaders across the nation whose stories of practice change have emboldened new approaches to interprofessional learning and work.

—**Joanne Cashman, EdD**
Senior Advisor, National Center for Systemic Improvement, and Former Director, IDEA Partnership, National Association of State Directors of Special Education Alexandria, VA

REFERENCES

Education for All Handicapped Children Act of 1975, Pub. L. 94–142, renamed the Individuals With Disabilities Education Improvement Act, codified at 20 U.S.C. §§ 1400–1482.

Every Student Succeeds Act, Pub. L. 114–95, 129 Stat. 1802 (2015).

Individuals With Disabilities Education Act Amendments of 1997, Pub. L. 105–117.

Introduction

Gloria Frolek Clark, PhD, OTR/L, BCP, SCSS, FAOTA; Joyce E. Rioux, EdD, OTR/L, SCSS; and Barbara E. Chandler, PhD, OTR/L, FAOTA

The *Philosophical Base of Occupational Therapy* (American Occupational Therapy Association [AOTA], 2017b, p. 1) states, "The focus and outcome of occupational therapy are clients' engagement in meaningful occupations that support their participation in life situations."

The first edition of *Best Practices for Occupational Therapy in Schools* (Frolek Clark & Chandler, 2013) served as a single source of current school occupational therapy topics. It described best practices in how occupational therapy practitioners could support students' engagement in meaningful school occupations. Before its publication, little had been written about the role of occupational therapy in schools on many of these topics. The book served to fill this gap as national and international leaders immersed in school occupations and school practice conveyed their specialized knowledge and expertise in each chapter.

The occupational therapy profession's scope in schools has expanded, and thus the 2nd edition of this book adds new topics. In response to changes in several federal laws, the responsibilities of school occupational therapy practitioners are now interwoven at all levels of the school system. These responsibilities include services at the school district and building levels, participation on various school teams, and service provision with students in general education, students considered at risk for academic and behavior needs, students with a 504 plan, and students with an individualized education program (IEP). In addition to being related services (Individuals With Disabilities Education Improvement Act of 2004 [IDEA]; Pub. L. 108–446), occupational therapy practitioners are now specialized instructional support personnel under the 2015 reauthorization of the Elementary and Secondary Education Act of 1965 (Pub. L. 89–313), known as the Every Student Succeeds Act (ESSA; Pub. L. 114–95).

As a result of conversations with practitioners, parents, school administrators, and educational staff, many new topics have been added to this new edition. Previous chapters have been rearranged or absorbed into other chapters. All of the material in this book has been updated to acknowledge the changing landscape in school practice (e.g., emergent roles and responsibilities, emphasis on school improvement and accountability, new developments in research and evidence-based interventions, changes in federal laws and regulations). Table I.1 provides a quick overview of the book's layout. This edition expands on the 1st edition's original purpose and communicates the distinct value of occupational therapy in schools using language from the *Occupational Therapy Practice Framework: Domain and Process* (3rd ed.; AOTA, 2014).

AOTA's (2015) *Standards of Practice for Occupational Therapy* requires occupational therapy practitioners to be knowledgeable about evidence-based research and apply it ethically and appropriately to provide services that are consistent with best practices. Each chapter provides a summary of the evidence on the topic and links for additional information. In Appendix H, "Evidence-Based Practice and Occupational Therapy in Schools," the strength-of-evidence table used within AOTA and the one described in ESSA (U.S. Department of Education, 2016) are compared. School occupational therapy practitioners should understand both versions and be aware of evidence that supports their interventions in schools. Although these chapters summarize current research, ongoing rigorous research is still needed in many areas.

CONCLUSION

New education initiatives and laws have shaped general and special education and related services across the nation. We challenge occupational therapy practitioners to demonstrate occupational therapy's distinct value as an evidence-based profession and to be effective leaders in this setting by providing services at the systems, population, and individual levels. We hope this text promotes best school practices, education, research, and policy across the nation.

(Continued)

TABLE I.1.   Overview of Second Edition

SECTION	SUMMARY OF CONTENT	NEW TOPICS IN 2ND EDITION
I. Foundations of Occupational Therapy in Schools	History of occupational therapy in schools; using the *OTPF–3* (AOTA, 2014); laws; ethical reasoning; education and fieldwork that emphasizes school practice; role of the OTA; occupational therapy practitioners as administrators	Preparation to practice in schools; practitioners as administrators
II. Evidence-Guided Practices: System-Level Considerations to Support Participation	Advocacy; supporting access; supporting families; teaming; conflicts; workloads; program evaluation; Medicaid cost recovery, literacy and STEM skills, school health and wellness, school mental health, UDL, AT, transportation, and transition	Everyday advocacy; supporting family engagement; addition of STEM to literacy chapter; secondary transition split into planning for postsecondary settings and planning for independent living and workplace settings
III. Evidence-Guided Practices: Population-Level Considerations to Support Participation	MTSS; 504 plans; various IDEA educational disability categories	Chapter on ADHD; childhood trauma
IV. Evidence-Guided Practices: Service-Level Considerations to Support Participation	Evaluation and planning; intervention; group interventions; telehealth; services in nonpublic schools and homeschooling; documentation and data collection	Group interventions; telehealth; nonpublic schools and homeschooling
V. Evidence-Guided Practices: Supporting Occupations to Enhance Student Participation	ADLs; IADLs; school mealtimes; handwriting and written expression; reading; play, leisure, and extracurricular activities; driving; social participation	Written expression; reading
VI. Evidence-Guided Practices: Addressing Performance Skills to Enhance Student Participation	Cognition and EF; fine motor skills; motor skills; sensory processing skills; visual perception and visual–motor skills	
Appendixes	Future of occupational therapy in schools; sample occupational profile; sample occupational therapy intervention plan; templates for reviewing program documentation; examples of common assessment tools; evidence-based practice; professional liability; *Guidelines for Occupational Therapy Services in Early Intervention and Schools* (AOTA, 2017a).	All are new.

Note. ADHD = attention deficit hyperactiviy disorder; ADLs = activities of daily living; AOTA = American Occupational Therapy Association; AT = assistive technology; EF = executive functioning; IDEA = Individuals With Disabilities Education Improvement Act of 2004; MTSS = multi-tiered systems of support; OTA = occupational therapy assistant; *OTPF–3 = Occupational Therapy Practice Framework: Domain and Process* (3rd ed.); STEM = science, technology, engineering, and math; UDL = universal design for learning.

REFERENCES

American Occupational Therapy Association. (2014). Occupational therapy practice framework: Domain and process (3rd ed.). *American Journal of Occupational Therapy, 68*(Suppl. 1), S1–S48. https://doi.org/10.5014/ajot.2014.682006

American Occupational Therapy Association. (2015). Standards of practice for occupational therapy. *American Journal of Occupational Therapy, 64*(Suppl.), S106–S111. https://doi.org/10.5014/ajot.2010.64S106

American Occupational Therapy Association. (2017a). Guidelines for occupational therapy services in early intervention and schools. *American Journal of Occupational Therapy, 71*(Suppl. 2), 7112410010. https://doi.org/10.5014/ajot.2017.716S01

American Occupational Therapy Association. (2017b). Philosophical base of occupational therapy. *American Journal of Occupational Therapy, 71*(Suppl. 2), 7112410045. https://doi.org/10.5014/ajot.2017.716S06

Elementary and Secondary Education Act of 1965, Pub. L. 89–313, 20 U.S.C. §§ 2701–3386.

Every Student Succeeds Act, Pub. L. 114–95, 129 Stat. 1802 (2015).

Frolek Clark, G., & Chandler, B. (Eds.). (2013). *Best practices for occupational therapy in schools.* Bethesda, MD: AOTA Press.

Individuals With Disabilities Education Improvement Act of 2004, Pub. L. 108–446, 20 U.S.C. §§ 1400–1482.

U.S. Department of Education (2016). *Non-regulatory guidance: Using evidence to strengthen education investments.* Retrieved from https://ed.gov/policy/elsec/leg/essa/guidanceuseseinvestment.pdf

SECTION I.

Foundations of Occupational Therapy in Schools

Joyce E. Rioux, EdD, OTR/L, SCSS, and Barbara E. Chandler, PhD, OTR/L, FAOTA

KEY TERMS AND CONCEPTS

- Collaborative consultation
- Communities of practice
- Educationally relevant perspective

In these days, it is doubtful that any child may reasonably be expected to succeed in life if he is denied the opportunity of an education. Such an opportunity, where the state has undertaken to provide it, is a right that must be made available to all on equal terms.—Chief Justice Earl Warren, *Brown v. Board of Education of Topeka* (1954, p. 493)

OVERVIEW

The preceding words from the landmark U.S. Supreme Court case *Brown v. Board of Education of Topeka* (1954) provided the foundation for American educational reform. Although this case centered on civil rights, deeming it unconstitutional to separate students on the basis of race, the case decision became the impetus for integration and equal educational opportunity for all, regardless of race, gender, or ability. Realized impacts from this case, along with subsequent cases and laws, have had a cumulative effect on improving school systems. In addition, these profound social, economic, and political changes have strengthened occupational therapy's philosophical base for practice in which "all individuals have an innate need and right to engage in meaningful occupations throughout their lives" (American Occupational Therapy Association [AOTA], 2017b, p. 1).

HISTORICAL HIGHLIGHTS

Studying the historical contexts of school occupational therapy allows one to realize the meaningful and valuable contributions that occupational therapy practitioners[1]

[1]*Occupational therapy practitioner* refers to both the occupational therapist and the occupational therapy assistant. AOTA (2014a, p. S18) states, "The occupational therapist is responsible for all aspects of occupational therapy service delivery and is accountable for the safety and effectiveness of the occupational therapy service delivery process" and "must be directly involved in the delivery of services during the initial evaluation and regularly throughout the course of intervention.... The occupational therapy assistant delivers safe and effective occupational therapy services under the supervision of and in partnership with the occupational therapist."

make every day in the lives of students, families, and educational personnel. For example, practitioners are collaborating with others, analyzing the activity and environment to promote engagement and performance, effectively problem solving to enhance participation, collecting data to monitor student progress, co-teaching with educators, and contemplating future actions in the ever-evolving system of education.

Unequal Access to Education

In the United States, public education is regarded as a birthright that yields educated citizens who participate in preserving democracy and benefiting society (Yell et al., 1998). In accordance with the Tenth Amendment to the U.S. Constitution, state governments are responsible for education. Following suit, in the mid-1800s to early 1900s, states passed compulsory education laws (i.e., laws regarding mandated education). Despite these early laws, children with disabilities were not afforded the same opportunities—those schools that did form classes for students with disabilities were restrictive and, at times, custodial in nature.

Early legal records provide insight into some of the ill-perceived perceptions of this population. For example, in 1893 a Massachusetts student was expelled for being too "weak minded" to benefit from instruction, and in 1919, a Wisconsin student with cerebral palsy was excluded on the notion that he would "produce a depressing and nauseating effect" on others (*Beattie v. Board of Education of Antigo*, 1919).

During the 1900s, various hospitals and homes for children with disabilities included an educational component (McMurtrie, 1913). Quite often, a teacher would go to the ward or be employed by the home to provide teaching sessions to those children who were well enough to benefit from instruction. The focus might have been on primary subjects or common trade areas (e.g., basketry, benchwork, cabinetmaking, printing, stenography). In the 1920s, these same children might have received occupational therapy aimed at restoring or minimizing the impact of their disability on functional skills (Quiroga, 1995).

Copyright © 2019 by the American Occupational Therapy Association. All rights reserved. To reuse this content, contact www.copyright.com.
https://doi.org/10.7139/2019.978-1-56900-591-0.001

Disability Rights and Free Appropriate Public Education

During the 1930s and 1940s, parents and concerned citizens, in response to the deplorable conditions that children with disabilities had to endure in their schooling, banded together to form local advocacy groups—groups that later unified at the national level (e.g., the National Association of Retarded Citizens, known today as The Arc; Yell et al., 1998). The aim of these groups was to seek human treatment and equal access to education for children with disabilities. At the same time, the civil rights movement to end racial segregation was at the forefront.

As a result of *Brown v. Board of Education* (1954), in which equal protection based on the Fourteenth Amendment to the U.S. Constitution was extended to a class (i.e., a group of individuals—specifically, in this case, racial minorities), families, educators, and advocates challenged both state and federal governments for equal educational opportunities and access for their representative class—that is, children with disabilities (Colman, 1988).

A growing number of class action suits filed across the country gained momentum at the state level for new opportunities and access to education for children with disabilities (Yell et al., 1998). Points brought forth consisted of the concept that children with mental retardation could learn and that education should address not only academic experiences but also functional living experiences (e.g., learning to dress and feed oneself). Another legal case, *Mills v. Board of Education of District of Columbia* (as cited in Yell et al., 1998), charged that children with disabilities were denied access to education without due process.

Despite the success of these lawsuits, pushback occurred at the district level, claiming insufficient funds as well as inadequate space, materials, and training. By the start of the 1970s, most states had passed laws—although they varied from state to state—that children with disabilities were required to receive a public education. Unfortunately, *public education* for this group was not clearly defined.

At the federal level, efforts were taking place to protect people with disabilities, starting with the passage of Section 504 of the Rehabilitation Act of 1973, as amended (2008; Pub. L. 92–112), which stated that

> no otherwise qualified handicapped individual in the United States . . . shall solely by reason of his handicap, be excluded from the participation in, be denied the benefits of, or be subjected to discrimination under any activity receiving Federal financial assistance. (Section 504, 29 U.S.C. § 794[a])

Soon after, in 1974, an amendment to the Elementary and Secondary Education Act of 1965 (Pub. L. 89–313) authorized federal special education funding for states. Unfortunately, many felt that the act was not enforceable. Not until the passage of the Education for All Handicapped Children Act of 1975 (EHA; Pub. L. 94–142) did change occur. This law outlined that children with disabilities were

- Entitled to a free appropriate public education;
- In the least restrictive environment;
- Provided nondiscriminatory testing, evaluation, and placement procedures; and
- Afforded procedural due process rights.

States were required to submit their own state plan (i.e., outlined policies and procedures for implementing special education and related services) for approval and receipt of federal funding.

Occupational Therapy as a Related Service

EHA forever changed the face of public education in both the workforce and the student body. For occupational therapy practitioners, it greatly changed the work setting (public school) and profoundly altered how services were conceptualized and provided. Familiar with the expectations of medical or residential facilities but less sure of what to do in educational environments, occupational therapy practitioners entered school practice with little to guide them except past experience, professional standards, and the definition of occupational therapy as a related service under EHA:

> *Occupational therapy* means services provided by a qualified occupational therapist and includes:
> (A) Improving, developing, or restoring functions impaired or lost through illness, injury, or deprivation;
> (B) Improving ability to perform tasks for independent functioning if functions are impaired or lost; and
> (C) Preventing, through early intervention, initial or further impairment or loss of function. (Individuals With Disabilities Education Improvement Act [IDEA] of 2004, 34 CFR § 300.34[6][ii])

Provisions of the landmark EHA had to be in place by Fall 1977, which left little time for occupational therapy practitioners to develop an *educationally relevant perspective*—that is, a perspective to provide services that supported the student's educational program. As a result, the medical or clinical model was "taken to school." The initial starting point of evaluations and interventions was centered on students' disability versus ability (Rourk, 1996).

At first, this model worked well because teachers and others were seeking assistance with the wide variety of needs presented by this new population of students. Wheelchairs, feeding tubes, braces, splints, medications, and the like were intimidating. Most special needs students (*student with a disability* was not common language at that time) were taught in special education classrooms away from typically developing peers, and they usually had teachers with some experience or training in special education.

School personnel had a perception that related services should occur in a separate area with therapy equipment, similar to a clinical model. Most occupational therapy practitioners initially addressed component parts of the disability in these separate rooms: reducing postural tone, promoting tripod prehension, and eliminating fisted grasps. Students were pulled out of class and unfortunately missed out on the very "free appropriate public education" so recently made available to them.

In some states, occupational therapy practitioners were not invited to attend individualized education program (IEP) meetings to identify students' needs and goals, or they initially did not know that they should participate. Barbara Chandler recalls a special education administrator saying, "I don't know what you do, but I trust you to know. So, go out to the schools and do it." Across the United States, occupational therapy practitioners soon realized they had a great opportunity. However, what occupational therapy practitioners were expected and allowed to do varied greatly from state to state and from district to district. School systems struggled to meet EHA's mandates without having sufficient funds to do everything. Procedural compliance became more important than what students learned or where and how they were educated.

Training for School Practice

AOTA recognized the need to provide advanced specialized training to school occupational therapists and responded by rolling out a competency-based, educational "train-the-trainer" program titled *Training Occupational Therapists in Educational Management Systems* (Gilfoyle & Hays, 1980). The 8 modules of this program focused on
- Knowledge of educational laws and ethical practice;
- Theories and techniques of group decision making;
- Assessments used by occupational therapists and those commonly used by other disciplines;
- Development of the IEP;
- Supervision and training for technical assistants; and
- Systems program planning, including understanding the difference between the educational model and the clinical model from an administrative, theoretical, and practical perspective.

By the late 1980s, large numbers of occupational therapy practitioners worked in schools (AOTA, 1990). Some preservice programs even started to incorporate curricula aimed at preparing occupational therapy students for entry into school practice (Griswold & Strassler, 1995; Powell, 1994). Understanding the role of a related service provider in schools was important, and understanding that "functional outcomes [were] more likely when therapeutic strategies [were] part of the performance of functional life skills" (Dunn & Westman, 1995, p. 2) was a new concept.

Misunderstandings in Determining Need for Occupational Therapy

Not understanding that the determination of eligibility for special education allowed a student access to any related service, many school districts required occupational therapists to develop criteria to "qualify" students for occupational therapy services. Instead of drawing on the process already established by IDEA for determining eligibility for special education and the need for related services (§ 1414), occupational therapists attempted to develop criteria along with accompanying decision-making strategies. One proposed approach developed in Pennsylvania consisted of a rating scale for interpreting a student's functional levels combined with the therapist's clinical judgment to determine a student's intervention need (Farley et al., 1991). The rating scale appeared to align with the second edition of AOTA's (1989) *Uniform Terminology for Occupational Therapy* (the current edition at that time), with a focus on performance areas and components.

At this same time, some states relied on standardized assessment scores as the determining basis for receiving occupational therapy, whereas other states considered the
- Impact on students' daily life skills,
- Teachers' knowledge and skills to implement specialized programming, and
- Identified supports and barriers in the school environment.

In Iowa, where occupational therapy could be a stand-alone service on a student's IEP (considered support services that were specialized instruction or special education), an exit and entrance criteria form was developed to guide the team in decision making (Iowa Department of Education, 1988). Criteria centered on determining whether the problem interfered with students' participation in their educational program, aligned with occupational therapy's domain of practice, and required the expertise of the occupational therapist. Not until 1998, with the publication of School Function Assessment (Coster et al., 1998), did occupational therapists have a measure to examine what students needed to do in school (i.e., their levels of participation and performance across school environments and occupations).

Around this time, various service models and team programming were being considered to create successful learning environments for students (Campbell, 1987; Dunn, 1988, 1991). The notion of ***collaborative consultation*** was brought into play, in which educational team members were viewed as equal partners with diverse expertise aimed at identifying creative solutions to meeting student needs (Friend & Cook, 1992). Occupational therapy practitioners in Iowa schools even provided short-term interventions for struggling learners in general education using a model similar to the current multi-tiered systems of support (MTSS; Tilly et al., 1993).

Response to a Nation at Risk

In the 1980s, the National Commission on Excellence in Education (NCEE) acknowledged that educational reform of the public schools was necessary. The document *A Nation at Risk* (NCEE, 1983) was released, reporting that the state of public education in America was "lax and ineffective" (p. 1). Rather dire predictions of the future of the nation followed, along with calls for educational reform.

The response to these predictions was the development of curriculum standards in specific content areas, followed by tests to measure whether students had mastered the curriculum content and at what level. Occupational therapy practitioners were practicing in schools against the backdrop of an ever-changing curriculum. Understanding the curriculum, adjusting interventions, and supporting students for optimal participation in general education became a primary focus (http://www.corestandards.org).

Introduction of IDEA and Medicaid Cost Recovery

The 1990 reauthorization of EHA was renamed the Individuals With Disabilities Education Act, or IDEA (Pub. L. 101–476), reflecting people-first language. At this time, many occupational therapy practitioners embraced working toward educationally relevant outcomes. These practitioners supported students' education, understood and practiced in educationally relevant ways, participated in IEP meetings, spoke on a regular basis with teachers, and partnered with teachers in classrooms.

In the 1990s, Medicaid (Social Security Act of 1965; Pub. L. 89–97) funds were sought as a source of revenue for schools. The federal government had never fully funded IDEA, so Medicaid funds were seen as a cost recovery by many school districts. Along with Medicaid billing, ethical issues rose to the forefront (Royeen et al., 2000). School occupational therapy practitioners struggled to understand the impact and whether an educational or clinical perspective should be applied, given the new reimbursement source. Many occupational therapists felt pressured by their administration to make decisions about related services on the basis of whether Medicaid could be billed. Over time, most of these issues were clarified and resolved, and practice returned to an educational focus in compliance with IDEA.

AOTA Support

In 1988, AOTA hired the first pediatric program manager within its Practice Department. At that time, most of AOTA's support to pediatric practitioners focused on defining and implementing occupational therapy practitioners' roles in schools and early intervention. Across 25 years, AOTA conducted 5 surveys aimed at capturing the number of practitioners moving into school practice and ascertaining what they were doing. Eventually, a great deal of data was obtained and interpreted to establish guidance for school practitioners and occupational therapy educators, as well as to build AOTA's advocacy efforts in this practice area (Chandler, 1995).

In 1993, AOTA's School System Special Interest Section (SSSIS) was formally recognized to address the needs of those working under IDEA, both Parts B and C. During the IDEA reauthorization process (which resulted in the IDEA Amendments of 1997, Pub. L. 105–117), the SSSIS chairperson, Gloria Frolek Clark, provided testimony to the congressional subcommittee for reauthorization of IDEA about the role of occupational therapy in schools (Individuals With Disabilities Education, 1995). In 2008, SSSIS's name was changed to the Early Intervention and School Special Interest Section (EISSIS) to make explicit the full range of services provided under IDEA. Effective in 2018, AOTA's Special Interest Sections (SISs) were restructured in an effort to enhance member participation and expand leadership opportunities (AOTA, 2017c). Under this new structure, EISSIS has been renamed *Children and Youth* to reflect a broader focus and scope. This should prove helpful in building greater collaboration across occupational therapy practitioners working with children and youth in different practice settings.

In 1993, AOTA took a large step in advocacy with the Promoting Partnerships project, which conducted leadership seminars attended by 36 state teams of occupational therapists and state administrators. The project emphasized strategic planning to address issues of common concern in schools and early intervention. A positive outcome was realized along with continued collaboration efforts with other national and state organizations concerned with students with special needs.

Many occupational therapists who participated in this project continued to advise AOTA for several years as a resource cadre, working with lobbyists and a practice associate who focused on pediatrics. This collaboration continued when AOTA created a pediatric coordinator position in 2007 to advocate and promote the goals of the occupational therapy profession in relation to AOTA's *Centennial Vision* (AOTA, 2007).

A key external affiliate has been the IDEA Partnership, in which AOTA has joined with more than 50 national, state, and local organizations; parent advocacy groups; and technical assistance centers that support shared learning and implementation of IDEA (National Association of State Directors of Special Education, n.d.). Modeled after this concept, AOTA established volunteer pediatric workgroups known as *communities of practice,* which are groups of occupational therapy practitioners who agree to regularly interact, typically through virtual meetings, to solve a persistent problem or improve practice in an area important to them (Davis, 2012). Volunteer members in these communities work to develop resources, share perspectives from their state and local areas, and engage in IDEA Partnership activities.

With the 2002 publication of the first *Occupational Therapy Practice Framework (OTPF)*, practitioners gained an increased understanding of occupational engagement and its relationship to health, wellness, and life satisfaction. Some school practitioners systematically remodeled their practices based on the *OTPF* process (McKinley-Vargas & Thomas, 2008). In addition, occupational therapy practitioners embedded supportive practices in educational environments, making these interventions part of everyday classroom experiences. Since its 2002 release, *OTPF* has had 2 subsequent editions (AOTA, 2008, 2014b) in accordance with being "an ever-evolving document . . . [that is] reviewed on a 5-year cycle for usefulness and the potential need for further refinements or changes" (AOTA, 2014b, p. S2).

In 2011, the AOTA Commission on Practice published an official document titled *Occupational Therapy Services in Early Intervention and Schools* (AOTA, 2011). This document was subsequent to earlier versions (AOTA, 1998, 2004), and it provided information about various federal and state laws that affect practice and identified the role of occupational therapists working in these settings. In 2017, this document, renamed *Guidelines for Occupational Therapy in Early Intervention and Schools,* was expanded to reflect current influences (e.g., regulatory and legislative, professional, environmental, contextual) that affect practice and further expand occupational therapy's role in early intervention and schools (AOTA, 2017a). These documents have been written for occupational therapy practitioners as well as school staff and administrators, regulatory and policy-making bodies, and others who seek clarification on the role of occupational therapy in these settings.

In 2013, AOTA added a Specialty Certification in School Systems to its advanced and specialty certification offerings (AOTA, n.d.). This was an initial step in gaining national support and an opportunity for individual occupational therapists and occupational therapy assistants to validate their competence in school practice. The application is built on a reflective portfolio that aligns with AOTA's (2015b) *Standards for Continuing Competence* as applied to specialty practice in schools.

In 2013, to support school practitioners, AOTA held the first Specialty Conference for School Occupational Therapy Practitioners. A second conference was held 4 years later, and attendance was so overwhelming that AOTA plans to hold an annual specialty conference to meet the professional development needs of this group. The 2018 specialty conference, in alignment with the restructuring of AOTA's SISs, included topics on children and youth in an effort to provide professional development and connect pediatric practitioners across school, early intervention, clinical, and community settings.

School Practice in the 21st Century

In the 21st century, school occupational therapy practitioners work not only with individual students but also with groups of students, the educational team, schools, and districts. Their professional contributions often extend to students under IDEA (2004), Section 504 of the Rehabilitation Act of 1973 (as amended), and general education through MTSS. With the recent authorization of the Every Student Succeeds Act (2015; Pub. L. 114–195), school occupational therapy practitioners, now considered as specialized instructional support personnel, are positioned for an even greater presence and involvement at the systems level. Initiatives focused on effective teaching, promoting positive school climates, reducing barriers to learning, addressing mental health, and offering a continuum of supports open the doors for school practitioners to make a difference in students' education. For example, occupational therapy practitioners' expertise in mental health is being increasingly acknowledged as they explicitly use and share what they know and can do in this area. As schools begin to embrace mental health as a necessary component of what supports and facilitates education, practitioners are acknowledging the profession's mental health roots and addressing these needs (Bayzk, 2011).

Results of a salary and workforce survey published by AOTA in 2015 indicated that approximately 25% of occupational therapists and 18% of occupational therapy assistants work in early intervention and school settings (AOTA, 2015a). Occupational therapy practitioners face new challenges and opportunities in schools. The areas of expertise in occupational therapy are recognized and highly valued, especially regarding students with autism spectrum disorder, students with feeding issues, use of assistive technology, literacy needs, and universal design for learning. Occupational therapy has become a part of education—not *apart from* education—as school occupational therapy practitioners blend their interventions within school environments (e.g., recess, classroom, lunchroom).

Occupational therapy practitioners have an obligation to ensure evidence-based practice in schools (IDEA uses the term *scientific research-based intervention;* 34 C.F.R. § 300.307). Occupational therapy, like all professions, is being challenged to provide evidence that its interventions are effective. Although research in school practice is growing, a critical need to investigate the efficacy of what occupational therapy practitioners do in schools remains (see Appendix H, "Evidence-Based Practice and Occupational Therapy").

In 2016, AOTA completed 2 documents sharing occupational therapy's distinct value—one designed for family (AOTA, 2016a) and another for administrators and policymakers (AOTA, 2016b). These documents cite current research to support the roles of occupational therapy practitioners and can be used as guides when speaking with others about the profession's distinct value. In 2018, a preliminary report on the systematic review project between AOTA staff and occupational therapists and occupational therapy students was presented at AOTA's Annual Conference & Expo and at the 2018 Children & Youth Specialty Conference. The presenters focused on research

- On mental health, positive behavior, and social participation;
- To improve learning and academic achievement; and
- To improve ADLs, IADLs, play, leisure, work, rest, and sleep for children to young adults ages 5–21 years.

The critically appraised topics will be uploaded to AOTA's website for members to review and use in their practice.

Individuals in the profession can readily see that many needs and opportunities that occupational therapy can address are still present in schools. For exemplary occupational therapy practice to continue and grow, it is essential for occupational therapy educational programs to teach best practices in schools and provide enough preservice evidence-based content and fieldwork preparation for a practice area that employs one-fourth of the individuals in the profession.

The history of the profession can trace back to the start of occupational therapy practitioners working in schools with a sense of accomplishment and pride and can look forward with anticipation to what practitioners will continue to do so that students with disabilities can learn and participate in the occupations of school. For occupational therapy services to continue to be effective, best practices in schools must be identified, articulated, developed, acknowledged, taught, mentored, and used daily.

Looking Forward

Looking to the future, school occupational therapy will continue to evolve. In preparation, occupational therapy practitioners should develop leadership roles in schools, on school boards, and in school districts. They must continue to conduct well-designed, multisite randomized controlled studies with large sample sizes in the school setting to determine the effectiveness of interventions for various types of clients (e.g., MTSS, schoolwide models, classroom models, groups of students with similar conditions, individual students). In addition, high-quality education and fieldwork sites for training future occupational therapists and occupational therapy assistants will be essential, as well as ongoing professional development for current school occupational therapy practitioners in all their professional domains.

Last, practitioners must communicate the profession's distinct value in their daily interactions and take advantage of the many resources, networking opportunities, and supports afforded through AOTA membership. Please read Appendix A, "The Future of Occupational Therapy Practice," with information that is based on feedback from occupational therapy practitioners across the United States.

SUMMARY

Occupational therapy is an educationally necessary and relevant service linked to education and health. Occupational therapy practitioners need to be articulate and explicit about what they do (occupational therapy), what they support (engagement and participation in daily occupations), how they do it (through engagement in activities and occupations), why they do it (to promote access, learning, health, and performance), and where they do it (in the least restrictive environments and within natural settings and routines that are meaningful and important to students).

REFERENCES

American Occupational Therapy Association. (1989). Uniform terminology for occupational therapy (2nd ed.). *American Journal of Occupational Therapy, 48,* 808–815. https://doi.org/10.5014/ajot.43.12.808

American Occupational Therapy Association. (1990). *1990 member data survey.* Rockville, MD: Author.

American Occupational Therapy Association. (1998). Occupational therapy for individuals with learning disabilities. *American Journal of Occupational Therapy, 52,* 874–880. https://doi.org/10.5014/ajot.52.10.874

American Occupational Therapy Association. (2002). Occupational therapy practice framework: Domain and process. *American Journal of Occupational Therapy, 56,* 609–639. https://doi.org/10.5014/ajot.56.6.609

American Occupational Therapy Association. (2004). Occupational therapy services in early intervention and school-based programs. *American Journal of Occupational Therapy, 58,* 681–685. https://doi.org/10.5014/ajot.58.6.681

American Occupational Therapy Association. (2007). AOTA's *Centennial Vision* and executive summary. *American Journal of Occupational Therapy, 61,* 613–614. https://doi.org/10.5014/ajot.61.6.613

American Occupational Therapy Association. (2008). Occupational therapy practice framework: Domain and process (2nd ed.). *American Journal of Occupational Therapy, 62,* 625–683. https://doi.org/10.5014/ajot.62.6.625

American Occupational Therapy Association. (2011). Occupational therapy services in early childhood and school-based settings. *American Journal of Occupational Therapy, 65*(Suppl. 6), S46–S54. https://doi.org/10.5014/ajot.2011.65S46

American Occupational Therapy Association. (2014a). Guidelines for supervision, roles, and responsibilities during the delivery of occupational therapy services. *American Journal of Occupational Therapy, 68*(Suppl. 3), S16–S22. https://doi.org/10.5014/ajot.2014.686S03

American Occupational Therapy Association. (2014b). Occupational therapy practice framework: Domain and process (3rd ed.). *American Journal of Occupational Therapy, 68*(Suppl. 1), S1–S48. https://doi.org/10.5014/ajot.2014.682006

American Occupational Therapy Association. (2015a). *2015 AOTA salary and workforce survey.* Bethesda, MD: AOTA Press.

American Occupational Therapy Association. (2015b). Standards for continuing competence. *American Journal of Occupational Therapy, 69*(Suppl. 3), 6913410057. https://doi.org/10.5014/ajot.2015.696S06

American Occupational Therapy Association. (2016a). *Occupational therapy's distinct value: Children and youth: Resource for administrators and policy makers.* Retrieved from https://www.aota.org/~/media/Corporate/Files/Secure/Practice/Children/distinct-value-policy-makers-children-youth.PDF

American Occupational Therapy Association. (2016b). *Occupational therapy's distinct value: Children and youth: Resource for family engagement.* Retrieved from https://www.aota.org/Practice/Children-Youth/distinct-value.aspx

American Occupational Therapy Association. (2017a). Guidelines for occupational therapy services in early intervention and schools. *American Journal of Occupational Therapy, 71*(Suppl. 2), S1–S10. https://doi.org/10.5014/ajot.2017.716S01

American Occupational Therapy Association. (2017b). Philosophical base of occupational therapy. *American Journal of Occupational Therapy, 71*(Suppl. 2), 7112410045. https://doi.org/10.5014/ajot.716S06

American Occupational Therapy Association. (2017c). *SIS restructure pilot to enhance engagement and flexibility.* Retrieved from https://www.aota.org/Practice/Manage/SIS/restructure.aspx

American Occupational Therapy Association. (n.d.). *Specialty certification in school systems.* Retrieved from https://www.aota.org/Education-Careers/Advance-Career/Board-Specialty-Certifications/School-system.aspx

Bayzk, S. (Ed.). (2011). *Mental health promotion, prevention, and intervention with children and youth: A guiding framework for occupational therapy.* Bethesda, MD: AOTA Press.

Beattie v. Board of Ed. of Antigo, 169 Wis. 231, 232, 172 N. W. 153 (1919).

Brown v. Board of Education of Topeka, 347 U.S. 483 (1954).

Campbell, P. (1987). The integrated programming team: An approach for coordinating professionals of various disciplines in programs for students with severe and multiple handicaps. *Journal of the Association for Persons With Severe Handicaps, 21,* 107–116. https://doi.org/10.1177/154079698701200204

Chandler, B. (1995, March). The school-based practice survey: What do we do with the results? *School System Special Interest Section Newsletter, 2,* 2–4.

Colman, W. (1988). The evolution of occupational therapy in the public schools: The laws mandating practice. *American Journal of Occupational Therapy, 42,* 701–705. https://doi.org/10.5014/ajot.42.11.701

Coster, W., Deeney, T., Haltiwanger, J., & Haley, S. (1998). *School Function Assessment.* San Antonio, TX: Harcourt.

Davis, N. (2012, June). School-based practice: Collaborative partnerships in a complex system. *Early Intervention and School Special Interest Section Quarterly, 19*(2), 1–4.

Dunn, W. (1988). Models of occupational therapy service provisions in the school system. *American Journal of Occupational Therapy, 42,* 718–723. https://doi.org/10.5014/ajot.42.11.718

Dunn, W. (1991). Integrated related services. In L. Meyer, C. S. Peck, & L. Brown (Eds.), *Critical issues in the lives of people with severe disabilities* (pp. 353–377). Baltimore: Paul H. Brookes.

Dunn, W., & Westman, K. (1995, March). Current knowledge that affects school-based practice and an agenda for action. *School System Special Interest Section Newsletter, 2,* 1–2.

Education for All Handicapped Children Act of 1975, Pub. L. 94–142, renamed the Individuals With Disabilities Education Improvement Act, codified at 20 U.S.C. §§ 1400–1482.

Elementary and Secondary Education Act of 1965, Pub. L. 89–313, 20 U.S.C. §§ 2701–3386.

Every Student Succeeds Act, Pub. L. 114–95, 129 Stat. 1802 (2015).

Farley, S., Sarracino, T., & Howard, P. (1991). Development of a treatment rating in school systems: Service determination through objective measurement. *American Journal of Occupational Therapy, 45,* 898–906. https://doi.org/10.5014/ajot.45.10.898

Friend, M., & Cook, L. (1992). *Interactions: Collaboration skills for school professionals.* White Plains, NY: Longmans.

Gilfoyle, E., & Hays, C. (1980). *Training occupational therapists in educational management systems (TOTEMS).* Rockville, MD: Author.

Griswold, L., & Strassler, B. (1995). Fieldwork in schools: A model for alternative settings. *American Journal of Occupational Therapy, 49,* 127–132. https://dx.doi.org/10.5014/ajot.49.2.127

Individuals With Disabilities Education Act of 1990, Pub. L. 101–476, renamed the Individuals With Disabilities Education Improvement Act, codified at 20 U.S.C. §§ 1400–1482.

Individuals With Disabilities Education Act Amendments of 1997, Pub. L. 105–117.

Individuals With Disabilities Education: Hearings before the Subcommittee on Early Childhood, Youth, and Families, of the Committee on Economic and Educational Opportunities, 104th Cong. D795 (1995) (testimony of Gloria Frolek Clark).

Individuals With Disabilities Education Improvement Act of 2004, Pub. L. 108–446, 20 U.S.C. §§ 1400–1482.

Iowa Department of Education. (1988). *Iowa guidelines for educationally related occupational therapy services.* Des Moines, IA: Iowa State Department.

McKinley-Vargas, J., & Thomas, K. (2008). A framework for change. *OT Practice, 13*(11), 10–15.

McMurtrie, D. (1913). *Bibliography of the education and care of crippled children.* New York: Author.

National Association of State Directors of Special Education. (n.d.). *Welcome to IDEA partnership.* Retrieved from http://www.ideapartnership.org/

National Commission on Excellence in Education. (1983). *A nation at risk: The imperative for educational reform.* Washington, DC: U.S. Government Printing Office.

Powell, N. (1994). Content for educational programs in school-based occupational therapy from a practice perspective. *American Journal of Occupational Therapy, 48,* 131–137. https://doi.org/10.5014/ajot.48.2.130

Quiroga, V. (1995). *Occupational therapy: The first 30 years, 1900–1930.* Bethesda, MD: American Occupational Therapy Association.

Rehabilitation Act of 1973, Pub. L. 93–112, 29 U.S.C. §§ 701–7961.

Rourk, J. D. (1996). Nationally Speaking—Roles for school-based occupational therapists: Past, present, future. *American Journal of Occupational Therapy, 50,* 698–700. https://doi.org/10.5014/ajot.59.9.698

Royeen, C. B., Duncan, M., Crabtree, J., Richards, J., & Clark, G. F. (2000). Effects of billing Medicaid for occupational therapy services in the schools: A pilot study. *American Journal of Occupational Therapy, 54,* 429–433. https://doi.org/10.5014/ajot.54.4.429

Section 504 of the Rehabilitation Act of 1973, as amended, 29 U.S.C. § 794 (2008).

Social Security Act Amendments of 1965, Pub. L. 89–97, 42 U.S.C. §§ 1395–1395kkk1 (Medicare) and 42 U.S.C. §§ 1396–1396w5 (Medicaid).

Tilly, W. D. III, Grimes, J., & Reschly, D. (1993, September–December). Special education system reform: The Iowa story. *Communique,* pp. 18–19.

Yell, M. L., Rogers, D., & Rogers, E. L. (1998). The legal history of special education: What a long, strange trip it's been! *Remedial and Special Education, 19,* 219–228.

The *OTPF–3:* Communicating Occupational Therapy in Schools

2

Gloria Frolek Clark, PhD, OTR/L, BCP, SCSS, FAOTA, and Michelle Ponsolle-Mays, MS, OTR/L

KEY TERMS AND CONCEPTS

- Domain
- Occupation
- *OTPF–3*
- Outcomes
- Process
- Professional reasoning

OVERVIEW

School occupational therapy focuses on engagement in meaningful, important occupations that support access, learning, and participation in school. *Occupations* "refer to the everyday activities that people do as individuals, in families and with communities to occupy time and bring meaning and purpose to life. Occupations include things people need to, want to and are expected to do" (World Federation of Occupational Therapists, 2012, para. 2). Examples of occupations for students are listed in Table 2.1.

The *Occupational Therapy Practice Framework: Domain and Process* (OTPF; American Occupational Therapy Association [AOTA], 2002, 2008, 2014b) is a fluid, ever-evolving document that provides occupational therapy practitioners[1] with information detailing the integration of occupation throughout the occupational therapy process (Youngstrom, 2002). The *OTPF* describes occupational therapy's domain and process, and it is used in conjunction with the knowledge of the profession and evidence-based practices. Understanding this information is an essential component of effective occupational therapy, regardless of the setting. In school systems, occupational therapy practitioners use the *OTPF* to provide a structure for practice when developing occupation-based evaluations, interventions, and targeted outcomes (Levan, 2003; McKinley-Vargas & Thomas, 2008).

The current, 3rd edition of the *OTPF* (the **OTPF–3**) highlights the distinct value of occupation and occupational therapy in contributing to client health, well-being, and participation (AOTA, 2014b). Occupational therapy practitioners add value at multiple levels. The *OTPF–3* describes *clients*[2] as persons (individuals), groups (collectives of individuals, such as families or students), and populations (collectives of groups of individuals sharing similar characteristics or concerns). In schools, practitioners also interact at multiple levels. These levels may include the following:

- *Systems level:* Serving as a consultant for the state department of education (state level), being a lead occupational therapist for the school district (district level), serving on playground or curriculum committees (building or district level)
- *Group level (classrooms):* Co-teaching in general education classrooms, providing professional development for special education staff
- *Individual level:* Working with individual students through multi-tiered systems of support programs; working with students on a 504 plan, an individualized education program (IEP), or both.

The domain and process described in the *OTPF–3* are entwined to support the relationship among client, engagement, and the context and environment. The 5 areas of the domain are described in the "Essential Considerations" section, and the process (evaluation, intervention, and outcomes) is discussed later in the "Best Practices" section.

ESSENTIAL CONSIDERATIONS

The areas of occupational therapy knowledge and expertise are articulated in the domain of the occupational therapy profession. The overarching **domain** is "achieving health, well-being, and participation in life through engagement in occupation" (AOTA, 2014b, p. S4). These terms are defined as follows:

- *Health:* "A state of complete physical, mental, and social well-being, and not merely the absence of disease or

[1] *Occupational therapy practitioner* refers to both the occupational therapist and the occupational therapy assistant. AOTA (2014a, p. S18) states, "The occupational therapist is responsible for all aspects of occupational therapy service delivery and is accountable for the safety and effectiveness of the occupational therapy service delivery process" and "must be directly involved in the delivery of services during the initial evaluation and regularly throughout the course of intervention. . . . The occupational therapy assistant delivers safe and effective occupational therapy services under the supervision of and in partnership with the occupational therapist."

[2] For the purpose of this chapter, the word *client* is used to reflect the student, the family, educational staff, general education classroom, school district, and other persons or agencies seeking occupational therapy services.

Copyright © 2019 by the American Occupational Therapy Association. All rights reserved. To reuse this content, contact www.copyright.com.
https://doi.org/10.7139/2019.978-1-56900-591-0.002

TABLE 2.1. Occupations: School Examples

OCCUPATIONS	EXAMPLES FOR STUDENTS
ADLs	Showering, toileting and toilet hygiene, dressing, mealtime participation (e.g., feeding, eating, swallowing), functional mobility, care of personal devices (e.g., glasses, hearing aids, catheters), personal hygiene and grooming, sexual activity
Education	Formal educational participation (e.g., academic, nonacademic, extracurricular), informal personal education exploration and participation (e.g., acquire information related to personal interests)
IADLs	Care of pets, child rearing, communication management, driving and community mobility, financial management, health management and maintenance, home establishment and management, meal preparation and cleanup, religious and spiritual activities and expression, safety and emergency maintenance, shopping, use of technology
Leisure	Leisure exploration and participation
Play	Play exploration and participation
Social participation	Social interactions in the community, family, peer, friend
Rest and sleep	Obtaining adequate rest and sleep hygiene
Work	Employment interests and pursuits, employment seeking and acquisition, job performance, volunteer exploration and participation

Source. From "Occupational Therapy Practice Framework: Domain and Process (3rd Edition)," by the American Occupational Therapy Association, 2014, *American Journal of Occupational Therapy, 68*(Suppl. 1), S19–S21. Copyright © 2014 by the American Occupational Therapy Association. Adapted with permission.

infirmity" (adapted from the World Health Organization [WHO], 2006, p. 1, as cited in AOTA, 2014b, p. S4)

- *Well-being*: "A general term encompassing the total universe of human life domains, including physical, mental, and social aspects" (WHO, 2006, p. 211)
- *Participation*: "Involvement in a life situation" (WHO, 2001, p. 10)
- *Engagement in occupation*: "Performing occupations as the result of choice, motivation, and meaning within a supportive context and environment" (AOTA, 2014b, p. S4).

The *OTPF–3* identifies 5 areas of the domain that are equal in value and support engagement, participation, and health. These areas are listed in Table 2.2 (AOTA, 2014b).

Occupation-Based and Student-Centered Services

During the school day, students have multiple opportunities to be engaged in meaningful occupations and activities

TABLE 2.2. *OTPF–3* Aspects of the Domain: School Examples

DOMAIN	DESCRIPTION (AOTA, 2014B)	EXAMPLES
Occupations	See Table 2.1.	
Client factors	Capacities, characteristics, or beliefs that reside within the person and can influence their performance	- Student's or parent's belief regarding the importance of an education - Student's memory and attention - Student's loss of vision in one eye
Context and environment	*Context:* Interrelated conditions within and surrounding the student (personal, cultural, temporal, virtual) *Environment:* External physical and social conditions in which occupations occur	- *Context:* Age, gender, socioeconomic status, time of day, family and school customs, expectations of school, teletherapy - *Environment:* Physical and sensory qualities of the classroom or lunchroom; social relationships, expectations, and routines
Performance skills	Observable elements of action that have an implicit functional purpose (motor, process, social interactions)	- *Motor:* Manipulates, grips, endures - *Process:* Attends, initiates, adjusts - *Social interaction:* Approaches, regulates, takes turns, empathizes
Performance patterns	Patterns used in the process of engaging in occupations. Can support or hinder performance. Includes habits, routines, rituals, and roles	- *Habits:* Always hangs up coat, must eat the same foods for lunch or becomes upset - *Routines:* Follows morning routine independently, struggles with sequence of washing hands - *Rituals:* Joins friends for recess, rolls crayons all around desk before using them to color - *Roles:* Follows rules set by school building regarding lining up, enjoys being class comedian

Note. OTPF–3 = Occupational Therapy Practice Framework: Domain and Process (3rd ed.).

(e.g., reading, writing, playing outside during recess, navigating hallways, socially interacting with peers during lunch and class, getting on the bus for a school trip). When students cannot participate in their daily occupations, the occupational therapist may be asked to identify aspects that are potentially causing the occupational dysfunction.

To glean additional information, an occupational therapy evaluation can be conducted to understand what the client wants or needs to do (i.e., occupations), the supports and barriers to occupations, the context or environment of these occupations, and occupational risks (AOTA, 2014b; Coster, 1998). The focus of the evaluation should be on activities and occupations. For more information, see Chapter 40, "Best Practices in School Occupational Therapy Evaluation and Planning to Support Participation."

Professional Reasoning

Throughout the process of service provision, occupational therapy practitioners engage in professional reasoning. *Professional reasoning* is the "process used by practitioners to plan, direct, perform, and reflect on client care" (Boyt Schell et al., 2014, p. 1231). Through observation and interview, the occupational therapy practitioner identifies the supports and barriers within the person's performance, environment, or school system level (district, building, and classroom levels).

As occupational therapy practitioners gain an understanding of the dynamic relationship between the domain and the student's performance, they can identify and apply available evidence to interventions and modifications to facilitate participation in context. For example, pulling a student from the classroom results in the loss of access to instructional materials covered during that time. Providing services during the natural routine of the day when the student encounters educational demands enhances performance, fosters the student's problem-solving abilities, and demonstrates the distinct value of occupational therapy in schools.

Professional Responsibilities

Occupational therapists are licensed professionals who make recommendations or referrals to other professionals, as needed. The *Standards of Practice* (AOTA, 2015), as well as most state occupational therapy regulatory acts, require the referral of the client "to appropriate resources when the needs of the client can best be served by the expertise of other professionals or services" (p. 4). The occupational therapist has an ethical obligation to discuss with the team (e.g., parent, physician, IEP team member) any concern about a student's physical or mental health.

If an occupational therapy practitioner does not have the skills to provide evidence-based services to a student, then they must discuss this with their supervisor and develop a plan to provide these services. (*Note:* This does not refer to specific programs or interventions requested by the family. The practitioner is responsible for determining an appropriate evidence-based intervention for the student and for determining the effectiveness of this intervention.)

BEST PRACTICES

OTPF–3 **process** components include collaborative service provision with clients (e.g., evaluation, intervention, outcome monitoring), and the process occurs within the domain (AOTA, 2014b). "Only occupational therapy practitioners focus on the use of occupations to promote health, well-being, and participation in life" (AOTA, 2014b, p. S11). Whereas the process is covered in more detail in other sections, this chapter provides information about how to use the *OTPF–3* in practice.

Frame the Evaluation Process

Information gathered through record review and interview is used for developing the occupational profile (see Appendix B, "AOTA Occupational Therapy Profile Template"). AOTA developed an occupational profile template that can be used to gather and document information. Some funding sources, such as Medicaid, require that an occupational profile be completed as part of the evaluation (Centers for Medicare and Medicaid Services, 2017).

Complete the occupational profile

The first part of the evaluation process, gathering information for the occupational profile, provides an understanding of the purpose for seeking occupational therapy; the success of, or barriers to, the student's occupations; the personal interests and values (e.g., student enjoys using an iPad, playing sports, caring for a pet); occupational history (e.g., educational history, medical and health information); performance patterns that may support or interfere with occupations; specific information about the context or environmental supports and barriers; and what the student, teacher, or parent would like as the result of receiving occupational therapy.

Data collection is focused on identifying the student's academic, developmental, and functional needs (Individuals With Disabilities Education Improvement Act of 2004 [IDEA], Pub. L. 108–446), including barriers to and supports for participation in school occupations and activities. Data are collected and interpreted during the analysis of occupational performance.

Analyze occupational performance

The second part of the process is a synthesis of the information gathered through the occupational profile; observing the student's performance; when necessary, measuring specific aspects of the domain using formal or informal tools; selecting outcome measures; developing a hypothesis; and creating goals in collaboration with the client (e.g., student, family, educational staff).

Client: Individual student

The information gathered as part of the occupational profile provides a focus for the specific areas to be addressed. Family members are a critical part of the team and have information about the student that may be vital for decision making. It is essential for the occupational therapy practitioner to determine the supports and barriers in the curriculum (i.e., what is taught), instruction (i.e., how it is taught), and environment (i.e., where it is taught), because these interrelated factors have a strong influence on student participation.

Analysis of the student's performance during natural routines is an integral component of the identification of the supporting and inhibiting aspects of contextual factors, activity demands, client factors, performance skills, and performance patterns. The occupational therapist develops a hypothesis, gathers data through observation or assessments, and refines the hypothesis. Staying flexible and having a willingness to question what one is doing and why are important qualities to possess when demonstrating the value of occupational therapy (Candler et al., 2008). Considering multiple frames of reference allows the practitioner to structure the analysis and uncover the optimal approach to and discovery of goals to target improved occupational performance (Candler et al., 2008). Predetermining or not using a frame of reference would negatively affect this stage of the professional reasoning process.

In schools, goals are developed in collaboration with team members, including parents and the student when appropriate. The occupational therapist identifies the targeted participation and engagement outcomes and methods to measure change. Using best practices and current evidence, the intervention approach is identified.

Client: Groups or populations

Occupational therapy practitioners are often asked to provide assistance to the school district, in school buildings, or to specific classroom programs. The *OTPF–3* can be used as a template to guide the process.

Consider a school district's request for the occupational therapist to train faculty and staff. To learn more about the school demographics or personnel, the occupational therapist would begin by gathering the occupational profile through an interview with the person making the request. The information may include the reason for the request, information about the school, what is expected from the therapist, what has been attempted in the past, and so forth. The occupational therapist would analyze the information received and determine whether other data (e.g., whether students were sent to the office, common mental health conditions) are needed.

Careful analysis is made of client factors (e.g., values, beliefs), context and environment (e.g., cultural, personal, virtual, physical) of the agency, the demands of educational activities, and performance skills and performance patterns of school personnel and students. For example, some school districts have programs for students who exhibit aggressive and socially maladaptive behaviors.

Using the *OTPF–3*'s domain as a guide, the occupational therapist could identify potential areas of the program that would benefit from routine consultation, staff training, or co-teaching by an occupational therapy practitioner (e.g., self-care skills, work skills, social–emotional skills, self-regulation skills).

Establish Outcomes

Outcomes are identified before intervention begins and are the end result of the occupational therapy process. *Outcomes* describe what clients can achieve through occupational therapy intervention and are used to measure progress toward the desired engagement in valued occupations (AOTA, 2014b). Outcomes may be written as the student's IEP goal or listed on the occupational therapy intervention plan, and they can be used to determine the effectiveness of occupational therapy intervention. Table 2.3 lists some example outcomes of health, well-being, and participation in schools operationalized using the *OTPF–3*. Data collected during intervention would inform decisions about future services (e.g., whether to adjust intervention plans, continue monitoring, or recommend discontinuation).

TABLE 2.3.   Outcomes: Examples for Students and Staff

OUTCOME	EXAMPLES FOR PERSONS, GROUPS, AND POPULATIONS IN SCHOOLS
Occupational performance	▪ Students can safely climb on playground equipment ▪ Students can stock shelves in a cafeteria or grocery store
Prevention	▪ Students have proper seating and table arrangements to facilitate social interaction and academic participation ▪ Schoolwide bullying prevention program is implemented
Health and wellness	▪ Schoolwide healthy lunch program is in place ▪ Schoolwide positive mental health promotion program exists
Participation	▪ Student with intellectual disability is engaged in classroom computer activities ▪ School building modifications (e.g., automatic door openers, longer railings on stairs) allow access for students with physical disabilities ▪ Student with attention deficit hyperactivity disorder uses alternative seating options in class
Quality of life	▪ Student with multiple disabilities is fully included in general education with peer friendships and interactions ▪ A districtwide trauma-sensitive climate has been adopted
Role competence	▪ Student in middle school types their own notes during classes ▪ Student socially interacts and actively contributes to a group project with peers ▪ Staff use universal design for learning and differentiated instruction to optimize the participation of all students

Plan, Implement, and Review the Intervention

The intervention process includes 3 parts:
1. Development of the intervention plan,
2. Implementation of the intervention, and
3. Review of the intervention.

The intervention plan is developed in collaboration with the student, parent, and educational staff. Occupational therapists are responsible for the development, documentation, and implementation of the occupational therapy intervention plan, with input, when appropriate, from the occupational therapy assistant (AOTA, 2015). For more information on intervention in schools, see Chapter 41, "Best Practices in School Occupational Therapy Interventions to Support Participation."

Intervention plan

AOTA's *Standards of Practice for Occupational Therapy* (2015) state that intervention plans are required when providing occupational therapy services. When the client is a student, the intervention plan should be designed to indicate how the student's IEP goals will be met (e.g., enhance executive functions, train teachers in in-hand dexterity). The intervention plan is not the IEP; rather, the intervention plan documents occupational therapy objectives and measurable goals, time frames, intervention approaches, methods of service delivery (e.g., frequency and duration, types of interventions, persons providing intervention), potential discontinuation considerations, and recommendations or referrals to other professionals (AOTA, 2014b, 2018). For more information see Appendix C, "Occupational Therapy Intervention Plan."

Interventions are deliberately planned to facilitate engagement in occupations. Interventions may vary depending on the student's goals, grade or school expectations, and service provision model. Occupational therapy practitioners are encouraged to think systemwide first because the facilitation of successful environments for learning, effective instruction practices, and use of evidence-based curricula will have a greater impact on programmatic change for all students.

Intervention approaches and types

To meet the student's needs, the occupational therapist, with input from the occupational therapy assistant when appropriate, selects an intervention approach (see Table 2.4). *Approaches* "are specific strategies selected to direct the process . . . inform selection of practice models, frames of reference or treatment theories" (AOTA, 2014b, p. S33). Various combinations are used according to the needs of the client, family, relevant others, or caregivers. Focusing on the student's occupational performance (e.g., boarding the school bus safely, writing their name, completing prevocational activities), rather than on impairments, enhances performance skills and patterns through occupation and activities (Fisher, 1998) and may be less time consuming and more efficient in promoting participation.

Intervention implementation

After the intervention approach has been determined, the type of intervention for implementation is chosen to facilitate engagement in occupations with the outcome of promoting health and participation (see Table 2.5). As the interventions are implemented, the student's response is monitored (e.g., ongoing assessment of the student's progress to determine the effectiveness of intervention). When the client is the school district itself, monitoring may be a systematic ongoing collection of data supporting the organization's

---

TABLE 2.4. Occupational Therapy Approaches to Intervention in Schools

APPROACH	DESCRIPTION	EXAMPLES
Create, promote	Enrichment of context and environment, occupations, client factors, performance skills, or performance patterns (Dunn et al., 1998)	▪ Incorporating a universal design for learning in classrooms ▪ Recommending playground and supplies ▪ Creating opportunities for students to prepare for postsecondary transition
Establish, restore	Develop a skill, or restore a skill that has been impaired (Dunn et al., 1998)	▪ Designing a system to facilitate a student's independence in self-management of posttraumatic brain injury recovery
Maintain	Provide supports to preserve abilities, or performance will decrease	▪ Using a battery-operated wheelchair for independent mobility through school ▪ Programming a preset daily alarm to cue a young adult student to go to the nurse for their medication regimen
Modify (compensation, adaptation)	Revise activity or context to support performance (Dunn et al., 1998)	▪ Incorporating a daily visual schedule with icons to support independent performance of school jobs ▪ Introducing a push-button or keyed lock on a student's physical education locker so that the student can access belongings in a timely manner along with peers
Prevent	Prevent the occurrence or development of barriers to performance in context (Dunn et al., 1998)	▪ Adjusting work surface heights to facilitate adequate posture and endurance for academic tasks ▪ Instituting a schoolwide "no-lift" transfer policy for student bathroom needs

TABLE 2.5. Types of Occupational Therapy Interventions

CATEGORY	DESCRIPTION	EXAMPLES
Advocacy	Efforts to promote occupational justice and empower others to seek and obtain resources to participate in daily life occupations	▪ Act as an advisor for student-led LGBTQ clubs and activities on high school campus to promote awareness and inclusion ▪ Promote and support students as they self-advocate for reasonable accommodations
Education and training	Understanding (education) and facilitating skills to enhance performance (training)	▪ Teach students about emotional states and self-regulation strategies to enhance self-management
Group interventions	Facilitation of learning and skills through group dynamics and social interaction	▪ Co-lead a social skills group to teach and build students' awareness and practice of social interaction skills
Occupations and activities	Student-directed daily life activities that support identified goals (activities or occupations) to develop performance skills and performance patterns to enhance engagement and participation	▪ Students operate snack bar or school store activities to develop life skills such as money management, organization, and planning
Preparatory methods and tasks	Provided as part of an intervention session or concurrently with occupations or activities to prepare a student for occupations (e.g., splints, assistive technology, fabricated sensory environment)	▪ Student with cerebral palsy "warms up" on an exercise bike in the gym to enhance participation in physical education class

Note. LGBTQ = lesbian, gay, bisexual, transgender, queer.

Source. From "Occupational Therapy Practice Framework: Domain and Process (3rd Edition)," by the American Occupational Therapy Association, 2014, *American Journal of Occupational Therapy, 68*(Suppl. 1), S28–S31. Copyright © 2014 by the American Occupational Therapy Association. Adapted with permission.

goals (e.g., increase in number of elementary school students with physical disabilities playing on the playground equipment during recess, increase in number of students with anxiety demonstrating increased daily attendance rates).

Reviewing the intervention is a continuous process of reexamining the intervention plan, the progress toward the desired outcomes or IEP student goals, the effectiveness of services, and the progress toward occupational therapy outcomes. During this process, collaboration among occupational therapy practitioners, educational staff, parents, and the student, if applicable, should be ongoing.

Intervention review

On the basis of data collected during a student's occupational therapy intervention, the occupational therapist determines the need for continuation or discontinuation of services and makes this recommendation to the IEP team for their decision. Reevaluation of the student may occur at any time. For students who have an IEP, the reevaluation typically occurs before the student's annual IEP meeting (when additional data, not related to the IEP goal, are going to be gathered, parents need to be notified, and parental consent needs to be granted), during a 3-year review process, or when the student's goals established by the IEP team have been met. The occupational therapy intervention plan is then modified to reflect changes. The outcomes (which will have been chosen earlier) should be reviewed and modified as necessary. In addition, the occupational therapist has the responsibility to discuss with the IEP team the need for a referral to other professionals (either within or outside of the team) when appropriate.

SUMMARY

The *OTPF-3* describes the central tenets of occupational therapy and illustrates a distinct contribution to school

systems for students achieving health and participation in their occupations (AOTA, 2014b). The domain of occupational therapy and the process of service provision reflect the current knowledge of the profession. The process can readily be applied in school practice to remain occupation focused, client centered, contextual, and grounded in evidence.

As practitioners use the *OTPF-3* to guide occupational therapy practice in schools, they communicate their professional expertise and specialized skills. They do this by using a common language, working within a consistent format to promote the equality of opportunity required by IDEA and other regulations, and communicating to stakeholders the distinct value of occupational therapy in schools.

REFERENCES

American Occupational Therapy Association. (2002). Occupational therapy practice framework: Domain and process. *American Journal of Occupational Therapy, 56,* 609–639. https://doi.org/10.5014/ajot.56.6.609

American Occupational Therapy Association. (2008). Occupational therapy practice framework: Domain and process (2nd ed.). *American Journal of Occupational Therapy, 62,* 625–683. https://doi.org/10.5014/ajot.62.6.625

American Occupational Therapy Association. (2014a). Guidelines for supervision, roles, and responsibilities during the delivery of occupational therapy services. *American Journal of Occupational Therapy, 68*(Suppl. 3), S16–S22. https://doi.org/10.5014/ajot.2014.686S03

American Occupational Therapy Association. (2014b). Occupational therapy practice framework: Domain and process (3rd ed.). *American Journal of Occupational Therapy, 68*(Suppl. 1), S1–S48. https://doi.org/10.5014/ajot.2014.682006

American Occupational Therapy Association. (2015). Standards of practice for occupational therapy. *American Journal of*

Occupational Therapy, 64(Suppl.), S106–S111. https://doi.org /10.5014/ajot.2010.64S106

American Occupational Therapy Association. (2018). Guidelines for documentation of occupational therapy. *American Journal of Occupational Therapy, 72*(Suppl. 2), 7212410010. https://doi .org/10.5014/ajot.2018.72S203

Boyt Schell, B. A., Gillen, G., & Scaffa, M. (2014). Glossary. In B. A. Boyt Schell, G. Gillen, & M. Scaffa (Eds.). *Willard and Spackman's occupational therapy* (12th ed., pp. 1229–1243). Philadelphia: Lippincott Williams & Wilkins.

Candler, C., Frolek Clark, G., & Swinth, Y. (2008). School-based services: What does OT bring to the IFSP and IEP table? *Journal of Occupational Therapy, Schools, and Early Intervention, 1,* 17–23. https://doi.org/10.1080/19411240802060959

Centers for Medicare and Medicaid Services. (2017). *ICD–10– CM official guidelines for coding and reporting.* Retrieved from https://www.cms.gov/Medicare/Coding/ICD10/index.html

Coster, W. (1998). Occupation-centered assessment of children. *American Journal of Occupational Therapy, 52,* 337–344. https:// doi.org/10.5014/ajot.52.5.337

Dunn, W., McClain, L., Brown, C., & Youngstrom, M. (1998). The ecology of human performance. In M. E. Neistadt & E. B. Crepeau (Eds.), *Willard and Spackman's occupational therapy* (9th ed., pp. 525–535). Philadelphia: Lippincott Williams & Wilkins.

Fisher, A. (1998). Eleanor Clarke Slagle Lecture—Uniting practice and theory in an occupational framework. *American Journal of Occupational Therapy, 52,* 509–521. https://doi.org/10.5014/ajot .52.7.509

Individuals With Disabilities Education Improvement Act of 2004, Pub. L. 108–446, 20 U.S.C. §§ 1400–1482.

Levan, P. (2003, September). The *Framework* and school-based settings. *School System Special Interest Section Quarterly, 10,* 2–3.

McKinley-Vargas, J., & Thomas, K. (2008). A framework for change. *OT Practice, 13*(11), 10–15.

World Federation of Occupational Therapists. (2012). *Definition [of] occupation.* Retrieved from http://www.wfot.org/aboutus /aboutoccupationaltherapy/definitionofoccupationaltherapy .aspx

World Health Organization. (2001). *International classification of functioning, disability and health.* Geneva: Author.

World Health Organization. (2006). *Constitution of the World Health Organization* (45th ed.). Retrieved from http://www.who .int/governance/eb/who_constitution_en.pdf

Youngstrom, M. J. (2002). The *Occupational Therapy Practice Framework:* The evolution of our professional language. *American Journal of Occupational Therapy, 56,* 607–608. https://doi .org/10.5014/ajot.56.6.607

Laws That Affect Occupational Therapy in Schools · 3

Elizabeth Schneider, EdS, OTR/L, BCP, and Barbara E. Chandler, PhD, OTR/L, FAOTA

KEY TERMS AND CONCEPTS

- ADA Amendments Act of 2008
- Americans With Disabilities Act
- Annual Performance Report
- Child Abuse Prevention and Treatment Act
- Common Core State Standards
- DD Act
- Disability
- Every Student Succeeds Act
- Family Educational Rights and Privacy Act

- Healthy, Hunger-Free Kids Act of 2010
- 504 plan
- Free appropriate public education
- Individualized education program
- Individual with a disability
- Individuals With Disabilities Education Improvement Act of 2004
- Local educational agency
- Medicaid

- Program access
- Related services
- Social Security Amendments of 1965
- Special education
- Specialized instructional support personnel
- Specially designed instruction
- State Performance Plan
- Tech Act
- Travel training

OVERVIEW

The effective provision of school occupational therapy requires a solid understanding of the purpose of occupational therapy in this setting and of the rules and regulations governing the education of students with disabilities. In addition to understanding laws and regulations, occupational therapy practitioners[1] need to understand the purpose of public education. Having an understanding of such laws and regulations helps practitioners to understand a host of requirements, policies, and procedures that are central to their work.

It is important to note that specific laws and regulations in each state may differ slightly from each other. The laws and regulations provided by the federal government serve as a minimum standard for each state. In addition, each *local educational agency* (LEA) has its own policies, procedures, mission, and unwritten rules that dictate the implementation of educational service provision. This chapter helps occupational therapy practitioners understand the mission of public education as defined by the federal government. Practitioners are encouraged to seek additional information from their individual states and their LEAs regarding any mission, laws, regulations, policies, and procedures that may extend beyond those minimum requirements.

The education of all students is primarily the role of individual states; however, the federal government has stepped in to provide legislation, leadership, and funding for specific programs when it is in the national interest. To this end, according to the Center on Education Policy (2007), the federal government became involved in education for 4 major reasons:

1. To promote democracy,
2. To ensure equality of education,
3. To enhance national productivity, and
4. To strengthen national defense.

Funding for public schools comes largely from state and local governments. Federal funding for special programs makes up less than 10% of all education funding. School districts or LEAs are bound by federal and state laws; however, they are governed primarily by school boards made up of locally elected representatives. Each school board creates policies that dictate the administration and operation of schools within its boundaries. School board policies represent "a basic source of law for school personnel" (Essex 2012, p. 6), because they are legally defensible as long as they do not conflict with federal or state constitutions and law.

---

[1]*Occupational therapy practitioner* refers to both the occupational therapist and the occupational therapy assistant. AOTA (2014b, p. S18) states, "The occupational therapist is responsible for all aspects of occupational therapy service delivery and is accountable for the safety and effectiveness of the occupational therapy service delivery process" and "must be directly involved in the delivery of services during the initial evaluation and regularly throughout the course of intervention. . . . The occupational therapy assistant delivers safe and effective occupational therapy services under the supervision of and in partnership with the occupational therapist."

Copyright © 2019 by the American Occupational Therapy Association. All rights reserved. To reuse this content, contact www.copyright.com.
https://doi.org/10.7139/2019.978-1-56900-591-0.003

ESSENTIAL CONSIDERATIONS

Until the passage of the Elementary and Secondary Education Act of 1965 (ESEA; Pub. L. 89–313), states had primary control of education. Currently, because of the amount of funding from the federal government, states must adhere to many federal regulations, creating more consistency across the nation.

Goal of Public Education

According to the Common Core State Standards Validation Committee (2010), the goal of public education "is for all American children to graduate from high school ready for college, career pathways, and success in a global economy" (p. 1). The Council of Chief State School Officers and the National Governors Association Center for Best Practices launched the development of a set of core standards called the **Common Core State Standards** (CCSS) in 2009 (Common Core State Standards Initiative [CCSSI], 2018). The CCSS represent the knowledge and skills required for students to be successful in the 21st-century workforce. Although the federal government supported the development of CCSS, the primary driver of their development was individual states. The CCSS are not mandated by federal legislation; however, most states have voluntarily adopted the CCSS (CCSSI, 2018).

All students, regardless of disability or background, are expected to work toward rigorous state standards (the CCSS, in most states). Students with disabilities who have an individualized education program (IEP) are expected to have annual goals aligned to these standards or extended standards for students with severe cognitive disabilities (American Occupational Therapy Association [AOTA], 2014a). Occupational therapy practitioners should be familiar with the academic standards in their state and local districts to collaborate effectively with other educators and support student achievement of those standards.

Laws Enforced by the U.S. Department of Education

Four laws are discussed in this section: (1) the Individuals With Disabilities Education Improvement Act of 2004 (IDEA; Pub. L. 108–446); (2) the Every Student Succeeds Act (ESSA; 2015; Pub. L. 114–95); (3) the Family Educational Rights and Privacy Act of 1974 (FERPA; Pub. L. 93–380); and the Rehabilitation Act of 1973, as amended (2008; Pub. L. 93–112).

IDEA

IDEA was first enacted as the Education for All Handicapped Children Act (Pub. L. 94–142) in 1975. It is a special education law that provides children with disabilities the right to a **free appropriate public education** (FAPE) that meets their individual education and related service needs in the least restrictive environment (LRE; National Council on Disability, 2000).

IDEA is arguably the most important legislation for students with disabilities because it ensures that children with disabilities have access to an appropriate education.

It affirms the right of all children to attend public schools, regardless of the severity of their disability. Occupational therapy is an important component of a student's educational program when students need services to make meaningful progress in their educational program. An understanding of the basic provisions of IDEA is essential to practice effectively and ethically in schools. Although IDEA has four parts (i.e., A, B, C, D), this discussion concentrates on Part B, which addresses preschool- and school-age students.

Purpose. Under IDEA Part B, 4 overall purposes of the law are identified:

(a) To ensure that all children with disabilities have available to them a free appropriate public education that emphasizes special education and related services designed to meet their unique needs and prepare them for further education, employment, and independent living;
(b) To ensure that the rights of children with disabilities and their parents are protected;
(c) To assist States, localities, educational service agencies, and Federal agencies to provide for the education of all children with disabilities; and
(d) To assess and ensure the effectiveness of efforts to educate children with disabilities. (34 CFR § 300.1)

Eligibility. Eligibility for services under IDEA has 2 components: The student has a **disability** (e.g., meets criteria for at least 1 of the disability categories in IDEA) and has a need for specially designed instruction. A student may have a disability and not need specially designed instruction. These students may be eligible for supplemental aids and services under Section 504 of the Rehabilitation Act.

The categories of disability include almost all disabilities that students may have (i.e., autism, deaf-blindness, deafness, emotional disturbance, hearing impairment, intellectual disability, multiple disabilities, orthopedic impairment, other health impairment, specific learning disability, speech or language impairment, traumatic brain injury, visual impairment). This comprehensive language is intentional to promote consistency in eligibility across the United States.

Special education. **Special education** is defined as "specially designed instruction, at no cost to the parents, to meet the unique needs of a child with a disability, including . . . instruction in physical education" (IDEA, 34 CFR § 300.39[a] [ii]). The further description of **specially designed instruction** includes "adapting, as appropriate . . . the content, methodology or delivery of instruction . . . to ensure access of the child to the general education curriculum" (§ 300.39 [b][3][ii]).

In addition, of specific interest to occupational therapy practitioners are descriptions of **travel training**, which includes assisting students with disabilities in developing "an awareness of the environment in which they live" and learning the skills necessary to "move effectively and safely from place to place within that environment (e.g., in school, in the home, at work, in the community)" (IDEA, 34 CFR § 300.39 [b][4][i][ii]).

Related service. Occupational therapy is a related service to specially designed instruction. **Related services** are defined as "transportation and such developmental, corrective, and other supportive services as are required to assist a child with a disability to benefit from special education" (IDEA, 34 CFR § 300.34).

In most states, students must have special education services on their IEP to receive occupational therapy; however, some states define *occupational therapy* as specially designed instruction (e.g., special education). In these states, occupational therapy can be the only service on the student's IEP. Whether occupational therapy is a related service or specially designed instruction, supporting education for all students in all environments and school activities is the primary focus. Occupational therapy practitioners understand the occupations of school, daily demands, and expectations of students with special needs, allowing them to support these students and address their needs. IDEA also requires that interventions (e.g., special education and related services, supplementary aids and services) are based on "peer-reviewed research, to the extent practicable" (IDEA, 20 U.S.C. § 1414[d][1][A][IV]).

IEP. After a student has met the eligibility requirements, the team uses the information gathered (e.g., student's full and individual evaluation, reports shared by parents) to develop the student's IEP. The ***IEP*** outlines the program of services and supports that the IEP team commits to provide for, and with, the student. This team should include, at a minimum, the student's parents or guardian, a general education teacher, a special education teacher, a representative of the public agency involved who can provide information about the commitment of resources, a professional who can interpret the evaluation results (who may be one of the team members previously described), and others (e.g., related service personnel), as desired by the parent or agency. The student is also eligible (but not required) to attend the IEP meeting.

IDEA requires an IEP to have 8 components:
1. A statement of present levels of academic and functional performance (this statement also includes how the student's disability affects their involvement and progress in the general education curriculum and, for students who take alternate assessments aligned to alternate achievement standards, a description of benchmarks or short-term objectives)
2. A statement of measurable annual goals, including academic and functional goals
3. A description of how progress toward annual goals will be measured and when periodic progress reports will be provided to the family
4. A statement of special education services, related services, and supplementary aids and services, on the basis of peer-reviewed research to the extent practicable, that are provided to the student or on behalf of the student, as well as a statement of program modifications and supports for school personnel that are provided for the student (to be educated and participate with other students and to participate in extracurricular and nonacademic activities)
5. When applicable, an explanation of the extent to which a student will not participate with students without disabilities in the general education classroom and activities
6. A statement of any individual accommodations necessary to measure academic achievement and functional

performance on state- and districtwide assessments (e.g., if the student takes an alternative assessment, a statement must provide the reasoning and list the alternative assessment)
7. A projected date for beginning services and modifications and the anticipated frequency, location, and duration of these services and modifications
8. For children age 16 years (or younger, depending on state rules), a statement of appropriate measurable postsecondary goals (based on appropriate transition assessments in the areas of training, education, employment, and independent living skills, when applicable; modified from IDEA, 20 U.S.C. § 1414[d]).

The role of a related service provider is to support the specially designed instruction by supporting progress on one or more of the student goals identified on the IEP and any accommodations and modifications required by students to participate in their educational program.

When a team member's area of curriculum or related services will be discussed, IDEA requires that the team member attend the IEP meeting, unless "(i) The parent, in writing, and the public agency consent to the excusal; and (ii) The member submits, in writing to the parent and the IEP team, input into the development of the IEP prior to the meeting" (IDEA, 20 U.S.C. § 300.321[e][2][i][ii]). Attending the IEP meeting is critical because the student's needs are identified and discussed, the family's concerns and priorities are heard, strategies and ideas are shared, mutual understanding is realized, and the team commits to work together on behalf of the student. To provide effective services, the occupational therapist (and occupational therapy assistant, when applicable) should understand the specially designed instruction to support that educational program. Moreover, the IEP meeting is an ideal place for the occupational therapy practitioner to communicate to parents and other educators the purpose of occupational therapy services and discuss the generalization of skills and abilities addressed by occupational therapy.

In addition to the required annual meeting to develop or update the IEP, the IEP may be amended or modified if the parent and the public agency agree to do so, but all members of the IEP team must be informed of these changes (IDEA, 20 U.S.C. § 300.324[4][ii]).

Children with disabilities and their parents' rights. IDEA provides procedural safeguards for parents in the provision of a FAPE for their child with a disability. These safeguards include an opportunity
- To examine all records relating to their child;
- To participate in meetings regarding the identification, education, and educational placement of their child; and
- To obtain an independent educational evaluation.

Parents may request copies of progress-monitoring notes and data, assessments, and communication (including emails) on behalf of their child. Documentation and communication about a student should
- Be professional,
- Abide by the highest ethical standards,
- Use language that is supportive of the student's disability and circumstance, and
- Avoid personal judgments of the student, family, and educational staff.

Parents must provide written consent for their child's evaluation and special education and related services. With few exceptions, no formal assessments can be given or services provided to a student without these consents. Parents may withdraw their consent, in writing, at any time. The LEA must notify parents of any action proposed or refused by the school. For example, if an LEA does not believe that a service requested by parents on behalf of their student is necessary, the LEA needs to refuse the service and explain the reasons to the parents in writing. Parents of a child with a disability must receive a copy of the procedural safeguards (see IDEA, 20 U.S.C. § 1415[d], for exceptions).

Outcomes and accountability. IDEA requires state educational agencies (SEAs) to submit to the U.S. Department of Education (specifically, the Office of Special Education Programs [OSEP]) a *State Performance Plan,* which reports their baseline and goals for 20 indicators for Part B (preschool through graduation programs) for a 6-year period. SEA may set some of the target outcomes; however, some are set by OSEP, including the requirement that 100% of the students referred for an initial evaluation must receive this evaluation within 60 days (or whatever state time frame has been established) of the school's receiving parental written consent.

Every year, each SEA must submit an *Annual Performance Report* to OSEP, which indicates its performance on each of these indicators. Examples include the number of students with IEPs graduating, dropping out, participating in statewide assessments, and being expelled or suspended from schools. Data are reported regarding the percentage of time when students with IEPs are out of their general education classroom, including related services provided outside of any natural environment. School districts must also report on parent involvement (typically through parent survey). For more information about specific state plans and performance, readers are directed to their state's department of education website. (For a link to each state's website, go to https://bit.ly/2RqeBo5.) Also, more detailed information is available in the chapters throughout this book.

ESSA

ESSA, an education law, represents the 8th reauthorization of ESEA, which was originally passed in 1965 by President Lyndon Johnson as part of his administration's War on Poverty. ESEA provided additional funding to schools and districts with the poorest students for the purpose of improving education opportunities to students from low-income families. Without this funding, students from low-income areas typically attended schools that were poorly funded, which negatively affected their educational opportunities. ESEA provided more financial support for those low-income schools and districts.

ESSA continues to provide additional funding for schools with high levels of poverty and maintains requirements for accountability, including its requirement for annual testing in areas of reading, math, and science for certain grade levels; tracking of student performance and growth, especially for subgroups of students who are most at risk of poor performance (e.g., students from racial/ethnic minority groups, low-income students, English-language learners, students with disabilities); and targeting schools in the bottom 5% of overall performance or schools with poor performance in student subgroups for additional state support. ESSA allows states the flexibility to make their own goals and set their own consequences for schools and districts that do not meet those goals.

ESSA is important for occupational therapy practitioners for at least 2 reasons. First, ESSA requires that *specialized instructional support personnel* (SISP), including occupational therapy practitioners and other related service providers, be involved in program development, school climate initiatives, and the provision of testing accommodations (Parsons, 2015). This requirement opens the door for occupational therapy leadership and involvement in a wide range of school initiatives.

Second, ESSA mandates that students with disabilities have access to and participate in state assessments, with only 1% of students able to take an alternative assessment. Occupational therapy practitioners are frequently involved in the accommodations and modifications necessary for students with disabilities to participate in the annual testing process under ESSA and should collaborate with other educators regarding the identification and implementation of necessary accommodations.

FERPA

FERPA, a privacy law, addresses the privacy of student records in schools that receive funds from the federal government (i.e., the U.S. Department of Education). These rights of privacy rest with the parent until the child turns 18 years old or attends a postsecondary institution. Schools may charge a fee for copies of records. When parents (or the eligible student) believe that any information is misleading or inaccurate, they have a right to request corrections to these records. Evaluations conducted by occupational therapists are considered protected students' records. Email communications about a student may be considered part of that student's records. Intervention plans and notes may be considered part of the student's records, depending on state education laws or regulations of occupational therapy practice.

FERPA rules consider health information in files as "education records" and, therefore, not "protected health information" under the Health Insurance Portability and Accountability Act of 1996 (HIPAA; Pub. L. 104–191). However, if the schools are billing Medicaid, then they must be compliant with HIPAA as well. For example, schools must use a unique identification number, known as the National Provider Identifier (NPI), for billing Medicaid. The HIPAA transaction and code set standards relate to the electronic exchange of patient-identifiable, health-related information. Generally, schools use the *International Classification of Diseases, 11th Revision* (World Health Organization, 2018), or *Current Procedural Terminology* (*CPT*–10; American Medical Association, 2019) codes.

Rehabilitation Act of 1973

The Office of Civil Rights within the U.S. Department of Education oversees Section 504 of the Rehabilitation Act of 1973. This civil rights law protects qualified individuals from disability-based discrimination. An ***individual with a disability*** is "any person who: (i) has a mental or physical impairment that substantially limits one or more major life activity; (ii) has a record of such an impairment; or (iii) is regarded as having such an impairment" (34 C.F.R. § 104.3[j][1]). Major life activities include caring for oneself, walking, seeing, hearing, speaking, breathing, working, performing manual tasks, and learning. When a student with a disability does not qualify for specially designed instruction as defined in IDEA but requires some alteration in the school program or routine so that they can participate, Section 504 forbids the school, including parochial schools that receive federal funds, from denying students with disabilities an equal opportunity to receive services. Occupational therapists are ideal professionals to help develop and monitor 504 plans, and they should make school officials aware of their expertise in this area.

School building teams do not receive extra funding to develop and implement ***504 plans,*** which list the accommodations, modifications, or services that will be provided for an individual with a disability. Not providing these accommodations and modifications is a breach of federal civil rights law and can result in a significant loss of federal funds for school districts. (For further information see Chapter 27, "Best Practices in Supporting Students With a 504 Plan.")

Laws Enacted by the U.S. Department of Health and Human Services

Various units of the U.S. Department of Health and Human Services (DHHS) administer the following legislation: the Child Abuse Prevention and Treatment Act (CAPTA) Reauthorization Act of 2010 (Pub. L. 111–320), the Developmental Disabilities Assistance and Bill of Rights Act of 1975 (DD Act; Pub. L. 94–103), and the Assistive Technology Act of 2004 (Tech Act; Pub. L. 108–394). Within individual states, the state departments of health or social services may monitor these laws.

CAPTA Reauthorization Act of 2010

CAPTA programs are administered by the Administration on Children, Youth and Families (ACF) in the DHHS.

> The basis for government's intervention in child maltreatment is grounded in the concept of *parens patriae*—a legal term that asserts that government has a role in protecting the interests of children and in intervening when parents fail to provide proper care. (DHHS, 2010, p. 3)

CAPTA funds activities such as the coordination of programs related to child welfare; a national information clearinghouse for information related to child abuse and neglect; research and dissemination of findings; an interdisciplinary longitudinal study of children who have experienced abuse or neglect; and grants to states for child abuse and neglect prevention and intervention activities.

Personnel working in schools are mandatory reporters of instances of child abuse or neglect. Occupational therapy practitioners should know their obligations regarding training and reporting abuse or neglect.

DD Act

The DD Act was originally enacted as the Developmental Disabilities Services and Facilities Construction Amendments of 1970. The purpose of the ***DD Act*** is to

> assure that individuals with developmental disabilities and their families participate in the design of, and have access to, needed community services, individualized supports, and other forms of assistance that promote self-determination, independence, productivity, and integration and inclusion in all facets of community life. (42 U.S.C. 15001 § 101[b])

The DD Act has been reauthorized, with changes, multiple times. The act established state councils on developmental disabilities and required them to include a variety of members, including those who provide services to individuals with disabilities, such as occupational therapy practitioners. Protection and advocacy systems in each state have been influential in assisting people with disabilities in gaining access to appropriate provision of services, including in schools. The DD Act affects many individuals across the life course and in a wide variety of settings, from early intervention to group homes for elderly people. Occupational therapy practitioners in schools assist individuals whose services, especially during the transition to adult life, are governed by the DD Act.

Tech Act

The Tech Act was initially passed as the Technology-Related Assistance for Individuals With Disabilities Act of 1988 (Pub. L. 100–407). It was reauthorized in 1994, 1998, and then in 2004. The ***Tech Act*** is meant to "improve the provision of assistive technology to individuals with disabilities through comprehensive statewide programs of technology-related assistance, for individuals with disabilities of all ages" (Association of Assistive Technology Programs, 2016, p. 1). The Tech Act does not provide direct funding for assistive technology (AT) devices; rather, it maximizes access to such devices as well as to AT services in various community settings, including schools.

The definition of AT under IDEA (2004) has been adapted to focus on the needs of students with disabilities. IDEA (2004) requires a case-by-case review of each student's AT needs at the IEP meeting (20 U.S.C. 1412[a][1], 1412[a][12][b][i]). Occupational therapy practitioners are school leaders in AT needs and provision as well as in training students and teachers in use of AT devices. Occupational therapy practitioners should be familiar with AT and able to properly match student and device. Although programs resulting from Tech Act funding will look different in each state, occupational therapy practitioners may receive support and training in the area of AT as a result of this legislation. (See Chapter 21, "Best Practices in the Use of Assistive Technology to Enhance Participation.")

Laws Enforced by the U.S. Department of Justice

The Civil Rights Division of the U.S. Department of Justice enforces civil rights acts to prohibit discrimination.

Americans With Disabilities Act of 1990

Although the U.S. Department of Justice administers parts of the Americans With Disabilities Act of 1990 (ADA; Pub. L. 101–336), other federal agencies have responsibilities related to specific provisions within the ADA, including employment, public transportation, telephone relay services, proposed design guidelines, education, health care, and the workforce. The *ADA* and the *ADA Amendments Act of 2008* (Pub. L. 110–325) provide protections to individuals with disabilities in employment, state and local government, public accommodations, commercial facilities, transportation, and telecommunications. These protections are usually stated as rights of equal access and reasonable accommodations in employment and services provided by both public and private sectors.

ADA is a comprehensive civil rights law for individuals with disabilities. The Department of Justice enforces the following sections:

- Employment practices by units of state and local government (Title I)
- Programs, services, and activities of state and local governments (Title II)
- Public accommodations and commercial facilities (Title III).

Public schools are operated by state and local governments, so they are under Title II. The 2 key provisions of Title II are as follows: Public entities must provide program access, and this access must be in an integrated setting unless separate programs are necessary to ensure equal benefits or services. *Program access* under Title II means that school districts are required to operate their programs so that, when viewed in their entirety, they are accessible to and usable by people with disabilities. This requirement applies to all existing facilities (Pacer Center, 2013). However, although all new construction must be accessible, only parts of older buildings must be accessible.

Occupational therapists can provide guidance on ways to make multiple aspects of the school (e.g., curriculum, routines, learning tasks, facilities) accessible to students with disabilities and should assist in the problem-solving process with school teams. In addition, occupational therapy practitioners working with students in transition to adult life should be familiar with the following disability rights laws, because they apply to students and their families during transition: the Voting Accessibility for the Elderly and Handicapped Act of 1984 (Pub. L. 98–435), the Fair Housing Amendments Act of 1988 (Pub. L. 100–430), and the Architectural Barriers Act of 1968 (Pub. L. 90–480). Sources for general assistance include the ADA Information Line (https://www.ada.gov/infoline.htm) and the Regional Disability and Business Technical Assistance Centers (https://adata.org/).

Law Administered by the Centers for Medicare and Medicaid Services

The Centers for Medicare and Medicaid Services administers the Social Security Amendments of 1965 (Pub. L. 89–97). Medicaid is administered at the state level by different agencies, depending on the state.

Social Security Amendments of 1965

In response to millions of citizens with little to no access to health care or other supports, Congress passed the *Social Security Amendments of 1965,* far-reaching legislation that established Medicare (i.e., medical care for older adults) and *Medicaid* (i.e., aid for those in poverty and their children). These programs have changed over the years, and one change has been the ability to access federal Medicaid funds to recover costs for related services in schools. These related services must have a medical need in addition to an educational need for Medicaid funds to be appropriately accessed (see Chapter 16, "Best Practices in Medicaid Cost Recovery").

Federal, state, and local funds are used for education, and the amount from each of these sources varies across the country; however, most educational costs are covered by local and state funds. School systems are institutions of limited resources. Although IDEA authorized Congress to cover up to 40% of the cost of special education, Congress has only provided 14%–18%, on average (Council of Administrators of Special Education [CASE], 2016). Therefore, schools look for additional sources of funding to pay for special education services. Medicaid is one of these sources.

Medicaid began allowing payment for certain medically necessary services provided to children under the auspices of IDEA in 1988. Section 411(k)(13) of the Medicare Catastrophic Coverage Act of 1988 (Pub. L. 100–360) amended Section 1903(c) of the act to permit this type of Medicaid reimbursement. This mechanism of reimbursement allows school districts the ability to recover some of the costs of delivering medically necessary services to Medicaid-eligible students who have an IEP (CASE, 2016).

Many school districts (and some states) require occupational therapy practitioners to complete documentation to seek Medicaid reimbursement (including an occupational profile). The types of services and providers that are reimbursable can vary by state but typically include direct occupational therapy. States define *medical necessity* differently and have slightly different requirements for Medicaid. Some states assume that if occupational therapy services are included in an IEP, then the service is medically necessary. Other states may require a physician's prescription (Frolek Clark & Holahan, 2015). Regardless, decisions about the delivery of occupational therapy services should never be based on the potential for Medicaid reimbursement. The individual needs of the student with a disability in accessing the educational curriculum are the most important factor when determining service provision under IDEA. Documenting for services that were not delivered or services that students do not require constitutes fraud.

Law Administered by the U.S. Department of Agriculture

The U.S. Department of Agriculture administers the school lunch and breakfast programs, providing funding to school districts across the nation.

Healthy, Hunger-Free Kids Act of 2010

Originally authorized in 1946 as the National School Lunch Program, the *Healthy, Hunger-Free Kids Act of 2010* (Pub. L. 111–296) has expanded over the years, as needs have changed with the addition of the School Breakfast Program.

Occupational therapy practitioners may need to be involved in substitutions and modifications of school meals for students with disabilities. These modifications may involve changes to the food itself, alternative ways of consuming the food (e.g., intravenous or tube feeding), increased or decreased caloric needs, special plates and utensils, or foods to omit or increase. (Note that these services may also be important for homeless children; therefore, occupational therapy practitioners should become familiar with the provisions of the McKinney–Vento Homeless Assistance Act of 1987 [Pub. L. 100–77]. The U.S. Department of Agriculture, Food and Nutrition Service [2017] has additional information about school food programs.)

BEST PRACTICES

Providing occupational therapy services within the school system requires occupational therapy practitioners to develop many skills. Knowledge of laws allows occupational therapy practitioners to implement them for each student's benefit. Collaboration with others and the use of problem-solving skills, on the basis of knowing what is required and how it is supported, is essential for best practice in the schools.

Know the Laws

Knowing the provisions of the laws is important. The overarching bases for many school rules and procedures, especially those involving students with disabilities, are the laws that prescribe which services for students with special needs are to be provided, as well as how they are provided. Beyond a prescriptive process, these laws address inherent civil rights that must be adhered to and respected. It is important to note that state and local education laws can allow for more services to be provided to students with disabilities than are required by IDEA, but schools cannot provide fewer services than are required by IDEA. Understanding the role of the SISP is critical to building effective programs and services for all students.

Know the Educational System

In addition to understanding the laws and regulations governing services to students with disabilities, occupational therapy practitioners need to understand the mission, vision, goals, and strategic plan of the educational system (or systems) in which they work. Understanding the values of the community in which they work is also important. Such information will help occupational therapy practitioners understand how and why different LEAs and states choose to fund different initiatives and to implement laws and regulations in their own unique way. Moreover, occupational

therapy practitioners may need to alter their interactions to match the climate (e.g., the beliefs, values, and expectations of the people within a building or district), rules, classroom and curricular expectations, and social norms of each individual school, district, and state, or they may need to work to enhance the climate if a positive approach is needed.

Use Knowledge of Laws and Systems to Advocate for Students

Perhaps the corollary to knowing laws and educational organizations is negotiating systems to benefit students. When occupational therapy practitioners have a full understanding of the laws, regulations, and systemic structures that exist to benefit students with disabilities, they are better able to leverage that information to protect the rights and needs of parents and students with disabilities.

Help Families and Educational Staff Understand the Legal Context

The process for families entering and participating in their child's special education programming can be overwhelming. Likewise, the number of requirements just within the context of daily work with students can overwhelm educational staff. Occupational therapy practitioners who develop an understanding of local, state, and federal laws and regulations can help families and other educators navigate this tricky terrain. Families appreciate when the special education process is explained in a clear and practical manner.

Seek New Knowledge and Stay Updated

The knowledge base, as well as the perspective of what students with disabilities can accomplish, is changing and will continue to change. Laws are continually updated; regulations are continually revised. Occupational therapy practitioners cannot practice effectively and efficiently if they do not seek new knowledge and stay updated. Connecting with their state's department of education may be one way to stay updated on state-level changes to law and regulations. Occupational therapy practitioners should also stay updated on the actions of their local school board.

SUMMARY

Understanding the legal context of the educational environment is essential in the practice of occupational therapy in schools. Lack of knowledge in this area will be a barrier to effective and efficient service provision for students with disabilities. The legal context helps occupational therapy practitioners understand their roles and responsibilities in schools as well as the roles and responsibilities of other educators and administrators. In addition, knowledge of current legislation helps occupational therapy practitioners better advocate for children and families to receive the services necessary for participation in their educational programs.

REFERENCES

ADA Amendments Act of 2008, Pub. L. 110–325, 122 Stat. 3553.

American Medical Association (2019). *Current procedural terminology (ICD–10)*. Retrieved from https://commerce.ama-assn.org/store/catalog/productDetail.jsp?product_id=prod2870018&navAction=push

American Occupational Therapy Association. (2014a). *Frequently asked questions (FAQ): What should the occupational therapy practitioner know about the Common Core State Standards (CCSS)*. Bethesda, MD: Author. Retrieved from https://www.aota.org/~/media/corporate/files/secure/practice/children/faq-common-core-standards.pdf

American Occupational Therapy Association. (2014b). Guidelines for supervision, roles, and responsibilities during the delivery of occupational therapy services. *American Journal of Occupational Therapy, 68*(Suppl. 3), S16–22. https://doi.org/10.5014/ajot.2014.686S03

Americans With Disabilities Act of 1990, Pub. L. 101–336, 42 U.S.C. §§ 12101–12213. (2000).

Architectural Barriers Act of 1968, Pub. L. 90–480, 42 U.S.C. §§ 4151–4157.

Assistive Technology Act of 2004, Pub. L. 108–394, 29 U.S.C. §§ 3001–3007.

Association of Assistive Technology Programs. (2016). *Summary of Assistive Technology Act of 1998, as amended 2004 Public Law 108-364*. Retrieved from https://www.ataporg.org/ATActSummary

Center on Education Policy. (2007). *Why we still need public schools: Public education for the public good*. Washington, DC: Author.

Child Abuse Prevention and Treatment Act Reauthorization Act of 2010, Pub. L. 111–320, 42 U.S.C. § 5701.

Common Core State Standards Initiative. (2018). *Development process*. Retrieved from http://www.corestandards.org/about-the-standards/development-process/

Common Core State Standards Validation Committee. (2010, June). *Reaching higher: The Common Core State Standards Validation Committee*. Washington, DC: Author.

Council of Administrators of Special Education. (2016). *Lucky 21: Medicaid cost recovery in public schools*. Warner Robbins, GA: Author.

Developmental Disabilities Assistance and Bill of Rights Act of 1975, Pub. L. 94–103, 42 U.S.C. §§ 15001–15083.

Education for All Handicapped Children Act of 1975, Pub. L. 94–142, renamed the Individuals With Disabilities Education Improvement Act, codified at 20 U.S.C. §§ 1400–1482.

Elementary and Secondary Education Act of 1965, Pub. L. 89–313, 20 U.S.C. §§ 2701–3386.

Essex, N. L. (2012). *School law and the public schools: A practical guide for educational leaders* (5th ed.). Upper Saddle River, NJ: Pearson Education.

Every Student Succeeds Act, Pub. L. 114–95, 129 Stat. 1802 (2015).

Fair Housing Amendments Act of 1988, Pub. L. 100–430, 42 U.S.C. § 3601, 24 C.F.R. 100.

Family Educational Rights and Privacy Act of 1974, Pub. L. 93–380, 20 U.S.C. § 1232g, 34 C.F.R. Part 99.

Frolek Clark, G., & Holahan, L. (2015). In the Classroom—Medicaid FAQ for school occupational therapy practitioners. *OT Practice, 20*(20), 18–20.

Health Insurance Portability and Accounting Act of 1996, Pub. L. 104–191, 42 U.S.C. § 300gg, 29 U.S.C. §§ 1181–1183, and 42 U.S.C. §§ 1320d–1320d9.

Healthy, Hunger-Free Kids Act of 2010, Pub. L. 111–296, 124 Stat. 3183.

Individuals With Disabilities Education Improvement Act of 2004, Pub. L. 108–446, 20 U.S.C. §§ 1400–1482.

McKinney–Vento Homeless Assistance Act, Pub L. 100–77, 101 Stat. 482, 42 U.S.C. 11301 *et seq.* (1987).

Medicare Catastrophic Coverage Act of 1988, Pub. L. 100–360, 102 Stat. 683, 42 U.S.C. 1305, § 411.

National Council on Disability. (2000). *Back to school on civil rights*. Retrieved from https://www.ncd.gov/rawmedia_repository/7bfb3c01_5c95_4d33_94b7_b80171d0b1bc.pdf

Pacer Center. (2013). *ADA Q & A: Section 504 and postsecondary education*. Retrieved from http://www.pacer.org/publications/adaqa/504.asp

Parsons, H. (2015). *Bill to rewrite No Child Left Behind signed into law: What it means for OT*. Retrieved from https://www.aota.org/Advocacy-Policy/Congressional-Affairs/Legislative-Issues-Update/2015/no-child-left-behind-signed-law-every-student-succeeds-act.aspx

Rehabilitation Act of 1973, Pub. L. 93–112, 29 U.S.C. §§ 701-7961.

Section 504 of the Rehabilitation Act of 1973, as amended, 29 U.S.C. § 794. (2008).

Social Security Amendments of 1965, Pub. L. 89–97, 42 U.S.C. CFR §§ 1395–1395kkkl (Medicare) and 42 U.S.C. §§ 1396–1396w5 (Medicaid).

Technology-Related Assistance for Individuals With Disabilities Act of 1988, Pub. L. 100–407, amended as the Assistive Technology Act (2004), Pub. L. 108–364, 29 U.S.C. 3001.

U.S. Department of Agriculture, Food and Nutrition Service. (2017). *Accommodating children with disabilities in the school meal programs: Guidance for school food service professionals*. Washington, DC: Author. Retrieved from https://fns-prod.azureedge.net/sites/default/files/cn/SP40-2017a1.pdf

U.S. Department of Health and Human Services. (2010). *The Child Abuse Prevention and Treatment Act, including adoption opportunities and the Abandoned Infants Assistance Act, as amended by P.L. 111–320, the CAPTA Reauthorization Act of 2010*. Washington, DC: Author. Retrieved from http://www.acf.hhs.gov/sites/default/files/cb/capta2010.pdf

Voting Accessibility for the Elderly and Handicapped Act, Pub. L. 98–435, 52 U.S.C. § 20101 *et seq.* (1984).

World Health Organization. (2018). *International classification of diseases, 11th revision*. Retrieved from http://www.who.int/classifications/icd/en/

Best Practices in Ethical Reasoning for School Occupational Therapy Practitioners

4

Kathlyn L. Reed, PhD, MLIS, OTR, FAOTA, and Jean E. Polichino, OTR, MS, FAOTA

KEY TERMS AND CONCEPTS

- Ethics
- Stakeholder

OVERVIEW

Occupational therapy practitioners[1] who work in schools must adhere to various federal and state education rules and regulations as well as state licensure rules and regulations. The occupational therapy profession's official code of conduct provides further guidance (American Occupational Therapy Association [AOTA], 2015a, 2015b).

In *South Kingstown Sch. Dist., 113 LRP 19804* (2013), for example, the occupational therapist's evaluation of a child with autism spectrum disorder created concerns for the hearing officer reviewing the therapist's evaluation report. The therapist was found to have spent only an hour with the student. It was unclear whether the therapist had reviewed the student's records before the evaluation. In addition, the therapist was apparently unaware of the parent's concerns regarding the student's sensory functioning.

In his findings, the hearing officer wrote that the occupational therapy evaluation was not sufficiently comprehensive to identify all of the student's occupational therapy needs and, therefore, was not appropriate. The therapist's evaluation was out of compliance with federal regulations supporting the Individuals With Disabilities Education Improvement Act of 2004 (IDEA; Pub. L. 108–446) at 34 C.F.R. § 300.304(c)(4) and (6), which state that the evaluation must be sufficiently comprehensive to assess the child in all areas related to the suspected disability and must identify all of the child's special needs. From an ethical perspective, it appears that the therapist failed to adhere to the profession's principles of beneficence and justice. The legal and ethical violations by the therapist compromised the student's welfare (and proved expensive for the school district).

---

[1] *Occupational therapy practitioner* refers to both the occupational therapist and the occupational therapy assistant. AOTA (2014, p. S18) states, "The occupational therapist is responsible for all aspects of occupational therapy service delivery and is accountable for the safety and effectiveness of the occupational therapy service delivery process" and "must be directly involved in the delivery of services during the initial evaluation and regularly throughout the course of intervention. . . . The occupational therapy assistant delivers safe and effective occupational therapy services under the supervision of and in partnership with the occupational therapist."

Ethics is the discipline within philosophy that deals with what is good behavior on the basis of moral principles and practice ("Ethics," 2014). *Ethical reasoning* is used "to recognize, analyze, and clarify ethical problems that arise" (Doherty & Purtilo, 2016, p. 76). The focus is not on what could be done but on what should be done. An *ethical dilemma* occurs when there are "two (or more) morally correct courses of action that cannot both be followed" (Doherty & Purtilo, 2015, p. 66). *Ethical behavior* is the "enactment of ethical principles" (Purtilo et al., 2005, p. 14).

Ethical reasoning and practice constantly change in response to policy, political contexts, team structures, family and school demands, and workloads (Gallagher & Tschudin, 2010). The changes produce a complex environment with various challenges, including maintaining quality services with time and money constraints. Creating an ethical climate is critical (Kurfuerst & Yousey, 2012). A positive and acceptable ethical climate increases employee morale, commitment to the school district, and career engagement, and encourages staff retention (Shirey, 2005).

The *Occupational Therapy Code of Ethics (2015)* (hereinafter, the Code) is the profession's summary of ethical behavior, conduct, and practice. Its 2 purposes are to provide "aspirational Core Values that guide [practitioners] toward ethical courses of action in professional and volunteer roles" and to delineate "enforceable Principles and Standards of Conduct" (AOTA, 2015b, p. 1). Thus, the principles and standards are written to apply to all aspects of occupational therapy but must be interpreted in individual situations. This chapter addresses how the Code applies to practitioners providing occupational therapy services in schools.

ESSENTIAL CONSIDERATIONS

Essential considerations for ethical reasoning include understanding AOTA's ethics principles, categories of conflicts, and the barriers and supports present in school settings.

The Code

The Code asserts 6 ethics concepts organized into 6 principles. These principles are delineated in the Code (AOTA,

---

Copyright © 2019 by the American Occupational Therapy Association. All rights reserved. To reuse this content, contact www.copyright.com.
https://doi.org/10.7139/2019.978-1-56900-591-0.004

TABLE 4.1.   Principles From the *Occupational Therapy Code of Ethics (2015)*

PRINCIPLE AND DESCRIPTION	EXAMPLES	SCHOOL PRACTICE APPLICATIONS
Principle 1. Beneficence: "Occupational therapy personnel shall demonstrate a concern for the well-being and safety of the recipients of their services" (AOTA, 2015b, p. 2).	Requires taking action to help others by promoting good, by preventing harm, and by removing harm. The term *beneficence* connotes acts of mercy, kindness, and charity (Beauchamp & Childress, 2013); thus, actions that promote participation in educational activities should be the primary focus.	Instructional personnel implemented sensory strategies for students with ASD, including the use of weighted vests and blankets, without consulting the research literature for evidence of effectiveness or benefit to students with ASD or obtaining any formal training. On learning of this situation, the occupational therapist approached the campus principal to alert her to the research evidence, reviewed the precautions and inappropriate use, and offered to provide the needed training.
Principle 2. Nonmaleficence: "Occupational therapy personnel shall refrain from actions that cause harm" (AOTA, 2015b, p. 3).	"Obligates us to abstain from causing harm to others" (Beauchamp & Childress, 2013, p. 3). The obligation includes not imposing risks of harm, even when the potential risk is without malicious or harmful intent. Harm in educational settings may occur when students are denied participation in educational activities in which other students are engaged.	A student with behavioral challenges was having difficulty remaining in his seat. The occupational therapist discovered that the teacher was using another student's positioning chair and seat belt to restrict the student's mobility during instruction. The therapist shared her concerns with the teacher regarding the physical, social, and emotional risks of harm to the student as well as the legal prohibition of using positioning equipment for restraint.
Principle 3. Autonomy: "Occupational therapy personnel shall respect the right of the individual to self-determination, privacy, confidentiality, and consent" (AOTA, 2015b, p. 4).	Acknowledges a person's right to hold views, to make choices, and to take actions based on personal values and beliefs (Beauchamp & Childress, 2013). It also requires obtaining consent before initiation of occupational therapy services and protection of student's confidential information and records.	An 18-year-old high school student no longer wanted occupational therapy services as part of his transition IEP. His parents insisted the school continue to provide occupational therapy "in case something comes up." The occupational therapy practitioner reminded the IEP team that the student is of age for making his own (self-) determinations and reassured the team that occupational therapy was available should the IEP team, including the student, want assistance in the future.
Principle 4. Justice: "Occupational therapy personnel shall promote fairness and objectivity in the provision of occupational therapy services" (AOTA, 2015b, p. 5).	Relates to the fair, equitable, and appropriate treatment of persons (Beauchamp & Childress, 2013). Occupational therapy practitioners should respect all applicable laws, policies, rules, regulations, and standards related to their area of practice. The focus is on upholding the idea that all individuals have an equitable opportunity to achieve occupational engagement as an essential component of life (AOTA, 2015b).	A student was referred to occupational therapy because of concerns that his sensory processing may be the source of his behavioral difficulties. The occupational therapist performed an evaluation using interviews with the teacher and parents; observations in the classroom, cafeteria, and playground; and standardized testing, including data from school and home. She provided a fair, objective report of her findings, indicating that although the student processes sensory input differently from others in some areas, the responses did not present as affecting his participation in learning, self-help, and social activities, nor did they serve as a trigger for the unexpected behaviors.
Principle 5. Veracity: "Occupational therapy personnel shall provide comprehensive, accurate, and objective information when representing the profession" (AOTA, 2015b, p. 6).	This refers to comprehensive, accurate, and objective transmission of information and includes fostering the client's understanding of such information. The recipient of care or participant in research enters into a contract that includes a right to truthful information (Beauchamp & Childress, 2013). Parents and caregivers remain informed, and records should be complete and accurate.	The occupational therapy practitioner noticed that student documentation submitted by an occupational therapy colleague did not completely and accurately represent the time or activities provided by a colleague. She was concerned that the report should be comprehensive and accurate when it is submitted for Medicaid billing. She shared her concerns with her supervisor so that an investigation could be initiated.

(Continued)

TABLE 4.1. Principles From the *Occupational Therapy Code of Ethics (2015) (Cont.)*

PRINCIPLE AND DESCRIPTION	EXAMPLES	SCHOOL PRACTICE APPLICATIONS
Principle 6. Fidelity: "Occupational therapy personnel shall treat clients, colleagues and other professionals with respect, fairness, discretion, and integrity" (AOTA, 2015b, p. 7).	This refers to being faithful, which includes obligations of loyalty and of keeping promises and commitments (Veatch et al., 2010). This principle specifically addresses the need for practitioners to consistently balance their duties to service recipients and other stakeholders (e.g., individuals who have an interest in the success of an endeavor), who may influence ethical reasoning and professional practice (AOTA, 2015b).	As part of the early intervening team at her school, the occupational therapist recommended simple accommodations for students to enhance their participation and performance in curriculum activities. Teachers had not been implementing the recommendations in a matter that demonstrated integrity to student learning objectives. The therapist reached out to the teachers to seek understanding of their reticence to use the strategies and to determine whether she needed to provide training or model their use.

Note. AOTA = American Occupational Therapy Association; ASD = autism spectrum disorder; IEP = individualized education program.
Source. American Occupational Therapy Association (2015b).

2015b). Four of the principles are considered moral principles (Principles 1–4):

- Beneficence
- Nonmaleficence
- Autonomy
- Justice.

Two principles are viewed as standards of conduct that service providers should follow (Principles 5 and 6):

- Veracity
- Fidelity.

These moral principles and standards that occupational therapy practitioners in schools should follow are summarized in Table 4.1. The primary role of school occupational therapy practitioners with students in special education is to facilitate access to and participation in their individualized education program (IEP). The school occupational therapy practitioner also plays a role in increasing students' engagement and participation by assisting districts in preventing unnecessary referrals to special education. Occupational therapy services must be consistent with and support the educational mission. Thus, for example, the ethical Principle of Beneficence is best illustrated in school practice when occupational therapy services enable students to better perform their educational tasks and roles.

In school practice, adherence to these basic ethical principles encourages occupational therapy practitioners to ensure that their conduct is beyond reproach. Practitioners should avoid actions that would compromise or prevent student participation in educational activities and should actively support student self-determination. They should ensure that students and their parents or guardians understand their rights regarding consent for services and assure them of the confidentiality of provider interactions and documentation. Practitioners should make the effort to limit how health disparities and social inequality affect student outcomes.

Practitioners have an ethical obligation to know and follow all laws, rules, regulations, and policies that apply to school practice and should be sure that state or district policies, practice guidelines, and procedures ensure the protection of the recipients of occupational therapy. Respect should be demonstrated through truthfulness and accuracy in all actions, deeds, and communications.

Categories of Conflict

In educational settings, conflicts may arise around administrative directives, supervision, Medicaid billing, staffing, and resource allocation decisions. Clear lines of administrative supervision need to be established. Job descriptions will clarify the line of supervisory authority as well as the specific duties and responsibilities of occupational therapy practitioners.

Job descriptions need to be reviewed annually and updated as needed to ensure that they are an accurate and current reflection of the job. A convenient time for supervisors and their employees to review job descriptions is during the annual employee performance evaluation. Veracity, Principle 5 of the Code, states that occupational therapy practitioners shall "describe the type and duration of occupational therapy services accurately in professional contracts, including the duties and responsibilities of all involved parties" (AOTA, 2015b, p. 6).

Conflicts with administrative supervision and directives may also occur when rules and policies are written without adequate input from the people who have to carry them out. School administrators may not be familiar with occupational therapy and may have little understanding of what occupational therapy practitioners know and do. Occupational therapy practitioners need to take responsibility for ensuring that employers are aware of occupational therapy's ethical obligations as set forth in the Code and of the implications of those obligations for occupational therapy practice, policy, education, and research.

Third-party billing for services may also be a source of conflict for occupational therapy practitioners in schools. School systems often seek reimbursement for services, depending on how the student's services are classified. For example, when providing services for students who have disabilities, districts may seek cost recovery under the state's Medicaid program for schools. In some instances, they may bill private insurance or seek reimbursement from a state agency. Different sources of funding have different rules for documentation and submission of claims. Practitioners may find it frustrating to comply with the requirements, but it is an ethical responsibility under Principle 4, Justice.

Occupational therapy practitioners shall "ensure that documentation for reimbursement purposes is done in accordance with applicable laws, guidelines, and regulations" (AOTA, 2015b, p. 6).

In addition, the Code states that fees are to be collected "legally and justly in a manner that is fair, reasonable, and commensurate with services delivered" (AOTA, 2015b, p. 5). Occupational therapy practitioners whose schools bill third parties are also cautioned not to let the need for third-party funds drive the recommendations they make for student services (Royeen et al., 2000). The standard to determine whether occupational therapy should be part of the student's educational program is driven by educational need. Through the team process, consideration is given to the occupational therapy evaluation data as well as the student's academic, behavioral, self-help, and social goals for the IEP period. Together, the team members determine whether occupational therapy is needed for the student to benefit from special education, not whether third-party funds can be accessed.

If occupational therapy services for a student are desired by others to garner reimbursement, or if they appear unnecessary, then the occupational therapy practitioner uses the Principle of Fidelity: They will "use conflict resolution and internal and alternative dispute resolution resources as needed to resolve organizational and interpersonal conflicts, as well as perceived institutional ethics violations" (AOTA, 2015b, p. 7). Conversely, in accordance with the Principle of Justice, if the occupational therapy practitioner feels that services are needed but that others do not want them provided so as not to incur associated costs, then the practitioner will make efforts to "advocate for changes to systems and policies that are discriminatory or unfairly limit or prevent access to occupational therapy services" (AOTA, 2015b, p. 5).

Desired allocation of limited occupational therapy resources by stakeholders may be another source of conflict in school practice. Doherty and Purtilo (2016) define a *stakeholder* as "a person, group, or other entity that has a deep and compelling interest in a situation that it wants to protect" (p. 187). Stakeholders have a vested interest in the outcome of a situation or issue of concern and may include family members, school administrators, educators, school staff, providers of related services, private therapists, advocates, and the community as a whole. Stakeholders can be allies in ethical reasoning and decision making, or they may complicate the situation because of the interests that they want to promote or protect. Understanding the perspective and interests of stakeholders can assist in determining options and choices. The provision of occupational therapy requires professional time, supplies and materials, space, and equipment. All may be in short supply. Determining how to allocate the available resources requires consideration of the ethical Principle of Justice.

Conflicts Resulting From the Supervisory Relationship

Occupational therapists and occupational therapy assistants in schools will both experience ethical conflicts, but their views of the conflicts may differ on the basis of their unique professional perspectives. For example, supervision and the supervisory relationship will look different depending on each practitioner's role in the partnership. However, AOTA's (2014) *Guidelines for Supervision, Roles, and Responsibilities During the Delivery of Occupational Therapy Services* notes that both supervisors and practitioners have a responsibility for ensuring the success of the professional relationship. As stated in this document, professional standards specify that, to provide occupational therapy services, occupational therapy assistants should receive supervision from an occupational therapist. Together, they are responsible for collaboratively developing a plan for supervision (AOTA, 2014, p. S17).

Although state requirements vary regarding the specifics for supervision of occupational therapy assistants, the occupational therapist is, in all cases, responsible for all aspects of occupational therapy and is accountable for the safety and effectiveness of services. State occupational therapy licensure laws and regulations as well as state and local educational agency administrative directives should be consulted. Examples of supervisory methods include "direct face-to-face contact [such as] observation, modeling, . . . [co-treatment], discussions, teaching, and instruction" (AOTA, 2014, p. S17). "Examples of . . . indirect contact include phone conversations, written correspondence, and electronic exchanges" (p. S17).

In states in which supervision is specified, the ethical and legal responsibility is to follow the regulations. Where regulations are not spelled out, occupational therapy practitioners should collaboratively develop a working plan for supervisory relationships and review the plan at least annually. Whether 1 occupational therapist supervises one occupational therapy assistant or 1 occupational therapy assistant has multiple occupational therapist supervisors, a well-developed working plan is important. Considerations should include factors such as

- The amount of experience and competency level of the assistant;
- Any expertise or specialized training the assistant may have acquired, such as knowledge of assistive technology or feeding techniques;
- The complexity of students' disabling conditions and needs and of the intervention process; and
- The needs and requirements of each school setting.

The AOTA (2014) document on supervision provides the following guidance relevant to school practice:

- "The occupational therapist is responsible for all aspects of occupational therapy service delivery and is accountable for the safety and effectiveness of the occupational therapy service delivery process" (p. S18).
- "The occupational therapist must be directly involved in the delivery of services during the initial evaluation and regularly throughout the course of intervention, intervention review, and outcomes evaluation" (p. S18).
- "The occupational therapy assistant delivers occupational therapy services under the supervision of and in partnership with the occupational therapist" (p. S18).
- "It is the responsibility of the occupational therapist to determine when to delegate responsibilities to an occupational therapy assistant" (p. S19).

Barriers and Supports Within School Settings

Ethical conflicts and dilemmas can seem overwhelming. Providing support to staff dealing with ethical issues is essential. When the occupational therapist is the only therapist in the district or the only 1 assigned to a school or set of schools, a system of support is especially necessary. Taking steps in advance can reduce the barriers and increase the support system. Resources such as state occupational therapy rules and regulations (typically accessible on the Internet), the Code (AOTA, 2015b), and samples of effectively written documents may provide guidance. Activities that enhance support include the following:

- Developing a network of other school occupational therapy practitioners (e.g., district, state, and national), which may provide support when the need arises
- Establishing working relationships with occupational therapy practitioners working in nearby districts and with other related services practitioners in the same district, such as physical therapists and speech–language pathologists
- Building relationships with local administrative leaders and human resources personnel, and involving them when necessary in resolving ethical dilemmas
- Joining AOTA and accessing resources, including the pediatric program manager, the members of the Children and Youth Special Interest Section, and official AOTA guidelines and documents.

Emotional Distress and Ethical Dilemmas

It is common to experience emotional distress when dealing with ethical dilemmas. The practitioner may feel that something was done incorrectly, may experience self-doubt about their professional role, may be overwhelmed with decisions that need to be made, may feel that an individual is incompetent or not up to performing the job, or may experience anger directed at administrators and coworkers for allowing a situation to occur. To process emotional distress constructively, consider the following steps:

- Acknowledge the emotions and attempt to clarify the problem and determine possible solutions
- Identify whether the problem at hand is a legal problem (e.g., conflict with federal or state law), an employment problem (e.g., conflict with employment policies, procedures, and practices of your employer), or an ethical problem (e.g., violation of the code of conduct), keeping in mind that all 3 areas may be applicable in some cases
- When there is an ethical element to the issue, follow the suggested guidelines for ethical reasoning outlined in the next section.

BEST PRACTICES

Best practices for using the ethical reasoning process include developing partnerships with team members and documenting communication and actions related to occupational therapy services and any conflict that may have transpired. The following section presents strategies for dealing with ethical issues, an ethical reasoning process

for resolving ethical dilemmas, and guidance on what actions to take when the Code appears to be violated (AOTA, 2015b). Finally, occupational therapy practitioners are encouraged to gather additional resources on ethical reasoning and practice.

Develop Partnerships With Team Members

Decisions about occupational therapy services in special education are made in teams. It is important to collaborate with other team members and document those discussions. Doing so ensures that different professional perspectives are considered when issues arise, and that multiple perspectives factor into decision making when a course of action must be determined. For example, practitioners may encounter a parent who refuses to release medical information and restricts medical provider access regarding their child's health. Despite the child's unknown medical history, the occupational therapist might identify critical health concerns (e.g., gagging or choking during snack or lunch). This information must be immediately reported to the student's team, including the administrator, case manager, and school nurse. The team must determine steps to ensure a safe mealtime program for the student. In these instances, a team effort is often likely to produce successful outcomes for obtaining needed information.

For a student in regular education whose cognitive processing is slower than that of others or who is depressed and withdrawn, occupational therapy practitioners may find themselves advocating along with the parent in an early intervening effort to address the student's issues with simple accommodations or modifications. Clarifying the existence and impact of the student's "hidden" difficulties for other members of the team may provide insight that will assist instructional personnel with more effective delivery of curriculum content and may help prevent social isolation.

Document Communication and Actions

Conflicts may arise at any time. Documentation of therapy services (see Chapter 45, "Best Practices in School Occupational Therapy Documentation and Data Collection"), as well as phone calls and practitioner actions, may be key in resolving conflicts. Documentation should occur immediately after the occurrence and should succinctly articulate what transpired. Keep in mind that if no record of a phone call, service, or action exists, then there is no proof that it ever occurred. Such proof could become important when attempts are made to resolve a conflict.

Use Ethical Reasoning Process to Resolve Ethical Dilemmas

One method of resolving ethical dilemmas is to use a systematic method of ethical reasoning that is outlined in Table 4.2, which illustrates the ethical reasoning process used in the following case example:

A 6-year-old student has a congenital disorder that typically results in death before puberty. The student has been evaluated by the occupational therapist, who

TABLE 4.2. Application of Doherty and Purtilo's (2016) Ethical Reasoning Process for Resolving Ethical Dilemmas

STEPS	INFORMATION
1. Gather relevant information. Identify the major issue or essential problems using facts (data) that help to organize the thinking process.	Can occupational therapy services be withheld because of the beliefs or preferences of school personnel? Should occupational therapy services be provided to a student with a degenerative condition, particularly if resources are scarce?
2. Identify the type of ethical problem. Usually a concept described in Table 4.1 is the primary ethical concern, but there may also be secondary issues.	The Principles of Justice (fair treatment and an impartial share of the benefits of society) and Beneficence (protecting and defending the rights of others) are involved.
3. Use ethical theories or approaches to analyze the problem. • If the ethical issue is based on a duty, there is usually an actual or implied law, rule, regulation, policy, or procedure to be followed. • If the issue is based on a consequence, then the consequences can be identified and evaluated. Often, both occur together and can be evaluated together.	Here, the occupational therapy practitioner has a duty to treat the client with equality, fairness, and justice. The consequences should be based on need and not on factors such as age, race, ethnicity, economic status, or disability.
4. Explore the practical alternatives. Exploring practical alternatives allows for a discussion about options and choices. If one approach cannot be followed, perhaps another approach can be substituted. Occasionally, discussion of options allows a better choice to be made.	To meet the student's needs, consider strategically scheduling sessions, such as a 1-hour session the first 2 weeks of service for making initial modifications, and then a 30-minute session each grading period thereafter to make any needed adjustments as the student's condition progresses. This pattern ensures student participation in school activities. Work with the teacher to adapt new tasks related to curriculum content.
5. Complete the action. Implement the best choice of action.	Provide the service, problem solving continuously with the student and teacher.
6. Evaluate the process and outcomes. Evaluate the choice of action to determine whether the desired outcome was obtained.	Together with the teacher and student, collect data at predetermined intervals (e.g., every Tuesday) to monitor progress. Analyze the data, and adjust the intervention plan on the basis of the results.

recommends occupational therapy services to modify the classroom environment and curriculum activities to ensure continued participation in school. School personnel indicate in a written report that they think occupational therapy for this student is a waste of time and money. They ask the therapist not to recommend services. The therapist respectfully disagrees with her colleagues, explaining specifically how her services will help the student participate with peers (reflecting the ethical Principle of Justice), and restates her recommendations. She moves forward with presenting these recommendations at the IEP meeting.

If the aforementioned steps are followed, the desired outcome should occur. Sometimes the steps need to be repeated to obtain a satisfactory resolution to the ethical dilemma.

Take Action When Ethical Violations Are Suspected

If occupational therapy practitioners suspect that an ethical violation has occurred, then what course of action should be taken? First, as the ethical reasoning process previously discussed suggests, clarify the problem, and identify the ethical principle that may have been violated. Next, consider what steps can be taken to correct the violation. Often, the best approach is to talk with the person directly. Is the person aware that their actions appear to violate an ethical

principle? If the person does not know or realize that a violation has occurred, educating the person may solve the problem. If the person knows the violation is occurring but chooses not to correct their behavior, then the approach depends on administrative policies, which may include written notice to a supervisor or administrator.

Again, if the violation can be corrected within the institutional guidelines, that course of action should be pursued first. However, if the violation cannot be corrected within the facility or organization, then the next step is to contact the state regulatory board (SRB). Forms for filing complaints are usually available online or by calling the SRB. The online address or phone number may be on the license itself. The person making the complaint is often asked to identify what rule or regulation appears to be violated, so it is useful to have a copy of the regulations available to consult.

If the ethical violation is covered by the Code (AOTA, 2015b) and the occupational therapy practitioner is an AOTA member, then the AOTA Ethics Commission should be notified. The enforcement procedures for the Code (AOTA, 2015a) outline the process and include the form needed to file a complaint. A written statement should be attached that summarizes the facts and circumstances, including dates and events. If the person has maintained their certification with the National Board for Certification in Occupational Therapy (NBCOT), then NBCOT should also be notified. Information on how to file a complaint and related forms are available online at NBCOT's website (https://www.nbcot.org).

Gather Resources to Guide Ethical Reasoning and Practice

Occupational therapy practitioners should have access to documents (e.g., federal, state, local) that guide ethical reasoning and practice. These resources may be used to resolve ethical dilemmas. Most documents are available online. Practitioners should be knowledgeable about the federal, state, and district education laws and procedures. State regulations for billing Medicaid or other funding sources should be accessed by practitioners. All practitioners must follow their state credentialing regulations (e.g., licensure, practice act, rules).

SUMMARY

Ethical behavior is based on moral judgment. To facilitate ethical reasoning and help with decision making, professions organize moral judgment into codes of ethics. The AOTA Code is organized into 6 principles and standards of conduct: Beneficence, Nonmaleficence, Autonomy, Justice, Veracity, and Fidelity (AOTA, 2015b). These concepts form the structure for implementing the ethical reasoning process. Although issues in school practice may appear to be unique, the ethics concepts and the ethical reasoning process are the same for all areas of practice, policy, education, and research.

REFERENCES

American Occupational Therapy Association. (2014). Guidelines for supervision, roles, and responsibilities during the delivery of occupational therapy services. *American Journal of Occupational Therapy, 68*(Suppl. 3), S16–S22. https://doi.org/10.5014/ajot.2014.686S03

American Occupational Therapy Association. (2015a). Enforcement procedures for the *Occupational Therapy Code of Ethics. American Journal of Occupational Therapy, 69*(Suppl. 3), 6913410012. https://doi.org/10.5014/ajot.2015.696S19

American Occupational Therapy Association. (2015b). Occupational therapy code of ethics (2015). *American Journal of Occupational Therapy, 69*(Suppl. 3), 6913410030. https://doi.org/10.5014/ajot.2015.696S03

Beauchamp, T. L., & Childress, J. F. (2013). *Principles of biomedical ethics* (7th ed.). New York: Oxford University Press.

Doherty, R. F., & Purtilo, R. B. (2016). *Ethical dimensions in the health professions* (6th ed.). Philadelphia: Elsevier/Saunders.

Ethics. (2014). In *Merriam–Webster dictionary and thesaurus.* Springfield, MA: Author.

Gallagher, A., & Tschudin, V. (2010). Educating for ethical leadership. *Nurse Education Today, 30,* 224–227. https://doi.org/10.1016/j.nedt.2009.11.003

Individuals With Disabilities Education Improvement Act of 2004, Pub. L. 108–446, 20 U.S.C. §§ 1400–1482.

Kurfuerst, S., & Yousey, J. R. (2012). Leading with ethics: Creating an ethical climate in your occupational therapy department. *OT Practice, 17*(13), CE1–CE7.

Purtilo, R. B., Jenson, G. M., & Royee, C. G. (2005). *Educating for moral action: A source book in health and rehabilitation ethics.* Philadelphia: F. A. Davis.

Royeen, C. B., Duncan, M., Crabtree, J., Richards, J., & Frolek Clark, G. (2000). Effects of billing Medicaid for occupational therapy services in schools. *American Journal of Occupational Therapy, 54,* 429–433. https://doi.org/10.5014/ajot.54.4.429

Shirey, M. (2005). Ethical climate in nursing practice: The leader's role. *JONA's Healthcare Law, Ethics, and Regulation, 7*(2), 59–67.

South Kingstown Sch. Dist., 113 LRP 19804 (R.I. SEA Jan. 12, 2013).

Veatch, R. M., Haddad, A. M., & English, D. C. (2010). *Case studies in allied health ethics.* New York: Oxford University Press.

Best Practices in Preparing Students to Practice Occupational Therapy in Schools

Cynthia Clough, PhD, OT/L; Meredith P. Gronski, OTD, OTR/L, CLA; and Steven D. Taff, PhD, OTR/L, FNAP, FAOTA

5

KEY TERMS AND CONCEPTS

- Basic principles of adult learning
- Instructional design
- Occupational therapy education

OVERVIEW

Executing best practices in preparing students[1] to practice occupational therapy in schools is critical to supporting the nearly 25% of occupational therapists and 18% of occupational therapy assistants who work in an early childhood or school practice setting (American Occupational Therapy Association [AOTA], 2015c). Given this volume, future occupational therapy practitioners[2] require a solid preservice education to prepare for this setting.

An entry-level ***occupational therapy education*** prepares future practitioners to address the occupational needs of individuals, groups, communities, and populations (Accreditation Council for Occupational Therapy Education [ACOTE®], 2018). Policies guiding practice dictate that occupational therapy practitioners, as related service professionals, must demonstrate professional role performance and conduct aligned with the best available evidence. Essential to this is the ability to differentiate the educational model of practice from the traditional medical model. The future of occupational therapy's professional role identity in schools is dependent on the effective preparation of students to recognize the many roles that occupational therapy has beyond direct, restorative, and developmental intervention.

Occupational therapy practitioners in schools work with children and youth, parents, caregivers, educational staff, team members, and district administrators to facilitate a child's participation in purposeful and meaningful daily life and school activities (AOTA, 2014). To be effective, students must obtain knowledge of the physical, adaptive, cognitive, behavioral, social, and mental health factors that can affect a child's participation. In addition, students must learn to negotiate interdisciplinary team communication; abide by federal, state, district, and local policies; and maintain a high level of professional advocacy to ensure that the distinct value of occupational therapy in schools is known and used. This chapter discusses the dynamic interaction of context and process in the academic portion of occupational therapy education that is specific to preparing students to practice occupational therapy in schools.

ESSENTIAL CONSIDERATIONS

As occupational therapy educators design courses, modules, or learning activities to prepare students for school practice, they also need to consider effective course design methods, multilayered assessment practices, overall position of content within the educational program's curriculum, and how adult learners approach and integrate knowledge.

Academic Preparation for Entry-Level School Practice

Various degree levels, pedagogical strategies, curriculum designs, and course structures are used in occupational therapy education to develop learners into competent and compassionate professional practitioners. Ultimately, occupational therapy education cultivates professional reasoning skills and the integration of professional values, theories, evidence, ethics, and skills within both didactic and fieldwork components. AOTA's (2015b) Commission on Education outlined fundamental beliefs that an occupational therapy "education promotes clinical reasoning and the integration of professional values, theories, evidence, ethics, and skills" (p. 1).

Moreover, the occupational therapy curriculum must incorporate
- Active learning strategies within and beyond the didactic classroom,

---

[1]To avoid confusion between children in public schools and persons attending college programs, in this chapter, the term *student* refers to persons in occupational therapist or occupational therapy assistant education programs. The term *children* is used to refer to children or adolescents in school.

[2]*Occupational therapy practitioner* refers to both the occupational therapist and the occupational therapy assistant. AOTA (2014, p. S18) states, "The occupational therapist is responsible for all aspects of occupational therapy service delivery and is accountable for the safety and effectiveness of the occupational therapy service delivery process" and "must be directly involved in the delivery of services during the initial evaluation and regularly throughout the course of intervention. . . . The occupational therapy assistant delivers safe and effective occupational therapy services under the supervision of and in partnership with the occupational therapist."

Copyright © 2019 by the American Occupational Therapy Association. All rights reserved. To reuse this content, contact www.copyright.com.
https://doi.org/10.7139/2019.978-1-56900-591-0.005

- Collaborative processes that scaffold previous knowledge and experiences,
- Continuous evaluation and learner self-reflection, and
- A commitment to lifelong learning (AOTA, 2015b).

Clinical Model vs. Educational Model

Many occupational therapy education programs emphasize the clinical and rehabilitative model of practice. In addition, the vast majority of evaluation methods, reimbursement structures, and intervention strategies are discussed in terms of medical necessity for the recipient of occupational therapy. However, education programs must prepare future occupational therapy practitioners to support access, performance, and participation in the school and community settings.

Accreditation Standards in Occupational Therapy Education

ACOTE (2018) has developed minimum standards for each degree level within occupational therapy education. These standards guide the development of an entire curriculum. Best practices for preparing students as entry-level practitioners in schools must infuse content, learning experiences, and knowledge and skill outcomes across multiple courses. Although many occupational therapy and occupational therapy assistant programs have a course explicitly for pediatric content, integrating opportunities for school practice preparation throughout coursework is preferred.

For example, students across all levels of occupational therapy education are required to learn about the occupational development of children (Standard B.1.1) and the nature of the occupational roles of children in schools (Standard B.3.2); however, these concepts are most often presented early in the foundational course of the curriculum.

In contrast, the evaluation of a child's ability to perform ADLs, educational tasks, and leisure engagement in the context of a school day (Standard B.4.4), as well as using nonstandardized interviewing and observation techniques (Standard B.4.1), may be presented within the framework of a course devoted to assessment and evaluation. Finally, the design and implementation of evidence-based interventions (Standards B.5.2–B.5.14) may be incorporated into a course focused on pediatric interventions or may be designed as a module of another practice-based course. Occupational therapy education programs may also elect to fulfill ACOTE standards regarding program development (Standard B.7.9), supervision (Standard B.9.8), or leadership (Standard B.7.5) through lesson plans related to the practice of occupational therapy in schools.

Instructional Design and Learning Principles

Instructional design is the art of creating "instructional experiences which make the acquisition of knowledge and skill more efficient, effective, and appealing" (Merrill et al., 1996, p. 6). It moves beyond the "what" to teach and into the "how" to teach it. Although there are many approaches to instructional design, an in-depth exploration of any one of them is beyond the scope of this chapter. Most instructional design strategies use similar approaches (see Exhibit 5.1 for a sample approach with 8 basic steps and key questions at each stage).

EXHIBIT 5.1.   Sample Approach to Instructional Design

Step 1: Preassessment—How will *I find out* what learners already know about this topic?

Step 2: Anticipatory Set and Motivation—What will *I do* to connect learners with this topic? How will I engage their attention?

Step 3: Statement of Purpose—What will *I say* to explain the importance of learning this lesson?

Step 4: Instructor Modeling and Demonstration—What will *I do* to demonstrate to learners what is expected?

Step 5: Guided Practice—What will *we do* together to facilitate learners' understanding?

Step 6: Check for Understanding—What will *I ask* to uncover learners' understanding thus far?

Step 7: Independent Practice—What will *learners do* to internalize the knowledge?

Step 8: Closure—What will *learners say* or *do* to show what they learned?

Occupational therapy educators should consider this framework, whether in a one-time lecture or in a lab related to school-based practice, in modules in a school practice course or in individual assignments in a pediatric skills course. Understanding the needs of adult learners is critical when designing learning experiences that promote the acquisition of knowledge, skills, and professional behaviors for school practice. The **basic principles of adult learning** include the following concepts:

- Helping learners understand the *why,* not just the *what;*
- Learners being less dependent on educators and more self-directed;
- The importance of connecting knowledge and concepts to existing experiences; and
- Tapping in to learners' intrinsic motivation to learn and solve practical problems in everyday life (Brockett, 2015; Knowles et al., 2011).

Adult learners value hearing about others' ideas and lived experiences as well as learning through one-time presentations and professional learning communities (DuFour & Eaker, 1998). Bringing in school practitioners as guest lecturers or incorporating real-life scenarios to connect learning to school practice should aid this process. Students may benefit from being asked to develop an in-service for non–occupational therapy team members, modify or redesign an existing schoolwide program (e.g., regarding bullying, physical education, social skills), or execute a classroom resource around multi-tiered systems of support (MTSS) and positive behavioral supports (see Exhibit 5.2).

BEST PRACTICES

To adequately prepare occupational therapy students for school practice, educational programs need to build a curriculum starting with an understanding of performance expectations. These expectations center on content around education laws and regulations, evaluation processes, schools and families, least restrictive interventions, teaming, and leadership. See Appendix G, "How to Incorporate *Best Practices for Occupational Therapy in Schools, 2nd Edition.* Into a 16-Week Curriculum," for further information.

> **EXHIBIT 5.2.** Education Examples: Lecture and Lab
>
> **Scenario 1: One 2-hour lecture and one 3-hour lab**
> **Lecture Outline (example):**
>
> - Overview of practice influences and continuum of services from general education, Section 504, response to intervention, and IDEA (20 minutes)
> - Evaluating for eligibility in the school setting (25 minutes)
> - Overview of typical evidence-based interventions and modifications or accommodations used in the school setting (30 minutes)
> - Demonstration of goal writing and documentation for a school setting (IEP; 20 minutes)
> - Cases to highlight additional roles for occupational therapy in schools (e.g., consultant, in-service training, program development, literacy, mental health and wellness; 25 minutes)
>
> **Lab Activities (examples):**
>
> - Role-play an IEP meeting
> - Goal-writing practice with sample evaluation report
> - Role-play collaborative consultation with teacher
> - Case-based intervention plan development
> - Role-play teaching a strategy or AT use to a paraprofessional
>
> **Scenario 2: Weekly 3-hour course (3 credit hours, 16 weeks; labs included)**
>
> - **Week 1:** Influences on practice (laws, licensure)
> - **Week 2:** Applying the *OTPF–3* (AOTA, 2014) in schools
> - **Week 3:** Additional roles of OTs and OTAs in schools
> - **Week 4:** Working on educational teams
> - **Week 5:** Continuum of services (e.g., multi-tiered systems of support)
> - **Week 6:** Evaluation process: Determining strengths and needs
> - **Week 7:** Documentation and setting student goals
> - **Week 8:** Services on behalf of the student (e.g., accommodations, modifications, support to school personnel)
> - **Week 9:** Evidence-based interventions for all occupations in schools (e.g., literacy, self-care, play)
> - **Week 10:** Data-based decision making (e.g., progress monitoring)
> - **Week 11:** Transition planning
> - **Week 12:** Middle and high school special topics
> - **Week 13:** Conflicts and ethical decisions
> - **Week 14:** Behavior assessment and behavior intervention planning
> - **Week 15:** Professional development in schools
> - **Week 16:** School or districtwide program development
>
> *Note.* AOTA = American Occupational Therapy Association; AT = assistive technology; IDEA = Individuals With Disabilities Education Improvement Act of 2004; IEP = individualized education program; OTAs = occupational therapy assistants; *OTPF–3 = Occupational Therapy Practice Framework: Domain and Process* (3rd ed.); OTs = occupational therapists.

Develop Knowledge of Federal and State Education Laws and Regulations

Although the federal government passes education laws, each individual state has some autonomy in how laws are interpreted and applied at the individual state level. Some states may opt to have higher standard requirements than federal laws. As a result, variations exist across states in how education services are provided across school districts and schools and between individual teachers and their respective classrooms.

To support occupational therapy students' understanding of these variations, curriculum content must cover the interplay of federal laws, regulations, case laws, initiatives, and policies as well as changes that evolve over time and their impact on school practice. A plethora of laws and regulations guide practice in the school system (see Chapter 3, "Laws That Affect Occupational Therapy in Schools"). Content should also cover local governance by school boards, school administrative teams, the role of stakeholders, school funding mechanisms (e.g., taxpayer dollars, special education funding, Medicaid cost recovery), and

geographic and socioeconomic impact on student outcomes. In addition, occupational therapy educators should foster students' integration of professional resources to school practice (e.g., the *Occupational Therapy Framework: Domain and Process;* 3rd ed., or *OTPF–3* [AOTA, 2014] and *Guidelines for Occupational Therapy Services in Early Intervention and Schools* [AOTA, 2017]).

Apply the Occupational Therapy Evaluation Process to the Educational Setting

As the occupational therapy educator covers the service provision process that is operationalized in the *OTPF–3* (AOTA, 2014), attention can be focused more on moving from a foundational knowledge to application of skills—specifically, evaluation in the context of the educational setting. Occupational therapy students should understand their roles in evaluation, using their critical reasoning skills to assess clients (e.g., individuals, groups) in their natural contexts and to determine those areas that facilitate or restrict access and inclusive participation in academic, nonacademic, and functional skills within the domain of occupational therapy. All students should be able to implement evidence-based services that promote educationally necessary and educationally relevant interventions in the least restrictive environments.

Under IDEA (2004), the school occupational therapist may be included as a member of the initial individualized education program (IEP) team to determine whether a child has an educational disability and whether related services are needed for the student to benefit from special education. Although each request for an occupational therapy evaluation may include different questions to be answered through the evaluation process, a primary focus for evaluation is often aimed at better understanding the child's abilities, impairments, and challenges relative to participation and access to education.

Occupational therapy students need to gather data for the development of the occupational profile and analysis of occupational performance. Data may be gathered from interviews, record reviews, observations, and, when necessary, assessments (formal or informal). Occupational therapy students will need to have a foundational knowledge of the myriad measures available and how to select the most relevant ones to enhance participation skills in schools. To do so, occupational therapy students must acquire skills to evaluate assessment measures for potential bias, soundness of methodology, validity, reliability, and link to school participation and performance (Richardson, 2015).

Occupational therapy education programs need to provide students with the skills and tools to examine, adapt, and create physical, learning, and social environments that are accessible to all children (Schoonover & Grove, 2015). Occupational therapy practitioners often work with teams on the design and redesign of school spaces using principles of universal design (UD).

One example of an assignment that can help prepare occupational therapy students to think broadly about their role in school settings is incorporation of the redesign of indoor and outdoor school spaces to maximize opportunities for children of all ability levels to participate in school activities with peers. In such an assignment, occupational therapy students would use principles of UD to recommend updates to playground structures in ways that make physical access possible for students who are blind, use a wheelchair, have balance impairments, or simply have difficulty with highly coordinated motor tasks.

In addition, occupational therapy practitioners must ensure that the physical environment is accessible to individual students. Occupational therapy coursework should include case study assignments that require an analysis of fit between children's individual needs and their school environments. For example, recognizing that a child who has spina bifida may need access to a private bathroom and specialized space to receive health care during the school day will require occupational therapy students to contemplate the child's dignity, privacy, protected health information, and physical space accommodations.

To ensure that children have access to learning environments, occupational therapy students must develop skills to keep pace with continuously evolving assistive technology (AT) devices and equipment available to individuals with disabilities. As technology increases in complexity from low-tech tools such as pencil grippers and modified scissors to high-tech devices such as voice-activated environmental controls and eye-gaze technology, occupational therapy practitioners need to have the skills to acquire AT, monitor effectiveness, and ensure sustainability of use. This process requires advocacy for individual children and education on use and maintenance of devices for all members of the IEP team. Role playing and practicing education and training of high-tech and low-tech AT to laypersons can serve as useful lessons in preparing occupational therapy students for school practice.

Universal design for learning and differentiation of instruction are progressive movements in education that have increased teachers' capacity to reach the academic needs of all children in heterogeneous classrooms (Capper et al., 2000; Schoonover & Grove, 2015). Occupational therapy education programs must support the occupational therapist students' role in building the capacity of teachers to meet the needs of all children. Occupational therapists often work with general education teachers to differentiate classroom curricula to meet the learning needs of individual children whose academic performance falls outside the typical range of peers. Occupational therapy students who have the opportunity to practice modification of general education worksheets, workbooks, and assignments to align with an individual child's IEP goals will be prepared to support teachers in differentiating instruction for children identified with disabilities.

Environmental considerations for access and participation also include the social environment. Occupational therapy practitioners should be skilled in and advocate for a strengths-based, student-centered approach. Occupational therapy practitioners informed by social understandings of disability can take a lead role in advocating for children with disabilities to be fully included with nondisabled peers in all school activities (e.g., co-curricular activities, athletic programs, field trips, special school events).

Incorporate Contextual Considerations Across the Continuum of Education

A continuum of change occurs throughout a child's education with every transition and contextual progression (e.g., from elementary to middle and from middle to high school, from child to teenager and from teenager to young adult). In addition, contextual changes are experienced, including variations in school discipline policies, classroom structure and routines, school organization and daily schedules, and relationships with teachers and peers. Occupational therapy education programs need to include content regarding the developmental, emotional, and physical needs of children at each successive grade cluster. In addition, occupational therapy students must develop skills to fully assess the physical and social environments of various school contexts and to be prepared to advocate for children's access to classrooms, bathrooms with reasonable privacy, extracurricular activities (e.g., athletics, theater, band, art, clubs), and appropriate instruction.

The transition from high school to community life poses unique challenges for children with disabilities. IDEA

(2004) legislation has specific requirements of public schools and community organizations to meet individual children's and families' needs. Per IDEA, children with disabilities can receive special education and related services through age 21 years (although state law may vary). These transitional services require the occupational therapy practitioner to have knowledge of available community services, postsecondary education options, employment possibilities, leisure and social activities, public transportation, and housing options for young adults. Occupational therapy practitioners also need to be prepared to provide education and training to community employers, housing agencies, and other services or agencies. In addition, practitioners need to develop the skills to encourage young adults with disabilities to self-advocate and seek support services when necessary (Cleary et al., 2015). Anticipating these needs, occupational therapy education must prepare students for networking, program development, and life course planning.

Instruct Using Evidence to Inform Interventions for School Practice

Occupational therapy students need to learn how to assess and apply evidence that will inform interventions centered on optimizing a child's participation in school occupations. This process will require contemplating the child's abilities, environmental demands, and occupational expectations while critically analyzing those interventions that will likely produce the greatest impact.

In addition to intervention selection, occupational therapy students need thorough training for methodical collection of outcome measures. Formal data collection is becoming increasingly commonplace in schools because there are greater accountability demands related to efficacy of services (Bazyk & Cahill, 2015; Frolek Clark & Handley-More, 2017). Occupational therapy programs need to provide students with opportunities to engage in school documentation processes throughout their coursework to ensure that they understand the nature of team-based accountability and the terminology and expectations unique to school settings.

Address Interpersonal Skills and Collaboration as an Educational Team Member

Occupational therapy practitioners are integral members of district, building, and individual child teams. The occupational therapy curriculum that includes organizational theory, models of change, leadership, skills in teamwork and collaboration, and cultural responsiveness will serve to prepare practitioners for the many roles and responsibilities associated with these teams. Additional foci might encompass motivational interviewing, routine-based interviewing, navigation of challenging conversations, and reflective therapeutic use of self.

It is necessary that practitioners be able to interpret profession-specific terminology and understand each team member's role in supporting the child in their educational program. Without this, team members may become confused and unable to understand how to support the child

or, possibly, how occupational therapy can make a positive impact. Terminology must be distinctly defined and explained as it relates to practice in an educational model.

For example, task analysis has a different process and purpose for occupational therapy practitioners than for behavior analysts who may be working in the same classroom with the same child. Behavior analysts define *task analysis* as taking a complex task and breaking it down into small manageable steps. Occupational therapy practitioners further define it as the process of taking an occupation (or activity) and breaking it down to understand the many processes required (e.g., physical, cognitive, social). Behavior analysts teach the steps. Occupational therapy practitioners determine how to intervene (e.g., adapt, modify, create) to increase a child's participation. Understanding different professions' definitions of common terms allows occupational therapy practitioners to communicate the distinct value of occupational therapy in schools.

Under IDEA (2004), occupational therapy practitioners may be members of individual student teams. In this capacity, they need to work collaboratively with administrators, teachers, people from other disciplines, parents, and children—as well as, at times, representatives from community agencies, educational lawyers, and parent advocates. Occupational therapy students must acquire academic and interpersonal preparation to develop the skills to interact with the many professionals and individuals who are part of a child's team. This preparation includes recognizing various types of family structures, belief systems, roles, and cultural norms. Occupational therapy educators may consider inviting parents to supplement classroom instruction as guest speakers, either individually or in a panel format, to inspire occupational therapy students' consideration of parents' perspectives.

Occupational therapy practitioners also may serve as members of curriculum teams, school improvement initiatives, extracurricular organizations, and special program teams unique to a school or district. Occupational therapy and occupational therapy assistant education programs must prepare students for a wide range of team experiences and team roles.

Instruction in Documentation Skills Necessary for School Settings

Occupational therapy education programs need to prepare students for shared documentation and shared accountability for a child's educational outcomes. In addition, school practitioners need to understand educational and therapy documentation responsibilities from the perspective of federal and state legislation as well as occupational therapy licensing regulations and AOTA's best-practice documentation guidelines (Frolek Clark & Handley-More, 2017).

As in all practice settings, occupational therapy students need to be prepared to comply with professional documentation standards (e.g., evaluations, progress summaries, contact notes). In schools, occupational therapy practitioners have the added responsibility of communicating in parent-friendly terms. With this in mind, students need to be skilled in translating professional terminology and critical reasoning in their documentation so that parents,

EXHIBIT 5.3. Sample Learning Activity IEP Case Study

For this activity, occupational therapy educators provide a video of an occupational therapy practitioner conducting an evaluation with a child who has been referred for a full and individual educational evaluation.

The assignment begins with educators providing occupational therapy students with a written school referral and pertinent educational records. Students can then be directed to independently seek information on the diagnostic conditions being considered by the IEP team. Learning about the educational diagnostic criteria then leads students to the process of determining the evaluation methods that will contribute to answering the referral questions. With the recordings of parent and teacher interviews and the classroom and school observations, the assignment takes on a real-world feel. On the basis of the remaining questions, students can then clinically reason which assessment tools, if any, need to be administered.

While watching a recorded session in which an assessment is administered, students can score the results. This exercise would be followed by completion of a written evaluation summary to include an occupational profile, assessment results, interview data, and the occupational therapy interpretation of findings.

A mock IEP team meeting can then be conducted, with students and course educators taking on the roles of various team members. Students would then learn to develop an IEP document as an interprofessional team (with a parent being part of the team). This mock IEP document would contain a statement of the child's present level of performance, including strengths and needs; a plan for positive behavioral interventions and supports; AT needs; annual educational goals with plans to measure progress; and the school's commitment of services to ensure the child's access to education in the least restrictive environment. Students would also discuss how and when the child will be supported in co-curricular activities. The learning activity would conclude with a written occupational therapy intervention plan outlining interventions for an occupational therapy assistant.

This type of experiential assignment brings the opportunity for classroom discussion regarding the various ways in which parents may respond to the IEP process, interactions with team members from various professional backgrounds, negotiation and compromise regarding service needs, and advocacy for students and families as well as for the appropriate role of occupational therapy in an educational setting.

Note. AT = assistive technology; IEP = individualized education program.

other team members, and the school occupational therapy practitioner can integrate this information with that from other sources to determine a child's educational needs. Parents are part of the educational team and can assist in identifying when their child has an educational disability and, subsequently, in developing their child's IEP. The IEP outlines special education instruction and related service needs (e.g., occupational therapy). This is distinctly different from a clinical setting in which a SOAP (Subjective, Objective, Assessment, Plan) format might be used and the practitioner would determine therapy needs.

The development of educational goal and outcome statements is a critical aspect of the IEP process. The school occupational therapy practitioner, as a member of a child's team, must contribute to the development of meaningful, measurable, and achievable educational goals as well as outcome measures and progress reports. Occupational therapy students would benefit from learning how to develop subsequent data collection methods in tandem with learning how to write measurable goals.

A sample learning activity, described in Exhibit 5.3, incorporates role-playing an IEP meeting. Such a role play can be an effective means of helping students understand the differences between school documentation and traditional clinical documentation, as well as team decision making in these settings.

Provide an Understanding of Ethical Dilemmas

Part of the preparation for school practice should address ethical dilemmas in schools. Providing students with common scenarios in the school and having them use the AOTA (2015a) *Occupational Therapy Code of Ethics (2015)* as a foundation for their hypothetical actions will help prepare them for situations that may arise in the school.

Introduce System-Level Thinking as Applied to School Occupational Therapy

The domain of occupational therapy practice is broad and encompasses a wide range of populations with occupational needs (AOTA, 2014). School practitioners have done well to serve the needs of children who receive special education services under the auspices of IDEA. Therapy services have been broadening as occupational therapy practitioners go beyond one-to-one direct intervention with children. Occupational therapy practitioners have become instrumental in promoting the full participation of children with disabilities in general education experiences, engaging in general education initiatives associated with early intervening to prevent special education referrals, and using their skills to facilitate system-level efforts to support positive school climates (Bazyk & Cahill, 2015).

As school occupational therapy evolves and the needs of school children change, new ways of intervening on behalf of all children will emerge. This concept of system-level thinking should be introduced in occupational therapy programs so that occupational therapy practitioners will have the keen insight to look for opportunities and the resources to act. Two emerging practice foci—mental and behavioral health wellness and literacy achievement initiatives—have the potential to expand the role of occupational therapy practitioners in schools. In addition, recent AOTA discussions have been initiated to explore practitioners' potential as school leaders.

Address Emerging Roles of School Occupational Therapy Practitioners

Occupational therapy practitioners must be prepared to adapt to emerging roles as the climate of school practice continues to evolve. In school settings, occupational therapists may assume the roles of evaluator, consultant, trainer, contributor to strategic initiatives, and advocate. Occupational therapy assistants, under the supervision of the occupational therapist, may also assist in these functions. Identifying and distinguishing these roles will prepare students for occupational therapy practice in schools.

School practitioners serve the needs of children who receive special education services under the auspices of IDEA and promote the full participation of children with disabilities in general education as well as engage in MTSS to enhance academic and behavior performance for children in general education. They must be able to form effective partnerships by understanding the classroom routines, curriculum, literacy practices, available technology, and expectations across the school building or district. Students may benefit from being asked to develop an in-service or training for team members from other disciplines, modify or redesign an existing schoolwide program (e.g., bullying prevention, physical education instruction, social skills training), or execute a classroom resource around MTSS.

Mental and behavioral health wellness

Occupational therapy education programs must provide a strong base of knowledge regarding developmental mental health and wellness. This education should prepare occupational therapy practitioners to recognize the symptoms of mental health conditions in children and youth. Changes in a child's mental health typically manifest through behaviors that are often overlooked as age-related defiance, aloofness, or attention seeking. Occupational therapy students must be prepared to educate school personnel on the myriad manifestations of mental health conditions, to lead teams in addressing a child's underlying mental health needs, to refer to other professionals when required, and to support the families of children experiencing challenges with mental health (Bazyk & Cahill, 2015).

Children are increasingly being identified with experiencing trauma, social anxiety, depression, attachment disorders, attention deficit disorders, and other mental health conditions (Bitsko et al., 2016); occupational therapists have an opportunity to expand their services to address the occupational needs of these children. Occupational therapy programs must prepare practitioners to think innovatively so they can develop programs and group interventions that contribute to promoting mental health and wellness for student groups and individuals (Bazyk & Cahill, 2015). An example of a group intervention that an occupational therapy practitioner may facilitate in a school is one that promotes friendships and inclusion as part of an antibullying initiative. Occupational therapy practitioners also can work closely with school staff to monitor individual children who have a history of disruptions to their social–emotional stability or those who have a diagnosed mental health condition.

Educational programs should introduce concepts on relational discipline, restorative justice, and moral authority as relating to school discipline practices (Irby & Clough, 2015). This introduction will prepare occupational therapy students to apply a lens to examine practices, educate others, and advocate for effective school discipline policies that will not lead to retraumatization for students who have experienced trauma, abuse, or bullying. Some of the traditional consequence-based school discipline practices

have the potential to create, and even magnify, underlying student mental health problems (Shochet et al., 2006). Occupational therapy practitioners can best contribute to a positive student-centered school climate when they promote and engage in relationship building; restorative justice practices; and alternatives to traditional exclusion, suspension, and expulsion practices.

Literacy achievement

Occupational therapy education programs need to prepare occupational therapy practitioners in schools to evaluate student occupations broadly. Practitioners who can apply the principles of occupation to daily school events and activities will open new opportunities for occupational therapy practitioners to support student achievement and life skills development.

For example, by using an occupational therapy lens to evaluate student occupations, contemporary occupational therapists are shedding light on the interconnectedness of reading and participation in all daily life occupations (Grajo & Candler, 2016). Using the framework of occupational adaptation, Grajo and Candler (2016) highlighted the importance of functional reading skills. Moving the profession into innovative practices and interventions such as literacy achievement has the potential to affect all students.

School leadership

Occupational therapy practitioners have the potential to pursue leadership roles in schools. Practitioners prepared with an understanding of school leadership, school culture, team dynamics, educational policy, and the myriad initiatives that come and go in public education will be equipped to assume both formal and informal leadership roles on school teams. In most states, pathways to formal school leadership positions (e.g., principals, special education directors) as an occupational therapist are nonexistent to limited at best (Sauvigne-Kirsch, 2017). Occupational therapy students need to be prepared to advocate and build capacity for expansion of their roles within schools. This might include being actively involved in their state's occupational therapy associations or volunteering to support AOTA's efforts to protect, support, and expand the role of occupational therapy in school settings.

SUMMARY

Occupational therapy education programs need to prepare students for entry into school practice. The goal of setting a foundational knowledge and skills is to enhance the students' understanding of the requirements of the law and the rights of the child and family in the educational setting as well as the role of occupational therapy.

REFERENCES

Accreditation Council for Occupational Therapy Education. (2018). 2018 Accreditation Council for Occupational Therapy Education (ACOTE®) standards and interpretive guide. *American Journal of Occupational Therapy, 72*(Suppl. 2), 7212410005. https://doi.org/10.5014/72S217

American Occupational Therapy Association. (2014). Occupational therapy practice framework: Domain and process (3rd ed.). *American Journal of Occupational Therapy, 68*(Suppl. 1), S1–S48. https://doi.org/10.504/ajot/.2014.682006

American Occupational Therapy Association. (2015a). Occupational therapy code of ethics (2015). *American Journal of Occupational Therapy, 69*(Suppl. 3), 6913410030. https://doi.org/10.5014/ajot.2015.696S03

American Occupational Therapy Association. (2015b). Philosophy of occupational therapy education (2014). *American Journal of Occupational Therapy, 69*(Suppl. 3), 6913410052. https://doi.org/10.5014/ajot.2015.696S17

American Occupational Therapy Association. (2015c). *2015 salary and workforce survey: Executive summary.* Bethesda, MD: Author.

American Occupational Therapy Association. (2017). Guidelines for occupational therapy services in early intervention and schools. *American Journal of Occupational Therapy, 71*(Suppl. 2), 7112410010. https://doi.org/10.5014/ajot.2017.716S01

Bazyk, S., & Cahill, S. (2015). School-based occupational therapy. In J. Case-Smith & J. Clifford O'Brien (Eds.), *Occupational therapy for children and adolescents* (pp. 664–703). St. Louis: Elsevier.

Bitsko, R. H., Holbrook, J. R., Robinson, L. R., Kaminski, J. W., Ghandour, R., Smith, C., & Peacock, G. (2016). Health care, family, and community factors associated with mental, behavioral, and developmental disorders in early childhood—United States, 2011–2012. *MMWR Morbidity and Mortality Weekly Report, 65,* 221–226. https://doi.org/10.15585/mmwr.mm6509a1

Brockett, R. G. (2015). *Teaching adults: A practical guide for new teachers.* San Francisco: Jossey-Bass.

Capper, C. A., Frattura, E., & Keyes, M. W. (2000). *Meeting the needs of students of ALL abilities: How leaders go beyond inclusion.* Thousand Oaks, CA: Corwin Press.

Cleary, D., Persch, A., & Spencer, K. (2015). Transition to adulthood. In J. Case-Smith & J. Clifford O'Brien (Eds.), *Occupational therapy for children and adolescents* (pp. 727–746). St. Louis: Elsevier.

DuFour, R., & Eaker, R. (1998). *Professional learning communities at work: Best practices for enhancing student achievement.* Bloomington, IN: Association for Supervision and Curriculum Development.

Frolek Clark, G., & Handley-More, D. (2017). *Best practices for documenting occupational therapy services in schools.* Bethesda, MD: AOTA Press.

Grajo, L. C., & Candler, C. (2016). An Occupation and Participation Approach to Reading Intervention (OPARI) Part I: Defining reading as an occupation. *Journal of Occupational Therapy, Schools, and Early Intervention, 9*(1), 74–85. https://doi.org/10.1080/19411243.2016.1141082

Individuals With Disabilities Education Improvement Act of 2004, Pub. L. 108–446, 20 U.S.C. §§ 1400–1482.

Irby, D., & Clough, C. (2015). Consistency rules: A critical exploration of a universal principle of school discipline. *Pedagogy, Culture, and Society, 23,* 153–173. https://doi.org/10.1080/14681366.20214.932

Knowles, M. S., Holton, E. F. III., & Swanson, R. A. (2011). *The adult learner.* New York: Taylor & Francis.

Merrill, M. D., Drake, L., Lacy, M. J., & Pratt, J. A.; ID$_2$ Research Group. (1996). Reclaiming instructional design. *Educational Technology, 36*(5), 5–7.

Richardson, P. K. (2015). Use of standardized tests in pediatric practice. In J. Case-Smith & J. Clifford O'Brien (Eds.), *Occupational therapy for children and adolescents* (pp. 163–191). St. Louis: Elsevier.

Sauvigne-Kirsch, J. (2017). Examining occupational therapists as potential special education leaders. *American Journal of Occupational Therapy, 71*(4, Suppl. 1), 7111510185. https://doi.org/10.5014/ajot.2017.71S1-PO3128

Schoonover, J. W., & Grove, J. E. A. (2015). Influencing participation through assistive technology and universal access. In J. Case-Smith & J. Clifford O'Brien (Eds.), *Occupational therapy for children and adolescents* (pp. 525–559). St. Louis: Elsevier.

Shochet, I. M., Dadds, M. R., Ham, D., & Montague, R. (2006). School connectedness is an underemphasized parameter in adolescent mental health: Results of a community prediction study. *Journal of Clinical Child and Adolescent Psychology, 35,* 170–179. https://doi.org/10.1207/s15374424jccp3502_1

Best Practices in School Occupational Therapy Fieldwork

6

Rebecca Nicholson, OTD, OTR/L

KEY TERMS AND CONCEPTS

- Academic fieldwork coordinator
- Collaborative learning model
- Fieldwork educator
- Fieldwork student
- Interprofessional education
- Level I fieldwork
- Level II fieldwork
- Memorandum of understanding
- Problem-based learning
- Professional reasoning

OVERVIEW

Schools continue to be one of the largest practice settings for occupational therapy practitioners[1] (American Occupational Therapy Association [AOTA], 2015b). Their role is to optimize students' participation in the activities common to the education setting, which can include academics, functional performance activities, and work and community preparation. School environments (e.g., classroom, bus, cafeteria, work site) provide rich learning opportunities to understand developmental challenges, the complexities of students with medically fragile conditions, and the impact of mental health conditions in authentic contexts.

Occupational therapy *fieldwork students* (FWSs) can complete Level I and Level II fieldwork in school settings. A *Level I fieldwork* experience in a school provides FWSs with an introduction to this specialty setting and possibly an opportunity to apply classroom learning. *Level II fieldwork* is designed to provide an in-depth experience in the provision of occupational therapy with clients (e.g., students, classrooms, small groups).

It is important to understand the terms used in this chapter to differentiate various persons involved with fieldwork activities:

- FWS (may be an occupational therapy or occupational therapy assistant student on fieldwork)
- *Fieldwork educator* (FWE; person who supervises students on fieldwork at this setting)
- *Academic fieldwork coordinator* (AFWC; person at the academic institution who coordinates fieldwork placement of students).

The FWE in the school setting provides occupational therapy FWSs with ample opportunities for active participation, application of classroom learning, and preparation as entry-level practitioners.

ESSENTIAL CONSIDERATIONS

When developing a fieldwork program, the FWE should compile resources, gain knowledge of the fieldwork requirements, and identify FWE competencies to prepare for the fieldwork experience and support the FWS. The AOTA website (https://www.aota.org) has resources that can make this process easier.

Understanding Fieldwork Requirements

Fieldwork is the opportunity for FWSs to apply the knowledge they have acquired in the academic setting. The Accreditation Council for Occupational Therapy Education (ACOTE®) requires academic institutions to ensure that fieldwork is "integral to the program's curriculum design" (ACOTE, 2012, p. S34). Fieldwork also "must include an in-depth experience in delivering occupational therapy services to clients, focusing on application of purposeful and meaningful occupations and research, administration, and management of occupational therapy services" (p. S34). ACOTE (2012) established standards[2] for the length of time required for fieldwork and the type of supervision required for FWSs. Table 6.1 provides supervision and time requirements for fieldwork.

---

[1]*Occupational therapy practitioner* refers to both the occupational therapist and the occupational therapy assistant. AOTA (2014a, p. S18) states, "The occupational therapist is responsible for all aspects of occupational therapy service delivery and is accountable for the safety and effectiveness of the occupational therapy service delivery process" and "must be directly involved in the delivery of services during the initial evaluation and regularly throughout the course of intervention. . . . The occupational therapy assistant delivers safe and effective occupational therapy services under the supervision of and in partnership with the occupational therapist."

[2]ACOTE standards approved in 2018 are effective July 31, 2020. The 2012 standards are in effect as of publication.

Copyright © 2019 by the American Occupational Therapy Association. All rights reserved. To reuse this content, contact www.copyright.com. https://doi.org/10.7139/2019.978-1-56900-591-0.006

TABLE 6.1. Supervision and Time Requirements for FWSs

REQUIREMENTS	OCCUPATIONAL THERAPY FWSs	OCCUPATIONAL THERAPY ASSISTANT FWSs
Level I time requirement	No required amount of time	No required amount of time
Level I supervision	Occupational therapist, occupational therapy assistant, or qualified person with at least 1 year of experience[a]	Occupational therapist, occupational therapy assistant, or qualified person with at least 1 year of experience[a]
Level II time requirement	Minimum 24 weeks full-time	Minimum 16 weeks full-time
Level II supervision	Licensed occupational therapist with minimum 1 year of experience	Licensed occupational therapist or occupational therapy assistant with minimum 1 year of experience
Level II innovative model time requirement	Minimum 24 weeks full-time	Minimum 16 weeks full-time
Level II innovative model supervision	Licensed occupational therapist with minimum 3 years' experience; direct on-site minimum 8 hours per week	Licensed occupational therapist with minimum 3 years' experience; direct on-site minimum 8 hours per week
Doctoral capstone time requirement[a]	Minimum 14 weeks full-time; 112 of 560 hours can be off-site	Not applicable
Doctoral capstone or baccalaureate project supervision[a]	Occupational therapy or non–occupational therapy subject matter expert[b] in area of project content	Baccalaureate project, if applicable, must have individualized specific objectives

Note. Requirements are based on Accreditation Council for Occupational Therapy Education (2012, 2018) standards. FWSs = fieldwork students.
[a]Based on Accreditation Council for Occupational Therapy Education (2018) standards.
[b]Qualified personnel may include teachers, social workers, psychologists, and physical therapists.

Collaborating With Educational Personnel

One model that is prevalent in the academic setting designed to prepare FWSs for practice is ***problem-based learning,*** a teaching method that involves group collaboration to develop critical thinking skills in students. Students take responsibility for analyzing problems and researching evidence to implement a client-centered approach to address the client's needs (Duch et al., 2001). Faculty may find it helpful to collaborate with community partners on assignments associated with this model. School practitioners may be well positioned to contribute actual case scenarios. Research supports the use of problem-based learning in academic settings to develop skills in problem solving that will be beneficial in practice settings (Schmidt et al., 2011). Problem-based learning promotes the use of evidence-based practice (Hanson, 2015; Van Lew & Singh, 2010) and increases FWSs' responsibility, comprehension, and retention of information (Schmidt et al., 2011).

Sadlo (2014), an educator in the United Kingdom, has developed an e-learning master class geared toward the use of problem-based learning in fieldwork programs that emphasize professional reasoning. ***Professional reasoning,*** a widely recognized component of occupational therapy, is the process of planning, directing, performing, and reflecting on client care (Boyt Schell, 2014). Using the framework for professional reasoning outlined by Boyt Schell, faculty from the institution and the FWE can create valuable learning activities for a specific case during fieldwork.

Itinerant Practice and Academic Calendar

School practice may require travel to multiple sites, which can create a schedule that considers multiple factors and collaboration with a wide range of educational teams. When FWSs start their fieldwork at the beginning of the school year, they may be able to participate in creating the master schedule. FWSs who start at other times of the school year should be provided with opportunities to make schedule adjustments, gain independence in time management, and navigate the complexities of itinerant practice. The FWEs can document and share with the FWS step-by-step procedures they have found useful in their setting.

FWE Professional Development and Continued Competence

AOTA's (2015c) *Standards for Continuing Competence* outlines 5 areas that practitioners—and, more pertinent to this chapter, FWEs—should contemplate:

- Knowledge
- Critical reasoning
- Interpersonal skills
- Performance skills
- Ethical practice.

These key standards will help new FWEs recognize their capacity to provide a valuable learning experience for the FWS in school practice (Costa, 2007).

An additional resource is the AOTA (2009a) *Self-Assessment Tool for Fieldwork Educator Competency.* This tool is useful in providing guidance for the FWE's own professional development. Table 6.2 summarizes an application of these documents as applied to school FWEs.

To prepare occupational therapy practitioners to become FWEs, AOTA has developed the Fieldwork Educator Program (Johnson & Stutz-Tanenbaum, 2009). Trainers provide a 2-day course examining topics such as administration,

TABLE 6.2. Standards for Continued Competence and School Practice Examples

COMPETENCE AND GENERAL DESCRIPTION	SCHOOL PRACTICE EXAMPLE
Knowledge • Structure fieldwork to build the FWS's professional development • Recognize different styles of adult learning and collaborative learning approaches • Understand legalities, contracts, and supervision models	• Structure the fieldwork to provide an FWS with well-rounded experiences and active learning in evaluation, consultation with the educational team, and IEP development • Provide supervision that facilitates an understanding of educational laws and decision making for service provision
Critical reasoning • Evaluate and share fieldwork literature • Apply theoretical, evidence-based, and outcome-data decision making • Assess FWS and team dynamics • Facilitate a continuum of professional development	• Review and discuss articles on professional reasoning with the FWS (Sadlo, 2014; Unsworth & Baker, 2016) • Promote daily reflection in professional reasoning and interactions
Interpersonal skills • Create a positive learning environment • Foster a working relationship with the FWS that optimizes learning potential • Resolve differences respectfully • Communicate observed strengths of the FWS • Provide constructive feedback for areas of improvement	• Help the FWS build comfort in the school environment • Facilitate the FWS's ability to communicate with education personnel • Model professional interactions in meetings • Provide the FWS with responsibilities for communicating with teachers and parents • Discuss articles regarding collaborative consultation in an educational setting (Boshoff & Stewart, 2013; Kennedy & Stewart, 2011; Shasby & Schneck, 2011)
Performance skills • Design and adapt fieldwork to promote the FWS's competence and entry-level knowledge and skills • Outline learning objectives, on-the-job assignments, and meaningful activities • Evaluate the FWS's performance • Document learning outcomes	• Review site-specific objectives for school practice • Partner with the FWS to develop specific activities and goals outlined in the fieldwork performance evaluation form • Refer to resources for school-specific objectives
Ethical practice • Model ethical principles • Apply ethical reasoning when navigating complex situations • Ethically resolve any fieldwork issues that surface	• Review articles on evaluation practices from the parents' perspective in preparation for team meetings (Cavendish & Conner, 2018; Cheatham et al., 2012; Chu, 2017; Holzmueller, 2005) • Inform FWS of state mandatory reporting of child abuse, and share resources • Describe Medicaid cost-recovery regulations • Discuss AOTA's (2015a) *Occupational Therapy Code of Ethics*

Note. AOTA = American Occupational Therapy Association; FWS = fieldwork student; IEP = individualized education program.

education, supervision, and evaluation. The course is intended to build practitioners' in-depth knowledge regarding the role of the FWE as well as strategies to promote the use of evidence in practice and application of theories and professional reasoning. For information about hosting or attending, visit the AOTA website at https://www.aota.org /Education-Careers/Fieldwork/Workshop.aspx.

Models of Supervision

Most often, FWEs supervise FWSs using an apprentice model of 1 FWS assigned to a single supervisor. Occasionally, supervision may be divided across 2 FWEs. When this model is used, communication between FWEs is critical to ensure that feedback to the FWS is consistent. In addition, FWEs should work closely with the AFWC in identifying FWSs who will likely thrive within this model.

The demand for high-quality fieldwork has steadily increased over the years, creating an impetus for the development of alternative group supervision models. Costa (2007) described a ***collaborative learning model*** as

an innovative approach to fieldwork supervision. In this model, 2 or more FWSs are assigned to 1 FWE. The fieldwork is then structured to promote collaborative learning among the pair or group of FWSs in partnership with the FWE (Cohn et al., 2001).

Johnson and Johnson (1999) outlined the keys to group supervision models as
- Positive interdependence,
- Individual and group accountability,
- Group interaction,
- Interpersonal and teamwork skills, and
- Group processing.

More recently, researchers have built on the work of Johnson and Johnson to provide a detailed structure for the collaborative learning models (Covington et al., 2017; Hanson & DeIuliis, 2015). These investigators described the importance of FWSs' gaining experience in teamwork, reviewing literature on successful teaming, and completing self-evaluations as learners and teachers before the fieldwork placement. Before placing FWSs in settings that use this model, the AFWC should work closely with program faculty to determine those individuals who have successfully demonstrated effective teaming practices in the classroom.

Using Technology to Support FWSs

Telesupervision and teleconsultation may prove useful approaches in school fieldwork programs (Nicholson et al., 2014). Such an approach has several benefits for FWSs (Criss, 2013; Nagarajan et al., 2016):

- Increased confidence
- Improved clinical reasoning
- Increased understanding of the profession.

In a recent pilot study, researchers found that the use of teleconsultation in a rural school practice increased collaboration between faculty and FWEs (Nicholson et al., 2014). In addition, participants reported that teleconferencing was more efficient and provided more in-depth discussion than use of email or phone conversations.

Interprofessional Education

In the current health care climate, **interprofessional education** is a priority for health professions (Shrader et al., 2015, 2016; Willgerodt et al., 2015). These interprofessional programs have been developed according to the guidelines from the *Core Competences in Interprofessional Education* (Interprofessional Education Collaborative Expert Panel, 2016). Even though these competencies are geared toward medical professions, the key principles are applicable to school settings. School practice provides FWSs with an opportunity to implement the principles of interprofessional collaboration when participating on educational teams. Research from a recent study (Strong et al., 2016) identified that FWSs reported increased confidence in their own discipline as they engaged in interprofessional discussions and reflective activities with persons from other professions.

BEST PRACTICES

When starting or adjusting a fieldwork program, school occupational therapy practitioners, in collaboration with the AFWC, should put steps in place to explore feasibility and logistics, prepare for an FWS, and promote and model best practices.

Begin Initial Groundwork

Determining whether to institute a fieldwork program requires some initial groundwork and exploration by the school occupational therapy department or, in some cases, the individual school practitioner. This initial work requires analyzing the facility, collaborating with academic programs, and fulfilling legal responsibilities.

Analyze the facility

Start by identifying the facility's philosophy, mission, and vision; recognizing practitioners interested in becoming FWEs; outlining key opportunities and resources in the facility; and obtaining administrative support for a fieldwork program.

Philosophy, mission, and vision. Determine whether the facility's philosophy, mission, and vision align with the work of preparing future practitioners. In addition, outline the overall philosophy of the school's occupational therapy services. Save any materials that you gather or develop; these might be fitting to include in a student manual should you decide to develop a fieldwork program. These materials will help outline distinct differences between your setting and other settings (e.g., educational vs. clinical).

Recognize practitioners interested in becoming FWEs. In some cases, the occupational therapy supervisor initiates the discussion to determine those occupational therapy practitioners interested in participating in a fieldwork program. In other instances, the occupational therapy practitioner may initiate the exploration. The supervisor and practitioners examine their own strengths and needs for becoming FWEs. Practitioners who have an interest in participating in fieldwork education will find it helpful to complete the *Self-Assessment Tool for Fieldwork Educator Competency* (AOTA, 2009a).

Outline key learning opportunities and resources in the facility. The FWEs should identify learning opportunities and resources (e.g., information on school practice, site-specific practices) that would be valuable to FWSs. Activities such as spending a day in a special education or general education classroom working alongside the teacher or working with other disciplines provide FWSs with better perspectives in understanding the roles of other disciplines. FWEs should consider ensuring that FWSs can participate in individualized education program meetings, staff meetings, and in-service sessions to give them a realistic picture of school practice.

Obtain administrative support for a fieldwork program. To initiate a fieldwork experience, the occupational therapy practitioner must first obtain administrative support from the school and school district for the development of the fieldwork program. Administrators may be hesitant to support the concept of a fieldwork program if they do not recognize the value (e.g., the value in recruiting and retaining occupational therapy practitioners) and the professional responsibility of an occupational therapy practitioner to participate in fieldwork supervision.

Administrators need to recognize that the FWE will require additional time allotted for supervisory tasks. Citing studies such as the one conducted by Ozelie et al. (2018) may help in communicating this need and the benefits. Ozelie et al. (2018) found that FWEs worked an additional 25 minutes per day on average. The researchers also discovered that despite the additional time, participants reported benefits in supervising FWSs, including the opportunity to share practice knowledge and to stay up to date with current content being taught in occupational therapy programs. Administrators are often concerned about the impact on therapists' productivity when they are supervising students. Ozelie et al. (2015) found that a significant difference in productivity did not exist between pediatric therapists with and without FWSs.

Collaborate with the academic institution

After analyzing the facility, proceed to connect with AFWCs at academic institutions, designate a fieldwork site contact, become familiar with the curriculum of the chosen academic institution, and develop a plan for ongoing communication with the AFWC.

Connect with AFWCs at academic institutions to determine the best fit. Connect with the AFWC to determine the best fit between the higher education curriculum and the potential fieldwork program. Securing contracts with institutions that are compatible with the philosophy of the school setting is important. Other pragmatic considerations include the length of the fieldwork experiences, the time of year when the rotations occur, and the number of slots reasonably available.

Designate a fieldwork program contact. Securing fieldwork sites is the job of the AFWC. However, the importance of the fieldwork designee responsible for coordinating assignments in the school setting cannot be overemphasized. The profession is experiencing shortages in almost every area of practice, and school placements are no exception (Roberts & Simon, 2012). The designee needs to have an effective and efficient method of identifying school practitioners who are ready, willing, and able to supervise FWSs.

In addition, the designee needs to fully understand FWE eligibility requirements. When a breakdown in the system occurs, the potential for error grows (e.g., practitioners are not aware of FWSs' placements, emails go unanswered, mismatched assignments are made, eligible FWEs miss out on opportunities). The designee needs to make sure that lines of communication are well established to ensure that practitioners interested in participating are notified as well as administrative staff who will be responsible for facilitating the completion of paperwork that the setting requires.

To create a successful fieldwork experience, all parties involved need to have a clear understanding of the administrative, didactic, and ethical components associated with fieldwork. The academic institution must provide resources to support the FWE and be available to collaborate as needed. The school system must create materials to support FWSs that are tailored to the particular site. A successful partnership between the 2 entities helps to promote the use of evidence-based strategies by providing access to current literature and addressing the pragmatics of incorporating evidence into school practice.

Become familiar with the curriculum of the chosen academic institution. The AFWC provides information regarding the scope and sequence of the curriculum as well as opportunities to participate in teaching activities and continuing education opportunities that may be available to FWEs. In addition, the AFWC can provide information about assignments that FWSs will be required to complete during their fieldwork experience.

Fieldwork is an integral part of the curriculum, and the academic institution is obligated to ensure that education in the fieldwork setting is aligned with the curriculum of the institution (ACOTE, 2012). The AFWC assumes the responsibility for monitoring the effectiveness of the preparation by reviewing the *Level I Fieldwork Competency Evaluation for OT and OTA Students* (AOTA, 2017b) and the *Student Evaluation of the Fieldwork Experience* (AOTA, 2016b). The AFWC also routinely provides on-site visits, virtual check-ins, communications, and continuing education opportunities specific to fieldwork for practitioners.

These traditional methods of monitoring preparation are helpful to the academic institution. However, educators in the academic program should not assume the role of expert when developing materials related to school practice. Instead, a reciprocal collaboration between the academic program and the fieldwork site should be fostered. To that end, faculty should take the opportunity to collaborate with school practitioners in the development of course materials. This demonstrates the faculty's recognition of the FWE as a valued partner in FWS preparation and as a sharer of practical experience in the school setting.

In addition to faculty's facilitating input from the FWE on course materials, collaborating on assignments in the classroom and on fieldwork serves to strengthen the connection between didactic and fieldwork education. FWSs and the FWE can provide important feedback regarding the usefulness of course materials and assignments in supporting the fieldwork experience. In addition, FWEs might provide valuable insights into curriculum development, serve as guest lecturers, or become adjunct faculty, which would further strengthen the partnership between the academic institution and the fieldwork program.

One of the most important pieces of the fieldwork experience is to have a competent and willing fieldwork supervisor in the school. All practitioners should supervise students during Level I and Level II fieldwork to advocate for the profession and as a part of professional responsibility. School practitioners interested in developing a fieldwork practice should contact the AFWC at a university of interest or an academic institution in their area to obtain support and guidance in developing their skills as a fieldwork supervisor.

Fulfill legal responsibilities

Once the practitioner obtains administrative support for developing the fieldwork program, the administrative entity of the school and academic setting must collaborate to complete a memorandum of understanding (MOU). The *MOU* is an agreement between the fieldwork site and the academic setting that describes in writing the expectations and responsibilities of all parties. It is a nonbinding document that describes, for example, the responsibilities and qualifications of the supervisor, the requirement for liability insurance for students, and any other specific details required by the fieldwork site or the academic setting. The agreement also outlines the duration of the agreement and notification requirements should either party wish to terminate the contract.

Completing the MOU may be a lengthy process, depending on the procedures of the local school district and the legal department in the academic setting. It is important to initiate this process with ample time to ensure that the MOU is in place well in advance of initiation of the fieldwork experience. In addition to the MOU, the school setting must also complete the AOTA (2017a) *Fieldwork Data Form* so that the academic setting has up-to-date information about the setting and the therapists involved in fieldwork education.

The academic setting, under the guidance of the AFWC, collaborates with the school system to establish and implement the fieldwork experience. The AFWC is responsible for establishing and maintaining relationships with the FWEs. The AFWC works closely with the school system to ensure that all legal documents for the academic institution and those required by the school system are completed before the FWS can begin the school placement. The AFWC provides resources and training to the FWE as needed to facilitate competency and confidence in supervisors. The AFWC and the designee collaborate to determine scheduling and the type of fieldwork experience that will take place.

Prepare the Fieldwork Program

When preparing your fieldwork program, best practice is to review AOTA documents and develop a fieldwork manual.

Review AOTA documents

Reviewing current AOTA documents will prepare FWEs to articulate best practice and provide them with resources to lean on when fielding questions. These documents may include the following:

- *ACOTE Standards* (ACOTE, 2012, 2018)
- *Occupational Therapy Practice Framework: Domain and Process* (3rd ed.; AOTA, 2014b)
- *Standards of Practice for Occupational Therapy* (AOTA, 2015d)
- *Guidelines for Documentation of Occupational Therapy* (AOTA, 2018)
- *Occupational Therapy Code of Ethics* (AOTA, 2015a)
- *Guidelines for Supervision, Roles, and Responsibilities During the Delivery of Occupational Therapy Services* (AOTA, 2014a)
- *Occupational Therapy Fieldwork Education: Value and Purpose* (AOTA, 2016a).

Develop a fieldwork manual

The fieldwork manual should include site-specific learning and performance objectives, a schedule of FWS responsibilities, and site-specific resources. For more information, see the AOTA website (https://bit.ly/2QxZwU4) for recommended content for the fieldwork manual.

Set site-specific objectives

To facilitate the success of the fieldwork experience, the fieldwork site needs to develop site-specific objectives to measure FWSs' performance. These objectives provide the FWS with a structure for achieving competence in key tasks in the setting. Site-specific objectives developed for school practice (Tucker et al., 2003) are available for download and revision on the AOTA website at https://bit.ly/2RrJqZt.

Outline a week-by-week schedule of responsibilities

Although FWSs are familiar with an educational setting, the roles, responsibilities, and unique aspects of the specific site may be less apparent. The FWE must ensure that the FWS understands the role of occupational therapy in general education and special education. A list of responsibilities for building the FWS's practical experience across the fieldwork placement will be beneficial.

Provide site-specific resources and school practice resources

The process of developing the fieldwork manual often helps the fieldwork supervisor systematically think through the entire fieldwork experience and identify areas needing further attention before a student is accepted. FWEs need to provide information specific to guidelines and regulations for offering accommodations to FWSs in the educational setting (Christensen et al., 2011). FWSs should be given resources, such as Common Core State Standards Initiative (2010) as well as the Individuals With Disabilities Education Improvement Act of 2004 (IDEA; Pub. L. 108–446).

Assume the FWE Role

In the FWE role, the school occupational therapy practitioner not only models best practice in day-to-day activities (e.g., scheduling, evaluation, intervention, teaming) but also takes on the responsibility of being an innovator, scholar, leader, integrator, and mentor in school practice (AOTA, 2009b).

Innovator

An *innovator* looks ahead and seeks opportunities to meet future client needs. In schools, this can present when new referrals are made, evaluations are conducted, professional reasoning is applied, and recommendations are formed to present to the team. Recommendations that consider the least restrictive environment, contextual application, and universal design for learning may lead to innovative approaches that address the needs not only of the individual student but also of all students (e.g., creating a playground club to promote participation and discover ways to optimize a student's strengths in play and minimize motor coordination barriers). FWSs can learn to take on the responsibility of looking for opportunities, researching literature, designing creative interventions, collaborating with others, and addressing logistics for change.

Scholar

A *scholar* seeks, applies, translates, and contributes to the body of knowledge to affect client outcomes. With the focus of IDEA (2004) and the Every Student Succeeds Act (2015; Pub. L. 114–95) on the use of interventions grounded in research, school occupational therapy practitioners should naturally model the need to stay on top of the latest research, methods to collect data, and the best ways to monitor student progress to ensure that targeted outcomes will be attained. The FWS should follow this practice and should be expected to share research with others, communicate student outcomes in parent-friendly terms, and find ways to contribute to the body of knowledge for school practice (e.g., write an article for the parent–teacher organization newsletter, create a tip sheet for parents on setting up a homework area, provide an in-service session on school occupational therapy).

Leader

A *leader* examines trends across time (i.e., past, present, future); is solution focused; and collaborates, inspires, and encourages others to look ahead. Starting a fieldwork program is a form of leadership. When developing the fieldwork manual, the FWE looks at trends, examines their own practice, explores the many resources available, and collaborates with others in the process. The FWS uses the fieldwork manual as a guide but should also be involved in providing suggestions for revisions, additions, or clarifications as needed. This begins their process of looking back, examining the present, and contemplating their preparation for school practice.

Integrator

An *integrator* uncovers different directions or differences in opinion and seeks to build relationships and connections to lead to new understandings. In schools, this may come about if each team member examines a situation through their profession-specific lens versus the collective lens of the team. The skills to effectively articulate a point of view, listen to others, and discover the best options as a team are expected in school practice.

With this in mind, FWSs may benefit from reviewing research from Canada on the school practice model Partnering for Change (Missiuna et al., 2012, 2015). This model focuses on collaboration and coaching in the classroom to increase students' participation in their education. FWSs should also be prepared to answer the question, How do you define occupational therapy in schools? FWSs must be able to communicate occupational therapy's role in schools, identify the different foci of clinical and educational models, and outline examples to support their definition.

Mentor

A *mentor* "inspires, encourages, influences, challenges, and facilitates the growth and development of others" (AOTA, 2009b, p. 805). In this capacity, FWEs are not only mentors to the FWSs but also role models for fellow colleagues. During the fieldwork experience, FWEs will most likely mentor students through ethical dilemmas, advocate for student needs, address interpersonal challenges that may arise in a complex situation, and recognize positive change. Having the FWS draw on and apply the knowledge and skills they acquired in their preservice education, look for additional resources, and consider actions to address to real-world situations will prepare them for the continuum of professional development.

SUMMARY

As one of the largest employers of occupational therapy practitioners, schools should be considered a fieldwork opportunity at all levels of practice. It is imperative that school practitioners actively participate in the education of FWSs to provide the unique learning opportunities that will enable FWSs to gain competence in the provision of educationally related services. School practitioners who have not yet initiated a fieldwork education program should make connections with an occupational therapy academic institution in their region for support in establishing a fieldwork program. Occupational therapy practitioners who have an established fieldwork program should contact AOTA about sponsoring a FWE Training Workshop to ensure best practices in fieldwork education.

REFERENCES

Accreditation Council for Occupational Therapy Education. (2012). 2011 Accreditation Council for Occupational Therapy Education (ACOTE®) standards. *American Journal of Occupational Therapy, 66*(6, Suppl.), S6–S74. https://doi.org/10.5014/ajot.2012.66S6

Accreditation Council for Occupational Therapy Education. (2018). 2018 Accreditation Council for Occupational Therapy Education (ACOTE®) standards and interpretive guide. *American Journal of Occupational Therapy, 72*(Suppl. 2), 7212410005. https://doi.org/10.5014/ajot.2018.72S217

American Occupational Therapy Association. (2009a). *Self-Assessment Tool for Fieldwork Educator Competency.* Retrieved from https://health.utah.edu/occupational-recreational-therapies/docs/fieldwork/selfassessmentfwedcompetency.pdf

American Occupational Therapy Association. (2009b). Specialized knowledge and skills of occupational therapy educators of the future. *American Journal of Occupational Therapy, 63,* 804–818. https://doi.org/10.5014/ajot.63.6.804

American Occupational Therapy Association. (2014a). Guidelines for supervision, roles, and responsibilities during the delivery of occupational therapy services. *American Journal of Occupational Therapy, 68*(Suppl. 3), S16–S22. https://doi.org/10.5014/ajot.2014.686S03

American Occupational Therapy Association. (2014b). Occupational therapy practice framework: Domain and process (3rd ed.). *American Journal of Occupational Therapy, 68*(Suppl. 1), S1–S48. https://doi.org/10.5014/ajot.2014.682006

American Occupational Therapy Association. (2015a). Occupational therapy code of ethics (2015). *American Journal of Occupational Therapy, 69*(Suppl. 3), 6913410030. https://doi.org/10.5014/ajot.2015.696S03

American Occupational Therapy Association. (2015b). Salary and workforce survey. *OT Practice, 20*(11), 7–11.

American Occupational Therapy Association. (2015c). Standards for continuing competence. *American Journal of Occupational Therapy, 69*(Suppl. 3), 6913410055. https://doi.org/10.5014/ajot.2015.696S16

American Occupational Therapy Association. (2015d). Standards of practice for occupational therapy. *American Journal of Occupational Therapy, 69*(Suppl. 3), 6913410057. https://doi.org/10.5014/ajot.2015.696S06

American Occupational Therapy Association. (2016a). Occupational therapy fieldwork education: Value and purpose. *American Journal of Occupational Therapy, 70*(Suppl. 2), 7012410060. https://doi.org/10.5014/ajot.2016.706S06

American Occupational Therapy Association. (2016b). *Student evaluation of the fieldwork experience.* Retrieved from https://www.aota.org/Search.aspx#q=student%20evaluation%20of%20the%20fieldwork%20experience&sort=relevancy

American Occupational Therapy Association. (2017a). *AOTA fieldwork data form*. Retrieved from https://www.aota.org /Search.aspx#=Fieldwork%20Data%20Form&sort=relevancy

American Occupational Therapy Association. (2017b). *Level I fieldwork competency evaluation for OT and OTA students*. Retrieved from https://www.aota.org/~/media/Corporate/Files /EducationCareers/Educators/Fieldwork/LevelI/Level -I-Fieldwork-Competency-Evaluation-for-ot-and-ota-students .pdf

American Occupational Therapy Association. (2018). Guidelines for documentation of occupational therapy. *American Journal of Occupational Therapy, 72*(Suppl. 2), 7212410010. https://doi .org/10.5014/ajot.2018.72S203

Boshoff, K., & Stewart, H. (2013). Key principles for confronting the challenges of collaboration in educational settings. *Australian Occupational Therapy Journal, 60*, 144–147. https://doi .org/10.1111/1440-1630.12003

Boyt Schell, B. A. (2014). Professional reasoning in practice. In E. B. Crepeau, E. S. Cohn, & B. A. Boyt Schell (Eds.), *Willard and Spackman's occupational therapy* (12th ed., pp. 384–397). Philadelphia: Lippincott Williams & Wilkins.

Cavendish, W., & Connor, D. (2018). Toward authentic IEPs and transition plans: Student, parent, and teacher perspectives. *Learning Disability Quarterly, 41*(1), 32–43. https://doi .org/10.1177/073194871668468

Cheatham, G. A., Hart, J. E., Malian, I., & McDonald, J. (2012). Six things to never say or hear during an IEP meeting: Educators as advocates for families. *Teaching Exceptional Children, 44*(3), 50–57. https://doi.org/10.1177/004005991204400306

Christensen, L., Carver, W., VanDeZande, J., & Lazarus, S. (2011). *Accommodations manual: How to select, administer, and evaluate use of accommodations for instruction and assessment of students with disabilities*. Washington, DC: Council of Chief State School Officers.

Chu, S. (2017). Supporting children with special educational needs (SEN): An introduction to a 3-tiered school-based occupational therapy model of service delivery in the United Kingdom. *World Federation of Occupational Therapists Bulletin, 73*(2), 107–116. https://doi.org/10.1080/14473828.2017.1349235

Cohn, E., Dooley, N., & Simmons, L. (2001). Collaborative learning applied to fieldwork education. *Occupational Therapy in Health Care, 15*, 69–83. https://doi.org/10.1080/J003v15n01_08

Common Core State Standards Initiative. (2010). *Common Core state standards for English language arts and literacy in history/ social studies, science, and technical subjects*. Washington, DC: National Governors Association. Retrieved from http://www .corestandards.org/wp-content/uploads/ELA_Standards1.pdf

Costa, D. M. (2007). Fieldwork issues: Fieldwork educator readiness. *OT Practice, 12*(20), 20–22.

Covington, K., Odom, C., Heflin, S., & Gwyer, J. (2017). Student team learning in practice (STEPs): An integrated clinical education collaborative model. *Journal of Physical Therapy Education, 31*(2), 18–29.

Criss, M. J. (2013). School-based telerehabilitation in occupational therapy: Using telerehabilitation technologies to promote improvements in student performance. *International Journal of Telerehabilitation, 5*(1), 39–46. https://doi.org/10.5195 /ijt.2013.6115

Duch, B. J., Groh, S. E., & Allen, D. E. (Eds.). (2001). *The power of problem-based learning*. Sterling, VA: Stylus.

Every Student Succeeds Act, Pub. L. 114–95, 129 Stat. 1802. (2015).

Hanson, D. J., & DeIuliis, E. D. (2015). The collaborative model of fieldwork education: A blueprint for group supervision of students. *Occupational Therapy in Health Care, 29*, 223–239. https://doi.org/10.3109/07380577.2015.1011297

Holzmueller, R. P. (2005). Therapists I have known and (mostly) loved. *American Journal of Occupational Therapy, 59*, 580–587. https://doi.org/10.5014/ajot.59.5.580

Individuals With Disabilities Education Improvement Act of 2004, Pub. L. 108–446, 20 U.S.C. §§ 1400–1482.

Interprofessional Education Collaborative Expert Panel. (2016). *Core competencies for interprofessional collaborative practice: 2016 update*. Washington, DC: Interprofessional Education Collaborative.

Johnson, C., & Stutz-Tanenbaum, P. (Eds.). (2009). *Fieldwork educator certification program manual*. Bethesda, MD: American Occupational Therapy Association.

Johnson, D. W., & Johnson, R. T. (1999). *Learning together and alone: Cooperative, competitive and individualistic learning*. Boston: Allyn & Bacon.

Kennedy, S., & Stewart, H. (2011). Collaboration between occupational therapists and teachers: Definitions, implementation and efficacy. *Australian Occupational Therapy Journal, 58*, 209–214. https://doi.org/10.1111/j.1440-1630.2011.00934.x

Missiuna, C., Pollock, N., Campbell, W., Dix, L., Whalen, S. S., & Stewart, D. (2015). Partnering for change: Embedding universal design for learning into school-based occupational therapy. *Occupational Therapy Now, 17*(3), 13–15.

Missiuna, C. A., Pollock, N. A., Levac, D. E., Campbell, W. N., Sahagian Whalen, S. D., Bennett, S. M., . . . Russell, D. J. (2012). Partnering for change: An innovative school-based occupational therapy service delivery model for children with developmental coordination disorder. *Canadian Journal of Occupational Therapy, 79*, 41–50. https://doi.org/10.2182 /cjot.2012.79.1.6

Nagarajan, S., McAllister, L., McFarlane, L., Hall, M., Schmitz, C., Roots, R., . . . & Lam, M. (2016). Telesupervision benefits for placements: Allied health students' and supervisors' perceptions. *International Journal of Practice-Based Learning in Health and Social Care, 4*(1), 16–27. https://doi.org/10.18552/ijpblhsc.v4i1.326

Nicholson, R., Bassham, L., Chapman, A., & Fricker, D. (2014). Telecommunication for collaboration between occupational therapy fieldwork and academic settings. *Technology Special Interest Section Quarterly, 24*(1), 1–4.

Ozelie, R., Hansen, P., Liguzinski, J., Saylor, A., & Woodcock, E. (2018). Occupational therapy Level II fieldwork impact on clinicians: A preliminary time study. *Occupational Therapy in Health Care, 32*, 61–71. https://doi.org/10.1080/07380577.2017.1421800

Ozelie, R., Janow, J., Kreutz, C., Mulry, M. K., & Penkala, A. (2015). Supervision of occupational therapy Level II fieldwork students: Impact on and predictors of clinician productivity. *American Journal of Occupational Therapy, 69*, 6901260010. https://doi.org/10.5014/ajot.2015.013532

Roberts, M. E., & Simon, R. L. (2012). Fieldwork challenge 2012. *OT Practice, 17*(6), 20.

Sadlo, G. (2014). Using problem-based learning during student placements to embed theory in practice. *International Journal of Practice-Based Learning in Health and Social Care, 2*(1), 6–19. https://doi.org/10.11120/pblh.2014.00029

Schmidt, H. G., Rotgans, J. I., & Yew, E. H. (2011). The process of problem-based learning: What works and why. *Medical Education, 45,* 792–806. https://doi.org/10.1111/j.1365-2923.2011.04035.x

Shasby, S., & Schneck, C. (2011). Commentary on collaboration in school-based practice: Positives and pitfalls. *Journal of Occupational Therapy, Schools and Early Intervention, 4,* 22–33. https://doi.org/10.1080/19411243.2011.573243

Shrader, S., Hodgkins, R., Laverentz, D., Zaudke, J., Waxman, M., Johnston, K., & Jernigan, S. (2016). Interprofessional Education and Practice Guide No. 7: Development, implementation, and evaluation of a large-scale required interprofessional education foundational programme. *Journal of Interprofessional Care, 30,* 615–619. https://doi.org/10.1080/13561820.2016.1189889

Shrader, S., Mauldin, M., Hammad, S., Mitcham, M., & Blue, A. (2015). Developing a comprehensive faculty development program to promote interprofessional education, practice and research at a free-standing academic health science center. *Journal of Interprofessional Care, 29,* 165–167. https://doi.org/10.3109/13561820.2014.940417

Strong, J., Chipchase, L., Allen, S., Eley, D. S., McAllister, L., & Davidson, B. (2016). Interprofessional learning during an international fieldwork placement. *International Journal of Practice-Based Learning in Health and Social Care, 2*(2), 27–39. https://doi.org/10.11120/pblh.2014.00032

Tucker, D., Honea, D., & Ledet, L. (2003). *School setting site objectives.* Retrieved from http://www.aota.org/Educate/EdRes/Fieldwork/SiteObj.asp

Unsworth, C., & Baker, A. (2016). A systematic review of professional reasoning literature in occupational therapy. *British Journal of Occupational Therapy, 79,* 5–16. https://doi.org/10.1177/0308022615599994

Van Lew, S., & Singh, N. (2010). Integrating the *Centennial Vision* into an evidence-based fieldwork-learning experience. *Occupational Therapy in Health Care, 24*(1), 68–73. doi:10.3109/07380570903410852

Willgerodt, M. A., Abu-Rish Blakeney, E., Brock, D. M., Liner, D., Murphy, N., & Zierler, B. (2015). Interprofessional Education and Practice Guide No. 4: Developing and sustaining interprofessional education at an academic health center. *Journal of Interprofessional Care, 29,* 421–425. https://doi.org/10.3109/13561820.2015.1039117

Best Practices for Occupational Therapy Assistants in Schools

Meghan E. Spielman, COTA/L

7

KEY TERMS AND CONCEPTS

- Collaborative partnership
- Continuing competence
- Documentation
- Intervention plan
- Occupational profile
- Supervision
- Therapeutic use of self

OVERVIEW

Under the supervision of occupational therapists, occupational therapy assistants have been providing services in school systems since 1975, when the Education for All Handicapped Children Act (Pub. L. 94-142) was passed by the U.S. Congress (Frolek Clark & Chandler, 2013). According to the American Occupational Therapy Association's ([AOTA's], 2015d) workforce survey, the percentage of occupational therapy assistants working in school systems and responding to the survey was 15.2% as of 2015, making it the second most common practice area for occupational therapy assistants.

AOTA defines an *occupational therapy assistant* as a person licensed in the practice of occupational therapy who provides occupational therapy services "under the supervision of and in partnership with occupational therapists" (AOTA, 2014a, pp. S16–S17). Clearly, this definition delineates a different role than the fully autonomous *occupational therapist*. Therefore, occupational therapy assistants must never identify themselves as occupational therapists; that would be a breach of AOTA's (2015a) *Occupational Therapy Code of Ethics*.

To practice as an occupational therapy assistant, candidates must first meet multiple educational requirements. These qualifications are found in AOTA's (2015c) *Standards of Practice for Occupational Therapy* and include the following:

- Graduation from an occupational therapy assistant program accredited by the Accreditation Council for Occupational Therapy Education or predecessor organizations
- Successful completion of a supervised fieldwork experience
- Receipt of a passing grade on the entry-level examination for occupational therapy assistants approved by the governing state occupational therapy regulatory board or agency
- Fulfillment of state requirements for licensure, certification, or registration.

All 50 states, the District of Columbia, and Puerto Rico require the licensure of occupational therapy assistants (AOTA, 2018b). To obtain a state license, occupational therapy assistants must pass the National Board for Certification in Occupational Therapy occupational therapy assistant certification examination. On passing the exam, the occupational therapy assistant may choose to carry the designation of *certified* (i.e., use the credential C̲OTA). The maintenance of this certification is voluntary except in 1 state.

Most states address the occupational therapy assistant's role and practice standards through their respective regulations and guidelines. For this reason, it is essential that practitioners be well versed in their state's practice act as well as their local district's implementation of set requirements. AOTA has released several documents pertaining to state regulations, including compiled lists of statutes from each state regarding the supervision of occupational therapy assistants, qualifications and licensure requirements, and the occupational therapy scope of practice (AOTA, 2014a, 2014c, 2015a, 2015b, 2015c, 2017).

As occupational therapy becomes a more widely recognized profession, the demand for occupational therapy practitioners[1] continues to rise, especially in the school systems, where the role of occupational therapy has expanded from a clinical model to a much broader educational model (Chandler, 2013). As workloads increase and occupational therapy practitioners participate in more systemwide initiatives, the need arises for occupational therapy assistants to become a larger part of the school community.

---

[1]*Occupational therapy practitioner* refers to both the occupational therapist and the occupational therapy assistant. AOTA (2014a, p. S18) states, "The occupational therapist is responsible for all aspects of occupational therapy service delivery and is accountable for the safety and effectiveness of the occupational therapy service delivery process" and "must be directly involved in the delivery of services during the initial evaluation and regularly throughout the course of intervention. . . . The occupational therapy assistant delivers safe and effective occupational therapy services under the supervision of and in partnership with the occupational therapist."

Copyright © 2019 by the American Occupational Therapy Association. All rights reserved. To reuse this content, contact www.copyright.com.
https://doi.org/10.7139/2019.978-1-56900-591-0.007

There are many benefits to hiring occupational therapy assistants in a school district. Under the supervision of the occupational therapist, occupational therapy assistants have the ability to provide services at many levels, including direct and group instruction (building level); consultation with teachers and staff (building and district levels); attendance at various meetings (building and district level); assistance with the evaluation process (building level); and participation at a systemwide level alongside their colleagues and supervisors (district and state level). In addition, having occupational therapy assistants in a district provides a unique opportunity for students to work with more than one practitioner. With the plurality of expert eyes and minds, collaboration increases, and students receive more well-rounded services.

Working together with occupational therapists, team members, classroom teachers, and the families and students they serve, occupational therapy assistants are in the trenches, devoting their days to working directly with students to enable them to fully participate in school environments. Not only do occupational therapy assistants provide intervention on a daily basis, they may also contribute to almost every portion of the occupational therapy process, from evaluation to discontinuation of services, under the supervision of the occupational therapist. This chapter explores the role of occupational therapy assistants and gives an in-depth look at how they contribute to students and school systems across the United States.

ESSENTIAL CONSIDERATIONS

There are several considerations for occupational therapy assistants working in schools. Occupational therapy assistants are legally required to work under the supervision of occupational therapists; therefore, all practitioners must have an understanding of what is to be expected from this partnership. In addition, occupational therapy assistants should be familiar with the laws and regulations concerning their scope of practice, including roles and responsibilities, documentation, and professional development requirements.

National, State, and Local Laws and Policies

Occupational therapy practitioners must have a proficient awareness of the laws, policies, and regulations that surround them, not only at the national level but also at the state, district, and building levels. To ensure effective and best practice, occupational therapy assistants should know the difference between individualized education programs (IEPs) and Section 504 plans as well as how they are able to contribute to each process. The official professional documents developed by AOTA are excellent resources for both occupational therapists and occupational therapy assistants looking to grow their foundational knowledge of the profession.

Role and Responsibilities of OTAs in Schools

Depending on state regulations, each district may vary slightly in its expectations of the occupational therapy assistant's role, but many responsibilities are consistent nationwide. Exhibit 7.1 provides a sample job description for occupational therapy assistants working in a school system.

Partnership of the OT and OTA

Under the supervision of the occupational therapist, the occupational therapy assistant carries numerous responsibilities (AOTA, 2014a). This partnership is of utmost importance, first because it is legally required and second because it ensures accountability for both practitioners. Although the occupational therapist is ultimately responsible for the occupational therapy process, a successful collaboration between the occupational therapist and occupational therapy assistant is necessary.

The most vital factor to note about occupational therapy assistants and supervising occupational therapists is that the relationship is a *collaborative partnership.* Occupational therapists should not dictate what the occupational therapy assistant should do because this would be a misuse of the assistant's role. In contrast, practitioners should work together to develop a collaborative plan for supervision. Occupational therapy assistants build their knowledge and skills, using them to contribute to the decision-making process to optimize student outcomes. Supervision should provide an opportunity for occupational therapy assistants to expand their expertise as well as learn from and share insight with the supervising occupational therapist.

Supervision is not merely a one-sided partnership in which the occupational therapy assistant is the only beneficiary. Rather, it ought to be a continually occurring and interactive process that promotes the professional growth of those involved. A healthy working relationship between the supervisor and supervisee is crucial and, ideally, should be based on trust and an understanding of each practitioner's qualifications. The focus of the partnership should make certain that students' needs are prioritized and that services are provided in an ethical and effectual manner.

Supervision Methods

According to AOTA (2014a), *supervision* is defined as "a process aimed at ensuring the safe and effective delivery of occupational therapy services" (p. S16). Although the occupational therapist is ultimately responsible for providing sufficient supervision, it is the duty of the occupational therapy assistant to seek out the appropriate amount of supervision (AOTA, 2014a). The specifics surrounding supervision, such as the regularity, techniques, and subject matter, are dependent on a variety of factors. AOTA (2014a) has provided 6 principles to guide supervision practices:

> The specific frequency, methods, and content of supervision may vary and are dependent on the (a) complexity of client needs, (b) number and diversity of clients, (c) knowledge and skill level of the occupational therapist and the occupational therapy assistant, (d) type of

EXHIBIT 7.1. Sample Job Description for an Occupational Therapy Assistant in a School

Purpose Statement:
The OTA works under the supervision of an OT to enhance student participation in the educational environment by providing occupational therapy services, including direct intervention and consultation, on the basis of student need. The holder of this position reports to the supervising OT and appointed department director.

General Responsibilities:
- Assists and contributes to screenings and evaluations by providing information regarding students to the OT
- Contributes to creating measurable goals with the OT and IEP team
- Collaborates with the OT to develop intervention plans and develop interventions in students' school context and routine to enhance participation in their educational program
- Provides direct and indirect occupational therapy services to students in accordance with IEP or 504 plans
- Completes documentation, including data collection, on therapy services (e.g., contact notes, progress reports, updated IEPs, Medicaid billing)
- Communicates information regarding student progress and suggested recommendations to appropriate individuals (e.g., students, families, educational staff, administrators)
- Consults with OTs, teachers, paraeducators, PTs, SLPs, and other members of the educational team regarding student needs
- Attends meetings (e.g., IEP meetings, parent–teacher conferences, team meetings) for the purpose of conveying and obtaining information regarding student progress (all decisions must be made by the OT)
- Provides training to paraeducators regarding specifically assigned tasks
- Participates in supervisory activities with the OT, advocating for more supervision when needed
- Supervises OTA fieldwork students
- Participates in and, when appropriate, facilitates education and training through in-service sessions for school personnel.

Skills, Knowledge, and Abilities:
- Graduated from an accredited OTA program, after completion of all educational and supervised fieldwork requirements
- Holds current licensure in the state of desired employment
- Has excellent interpersonal, organizational, and communication skills

Working Conditions:
Travel between school buildings is required. Physical demands include moving therapy equipment and assisting with transfer of students on and off equipment as well as bending, crawling, kneeling, and moving on and off the floor.

Note. IEP = Individualized education program; OT = occupational therapist; OTA = occupational therapy assistant; PT = physical therapist; SLP = speech–language pathologist.

practice setting, (e) requirements of the practice setting, and (f) other regulatory requirements. (p. S17)

To ensure efficient and ethical service implementation, practitioners must thoroughly consider each of the 6 principles when determining how to carry out the supervision process. State laws must also be followed. Certain states provide detailed requirements on how supervision should be implemented, whereas others have no relevant policies. AOTA has provided a document on its website listing each state's supervision regulations, which is helpful for all practitioners seeking to become more familiar with the laws in their state of employment (see https://bit.ly/2rlkMOG).

A variety of media can be used for supervision, including direct face-to-face contact and indirect contact. Examples of each can be found in Table 7.1. Given the various means available to accomplish effective supervision, practitioners must have an understanding of what methods work best for their individual learning styles as well as what is manageable within their workload.

Identifying Competence for Service Provision

Competency for gathering and sharing assessment data is established with the supervising occupational therapist through a variety of measures and considerations. The first

TABLE 7.1. Methods Used to Perform Occupational Therapy Supervision

TYPE OF CONTACT	EXAMPLES
Direct (face-to-face) contact	"Including, but not limited to, observation, modeling, client demonstration, discussions, teaching, web-based apps (depending on the amount of privacy and confidentiality required), and instruction" (AOTA, 2014a, p. S17)
Indirect contact	"Including, but not limited to, phone conversations, written correspondence, and electronic exchanges" (AOTA, 2014a, p. S17)

Note. AOTA = American Occupational Therapy Association.

action the occupational therapist should take is to simply converse with the occupational therapy assistant. Listening to the occupational therapy assistant talk about the process of occupational therapy, the students, their interventions, and how they interpret daily experiences gives the occupational therapist valuable insight into the occupational therapy assistant's knowledge and skill base.

In addition to these conversations, the supervising occupational therapist should make observations across the educational environment. When talking with and observing the occupational therapy assistant, the occupational therapist should contemplate several considerations and questions: How is the professional judgment of the occupational therapy assistant displayed? What methodology drives their decisions? When performing an entry-level task, do they meet the minimum requirement or go beyond the expectations? When administering an assessment, does the occupational therapy assistant follow the instructions and gather the needed information? Do they exercise professionalism when interacting with students, parents, and staff? Do they utilize therapeutic use of self?

Assessing the occupational therapy assistant's competence will drive the supervision process, which requires each practitioner to become familiar with their partner's strengths and weaknesses and, subsequently, provide the necessary amount of support. A change in supervisors may necessitate the reestablishment of practice competence with the new supervising occupational therapist. When the supervision process is executed appropriately and communication is prioritized, the resulting partnership should provide ample opportunity for the occupational therapist to determine the knowledge and skill the occupational therapy assistant possesses and applies.

Supervision Challenges

Despite efforts to create a supervision model that works for all occupational therapy practitioners in a given school district, challenges often arise that hinder effective supervision practices. One of the most common difficulties practitioners encounter is a lack of time. As practitioners face growing workloads, responsibilities at multiple locations, and ever-present funding concerns that result in layoffs, the result is decreased time for supervisory activities. These constraints plague not only the regular school year but also the summer months. If an occupational therapy assistant provides services during extended school-year programs (i.e., programs that occur outside of the district's school calendar), the district must also hire an occupational therapist to ensure that supervision is readily available.

Another challenge in supervisory relationships that can be the most difficult to overcome is strained relationships. A wide spectrum of mistreatment from both levels of the profession may exist, often stemming from a misunderstanding of roles. For example, an occupational therapist may expect too little or too much from the occupational therapy assistant, especially when they are unfamiliar with the role. Another example is an occupational therapy assistant's assuming too much responsibility (e.g., independently completing evaluations or referring a student for services) or not enough, both of which can be unethical and, in some occurrences, illegal.

These examples demonstrate a misuse of the occupational therapy assistant's role and can lead to extremely tense exchanges between the occupational therapist and occupational therapy assistant. Open communication and respect are 2 main components required in successful supervisory relationships. This is especially true when practitioners have significant differences in their experience levels. For instance, when an occupational therapy assistant with 20 years of experience in a school setting is assigned a supervisor who is new to school practice, supervision activities may need to occur more often as the therapist settles into the new environment and builds their knowledge base. Likewise, an occupational therapy assistant who is entering a school setting for the first time or one who is appointed an intense, heavy workload will likely require more supervision to effectively manage such demands.

In an effort to decrease or altogether avoid difficult relationships, it is paramount that the occupational therapist and the occupational therapy assistant not only have a thorough understanding of each level's scope of practice but also exude respect for each other in the process. Regardless of time restraints, service locations, and practitioner experience, it is imperative that expectations surrounding supervision be clear, from how supervision is to be structured to what each practitioner is responsible for, as well as how the supervisory activities will be recorded.

Supervision Documentation

It is strongly recommended, even required in certain states, that supervisory activities be documented. Suggestions concerning the content of such documentation include frequency of contact, the method in which the supervision was administered, what was discussed, evidence to support practitioner competency, and names and qualifying credentials of those involved in the process (AOTA, 2014a). Ideally, supervision logs should be simple to maintain, documenting fundamental information such as the date, conversation points (including students discussed, if applicable), and the outcome of the meeting. Intervention plans may also be included in the documentation process. To ensure accountability, both practitioners should sign and retain copies of the supervision documentation, whether electronic or handwritten (Frolek Clark & Handley-More, 2017). Practitioners must be aware of their state and facility's regulations related to all documentation, including supervision and service provision.

Professional Development and Continuing Competence

Many states have continuing competence requirements that practitioners need to meet to uphold licensure, a summary of which can be found on AOTA's website (see https://bit.ly/2rmINoL). However, apart from state standards, it is expected that all practitioners participate in continuing education and professional development to advance their competence in the field of occupational therapy. AOTA's Commission on Continuing Competence and Professional Development described *continuing competence* as a "dynamic and multidimensional process in which . . .

[practitioners] develop and maintain the knowledge, . . . skills, . . . and abilities . . . necessary to perform current and future roles and responsibilities within the profession" (AOTA, 2015b, p. S103). This document lists 5 standards for developing competence, including knowledge, critical reasoning, interpersonal skills, performance skills, and ethical practice (AOTA, 2015b). Regardless of how many years they have spent in the field, all occupational therapists and occupational therapy assistants must seek out learning opportunities to grow their knowledge and skills in those areas of competence.

It is especially important for occupational therapy assistants to develop competence in areas related to their practice area. In school systems, such areas could include understanding curricula and instruction, using observation methods for assessment, developing programs, or implementing evidence-based practices for students with specific conditions. Examples of professional development activities might include formal learning, independent learning (e.g., review of evidence-based articles), and mentorship by a more experienced practitioner. AOTA (2014b) also has provided a toolkit for starting a journal club that can center on current trends in literature applicable to school practice for occupational therapy assistants.

An additional opportunity for school occupational therapy assistants is to seek a Specialty Certification in School Systems. This peer-reviewed process enables applicants who have acquired the minimum requirements (e.g., 2,000 hours in occupational therapy assistant practice, with 600 hours specific to schools in the past 5 years) to validate their level of specialization and commitment to school practice by gaining nationally recognized credentials (AOTA, 2018a). Whether it takes the form of pursuing additional credentials or simply attending courses to increase one's knowledge about a specific topic, professional development is vital for all practitioners because it increases competence, promotes advancement of skills, and informs best practice.

BEST PRACTICES

On the establishment of competence, occupational therapy assistants have the ability to be involved in nearly every part of the occupational therapy process, from screening to discontinuation of services. Because state regulations vary, practitioners are strongly encouraged to check their respective state's laws.

Always Document Services

According to Frolek Clark and Handley-More (2017), *documentation,* the process of recording the provision of occupational therapy services, must "provide a trail of data that supports service delivery by occupational therapy practitioners" (p. xiii) Therefore, when occupational therapy assistants provide services to students, it is their responsibility to document the intervention as well as the outcome of the session. In an effort to ensure best practice and oversight of services, documentation completed by the occupational therapy assistant should be reviewed and signed by the supervising occupational therapist. The methods used to document differ by district and, at times,

by building, but all practitioners must be familiar with and follow through with what is expected of them by way of documentation, including policies related to Medicaid reimbursement. (For more information on this topic, see Chapter 16, "Best Practices in Medicaid Cost Recovery," and Chapter 45, "Best Practices in School Occupational Therapy Documentation and Data Collection.")

Contribute to Screenings

In states in which occupational therapy services can be provided to students in general education, the occupational therapist must be directly involved and initiate the process. After initial contact with the student, the occupational therapist may delegate activities to the occupational therapy assistant as part of the screening process, such as file review, observation of the student's performance in a variety of environments, and collection of work samples. Although the occupational therapy assistant contributes information to the process, the occupational therapist is responsible for identifying instructional strategies that might benefit the student.

Assist in Evaluations in School Contexts and Routines

As with all aspects of occupational therapy service provision, the occupational therapist is responsible for the evaluation process (AOTA, 2014a). This process begins with the *occupational profile* (i.e., a summary of the student's experiences; interests; needs; medical, educational, and job histories). After competence has been established and where state professional laws allow, the occupational therapy assistant can contribute by gathering data and providing reports of observations to the occupational therapist (AOTA, 2015b). The data are analyzed by the occupational therapist with input from the occupational therapy assistant. The evaluation report, written by the occupational therapist with contributions from the occupational therapy assistant, may recommend occupational therapy services to the IEP team.

The team then uses data from all of the reports to determine whether a student is eligible for special education and related services (e.g., occupational therapy). In addition, the team determines the student's strengths, needs, and services, using this information to develop student goals. Using data from the occupational therapy evaluation as well as input from the occupational therapist, the team ascertains whether services are necessary for students to benefit from their educational program.

The occupational therapy assistant may attend the IEP meeting under the direction of the occupational therapist but is not to make final decisions about occupational therapy services. Once the IEP is finalized, the occupational therapy assistant collaborates with the occupational therapist and clients (e.g., student, parent, teacher) to develop the *intervention plan*. This plan is an occupational therapy document that describes the occupational therapy practitioner's actions (e.g., similar to a teacher's lesson plan) and designates aspects to the occupational therapy assistant, with supervision required from the occupational therapist.

Provide Intervention

In accordance with AOTA guidelines and state professional laws, occupational therapy assistants carry out the aspects of occupational therapy intervention delegated to them by the supervising occupational therapist. In collaboration with the occupational therapist, the occupational therapy assistant may select, implement, and make modifications to the interventions consistent with demonstrated competence levels established with the supervising therapist (AOTA, 2014a).

Services must be provided in the student's least restrictive environment, per the Individuals With Disabilities Education Improvement Act of 2004 (Pub. L. 108–446). Such environments could include general education classrooms, cafeterias, hallways, playgrounds, and art or music classrooms (AOTA, 2017). If a student is unable to receive services in these sites because of specific needs, occupational therapy practitioners must work together with the IEP team to make decisions regarding service location and justify the reason accordingly on the student's IEP. (For more information on least restrictive environments and IEP requirements, see Chapter 3, "Laws That Affect Occupational Therapy in Schools").

Regardless of service location, the occupational therapy assistant must be knowledgeable about evidence-based research and apply this information to everyday practice (AOTA, 2015b, 2015c). Interventions should be directed at meeting the student's IEP goals, with the occupational therapy evaluation guiding the intervention process using evidence-based practices (AOTA, 2014c).

Another critical aspect to consider is how a practitioner's attitude, personality, and skill level contribute to the intervention process. Occupational therapists and occupational therapy assistants must work together to create manageable workloads and, when dividing caseloads and service provision, consider their own competencies and personalities and subsequently match those strengths to individual students. *Therapeutic use of self,* the practice of using one's strengths and personality to cultivate meaningful therapeutic relationships, is a fundamental element of occupational therapy that allows practitioners to build and maintain relationships with students by using clinical reasoning, empathy, and a collaborative approach, all while keeping the student as the central priority (AOTA, 2014c). Because occupational therapy assistants are in continuous contact with students, staff, and families, it is crucial for them to exhibit therapeutic use of self.

Occupational therapy practitioners frequently interact with students and families when they are most vulnerable. Developing high-quality, professional relationships should be viewed as an indispensable component of the occupational therapy process because it increases the effectiveness of the intervention provided (AOTA, 2014c). Good rapport is essential for optimal outcomes.

Target IEP Goals

To measure the efficacy of occupational therapy services, providers must collect data to show the student's rate of progress. The data occupational therapy assistants record in their documentation are a formative factor used to determine whether and when changes need to be made to the IEP.

Although it depends on the local educational agency's policies, an occupational therapy assistant typically has the ability to contribute to progress reports about performance on students' IEP goals, under the supervision of the occupational therapist. Once competency is established, the occupational therapy assistant is also able to attend and report at IEP meetings without the occupational therapist present, but they must not change what the supervising therapist recommended before the meeting's commencement. If it is anticipated that multiple questions may arise from family members or considerable decisions may need to be made, both the occupational therapist and the occupational therapy assistant should consider attending the meeting.

When a student no longer requires occupational therapy services, the occupational therapy assistant may contribute to a discontinuation plan by providing information and documentation to the supervising occupational therapist that relates to the student's performance, needs, and goals (AOTA, 2015c). Identical to the other stages of the occupational therapy process, the conclusion involves the occupational therapist and occupational therapy assistant working collaboratively to ensure best practice and positive outcomes.

SUMMARY

Under the supervision of and in collaboration with occupational therapists, occupational therapy assistants have been providing occupational therapy services to students in school systems for more than 4 decades. Using their personality, strength, and skill level, occupational therapy assistants contribute to the occupational process, from screening to discontinuation of services. Delegated aspects of occupational therapy may include implementing intervention plans, documenting progress, and participating in supervisory activities for occupational therapy assistant students. Occupational therapy assistants are required to be conversant in national laws, state and district regulations, and professional standards concerning their role and the delivery of occupational therapy services.

The multifaceted role of occupational therapy assistants provides opportunities for them to advocate for this level of the profession and secure a greater voice not only in the field of occupational therapy but in school systems as well.

REFERENCES

American Occupational Therapy Association. (2014a). Guidelines for supervision, roles, and responsibilities during the delivery of occupational therapy services. *American Journal of Occupational Therapy, 68*(Suppl. 3), S16–S22. https://doi10.5014/ajot.2014.686S03

American Occupational Therapy Association. (2014b). *Journal club toolkit.* Retrieved from https://www.aota.org/Practice/Researchers/Journal-Club-Toolkit.aspx

American Occupational Therapy Association. (2014c). Occupational therapy practice framework: Domain and process (3rd ed.). *American Journal of Occupational Therapy, 68*(Suppl. 1), S1–S48. https://doi.org/10.5014/ajot.2014.682006

American Occupational Therapy Association. (2015a). Occupational therapy code of ethics (2015). *American Journal of Occupational Therapy, 69*(Suppl. 3), 6913410030. https://doi.org/10.5014/ajot.2015.696S03

American Occupational Therapy Association. (2015b). Standards for continuing competence. *American Journal of Occupational Therapy, 64*(6, Suppl.), S103–S105. https://doi.org/10.5014/ajot.2010.64S103

American Occupational Therapy Association. (2015c). Standards of practice for occupational therapy. *American Journal of Occupational Therapy, 69*(Suppl. 3), 6913410057. https://doi.org/10.5014/ajot.2015.696S06

American Occupational Therapy Association. (2015d). *Work setting trends for occupational therapy: How to choose a setting.* Retrieved from https://www.aota.org/Education-Careers/Advance-Career/Salary-Workforce-Survey/work-setting-trends-how-to-pick-choose.aspx

American Occupational Therapy Association. (2017). Guidelines for occupational therapy services in early childhood and schools. *American Journal of Occupational Therapy, 71*(Suppl. 2), 7112410010. https://doi.org/10.5014/ajot.2017.716S01

American Occupational Therapy Association. (2018a). *Board and specialty certifications.* Retrieved from https://www.aota.org/Education-Careers/Advance-Career/Board-Specialty-Certifications.aspx

American Occupational Therapy Association. (2018b). *How to get a license.* Retrieved from https://www.aota.org/Advocacy-Policy/State-Policy/Licensure/How-To.aspx

Chandler, B. E. (2013). History of occupational therapy in the schools. In G. Frolek Clark & B. E. Chandler (Eds.), *Best practices for occupational therapy in schools* (pp. 1–14). Bethesda, MD: AOTA Press.

Education for All Handicapped Children Act of 1975, Pub. L. 94–142, renamed the Individuals With Disabilities Education Improvement Act, codified at 20 U.S.C. §§ 1400–1482.

Frolek Clark, G., & Chandler, B. E. (Eds.). (2013). *Best practices for occupational therapy in schools.* Bethesda, MD: AOTA Press.

Frolek Clark, G., & Handley-More, D. (2017). *Best practices for documenting occupational therapy services in schools.* Bethesda, MD: AOTA Press.

Individuals With Disabilities Education Improvement Act of 2004, Pub. L. 108–446, 20 U.S.C. §§ 1400–1482.

Best Practices for School Occupational Therapy Practitioners as Administrators

8

Patricia Laverdure, OTD, OTR/L, BCP, and Jean E. Polichino, OTR, MS, FAOTA

KEY TERMS AND CONCEPTS

- Change implementation plan
- Divisional structure
- Employee performance appraisal
- Functional structure
- Human resources professional
- Hybrid structure
- Leadership self-efficacy
- Local educational agency
- Mediation
- Performance expectations
- Program evaluation
- State educational agency

OVERVIEW

In educational settings, occupational therapy is provided across a complex and hierarchical organization designed to prepare students to be contributing members of society. The administration of public education is the responsibility of a superintendent hired by the local educational agency (LEA) board of trustees (i.e., school board). The **LEA** is the local governmental authority that administers public education in a specific jurisdiction. The school board delegates authority to the superintendent to administer and manage the LEA in accordance with school board policy and in compliance with the legal requirements of the state's department of education (i.e., *state educational agency* [SEA], the subdivision of state government charged with implementing federal and state education policy and supervising LEA adherence to these policies; Hoyle et al., 2005).[1]

According to the Department for Professional Employees (2016) of the American Federation of Labor and Congress of Industrial Organizations, the superintendent and their designees provide essential leadership to ensure smooth day-to-day operations in educational institutions. Administrative and management activities typically include capacity assessment and development, oversight of personnel and their assignments, execution of program responsibilities and implementation of services, and management of fiscal and material resources (Richmond & Powers, 2009).

Occupational therapists possess the knowledge, performance skills, critical and ethical reasoning, and interpersonal abilities (American Occupational Therapy Association [AOTA], 2013) necessary to fill critical administrative and management roles in educational settings and are doing so with increasing regularity and success (Sauvigne-Kirsch,

2017). With an advanced academic degree and additional training, occupational therapy assistants may be prepared to fulfill administrative and management roles in educational settings as well. However, although occupational therapy assistants serving in administrative roles can effectively provide administrative supervision of the workforce, they must adhere to the clinical supervisory regulations of the state's practice act. Although most occupational therapy practitioners[2] identify administrative and managerial responsibilities in their roles in educational settings (AOTA, 2013), occupational therapy practitioners serving in formal administrative roles in educational institutions remain rare.

A recent study identified numerous barriers that limit occupational therapy practitioners from acquiring administrative positions (Sauvigne-Kirsch, 2017). Most notably, the findings suggested that the lack of clear pathways to obtaining SEA educational administrator credentials often prevents occupational therapy practitioners from advancing their career in educational systems.

Despite these challenging realities, when there are no explicit legal or procedural prohibitions, occupational therapy practitioners have been able to secure administrative positions in LEAs, centers, and schools. In some cases, occupational therapy practitioners serving in administrative roles oversee large departments of occupational, physical, and speech–language therapy programs (Sauvigne-Kirsch, 2017). In others, occupational therapy practitioners hold positions in

---

[1]Although some states provide special education and related services through multiple educational agencies, which may cover one or multiple districts in the state, for the purpose of this chapter, only the LEA organization is discussed.

[2]*Occupational therapy practitioner* refers to both the occupational therapist and the occupational therapy assistant. AOTA (2014a, p. S18) states, "The occupational therapist is responsible for all aspects of occupational therapy service delivery and is accountable for the safety and effectiveness of the occupational therapy service delivery process" and "must be directly involved in the delivery of services during the initial evaluation and regularly throughout the course of intervention. . . . The occupational therapy assistant delivers safe and effective occupational therapy services under the supervision of and in partnership with the occupational therapist."

Copyright © 2019 by the American Occupational Therapy Association. All rights reserved. To reuse this content, contact www.copyright.com.
https://doi.org/10.7139/2019.978-1-56900-591-0.008

educational agencies that are not required to comply with state credentialing requirements (e.g., SEAs, educational cooperative arrangements, intermediate units). Finally, administrative roles have often been created and achieved through the assistance, mentorship, and advocacy of educators who advanced the work of the occupational therapy practitioner, particularly in special education programs and departments.

Entry-level administrative position titles include program specialist, coordinator or manager, and assistant director or director. Among those who have achieved advanced positions, it is interesting to note that many have advanced degrees in areas that complement or enhance their skill sets, such as administration and management, health care administration, educational leadership, and assistive technology. Others have achieved doctoral degrees in occupational therapy (AOTA, 2017b).

Serving in administrative roles and managing the delivery of occupational therapy services in the complex and ever-changing context of public education requires careful adherence to state and federal regulatory statute and policy; astute attention to the mission, vision, and core values of the educational institution; thorough oversight of service effectiveness, efficiency, outcomes, and security; and equitable balance of the interests of often competing stakeholders (Jacobs & McCormack, 2010). Occupational therapy administrators are champions of change. They serve as leaders who effectively challenge habits and beliefs, shift systems through times of uncertainty, and usher in adaptive change that improves the outcomes of those served (Heifetz & Linsky, 2002). Occupational therapy administrators in educational settings leverage their agency, relationships, and coherence making to ensure positive outcomes (Fullan, 2001).

ESSENTIAL CONSIDERATIONS

Occupational therapy practitioners who serve in administrative roles must understand the organizational structures and management models that are used in educational systems today. They are required to attend to the regulatory and sociocultural influences on practice and be able to respond with agility to change within systems.

Organizational Management Frameworks in Education

Several common structures of administrative operation can be found in public educational institutions today (Dunaway & Ausband, 2008; Honig, 2008; Hoy & Miskel, 2013; Spring, 1997). These operational structures are defined as either functional or divisional.

Functional structures are organized around key system functions or operations, such as human resources (HR), business and finance, facilities, instruction, and technology. Although services organized operationally within this structure are highly focused and performance and outcomes are easy to track, functions can be siloed and sluggish, and communication across functions and units is sometimes problematic.

Divisional structures, in contrast, are organized on the basis of product or service line, with each division independently performing all of the necessary functions to operate as separate business units. This structure allows for locally responsive and decentralized decision making but often results in poor integration, duplication of efforts, and communication barriers across divisions.

In recent years, school districts have increasingly adopted a *hybrid structure* that includes both functional and divisional operational approaches, maximizing the integration, flexibility, and agility attributes of both approaches and minimizing duplication and communication challenges (Honig, 2008). Ensuring that system activities, routines, and organizational structures align with LEA goals within available resource allocations (Spillane et al., 2011) and managing change in response to environmental influences are the overarching challenges of school administrators, regardless of the structure used (Fixsen et al., 2005).

Whether they use functional, divisional, or hybrid operational structures, LEA administrative personnel manage services in a complex system that is both political and instructional. They must also contend with myriad national, state, and local legal requirements and policies; cultural norms; and stakeholder interests (Murphy & Hallinger, 1988). In addition to the SEA and school board authorities, administrators balance the interests of a multitude of stakeholders, including students; parents; teachers; staff; and the social, educational, private educational, and medical communities. Balancing these interests requires the ability to build collaborative partnerships that focus on the educational and occupational outcomes of students and their families (Laverdure et al., 2017).

Managing Occupational Therapy Services

The role and responsibilities of the occupational therapy administrator are typically defined by the educational institution's job description and *performance expectations,* that is, the behaviors and actions required by the job. Performance expectations may be explicitly shared through assignments and directives, but in almost all cases they are aligned with the institution's strategic mission and goals and documented in the administrator's performance evaluation. Common administrator activities include evaluating the capacity and outcomes of the program, its services, and its opportunities; developing, marketing, and implementing service delivery plans; making decisions; and resolving conflicts (Richmond & Powers, 2009).

Tasks routinely center around 3 key areas: budget, personnel, and practice management. Staying abreast of relevant legal and professional literature and ensuring the evidence basis of services delivered are critical components of the administrator role (Waite, 2016). Because the administrator overseeing occupational therapy services and personnel may not be an occupational therapy practitioner, it is important that administrators and occupational therapy practitioners work together to build knowledge of the role and value of occupational therapy in the school system. Documents that may facilitate this conversation include the following:

- *Guidelines for Occupational Therapy Services in Early Intervention and Schools* (AOTA, 2017a)
- *Guidance for Performance Evaluation of School Occupational Therapists* (AOTA, 2013)
- *Occupational Therapy's Distinct Value—Children and Youth: Resource for Administrators and Policy Makers* (AOTA, 2016)
- "Developing Quality Indicators for School Practice" (Laverdure et al., 2018).

In Fall 2017, AOTA initiated an advocacy effort to assist occupational therapy practitioners working in school settings to access leadership and administrative positions. AOTA sent a letter to all SEA superintendents of education and SEA directors of special education, seeking a means to enable "practitioners who are experienced and committed to school-based practice to move up the career ladder in educational systems" (Schefkind, 2017, p. 1). The AOTA State Leaders in Schools Community of Practice is developing tools and resources to educate occupational therapy practitioners and stakeholders about the attributes and benefits of school leadership and advancement, and has encouraged occupational therapy practitioners to advocate for action on this issue in their state (AOTA, 2017b).

Educational Laws and Regulations

In educational settings, occupational therapy administrators must understand federal laws and regulations that govern public education and state policies that are enacted to implement them (AOTA, 2017a; Laverdure et al., 2016). Explicit and clear occupational therapy procedures must be in place to support provider compliance with these regulations. Local education policy, occupational therapy procedures, and the laws that inform them must be internalized to ensure that the expectations for professional behavior and the provision of services to students and teams are well understood and executed.

Administrative decision making, control strategies, and oversight processes must be present so that breaches in compliance in areas such as individualized education program (IEP) implementation, progress monitoring and outcome measurement, and service documentation are consistent with federal, state, and local requirements. Efficient communication strategies for ensuring timely transmission and translation of information in this ever-changing environment are an essential function of the occupational therapy administrator. When tensions arise among or between legal and professional standards, the occupational therapy administrator ensures that SEA and LEA leaders and administrators collaborate to resolve the conflicts.

Trends in Leadership

Occupational therapy administrators must grapple with recurrent federal, state, and local regulatory reauthorization and judicial shifts; operational structures; education reform initiatives; emerging science; and stakeholder pressure for reproducible and cost-efficient outcomes. These shifting variables challenge administrators to lead change and innovation in school practice in ways that minimize variations in service delivery, inefficient processes and procedures, and waste that lead to inconsistent, unreliable, and costly outcomes. Change and innovation require administrators to usher in new practices, which often produces uncertainty and anxiety among personnel, disrupts processes (which may increase error in workflows and noncompliance), and affects client outcomes (Gosselin et al., 2015).

Leading change in the midst of increasing complexity takes time and requires agility (Allan et al., 2014). A well-designed *change implementation plan,* defined as the activities and roles to manage and control change during the execute-and-control stage of a project, balances the organizational press for innovation with the professional identity of diverse team members and the emotions and relationships that exist in that team (Allan et al., 2014; Andre & Sjovold, 2017).

Occupational therapy administrators can draw from a number of change implementation models that exist in the literature. Although these models vary in the type of innovation (setting, population, preventative or restorative, and targeted or holistic) and sequence, the process of change implementation is characterized similarly. Moullin et al. (2015), in their systematic review of change implementation models, suggested that occupational therapy administrators consider the following during the planning of change implementation in their school settings:

- The innovation to be implemented and the evidence that supports it
- The context in which the implementation is to occur
- The influencing facilitators and the barriers to change
- The process (stages and steps) of implementation
- The evaluations that will be used to measure change success.

Change and innovation ensure that occupational therapy services are vital and valued, and change management ensures that change and innovation are incorporated and integrated effectively and efficiently into practice.

In addition, occupational therapy leaders and administrators are increasingly advancing practice and influencing administrative policy at state, district, and campus levels from a public health framework (Bazyk et al., 2015). The public health framework enables occupational therapy administrators to examine challenges that exist throughout the system, identify resources and interventions that may prevent or mitigate the impacts of these challenges, and provide the maximum benefit for the largest number of clients at a systems level (Laverdure et al., 2016). Public health approaches address the risks facing all students in the system and establish strategies, programs, and curricula that reduce these risks (Wegner et al., 2014). Occupational therapy practitioners use public health approaches in early intervening services (multi-tiered systems of support), including response to intervention, mental health, bullying prevention, and health fitness services.

In alignment with the occupational therapy process (AOTA, 2014b), occupational therapy administrators design public health approaches using the following process:

- Data are systematically collected to identify the scope; characteristics; and academic, social, and participatory consequences of the challenge.
- Risk and protective factors (causes and correlates) and barriers to engagement are defined.
- Interventions are designed and implemented, and outcomes are assessed.
- Effective interventions are implemented on a larger scale, and the impacts, efficiencies, and cost-effectiveness are carefully monitored.

Public health approaches used by occupational therapy administrators enable programs to expose a large number of students to interventions that reduce risk; prevent social isolation, injury, illness, and disability; and promote inclusive engagement for all.

BEST PRACTICES

The responsibilities of the occupational therapy administrator in educational settings include managing human and fiscal resources, evaluating service delivery processes and outcomes, and identifying and marketing service opportunities. Collaborating with the multiple stakeholders to ensure mission compliance, goal achievement, and client satisfaction promotes best practice in occupational therapy administration.

Manage Human Resources

The complexity of education and employment law as well as the many personal and interpersonal issues that arise among personnel in public education can overwhelm even the most competent of administrators. Nurturing relationships with LEA *HR professionals* is essential. HR professionals provide leadership in areas such as organization development, strategic utilization of employees to serve business goals, and talent management and development. Their responsibilities encompass tasks like hiring, training, performance management, team building, rewards and loyalty programs, compensation, and pensions. The primary focus of the work of an HR professional is recruitment, performance evaluation, and compensation for personnel, which makes them important strategic partners in acquiring and managing the professional talent needed for success (Odden, 2011).

Once the right professionals are recruited for open positions, developing and maintaining their interest and motivation are of critical importance. Occupational therapy administrators are well advised to work together with HR professionals to provide clear performance standards and expectations to practitioners regarding job duties, offer support and strategies when personal or professional challenges affect job performance, ensure adherence to LEA disciplinary policies and procedures when job performance is substandard, and support positive growth experiences for the professional to maximize retention and minimize turnover. Although doing the right thing for all involved can be a daunting challenge, working in collaboration with the HR department before decision making in personnel issues is in the best interest of all involved. For the occupational therapy administrator, collaboration is the ideal approach for achieving protection of employee rights and securing a positive position for the LEA.

The HR department is also a valuable partner in administrative marketing efforts directed at recruiting occupational therapy practitioners in schools. Occupational therapy administrators leverage traditional and digital media connections, typically developed by the HR department, to advance recruitment efforts. The occupational therapy administrator's role in this partnership is to

- Provide specifics as to job features that are attractive to potential candidates (e.g., school-year calendar, professional development, mentoring, flexible work sites, diverse population) and
- Work with the HR department and LEA leadership to develop a compensation package that is competitive with other employers of therapy practitioners in the market.

Because HR recruitment activities in schools are focused primarily on attracting teachers, schools typically set the benchmarks for job requirements and salaries on the basis of other area LEAs. However, if LEAs want to attract and retain occupational therapists, they must evaluate school working conditions, salaries, and benefits against the medical marketplace as well (e.g., hospitals, outpatient and private practice facilities, home health agencies). Occupational therapy administrators must educate their HR team on the breadth and scope of the local competition and collect annual data to ensure that compensation packages remain competitive. Working with HR to devise innovative strategies, such as allowing job sharing of positions, providing housing, or offering repayment of all or a portion of student loans, can assist in attracting and retaining occupational therapy practitioners. Personnel shortages abound in occupational therapy school practice. Occupational therapy administrators and HR personnel can mitigate these challenges by collaborating to address these personnel issues.

In carrying out their duties, occupational therapy practitioners in schools are acting as agents of the LEA and therefore do not have significant personal legal exposure in school practice. However, should there be a claim of harm to a student or colleague as the result of actions (or a lack of action) on the part of the practitioners, there could be personal legal ramifications. It is unlikely that the LEA has insurance coverage that protects individual practitioners against claims of personal negligence or harm. Therefore, administrators should inform their personnel of the risks inherent in school practice and ensure that personnel know how to access vendors who provide insurance against malpractice claims (see Appendix I, "Importance of Professional Liability Insurance").

Due process under the Individuals With Disabilities Education Improvement Act of 2004 (Pub. L. 108–446) allows for legal remedies for students (and those representing students' interests) as well as for LEAs that are dissatisfied with aspects of the IEP process, program, or services identified and implemented for a student. Systems for the provision of due process are overseen by SEAs. *Mediation,* defined as intervention between conflicting parties to promote reconciliation, settlement, or compromise, is typically offered to the parties when there is a filing for due process.

If mediation is not used or if the outcome of mediation does not resolve the issue, adjudication through a hearing process overseen by a state-appointed hearing officer is offered. Parties engage attorneys or advocates, who submit documents supporting their point of view, and the hearing officer hears assertions from witnesses from each party supporting their relative positions. The hearing officer takes the testimony under consideration and then issues findings that stipulate their conclusions and directives for actions or the payment of fees.

At times, due process findings do not resolve the conflict, and cases are adjudicated through the judicial system of courts. It is important that occupational therapy administrators stay informed of the court decisions and prepare to address practice compliance with prevailing court decisions (Laverdure, 2018).

In recent years, there has been an uptick in adjudication of complaints of discrimination by the Office of Civil

Rights in the U.S. Department of Education. When the Office of Civil Rights takes a case, the complaint is investigated, and an effort is made to negotiate a resolution of the issue among the parties involved. Due process includes an option for appeals, which could include court action. Occupational therapy may be among the issues of concern, and occupational therapy practitioners and administrators may be asked to submit data or testify during the due process hearing. Administrators must provide information and leadership to guide the occupational therapy practitioners through the legal action, which may include responding to a subpoena for documents or providing testimony.

One area that can be challenging for both occupational therapy administrators and occupational therapy practitioners is how to reconcile federal, state, and local education policies with occupational therapy practice acts and rules when they appear to be in conflict. Conflicts may arise regarding evaluation or assessment procedures, the provision of student services (including early intervening services, e.g., response to intervention), and the documentation of those services (AOTA, 2017a). Requirements for serving students who are Medicaid eligible may also be a factor (Frolek Clark & Holahan, 2015). State law and regulations, including the intersection of occupational therapy licensure and local public education policies, must be carefully reviewed, and resolution must be sought with the relevant governing agencies (e.g., the SEA and the state licensing authority). This is most effectively done by those who administer occupational therapy in educational settings, because it is the responsibility of the administrator to clearly communicate needed guidance to the occupational therapy team and relevant stakeholders in the LEA regarding how to move forward.

Promote Continued Competence Across the Workforce

Although safeguarding compliance with legal mandates and applicable regulations is a primary responsibility of school administrators, ensuring an educated workforce is an imperative and integral component (Hollenbeck, 2010; Laverdure, 2014). Occupational therapy administrators are responsible for initial orientation and ongoing professional development about the legal influences on practice for the personnel under their supervision. DuPrey et al. (2017) suggested that well-constructed orientation and training programs can improve occupational therapy practitioners' knowledge and productivity; prepare them to be active contributors to the practice setting; reduce anxiety and service delivery errors and clinical adverse effects; reduce noncompliance with regulatory standards; and reduce recruitment, training, and turnover costs.

An effective continuing education program in occupational therapy requires a collaborative and open learning environment that promotes a culture of continuing competence, workplace monitoring, and expectation for practice. Change that produces consistent student outcomes is built around the following key principles (Laverdure, 2014):

- A strong theoretical orientation and solid base of practice knowledge
- A foundation for collaborative client-centered and occupation-based practice

- A thorough understanding of how to access and analyze scientific evidence
- Effective data-based decisional capacity
- Personal motivation, commitment to lifelong learning, and engagement in reflective practices.

Administrators and practitioners alike must take advantage of professional association resources, legal sources, government news feeds, and other relevant sources to ensure that practitioners are informed and complying with all requirements (Hollenbeck, 2010; Laverdure, 2014).

Support and Inspire Staff

In addition to supporting the practice competence of those whom they supervise, occupational therapy administrators must establish an individual, organizational, or system-level leadership plan to facilitate strategic leadership development within the team and organization. Leadership within organizations is crucial and contributes to effective and efficient intervention and practice advancement; partnerships and collaboration that promote innovation and entrepreneurialism; advanced problem-solving and decisional capacity; and the development of an organizational culture that enhances the engagement of personnel through reflective analysis (Fitzgerald & Schutte, 2010). As with change theory, the occupational therapy administrator has many leadership theories to draw from when facilitating the leadership development of the team.

Building *leadership self-efficacy,* or the confidence individuals have in their own capabilities to lead, precedes the development of leadership competency. Paglis and Green (2002) posited that leadership self-efficacy is

> a person's judgment that he or she can successfully exert leadership by setting a direction for the work group, building relationships with [colleagues] in order to gain commitment to change goals, and working with them to overcome obstacles to change. (p. 217)

The occupational therapy administrator builds leadership self-efficacy by facilitating collaborative relationships and engaging staff in opportunities for self-discovery in which they find answers to complex practice and process problems. Staff grow as leaders when they are nudged out of their comfort zone and empowered to take risks (Machida & Schaubroeck, 2011). Mentoring and inspiring leaders in the organization extend the influence of the occupational therapy administrator on the organization and the advancement of practice (Gilfoyle et al., 2011).

Appraise Employee Performance

Employee performance appraisal is often an important responsibility of the occupational therapy administrator. *Employee performance appraisal* is a process—often combining both written and oral elements—whereby management evaluates and provides feedback on employee job performance, including steps to improve or redirect activities as needed. The HR department often plays a part in the development of formative and summative assessment tools as well as in the development of procedures to outline their implementation. Performance appraisal can be a powerful means of recognizing an occupational therapy practitioner's effort and contribution and can provide a foundation for promoting continued professional growth (AOTA, 2013).

The literature suggests that occupational therapy practitioners practicing in school settings often report no supervision or find their work overseen by administrators who are not occupational therapy practitioners (Hollenbeck, 2010). Inappropriate appraisal occurs when processes and tools used were designed to appraise instructional personnel (these tools are often developed to evaluate teacher performance). Administrators evaluating occupational therapy practitioners' performance are responsible for ensuring that the process and tools used accurately reflect

- Current professional practice domain and process, as described in the *Occupational Therapy Practice Framework: Domain and Process* (3rd ed.; AOTA, 2014b);
- Thorough understanding of the roles and responsibilities of occupational therapy practitioners in school settings (AOTA, 2017a);
- Core competencies in occupational therapy practice (Laverdure et al., 2018);
- Job expectations, as specified in the job description (AOTA, 2013);
- Occupational therapy practices most likely to yield student success in schools, on the basis of current published evidence from occupational therapy and other relevant professional publications (Handley-More et al., 2013); and
- Current best practices in schools, as articulated in the professional literature (Laverdure & Rose, 2012).

Formal performance appraisal meetings should occur at regular intervals and reflect the analysis of data from multiple sources and artifacts. For example, such meetings could draw on observations, work products (e.g., evaluation reports and documentation of student progress), and reports from building-level personnel, including IEP team leaders (AOTA, 2013). The roles and competencies of occupational therapy practitioners should be carefully considered in the appraisal process (AOTA, 2013).

Implement Program Evaluation and Development to Enhance Quality of Services

An essential function of the occupational therapy administrator is *program evaluation* and development. This evaluation is a systematic method for collecting, analyzing, and using information to answer questions about projects, policies and programs, particularly about their effectiveness and efficiency. Evaluating the quality of the program and the services provided and analyzing program data inform programmatic goals and ensure the quality of service delivery. The administrator can use this information to make necessary changes in service delivery and program processes.

Occupational therapy administrators and occupational therapy practitioners must consider both student outcomes (intervention effectiveness, student participation, change in risk factors, and student satisfaction) and program outcomes (utilization of services, cost-effectiveness, efficiency and effectiveness of personnel, referral appropriateness, and marketing results). In designing program evaluation measures, the occupational therapy administrator and occupational therapy practitioners must consider how the student or program outcomes will be evaluated, what data will be collected and by whom, how the data will be analyzed, and how and with whom the data will be shared. Formative assessment processes that begin early and are performed continually throughout the program can produce data that are useful in identifying where problems are influencing outcomes and how to intervene quickly to make improvements. Similarly, occupational therapy administrators can implement summative assessments to evaluate the impacts of the program and determine whether the program met the intended purposes and goals.

Program evaluation data are used to inform budgeting and allocation plans, distribution of labor hours, productivity requirements, marketing plans, and strategic planning. In addition, program evaluation data are essential for the implementation of new processes and programs. The key steps involved in the development of new processes and program are as follows:

- Identify the project's purpose and aims
- Identify the team that will support the development of the project:
  - What are the key competencies required to enact the project plan?
  - What resources will the team need to enact the project plan?
  - How will the team will communicate and make decisions?
- Empower the team to set specific goals and objectives and determine the timelines of the project (i.e., ensure that goals are specific, measurable, agreeable and attainable, realistic and relevant, time based)
- Identify project task steps in alignment with the specific goals, objectives, and time lines (i.e., what resources will be necessary for each of the task steps?)
- Identify formative and summative measures of project success.

The development of plans for improvement in occupational therapy programs and processes requires administrators and occupational therapy practitioners to consider how innovation and change will be sustained. Program sustainability requires the demonstration of positive outcomes, a trained and sustainable workforce, stakeholder engagement and partnership, and a plan for careful utilization of resources.

Manage Fiscal Resources

Funding for public schools is derived from federal, state, and local tax appropriations and occasionally through discretionary grant sources. School boards are charged with developing long-range fiscal plans and annual operating budgets and appropriating funds within the parameters of federal, state, and local regulations. The occupational therapy administrator contributes to the fiscal process by projecting budgetary needs for consideration by the superintendent and the school board.

The LEA's fiscal goals and objectives for the coming year serve as the foundation for the occupational therapy administrator's budget proposal. For each fiscal cycle, the occupational therapy administrator reviews budget data and historical trends in fiscal needs across all budget categories assigned to occupational therapy services to determine continued utility and value. Additional environmental scanning to identify program and service strengths, weaknesses, opportunities, and threats (i.e., SWOT analysis) and thorough needs assessments are important tools for identifying factors that may influence operations and fiscal needs and affect budget planning. Moreover, such analysis can provide essential data required to justify spending projections in the coming years.

Data analysis related to salary categories (e.g., skilled and unskilled personnel positions, requests for salary increases) and nonsalary categories (e.g., professional development, equipment, technology, assessments, materials, supplies) is conducted to inform budget planning. In addition, data must be collected, analyzed, and reported to support requests for new positions or projects. Data are typically entered by each department or service into budgeting software provided by the LEA so that decision makers can view requests from a comprehensive perspective.

Once final budget decisions have been made and funds appropriated, the occupational therapy administrator must manage the funds allocated for occupational therapy services. Systems for decision making and control must be in place to ensure appropriate use of funds in accordance with LEA personnel and purchasing priorities, policies, and procedures. Documentation of expenditures during the budget year must adhere to procedural requirements of the LEA budget manager, typically through digital tools in compliance with general accounting principles.

SUMMARY

Occupational therapy administrator roles offer expanding opportunities for occupational therapy practitioners to strengthen partnerships and leverage leadership to increase understanding of the outcomes of occupational therapy services. These roles also present opportunities to drive policy decisions in schools and states; advance practice; and improve outcomes for students, families, and school teams.

While maintaining focus on the services to clients, occupational therapists as administrators balance the needs and interests of stakeholders to design, implement, and evaluate the delivery of occupational therapy services in school settings and improve service delivery processes. Occupational therapists as administrators are responsible for the management and administration of human, fiscal, and material resources in school settings. In addition, they ensure compliance with federal, state, and local educational requirements, and maintain the effectiveness and efficiency of occupational therapy services. Occupational therapy practitioners in school practice have the responsibility and the opportunity to proactively shape a future with greater representation of occupational therapy practitioners in administrative positions in school settings.

REFERENCES

Allan, H. T., Brearley, S., Byng, R., Christian, S., Clayton, J., Mackintosh, M., . . . Ross, F. (2014). People and teams matter in organizational change: Professionals' and managers' experiences of changing governance and incentives in primary care. *Health Services Research, 49,* 93–112. https://doi.org/10.1111/1475-6773.12084

American Occupational Therapy Association. (2013). *Guidance for performance evaluation of school occupational therapists.* Retrieved from https://www.aota.org/~/media/Corporate/Files/Practice/Children/Performance-Evaluation-School-based-Therapists10-31-13.pdf

American Occupational Therapy Association. (2014a). Guidelines for supervision, roles, and responsibilities during the delivery of occupational therapy services. *American Journal of Occupational Therapy, 68*(Suppl. 3), S16–S22. https://doi.org/10.5014/ajot.2014.686S03

American Occupational Therapy Association. (2014b). Occupational therapy practice framework: Domain and process (3rd ed.). *American Journal of Occupational Therapy, 68,* S1–S48. https://doi.org/10.5014/ajot.2014.682006

American Occupational Therapy Association. (2016). *Occupational therapy's distinct value—Children and youth: Resource for administrators and policy makers.* Retrieved from https://www.aota.org/~/media/Corporate/Files/Secure/Practice/Children/distinct-value-policy-makers-children-youth.PDF

American Occupational Therapy Association. (2017a). Guidelines for occupational therapy services in early intervention and schools. *American Journal of Occupational Therapy, 71,* 7112410010. https://doi.org/10.5014/ajot.2017.716S01

American Occupational Therapy Association. (2017b). *Pediatric virtual chat: School leadership* [Online forum transcript]. Bethesda, MD: Author, Pediatric Program.

Andre, B., & Sjovold, E. (2017). What characterizes the work culture at a hospital unit that successfully implements change: A correlation study. *BMC Health Services Research, 17,* 486–493. https://doi.org/10.1186/s12913-017-2436-4

Bazyk, S., Demirjian, L. Laguardia, T., Thompson-Repas, K., Conway, C., & Michaud, P. (2015). Building capacity of occupational therapy practitioners to address the mental health needs of children and youth: A mixed-methods study of knowledge translation. *American Journal of Occupational Therapy, 69,* 6906180060. https://doi.org/10.5014/ajot.2015.019182

Department for Professional Employees. (2016). *School administrators: An occupational overview* [Fact sheet]. Retrieved from http://dpeaflcio.org/programs-publications/issue-fact-sheets/school-administrators-an-occupational-overview/

Dunaway, D., & Ausband, L. (2008). An analysis of the organizational patterns of North Carolina school districts. *Academic Leadership, 6*(3), Art. 4. Retrieved from https://scholars.fhsu.edu/alj/vol6/iss3/4

DuPrey, J., Laverdure, P., Lynn, J., Smith, L. C., & Swope, K. (2017). Beyond the badge: Supporting the orientation and training of new employees across practice settings. *OT Practice, 22*(17), 8–13.

Fitzgerald, S., & Schutte, N. (2010). Increasing transformational leadership through enhancing self-efficacy. *Journal of Management Development, 29,* 495–505. https://doi.org/10.1108/02621711011039240

Fixsen, D. L., Naoom, S. F., Blase, K. A., Friedman, R. M., & Wallace, F. (2005). *Implementation research: A synthesis of the literature* (Florida Mental Health Institute Publication No. 231). Tampa: Louis de la Parte Florida Mental Health Institute, National Implementation Research Network, University of South Florida.

Frolek Clark, G., & Holahan, L. (2015). Medicaid FAQ for school occupational therapy practitioners. *OT Practice, 20*(20), 18–20.

Fullan, M. (2001). *Leading in a culture of change.* San Francisco: Jossey-Bass.

Gilfoyle, E., Grady, A., & Nielson, C. (2011). *Mentoring leaders.* Bethesda, MD: AOTA Press.

Gosselin, T., Ireland, A., Newton, S., & O'Leary, C. (2015). Practice innovations, change management, and resilience in oncology care settings. *Oncology Nursing Forum, 42,* 683–687. https://doi.org/10.1188/15.ONF.683-687

Handley-More, D., Hollenbeck, J., Orentlicher, M. L., & Wall, E. (2013, September). Education reform initiatives and school-based practice. *Early Intervention and School Special Interest Section Quarterly, 20*(3), 1–4.

Heifetz, R., & Linsky, M. (2002). *Leadership on the line.* Boston: Harvard Business Review Press.

Hollenbeck, J. (2010). Supporting the competency needs of school-based occupational therapists in school-based practice through development of a web-based resource. *Journal of Occupational Therapy, Schools, and Early Intervention, 3,* 239–254. https://doi.org/10.1080/19411243.2010.514839

Honig, M. I. (2008). District central offices as learning organizations: How sociocultural and organizational learning theories elaborate district central office administrators' participation in teaching and learning improvement efforts. *American Journal of Education, 114,* 627–664. https://doi.org/10.1086/589317

Hoy, W., & Miskel, C. (2013). *Educational administration: Theory, research, and practice* (9th ed.). New York: McGraw-Hill.

Hoyle, J. R., Bjork, L. G., Collier, V., & Glass, T. (2005). *The superintendent as CEO.* Thousand Oaks, CA: Corwin Press.

Individuals With Disabilities Education Improvement Act of 2004, Pub. L. 108–446, 20 U.S.C. §§ 1400–1482.

Jacobs, K., & McCormack, G. (Eds.). (2010). *The occupational therapy manager* (5th ed.). Bethesda, MD: AOTA Press.

Laverdure, P. (2014). Considerations for the development of expert practice in school-based occupational therapy. *Journal of Occupational Therapy, Schools, and Early Intervention, 7,* 225–234. https://doi.org/10.1080/19411243.2014.966016

Laverdure, P. (2018). Some *benefit* or *some* benefit. *Journal of Occupational Therapy, Schools, and Early Intervention, 11,* 1–6. https://doi.org/10.1080/19411243.2018.1396015

Laverdure, P., Cosbey, J., Gaylord, H., & Le-Compte, B. (2017). Providing collaborative and contextual service in school contexts and environments. *OT Practice, 22*(15), CE-1–CE-8.

Laverdure, P., McCann, M., McLoone, H., Moore, L., & Reed, L. (2018). Developing quality indicators for school practice. *Journal of Occupational Therapy, Schools, and Early Intervention.* Advance online publication. https://doi.org/10.1080/19411243.2018.1496871

Laverdure, P., & Rose, D. (2012). Providing educationally relevant occupational and physical therapy services. *Physical and Occupational Therapy in Pediatrics, 32,* 347–354. https://doi.org/10.3109/01942638.2012.727731

Laverdure, P., Seruya, F. M., Stephenson, P., & Cosbey, J. (2016, May). Paradigm transitions in pediatric practice: Tools to guide practice. *SIS Quarterly Practice Connections, 1*(2), 5–7.

Machida, M., & Schaubroeck, J. (2011). The role of self-efficacy beliefs in leader development. *Journal of Leadership and Organizational Studies, 18,* 459–468. https://doi.org/10.1177/1548051811404419

Moullin, J. C., Sabater-Hernández, D., Fernandez-Llimos, F., & Benrimoj, S. I. (2015). A systematic review of implementation frameworks of innovations in healthcare and resulting generic implementation framework. *Health Research Policy Systems, 13*(1), 16. https://doi.org/10.1186/s12961-015-0005-z

Murphy, J., & Hallinger, P. (1988). Characteristics of instructionally effective school districts. *Journal of Educational Research, 81,* 175–181. https://doi.org/10.1080/00220671.1988.10885819

Odden, A. (2011, April 1). Manage "human capital" strategically. *Education Week.* Retrieved from https://www.edweek.org/ew/articles/2011/04/01/kappan_odden.html

Paglis, L., & Green, S. (2002). Leadership self-efficacy and managers' motivation for leading change. *Journal of Organizational Behavior, 23,* 215–235. https://doi.org/10.1002/job.137

Richmond, T., & Powers, T. (2009). *Business fundamentals for the rehabilitation professional.* Thorofare, NJ: Slack.

Sauvigne-Kirsch, J. (2017). Promoting school administrators. *OT Practice, 22*(6), 7–9.

Schefkind, S. (2017, August 15). [Letter to state superintendents of education and/or state directors of special education]. Pediatric Program, American Occupational Therapy Association, Bethesda, MD. Retrieved from https://www.aota.org/~/media/Corporate/Files/Practice/Children/Resources/AOTA-School-Leadership-Track-Both-20170814.pdf

Spillane, J. P., Parise, L. M., & Sherer, J. Z. (2011). Organizational routines as coupling mechanisms: Policy, school administration, and the technical core. *American Educational Research Journal, 48,* 586–619. https://doi.org/10.3102/0002831210385102

Spring, J. (1997). *The American school 1642–1999* (4th ed.) New York: McGraw-Hill.

Waite, A. (2016). Leading the way: Occupational therapy leaders map out their varying paths to success. *OT Practice, 21*(10), 19–22.

Wegner, L., Caldwell, L., & Smith, E. (2014). A public health perspective of occupational therapy: Promoting adolescent health in school settings. *African Journal for Physical, Health Education, Recreation and Dance, 20,* 480–491. https://hdl.handle.net/10520/EJC155179

SECTION II.

Evidence-Guided Practices: System-Level Considerations to Support Participation

Best Leadership Practices Through Everyday Advocacy

Sandra Schefkind, OTD, OTR/L, FAOTA

9

KEY TERMS AND CONCEPTS

- Advocacy
- Community of practice
- Empowerment
- Leader
- Meaningful benefit of service
- Mobilization
- Needs assessment
- Representation

OVERVIEW

Past American Occupational Therapy Association (AOTA) President Ginny Stoffel (2014) coined the phrase, "Every member is a leader" (p. 633), and current AOTA President Amy Lamb (2016) reflected that "every member . . . [should] be a leader in his or her daily work" (p. 3). A **leader** is not designated by position or by a credential. Leaders empower others to reach their potential. When occupational therapy practitioners seek out opportunities to advocate for their clients or for their services, they demonstrate leadership. Some key characteristics of leaders are credibility, trustworthiness, experience, and dynamism (Kouzes & Posner, 2007).

Advocacy cannot be relegated to a limited number of practitioners[1] or representatives. Instead, we must use a growth mindset when considering our personal path and local responsibility to champion services and to articulate value. Every school occupational therapy practitioner is a leader who should advance, lead, and advocate (AOTA, 2017b). As Kouzes and Posner (2007) asserted, "In this dynamic and global environment, only adaptive individuals and organizations will thrive. This means leaders must . . . meet the changing demands of . . . clients . . . and other stakeholders" (p. 256). This chapter provides information to increase our advocacy and leadership in the school setting, regardless of title or administrative position (Sauvigne-Kirsch, 2017).

---

[1]*Occupational therapy practitioner* refers to both the occupational therapist and the occupational therapy assistant. AOTA (2014b, p. S18) states, "The occupational therapist is responsible for all aspects of occupational therapy service delivery and is accountable for the safety and effectiveness of the occupational therapy service delivery process" and "must be directly involved in the delivery of services during the initial evaluation and regularly throughout the course of intervention" (p. S18). "The occupational therapy assistant delivers safe and effective occupational therapy services under the supervision of and in partnership with the occupational therapist."

ESSENTIAL CONSIDERATIONS

The *Occupational Therapy Practice Framework: Domain and Process* (3rd ed., or *OTPF–3;* AOTA, 2014c) defines **advocacy** as "efforts directed toward promoting occupational justice and empowering clients to seek and obtain resources to fully participate in daily life occupations. The outcomes of advocacy and self-advocacy support health, well-being, and occupational participation at the individual or systems level" (p. S30). The Center for Society Orientation (CSO; 2013) defines advocacy as the "practical use of knowledge for purposes of social changes" (para. 1) and divides it into 3 types of activities that can be applied to school practice:

1. **Representation** is to speak on behalf of oneself and on behalf of the interests of others for whom one is advocating (CSO, 2013). School occupational therapy practitioners can engage children, youth, families, and education personnel in school programs and exchange successful practice and advocacy stories (e.g., developing new student programs using occupational therapy services, educating others about outcomes of effective occupational therapy, sharing tips on how to lobby for expanded school services).

2. **Mobilization** involves including others in one's base of support, establishing common goals, and taking action (CSO, 2013). For example, using the evidence-based journal club toolkit (AOTA, 2014a), school occupational therapy practitioners can establish an interprofessional or discipline-specific network to exchange and to review articles. Developing a journal club is one effective mobilization strategy to activate practitioners.

3. **Empowerment** includes a belief in one's right to be heard and a recognition that one has an ability to influence change. It expands a sense of ownership and responsibility to address issues (CSO, 2013). When a school occupational therapy practitioner proposes a pilot program to the principal or offers an in-service to the school's parent–teacher organization, the practitioner demonstrates leadership for the profession.

Copyright © 2019 by the American Occupational Therapy Association. All rights reserved. To reuse this content, contact www.copyright.com.
https://doi.org/10.7139/2019.978-1-56900-591-0.009

The *OTPF–3* (AOTA, 2014c) provides a unifying theoretical construct, and *Occupational Therapy's Distinct Value: Children and Youth* (AOTA, 2018c) offers evidence-supported themes to communicate. In addition, the *Guidelines for Occupational Therapy Services in Early Intervention and Schools* (AOTA, 2017a) is a key resource describing the role of the school occupational therapy practitioner. These important AOTA documents help practitioners to recognize their contributions, but practitioners must also modify their language to "common speak." Practitioners must simplify and customize messaging to the intended audience (i.e., teachers, parents). School occupational therapy practitioners must understand education priorities and jargon and then connect their language and theoretical constructs accordingly.

Customizing language to fit an educational setting is an essential component of a personal leadership implementation plan. Stakeholders will learn more about the "value added" of school occupational therapy as practitioners seize opportunities to demonstrate and to discuss participation. Advocating and leading are about making connections (Cross, 1999), with occupational value revealed not just for students but for the full school community.

As we engage in essential interprofessional practices (AOTA, 2015), we must be able to articulate our distinct contributions to the team. In her 2016 Presidential Address, Lamb said that "it is essential that we advocate for occupational therapy and show the value we bring to enhancing the quality of life of those we serve" (p. 3). Communicating the distinct value of our discipline is increasingly important to build awareness of the profession in reaching goals. When advocacy efforts are successful, there may be stronger interprofessional collaborations and greater understanding and respect of distinct school roles. This, in turn, could lead to greater job satisfaction and enhance workforce recruitment and retention efforts, thereby ameliorating personnel shortages.

Expressing Professional Value

School occupational therapy practitioners lead by expressing professional value in achieving educational state accountability measures as well as contributing to individual student and school goals. In this way, practitioners connect educational and occupational objectives and terminology and share contributions as key team members. As Hanft et al. (2013) asserted, "Collaborative teaming depends on . . . fram[ing] a common vision and promot[ing] joint decision-making" (p. 153). Table 9.1 compares and connects some education and occupational goals and terms.

Changing Our Mindset

Research suggests that a fixed mindset may limit our ability to advance (Haimovitz & Dweck, 2017). Reframing and expanding our beliefs through a growth mindset about our role in schools is imperative. With a growth mindset, we can overcome challenges through work and a focus on education and advancement. We must articulate that we are a key provider, supporting participation throughout the school population, and well integrated within an educational team. We support instruction so students participate and succeed. We understand that groups (e.g., classrooms) and systems (e.g., building and district committees) may also be our clients and need our professional expertise (e.g., problem solving, resources, education, modifications). Exhibit 9.1 shares a study about enhancing the leadership role for school occupational therapy practitioners.

TABLE 9.1.   Accountability Language

EDUCATIONAL GOALS AND LANGUAGE	OCCUPATIONAL GOALS AND LANGUAGE	INTERSECTING GOALS AND LANGUAGE FOR ADVOCACY
Meeting postsecondary goals and transition indicators	Meaningful participation in current and future occupations (e.g., work, education, leisure, ADLs, IADLs such as community mobility)	Occupational therapy is a skilled service to build life and work readiness skills for college, career, and community integration.
Supporting Every Student Succeeds Act (Pub. L. 114–95) accountability indicators for school health and safety	Occupational performance in school routines	Occupational therapy practitioners support healthy and safe school participation of all students (general and special education) throughout the school day and across environments (e.g., classroom, playground, bus, cafeteria).
Achieving proficiency in literacy: Meeting state curriculum standards for reading and writing	Literacy as an occupation	Occupational therapy practitioners support differentiated instruction and curricular design for diverse learners. They also support development of functional literacy skills (e.g., adhering to street and school signs, communicating needs, turning pages of a book, managing homework).
Identifying the contribution of individual members of the school team: Addressing mental, academic, and physical needs for learning	Occupational therapy practitioners consider the person, activities or occupations, and the environment during evaluation and intervention.	Through inclusive, integrated service, school occupational therapy practitioners address contextualized learning and school participation. They are key contributors to all teams because of their holistic, collaborative approach and their emphasis on function.

EXHIBIT 9.1. An Advocacy and Leadership Study

During the 2-year Ohio Occupational Therapy Transition Outcomes Study, school OT practitioners reflected on their role in offering innovative occupation-based services (Gooch et al., 2015). Through peer groups, workshops, and journaling, 14 OT practitioners reviewed their interventions with 49 students with high-incidence disabilities to address work and life skills for independent living. Practitioners also considered their interactions with district superintendents, special education directors, and high school principals to discuss the value of an OT practitioner as a key member of a student's transition-planning team.

The school OT practitioners reviewed the practitioner's role in transition-building activities, such as portfolio design, IEP and disability knowledge development, job tours, job search skills, cooking, budgeting, and community outings. In addition, they held issue discussions on such topics as friendships, support networks, bullying, and self-advocacy. A qualitative analysis of the theoretical descriptions resulted in a cost-effective model and change (i.e., changes in roles, schedules, and teaming) in how OT could optimally address the transition needs of students.

Note. IEP = individualized education program; OT = occupational therapy.

BEST PRACTICES

Occupational therapy practitioners should customize their leadership strategies to targeted audiences for increasing the impact of and understanding about the value of the profession. Following is a list of advocacy strategies that practitioners can institute at a state or local level.

Use the *OTPF–3* to Apply the Full Scope of Occupational Therapy Practice

The school occupational therapy practitioner must demonstrate knowledge and skills in addressing both mental and physical health and safety as well as in facilitating participation in daily activities (AOTA, 2014c). The practitioner must articulate that occupational therapy is a skilled, essential school service because it supports and improves outcomes for students. Under the Every Student Succeeds Act (2015; Pub. L. 114–95); usually abbreviated as ESSA), with significant state interpretation, occupational therapy practitioners are designated as specialized instructional support personnel and may offer supports through general education initiatives (e.g., multi-tiered systems of support [MTSS], positive behavioral intervention and supports). Using a public health approach of prevention and promotion as well as intervention, occupational therapy can support state ESSA implementation plans by addressing the academic and social needs of all students, including those at risk, whole classrooms, and entire school populations.

Use a Systems Approach

Occupational therapy practitioners should consider their service as a means to create positive change along a continuum of organizational needs. It is essential that the occupational therapy practitioner understand the strengths and needs of the system before advocating for changes. The practitioner may advocate for services or new programs that will benefit individual students, groups of students, or the whole school population. Advocacy efforts can be self-directed (e.g., when the school practitioner collaborates with teachers) as well as client directed (e.g., when the practitioner assists students to make their own requests during an individualized education program [IEP] meeting; Frolek Clark, 2016).

Sharing our value within a continuum of service provision from general to special education is essential. For example, AOTA (2017c) offered a school mental health toolkit that aligns with MTSS. These information sheets can be distributed to parents, principals, and administrators. Occupational therapy practitioners may assist school districts in meeting state accountability measures determined through the State Systemic Improvement Plan (SSIP) and through the State Identified Measurable Result (SIMR; AOTA, 2018a).

A resource for occupational therapy practitioners is the National Center for Systemic Improvement (NCSI; see https://ncsi.wested.org/). NCSI provides state technical assistance to shape and to assess school practice for quality and for compliance. Practitioners should review and apply NCSI state resources (e.g., rubrics) to their local practice.

Use a Business Model

Although occupational therapy is a profession, health care is becoming more of a business (Pearl, 2015). In the business of learning, the benefits of school occupational therapy services must be an asset, not a liability. The benefits, measured by outcomes, are weighed against workforce investment costs (e.g., salary, professional development). If practitioners' interventions improve attainment of targeted educational goals, then occupational therapy is a good return on investment.

The Triple Aim of health care is to improve the patient experience, to reduce costs, and to improve quality (Metzler et al., 2012). Linked aims for "quality improvement" in health care include better patient health, better patient care, and better professional development (i.e., learning; Batalden & Davidoff, 2007). A similar approach must be applied in educational settings. In addition to improving students' discrete performance skills, the school practitioner must articulate the *meaningful benefit of service* to improve learning and life skills, improve graduation rates, and increase school health and safety.

Service may reduce overall risks or costs associated with poor attendance, due process, and dropout. School occupational therapy can be linked to better student and family engagement or experience. Occupational therapy facilitates the achievement of accountability measures in SSIP and indicators such as the SIMR to reach specific transition goals, support development of socioemotional skills, and develop specific literacy skills by 3rd grade (AOTA, 2018a, 2018b, 2018d).

When considering the school as the client, occupational therapists must identify the school's needs by conducting an occupational profile (e.g., concerns, goals) to learn more about the school. The *needs assessment* should explore the school mission, vision, barriers, and strengths and give a profile of student demographics and daily routines. If the school enrolls a large population of students with autism who need social skills training, for example, then the practitioner might develop social groups for peer mentoring in the cafeteria to improve social participation in the school mealtime routine. To reduce bullying and diversify play opportunities on the playground, the practitioner might offer recess promotion strategies (AOTA, 2017c).

Provide Service Through Contextualized, Evidence-Based Interventions

Providing effective services in the natural or least restrictive environment (e.g., classroom, playground) aligns with mandates in the Individuals With Disabilities Education Improvement Act of 2004 (Pub. L. 108–446). Integrated, inclusive practice offers value for the student because it captures authentic demands and needs. It offers value for the practitioner as well. Research indicates that more teacher collaborations occur with closer work zone proximities (Spillance et al., 2017). When an occupational therapy practitioner offers a strategy or modification in the classroom, a "value-added" or quality demonstration occurs. This clarifies for our key stakeholders (e.g., the educator, paraeducator, principal) the profession's distinct value and provides opportunity for teaming.

Effective, quality inclusive practice is evidence and outcome based, innovative, person centered, and strength based (AOTA, 2018d). There are benefits for students and for the profession when the educator observes the high quality of occupational therapy being provided with staff and students. More collaborations and a greater mutual respect and understanding may ensue (Casillas, 2010).

Build Leaders Through Communities of Practice

A *community of practice* (CoP) is an effective, evidence-based approach to meet all 3 advocacy goals of representation, mobilization, and empowerment. CoPs can be defined as "groups of people who share a concern, a set of problems, or a passion about a topic, and who deepen their knowledge and expertise in this area by interacting on an ongoing basis" (Wenger et al., 2002, p. 4). The mere act of bringing together (i.e., convening) diverse stakeholders for discussion and for action is a leadership strategy.

A CoP offers an effective network for occupational therapy knowledge translation and mentorship (Cramm et al., 2013). It is a social learning approach of building identity and capacity that cultivates advocacy and leadership. Exchanging research-based articles and information on discussion boards is not enough to bring about change. The ongoing discussion and reflection in the CoP lead to new shared work as well as professional growth. Some research suggests that CoPs of occupational therapy practitioners can advance their occupation-based knowledge, beliefs, and actions associated with literacy and mental health (Bazyk et al., 2015; Grajo & Candler, 2017).

The CoP offers authentic stakeholder engagement, not management (Cashman et al., 2014). The leading by convening approach, based on CoP principles, is well documented in the education literature (Cashman et al., 2014). A CoP builds social capital as networks and relationships strengthen. Discipline-specific and interprofessional CoPs can be launched. Occupational therapy practitioners can organize by building and expanding in CoPs.

Engage and educate through shared stories

Storytelling can be an effective knowledge-sharing strategy (Swap et al., 2015). A brief case vignette helps to illustrate the value of the profession and helps to build understandings. Stories offer opportunities for role-playing, learning, and modeling. The AOTA website offers school stories demonstrating use of the occupational profile (https://bit.ly/2BTmNYn) as well as a template to submit your pediatric practice stories (https://bit.ly/2BW2w4z).

Advocate for occupational therapy through community actions

Earnest et al. (2010) wrote that "advocacy . . . requires more than helping individual patients get the services they need; it requires working to address the root causes of the problems they face" (p. 63). Innovative programming and leadership opportunities can emerge when we mobilize in the community and connect our words and deeds to social issues. Literacy relates to work attainment; emotional regulation relates to positive behaviors and community living.

The occupational therapy practitioner could seek permission from the school administrators to build networks in the community and to heighten visibility of services. The school occupational therapy practitioner might consider volunteering to support social change in the local community (e.g., homeless shelters, book drive for library). Because poverty, as experienced through homelessness, may impede children's occupational engagement and learning (Rybski et al., 2016), the school occupational therapy practitioner's volunteerism connects occupational and social justice.

Use a Clear and Succinct Message About Occupational Therapy

Formulate a consistent, brief, and targeted communication message that is free of jargon. This language should match the knowledge, literacy level, and motivations of the listener. See Exhibit 9.2.

EXHIBIT 9.2. An Advocacy–Leadership Story

In Dayton, Ohio, an intervention specialist felt that a high school student with a specific learning disability could not be successful in a nursing program because the specialist believed it was too academically challenging. The OTA advocated for the student to be placed in the vocational school nursing assistant program on a trial basis. The OT and OTA set up adaptations and accommodations in the curriculum by chunking content, adding graphs and images, and recommending oral exams and projects for expressing knowledge. During individual therapy time, the occupational therapy practitioners focused on helping the student build study skills by using graphic organizers, timers, and other customized strategies specific to the student's learning preferences. The student graduated from the vocational program and was accepted into the neighborhood community college, where she received her associate's degree in nursing. Currently she is enrolled in a college program to earn her bachelor of science in nursing.

Note. OT = occupational therapist; OTA = occupational therapy assistant.

| EXHIBIT 9.3. | 60-Second Speech to Advocate for Innovative Programming: A Strategy to Promote Occupational Therapy |

- Share your name and where you work or live. Distribute your business card if you have one.
- Describe the educational issue that the school or community is facing (e.g., incidences of bullying on the playground, high turnover rates of school staff, number of students who do not meet literacy standards by 3rd grade, poor graduation rate).
- Humanize the issue by telling a brief story that illustrates the impact of the problem (e.g., high workload results in missed services, increased costs).
- Cite a study with findings that align with your goals.
- Describe what you would like to pilot to address the problem and what goals will be met.
- State why you, as an OT or OTA, are well suited to meet this need in a collaborative team.
- Distribute two documents: (1) a fact sheet describing the issue and connections to the role of occupational therapy and (2) your proposal to address the issue (which should include your contact information).

Note. OT = occupational therapist; OTA = occupational therapy assistant.

One local advocacy strategy is to prepare a "60-second speech" that can be delivered to stakeholders, such as parents and administrators (see Exhibit 9.3; Tomajan, 2012). Although other stakeholders may not inherently understand or care about the role of the occupational therapy practitioner, they do care about the shared problem and the potential to find a solution. Instead of advocating directly for more occupational therapy practitioners, one strategy is to advocate for an identified, widely accepted school need or occupational problem that needs to be addressed. This allows indirect advocacy for the profession as a key contributor to remediate the problem. The proposed solution might include new occupational therapy programming or an alternative methodology. A fact sheet, tip sheet, or infographic can be distributed to reinforce the message.

Build Connections

To be leaders in the school, occupational therapy practitioners must build social relationships so that they are woven into the fabric of the school. The principal and office staff must recognize practitioners by face and name, and they must have their contact information. Educators should associate practitioners' role and service with quality, compassion, and positive actions and collaborations. Parents should be familiar with occupational therapy services and practitioners' position through interactions at Back to School Night, IEP meetings, and Parent–Teacher Organization in-services. If practitioners are accessible and visible in the school, they will have more potential exchanges and opportunities for partnering.

Occupational therapy practitioners must be well positioned to join interprofessional teams and programs and must be available for troubleshooting and problem solving. Practitioners will be viewed as a valuable resource for development and innovation. "Influence and connections are social capital. A person or entity who has 'good social capital' can ask favors, influence decisions, and communicate efficiently. Social capital is of primary importance in politics, business, and community organizing" (Roland & Landua, 2011, "Social Capital," para. 2).

Use AOTA Resources

The school practice area of the AOTA website (see https://bit.ly/2aqUIcr) has bundled resources together on topics such as school leadership, ethics, accountability, and inclusion. It includes brochures for sharing with administrators and presentations for presenting an in-service. Specific materials on workload, universal design for learning, and literacy are available.

A school mental health toolkit and childhood occupations toolkit provide resources to share about our role under a public health approach and for supporting everyday routines at school and at home. Evidence-based practice resources provide current information on interventions for a variety of conditions and settings. These resources provide leadership action steps for your consideration.

SUMMARY

Each of us is an advocate and a leader to support students to achieve a healthy and productive life. Advocacy takes many forms, and it is strategic in nature. We must seize opportunities to demonstrate our leadership for occupational change. We must share how we support short- and long-range goals for a student as well as for a school and a state. We must align our knowledge and skills with education theory and terminology. We must also strengthen alliances with the education community, including schools, businesses, families, and youth. We address both the mental and the physical components of student participation. We must capitalize on our everyday inclusive, integrated practices to build social and technical connections to our work and to our profession.

REFERENCES

American Occupational Therapy Association. (2014a). *AOTA journal club toolkit.* Retrieved from https://www.aota.org/Practice/Researchers/Journal-Club-Toolkit.aspx

American Occupational Therapy Association. (2014b). Guidelines for supervision, roles, and responsibilities during the delivery of occupational therapy services. *American Journal of Occupational Therapy, 68*(Suppl. 3), S16–S22. https://doi.org/10.5014/ajot.2014.686S03

American Occupational Therapy Association. (2014c). Occupational therapy practice framework: Domain and process (3rd ed.). *American Journal of Occupational Therapy, 68*(Suppl. 1), S1–S48. https://doi.org/10.5014/ajot.2014.682006

American Occupational Therapy Association. (2015). Importance of interprofessional education in occupational therapy curricula. *American Journal of Occupational Therapy, 69*, 691341020. https://doi.org/10.5014/ajot.2015.696S02

American Occupational Therapy Association. (2017a). Guidelines for occupational therapy services in early intervention and schools. *American Journal of Occupational Therapy, 71*, 7112410010. https://doi.org/10.5014/ajot.2017.716S01

American Occupational Therapy Association. (2017b). *Promoting school leadership.* Retrieved from https://www.aota.org

/Practice/Children-Youth/School-based/Resources/Promoting-School-Leadership.aspx

American Occupational Therapy Association. (2017c). *School mental health toolkit.* Retrieved from https://www.aota.org/Practice/Children-Youth/Mental%20Health/School-Mental-Health.aspx

American Occupational Therapy Association. (2018a). *Being accountable in schools.* Retrieved from https://www.aota.org/practice/children-youth/school-based/resources/accountable.aspx

American Occupational Therapy Association. (2018b). *Literacy.* Retrieved from https://www.aota.org/Practice/Children-Youth/literacy.aspx

American Occupational Therapy Association. (2018c). *Occupational therapy's distinct value: Children and youth.* Retrieved from https://www.aota.org/~/media/Corporate/Files/Secure/Practice/Children/distinct-value-policy-makers-children-youth.PDF

American Occupational Therapy Association. (2018d). *Promoting inclusion of both clients and practitioners in natural settings.* Retrieved from https://www.aota.org/Practice/Children-Youth/School-based/Resources/Promoting-Inclusion-Clients-Practitioner-Natural-Settings.aspx

Batalden, P. B., & Davidoff, F. (2007). What is "quality improvement" and how can it transform healthcare? *Quality and Safety in Health Care, 16*(1), 2–3. https://doi.org/10.1136/qshc.2006.022046

Bazyk, S., Demirjian, L., LaGuardia, T., Thomapson-Repas, K., Conway, C., & Michaud, P. (2015). Building capacity of occupational therapy practitioners to address the mental health needs of children and youth: A mixed-methods study of knowledge translation. *American Journal of Occupational Therapy, 69,* 6906180060. https://doi.org/10.5014/ajot.2015.019182

Cashman, J., Linehan, P., Purcell, L., Rosser, M. Schultz, S., & Skalski, S. (2014). *Leading by convening: A blueprint for authentic engagement.* Alexandria, VA: National Association of State Directors of Special Education.

Casillas, D. (2010, June). Teachers' perceptions of school-based occupational therapy consultation: Part II. *Early Intervention and School Special Interest Section Quarterly, 17*(2), 1–4.

Center for Society Orientation. (2013). *Advocacy and lobbying.* Retrieved from http://www.cod.rs/en/what-we-do/advocacy-and-lobbying/

Cramm, H., White, C., & Krupa, T. (2013). From periphery to player: Strategically positioning occupational therapy within the knowledge translation landscape. *American Journal of Occupational Therapy, 67,* 119–125. https://doi.org/10.5014/ajot.2013.005678

Cross, P. K. (1999). *Learning is about making connections* [Cross Papers No. 3]. Laguna Hills, CA: League for Innovation in the Community College. Retrieved from https://eric.ed.gov/?id=ED432314

Earnest, M. A., Wong, S. L., & Federico, S. G. (2010). Perspective: Physician advocacy: What is it and how do we do it? *Academic Medicine, 85*(1), 63–67. https://doi.org/10.1097/ACM.0b013e3181c40d40

Every Student Succeeds Act, Pub. L. No. 114–95, 129 Stat. 1802 (2015).

Frolek Clark, G. (2016). Collaborating within the *Paces:* Structures and routines. In B. Hanft & J. Shepherd (Eds.), *Collaborating for student success* (2nd ed., pp. 177–208). Bethesda, MD: AOTA Press.

Gooch, K., Miller, P., Spence, A., Toland, A., & Pierce, P. (2015). The Ohio Occupational Therapy Transition Outcomes Study: A three-year description of secondary transition services. *American Journal of Occupational Therapy, 69,* 6911520173. https://doi.org/10.5014/ajot.2015.69S1-RP207A

Grajo, L. C., & Candler, C. (2017). The Occupation and Participation Approach to Reading Intervention (OPARI): A community of practice study. *Journal of Occupational Therapy, Schools, and Early Intervention, 10,* 90–99. https://doi.org/10.1080/19411243.2016.1257967

Haimovitz, K., & Dweck, C. S. (2017). The origins of children's growth and fixed mindsets: New research and a new proposal. *Child Development, 88,* 1849–1859. https://doi.org/10.1111/cdev.12955

Hanft, B., Shepherd, J., & Read, J. (2013). Best practices in collaborating on school teams. In G. Frolek Clark & B. Chandler (Eds.), *Best practices for occupational therapy in schools* (pp. 151–161). Bethesda, MD: AOTA Press.

Individuals With Disabilities Education Improvement Act of 2004, Pub. L. 108–446, 20 U.S.C. §§ 1400–1482.

Kouzes, J. M., & Posner, B. Z. (2007). *The leadership challenge* (4th ed.). San Francisco: Wiley.

Lamb, A. J. (2016). The power of authenticity. *American Journal of Occupational Therapy, 70,* 7006130010. https://doi.org/10.5014/ajot.2016.706002

Metzler, C. A., Hartmann, K. D., & Lowenthal, L. A. (2012). Health Policy Perspectives—Defining primary care: Envisioning the roles of occupational therapy. *American Journal of Occupational Therapy, 66,* 266–270. https://doi.org/10.5014/ajot.2010.663001

Pearl, R. (2015). *5 tips for breaking into the business of health care.* Retrieved from https://www.forbes.com/sites/robertpearl/2014/07/17/5-tips-for-breaking-into-the-business-of-health-care/#2ddf118f1107

Roland, E., & Landua, G. (2011). *8 forms of capital.* Retrieved from http://www.appleseedpermaculture.com/8-forms-of-capital/

Rybski, D., Huston, C., & Israel, H. (2016). Need for social skills intervention in preschool children who experience poverty as homeless or housed. *American Journal of Occupational Therapy, 70,* 7011505174. https://doi.org/10.5014/ajot.2016.70S1-PO7055

Sauvigne-Kirsch, J. (2017). Examining occupational therapists as potential special education leaders. *American Journal of Occupational Therapy, 71,* 7111510185. https://doi.org/10.5014/ajot.2017.71S1-PO3128

Spillance, J. P., Shirrell, M., & Sweet, T. M. (2017). The elephant in the schoolhouse: The role of propinquity in school staff interactions about teaching. *Sociology of Education, 90,* 149–171. https://doi.org/10.1177/0038040717696151

Stoffel, V. C. (2014). Attitude, authenticity, and action: Building capacity. *American Journal of Occupational Therapy, 68,* 628–635. https://doi.org/10.5014/ajot.2014.686002

Swap, W., Leonard, D., Shields, M., & Abrams, L. (2015). Using mentoring and storytelling to transfer knowledge in the workplace. *Journal of Management Information Systems, 18*(1), 95–114. https://doi.org/10.1080/07421222.2001.11045668

Tomajan, K. (2012). Advocating for nurses and nursing. *Online Journal of Issues in Nursing, 17*(1), Article 4.

Wenger, E., McDermott, R., & Snyder, W. M. (2002). *Cultivating communities of practice: A guide to managing knowledge.* Boston: Harvard Business School Press.

Best Practices in Supporting Student Access to School Environments, Programs, and Support

Gloria Frolek Clark, PhD, OTR/L, BCP, SCSS, FAOTA, and Barbara E. Chandler, PhD, OTR/L, FAOTA

10

KEY TERMS AND CONCEPTS

- Context
- Cultural context
- Environment
- Extended school year services
- Homebound services
- Individualized emergency evacuation plan
- Least restrictive environment
- Multi-tiered systems of support
- Personal context
- Physical environment
- Reasonable modifications
- Social environment
- Telehealth
- Temporal context
- Universal design for learning
- Virtual context

OVERVIEW

Although equality is stressed in the Individuals With Disabilities Education Improvement Act of 2004 (IDEA; Pub. L. 108–446), Section 504 of the Rehabilitation Act of 1973, as amended (2008; Pub. L. 92–112), and the Every Student Succeeds Act (ESSA; 2015; Pub. L. 114–195), the fundamental implementation of these laws rests on access. Students with disabilities as well as those without disabilities must have access to

- School environments;
- Educational programs with peers;
- Effective curriculum and instruction, supports, and modifications;
- School meals; and
- Occupational therapy, when needed, to benefit from and participate in the education provided by public schools.

Many education and civil rights laws guarantee access for children (i.e., students) who meet eligibility for having a disability, as defined in the specific laws. IDEA (2004) ensures that "children with disabilities and the families of such children [have] access to a free appropriate public education and [improved] educational results for children with disabilities" (§ 1400[c][3]). IDEA requires that special education and related services be provided in the least restrictive environment (LRE; § 300.114). As much as possible, children with disabilities have a right to be included with children without disabilities.

ESSA (the most recent reauthorization of the Elementary and Secondary Education Act of 1965 [Pub. L. 89–313]) also safeguards equal access to education for students with high needs. In addition, Section 504 of the Rehabilitation Act of 1973 (as amended, 2008) ensures that people with disabilities will not be discriminated against by reason of disability by any programs or activities receiving federal funds (i.e., programs must provide access with reasonable accommodation to people with disabilities and guarantee client participation in the rehabilitation decision-making process). This applies to eligible students who do not require specifically designed instruction under IDEA but may need accommodations and modifications for access (see Chapter 27, "Best Practices in Supporting Students With a 504 Plan").

The Assistive Technology Act of 2004 (Pub. L. 108–364) promotes access to assistive technology (AT) for persons with disabilities. The Carl D. Perkins Vocational and Applied Technology Education Act of 2006 (Pub. L. 109–270) requires that vocational education for students with disabilities is provided in an LRE and, when appropriate, is a part of the individualized education program (IEP). The ADA Amendments Act of 2008 (Pub. L. 110–325) prohibits discrimination on the basis of disability and provides for the rights of equal access and reasonable accommodation in employment and services provided by both private and public sectors.

Citing Section 504 of the Rehabilitation Act of 1973, ADA, and IDEA, the U.S. Department of Agriculture (2017) outlined nondiscrimination language requiring schools to provide reasonable modifications to ensure students' access to school meals. **Reasonable modifications** to accommodate students with disabilities may include special meals offered at no extra cost when necessary to a student's diet (some states require a written statement from a licensed health care professional, e.g., a physician, nurse practitioner).

In addition to participating in schoolwide programs for all students (e.g., universal design for learning, multi-tiered systems of support [MTSS], positive behavioral interventions and supports, school mental health), occupational

Copyright © 2019 by the American Occupational Therapy Association. All rights reserved. To reuse this content, contact www.copyright.com.
https://doi.org/10.7139/2019.978-1-56900-591-0.010

therapy practitioners[1] promote access (e.g., physical, academic, social) in schools for students who have disabilities or are at risk for disabilities in a variety of ways. They facilitate access to the environment (e.g., opening doors, getting on the bus), a supportive school climate (e.g., staff willing to make accommodations and include the student), educational programs with peers (e.g., inclusive programs, therapy interventions), effective curriculums and instruction (e.g., in schools, community, homebound services), school meals, and occupational therapy, when needed for the student to participate in educational and other activities at school.

ESSENTIAL CONSIDERATIONS

School occupational therapy practitioners have an essential role in enhancing students' access to, engagement with, and participation in their educational program. They understand context and environment and apply a holistic, person-centered focus, as expressed in the *Occupational Therapy Practice Framework: Domain and Process* (3rd ed.; *OTPF–3*; American Occupational Therapy Association [AOTA], 2014b).

As Dunn et al. (1994) wrote, "A person does not exist in a vacuum; the physical environment as well as social, cultural, and temporal factors all influence behavior" (p. 595). Occupational therapy practitioners might use the Ecology of Human Performance Conceptual Framework (Dunn et al., 2003) or the Person–Environment–Occupation Framework (Dunbar, 2007) to consider how the context or environment and the activities or occupations affect the student's occupational performance.

Practitioners realize that a change to any one aspect (e.g., environment, activity, person) can result in changes to other aspects and can affect students' access, engagement, and participation. During the occupational therapy evaluation, the occupational therapist needs to complete a skilled observation to identify the effect that supports and barriers in the context or environment and the activities or occupation have on students' occupational performance.

Access to School Contexts and Environments

The *OTPF–3* (AOTA, 2014b) defines **context** as "a variety of interrelated conditions within and surrounding the client that influence performance" (p. S42). These conditions include cultural, personal, temporal, and virtual aspects. **Environment** is "the external physical and social conditions that surround the client and in which the client's daily life occupations occur" (p. S42). Occupational therapy

practitioners must consider the supports and barriers of the school context and environment as they affect student access and participation. For example, is the student with muscular dystrophy expected to climb stairs to a 3rd-floor classroom 4 times a day, or can the class be moved to the 1st floor?

Cultural context

Cultural context refers to customs, beliefs, choices, and expectations that are acceptable in the student's school and home community. School rules and expectations reflect the school district's values and beliefs and are cultural contexts. Administration and school staff who value all students as learners and important members of the school are reflected by a positive and supportive school climate in which diversity and levels of achievement are promoted.

A positive school climate promotes healthy relationships, school connectedness, and dropout prevention (Centers for Disease Control and Prevention, 2011). Researchers have found that providing assistance on an as-needed basis, rather than assuming that students with disabilities are "not able," reflects acceptance and builds independence and self-advocacy skills (Richardson, 2002; Snell et al., 2000). The values and beliefs in the home and community are often reflected in the school. Occupational therapy practitioners should be knowledgeable about the school culture and promote supportive school climates through education and training.

Personal context

Personal context is not part of the health condition; rather, it refers to the individual's age, gender, educational level, and so forth (World Health Organization, 2001). The *OTPF–3* (AOTA, 2014b) provides a lens to consider the values, beliefs, and spirituality of the individual. This information is necessary for decision making. For example, a high school student who reads at the 2nd-grade level and believes school is not important has different needs than a student who performs at grade level.

Temporal context

History, rhythm of an activity, duration, routines, sequence, and time of daily occupations are included in **temporal context.** These temporal aspects are powerful parts of a school day. Often, adults can recall what time the school bus picked them up or when their school bell rang for dismissal. If temporal aspects were not followed, then consequences resulted.

Occupational therapy practitioners working in schools must understand the student's schedule and how routines and time of day can affect the student's performance. For example, research has shown that sleep patterns of high school students do not support early-morning readiness for learning. Schools that changed their start time to after 8:00 a.m. found improvements in high school students' enrollment, attendance, and alertness, along with a decrease in depression (National Sleep Foundation, n.d.). In addition, Purohit et al. (2016) found preliminary support that middle and high school students reap long-term health benefits when provided breaks (e.g., movement or yoga breaks) throughout their school day.

---

[1]*Occupational therapy practitioner* refers to both the occupational therapist and the occupational therapy assistant. AOTA (2014a, p. S18) states, "The occupational therapist is responsible for all aspects of occupational therapy service delivery and is accountable for the safety and effectiveness of the occupational therapy service delivery process" and "must be directly involved in the delivery of services during the initial evaluation and regularly throughout the course of intervention. . . . The occupational therapy assistant delivers safe and effective occupational therapy services under the supervision of and in partnership with the occupational therapist."

Students with disabilities might have additional problems with temporal aspects as a direct result of their disability. For example, 48% of students with physical disabilities report sleep problems, compared with only 5%–10% of students without disabilities (Hemmingsson et al., 2008). Students with health issues might have to miss certain classes because of daily needs (e.g., catheterization, medication). Still others might have to arrive late to class or leave early as a result of transportation schedules. These time deviations restrict their participation in the full complement of school activities.

Virtual context

Technology has changed education and social interactions in a manner referred to as *virtual context.* Students now attend virtual schools, receive therapy through telehealth, and engage with others through social media (e.g., blogs, texts, chat rooms). School staff use video conferencing to attend meetings and trainings without spending hours driving to a location.

Many occupational therapy practitioners use a *telehealth* model—interactive technology in real time—to provide services to students and educational staff. A 2013 AOTA Position Paper outlined that "occupational therapy practitioners use telehealth as a service delivery model to help clients develop skills; incorporate assistive technology and adaptive techniques; modify work, home, or school environments; and create health-promoting habits and routines" (p. S69).

Evaluation and interventions can be conducted through a telehealth model when appropriate for the client (e.g., school district, student, teacher, family). Any occupational therapy practitioner considering the use of a telehealth model should contact their state occupational therapy regulatory board to determine whether there are any restrictions in their state regulations. (See Chapter 43, "Best Practices in Providing Telehealth to Support Participation.")

Physical environment

"Successful environmental participation depends on the complex interplay between individual skills and environmental demands" (Kientz & Dunn, 2012, p. 196). Access to the *physical environment* of schools occurs multiple times and in multiple ways throughout the student's day. Getting on a bus, stepping onto the curb or sidewalk, opening a door or bathroom stall, climbing stairs, using swings, or leaving the building in case of an emergency or drill are examples of how students must physically access school environments. Accommodations (i.e., strategies to assist with meeting standard expectations, such as additional time) or modifications (i.e., making changes to the environment, such as a ramp) might be necessary so all students have equal access. Occupational therapy practitioners have the knowledge and expertise to assist school districts in making environmental accommodations and modifications to enhance access for students with disabilities.

One of the most important contributions that occupational therapy practitioners can provide is to assist the school in developing an *individualized emergency evacuation plan* for each student who cannot leave the building

independently (Asher & Pollak, 2009). This plan outlines the procedures to follow in case of an emergency (e.g., who is responsible for transporting the student outside, who is the backup person in case the first person is ill, which exit must be used because of accessibility).

Safety for students and staff during emergencies is important. Students with unique needs might require alternative plans for emergency evacuation situations (e.g., fire, tornado, earthquake, lockdown). Preplanning and secondary plans (in case a key person is absent or unavailable) are critical and essential for student safety and the safety of those who might assist the student in an emergency.

Social environment

Social environment includes the "presence of, relationships with, and expectations of persons, groups, and populations with whom the student has contact" (AOTA, 2014b, p. S45). Schools provide incredible opportunities for socialization. The 2 most important questions a young child wants answered before school starts are "Who is my teacher?" and "Who is in my class?"

The social environment is especially important for students with physical disabilities, who often have adults nearby. Coster and Haltiwanger (2004) observed that adults and peers provided multiple occurrences of unnecessary help without the student's request, thus contributing to dependence and decreasing the student's opportunity to work with other students on assignments, group projects, and presentations.

In addition, interactions with adults often prevented the student from playing and interacting with peers. Moreover, students with physical disabilities were frequently positioned as onlookers rather than active participants in play interactions. Richardson (2002) found that students with disabilities were often given help, but expectations and opportunities for these students to return the help were few.

Interventions by school occupational therapy practitioners should facilitate engagement and participation with peers, not separation. Training school staff to use strategies that support students in their social interactions with other students is essential. Students should negotiate interactions on their own.

Access to Educational Programs With Peers

Occupational therapy services must adhere to the *LRE* mandate in IDEA, which states,

> Special classes, special schooling, or other removal of children with disabilities from the regular educational environment occurs only if the nature or severity of the disabilities is such that education in regular classes with the use of supplementary aids and services cannot be achieved satisfactorily. (IDEA, 2004, § 300.114[a][2][ii])

Any time students are removed from their regular (i.e., general education) class, it must be documented and justified on the IEP. These data are collected by the state departments of education and reported to the Office of Special

Education Programs. Sanctions occur when states restrict access to the student's LRE.

Many occupational therapy practitioners are not removing students from their general education class but are working in the classroom to promote students' skills and participation. Models such as coplanning and coteaching along with classroom groups are being used in general education classrooms. In addition to providing services to enhance the students' participation in their educational program, practitioners are also providing suggestions for program accommodations, modifications, or supports for school personnel to allow the students with a disability to participate in extracurricular and other nonacademic activities (IDEA, 2004, §300.320) and extracurricular athletic activities (U.S. Department of Education, 2013).

Extended school year services

Extended school year services are individualized special education or related services that are provided to a student with a disability that extend beyond the typical school year. The IEP team determines whether the student meets eligibility for this determination, including likelihood of regression, slow recoupment of knowledge, and predictive data, on the basis of professional opinion. Public agencies may not limit extended school year services to particular categories of disability or limit the amount, type, or duration of services.

Homebound services

School districts are required to provide **homebound services,** which are educational services that occur in the student's home or hospital, when a student will be absent for an extended length of time (determined by each state education law). Because of physical or mental health or medical conditions, some students cannot attend school (e.g., student with a depressed immune system, student with cerebral palsy who had hip surgery, student with school phobia). The IEP team generally requests a written statement from the student's physician to verify that the student cannot attend school and that homebound services will not affect the student's recovery or health. IEPs generally need to be revised to align with the student's educational needs in the new setting.

Homebound educational services are provided by teachers. It is not appropriate for homebound educational services to be the sole responsibility of the school occupational therapy practitioner. The practitioner may provide services according to the student's revised IEP and consult with the teacher or visit the student in the home regarding interventions, such as positioning and AT devices to enhance participation in academic activities. The practitioner may also collaborate with occupational therapy practitioners from the medical community who are providing therapy in the home.

Home school or nonpublic school

Families may choose to home school their child with a disability or send them to a nonpublic (e.g., parochial) school.

In some states, students may be dually enrolled, meaning they can access school district resources (e.g., textbooks, classes, extracurricular activities, standardized testing) and obtain most of their education at home. Occupational therapy practitioners should refer to their state department of education rules and policies regarding related services for students who attend home school or a nonpublic school. (See Chapter 44, "Best Practices in Providing Services in Nonpublic Schools and Homeschooling.")

Access to Effective Instruction and Curriculum

As part of the evaluation to determine eligibility for special education, the team has to determine that a student's performance was not based on lack of appropriate instruction (e.g., reading and math) or on limited English proficiency. For example, a student's handwriting might be a concern, yet the student did not receive handwriting instruction because it was not provided in the curriculum or they missed instruction because of medical or behavior needs. In these instances, the school must first provide appropriate instruction before determining eligibility for special education programming and related services.

Many schools provide assistance to students at risk for learning and behavior through **MTSS,** which is a continuum of services for students from core education in general education to specialized instruction in special education (see Chapter 26, "Best Practices in Multi-Tiered Systems of Support"). IDEA does not support removal of a student from a general education classroom solely because they need modifications to the general education curriculum (IDEA, 2004, § 300.116[a][2]).

School districts should be familiar with and incorporate **universal design for learning** (UDL), an initiative to provide multiple means of actions and expression (e.g., flexible opportunities for demonstrating skills), representation (e.g., more than one example is allowed), and engagement (e.g., various levels of challenge, learning context) for all students (see Chapter 20, "Best Practices in Universal Design for Learning"). Schools rely on assistance from occupational therapy practitioners to identify and suggest AT and software that will assist student participation and learning (see Chapter 21, "Best Practices in the Use of Assistive Technology to Enhance Participation").

Access to School Meals

The U.S. Department of Agriculture (2017) has nondiscrimination requirements that require schools to provide reasonable modifications to ensure student access to meals. Reasonable modifications to accommodate students with disabilities may include special meals at no extra cost when a student's diet is restricted for medical reasons. The U.S. Department of Agriculture (2017) requires schools to provide reasonable modifications so students with disabilities can access school meal programs. As part of this process, a licensed health care professional (e.g., physician, nurse practitioner) provides a written statement that describes dietary restrictions. For example, substitutions may be necessary because some foods cannot be safely modified for the student (e.g., tacos) or the student has allergies or requires a special diet.

School teams document these modifications or substitutions on appropriate documents (e.g., health records, 504 plan, IEP). The dietitian or physician can provide input on caloric intake and medical needs, and the occupational therapy practitioner can be a resource for the team on the types of modifications to food and drink (e.g., thickened liquids, blended or mashed foods). Seating position and location in the cafeteria may also be important to ensure the student is safe and has social access to peers during meals.

Access to Occupational Therapy

To be eligible to receive special education and related services, a student must have one of the disabilities listed in IDEA and need special education services (IDEA, 2004, § 300.08[a][2]). A student may be advancing from grade to grade or even be in gifted classes yet still be eligible for special education (U.S. Department of Education, 2010). For example, a student in a gifted class may have autism and need social skills training. In some states (e.g., Iowa, Washington), occupational therapy is considered special education and may be the only service on the student's IEP.

Hocking (2001) found that occupational therapists who evaluated performance components (e.g., fine motor skills, visual–motor skills) tended to focus intervention on those components rather than on enhancing the student's participation in activities in the educational context (e.g., writing in a journal, playing on the playground). Evaluation should include observation of the student's engagement in school activities and daily routines that allows the occupational therapist to determine supports and needs in the environment, curriculum, instruction, and student performance (see Chapter 40, "Best Practices in School Occupational Therapy Evaluation and Planning to Support Participation").

Occupational therapy practitioners should focus intervention on enhancing the student's access and opportunities to participate and be engaged in the same routines as peers. A continuum of service options should be considered and may include
- Providing resources to the team or educational staff;
- Modifying or adapting the environment for successful engagement and participation;
- Working directly with the student; and
- Training, consulting, or educating others on behalf of the student in strategies (which may include use of equipment) that will enable the student to benefit from the educational program.

See Chapter 41, "Best Practices in School Occupational Therapy Interventions to Support Participation."

Supporting participation through engagement in school activities and daily routines allows the student to be a part of their class rather than developing skills in an isolated manner. Moreover, how the environment or context and the task or occupation affect the student's occupational performance should be considered. Research has linked improvements in occupational performance with modifications in environments and educational tasks (Dietz et al., 2002; Handley-More et al., 2003).

BEST PRACTICES

Occupational therapy practitioners facilitate access for students during their school routines and in their student role. Strategies for enhancing access include identifying barriers to access, changing the activity or environment, and providing services when needed.

Identify Barriers to Access

Occupational therapy practitioners must understand the school system (e.g., physical, cultural, values) in which they work to recognize barriers for students. Students should have access to the context and environment, a positive school climate, educational programming with peers, quality curriculum and instruction, school meals, and occupational therapy services. Barriers to accessing any one of these elements should be explored. On the basis of the student's program and daily routine, systematically observing every part of a building (e.g., corridors, bathrooms, classrooms, science labs, locker rooms) is essential to identify environmental barriers and to make informed recommendations about ways to address them.

When considering accessibility, the practitioner should observe students as they follow their schedule and take part in the routines of the day. A determination can then be made as to whether students have access to and can participate in activities across school environments. Observations of students' natural routines, such as their ability to open their locker, use the bathroom, move through the cafeteria, and carry books to their next class, can provide the occupational therapy practitioner with information about the interaction among the students, context or environment, and activity or occupation.

Coding the data collected according to the time of day, location, environmental factors (e.g., unable to move to access water fountain), or activity demands (e.g., unable to use scissors to cut paper) provides additional information. For example, a first-grade student who uses crutches may spend recess on the playground talking to adults because she cannot play on the equipment. Observation by the occupational therapy practitioner may lead to modifications of playground equipment that result in increased social participation for the student. Assisting in intervention planning, targeting meaningful outcomes, and collecting data (e.g., number of times a student responds to peers) is important.

Egilson and Traustadottir (2009) used the School Function Assessment (Coster et al., 1998) and School Setting Interview (Hemmingsson et al., 2005) to collect information from 14 students with physical disabilities, 17 parents, and 18 teachers. Findings revealed that students' participation was affected by the interaction among student, environmental aspects, and educational tasks. The interactive effects versus the individual components had the greatest impact on students' participation. With this in mind, occupational therapy evaluations should identify the interactive effects and outline interventions that support students' access to and participation in all experiences in the educational environment.

Change the Environment or Activity to Promote Access

Changing the environment or activity first is more effective and successful than changing the student. A student's disabilities or conditions might not be changeable or change might not occur until far into the future, which thus affects immediate access. For example, a middle school student with poor motor control may be unable to manage showering in the locker room by himself. Focusing interventions on the student acquiring motor control would be far reaching and ultimately restrict his participation. Instead, through collaboration with others, the school occupational therapy practitioner could facilitate changes in the context or environment, task or activity, and person to facilitate the student's independence in this activity.

Context or environment

Environments that enhance the student's ability to benefit from their educational program are necessary. For a student to participate fully in the educational experience, they must have both capacity and opportunity; however, environments can afford or restrict that opportunity. Specific physical barriers (e.g., narrow hallways, heavy doors, small bathrooms, inaccessible classroom levels) to participation are evident in most schools. Buildings are routinely accessible, yet cluttered hallways and classrooms become obstacles for students with disabilities. The distance between classrooms or their location may also decrease accessibility. The principles of UDL are essential to consider for structural and other modification recommendations.

Research on barriers in physical and social aspects of schools revealed that they were primarily caused by the organization and use of the classroom environment or school activities (Hemmingsson & Borell, 2002). For example, holding the pep rally in the accessible gymnasium rather than on the football field may increase participation by students with special mobility needs. A positive school climate treats all children as equals, believes they are all capable of learning, and provides students with the best opportunities possible for academic success (Hemmingsson & Borell, 2002).

The following suggestions are helpful for occupational therapy practitioners to improve the school environment:
- Identify barriers and supports in the physical and social environment
- Collaborate with other team members to identify priorities and solutions for accessibility in the student's program (major environmental challenges are often recess, field trips, transportation, and physical education; Egilson & Traustadottir, 2009)
- Support educational staff in creating a positive environment for the student.

Activities

Activity analysis and modification is an area of expertise for occupational therapy practitioners. It requires that the occupational therapy practitioner understand what is currently occurring in the classroom, what the expected performance and outcomes are, and how peers are performing. Recommendations for practitioners include the following:
- Consider activity and occupational demands listed in the *OTPF–3* (AOTA, 2014b): objects and their properties, space demands, social demands, sequence and timing, required actions and performance skills, required body functions, and required body structures (one study found that teachers were more resistant to changing physical aspects of educational activities than cognitive or behavioral demands of tasks; Majnemer et al., 2010).
- Educate teachers and parents on how to create opportunities for students with disabilities to optimally participate in their daily occupations and routines.
- Encourage teachers to use a variety of instructional strategies to teach concepts and to allow a variety of ways for students to demonstrate competence in knowledge (e.g., UDL, differentiated instruction).
- Modify materials, assignments, and teaching strategies when necessary to meet individual students' needs (when the teacher does not understand how to adapt or modify curriculum or settings, the need for additional adult assistance for students increases; Giangreco & Broer, 2005).
- Make recommendations for evaluation modifications, including state and district tests, when needed.
- Match AT to the student's needs.
- Although students cannot be denied participation in field trips or class events on the basis of their disability, parents may opt their child out for safety or health reasons. If this is the case, then suggest alternative activities to build the student's experiences and opportunities (e.g., similar social or physical attributes).
- Encourage reciprocal interactions between students with disabilities and their peers to foster friendships and allow students with disabilities to "give back."
- Participate as part of the transportation team in the school district, and provide suggestions for transportation so that students are transported safely (see Chapter 22, "Best Practices in Safe Transportation").

Provide Services on Behalf of or With the Student

Some students require access to occupational therapy services to benefit from their educational programs. Practitioners support the student's health and learning through strategies such as
- Proper positioning;
- Consideration of fatigue, pain, and effects of medication;
- Use of AT; and
- Support for the student's participation in their activities and occupations.

Access to the educational program includes participation in the natural context and routine of the school. Direct services with the student outside of the natural context are restrictive and should be used only when necessary and with a plan to integrate the student back into the natural context and routine. Services on behalf of the student (e.g., training others, changing the environment, changing the task) may be more beneficial in enhancing the student's participation in their educational program. Occupational therapy practitioners must advocate for access to services that enhance participation.

SUMMARY

Occupational therapy practitioners working in schools must understand the school context and environment, expected tasks, and students' ability to participate in their educational program. School occupational therapy practitioners are in a position to advocate for students, especially for physical and social accessibility. Students' ability to participate physically and socially during educational routines with peers has a profound impact on all students.

REFERENCES

American Occupational Therapy Association. (2018). Telehealth in occupational therapy. *American Journal of Occupational Therapy, 67*(6, Suppl.), S69–S90. https://doi.org/10.5014/ajot.2013.67S69

American Occupational Therapy Association. (2014a). Guidelines for supervision, roles, and responsibilities during the delivery of occupational therapy services. *American Journal of Occupational Therapy, 68*(Suppl. 3), S16–S22. https://doi.org/10.5014/ajot.2014.686S03

American Occupational Therapy Association. (2014b). Occupational therapy practice framework: Domain and process (3rd ed.). *American Journal of Occupational Therapy, 68*(Suppl. 1), S1–S48. https://doi.org/10.5014/ajot.2014.682006

ADA Amendments Act of 2008, Pub. L. 110–325, 122 Stat. 3553.

Asher, A., & Pollak, J. (2009). Planning emergency evacuations for students with unique needs: Role of occupational therapy. *OT Practice 14*(21), CE1–CE8.

Assistive Technology Act of 2004, Pub. L. 108–364, 118 Stat. 1707.

Carl D. Perkins Vocational and Applied Technology Education Act of 2006, Pub. L. 109–270, 120 Stat. 683.

Centers for Disease Control and Prevention. (2011). *School violence: Prevention.* Retrieved from http://www.cdc.gov/violenceprevention/youthviolence/schoolviolence/prevention.html

Coster, W., Deeney, T., Haltiwanger, J., & Haley, T. (1998). *School Function Assessment: User's manual.* San Antonio: Psychological Corporation.

Coster, W., & Haltiwanger, J. (2004). Social–behavioral skills of elementary students with physical disabilities included in general education classrooms. *Remedial and Special Education, 25*, 95–103. https://doi.org/10.1177/07419325040250020401

Dietz, J., Swinth, Y., & White, O. (2002). Powered mobility and preschoolers with complex developmental delays. *American Journal of Occupational Therapy, 56*, 86–96. https://doi.org/10.5014/ajot.56.1.86

Dunbar, S. (2007). *Occupational therapy models for intervention with children and families.* Thorofare, NJ: Slack.

Dunn, W., Brown, C., & McGuigan, A. (1994). The ecology of human performance: A framework for considering the effect of context. *American Journal of Occupational Therapy, 48*, 595–607. https://doi.org/10.5014/ajot.48.7.595

Dunn, W., Brown, C., & Youngstrom, M. J. (2003). Ecological model of occupation. In P. Kramer, J. Hinojosa, & C. Royeen (Eds.), *Perspectives in human occupation: Participation in life* (pp. 222–263). Baltimore: Lippincott Williams & Wilkins.

Egilson, S. T., & Traustadottir, R. (2009). Participation of students with physical disabilities in the school environment. *American Journal of Occupational Therapy, 63*, 264–272. https://doi.org/10.5014/ajot.63.3.264

Elementary and Secondary Education Act of 1965, Pub. L. 89–313, 20 U.S.C. §§ 2701–3386.

Every Student Succeeds Act, Pub. L. No. 114–195, 129 Stat. 1802 (2015).

Giangreco, M., & Broer, S. (2005). Questionable utilization of paraprofessionals in inclusive schools: Are we addressing symptoms or causes? *Focus on Autism and Other Developmental Disabilities, 20*, 10–26. https://doi.org/10.1177/10883576050200010201

Handley-More, D., Dietz, J., Billingsley, F., & Coggins, T. (2003). Facilitating written work using computer word processing and word prediction. *American Journal of Occupational Therapy, 57*, 139–151. https://doi.org/10.5014/ajot.57.2.139

Hemmingsson, H., & Borell, L. (2002). Environmental barriers in mainstream schools. *Child Care Health and Development, 28*(1), 57–63. https://doi.org/10.1046/j.1365-2214.2002.00240.x

Hemmingsson, H., Egilson, S., Hoffman, O., & Kielhofner, G. (2005). *The School Setting Interview* (3rd ed.). Nacka: Swedish Association of Occupational Therapists.

Hemmingsson, H., Stenhammar, A. M., & Paulsson, K. (2008). Sleep problems and the need for parental night-time attention in children with physical disabilities. *Child Care, Health, and Development, 35*(1), 89–95. https://doi.org/10.1111/j.1365-2214.2008.00907.x

Hocking, C. (2001). The Issue Is—Implementing occupation-based assessment. *American Journal of Occupational Therapy, 55*, 463–469. https://doi.org/10.5014/ajot.55.4.463

Individuals With Disabilities Education Improvement Act of 2004, Pub. L. 108–446, 20 U.S.C. §§ 1400–1482.

Kientz, M., & Dunn, W. (2012). Evaluating the effectiveness of contextual intervention for adolescents with autism spectrum disorders. *Journal of Occupational Therapy, Schools, and Early Intervention, 5*, 196–208. https://doi.org/10.1080/19411243.2012.737271

Majnemer, A., Shevell, M., Law, M., Poulin, C., & Rosenbaum, P. (2010). Level of motivation in mastering challenging tasks in children with cerebral palsy. *Developmental Medicine and Child Neurology, 52*, 1120–1126. https://doi.org/10.1111/j.1469-8749.2010.03732.x

National Sleep Foundation. (n.d.). *School start time and sleep.* Retrieved from http://www.sleepfoundation.org/article/sleep-topics/school-start-time-and-sleep

Purohit, S., Pradhan, B., & Nagendra, H. (2016). Effect of yoga on EUROFIT physical fitness parameters on adolescents dwelling in an orphan home: A randomized control study. *Vulnerable Children and Youth Studies, 11*(1), 33–46. https://doi.org/10.1080/17450128.2016.1139764

Rehabilitation Act of 1973, Pub. L. 93–112, 29 U.S.C. §§ 701–7961.

Richardson, P. (2002). The school as social context: Social interaction patterns of children with physical disabilities. *American Journal of Occupational Therapy, 56*, 296–304. https://doi.org/10.5014/ajot.56.3.296

Section 504 of the Rehabilitation Act of 1973, as amended, 29 U.S.C. § 794 (2008).

Snell, D., Janney, R., & Colley, K. (2000). Approaches for facilitating positive social relationships. In M. E. Snell & R. Janney (Eds.),

Social relationships and peer support (pp. 35–77). Baltimore: Brookes.

U.S. Department of Agriculture. (2017). *Accommodating children with disabilities in the school meal programs: Guidance for school food service professionals.* Washington, DC: Author. Retrieved from https://fns-prod.azureedge.net/sites/default/files/cn/SP40-2017a1.pdf

U.S. Department of Education. (2010). *Opinion letter to redacted regarding children with "high cognition" who have disabilities.* Retrieved from https://www2.ed.gov/policy/speced/guid/idea/letters/2010-1/redacteda011310eval1q2010.pdf

U.S. Department of Education. (2013). *USDE clarified schools' obligation to provide equal opportunity.* Retrieved from http://www.ed.gov/news/press-releases/us-department-education-clarifies-schools-obligation-provide-equal-opportunity-s

World Health Organization. (2001). *International classification of functioning, disability and health.* Geneva: Author.

Best Practices in Supporting Family Engagement in Schools

11

Sarah E. Fabrizi, PhD, OTR/L, and Elizabeth O. Morejon, OTD, OTR/L, C–SIPT

KEY TERMS AND CONCEPTS

- Advocacy
- Cultural and linguistic competence
- Cultural and linguistic diversity
- Every Student Succeeds Act
- Family engagement in school
- Family–school–community partnership
- Justice
- Occupational justice
- Social justice

OVERVIEW

Students who need services and support in schools are increasing both in number and in diversity, and professionals working in schools must be prepared to meet the unique needs of these students and their families. More than 6.5 million children, 13% of all public school students ages 3–21 years, received special education services in 2015–2016 (National Center for Education Statistics, 2017). A 2016 study (Kena et al., 2016) found that a considerable number of students with disabilities who were served under the Individuals With Disabilities Education Improvement Act of 2004 (IDEA; Pub. L. 108–446) were minorities. The highest number were listed as American Indian or Alaska Native (17%), followed by

- Black (15%),
- White (13%),
- Of 2 or more races (13%),
- Hispanic (12%),
- Pacific Islander (12%), and
- Asian (7%; Kena et al., 2016).

Families play a critical role in the health and well-being of their children, and the impact of this relationship is seen in the performance of children during their school years. *Family engagement in school* refers to families, educators, and communities working together to support and improve the learning, development, and health of children and adolescents in meaningful and culturally respectful ways (Weiss et al., 2018). The National Policy Forum for Family, School, and Community Engagement stated that family, school, and community engagement in education should be an essential strategy in building a pathway to college and career readiness in today's competitive global society (Weiss et al., 2010).

Family–School–Community Partnership

Engaging families in their child's school life is a protective factor that decreases or eliminates other risks and predicts success in school and life. Essentially, enhancing family engagement in the education of school-age children can improve both health and educational outcomes throughout the child's lifetime.

There has been an ongoing effort to include families not only as recipients of services but also as partners in school and community success. Research demonstrates that initiatives that take on a partnership, often called a *family–school–community partnership,* create a shared responsibility for the education and development of children, which establishes the culture for family engagement to thrive (Mapp & Kuttner, 2013). A growing body of evidence suggests that family–professional partnerships that support family engagement in school improve the social–emotional development and academic success of all children. This improvement is especially found among children with disabilities under IDEA and Section 504 of the Rehabilitation Act of 1973 (Pub. L. 93–112).

Epstein (2016) identified 6 components of parent involvement:
1. Fulfilling parenting and basic obligations,
2. Facilitating communication between home and school,
3. Volunteering in school activities,
4. Helping the child learn at home and complete homework,
5. Including the family as a partner in school decisions, and
6. Collaborating with the community and school outreach.

Sheehey and Sheehey (2007) offered suggestions for building partnerships from their perspective as parents of a child with severe disabilities and as educators (see Exhibit 11.1).

IDEA states that both the parents or caregivers and the child are essential members of the individualized education program (IEP). The *Every Student Succeeds Act* (ESSA; 2015; Pub. L. 114–195) provides inclusive opportunities for parent and family engagement by mandating states to get input from parents and families as they create education plans:

(f) ACCESSIBILITY. In carrying out the parent and family engagement requirements of this part, local educational agencies and schools, to the extent practicable, shall

---

Copyright © 2019 by the American Occupational Therapy Association. All rights reserved. To reuse this content, contact www.copyright.com.
https://doi.org/10.7139/2019.978-1-56900-591-0.011

EXHIBIT 11.1.   Suggestions for Family–School–Community Partnerships

PARENTS	PROFESSIONALS
Keep asking for information that is understandable to you.	Provide information that is understandable, and assist with advocacy.
Share with professionals about your family's and child's needs and strengths.	Ensure that all team members know each other and their relationship to the family and child.
Share your feelings about assuming the role of teacher or therapist.	Be responsive to parents' fears about assuming other roles.
Showcase your child by sharing stories about your child's strengths and what you want them to learn.	Focus on the child's strengths while acknowledging needs that are important to the parents.
Be available while also taking time to engage in stress-relieving activities.	Communicate with parents using a communication form suggested by the parents.
Ask about skills for your child, provide suggestions, and be open to other suggestions.	Explain the importance of a skill, and provide informal opportunities for parents to share.
Keep your child as the focus while you share your expectations and express support.	Acknowledge the level of involvement chosen by parents, allow parents to share information, and reflect on your own values and beliefs.

Source. From "Elements for Successful Parent–Professional Collaboration: The Fundamental Things Apply as Time Goes By," by P. H. Sheehey and P. E. Sheehey, 2007, *TEACHING Exceptional Children Plus, 4*(2), Article 3, p. 5. Copyright © 2007 by P. H. Sheehey and P. E. Sheehey. Adapted with permission.

provide opportunities for the informed participation of parents and family members (including parents and family members who have limited English proficiency, parents and family members with disabilities, and parents and family members of migratory children), including providing information and school reports required under section 1111 in a format and, to the extent practicable, in a language such parents understand. (129 Stat. 1871)

Family engagement is a quality indicator in ESSA with a substantial focus on positive outcomes. The intent of the language change was to capture the difference between the "doing to" implications of involvement and the "doing with" possibilities of engagement. Families who are involved support the agenda of the professionals and school, whereas families who are engaged work together with their schools and communities (Michigan Department of Education, 2011).

Fostering parent and family engagement is not only a mandate of the law but also an important role of *occupational therapy practitioners*[1] working in schools. Characteristics of the family that practitioners need to take into consideration when engaging in partnerships include

- The family's size and form,
- Cultural background,
- Socioeconomic status (SES), and
- Geographic location (Turnbull et al., 2015).

Occupational therapy practitioners, given their mandate to be client and family centered, have the knowledge and skills

to facilitate effective family–school–community partnerships that support family engagement in schools and their surrounding communities.

ESSENTIAL CONSIDERATIONS

This section presents an overview of parent and family engagement related to the role of the occupational therapy practitioner in schools with regard to

- The impact of engagement on the occupation and participation of the child and the family,
- Potential barriers to family engagement, and
- Professional preparation and training.

Role of the Occupational Therapy Practitioner

Occupational therapy practitioners have an important role in health promotion and prevention, social and occupational justice, and facilitation of engagement in occupations that are meaningful to the people served across settings. Every school occupational therapy practitioner has the responsibility to serve clients (e.g., students, parents, school staff, school district) ethically and to provide services in a respectful manner.

The Principle of *Justice,* as defined in the *Occupational Therapy Code of Ethics (2015)* (AOTA, 2015a), describes an obligation to look beyond race, ethnic background, sexual preference, and SES to provide fair and equitable services that address the best interests of the child and family. Every family has a right to be included and to have their concerns adequately addressed.

The *Occupational Therapy Practice Framework: Domain and Process* (3rd ed.; AOTA, 2014b) highlights the need for occupational therapy practitioners to be mindful of the influence that cultural context has on the client's identity and activity choices. In the *Standards for Continuing Competence* (AOTA, 2015b), Standard 3: Interpersonal Skills states that occupational therapy practitioners

must demonstrate . . . cultural competence through effective interaction with people from diverse backgrounds;

---

[1] *Occupational therapy practitioner* refers to both the occupational therapist and the occupational therapy assistant. AOTA (2014a, p. S18) states, "The occupational therapist is responsible for all aspects of occupational therapy service delivery and is accountable for the safety and effectiveness of the occupational therapy service delivery process" and "must be directly involved in the delivery of services during the initial evaluation and regularly throughout the course of intervention. . . . The occupational therapy assistant delivers safe and effective occupational therapy services under the supervision of and in partnership with the occupational therapist."

integration of feedback from clients, supervisors, and colleagues to modify one's behavior and therapeutic use of self; [and] collaboration with consumers, families, and professionals to attain optimal consumer outcomes. (p. 2)

Social justice addresses the impact of social inequalities affecting daily occupations (Braveman & Bass-Haugen, 2009). In school, social justice can influence not only policy and curriculum but also parent engagement and can include complex issues, such as poverty and racism.

Occupational justice is the right of every individual to be able to meet basic needs and to have equal opportunities and life chances for engagement in diverse and meaningful occupation (AOTA, 2014b). A lack of access to basic human occupations can lead to occupational deprivation and alienation, causing risky behavior and even leading to school dropout (Marczuk et al., 2014).

Impact of Family Engagement on the Child and Family

Family engagement in the child's school life is beneficial to both the physical and the mental health of the child. When parents team with educators, their children generally have better academic performance and higher achievement (Jeynes, 2003, 2007), including more consistent attendance and homework completion and better test scores and grades.

The strongest evidence supports the importance of family engagement for young children's literacy and math skills (Van Voorhis et al., 2013). Across all 50 studies in a meta-analysis, parental involvement in middle school was positively associated with child achievement (Hill & Tyson, 2009). A meta-analysis (Castro et al., 2015) highlighted parents' academic expectations, communication of school activities between parent and child, and the development of reading habits as effective methods for engagement that resulted in child achievement.

The behavior of the child, at home and in school, is influenced by the engagement of the family. The literature has consistently reported that children with parents who are highly involved in school have fewer reported behavior problems (Hill & Tyson, 2009; McCormick et al., 2013). Pear et al. (2015) used a randomized controlled trial design to explore the effectiveness of a school readiness intervention for transitioning kindergartners with developmental disabilities and behavioral difficulties. Results from the study demonstrated that an intervention program that included parenting and parental involvement improved both the self-regulation of children and the parenting skills of caregivers.

Parent engagement also provides many positive opportunities for the social and emotional development of the child. Early parent engagement during the preschool and kindergarten years supports skill development for making friends and getting along with others (Bierman et al., 2017). Additional benefits of parent engagement for the school-age child include promoting social–emotional skills, positive social behavior, social confidence, and self-esteem (Bazyk & Arbesman, 2013; Brandt et al., 2014; Van Voorhis et al., 2013). Social–emotional learning programs, now used in many schools, are more effective when they cross over to both school and home environments (Albright et al., 2011).

Parents and families are a child's first and most influential teachers. The family system creates the foundation for learning, and parents and other caregivers are role models for learning as exciting and meaningful. Parent engagement in school increases parental responsiveness to the child's learning needs, builds parents' confidence in their parenting skills, and gives families a better understanding of and a stronger commitment to the school and educational team.

Parents' role in their child's learning changes as the child grows. In the early childhood years, parents are more likely to attend meetings and events and to volunteer at their child's school; this involvement generally decreases into middle and high school (Fette et al., 2009; Noel et al., 2013). Part of this decline may be the environment of the upper school, parents' confidence with the subject matter, or the false perception that older children do not want their parents involved at school (Hornby, 2011).

The benefits of parent engagement do extend well beyond the early childhood years into middle and high school. Families who come from a disadvantaged background, such as those with lower SES, have demonstrated particularly beneficial outcomes from school involvement (Benner et al., 2016). Parents from diverse backgrounds can become more engaged with their children when given direction, and when families are engaged, the children do better in school (Van Voorhis et al., 2013).

Potential Barriers to Family Engagement

It is unrealistic and ineffective to assume that the responsibility of educating children should be divided between parents and schools, so that the school only addresses the academic needs of children and families are limited to fostering social and emotional development. Although the importance of family engagement is clear, knowledge about how this information applies to parents of children with disabilities is lacking, with much of the focus on parent involvement described in terms of the IEP meeting (Goldman & Burke, 2017).

Caregiving of any child can be stressful, but parents of a child with a developmental delay or learning disorder are likely to experience increased stress, difficulty coping, and decreased self-efficacy (Bazyk & Arbesman, 2013; Fingerhut et al., 2013). Every day is an accumulation of not only what happens in the morning, after school, or in the community but also how the parent and the family find balance in the joys and challenges of everyday life. Even with additional barriers, families who establish and maintain a normal routine and feel connected to each other and to their schools and community can build resilience (Blacher et al., 2013; Breitkreuz et al., 2014).

In a survey conducted by the Family–School–Community Partnership Practice Group (Fette et al., 2009), families described barriers to building family–school–community partnerships around 2 major themes: (1) family barriers to engagement and (2) system barriers to engagement. *Family barriers* included a lack of resources (e.g., time, finances, transportation) that support involvement in the school (Turnbull et al., 2015). Fear, mistrust, and past negative experiences in the school can give families the impression that there is no value in participating at school and that involvement will not have any impact (Fette et al., 2009;

Wolfe & Duran, 2013). *System barriers* that preclude parents from engaging in their child's education can include stigma, a negative attitude, and a lack of adequate staff training on how to facilitate collaboration between school staff and parents (Fette et al., 2009). Cultural and language differences between families and school staff can also be a barrier to family engagement.

Cultural and linguistic diversity (CLD) is a term used to refer to students who do not fluently speak English, who are learning English, and who come from homes and communities in which a language other than English is spoken. The term also encompasses students of a different ethnicity or race (Gonzalez et al., 2011). Parents from CLD backgrounds encounter additional difficulties compared with non–CLD parents. In 1 review, the main themes that emerged as barriers to parental engagement were excessive use of professional jargon, insufficient information, the cultural awareness of professionals, a lack of respect for the parent, and perceived negativity toward the child (Wolfe & Duran, 2013).

Professional Preparation and Training

Cultural and linguistic competence refers to the ability to work effectively with individuals and families from different cultural and ethnic backgrounds while communicating information in a manner that is easily understood by diverse groups (Bjoralt et al., 2009). The United States has a growing number of CLD and minority populations, with 47% of school-age students in special education coming from families with CLD backgrounds (National Center for Education Statistics, 2017). These students also come from diverse social, cultural, and economic backgrounds (Gonzalez et al., 2011).

One concern, although it is not a professional crisis, is that a disproportionate number of occupational therapy practitioners are not from CLD backgrounds:

- 87% are White,
- 5% are African American, and
- 4% are Hispanic (U.S. Department of Health and Human Services, 2015).

Muñoz (2007) suggested that educational programs should address the need to increase the diversity of health care personnel. Occupational therapy practitioners need to expand their knowledge and expertise to work effectively with vulnerable families to become culturally competent professionals (Hinojosa et al., 2002; Suarez-Balcazar et al., 2009).

BEST PRACTICES

Family engagement depends on an ongoing, reciprocal, strengths-based partnership among the parent, the student, and the educational team at the school. With all states now focused on family engagement in the school as a requirement of the law, occupational therapy practitioners are well positioned to promote family engagement by creating a welcoming environment and establishing a therapeutic relationship using cultural competence and respect, involving the parent in the entire occupational therapy process through advocacy and education, and building and sustaining an effective mode for communication. The following practices provide practical methods and strategies for occupational therapy practitioners to support family engagement in schools and communities.

Establish a Therapeutic Relationship

The first step in building a therapeutic relationship is activating the principles of partnership (Turnbull et al., 2015). To be successful, practitioners must respect the family by listening carefully and responding to the family's priorities (Fette et al., 2009). Occupational therapy practitioners can empower families to self-advocate for involvement by asking, "What are your hopes for your child" "What educational outcomes are important to you?" or "What do you see as getting in the way of your child's learning and participation at school?"

Occupational therapy practitioners can create a welcoming environment by seeking out information about the unique background of each family using open-ended questions. Encourage the family to describe the home environment, regular routines, and resources available to them. This can even be done with a simple "getting to know you" form or email sent to the family for the parent and child to complete together.

Practitioners should recognize that every family has a range of engagement that is possible for them, and a great place to start is with the identified strengths of the family. What does this family do really well, especially with regard to supporting their child's learning? Establish that involvement is wanted, needed, and expected as the family receives services throughout the child's time in school and during transition. Practitioners can do this by validating the parent's concerns and seeking feedback in the information-gathering and decision-making process. See Table 11.1 for a summary

TABLE 11.1. Methods and Strategies to Increase Family Engagement	
METHOD	**EXAMPLES OF STRATEGIES**
Partnership	Recognize families' expertise; build on child and family strengths; purposefully, intentionally, and explicitly ask for family input; include families as part of a collaborative, responsive team
Respect and trust	Value families' wishes; learn about the family culture and priorities; honor cultural diversity; build family confidence and competence through targeted family-driven education
Communication	Make a connection early and throughout the process; identify the mode of communication preferred by the family; provide culturally appropriate oral and written language at their reading level; listen to families' opinions and include them in decision making; ask preference for communication style; provide options; have students share back with families

Sources. Fette et al. (2009) and Turnbull et al. (2015).

of strategies to support family engagement, adapted from suggestions by Turnbull et al. (2015) and Fette et al. (2009).

Encourage Family Engagement During the Evaluation Process

The assessment materials used during evaluation must not discriminate on the basis of race or culture and must be administered in the student's native language or other method of communication to obtain accurate information on the student's academic and functional performance at school. In addition to IDEA, ESSA Section 1116, Subsection (b), stipulates that parents, school staff, and students have shared responsibility and must build partnerships to ensure that the student meets the state's high standards for academic achievement.

Despite what is written in law, parent and family engagement in the occupational therapy initial evaluation process in the educational setting is considered rare (Fingerhut et al., 2013). A considerable amount of money is spent annually ($146.5 million) in mediation and litigation regarding support and services for children (Chambers et al., 2003), and that amount appears to be rising (Granelli & Sims, 2018). Preventive strategies, such as developing skills and knowledge of working partnerships between parents and district personnel, could help offset the cost of conflict resolution (Mueller, 2015).

Best practice in evaluation includes partnering with parents to prevent conflict and use time and resources to support student success. The relationship should be collaborative, respectful, and caring. It should also address the needs of families from CLD backgrounds. The self-reflection questions in Exhibit 11.2 may serve as a guide during the evaluation process and intervention planning.

Encourage family engagement with intervention planning and implementation

Occupational therapy practitioners should consider methods of communicating, educating parents, and supporting advocacy efforts by parents for their children with disabilities.

Effective communication

Effective communication is essential not only for building the family–school–community partnership but also for successful parent education and sustaining family engagement. Communication involves both the verbal (e.g., phone calls, video conferencing, face-to-face meetings) and the written exchanges (e.g., text message, notebooks, newsletters) shared among members of the educational team.

Occupational therapy practitioners should foster communication with the family and, when feasible, adapt their communication style to that preferred by the family (Benson et al., 2015; Novak, 2011), adhering to confidentiality requirements and district policy. Occupational therapy practitioners should be responsive to families and share information about how frequently updates on progress will be given. Depending on the family, determine the amount of information to be shared, with a focus on helpful and practical strategies for the family to support their child.

Family education

For parents to engage, they need to believe that their actions will improve their child's learning and well-being. Self-determination theory may be used to achieve engagement of parents and children in the occupational therapy process (D'Arrigo et al., 2017). According to the self-determination theory framework, autonomy, relatedness, and competence facilitate motivation. In addition to motivation, families need to believe that the intervention plan is manageable (King et al., 2014). Providing choices, making connections, and helping families feel mastery are essential to optimize motivation and enhance engagement.

The majority of the literature on parent involvement for students with disabilities focuses on parent involvement in IEP meetings. Best practices include not only collaborating with parents before and during IEP meetings but also providing additional opportunities, such as observing and volunteering in the school (Goldman & Burke, 2017). When describing parents' perceptions of school occupational therapy, Benson et al. (2015) discovered that parents want to know what is being done with their child during the intervention and what

---

EXHIBIT 11.2.   Self-Reflection Questions and Strategies

SELF-REFLECTION QUESTIONS FOR EVALUATION

- Have I reached out to the parent or family of the student to provide them an opportunity to share their concerns and family needs (Benson et al., 2015; Egilson, 2011)?
- Have I considered assessment methods that address engagement and participation in occupations (e.g., social participation, academics, self-care) in different contexts in the school?
- Have I conducted an evaluation and used assessment materials that are nondiscriminatory on the basis of race or culture in accordance with the law?
- Have I addressed the cultural and linguistic needs of the family, used interpreters when contacting the family, or administered assessment and checklists in their native language (Wolfe & Duran, 2013)?
- Have I considered the future needs of the student in school and family impact (Egilson, 2011)?

SELF-REFLECTION STRATEGIES FOR IDENTIFYING STUDENT GOALS AND INTERVENTION PLANNING

- Have I respected and addressed the concerns voiced by the family (Benson et al., 2015)?
- Are the goals realistic and individualized to the student and driven by family priorities as well as school expectations (Benson et al., 2015)?
- Did I consider the family's cultural and linguistic diversity when I communicated with them (Bazyk et al., 2015; Muñoz, 2007)?
- Is my relationship with this family based on trust, respect, equality, and commitment (Turnbull et al., 2015)?
- If there is a conflict, did I ask the family to explain so I could understand their values and beliefs regarding this area?

| EXHIBIT 11.3. | Resources for Family Engagement, Cultural and Linguistic Competence, and Assessment Tools |

RESOURCES FOR FAMILY ENGAGEMENT

- The Center for Appropriate Dispute Resolution in Special Education: https://www.cadreworks.org/resources/data-resources
- Family Voices: http://www.familyvoices.org/work
- Family and Community Engagement: https://www.ed.gov/parent-and-family-engagement
- Family Engagement Resource Providers Project: https://y4y.ed.gov/tools/#family
- Global Family Research Project: https://globalfrp.org
- National Association for the Education of Young Children: https://www.naeyc.org/resources/topics/family-engagement/principles
- National Center on Parent, Family, and Community Engagement: https://eclkc.ohs.acf.hhs.gov/about-us/articlenational-center-parent-family -community-engagement-ncpfce

RESOURCES FOR CULTURAL AND LINGUISTIC COMPETENCE

- Coalition of Occupational Therapy Advocates for Diversity: https://www.cotad.org
- Family Run Executive Director Leadership Association organizational and school tool for assessing capacity to engage families from diverse backgrounds: http://www.fredla.org/wp-content/uploads/2015/09/AECF-EngagingParentsDevelopingLeaders-2016.pdf
- Life Participation for Parents® (Fingerhut, 2005; available in Spanish): http://veipd.org/earlyintervention/wp-content/uploads/2012/12/Life -Participation-for-Parents-and-description.pdf
- Multicultural competency—American Occupational Therapy Association's Cultural Competence Tool Kits: available to members at https://www.aota .org/Practice/Manage/Multicultural/Cultural-Competency-Tool-Kit.aspx
- National Center for Cultural Competence, Georgetown University: https://nccc.georgetown.edu/assessments/

RESOURCES FOR ASSESSMENT TOOLS ON PARENTAL PERCEPTIONS AND SATISFACTION

- University of North Dakota, School of Medicine and Health Sciences, Occupational Therapy Program: https://med.und.edu/occupational-therapy /cultural-competency/index.cfm

they can do at home to support their child. Family education should be based on the families' priorities and concerns.

A grounded theory study conducted by Novak (2011) concluded that parents view home programs as an extension of school interventions that strengthen the therapist–parent partnership. Continued opportunities for the student to practice activities and skills at home maximize the student's progress. Learning occurs best in natural routines and environments, so home opportunities should include routines to enhance learning.

Family advocacy

Advocacy is defined as partners working together to solve a problem. Advocacy can occur at various levels. An occupational therapy practitioner works with school teams to identify resources and provide supports to all families.

Schoolwide advocacy efforts may target the barriers to parent engagement specific to the needs of the community. Practitioners should also consider financial resources, culture and language barriers, parents' schedules, and how comfortable families feel at the school. Development of culturally responsive approaches is correlated with increased parental and family engagement (Wolfe & Duran, 2013).

The physical presence of the occupational therapy practitioner is a necessary component of advocacy at the school, at IEP meetings, and even in the community. Occupational therapy practitioners may include resource and support information on the school's web page, newsletters, a bulletin board display, or informational family meetings on relevant topics. The parents and the educational team can support students at all levels to be self-advocates by understanding their own needs and participating in identifying and monitoring IEP goals. Exhibit 11.3 contains resources for family engagement.

SUMMARY

Occupational therapy practitioners have the opportunity and responsibility to promote and support family engagement in schools and communities. Because of the increasing diversity in families, occupational therapy practitioners need to have the initial and ongoing professional training and self-reflection to provide culturally and linguistically competent care. Practitioners may advocate for systemwide capacity to engage families while supporting families to become advocates in their child's learning and participation during the school-age years and beyond. Best practices to engage parents are key for not only effective occupational therapy interventions in the school but also the health and well-being of the family and student throughout the lifetime.

REFERENCES

Albright, M. I., Weissberg, R. P., & Dusenbury, L. A. (2011). *School–family partnership strategies to enhance children's social, emotional, and academic growth.* Retrieved from https://www .cde.state.co.us/cdesped/school-familypartnershipstrategies

American Occupational Therapy Association. (2014a). Guidelines for supervision, roles, and responsibilities during the delivery of occupational therapy services. *American Journal of Occupational Therapy, 68*(Suppl. 3), S16–S22. https://doi.org/10.5014 /ajot.2014.686S03

American Occupational Therapy Association. (2014b). Occupational therapy practice framework: Domain and process (3rd ed.). *American Journal of Occupational Therapy, 68*(Suppl. 1), S1–S48. https://doi.org/10.5014/ajot.2014.682006

American Occupational Therapy Association. (2015a). Occupational therapy code of ethics (2015). *American Journal of Occupational Therapy, 69*(Suppl. 3), 6913410030. https://doi.org /10.5014/ajot.2015.696S03

American Occupational Therapy Association. (2015b). Standards for continuing competence. *American Journal of Occupational Therapy, 69*(Suppl. 3), 6913410055. https://doi.org/10.5014/ajot.2015.696S16

Bazyk, S., & Arbesman, M. (2013). *Occupational therapy practice guidelines for mental health promotion, prevention, and intervention for children and youth.* Bethesda, MD: AOTA Press.

Bazyk, S., Demirjian, L., LaGuardia, T., Thompson-Repas, K., Conway, C., & Michaud, P. (2015). Building capacity of occupational therapy practitioners to address the mental health needs of children and youth: A mixed-methods study of knowledge translation. *American Journal of Occupational Therapy, 69,* 6906180060. https://doi.org/10.5014/ajot.2015.019182

Benner, A. D., Boyle, A. E., & Sadler, S. (2016). Parental involvement and adolescents' educational success: The roles of prior achievement and socioeconomic status. *Journal of Youth and Adolescence, 45,* 1053–1064. https://doi.org/10.1007/s10964-016-0431-4

Benson, J., Elkin, K., Wechsler, J., & Byrd, L. (2015). Parent perceptions of school-based occupational therapy services. *Journal of Occupational Therapy, Schools, and Early Intervention, 8,* 126–135. https://doi.org/10.1080/19411243.2015.1040944

Bierman, K. L., Morris, P. A., & Abenavoli, R. M. (2017). *Parent engagement practices improve outcomes for preschool children.* Retrieved from https://www.rwjf.org/content/dam/farm/reports/issue_briefs/2017/rwjf432769

Bjoralt, K., Henson, K., & Fox, L. (2009). *OT cultural competence website.* Retrieved from https://commons.und.edu/ot-grad/23

Blacher, J., Begun, G. F., Marcoulides, G. A., & Baker, B. L. (2013). Longitudinal perspectives of child positive impact on families: Relationship to disability and culture. *American Journal on Intellectual and Developmental Disabilities, 118,* 141–155. https://doi.org/10.1352/1944-7558-118.2.141

Brandt, N. E., Glimpse, C., Fette, C., Lever, N. A., Cammack, N. L., & Cox, J. (2014). Advancing effective family–school–community partnerships. In M. D. Weist, N. A. Lever, C. P. Bradshaw, & J. S. Owens (Eds.), *Handbook of school mental health* (pp. 209–221). Boston: Springer.

Braveman, B., & Bass-Haugen, J. D. (2009). Social justice and health disparities: An evolving discourse in occupational therapy research and intervention. *American Journal of Occupational Therapy, 63,* 7–12. https://doi.org/10.5014/ajot.63.1.7

Breitkreuz, R., Wunderli, L., Savage, A., & McConnell, D. (2014). Rethinking resilience in families of children with disabilities: A socioecological approach. *Community, Work and Family, 17,* 346–365. https://doi.org/10.1080/13668803.2014.893228

Castro, M., Exposito-Casas, E., Lopez-Martin, E., Navarro-Ascencio, E., & Gaviria, J. L. (2015). Parental involvement on student academic achievement: A meta-analysis. *Educational Research Review, 14,* 33–46. https://doi.org/10.1016/j.edurev.2015.01.002

Chambers, J. G., Harr, J. J., & Dhanani, A.; Special Education Expenditure Project. (2003). *What are we spending on procedural safeguards in special education, 1999–2000?* Washington, DC: American Institute for Research. Retrieved from https://www.air.org/sites/default/files/SEEP4-What-Are-We-Spending-Procedural-Safeguards.pdf

D'Arrigo, R., Ziviani, J., Poulsen, A. A., Copley, J., & King, G. (2017). Child and parent engagement in therapy: What is the key? *Australian Occupational Therapy Journal, 64,* 340–343. https://doi.org/10.1111/1440-1630.12279

Egilson, S. T. (2011). Parent perspectives of therapy services for their children with physical disabilities. *Scandinavian Journal of Caring Sciences, 25,* 277–284. https://doi.org/10.1111/j.1471-6712.2010.00823.x.

Epstein, J. L. (2016). Framework of six types of involvement. In D. L. Couchenour & K. Chrisman (Eds.), *Encyclopedia of contemporary early childhood education* (pp. 610–613). Thousand Oaks, CA: Sage.

Every Student Succeeds Act, Pub. L. No. 114–95, 129 Stat. 1802 (2015).

Fette, C. V., Glimpse, C. R., Rodarmel, S. L., Carter, A., Derr, P., Fallon, H., & Miller, K. (2009). Spatiotemporal model of family engagement: A qualitative study of family-driven perspectives on family engagement. *Advances in School Mental Health Promotion, 2*(4), 5–19. https://doi.org/10.1080/1754730X.2009.9715712

Fingerhut, P. E. (2005). *Life Participation for Parents®.* Retrieved from http://veipd.org/earlyintervention/wp-content/uploads/2012/12/Life-Participation-for-Parents-and-description.pdf

Fingerhut, P. E., Piro, J., Sutton, A., Campbell, R., Lewis, C., Lawji, D., & Martinez, N. (2013). Family-centered principles implemented in home-based, clinic-based, and school-based pediatric settings. *American Journal of Occupational Therapy, 67,* 228–235. https://doi.org/10.5014/ajot.2013.006957

Goldman, S. E., & Burke, M. M. (2017). The effectiveness of interventions to increase parent involvement in special education: A systematic literature review and meta analysis. *Exceptionality, 25*(2), 97–115. https://doi.org/10.1080/09362835.2016.1196444

Gonzalez, R. J., Pagan, M., Wendell, L., & Love, C. (2011). *Supporting ELL/culturally and linguistically diverse students for academic achievement.* Rexford, NY: International Center for Leadership in Education. Retrieved from https://www.brown.edu/academics/education-alliance/teaching-diverse-learners/sites/brown.edu.academics.education-alliance.teaching-diverse-learners/files/uploads/ELL%20Strategies%20Kit_Intl%20Ctr%20for%20Leadership%20in%20Educ%202011.pdf

Granelli, L. J., & Sims, B. L. (2018, October). *Special education disputes—Litigate or settle: That is the question* (E. J. Sarzynski, Moderator). Presented at the 22nd Annual Pre-Convention School Law Seminar, New York. Retrieved from https://www.nyssba.org/clientuploads/nyssba_pdf/Events/precon-law-2018/06-special-ed-disputes-outline.pdf

Hill, N. E., & Tyson, D. F. (2009). Parental involvement in middle school: A meta-analytic assessment of the strategies that promote achievement. *Developmental Psychology, 45,* 740–763. https://doi.org/10.1037/a0015362

Hinojosa, J., Sproat, C. T., Mankhetwit, S., & Anderson, J. (2002). Shifts in parent–therapist partnerships: Twelve years of change. *American Journal of Occupational Therapy, 56,* 556–563. https://doi.org/10.5014/ajot.56.5.556

Hornby, G. (2011). *Parental involvement in childhood education.* New York: Springer.

Individuals With Disabilities Education Improvement Act of 2004, Pub. L. 108–446, 20 U.S.C. §§ 1400–1482.

Jeynes, W. H. (2003). A meta-analysis: The effects of parental involvement on minority children's academic achievement. *Education and Urban Society, 35,* 202–218. https://doi.org/10.1177/0013124502239392

Jeynes, W. (2007). The relationship between parent involvement and urban secondary school achievement: A meta-analysis.

Urban Education, 42(1), 82–110. https://doi.org/10.1177/0042085906293818

Kena, G., Hussar, W., McFarland, J., De Brey, C., Musu-Gillette, L., Wang, X., . . . Barmer, A. (2016). *The condition of education 2016* (NCES 2016-144). Washington, DC: National Center for Education Statistics. Retrieved from https://files.eric.ed.gov/fulltext/ED565888.pdf

King, G., Currie, M., & Petersen, P. (2014). Child and parent engagement in the mental health intervention process: A motivational framework. *Child and Adolescent Mental Health, 19*, 2–8. https://doi.org/10.1111/camh.12015

Mapp, K. L., & Kuttner, P. J. (2013). *Partners in education: A dual capacity-building framework for family–school partnerships.* Retrieved from https://www2.ed.gov/documents/family-community/partners-education.pdf

Marczuk, O., Taff, S. D., & Berg, C. (2014). Occupational justice, school connectedness, and high school dropout: The role of occupational therapy in meeting the needs of an underserved population. *Journal of Occupational Therapy, Schools, and Early Intervention, 7*, 235–245. https://doi.org/10.1080/19411243.2014.966018

McCormick, M. P., Cappella, E., O'Connor, E. E., & McClowry, S. G. (2013). Parent involvement, emotional support, and behavior problems. An ecological approach. *Elementary School Journal, 114*, 277–300. https://doi.org/10.1086/673200

Michigan Department of Education. (2011). *Collaborating for success: Parent engagement toolkit.* Retrieved from https://www.michigan.gov/documents/mde/4a._Final_Toolkit_without_bookmarks_370151_7.pdf

Mueller, T. G. (2009). IEP facilitation: A promising approach to resolving conflicts between families and schools. *Teaching Exceptional Children, 41*(3), 60–67. https://doi.org/10.1177/004005990904100307

Mueller, T. G. (2015). Litigation and special education: The past, present, and future direction for resolving conflict between parents and school districts. *Journal of Disability Policy Studies, 26*, 135–143. https://doi.org/10.1177/1044207314533382

Muñoz, J. P. (2007). Culturally responsive caring in occupational therapy. *Occupational Therapy International, 14*, 256–280. https://doi.org/10.1002/oti.238

National Center for Education Statistics. (2017). *Table 204.50: Children 3 to 21 served under Individuals With Disabilities Education Act (IDEA), Part B, by age group and sex, race/ethnicity, and type of disability: 2015–16.* Retrieved from https://nces.ed.gov/programs/digest/d17/tables/dt17_204.50.asp

Noel, A., Stark, P., Redford, J., & Zukerberg, A. (2013). *Parent and family involvement in education, from the National Household Educations Surveys Program of 2012* (NCES 2013-028). Retrieved from https://nces.ed.gov/pubs2013/2013028rev.pdf

Novak, I. (2011). Parent experience of implementing effective home programs. *Physical and Occupational Therapy in Pediatrics, 31*, 198–213. https://doi.org/10.3109/01942638.2010.533746

Pear, K. C., Kim, H. K., Healey, C. V., Yoerger, K., & Fisher, P. A. (2015). Improving child self-regulation and parenting of pre-kindergarten children with developmental disabilities and behavioral difficulties. *Prevention Science, 16*, 222–232. https://doi.org/10.1007/s11121-014-0482-2

Rehabilitation Act of 1973, Pub. L. 93–112, 29 U.S.C. §§ 701–796l.

Sheehey, P. H., & Sheehey, P. E. (2007). Elements for successful parent–professional collaboration: The fundamental things apply as time goes by. *TEACHING Exceptional Children Plus, 4*(2), Article 3. Retrieved from https://files.eric.ed.gov/fulltext/EJ967473.pdf

Suarez-Balcazar, Y., Rodawoski, J., Balcazar, F., Taylor-Ritzler, T., Portillo, N., Barwacz, D., & Willis, C. (2009). Perceived levels of cultural competence among occupational therapists. *American Journal of Occupational Therapy, 63*, 498–505. https://doi.org/10.5014/ajot.63.4.498

Turnbull, A., Turnbull, R., Erwin, E., Soodak, L., & Shogren, K. (2015). *Families, professionals, and exceptionality: Positive outcomes through partnerships and trust* (7th ed.). Columbus, OH: Pearson/Merrill Prentice Hall.

U.S. Department of Health and Human Services. (2015). *Sex, race, and ethnic diversity of U.S. health occupations (2010–2012).* Retrieved from https://bhw.hrsa.gov/sites/default/files/bhw/nchwa/diversityushealthoccupations_2012.pdf

Van Voorhis, F. L., Maier, M. F., Epstein, J. L., Lloyd, C. M., & Leung, T. (2013). *The impact of family involvement of the education of children ages 3 to 8. A focus on literacy and math achievement outcomes and social–emotional skills.* Retrieved from http://www.mdrc.org/publication/impact-family-involvement-education-children-ages-3-8

Weiss, H., Lopez, M. E., & Caspe, M. (2018). *Leading family engagement in early learning: A supplemental guide.* Retrieved from https://globalfrp.org/Articles/Leading-Family-Engagement-in-Early-Learning-A-Supplemental-Guide

Weiss, H. B., Lopez, M. E., & Rosenberg, H. (2010). *Beyond random acts: Family, school, and community engagement as an integral part of education reform.* Retrieved from http://www.thelearningcoalition.org/wp-content/uploads/2012/10/Beyond%20Random%20Acts%20Family,%20School,%20and%20Community%20Engagement%20as%20an%20Integral%20Part%20of%20Education%20Reform.pdf

Wolfe, K., & Duran, L. K. (2013). Culturally and linguistically diverse parents' perceptions of the IEP process: A review of current research. *Multiple Voices for Ethnically Diverse Exceptional Learners, 13*(2), 4–18. https://doi.org/10.5555/muvo.13.2.y452140732mlg231

Best Practices in Collaborating on School and Community Teams

Jayne Shepherd, MS, OTR/L, FAOTA; Barbara Hanft, MA, OTR, FAOTA; and Jo Smith Read, PhD

12

KEY TERMS AND CONCEPTS

- Coach
- Collaboration
- Collaborative team
- Communities of practice
- Conflict
- Conflict resolution
- Knowledge translation
- Mentor
- Professional learning communities
- Social media
- Stand-alone team supports
- System-level supports
- Team operations
- Team supports

OVERVIEW

The *Occupational Therapy Practice Framework: Domain and Process* (3rd ed., or *OTPF–3*; American Occupational Therapy Association [AOTA], 2014b) promotes collaboration with individuals or groups (including education teams) to evaluate students, develop goals, and implement intervention. Schools are complex organizations with multiple teams collaborating to educate and prepare all students for a productive life after graduation, regardless of their learning strengths and challenges and their sociocultural status. A school team that collaborates and shares their knowledge, experience, and interpersonal skills is the collective responsibility of administrators, education and related services staff, and families (Friend & Cook, 2017; Hanft & Shepherd, 2016).

Federal law mandates occupational therapy for eligible students with disabilities as related services, supplementary aids and services, and assistive technology (Individuals With Disabilities Education Improvement Act of 2004 [IDEA]; Pub. L. 108–446). Services and supports "on behalf of the child" (34 C.F.R. §300.320[a][4]) can be provided with parents and teachers to educate specific students. Funds may also be used to develop and provide early intervening services (34 C.F.R. §300.226) for all students from kindergarten through high school, typically through a multi-tiered systems of support (MTSS) model based on a continuum of instruction and intervention (Frolek Clark, 2016).

Additional provisions of IDEA establish an expectation for team collaboration during evaluation, eligibility determination for special education and related services, and individualized education program (IEP) planning and implementation in the least restrictive environment. Whenever postsecondary goals and transition services are considered, students themselves must be involved in the IEP team decision-making process.

Two other federal laws, Section 504 of the Rehabilitation Act of 1973, as amended (2008; Pub. L. 93–112) and the ADA Amendments Act of 2008 (Pub. L. 110–325), require schools to provide equal access to education for students with a physical or mental impairment that substantially limits at least 1 major life activity. Occupational therapists may participate on school teams to help identify eligible students with disabilities and develop an individualized 504 plan specifying necessary accommodations, modifications, and services to ensure equal access to education (U.S. Department of Education, Office of Civil Rights, 2010).

Under the Every Student Succeeds Act (2015; Pub. L. 114–195), services are available for educational staff and students in general education to improve their academic and behavioral outcomes. State and local educational agencies are charged with conducting timely and meaningful consultation with specialized instructional support personnel, including occupational therapy practitioners,[1] to provide services with "at-risk" students and contribute to proactive, schoolwide initiatives (e.g., positive behavioral interventions and supports). Specialized instructional support personnel may also provide professional development and training programs for teachers and other staff (AOTA, 2017a).

Through leading and participating on school teams, occupational therapy practitioners form partnerships with education colleagues and families to ensure that all students learn and interact with their typically developing peers. For students with disabilities, the goal is to participate to the "maximum extent appropriate" (IDEA, 2004, 34

---

[1]*Occupational therapy practitioner* refers to both the occupational therapist and the occupational therapy assistant. AOTA (2014a, p. S18) states, "The occupational therapist is responsible for all aspects of occupational therapy service delivery and is accountable for the safety and effectiveness of the occupational therapy service delivery process" and "must be directly involved in the delivery of services during the initial evaluation and regularly throughout the course of intervention. . . . The occupational therapy assistant delivers safe and effective occupational therapy services under the supervision of and in partnership with the occupational therapist."

Copyright © 2019 by the American Occupational Therapy Association. All rights reserved. To reuse this content, contact www.copyright.com.
https://doi.org/10.7139/2019.978-1-56900-591-0.012

C.F.R. § 114[a]). Understanding collaboration as an interactive team process supported by specific team roles and communication skills is essential.

Evidence substantiates that collaborative occupational therapy services and supports provided in inclusive environments are as effective as traditional one-to-one therapy services in evaluation, goal development, intervention, and reevaluation. The benefits include

- Students master specific skills and lessons, fulfill meaningful school roles and occupations, and engage in daily routines with peers (Hanft & Shepherd, 2016).
- Educators expand and integrate innovative learning strategies and supports into daily school lessons and activities (Handley-More et al., 2013; Laverdure et al., 2017).
- All partners share knowledge, resources, and accountability to build capacity and ensure that students progress to reach goals (Frolek Clark, 2016).

ESSENTIAL CONSIDERATIONS

Collaboration flourishes in health and education settings when partners work together to achieve specific, mutually agreed-on outcomes (Orentlicher et al., 2014). The World Health Organization (2010) acknowledged the importance of interprofessional collaboration in developing and maintaining effective working relationships with learners, practitioners, patients, clients, families, and communities to achieve optimal health outcomes. In addition, entry-level curricula in health science and medical professions emphasize developing skill sets in interprofessional collaborative practices through shared learning among preprofessional students to enhance client outcomes from intervention provided in education and health settings (AOTA, 2015; Cox et al., 2016).

In education settings, *collaboration* is defined as "an interactive team process that focuses student, family, education, and related services partners on enhancing the academic achievement and functional performance of all students in education lessons and school activities" (Hanft & Shepherd, 2016, p. 4). A school community consists of various academic, social, vocational, and extracurricular environments in which students socialize and learn, both at school and in other community settings (e.g., field trips, job sites). These environments provide natural contexts for team members to consider the explicit and implicit professional, cultural, and social expectations that influence how effectively they are working, or could work, together (Bazyk & Case-Smith, 2015; Casillas, 2010; Hanft & Shepherd, 2016).

Collaboration is both an art and a science. It should be considered not a service model but rather a team practice that may be identified on a student's IEP as indirect time provided "on behalf of the child." As an umbrella term describing how team members interact, *collaboration* is variously described in the literature as collaborative consultation, coteaching, mentoring, coaching, professional learning communities, and transdisciplinary teaming (Friend & Cook, 2017; Hanft & Shepherd, 2016; Kampwirth & Powers, 2012; Villa & Thousand, 2016, 2017).

Collaboration deemphasizes a practitioner's role as "fixer" or "expert," which is central to traditional forms of consultation. Instead, team members are actively engaged in identifying and evaluating intervention strategies and building their knowledge of students' strengths and challenges (Bazyk & Case-Smith, 2015). Research regarding teamwork in education settings has identified 6 core characteristics that help build an effective structure to promote effective collaboration by defining its membership (Friend & Cook, 2017; Hanft & Shepherd, 2016; Knackendoffel et al., 2018):

- Purpose,
- Communication,
- Culture,
- Roles,
- Responsibilities, and
- Actions.

These characteristics are not distinct, and they overlap to build a framework or structure that sustains collaborative interaction among all partners over time. The art of collaboration is a function of how effectively occupational therapy practitioners and their partners communicate and interact to select and blend hands-on services for students with team- and system-level supports in the daily context of meaningful school lessons and activities (Hanft & Shepherd, 2016; Laverdure et al., 2017). The science of collaboration focuses partners on identifying and using evidence judiciously to inform their decision making regarding student programming, as well as team operations and management (Handley-More et al., 2013).

Challenges to collaborative and contextual services fall into 3 categories:

- *Interpersonal:* Frequent changes in team membership, stakeholder receptivity to change or self-assessment, team relationships and communication styles, knowledge about collaborative services and supports, and willingness of students to participate in services in natural environments (Benson et al., 2016)
- *Routines and interactions:* Time and structure to meet and communicate; caseload instead of workload philosophy; and unclear team operations, including decision making or conflict resolution procedures (Friend & Cook, 2017; Swinth, 2016)
- *Environment and contexts:* Physical, social, or cultural environments; workplace culture or standards; and virtual supports for communication and professional learning (Hanft & Shepherd, 2016).

The following best practices minimize these barriers to effective collaboration by promoting team relationships, contextual services, and supports.

BEST PRACTICES

When contributing to education teams, occupational therapy practitioners assume 3 collaborative roles:

1. Contextually based, direct services for students, always paired with team supports;
2. Team supports on behalf of students; and
3. System supports.

Team supports are the strategies partners use and the interactions they engage in to assist each other to competently facilitate their students' academic achievement and participation in school. Team supports may identify student learning and behavior challenges, conduct trials of possible interventions, model selected strategies, and monitor student progress. Examples of contextually based direct services with team supports include

- Assessing students' baseline handwriting performance and coaching classroom staff on using adapted materials or assistive-technology devices (Case-Smith, Weaver, & Holland, 2014);
- Developing work readiness and transition skills with middle school students through direct services at work sites and coaching IEP teams, including parents (Hollenbeck et al., 2015); and
- Creating jobs for elementary students with autism using direct services with team supports to promote socialization and productive role fulfillment (Schwind, 2017).

Stand-alone team supports provided through coteaching, consultation, coaching, and other collaborative practices are often considered an appropriate education service on their own. Examples of stand-alone team supports include

- Jointly implementing and monitoring intervention with educators through coteaching and problem solving (Cahill & Lopez-Reyna, 2013),
- Coaching team members to implement evidence-based practices in daily instruction and school routines (Reed & Bowser, 2012), and
- Supporting classroom instruction by assisting a teacher to implement recommendations from a school assistive technology team (Schoonover, 2014).

Occupational therapy practitioners also provide ***system-level supports*** by sharing their professional expertise with school committees and initiatives to benefit a specific student population or grade in the school, across a school district, or at the state level (AOTA, 2012; Frolek Clark, 2016). Examples of system-level supports include the following:

- Designing and implementing an interdisciplinary social participation program for all students (Bazyk et al., 2015)
- Expanding staff knowledge and skills in educating students with autism spectrum disorder through a statewide professional development program (Case-Smith, Fristad, & Weaver, 2014)
- Developing Tier 1 programs to improve general education kindergarten students' motor skills in ways that support academic achievement (Ohl et al., 2013).

Promote Teamwork as Part of Contextually Based Services and Supports

A ***collaborative team*** has a definable membership with voluntary, active participation from all members. Members' equality and respect for one another provide an incentive for sharing resources and knowledge. Their commitment to a shared purpose motivates all partners to work together to provide effective education programs and contextual services for all students as well as team and system supports for their peers and school district.

Collaborative teams value their members and recognize that each contributes unique skills and knowledge to consider during collective decision making. Joint responsibility for outcomes related to team decisions creates interdependence among members and decreases disciplinary boundaries and turf conflicts. It also forestalls potential conflicts

by considering, at regular intervals, whether a team is effectively meeting students' and members' goals.

Collaborative teams also build trusting, respectful relationships between individuals and stakeholders that are focused on a common goal or vision. Building relationships among individuals who are often on many different teams requires careful analysis of team operations, cultural expectations, knowledge and experience levels, and interpersonal styles of stakeholders. When relationships are strong, school personnel learn from each other and communicate their distinct roles and responsibilities so team members know whom to talk to and when (Capizzi & Da Fonte, 2012; Casillas, 2010; Hanft & Shepherd, 2016).

Contextual services and supports, including evaluation, intervention, and team interaction, are provided daily in school routines, activities, and environments (Laverdure et al., 2017). Student participation and outcomes are enhanced when occupational therapy practitioners provide collaborative services across the life course, blending direct, team, and system supports in a student's everyday school lessons and activities (Case-Smith, Weaver, & Holland, 2014; Dunn et al., 2012; Hanft & Shepherd, 2016; Missiuna et al., 2012; Ohl et al., 2013).

The term *collaborative* describes 1 of the 4 core tenets in AOTA's (2017b) *Vision 2025*: "Occupational therapy excels in working with clients and within systems to produce effective outcomes" (p. 1). Collaboration between educators and administrators leads to improved school outcomes (Anig, 2015). Educators' preference for team collaboration is also consistent with the *OTPF–3* and research that promotes contextualized student learning and functioning in meaningful routines, occupations, and familiar environments (AOTA, 2017a; Benson et al., 2016; Casillas, 2010; Shasby & Schneck, 2011).

Educators request that occupational therapy practitioners delineate their role and scope of practice for school teams, find more time for collaboration, recognize classroom context needs and constraints, and use reciprocal communication and knowledge transfer (Benson et al., 2016; Casillas, 2010; Huang et al., 2011; Truong & Hodgets, 2017). By collaborating with administrators and other stakeholders, occupational therapy practitioners have more opportunities to advocate for policies that support communication and collaboration, such as workload versus caseload, time to meet, work standards, professional development, and the use of technology for communication and team development (AOTA et al., 2014; Benson et al., 2016; Laverdure et al., 2017).

Include Students and Families as Equal Team Members

Families know their child's personality, history, and behavior; students often provide vital insights about their interests and challenges in school lessons and interactions with peers. Both partners have expectations about a student's learning and participation in school activities that need to be considered during IEP development and implementation (Hanft et al., 2012; Knackendoffel et al., 2018).

As equal team members, families (and key caregivers, e.g., child care providers) express opinions; ask questions;

and participate in team roles, operations, decision making, and data collection processes. Parents desire

- Flexible planning and processes;
- Communication that is understandable, hopeful, honest, and respectful;
- Support and coaching when they are advocating for their child or learning new strategies; and
- Manageable recommendations that are not a burden on their time and energy (An & Palisano, 2014; Mueller & Buckley, 2014; Tucker & Schwartz, 2013).

Families benefit from preparation in making educational decisions, and they should have some knowledge of evidence-based research, experience-based knowledge, and current policy to contribute suggestions and make collaborative decisions with team members (Turnbull et al., 2010).

Establish Team Operations

Given that occupational therapy practitioners work in multiple teams and schools on an itinerant basis and identify different rules and guidelines for each team, they have limited time and contact with team members for communication, problem solving, or mentoring (Benson et al., 2016; DuPrey et al., 2017; Hanft & Shepherd, 2016). Defined roles and operations help teams stay on track and address and possibly prevent challenges before they occur (Friend & Cook, 2017).

Team operations include everyday practices—that is, team rules and guidelines for roles and tasks—the team uses to meet goals efficiently. Roles and tasks are assigned by consensus related to team members' knowledge and ability to contribute to a task. Typical roles to streamline team meetings are

- Facilitator or leader,
- Scribe or recorder of team decisions,
- Timekeeper to monitor time and agenda items,
- Jargon buster to encourage the use of easily understandable words, and
- Reflector who gives feedback about team interaction and operations (Villa & Thousand, 2017).

The team gives equal footing to all team members when making decisions or defining expectations for team operations. At the outset, the team should define agendas, schedules, timelines, flexible communication methods and expectations, collective decision making, periodic review of the team process, and methods to provide professional development and resolve conflict (Friend & Cook, 2017; Hanft & Shepherd, 2016; Knackendoffel et al., 2018). Checklists for considering how well team members interact and communicate with one another, conduct meetings, and solve problems together are available (Hanft & Shepherd, 2016; Villa & Thousand, 2016, 2017).

Share Knowledge and Resources

Collaborative teams share resources, and members translate knowledge with each other respectfully to address their ongoing professional development (Friend & Cook, 2017; Hanft & Shepherd, 2016; Knackendoffel et al., 2018). Team membership changes frequently, given that more than 50% of new educators leave classroom teaching within 5 years (Gray & Taie, 2015). One key reason cited by these educators is limited professional development and opportunities

to learn from their colleagues (Kaiser, 2011). In addition, occupational therapy practitioners and other related service providers may be reassigned to new schools or programs each year, which can initiate requests for additional training and information to meet the learning challenges of different student populations.

Knowledge translation is the "creation, synthesis, and dissemination of research evidence in a user-friendly and accessible way that is relevant and meaningful for youth, families and health care providers" (CanChild, 2016, para. 4). When a team is researching evidence-based practice and translating knowledge, the following 5 questions can help focus discussion among team members (Hanft & Shepherd, 2016):

1. What do we need to know to ensure that students achieve their outcomes?
2. What do we already know, and who might have the role, experience, or expertise related to this knowledge?
3. Who can best instruct or share this knowledge with other team members?
4. How should we share this knowledge, applying adult learning principles (Knowles et al., 2015)?
5. When and where will we share, implement, and follow up on newly acquired knowledge?

Use Multiple Approaches to Share Knowledge

Team members use self-assessment and reflection to evaluate their own competence in providing collaborative and contextual practice by analyzing interactions, instructions, intervention practices, and unexpected outcomes (Bannigan & Moores, 2009; Epstein et al., 2008; Laverdure, 2016; Stephenson et al., 2017). Data-based self-assessment techniques may include

- Focused prompts for self-reflection,
- Professional development tools,
- Competency checklists,
- Videotaping of interventions or team meetings (when agreed on), and
- Reviews by another party for feedback (Bannigan & Moores, 2009; Laverdure, 2016; Laverdure et al., 2016).

Mentoring and coaching can serve to guide individuals, teams, and school districts in acquiring or refining skills and knowledge. Coaches and mentors are grounded in basic principles of collaboration: trust, clear communication, and shared problem solving based on individual or team-identified goals (Aguilar, 2013; Gilfoyle et al., 2011).

Differences between coaching and mentoring lie in methodology. A ***coach*** focuses on a partner's reflection and self-discovery to enhance learning and performance (Hanft & Shepherd, 2016; Rush & Shelden, 2011). ***Mentors*** typically support their protégés (e.g., novice teachers, therapists) by sharing knowledge, experiences, and networking opportunities, along with providing advice and counseling when challenges arise.

Aguilar (2013) suggested that coaches and mentors use an approach of observing, listening, responding, and planning to support and build a protégé's or partner's knowledge and skills. Occupational therapy practitioners may request a coach or mentor or may be invited (or expected) to assume the role of coach or mentor to another team member. In 1 study, school practitioners participating in a peer mentoring program improved their competence in collaborative practice when they had specific peer support, personal goals, and timelines (Bucey & Provident, 2017).

Communities of practice (CoPs) are informal or formal groups of individuals who share a passion or interest related to their work duties, interests, and desires to improve professional knowledge and student learning (Wenger, 2013). Members can collaborate through regular virtual or in-person interactions and share knowledge and resources across disciplines (Barry et al., 2017; Bazyk et al., 2015; Wilding et al., 2012).

Professional learning communities (PLCs) are more formal collaborations in which team members regularly meet; develop individualized learning plans; and learn together through reading, demonstrations, actual practice, and reflection (Missiuna et al., 2012). The structure and support provided by administrators contributes to the success of CoPs and PLCs (Dooner et al., 2008; Lippy & Zamora, 2012).

CoPs and PLCs may also use closed-group social media to enhance their learning. ***Social media*** is defined as technology-generated virtual communities and networks to share ideas, opinions, or information. Individuals or groups with common interests ask for advice or make recommendations for articles, books, or best practice through various media, such as Facebook, AOTA's CommunOT, Instagram, Pinterest, Twitter, Messenger, or organizational intranets.

Develop Effective Interpersonal Skills

Role clarity and effective interpersonal skills are especially important for collaborative teams (Glennon, 2011). Teams often spend more time developing and implementing goals than they spend communicating among team members to evaluate their roles, team operations, and how instructional strategies affect student outcomes (Laverdure et al., 2017).

Teams experience 5 predictable and inevitable stages of team development:
1. Forming,
2. Storming,
3. Norming,
4. Performing, and
5. Adjourning (Egolf & Chester, 2013).

Understanding the typical interpersonal dynamics and challenges of each stage is advantageous for team members so they may recognize developmental sources of conflict and discuss how to move forward.

Interpersonal skills include effective communication and conflict resolution, empathy, self-awareness, self-discipline, and flexibility in using the therapeutic use of self to meet the needs of a situation (i.e., context) or person (Taylor, 2008). How a team solves problems, makes decisions, and implements selected strategies is largely dependent on how individual members use their interpersonal and communication skills to develop and maintain trust, respect, and positive relationships.

Awareness of and respect for individual collaborative styles and communication preferences are essential for open communication (Conderman et al., 2009). All team members need to convey competence and confidence, provide timely follow-up, and apply the principles of adult learning in their interactions. As Kampwirth and Powers (2012)

wrote, "Having all the expert content in the world . . . is of no use if the consultant does not know how to relate it to the consultee as an adult learner–collaborator" (p. 117).

Effective communication skills are essential for collaborative interaction and include
- Listening actively (e.g., paraphrasing and restating),
- Asking open-ended questions to clarify or prompt reflection,
- Inviting constructive feedback,
- Using jargon-free language when sharing knowledge or explaining why a possible strategy might work,
- Elaborating on ideas,
- Summarizing a discussion, and
- Using positive nonverbal body language (Casillas, 2010; Hanft & Shepherd, 2016; Manor-Binyamini, 2011).

Clear, concise, and individualized observations; verbal and written information; and strategies enhance a student's or team member's learning, role, and socialization (Hanft & Shepherd, 2016). Specific, jargon-free instructions regarding why, how, and when to use a strategy as well as time to give and receive feedback are essential for successful implementation of strategies (Capizzi & Da Fonte, 2012). When goals and progress are collectively determined and monitored by the team, education decision making is enhanced (Laverdure et al., 2017).

Resolve Conflicts

Disagreement is inevitable and expected among partners who share responsibility for student outcomes and team operations, even when members have excellent interpersonal skills. Collaborative partners openly address conflict and recognize when to encourage colleagues and parents to identify what is working rather than declare expert solutions to resolve differences or direct a team member to refine instructional strategies.

Miscommunication may arise from team members' perceived loss of control over their classroom, workspace, materials, or familiar teaching routines and procedures. Effective problem solving includes working toward joint understanding of each partner's point of view, generating many solutions to address issues, and weighing the strengths and weaknesses of all solutions generated before choosing one. Hanft and Shepherd (2016) discussed communication strategies and provided checklists for coping with challenging interactions.

Conflict is a perceived or active disagreement between 2 or more team members, usually related to value, opinion, principles, or failure to understand each other's point of view (i.e., absence of or misperceived knowledge translation; Fisher & Shapiro, 2005). It is usually emotional, with mistrust, anger, fear, frustration, or past negative experiences influencing interactions (Martin, 2010). These negative feelings impede the team's primary function to optimize student outcomes (Boshoff & Stewart, 2013; Martin, 2010). Miscommunication, lack of knowledge transfer, or hurt emotions might need discussion before the team moves forward.

Conflict resolution includes engaging in joint problem-solving procedures, defusing challenging behaviors, learning to negotiate, and focusing on the core concern of members to assist teams in handling conflict. When the emotional concerns (e.g., affiliation, appreciation, autonomy, role, status) of team members are recognized and addressed, then opinions are heard, and a willingness to listen, compromise, or agree to disagree may occur (Boshoff & Stewart, 2013; Fisher & Shapiro, 2005; Hanft & Shepherd, 2016; Martin, 2010).

SUMMARY

When a set of interdependent individuals with unique skills and perspectives interact to achieve their mutual goal of providing students with effective education programs and services, they are considered to function as a team. Collaboration, an interactive team process including the student, family, school, and community partners, incorporates the best practices identified in this chapter to provide effective, contextual-based service and supports by doing the following:

- Building relationships with all stakeholders; evaluating and promoting interpersonal skills; and managing disagreements and conflict with trust, respect, and joint accountability;
- Conducting personal self-assessment and reflection on collaborative and contextual practice, that is, analyzing strengths, needs, and interests in learning along with planning and developing measurable goals for improvement;
- Sharing knowledge and learning with the team by using evidence-based readings, observations, and practices along with engaging in self-reviews and team peer reviews, mentorship, coaching, CoPs, PLCs, and virtual supports;
- Evaluating team operations and asking questions: Are operations defined, mutually agreed on, and reevaluated periodically? What works at each stage of team development? and
- Advocating to administration for collaboration time, a workload model, collaborative practice and professional development supports, and standards of practice.

REFERENCES

ADA Amendments Act of 2008, Pub. L. 110–325, 122 Stat. 3553.

Aguilar, E. (2013). Directive coaching conversations. In E. Aguilar (Ed.), *The art of coaching: Effective strategies for school transformation* (pp. 195–209). San Francisco: Jossey-Bass.

American Occupational Therapy Association. (2012). *AOTA practice advisory on occupational therapy response to intervention*. Bethesda, MD: Author.

American Occupational Therapy Association. (2014a). Guidelines for supervision, roles, and responsibilities during the delivery of occupational therapy services. *American Journal of Occupational Therapy, 68*(Suppl. 3), S16–S22. https://doi.org/10.5014/ajot.2014.686S03

American Occupational Therapy Association. (2014b). Occupational therapy practice framework: Domain and process (3rd ed.). *American Journal of Occupational Therapy, 68*(Suppl. 1), S1–S48. https://doi.org/10.5014/ajot.2014.682006

American Occupational Therapy Association. (2015). Importance of interprofessional education in occupational therapy curricula. *American Journal of Occupational Therapy, 69,* 691341002. https://doi.org/10.5014/ajot.2015.696S02

American Occupational Therapy Association. (2017a). Guidelines for occupational therapy services in early intervention and schools. *American Journal of Occupational Therapy, 71*(Suppl. 2), 711241001. https://doi.org/10.5014/ajot.2017.716S01

American Occupational Therapy Association. (2017b). Vision 2025. *American Journal of Occupational Therapy, 71,* 7103420010. https://doi.org/10.5014/ajot.2017.713002

American Occupational Therapy Association, American Physical Therapy Association, & American Speech–Language–Hearing Association. (2014). *Workload approach: A paradigm shift for positive impact on student outcomes.* Retrieved from http://www.aota.org/~/media/Corporate/Files/Practice/Children/APTA-ASHA-AOTA-Joint-Doc-Workload-Approach-Schools-2014.pdf

An, M., & Palisano, R. (2014). Family–professional collaboration in pediatric rehabilitation: A practice model. *Disability Rehabilitation, 36,* 434–440. https://doi.org/10.3109/09638288.2013.797510

Anig, G. (2015). How we know collaboration works. *Educational Leadership, 72*(5), 30–35.

Bannigan, K., & Moores, A. (2009). A model of professional thinking: Integrating reflective practice and evidence-based practice. *Canadian Journal of Occupational Therapy, 5,* 342–350. https://doi.org/10.1177/000841740907600505

Barry, M., Kuijer-Siebelink, W., Nieuwenhuis, L., & Scherpbier-deHaan, N. (2017). Communities of practice: A means to support occupational therapists' continuing professional development. *Australian Occupational Therapy Journal, 64,* 185–193. https://doi.org/10.1111/1440-1630.12334

Bazyk, S., & Case-Smith, J. (2015). School-based occupational therapy. In J. Case-Smith & J. O'Brien (Eds.), *Occupational therapy for children* (7th ed., pp. 664–703). St. Louis: Elsevier.

Bazyk, S., Demirjian, L., LaGuardia, T., Thompson-Repas, K., Conway, C., & Michaud, P. (2015). Building capacity of occupational therapy practitioners to address the mental health needs of children and youth: A mixed-methods study of knowledge translation. *American Journal of Occupational Therapy, 69,* 690618006. https://doi.org/10.5014/ajot.2015.019182

Benson, J. D., Szucs, K. A., & Mejasic, J. J. (2016). Teachers' perceptions of the role of occupational therapist in schools. *Journal of Occupational Therapy, Schools, and Early Intervention, 9,* 290–301. https://doi.org/10.1080/19411243.2016.1183158

Boshoff, K., & Stewart, H. (2013). Key principles of confronting the challenges of collaboration in education settings. *Australian Occupational Therapy Journal, 60,* 144–147. https://doi.org/10.1111/1440-1630.12003

Bucey, J., & Provident, I. (2017). Strengthening school-based occupational therapy through peer mentoring. *Journal of Occupational Therapy, Schools, and Early Intervention, 10,* 87–105. https://doi.org/10.1080/19411243.2017.1408444

Cahill, S., & Lopez-Reyna, N. (2013). Expanding school-based problem solving teams to include occupational therapists. *Journal of Occupational Therapy, Schools, and Early Intervention, 6,* 314–325. https://doi.org/10.1080/19411243.2013.860763

CanChild. (2016). *Research in practice: Knowledge translation and exchange.* Retrieved from https://www.canchild.ca/en/research-in-practice/knowledge-translation-exchange

Capizzi, A. M., & Da Fonte, M. A. (2012). Supporting paraeducators through a collaborative classroom support plan. *Focus on Exceptional Children, 44*(6), 1–16. https://doi.org/10.17161/foec.v44i6.6685

Case-Smith, J., Fristad, M., & Weaver, L. (2014). A systematic review of sensory processing interventions for children with autism spectrum disorders. *Autism, 19,* 133–148. https://doi.org/10.1177/1362361313517762

Case-Smith J., Weaver, L., & Holland, T. (2014). Effects of a classroom-embedded occupational therapist–teacher handwriting program for first-grade students. *American Journal of Occupational Therapy, 68,* 690–698. https://doi.org/10.5014/ajot.2014.011585

Casillas, D. (2010, June). Teachers' perceptions of school-based occupational therapy consultation: Part II. *Early Intervention and School Special Interest Section Quarterly, 17*(2), 1–4.

Conderman, G., Johnston-Rodriguez, S., & Hartman, P. (2009). Communicating and collaborating in co-taught classrooms. *TEACHING Exceptional Children Plus, 5*(5), Article 3.

Cox, M., Cuff, P., Brandt, B., Reeves, S., & Zierler, B. (2016). Measuring the impact of interprofessional education on collaborative practice and patient outcomes. *Journal of Interprofessional Care, 30*(1), 1–3. https://doi.org/10.3109/13561820.2015.1111052

Dooner, A., Mandzuk, D., & Clifton, R. (2008). Stages of collaboration and the realities of professional learning communities. *Teaching and Teacher Education, 24,* 564–574. https://doi.org/10.1016/j.tate.2007.09.009

Dunn, W., Cox, J., Foster, L., Mische-Lawson, L., & Tanquary, J. (2012). Impact of a contextual intervention on child participation and parent competence among children with autism spectrum disorders: A pretest–posttest repeated-measures design. *American Journal of Occupational Therapy, 66,* 520–528. https://doi.org/10.5014/ajot.2012.004119

DuPrey, J., Laverdure, P., Lynn, J., Smith, L. C., & Swope, K. (2017). Beyond the badge: Supporting the orientation and training of new employees across practice settings. *OT Practice, 22*(17), 8–13.

Egolf, D., & Chester, S. (2013). *Forming, storming, norming, performing: Successful communication in groups* (3rd ed.). Lincoln, NE: Universe.

Epstein, R., Siegel, D., & Silberman, J. (2008). Self-monitoring in clinical practice: A challenge for medical educators. *Journal of Continuing Education Health Professions, 28*(1), 5–13. https://doi.org/10.1002/chp.149

Every Student Succeeds Act, Pub. L. 114–195, 129 Stat. 1802 (2015–2016).

Fisher, R., & Shapiro, D. (2005). *Beyond reason: Using emotions as you negotiate.* New York: Viking Penguin.

Friend, M., & Cook, L. (2017). *Interactions: Collaboration skills for school professionals* (8th ed.). Boston: Pearson Education.

Frolek Clark, G. (2016). Collaborating within the *Paces*: Structures and routines. In B. Hanft & J. Shepherd (Eds.), *Collaborating for student success* (2nd ed., pp. 177–208). Bethesda, MD: AOTA Press.

Gilfoyle, E., Grady, A., & Nielson, C. (2011). *Mentoring leaders: The power of storytelling for building leadership in health care and education.* Bethesda, MD: AOTA Press.

Glennon, T. (2011). Human factors: Just as important as knowledge factors in collaborative experiences. *Journal of Occupational Therapy, Schools, and Early Intervention, 4,* 13–21. https://doi.org/10.1080/19411243.2011.581873

Gray, L., & Taie, S. (2015). *Public school teacher attrition and mobility in the first five years: Results from the first through fifth waves of the 2007–08 Beginning Teacher Longitudinal Study* (NCES 2015-337). Washington, DC: National Center for Education Statistics, U.S. Department of Education. Retrieved from https://nces.ed.gov/pubs2015/2015337.pdf

Handley-More, D., Wall, E., Orentlicher, M., & Hollenbeck, J. (2013, June). Working in early intervention and school settings: Current views of best practice. *Early Intervention and School Special Interest Section Quarterly, 20*(2), 1–4.

Hanft, B., & Shepherd, J. (Eds.). (2016). *Collaborating for student success* (2nd ed.) Bethesda, MD: AOTA Press.

Hanft, B., Shepherd, J., & Read, J. (2012). Pediatric therapy teams: How many perspectives are on the team? In S. J. Lane & A. Bundy (Eds.), *Kids can be kids: A childhood occupations approach* (pp. 273–292). Baltimore: F. A. Davis.

Hollenbeck, J., Orentlicher, M., & Handley-More, D. (2015, September). Expanding roles, expanding impact: Supporting work readiness in middle school. *Early Intervention and School Special Interest Quarterly, 22*(3), 1–3.

Huang, Y., Peyton, C., Hoffman, M., & Pascua, M. (2011). Teacher perspectives on collaboration with occupational therapists in inclusive classrooms: A pilot study. *Journal of Occupational Therapy, Schools, and Early Intervention, 4,* 71–89. https://doi.org/10.1080/19411243.2011.581018

Individuals With Disabilities Education Improvement Act of 2004, Pub. L. 108–446, 20 U.S.C. §§ 1400–1482.

Kaiser, A. (2011). *Beginning teacher attrition and mobility: Results from the first through third waves of the 2007–08 Beginning Teacher Longitudinal Study* (NCES 2011-318). Washington, DC: National Center for Education Statistics, U.S. Department of Education. Retrieved from https://nces.ed.gov/pubs2011/2011318.pdf

Kampwirth, T., & Powers, K. (2012). *Collaborative consultation in the schools* (4th ed.). New York: Prentice Hall.

Knackendoffel, K., Dettmer, P., & Thurston, L. (2018). *Consultation, collaboration, and teamwork for students with special needs* (8th ed.). Boston: Pearson.

Knowles, M., Holton, E., & Swanson, R. (2015). *The adult learner* (8th ed.) New York: Routledge.

Laverdure, P. (2016). Using reflection to advance professional expertise: A novice-to-expert trajectory. *OT Practice, 22*(4), 8–11.

Laverdure, P., Cosbey, J., Gaylord, G., & LeCompte, B. (2017). Providing collaborative and contextual service in school contexts and environments. *OT Practice, 22*(15), CE1.

Laverdure, P., Seruya, F., Stephenson, P., & Cosbey, J. (2016, June). Paradigm transitions in pediatric practice: Tools to guide practice. *SIS Quarterly Practice Connections, 1*(2), 5–7.

Lippy, D., & Zamora, E. (2012). Implementing effective professional learning communities with consistency at the middle school level. *National Forum of Educational Administration and Supervision Journal, 29*(3), 51–74.

Manor-Binyamini, I. (2011). A model of ethnographic discourse analysis for an interdisciplinary team. *Journal of Pragmatics, 43,* 1997–2011. https://doi.org/10.1016/j.pragma.2010.12.011

Martin, N. (2010). *Supporting the IEP: A facilitator's guide.* Baltimore: Brookes.

Missiuna, C., Pollock, N., Levac, D., Campbell, W., Sahagian Whalen, S., Bennett, S., & Russell, D. (2012). Partnering for change: An innovative school-based occupational therapy service delivery model for children with developmental coordination disorder. *Canadian Journal of Occupational Therapy, 79,* 41–50. https://doi.org/10.2182/cjot.2012.79.1.6

Mueller, T., & Buckley, P. (2014). The odd man out: How fathers navigate the special education system. *Remedial and Special Education, 35*(1), 40–49. https://doi.org/10.1177/0741932513513176

Ohl, A., Graze, H., Weber, K., Kenny, S., Salvatore, C., & Wagreich, S. (2013). Effectiveness of a 10-week Tier 1 response to intervention program in improving fine motor and visual–motor skills in general education kindergarten students. *American Journal of Occupational Therapy, 67,* 507–514. https://doi.org/10.5014/ajot.2013.008110

Orentlicher, M., Handley-More, D., Ehrenberg, R., Frenkel, M., & Markowitz, L. (2014, June). Interprofessional collaboration: A review of current evidence. *Early Intervention and School Special Interest Section Quarterly, 21*(2), 1–3.

Reed, P., & Bowser, G. (2012). Consultation, collaboration, and coaching: Essential techniques for integrating assistive technology use in schools and early intervention programs. *Journal of Occupational Therapy, Schools, and Early Intervention, 5,* 15–30. https://doi.org/10.1080/19411243.2012.675757

Rehabilitation Act of 1973, Pub. L. 93–112, 29 U.S.C. §§ 701–7961.

Rush, D., & Shelden, M. (2011). *The early childhood coaching handbook.* Baltimore: Brookes.

Schoonover, J. (2014, September). Interdisciplinary collaboration with assistive technology in schools. *Technology Special Interest Section, 24*(3), 1–3.

Schwind, D. (2017). Using typical school routines to build transition skills: A paradigm shift in community-based instruction. *OT Practice, 22*(6), 10–13.

Section 504 of the Rehabilitation Act of 1973, as amended, 29 U.S.C. § 794. (2008).

Shasby, S., & Schneck, C. (2011). Commentary on collaboration in school-based practice: Positives and pitfalls. *Journal of Occupational Therapy, Schools, and Early Intervention, 4,* 22–33.

Stephenson, P., Laverdure, P., Seruya, F. M., & Cosbey, J. (2017). Not just for children: Facilitating behavior change in school-based practice. *SIS Quarterly Practice Connections, 2*(4), 2–4.

Swinth, Y. (2016). Collaboration in action: The nitty gritty. In B. Hanft & J. Shepherd (Eds.), *Collaborating for student success* (2nd ed., pp. 209–242). Bethesda, MD: AOTA Press.

Taylor, R. R. (2008). *The intentional relationship: Occupational therapy and use of self.* Philadelphia: F. A. Davis.

Truong, V., & Hodgets, S. (2017). An exploration of teacher perceptions toward occupational therapy and occupational therapy practices: A scoping review. *Journal of Occupational Therapy, Schools, and Early Intervention, 10,* 121–136. https://doi.org/10.1080/19411243.2017.1304840

Tucker, V., & Schwartz, I. (2013). Parents' perspectives of collaboration with school professionals: Barriers and facilitators to successful partnerships in planning for students with ASD. *School Mental Health, 5*(1), 3–14. https://doi.org10.1007/s12310-012-9102-0

Turnbull, A., Zuna, N., Hong, J., Hu, X., Kyzar, K., Ohremski, S., & Stowe, M. (2010). Knowledge-to-action guides: Preparing families to be partners in making educational decision. *Exceptional Children, 42*(3), 42–53. https://doi.org/10.1177/004005991004200305

U.S. Department of Education, Office of Civil Rights. (2010). *Free appropriate education for students with disabilities: Section 504 of the Rehabilitation Act of 1973.* Washington, DC: Author.

Villa, R., & Thousand, J. (2016). *The Inclusive Education Checklist: A self-assessment of best practices.* Naples, FL: National Professional Resources.

Villa, R., & Thousand, J. (2017). *Leading an inclusive school: Access and success for all children.* Alexandria, VA: Association for Supervision and Curriculum Development.

Wenger, E. (2013). *Cultivating communities of practice: A quick start-up guide.* Retrieved from https://www.slideshare.net/powerhouse1/start-up-guidepdf

Wilding, C., Curtin, M., & Whiteford, G. (2012). Enhancing occupational therapists' confidence and professional development through a community of practice scholars. *Australian Occupational Therapy Journal, 59,* 312–318. https://doi.org/10.1111/j.1440-1630.2012.01031.x

World Health Organization. (2010). *Framework for action on interprofessional education and collaborative practice.* Geneva: Author.

Best Practices in Resolving Conflicts in Schools

Elizabeth Goodrich, OTR, ATP, PhD, FAOTA

13

KEY TERMS AND CONCEPTS

- Agenda
- Assume goodwill
- Broaden-and-Build Theory
- Closed-ended question
- Conflict
- Conflict resolution
- Documentation
- Due process complaint
- Empathetic listening
- Equal communication
- Facilitation
- Formal complaint
- Goals
- Ground rules
- Independent educational evaluation
- Mediation
- Neutral facilitator
- Nonverbal communication
- Open-ended question
- Parking lot
- Permissive question
- Physical environment
- Positive psychology process

OVERVIEW

Conflict is a natural part of the human experience. It cannot be avoided. However, it can be an opportunity for growth and development—that is, an evolutionary experience.

Some components of conflict for school occupational therapy practitioners[1] are unique because of local, state, and federal regulations that lead to misconceptions in the role of occupational therapy, the team process for decision making, and the differentiation in services from clinical or medical settings. When faced with conflict, school practitioners can facilitate a positive growth experience for all when they have skills to address conflict, are knowledgeable and engaged participants in the conflict resolution process, and engage others in the very same process.

Conflict Is an Opportunity

Experts (Anderson et al., 2011; Xu et al., 2011) have described *conflict* as experienced across various contexts (interpersonal, managerial, political, and international relationships) and occurring on a continuum of severity involving at least one relationship or issue and opposing perception, interest, or

---

[1]*Occupational therapy practitioner* refers to both the occupational therapist and the occupational therapy assistant. The American Occupational Therapy Association (AOTA; 2014, p. S18) states, "The occupational therapist is responsible for all aspects of occupational therapy service delivery and is accountable for the safety and effectiveness of the occupational therapy service delivery process" and "must be directly involved in the delivery of services during the initial evaluation and regularly throughout the course of intervention. . . . The occupational therapy assistant delivers safe and effective occupational therapy services under the supervision of and in partnership with the occupational therapist."

understanding. The severity of a conflict is described in terms of behaviors that people encounter as they experience the conflict.

Carruthers and Carruthers (1996) stated that "conflict can be a growth-enhancing experience if understood in theory, respected in attitude, and managed properly in behavior" (p. 354). Conflict provides opportunity for new learning and emotional growth. One enters conflict with a perspective that may broaden when one has been forced to more deeply explore one's view. Considering others' perspectives that might conflict with one's own reflects emotional intelligence and maturity. As with any maturational process, practice in the skill facilitates growth.

Conflict Differs in Schools

Conflicts experienced by occupational therapy practitioners in schools vary from those experienced in clinical settings primarily because of the different local, state, and federal regulations that affect services in each setting. In a clinical setting, occupational therapy practitioners typically provide a service to remediate or habilitate the degree of impairment that a child experiences as a result of disability or impairment in the context of daily life activities.

In an educational setting, however, occupational therapy services are more focused on how to improve students' level of participation in their educational program (e.g., academic, behavioral, functional). The local, state, and federal regulations affording these services alter the stakeholders, the roles of stakeholders, and the authority of stakeholders to affect change processes as conflict is experienced.

For example, the Individuals With Disabilities Education Improvement Act of 2004 (IDEA; Pub. L. 108–446) provides parents and their child who has a disability with rights, including but not limited to the right to a publicly funded full and individual evaluation and the right to disagree and

---

Copyright © 2019 by the American Occupational Therapy Association. All rights reserved. To reuse this content, contact www.copyright.com.
https://doi.org/10.7139/2019.978-1-56900-591-0.013

progress into mediation or due process. Federal and state accountability measures encourage school administrators to resolve conflict without progressing into formal processes, which can influence an administrator with little knowledge about occupational therapy regulations and practices to make assumptions on how to best resolve conflicts involving these services. Local policies structuring authority, financial decision making, and employment practices can bring additional stakeholders into a conflict resolution process.

Although conflict is often inevitable, options for dispute and conflict resolution processes in schools are becoming more prevalent and effective. According to the Center for Appropriate Dispute Resolution in Special Education (CADRE; 2017), between 2004–2005 and 2014–2015, the reported rate of filed due process complaints in the United States and outlying areas decreased. Moreover, of those filed complaints, fewer than 20% required a fully adjudicated hearing.

CADRE (2017) also reported that the number of mediation requests—although considerably less than filed due process complaints—has increased. Although the influencing variables are not fully understood, one might wonder whether the implementation of early dispute resolution options and conflict management approaches have been the impetus for change.

Conflict Resolution as a Necessary Skill

Occupational therapy practitioners serving students with disabilities in schools will find conflict resolution a critical skill for successful job performance. *Conflict resolution* consists of purposeful actions designed to bring resolution (not necessarily agreement) to a conflictual situation. Initial strategies are used to preempt conflict; nonetheless, when conflict arises, the practitioner needs to customize a core set of strategies to address the situation. Through this process, the practitioner customizes this set of strategies to the current situation and thereby evolves in professional practice.

Conflicts experienced in supporting students with disabilities can bruise a practitioner's confidence, but there are multiple resources for addressing conflict. AOTA (2015) stated in its *Occupational Therapy Code of Ethics* that "occupational therapy personnel shall use conflict resolution and/or alternative dispute resolution resources to resolve organizational and interpersonal conflicts as well as perceived institutional ethics violations" (p. 7). (For more information, see Chapter 4, "Best Practices in Ethical Reasoning for School Occupational Therapy Practitioners.")

Sources of Conflict

Mueller et al. (2008) identified 5 common sources of conflict in special education:
1. Design of services,
2. Provision of services,
3. Relationship issues,
4. Constraints (e.g., restricted resources), and
5. Knowledge (e.g., lack of educational training).
Although Mueller and colleagues were addressing the bigger picture of special education, these same 5 sources of conflict can be applied to occupational therapy as a related service under IDEA.

Design of services

Traditionally, the occupational therapy evaluation informs the design of services. In school practice, the team considers the results of the occupational therapy evaluation along with other sources of data to determine the design of services—in this case, the student's individualized education program (IEP). Conflict can occur when there is disagreement among team members on how to design services.

Provision of services

The provision of occupational therapy as documented on the student's IEP is the responsibility of the occupational therapist. Conflict can occur when there is disagreement with the therapist's recommendations, including the goals the services are to address as well as the time, frequency, and duration of services needed to address the goals.

Conflict can also occur with the provision of services because of variations in the student's school schedule (e.g., field trips, absences, special programs) or variations in the student's ability to benefit from the service (e.g., fatigue, episodes of emotional or behavioral challenges). Because the services are specified in a legal document (i.e., IEP) and are developed through a legal process (i.e., IEP process), the school district is bound to demonstrate the provision of services.

Practitioners may experience circumstances in which they feel that it is not in the best interest of the student to provide the services at that time or that services conflict with state occupational therapy practice acts (licensure). This can create conflict between the recommendations made through a legally binding process and the service provider's professional judgment or state regulations.

Relationship issues

Relationship issues can be a source of conflict for the occupational therapy practitioner because of the differences in perspectives of a professional trained in an education program and a professional trained in a health science program. Ineffective teams may result in poor relationships among team members, which can add to conflict.

Family members are a part of this team, so establishing contact and building relationships are essential for trust and respect to develop. Communication options include phone calls, email, notes sent home, and face-to-face contact.

Cultural differences can affect relationships and communications. Even for individuals in a common culture, words can
- Carry different connotations (e.g., the word *disability* may be interpreted as an insult as opposed to a means of understanding the needs of a child);
- Be understood with varying levels of emphasis (e.g., reference to a legal regulation may be seen as a requirement to some and a negotiable point to others); and
- Generate varying emotions (e.g., referring to a child as "the child" as opposed to by name may seem to show a disconnection from the child as a person).

Constraints

Constraints can be a source of conflict caused by working in an underfunded system with limited qualified personnel to provide services. The time an occupational therapist can spend to thoroughly investigate and understand a teacher's objectives for a student or the concerns a parent might have can be affected by the demands of their overall workload or the need to comply with regulated evaluation timelines.

Knowledge

Lack of knowledge can be a source of conflict. Not understanding what occupational therapy has to offer or what the teacher or parent are accomplishing or dealing with in the classroom can cause conflicts among team members. Practitioners should educate the local educational agency (LEA) and teams on the role of occupational therapy.

Common Conflicts Specific to Occupational Therapy

Some common reasons conflict may occur specifically in relation to occupational therapy services in schools include
- Team members disagreeing with the occupational therapist's evaluation or recommendations for services,
- Team members or parents misunderstanding the role of the school occupational therapy practitioner, and
- Administrators making decisions that conflict with state occupational therapy regulations or the occupational therapy practitioner's professional judgment.

Other issues that can create misunderstanding are political, financial, and ethical dilemmas. For example, a school administrator, seeing an area of disagreement that could lead to a formal conflict resolution process, might seek to influence the decision to provide occupational therapy services in lieu of allowing the conflict to develop further. A driving factor in this decision might be to maintain or build rapport with the family or to forgo the expense of a formal complaint process.

Sometimes issues arise out of fear or lack of resources. As health care in the United States undergoes significant change processes, parents may become fearful that their child's complement of needs will not be met because of changes in insurance or the unavailability of a clinical practitioner.

ESSENTIAL CONSIDERATIONS

Essential considerations for occupational therapy practitioners working in schools include understanding conflict resolution, common conflicts that might arise while they are working within legal requirements, and the impact of the public nature of public education on conflict resolution.

Conflict Resolution Under IDEA

When conflict occurs in the context of providing services under IDEA, the law protects the rights of children with disabilities by offering 3 options for formal conflict resolution:
1. Formal complaint to the state educational agency (SEA),
2. Mediation, and
3. Due process.

Formal complaint

An individual or an organization may file a *formal complaint* with the SEA, stating that the LEA has violated a requirement of IDEA. This complaint process is a complaint not against a specific individual but against the LEA. In the complaint process, the complainant states the facts on which the complaint is based, the identifying information for the complainant, and the identifying information for the student (e.g., when the complaint affects a specific student vs. all students). The complainant also provides a proposed resolution to the problem and gives a copy to the LEA as well as the SEA. A complaint must be filed within a year of an alleged violation (IDEA, 2004, 34 C.F.R. § 300.153).

Mediation

Before filing a formal complaint, or as a step to resolve a formal complaint before going to a due process hearing, each LEA must provide an option for dispute resolution through *mediation*. This is a voluntary process for both parties involved in the dispute (i.e., LEA and complainant). Dispute resolution does not deny or delay a parent's right to a hearing.

A mediator who is trained in effective mediation techniques and is identified by the SEA as a qualified mediator conducts the process. If a parent declines to participate in a mediation process, then the LEA may offer an opportunity to voluntarily meet with a disinterested party who can explain the benefits and encourage the use of a mediation process to resolve the dispute. The cost of the mediation process is incurred by the state (IDEA, 2004, § 300.506).

Due process

A *due process complaint* can be filed by either party or the attorney representing a party and must remain confidential. A hearing officer assigned by the SEA responds to the complaint, and if it meets the requirements, it may proceed into a due process hearing conducted by the hearing officer. In this process, both the complainant and the LEA have legal representation (IDEA, 2004, § 300.508).

Conflict Resolution Strategies

When a parent or adult student activates conflict resolution channels, the pending conflict process can be stressful for practitioners, affecting their overall job satisfaction and sometimes their perception of their own competence to effectively provide services in the school setting. The following strategies may help an occupational therapy practitioner move through the process more efficiently.

Assume goodwill

Occupational therapy practitioners are experts in problem analysis; therefore, their natural response to conflict is to analyze the components of the conflict to find solutions. Many conflicts experienced in school systems are driven by processes that are outside the occupational therapy practitioner's direct control (e.g., IEP team decisions, public regulations). Therefore, it is important to recognize that conflict is often not personal. The conflict might feel personal, but it is typically rooted in miscommunication or misunderstanding.

A key strategy to keeping a professional perspective amid conflict is to **assume goodwill.** Human nature might cause a difference of opinion to be interpreted as a personal attack or evidence of an ulterior motive, but assuming goodwill amid differences means always valuing and respecting the opinions of others, even in a disagreement. Someone assuming goodwill makes an intentional effort to foster positive emotions.

Conoley and Conoley (2010) proposed that given the multitude of adult relationships that are juggled in the provision of special education services (e.g., teacher to teacher, teacher to paraeducator, teacher to home caregiver), positive psychology processes mediate the influences of collaboration. A **positive psychology process** fosters positive emotions in individuals that encourage broadened thinking and openness to new ideas, instead of a flight-or-fight response that might occur with a negative thought process.

Conoley and Conoley (2010) referenced Fredrickson's (1998, 2001) Broaden-and-Build Theory as a means to "insert more energy, optimism, creativity, and hope in the work of educators" (p. 77). **Broaden-and-Build Theory** posits that people broaden their repertoire of thoughts and actions when they receive positive emotional responses. The broadened repertoire of thoughts and actions then increases the opportunity for a person to provide a well-informed, optimistic, and compassionate response.

This theoretical perspective teaches the professional to "spiral up" with positive responses in adult relationships to build collaborative relationships. Conflict resolution begins with relationships in which respect and trust can be nourished and developed. Whether the occupational therapy practitioner is new to the team or has long-term relationships with team members, the key is to allow respect and trust to grow in these relationships.

Include the student's family as a critical member of the team by establishing ongoing communication with them during the year. Throughout the relationship, if the occupational therapy practitioner can maintain a perspective of assuming goodwill in every step of the process, then respect and trust have an opportunity to grow even in the face of disagreement.

See conflict as an opportunity for growth

Seeing conflict as an opportunity to grow is important not only for the occupational therapy practitioner but also for all stakeholders involved. Conflict is not as simple as right and wrong or good and bad but is a complex web of interests, understandings, relationships, and emotions. Demonstrating an understanding of these complexities through well-structured problem analysis, the occupational therapy practitioner can be a strong asset to the conflict resolution process. This approach not only develops the practitioner's skills but also facilitates growth among all stakeholders. Most experienced practitioners can recall at least 1 challenging conflict resolution process in their career that afforded them the most professional growth.

Seek understanding

Disagreement does not typically occur because of one incident or one meeting. The complexities of providing special education and related services are challenging for the entire team. Such complexity sets the stage for misunderstanding and miscommunication, common precursors to disagreement. Seeking understanding, particularly by asking clarifying questions, can help avoid or rectify disagreement.

A common conflict arises from the lack of understanding of the role of occupational therapy in a school environment versus a clinical setting (Goodrich et al., 2012). Although these are both occupational therapy settings, the laws and regulations that define practice are different. Under IDEA, the intent of school services is to help the student benefit from educational programming. School occupational therapy practitioners provide services in the least restrictive environment to enhance the student's participation in school activities.

The teacher is responsible for the student's education through instruction in the curriculum; related service personnel support the student's ability to participate in and benefit from instruction, depending on the concerns. Therefore, the occupational therapy practitioner, teacher, and entire IEP team need to truly understand a concern by asking clarifying questions such as "What would you like to see the student doing a year from now?" and "What occupational therapy services are needed to support the teacher and the student in meeting these goals?" These types of questions can help the IEP team break down the concern to specific skill sets that they can then target with the right support for development. Clarifying questions facilitate the team process.

Focus on the student

Many times amid planning for the student, the focus of the conflict is diverted to other concerns. For example, a family might expect that their child, who was discontinued from private therapy services, will now receive occupational therapy from the school district. Similarly, a family might be surprised to hear that their child, who received special education services and occupational therapy in their previous state, is no longer eligible for the same services according to the new state's educational laws.

The IEP team's root concerns in both of these circumstances must be determining eligibility for special education to meet the needs of the student at school and deciding whether the student needs related services (e.g., the expertise of an occupational therapist). The IEP team keeps its focus on the student by clearly identifying student-specific strengths and needs, developing a student goal that can be achieved within the IEP period, and identifying supports that are anticipated to allow students to achieve their goals.

Impact of the Public Nature of Public Education on Conflict Resolution

As the occupational therapy practitioner addresses conflictual situations in public schools, it is important to recognize the public nature of public education. This is not to say that this perspective should change how the practitioner works through a conflictual situation. Instead, it emphasizes the necessity of maintaining a professional and student-centered process.

A free appropriate public education is a right in the United States. What is "appropriate" varies depending on the perspective of a wide range of stakeholders. Many times, conflict in public education is a difference in defining *appropriate* for one or more students.

For example, the series of articles "Denied: Houston Schools Systemically Blocked Disabled Kids From Special Ed" (Rosenthal & Barned-Smith, 2016) created a national outrage over practices that were actually intended to ensure that students with disabilities had access to multi-tiered systems of support (MTSS). There were many sides to this story, yet the public story, once published, halted a change process that would have ensured that students with disabilities had access to MTSS. This halt was intended to allow time to reassess the concerns of stakeholders who felt underserved in the change process.

Although this conflict was not specific to occupational therapy, it provides an example of how practice in schools is a component of a larger entity. It is not only a service area but also part of a district, a state, and a national system, each with practices and policies. As public systems, these practices and policies can have greater impact.

School occupational therapy practitioners providing services will experience times when conflict is bigger than their immediate service. Responding to these conflicts is no different than responding to localized conflicts: Assume goodwill, see conflict as an opportunity for growth, seek understanding, and focus on the student.

BEST PRACTICES

Occupational therapy practitioners will experience conflicts during their work. Being prepared is important. Practitioners need to learn ways to effectively prepare for and deal with conflicts that arise.

Effectively Use Communication and Documentation

The best conflict resolution strategy is to be proactive in understanding and addressing the conflict before it requires more formal processes. Tools that occupational therapy practitioners have at their immediate disposal are communication and documentation. In addition, establishing system-level supports that provide stakeholders with ready access to a practitioner provides a proactive support-building confidence that when a need arises, it will be addressed in a timely and efficient manner.

Communication

Frequently, consistently, and effectively communicating with teams (e.g., building teams, IEP teams) is not only an element of effective service but is also a proactive measure to head off conflict. Blue-Banning et al. (2004) listed 5 actions necessary for effective communication between professionals and parents:
1. Be friendly.
2. Listen.
3. Be clear.
4. Be honest.
5. Provide information.

This is true not only for effective communication between professionals and parents but also across the whole team supporting a student. In addition, be timely. The entire team should have the ability to access the occupational therapy practitioner and receive a timely response (e.g., within 24 hours).

When effectively communicating with teams, including families, it is important to understand cultural differences and individual preferences regarding method of communication (e.g., face to face, texting, email, phone, web-based methods), style (e.g., verbal, nonverbal), and reading level (e.g., "health literacy"; some families might not be proficient in English or read past the 5th-grade level). When meeting new team members for the first time, inquire about their preferred methods of communication.

Effective communication is a combination of verbal and nonverbal communication. Verbal communication may include reflecting feeling or content and effective questioning. Reflecting feelings acknowledges the feelings of the person speaking and demonstrates empathy. To reflect feelings, the occupational therapy practitioner may summarize or restate the speaker's feelings, indicating that they recognize those feelings. This gives an opportunity to correct misunderstandings.

Reflecting content, or the facts, summarizes information, which allows room for clarification. Effective questioning is used to gain information. Questions may be *permissive* (e.g., "In order to understand your concern, may I ask some questions?"), *open ended* (e.g., "Help me understand what you are expecting from occupational therapy services"), or *closed ended* (e.g., "Does your child exhibit this behavior at home?"). Be cautious when asking "why" questions because they may be perceived as probing or judging.

Nonverbal communication includes listening with the intent to understand the other person. Covey (1990) described *empathetic listening* as not only hearing the spoken words but also listening with your ears, eyes, and heart for the person's feelings, behavior, and perceptions. Listening does not mean you agree but that you are trying to understand the other person's experiences and feelings.

Other nonverbal communication that influences relationships and decisions includes facial expressions, eye contact, body posture, gestures, and personal space. Having your arms crossed, refusing eye contact, or smiling during a family's description of their concerns for their child may convey to the family a lack of professionalism or interest. Notice the nonverbal communication used by others, and find a comfortable way to show you are interested.

Documentation

The second tool occupational therapy practitioners have at their disposal in dealing with conflict is documentation. *Documentation* creates a record of the services provided; it includes evaluations, service contacts, progress reports, and discontinuation summaries (AOTA, 2018).

Occupational therapy practitioners working in schools have to understand that documents they produce (even a sticky note or an email) are potentially a public record and can be subpoenaed in a due process hearing or other formal legal action. An email (or sticky note) is part of a student's education record if it personally identifies a student and is maintained by the district (*S. A. by L. A. and M. A. v. Tulare County Office of Education,* 2009). The occupational therapy practitioner should record information with the idea that all documents may be seen by others and used as a foundation for decisions. (See Chapter 45, "Best Practices in School Occupational Therapy Documentation and Data Collection.")

Provide MTSS and Systems-Level Thinking

A proactive strategy gaining a greater focus in schools is providing MTSS and systems-level thinking to address the needs of not only those students with IEPs but all students. This strategy allows the opportunity to positively affect students' participation in school activities, address common challenges that surface in system processes, and streamline services.

For example, Goodrich et al. (2012) reported on examining an issue with inappropriate referrals for occupational therapy evaluations by establishing a prereferral screening. As defined by IDEA (2004), a *screening* is used to determine appropriate instructional strategies for curriculum implementation. As this practice became an integrated part of the school district, parents, teachers, and therapy practitioners gained confidence that students' needs would be addressed efficiently and effectively.

In another example, occupational therapy practitioners can bring a highly valued lens to the challenges some students experience with handwriting development. Many times, these challenges are not unique to a student or specific to disability but associated with a lack of effective instruction (e.g., the curriculum no longer includes handwriting instruction, the instruction does not align with best practice for the student population). Applying a systems-level solution, an occupational therapist might join a teacher (with administrative approval) and coteach handwriting. In addition to building capacity with the teacher, this can become an effective use of the therapist's time and expertise to meet the needs of a student population rather than one student at a time.

Gain Understanding of the Processes

The IEP process is complex, is driven by state and federal regulations, and requires team collaboration. School occupational therapy practitioners need to build their understanding and fully participate in the IEP process. In addition, they can help support parents and students to participate in the IEP process. Burke et al. (2017) described how parents of students with disabilities experienced high levels of stress when participating in an IEP meeting. They found that when parents used mindfulness strategies, their stress was reduced during IEP meetings, and they developed better relationships with school personnel.

Conflict is not experienced in isolation. The whole team experiences conflict through different lenses and with varying levels of knowledge, resilience, and experience. Meneghel et al. (2016) reported on the necessity of enthusiasm, optimism, satisfaction, comfort, relaxation, and resilience for successful team processes. It only takes one person on the team to seed positive emotions and build team resilience. Professional development areas may include the IEP process, mindfulness strategies, IEP facilitation, mediation, effective communication skills, and special education law.

Facilitated IEP process

A common process that is used across the United States to resolve conflicts that occur during development of IEP is *facilitation* (CADRE, 2002). Mueller (2009) provided 7 essential components of a successful IEP facilitation:
1. Neutral facilitator,
2. Agenda,
3. Goals,
4. Ground rules,
5. Physical environment,
6. Equal communication, and
7. Parking lot.

Each component helps keep the focus on the purpose of the meeting: developing an IEP for the student. The **neutral facilitator** does not run the meeting but is solely there to redirect the meeting when the discussion loses focus. The **agenda** is typically designed to follow the process of developing an IEP, as outlined in IDEA. SEAs commonly publish an agenda for IEP teams to follow, but during a facilitated IEP meeting, the team typically creates an agenda together that all agree to before the meeting.

The **goals** proposed by team members are designed to focus the meeting on the needs of the student through the lens of each team member. **Ground rules** are rules of the meeting procedure that are agreed to by all in attendance. These rules are typically referenced several times during the meeting. The **physical environment** is set up to facilitate open communication and collaboration. A common design is to have all in attendance seated around a large table.

The facilitator also uses strategies to encourage opportunities for **equal communication** from all participants—for example, by requesting an opinion from a quiet participant or asking a more verbal participant to allow others to respond to a discussion. The **parking lot** is a strategy whereby issues that arise during the meeting are written down and addressed at a designated time in the meeting agenda.

As a participant in a facilitated IEP meeting or other conflict resolution process, the occupational therapy practitioner should actively engage by assuming goodwill, asking clarifying questions, and keeping the focus on the student. For example, when an occupational therapy practitioner disagrees with the service recommendations being considered for a student by the IEP team, they assume a perspective of goodwill and ask clarifying questions to understand the concern. This new information may help the entire team better understand the student's needs. This process could even lead to identifying a student's need that is better addressed by another support or service.

Discussion needs to occur as a part of an effective IEP team process to ensure that the focus remains on the student's needs and best resources to support the student. If their needs are unclear or if the team cannot provide the information needed for IEP decisions, then further assessment may need to be completed, additional data collected on a specific skill set for the student, or a support added for a trial period (e.g., an adaptive strategy, assistive technology device, training for the classroom personnel).

Independent educational evaluations

When a disagreement with the occupational therapist's recommendations is not resolved in the context of the IEP process, IDEA includes an option for a family to request an *independent educational evaluation* (IEE) to provide a second opinion of the student's need for service. The IEE process is an opportunity to gain additional information for the IEP team to consider.

In accordance with federal regulations, the independent evaluator in most cases addresses the same areas identified through the IEP process (e.g., evaluate the student in all areas of the suspected disability; IDEA, 2004, 34 CFR § 300.502[e][1]). When a parent disagrees with the occupational therapy evaluation conducted by the LEA because it did not include areas they desired, then the IEE may address additional areas. The LEA may have a list of independent evaluators who meet their IEE criteria. The parent may choose from this list or identify an evaluator who meets the LEA's IEE criteria. Criteria set by the LEA may outline, for example, the qualifications of the examiner, the location of the evaluation, and the maximum allowable cost.

The IEE is different from a clinical evaluation and should be completed by an occupational therapist with training and experience in school practice. The IEE should take place in the educational environment where the student's IEP is provided, and it should include the following criteria:

- Review of the student's progress and pertinent educational history;
- Interview with the student's teacher or other significant persons regarding the student's educational program;
- Documented procedures and testing materials used during the IEE (e.g., observations; assessment measures administered; the occupational therapist's interpretation of the student's performance, including identified strengths and needs at school);
- An impact statement of the student's performance on their ability to benefit from general education; and
- Recommendations to the team for supports, strategies, or tools to address the student's identified needs, measurable goals, and objectives and benefit from their educational program.

Formal conflict resolution procedures

At times, disagreements progress into formal conflict resolution procedures. These formal proceedings can require quite a bit of preparation time for all involved. In most circumstances, LEAs engage professional legal counsel to assist in the process and provide occupational therapy practitioners with appropriate direction specific to the case. Effective documentation practices are critical. Resources are typically available through SEAs for formal conflict resolution procedures.

Actions speak louder than words

Strategies to resolve conflict have common components. Mueller and Piantoni (2013) identified 7 key action-based strategies school administrators should use to prevent and resolve conflict that specifically address conflict between families of students with disabilities and school personnel.

These actions are consistent for the whole team:
1. Establish communication.
2. Provide parent support.
3. Level the playing field.
4. Intervene at the lowest level possible.
5. Maintain the focus on the child.
6. Find a middle ground.
7. Understand perspectives.

Although these actions are proposed for school administrators, occupational therapy practitioners in school practice would be wise to adhere to and support them.

SUMMARY

In school practice, typical conflicts differ from conflicts experienced in other occupational therapy settings. Learning to effectively address conflicts experienced in school practice can facilitate professional growth. Amid conflict, the occupational therapy practitioner is encouraged to assume goodwill, see conflict as an opportunity for growth, ask clarifying questions, and focus on the student. The occupational therapy practitioner's skill in problem-solving analysis is an asset to the team in addressing conflict.

Effective communication and documentation practices are key tools to heading off conflict. In addition, supporting the system can proactively build confidence that services can be provided while meeting the student's needs in the most efficient and effective manner. Moreover, it establishes positive relationships before conflict arises. These practices can shift a potential reactionary process from conflict to a positive proaction.

To work through conflict, IEP teams may engage in facilitated IEP processes or may seek an IEE to support the conflict resolution process before it turns into a more formal process. In all cases, the occupational therapy practitioner's role is to actively participate and help the IEP team gain the information necessary to make the best decisions in developing the student's IEP.

REFERENCES

American Occupational Therapy Association. (2014). Guidelines for supervision, roles, and responsibilities during the delivery of occupational therapy services. *American Journal of Occupational Therapy, 68*(Suppl. 3), S16–S22. https://doi.org/10.5014/ajot.2014.686S03

American Occupational Therapy Association. (2015). Occupational therapy code of ethics (2015). *American Journal of Occupational Therapy, 69*(Suppl. 3), 6913410030. https://doi.org/10.5014/ajot.2015.696S03

American Occupational Therapy Association. (2018). Guidelines for documentation of occupational therapy. *American Journal of Occupational Therapy, 72*(Suppl. 2), 7212410010. https://doi.org/10.5014/ajot.2018.72S203

Anderson, S. R., Anderson, S. A., Palmer, K. L., Mutchler, M. S., & Baker, L. K. (2011). Defining high conflict. *American Journal of Family Therapy, 39*(1), 11–27. https://doi.org/10.1080/01926187.2010.530194

Blue-Banning, M., Summers, J., Frankland, H., Nelson, L., & Beegle, G. (2004). Dimensions of family and professional partnerships: Constructive guidelines for collaboration. *Exceptional Children, 70*, 167–184. https://doi.org/10.1177/001440290407000203

Burke, M. M., Neilson, C., & Neece, C. L. (2017). Parent perspectives of applying mindfulness-based stress reduction strategies to special education. *Intellectual and Development Disabilities, 55,* 167–180. https://doi.org/10.1352/1934-9556-55.3.167

Carruthers, W. L., & Carruthers, B. (1996). Conflict resolution as curriculum: A definition, description, and process for integration in core curricula. *School Counselor, 43,* 345–374.

Center for Appropriate Dispute Resolution in Special Education. (2002). *Facilitated IEP meetings: An emerging practice.* Eugene, OR: Author. Retrieved from https://eric.ed.gov/?id=ED483194

Center for Appropriate Dispute Resolution in Special Education. (2017). *IDEA Data Brief: Due process complaints/hearings.* Retrieved from http://www.cadreworks.org/sites/default/files/resources/CADRE%20DPC%20Brief_WebFinal_6.2017.pdf

Conoley, J., & Conoley, C. (2010). Why does collaboration work? Linking positive psychology and collaboration. *Journal of Educational and Psychological Consultation, 20,* 75–82. https://doi.org/10.1080/10474410903554902

Covey, S. (1990). *The seven habits of highly effective people: Restoring the character ethic.* New York: Fireside/Simon & Schuster.

Fredrickson, B. L. (1998). What good are positive emotions? *Review of General Psychology, 2,* 300–319. https://doi.org/10.1037/1089-2680.2.3.300

Fredrickson, B. L. (2001). The role of positive emotions in positive psychology: The Broaden-and-Build Theory of positive emotions. *American Psychologist, 56,* 218–226. https://doi.org/10.1037/0003-066X.56.3.218

Goodrich, B., Hawkins, J., Burridge, A., & White, C. (2012). Facilitating appropriate referrals for related services in schools. *Journal of Occupational Therapy, Schools, and Early Intervention, 5,* 221–238. https://doi.org/10.1080/19411243.2012.737282

Individuals With Disabilities Education Improvement Act of 2004, Pub. L. 108–446, 20 U.S.C. §§1400–1482.

Meneghel, I., Salanova, M., & Martinez, I. (2016). Feeling good makes us stronger: How team resilience mediates the effect of positive emotions on team performance. *Journal of Happiness Studies, 17,* 239–255. https://doi.org/10.1007/s10902-014-9592-6

Mueller, T. (2009). IEP facilitation: A promising approach to resolving conflicts between families and schools. *Teaching Exceptional Children, 41,* 60–67. https://doi.org/10.1177/004005990904100307

Mueller, T., & Piantoni, S. (2013). Actions speak louder than words: How do special education administrators prevent and resolve conflict with families? *Journal of Special Education Apprenticeship, 2*(2), 1–15. Retrieved from http://josea.info/archives/vol2no2/vol2no2-1-FT.pdf

Mueller, T., Singer, G., & Draper, L. (2008). Reducing parental dissatisfaction with special education in two school districts: Implementing conflict prevention and alternative dispute resolution. *Journal of Educational and Psychological Consultation, 18,* 191–233. https://doi.org/10.1080/10474410701864339

Rosenthal, B. M., & Barned-Smith, J. (2016, December 27). Denied: Houston schools systemically block disabled students from special ed. *Houston Chronicle.* Retrieved from http://www.houstonchronicle.com/denied/6/

S. A. by L. A. and M. A. v. Tulare County Office of Education, E.D. Cal., Set. 24, 2009/Oct. 6, 2009, No. CV F 08–1215.

Xu, H., Kilgour, D., & Hipel, K. (2011). Matrix representation of conflict resolution in multiple-decision-maker graph models with preference uncertainty. *Group Decision and Negotiation, 20,* 755–779. https://doi.org/10.1007/s10726-010-9188-4

Joyce E. Rioux, EdD, OTR/L, SCSS, and Leslie L. Jackson, DrOT, MEd, OT/L, FAOTA

KEY TERMS AND CONCEPTS

- Bargaining agreement
- Caseload model
- Formal structure
- Free appropriate public education
- Guiding coalition
- Informal structure
- Practice guidelines
- Time study
- Workload analysis
- Workload approach
- Workload balance

OVERVIEW

The caseload versus workload conversation has been happening for quite some time. The dialogue has centered on the importance of accounting for workload variables when determining and managing occupational therapy staffing and programming in schools (American Occupational Therapy Association [AOTA] et al., 2014). The movement to embrace a workload approach has remained slow, and disparities continue to linger across states, districts, schools, and personnel (Polichino, 2017; Rogers & Rhoads, 2017). These disparities range from applying a traditional caseload approach to regulating caseload limits and affording time to address workload activities—that is, applying a workload approach.

Applying a traditional *caseload model*—an approach drawn from our medical counterparts that consists of seeing clients by appointment only and counting the number of cases seen for service—has considerable ramifications in school practice (Polichino & Jackson, 2014). Counting only those students mandated for direct service in accordance with their individualized education program (IEP) and packing the schedule with direct service sessions only runs the risk of high caseloads and insufficient time to manage all of the work required to meet students' needs (Jackson, 2013).

The inevitable downside of these risks is that the contributions of occupational therapy practitioners[1] become restricted and not valued by parents, school staff, administrators, or even practitioners themselves. This, in turn, can negatively affect the very same students whom practitioners are aiming to support and who need occupational therapy's complement of services to benefit from their education.

Caseload limits or caps for related service providers, including occupational therapists, have been regulated in a few states (e.g., Maine, Ohio, districts in Washington, Wisconsin; Maine Department of Education, 2015; Northshore Education Association & Northshore School District No. 417, 2016; Ohio Department of Education, 2014; Wisconsin State Legislature, 2016). The various pathways to establish these caseload caps have been through state legislation, department of education operating standards, and collective bargaining agreements. Each pathway has required the shared discussion of not only school occupational therapy practitioners but also educational colleagues, professional associations, and regulatory boards.

With the shared discussion in mind, AOTA, as part of the Individuals With Disabilities Education Association Partnership, joined the American Physical Therapy Association and the American Speech–Language–Hearing Association in a venture to discuss the mutual concern of caseload and workload for related service providers (AOTA et al., 2014). By coming together in this manner, the organizations aimed to address common concerns, compare approaches, weigh pros and cons, share resources, and contemplate next steps in driving change from caseload to workload.

The importance of accounting for workload variables when determining staffing has been described in a growing percentage of state practice guidelines for occupational therapy in schools (e.g., California, Connecticut, Georgia, Michigan, New York, North Carolina; AOTA, 2017b). Of these guidelines, some have included workload management forms, workload formulas, and recommendations to acknowledge contextual influences that affect workload demands. Despite the inclusion of workload references and resources, these guidelines do not hold the same weight as regulations for which penalties may be attached for

---

[1] *Occupational therapy practitioner* refers to both the occupational therapist and the occupational therapy assistant. AOTA (2014, p. S18) states, "The occupational therapist is responsible for all aspects of occupational therapy service delivery and is accountable for the safety and effectiveness of the occupational therapy service delivery process" and "must be directly involved in the delivery of services during the initial evaluation and regularly throughout the course of intervention. . . . The occupational therapy assistant delivers safe and effective occupational therapy services under the supervision of and in partnership with the occupational therapist."

Copyright © 2019 by the American Occupational Therapy Association. All rights reserved. To reuse this content, contact www.copyright.com.
https://doi.org/10.7139/2019.978-1-56900-591-0.014

violations. State practice guidelines are intended to be reference manuals to interpret existing law, detail best practice, and inform others on important issues (American Psychological Association, 2005).

Since the introduction of workload concepts, school occupational therapy has grown in complexity: legislation and regulatory influences, professional requirements, and environmental and contextual demands all need to be considered (AOTA, 2017a). In accordance with the Every Student Succeeds Act (ESSA; 2015; Pub. L. 114–195), school occupational therapy practitioners are now considered specialized instructional support personnel (SISP).

This recognition broadens the reach of occupational therapy in educational systems and opens avenues to further support effective teaching, promote positive school climates, reduce barriers to learning, address mental health, and be part of a continuum of support services for all students (e.g., serving on academic intervention teams, school mental health teams, and district professional development teams). Along with this opportunity comes a greater need and importance to advocate for a workload approach when determining occupational therapy staffing in schools and organizing the staff's work to optimize student outcomes.

ESSENTIAL CONSIDERATIONS

School practitioners and those pursuing a workload approach need to know what that approach entails, understand the current climate, recognize the interplay of influencing determinants, and appreciate that driving change can be a slow process.

Workload Approach

A *workload approach* is essentially a method used to determine minimum staffing requirements and management of occupational therapy (AOTA et al., 2014; Jackson, 2013; Polichino & Jackson, 2014). This approach takes into account not only direct intervention with students but also (and not limited to) conducting evaluations, planning interventions, and teaming with families and school personnel.

Implicit in each service lies a host of other activities that the practitioner must do to successfully accomplish each responsibility—for example, attending meetings, writing reports, monitoring student progress and outcomes, collecting data, conferring with team members, researching and ordering equipment, and serving on school committees. Each activity requires time to complete and may necessitate several sessions over time.

Evaluations may require an extended period of time to
- Travel to the school;
- Communicate with others about the referral;
- Conduct a record review;
- Interview teachers, parents, and students;
- Complete an occupational profile;
- Select evaluation methods on the basis of purpose;
- Observe the students in their natural routines and environments;
- Administer assessment tools when necessary;
- Interpret collected data;
- Clinically reason educational impact;

- Document results; and
- Share those results with the student's parents and educational team members.

Not only does each evaluation component require dedicated time, but it might also need to be completed over a specific window of time (e.g., 60 calendar days), as determined by federal law or state regulations. This requires the occupational therapist to prioritize tasks and scheduling (e.g., time management). The entire evaluation process could require 6–10 hours or longer, depending on the complexity of the evaluation.

In schools, occupational therapy practitioners provide services directly with students as well as on behalf of students (including indirect activities associated with these services), compliance activities to adhere to regulatory requirements, and services and supports for teachers and other staff (see Exhibit 14.1 for examples). In addition, depending on the length of the workday, the practitioner might need to allocate time for breaks and lunch so they can sustain productivity and energy levels throughout the day. Applying a workload approach requires that all services and activities distinct to a particular district or school be considered.

Caseloads, Workloads, and the Current Climate

A 2014 survey conducted by the National Coalition on Personnel Shortages in Special Education and Related Services revealed a national shortage of SISPs—which includes school occupational therapy practitioners in their capacity as related service providers under the Individuals With Disabilities Education Improvement Act of 2004 (IDEA; Pub. L. 108–446), building team support providers under Section 504 of the Rehabilitation Act of 1973, as amended (2008; Pub. L. 93–112), and SISPs under ESSA (2015). These shortages were coupled with unfunded occupational therapy positions as a result of district budget cuts. As a result, practitioners employed in schools without regulations or standards in place for caseload caps or manageable workloads might have been expected to carry the load and ultimately faced unmanageable demands, compliance dilemmas, and ethical predicaments.

In fact, a 2017 study on the impact of work demands on school services (Smith et al., 2017) supported this assertion. Findings included
- Increased work demands and expectations because of staff reductions and cutbacks in funding;
- Additional job duties and compliance with multi-tiered systems of support (MTSS) and supervision of occupational therapy assistants and fieldwork students;
- Oversight of program carryover and training others as well as lack of space, equipment, and materials;
- Use of new technology for billing and documentation; and
- Increased paperwork requirements.

Understand Workload Influences

When preparing to shift to a workload model, practitioners need to understand the multilayered influences that affect the occupational therapy workload in schools (Polichino

EXHIBIT 14.1. Common Roles, Responsibilities, and Activities of Occupational Therapy Practitioners in Schools

ROLES	
▪ Advocate	▪ Leader
▪ Case manager	▪ Researcher
▪ Collaborative team member	▪ Resource (Consultant)
▪ Educator and trainer	▪ Schoolwide systems of support
▪ Evaluator	▪ Service provider

RESPONSIBILITIES AND ACTIVITIES

Direct services with students

- Screenings and evaluations
  - Assist in universal screenings.
  - Conduct individual screenings (if allowed under state licensure laws).
  - Conduct full and individual initial evaluations.
  - Review files, interview, observe student, and administer assessments.
  - Reevaluate students.
  - Conduct transition evaluations.
- Interventions
  - Provide interventions along a continuum of service delivery options (multi-tiered systems of service):
    - *Tier 1:* Core instructional interventions (proactive for general population)
    - *Tier 2:* Targeted group interventions (grouped by same skill or strategy)
    - *Tier 3:* Intensive, individual interventions (in the natural context when appropriate).
  - Design and engage in early intervening services, response-to-intervention activities, school mental health, stop-bullying initiatives, positive behavioral intervention and support, and other schoolwide initiatives.
  - Educate and train staff.
- Outcomes
  - Collect data on student participation and performance during service provision.

Indirect services to implement IEP or intervention plan

- Teaming
  - Contribute to IEP and goal development as well as service planning.
  - Collaborate with team members to solve problems.
  - Consult with teachers and support teams.
  - Participate in parent–teacher conferences.
- Consulting
  - Design transition evaluations and goals.
  - Design or recommend adaptations to curriculum and delivery of instruction.
- Coordinating
  - Communicate with other providers (e.g., medical, educational, leisure).
  - Develop home programs, at parent request.
  - Refer to other professionals when appropriate.
- Educating and training
  - Provide in-services, trainings, and professional development to school staff, parents, and others.

(Continued)

EXHIBIT 14.1.   Common Roles, Responsibilities, and Activities of Occupational Therapy Practitioners in Schools *(Cont.)*

- Train teachers, staff, and parents in AT use.
- Monitoring
  - Check on the effectiveness of an instructional or intervention strategy.
  - Track a student's participation or performance at different intervals or across settings.

Indirect activities to promote student access and participation

- Analyze and engineer environments to increase opportunities for occupational performance.
- Participate in school improvement teams or district initiatives.
- Create opportunities and develop programs to optimize student participation.
- Program and maintain AT.

Compliance activities to adhere to laws, regulations, and professional standards

- Documentation
  - Write periodic student progress reports.
  - Write student evaluation reports.
  - Fulfill Medicaid documentation requirements.
  - Maintain service contact records, communication logs.
  - Record and analyze student performance data.
- Professional responsibilities
  - Stay current regarding regulations, practice standards, evidence, and interventions.
  - Attend mandatory staff meetings.
  - Participate in professional development.
  - Research basis for intervention and best practices.
- Travel between schools and sites and within each building
- Supervision
  - Supervise occupational therapy assistants and interns.
  - Supervise fieldwork students.
  - Oversee paraeducators implementing student-specific strategies or programs.

Note. AT = assistive technology; IEP = individualized education program.
Sources. American Occupational Therapy Association (2017a), American Speech–Language–Hearing Association (2002), Polichino and Jackson (2014), and Swinth (2008).

& Jackson, 2014). These influences might include federal law requirements, state regulatory practices, local district expectations, student needs, and professional responsibilities. Each of these layers has associated activity requirements that affect scheduling and time management. Understanding the demands that are unique to the school or district will provide context to the workload discussion around planning and management.

Scheduling and Common Workload Influences

Common workload influences that emerge in school practice center on scheduling and determining how to handle missed services, attend trainings, complete activities, and prioritize needs. The following considerations must be taken into account.

Make up missed or interrupted services

IDEA (2004) and Section 504 of the Rehabilitation Act of 1973, as amended, entitle eligible students with a disability to a ***free appropriate public education*** (FAPE). In 2017, the Supreme Court clarified FAPE under IDEA. The court established a bright-line rule to clarify that a public school "must offer an IEP reasonably calculated to enable a child to make progress appropriate in light of the child's circumstances" (*Endrew F. v. Douglas County School District,* 2017, 207).

For students who need occupational therapy as part of their IEP, services must be adequate, reasonably calculated to enable educational progress, and provided in accordance with the child's IEP. Missed or interrupted services—particularly when the child does not make appropriate progress—could constitute a denial of FAPE in certain situations and lead to a due process challenge. Some states and districts, such as the District of Columbia Public Schools (2013), have established standards for making up missed sessions.

Attend mandated trainings

State and local educational agencies may have stipulations that occupational therapy practitioners attend mandated trainings to ensure that they have the knowledge and competencies for working in school settings. Practitioners' attending training during the school day may result in students missing services required on their IEP.

Travel between sites, complete documentation, and monitor student outcomes

Depending on a given school or district, routine travel, site-specific paperwork and documentation, and frequent progress reporting may be required.

Manage complex needs of students

The number, age, and complex needs of students with disabilities can drive the volume of services and activities.

Provide services in accordance with the IEP

A student's IEP outlines what, where, and how services are to be provided. Scheduling these services, particularly contextually based interventions (i.e., in the student's environment during naturally occurring activities), requires that the practitioner have a targeted schedule to work with students during meaningful learning and school activities.

Build resources

When limited resources (e.g., documentation systems, technology access, personnel supports, assessment materials) impede the flow of work, then response time can be slowed, quality and creativity can be dampened, frustrations can be heightened, and job satisfaction can be depleted (Staats & Upton, 2011). Having time to build resources and improve processes contributes to long-term impact.

Know What Is Happening in Your Area

States and districts may have specific stipulations around caseload or workload calculations. Knowing these stipulations is critical. When conditions are not in place, explore whether local or national workload initiatives exist, and identify who is driving the initiative. Be familiar with different sources you can draw on (e.g., collective bargaining agreements; practice guidelines; organizational structures).

Collective bargaining agreements

In many school districts, caseload and workload are addressed in a ***bargaining agreement.*** This agreement, the result of negotiations between the employer (e.g., school district) and employees (e.g., labor union), spells out the conditions of employment and working conditions.

Federal and state laws, regulations, and judicial decisions govern collective bargaining (Cornell University Law School, Legal Information Institute, 2018). Depending on the district, occupational therapy practitioners may or may not be included in a collective bargaining agreement. It is incumbent on each practitioner to advocate with the appropriate collective bargaining unit for inclusion of occupational therapy and relevant work-related needs and issues.

Practice guidelines

Many states have developed ***practice guidelines*** that include stances on applying a workload approach when determining coverage needs. As described earlier, practice guidelines do not hold the same weight as regulations (i.e., they are not rules). However, they do have the backing and consensus of a collective group.

Guidelines are often developed by subject matter experts in the state and are frequently endorsed by state educational agencies and professional associations. When practitioners understand the expressed opinion in their state regarding workload, they can use that to start or continue the conversation in their region.

Organizational structure

Each school district—and, for that matter, each individual school in the district—has formal and informal organizational structures, each with a set of policies, procedures, and practices. In a ***formal structure,*** policies and procedures are published and clearly communicated to staff, with an established procedure in place for raising a grievance in the case of a labor disagreement. In an ***informal structure,*** rules and practices are unwritten. Veteran staff members are aware of the implicit rules and know when they have been violated.

These explicit and implicit organizational structures define what are and are not acceptable work behavior and practices (McCormack, 2011). Moreover, they can have a powerful impact on workflow and motivation (or lack thereof) for work productivity. Over time, occupational therapy practitioners begin to understand the formal and informal organizational structure of the schools they work in and settle into a norm of work behavior that is acceptable in the specific setting. When organizational structures challenge occupational therapy practice as regulated in the state's practice act (licensure), AOTA's ethical standards, and school practice governed by laws and regulations, then practitioners need to advocate for change.

Understand That Change Is Slow

When advocating for change from a caseload to a workload approach, practitioners need to understand the change process. To effect change, one must plan for and communicate it effectively. Kotter (2007) suggested that the change process goes through a series of phases that require considerable time and manpower. He recommended 8 sequential steps worthy of following and building momentum toward change.

1. Establish a great enough sense of urgency to make the status quo seem "more dangerous than launching into the unknown" (Kotter, 2007, p. 3). For example, practitioners can challenge the status quo by providing data on the adverse impact of insufficient time to make up missed sessions, to engage in professional reasoning, to involve parents, or to meet compliance requirements.
2. Build a powerful **guiding coalition.** Practitioners should formally seek out and connect with colleagues, school therapy leaders in their area, professional associations, and those within and outside the typical hierarchy of their work setting to rally together and drive change.
3. Create a vision—that is, a vision that is easily communicated, understood, and appealing. The vision might be a realistic formula for calculating staffing coverage or a statewide initiative for regulating caseload.
4. Communicate the vision by a factor of 10. Use as many venues as possible to clearly communicate the vision—in conversations, employee performance appraisals, newsletters, discussion boards, professional presentations, and so on.
5. Remove obstacles to the new vision. At times, an individual might stand in the way of change for one reason or another. When this occurs, a heart-to-heart conversation is in order so that the practitioner can understand their perspective and possibly uncover unrealized obstacles. During the conversation, it is wise to treat the person fairly while remaining consistent with the new vision.
6. Recognize short-term wins. Recall that change takes time, and pause to recognize short-term wins and the people who contributed.
7. Beware of declaring victory too soon. True change can take 5–10 years. A premature victory celebration can be disastrous. Resistors may spot an opportunity to stop change, and old approaches will creep back in.
8. Anchor change in the system. Change sticks when it becomes "the way we do things around here" (Kotter, 2007, p. 8). Communicate the connections and positive impact of the realized vision in shifting to the workload approach.

BEST PRACTICES

School occupational therapy practitioners provide a range of services and supports that help students access, benefit from, and participate in general education. A **workload analysis** is the process of identifying, tracking, and analyzing everything a practitioner must do to provide those services. In particular, the workload analysis ensures that the time needed to perform the required services and activities is consistent with the time available. Although this section is written from the perspective of guiding the individual practitioner, the information can be applied and will likely have a greater impact at the organizational and external levels.

Conduct a Workload Analysis

Although the following process for workload analysis is listed in a linear sequence, the occupational therapy practitioner should approach it in a circular order whereby steps are repeated, overlapped, or simultaneously conducted to gather rich data and propose reasoned solutions.

Step 1: List expected and anticipated roles, responsibilities, and activities

Before beginning efforts to document the occupational therapy workload, the practitioner should develop a comprehensive list of all roles, responsibilities, and activities necessary in their school setting (see Exhibit 14.1). While creating this list, the practitioner employed by the school or district is encouraged to review their job description; the practitioner who is contracted privately or through an agency should examine the established service agreement.

These documents should lend insight—at least in a general sense—into expected and anticipated roles, responsibilities, and activities. If they do not, then this is a time to have an open discussion with the individuals responsible for maintaining and updating these documents. Best practice is to review and update these documents annually at a minimum (e.g., on annual employee appraisal; Tyler, 2013).

By starting with the creation of a list, the practitioner should examine whether a **workload balance** exists. That is, does a balance exist to perform the required roles, responsibilities, and activities? The following questions may help guide the practitioner in this determination:

- What is the percentage of time allocated to each cluster of activities?
- Are resources available to perform the work (e.g., space, technology access, assessment tools, mentors)?
- Are streamlined processes and procedures in place for workflow efficiency (e.g., prereferral process, structured IEP meetings, lines of communication)?
- Do I have the knowledge and practice competence to fulfill expectations (e.g., AT, mealtime supports, diagnostic considerations)?

The answers to these questions provide an opportunity for reflection, discussion, and problem solving to set forth a plan for balancing the workload. For example, in developing a list and answering the questions, a practitioner might identify a deficit in practice knowledge surrounding assistive technology and, in turn, seek administrative support for time to receive mentorship.

Alternatively, in creating a list and reflecting on these questions, an occupational therapist might uncover that a consistent referral process is not in place, which thus demands excessive time to determine the referral source, concerns, and prereferral strategies trialed. By speaking with their supervisor, the therapist might have time allocated to draft a proposed process, with the ultimate gain of eliminating wasted time.

Last, an occupational therapy assistant might discover that computer access is not available at each assigned site, which would have a direct impact on their ability to complete required documentation. If they brought this to the administrator's attention, support might be provided, and a dedicated laptop might be assigned to the assistant to accomplish required documentation responsibilities.

Step 2: Schedule services and activities

Drawing from the roles, responsibilities, and activities list created in Step 1, draft a master schedule that accounts for all mandated services and subsequent activities. When drafting the schedule, be mindful of minimizing travel between sites and classrooms when possible. In addition, make every attempt to schedule services and activities and prioritize on the basis of common meeting days and classroom and school schedules. For instance, if School X has eligibility meetings on Tuesdays, then this is a preferred day to be on site. If School Y has several students with IEP goals for using materials (e.g., drawing, cutting, coloring) scheduled for art on Wednesdays, then this might be a highly preferred day for that school.

Having a well-thought-out master schedule is critical in determining whether work can be accomplished within the scheduled work hours. When flaws exist (e.g., provision of direct service does not allow time for paperwork or evaluation of new students), the occupational therapist should objectively assess and propose to the administrator options for how the workload can be managed. The occupational therapy assistant should do this in partnership with the occupational therapist. For example, the occupational therapist might prioritize services and activities, consider which students might benefit from grouping, defer nonessential tasks to others, establish a wait-list, or gain additional support.

As with the previous step, sharing anticipated problems with the administrator should help in determining viable solutions. If a viable solution cannot be reached, then the occupational therapist (partnering with the occupational therapy assistant when applicable) should further examine the challenge. If the challenge centers on insufficient time to schedule mandated services, then investigate whether local data exist that demonstrate how students are adversely affected by unmanageable workload conditions. These data can be useful to present in discussion with the administrator.

In the end, if ethical and reasoned solutions cannot be agreed on, then work with other school therapy practitioners, local union representatives, or professional organizations to address workload issues. In addition, move to capture a time study of a worked schedule (i.e., following the master schedule while documenting services missed, unplanned meetings, and episodic events that arise).

A *time study* is a snapshot of all student-related tasks and activities a practitioner actually completed over a specific period of time (e.g., 1 day, 2 weeks, 1 month). The data obtained from this study outline the services and activities that were provided as well as those that were not (Jackson, 2013; Polichino & Jackson, 2014). When conducting the time study, use set time increments (e.g., 15-minute intervals) to record what occurs at any given time. That is, document in detail each service and activity that occurred and the time frame in which it occurred, including driving, trips throughout the building, phone calls, and follow-up tasks. Each service and activity should be coded on the basis of categories, as referenced in the next step.

Step 3: Categorize services and activities

There are two lines of thought on when to categorize services and activities. One is to craft a system that allows the practitioner to simultaneously record and categorize activities and services provided using predetermined codes. This system might be more efficient and promote consistency when the goal is to capture time study data across multiple practitioners. Before rolling out such a system, practitioners should conduct a pilot test to correct systematic errors and clarify definitions as appropriate.

The other line of thought is to categorize services and activities once the time study is complete. This may offer the added benefit of revealing different themes, ideas, or events that surface and are more descriptive in understanding the data. For example, after looking at the data, one occupational therapist decided to apply lean principle concepts (Dennis, 2007). The schedule provided a map of the work week, which the therapist analyzed from the perspective of the following:

- *Actual work:* Value-added services during direct contact with students on educationally necessary and relevant outcomes
- *Auxiliary work:* Necessary services and activities that supported actual work, as described previously
- *Muda (i.e., waste):* Non–value-added or unnecessary activities or services for which adverse impact on student outcomes was not apparent (e.g., unnecessary wait time, trips, resource consumption).

No matter when or how services and activities are categorized, analysis of data should inform how time was actually spent in the process of meeting work demands.

Step 4: Analyze results

The data gathered during the workload analysis can help occupational therapy practitioners and their administrators assess workload balance. This is a time to refer back to Step 1 and contemplate the questions posed. In addition, practitioners should answer the following questions:

- Does sufficient time exist to accomplish what is supposed to be done?
- Are services and activities being provided in a timely manner?
- Are there trends or patterns that can provide insight into workload imbalances?

Analyzing the occupational therapy workload can help pinpoint patterns, the ratio between services and activities, and errors to workload assignments. Once the practitioner has collected, grouped, and analyzed the data, they can share information with the administrator to guide future decision making about the availability and provision of occupational therapy.

Implement Workload Planning and Management

Once data are collected and analyzed, the planning and management solutions can be explored. This exploration can occur at the individual practitioner level, the organizational level, or the external level. Bear in mind that changes enacted at one level may result in positive change or potential dilemmas at another level. Looking ahead and considering the interplay of the various levels may save frustrations and lead to better outcomes.

Individual level

When the goal is to put practices in place that can be controlled by the individual practitioner, then starting at this level may be easiest. Some practices might include ensuring that services are aligned for educational benefit, time management strategies are applied, and an ongoing process of improved practice competence occurs.

Educational benefit. Adhere to federal, state, and local regulations to consistently identify students who need occupational therapy to benefit from their educational program. Over- or underrecommending services is not best practice. Collaborate with other occupational therapists to determine the consistency of recommendations in the agency or state.

Services should be individualized to the student, which means that some services may be weekly, some twice a month, and some monthly or less often. Service times may vary as well (e.g., 30- or 45-minute sessions are based on a medical or clinical model and may not be appropriate for the activity in the education environment). Occupational therapists should review the provision of services across their caseload to ensure that the frequency and duration match the student's needs. Occupational therapy assistants should do this in partnership with the occupational therapist. When recommending changes to better meet the student's needs, the occupational therapist would apply current research-based methods and rigor in the selection of interventions, monitoring of students' progress, and choice of the least restrictive approaches that produce optimal outcomes.

Time management. Practitioners should use time management strategies such as prioritizing tasks and setting work goals, keeping a planner and allocating time for direct and indirect or administrative tasks in their schedule, and seeking help and delegating when necessary (Services for Australian Rural and Remote Allied Health [SARRAH], n.d.-b). In addition, practitioners should take the time to plan their workload individually, as a department, and as a team.

Organizational level

At this level, a group of practitioners or team of service providers might be shifting toward a workload approach. During this process, when sharing individual or group workload issues with principals, administrators, and others, practitioners should remain objective in all communications. They can use data collected during the time study or a copy of weekly schedules to communicate accurate information for decision making, and they can offer solutions for workload management. Strategies to better manage workloads include targeting focused efforts as well as broader initiatives among staff, improving worker effectiveness, and implementing program and practice changes (SARRAH, n.d.-a, n.d.-c).

Recruit and retain staff. Practitioners can encourage the use of revised hiring practices, such as improving worker–job match, offering higher salaries, and providing stipends. To retain staff, administrators can consider providing mentoring opportunities, job sharing or flexible time, and employee recognition and reward programs. Essential trainings, professional development, and advanced education opportunities should also be considered. Staff knowledge and passion can be capitalized on and used to create specialized jobs (e.g., AT, mealtime support team) and to efficiently allocate resources. Administrators can assign support staff to lessen paperwork and complete administrative tasks, thus lightening the workload for occupational therapy practitioners.

Worker effectiveness. Administrators should provide proper training and ensure that practitioners completely understand their assigned responsibilities. They should also confirm competencies and expect practitioners' involvement with new initiatives. Their supervision and supports (e.g., coaching, mentoring, counseling) should allow occupational therapy practitioners to build their specialized knowledge and skills for school practice. In addition, administrators should ensure that practitioners have access to current technology for documentation, decision making, and communication.

Implement program and practice changes. Occupational therapy practitioners should use collaborative teaming practices. They should also adopt early intervening and MTSS to promote successful performance of students in general education, which will decrease the number of referrals and the time required for evaluations. This will require administrative support to remove obstacles as practitioners implement a continuum of practice models.

Apply solution-focused thinking. Rural and remote settings can present particular workload challenges (SARRAH, n.d.-a) in addition to those already discussed in this chapter. These challenges include distance between schools, poorer child health status, lack of resources, higher levels of case variance and complexity, and limited access to specialist support. Each challenge can affect the available options for meeting the student's needs that are reasonably calculated to enable educational progress.

Occupational therapy practitioners who work in rural and remote areas have the potential to work with their supervisors and administrators to promote change and enact innovative workload management. Innovative workload management requires the practitioner to try new ways of looking at scenarios, to remain flexible, and to apply solution-focused thinking (SARRAH, n.d.-a). Solutions might center on delegating tasks when appropriate, using technology (e.g., telehealth, e-supervision, virtual meetings), instituting interprofessional collaboration, meeting staff education and training needs, and clustering (grouping) children on the basis of similar needs and expected outcomes.

External level

Driving change at the external level requires school practitioners to engage in active advocacy efforts and recruitment of stakeholders as well as grasp the political, professional, and social climate (refer to Chapter 9, "Best Leadership Practices Through Everyday Advocacy").

SUMMARY

Large workloads and excessive caseloads make it difficult for school occupational therapy practitioners to provide effective and meaningful services for students and schools. Manageable workloads can make a real difference in practitioners' skilled contributions to student programming; improve staff retention; and ultimately have a positive impact on outcomes for students, schools, and educational systems.

REFERENCES

American Occupational Therapy Association. (2014). Guidelines for supervision, roles, and responsibilities during the delivery of occupational therapy services. *American Journal of Occupational Therapy, 68*(Suppl. 3), S16–S22. https://doi.org/10.5014/ajot.2014.686S03

American Occupational Therapy Association. (2017a). Guidelines for occupational therapy services in early intervention and schools. *American Journal of Occupational Therapy, 71,* 7112410010. https://doi.org/10.5014/ajot.2017.716S01

American Occupational Therapy Association. (2017b). *OT and PT state guidelines for school-based practice.* Retrieved from https://www.aota.org/~/media/Corporate/Files/Secure/Practice/Children/State-Guidelines-School-Based-Practice-20170513.pdf

American Occupational Therapy Association, American Physical Therapy Association, & American Speech–Language–Hearing Association. (2014). *Workload approach: A paradigm shift for positive impact on student outcomes.* Retrieved from https://www.aota.org/-/media/corporate/files/practice/children/apta-asha-aota-joint-doc-workload-approach-schools-2014.pdf

American Psychological Association. (2005). *Determination and documentation of the need for practice guidelines.* Retrieved from https://www.apa.org/practice/guidelines/determination-documentation.pdf

American Speech–Language–Hearing Association. (2002). *A workload analysis approach for establishing speech–language caseload standards in the schools: Guidelines.* Retrieved from http://www.asha.org/policy/GL2002-00066/

Cornell University Law School, Legal Information Institute. (2018). *Collective bargaining.* Retrieved from www.law.cornell.edu/wex/collective_bargaining

Dennis, P. (2007). *Lean production simplified: A plain-language guide to the world's most powerful production system* (2nd ed.). Boca Raton, FL: CRC Press.

District of Columbia Public Schools. (2013). *Missed related service sessions, truancy, and due diligence guidelines.* Retrieved from https://dcps.dc.gov/sites/default/files/dc/sites/dcps/publication/attachments/GAGA-2015-R0046-AttachmentJ11MissedRelatedServiceSessionsTruancyandDueDiligenceGuidelines.pdf

Endrew F. v. Douglas County School District, 15-827 U.S.C. (2017).

Every Student Succeeds Act, Pub. L. 114–195, 129 Stat. 1802 (2015).

Individuals With Disabilities Education Improvement Act of 2004, Pub. L.108–446, 20 U.S.C. §§ 1400–1482.

Jackson, L. (2013). Best practices in determining school workloads. In G. F. Clark & B. E. Chandler (Eds.), *Best practices for occupational therapy in schools* (pp. 131–139). Bethesda, MD: AOTA Press.

Kotter, J. P. (2007, January). Leading change: Why transformation efforts fail. *Harvard Business Review, 85,* 2–9.

Maine Department of Education. (2015). *Chapter 101: Maine unified special education regulation birth to age twenty* (No. 05-071). Retrieved from https://mainedoenews.net/2017/08/30/revisions-to-chapter-101-maine-unified-special-education-regulations-birth-to-twenty/

McCormack, G. L. (2011). Historical and current perspectives of management. In K. Jacobs & G. L. McCormack (Eds.), *The occupational therapy manager* (5th ed., pp. 3–16). Bethesda, MD: AOTA Press.

National Coalition on Personnel Shortages in Special Education and Related Services. (2014). *Special education personnel shortages factsheet.* Retrieved from https://specialedshortages.org/wp-content/uploads/2014/03/NCPSSERS-Fact-Sheet.pdf

Northshore Education Association & Northshore School District No. 417. (2016). *Collective bargaining agreement.* Retrieved from https://www.washingtonea.org/file_viewer.php?id=2751

Ohio Department of Education. (2014). *Ohio Administrative Code Rules 3301-51-01 to 09, 11, and 12.* Retrieved from https://education.ohio.gov/getattachment/Topics/Special-Education/Federal-and-State-Requirements/Operational-Standards-and-Guidance/Ohio-Administrative-Code-Rules-3301-51-01-to-09-11-and-21.pdf.aspx

Polichino, J. (2017). *Caseload to workload: A data-driven approach to school-based OT and PT services.* Retrieved from https://www.occupationaltherapy.com/articles/caseload-to-workload-data-driven-3843

Polichino, J., & Jackson, L. (2014). *Transforming caseload to workload in school-based occupational therapy service.* Retrieved from https://www.aota.org/~/media/Corporate/Files/Secure/Practice/Children/Workload-fact.pdf

Rehabilitation Act of 1973, Pub. L. 93–112, 29 U.S.C. §§ 701–796l.

Rogers, S., & Rhoads, T. (2017). *Workloads and caseloads across the US: Challenge and opportunities for best practice in school settings.* Retrieved from https://douglasesd.k12.or.us/sites/douglasesd.k12.or.us/files/File/rsoi/ties-archive/workload-caseload-3-rogers.pdf

Section 504 of the Rehabilitation Act of 1973, as amended, 29 U.S.C. § 794 (2008).

Services for Australian Rural and Remote Allied Health. (n.d.-a). *Caseload management.* Retrieved from https://www.sarrah.org.au/content/caseload-management

Services for Australian Rural and Remote Allied Health. (n.d.-b). *Time management.* Retrieved from https://www.sarrah.org.au/content/time-management

Services for Australian Rural and Remote Allied Health. (n.d.-c). *Workload management.* Retrieved from https://www.sarrah.org.au/content/workload-management

Smith, R., Anthony, A., Gutierrez, J., Mugnolo, D., Ortega, J., & Talley, V. (2017). *Impact of work demands on school-based occupational therapy services* (Unpublished master's research project). Chicago State University, Chicago.

Swinth, Y. (2008). Collaboration in action: The nitty gritty. In B. Hanft & J. Shepherd (Eds.), *Collaborating for student success: A guide for school-based occupational therapy* (pp. 139–168). Bethesda, MD: AOTA Press.

Staats, B., & Upton, D. M. (2011). Lean knowledge work. *Harvard Business Review, 89*(10), 100–110.

Tyler, K. (2013). *Job worth doing: Update descriptions.* Retrieved from https://www.shrm.org/hr-today/news/hr-magazine/pages/0113-job-descriptions.aspx

Wisconsin State Legislature. (2016). *Chapter PI 11.24: Related service: Physical and occupational therapy.* Retrieved from https://docs.legis.wisconsin.gov/code/admin_code/pi/11/24

Best Practices in School Occupational Therapy Program Evaluation

Rebecca E. Argabrite Grove, MS, OTR/L, FAOTA

15

KEY TERMS AND CONCEPTS

- Assumptions
- Exploratory evaluation
- External factors
- Impact evaluation
- Implementation evaluation
- Logic model
- Outcome evaluation
- Performance measurement
- Process evaluation
- Progress monitoring
- Tier 1 intervention
- Tier 2 intervention
- Tier 3 intervention

OVERVIEW

The evolution of educational laws (e.g., Every Student Succeeds Act [ESSA], 2015, Pub. L. 114–95; Individuals With Disabilities Education Improvement Act of 2004 [IDEA], Pub. L. 108–446) has placed growing emphasis on accountability in school environments. Although ESSA and IDEA both require reporting of annual progress, the accountability and action necessary to ensure positive growth of all students differ. On a macro level, ESSA relies on statewide accountability systems that use multiple measures to demonstrate academic achievement, academic progress, graduation rates, English language proficiency, and both school quality and student success (U.S. Department of Education, 2016).

In contrast, IDEA mandates the provision of a free appropriate public education (FAPE) for individual students who receive specialized instruction and related services, including occupational therapy, in the least restrictive environment (LRE). The individualized education program (IEP) documents how students are provided with access to FAPE.

Over time, legal challenges pertaining to suspected denial of FAPE have served to clarify the evidence necessary to meet this requirement. In 2017, the U.S. Supreme Court issued a unanimous opinion in *Endrew F. v. Douglas County School District* (2017), clarifying that all students must be offered an IEP that is "reasonably calculated to enable a child to make progress appropriate in light of the child's circumstances" (U.S. Department of Education, 2017, p. 1). This ruling emphasized that evidence of progress in light of students' individual circumstances must be "more than *de minimis*" (p. 1).

Although state and local education agencies have flexibility to set goals and measurements of progress at a systems or organizational level, IEP teams make this determination for individual students. State systemic improvement plans required by IDEA, school improvement plans, and annual statewide assessments are common measures used for tracking both the progress and the achievement of students with disabilities.

However, these assessments often do not link outcomes to occupational therapy intervention, nor do they offer meaningful data regarding the quality of special education services or substantive information related to the contribution of occupational therapy to student performance and achievement. Despite the absence of a direct link to measurable occupational therapy outcomes, occupational therapy practitioners[1] have relied on professional documentation tools and resources to create their own accountability systems (Frolek Clark & Handley-More, 2017).

ESSA and IDEA have served to expand the roles and functions of the school occupational therapy practitioner (AOTA, 2016a, 2017b) from helping students with disabilities benefit from their education to working with students in general education to support full participation in the school environment in preparation for postsecondary opportunities. Evidence-based practices have now become a criterion for service provision that is directly linked to the attainment of student growth and outcomes.

As federal, state, and local education programs and budgets continue to be scrutinized and operate under fiscal, temporal, and human resources constraints, how do practitioners ensure that occupational therapy in schools meets policy standards while maintaining quality provision of cost-

---

[1] *Occupational therapy practitioner* refers to both the occupational therapist and the occupational therapy assistant. The American Occupational Therapy Association (AOTA; 2014a, p. S18) states, "The occupational therapist is responsible for all aspects of occupational therapy service delivery and is accountable for the safety and effectiveness of the occupational therapy service delivery process" and "must be directly involved in the delivery of services during the initial evaluation and regularly throughout the course of intervention. . . . The occupational therapy assistant delivers safe and effective occupational therapy services under the supervision of and in partnership with the occupational therapist."

Copyright © 2019 by the American Occupational Therapy Association. All rights reserved. To reuse this content, contact www.copyright.com.
https://doi.org/10.7139/2019.978-1-56900-591-0.015

effective services? How can school occupational therapy practitioners demonstrate the profession's distinct value (AOTA, 2016b) while serving as members of an interprofessional, collaborative education team?

Program evaluation can provide reliable, valid information about a specific program through the application of systematic methods to address questions regarding operations and results that help determine overall value on the basis of performance measures or outcomes (Hatry et al., 2015; Newcomer et al., 2015). Outcomes may be used to increase regulatory compliance, ensure accountability for use of public funds, improve the rigor of services provided, enhance consistency of implementation, and measure overall impact to support organizational capacity (Grob, 2015).

ESSENTIAL CONSIDERATIONS

It can be challenging to measure how occupational therapy practitioners make direct contributions to educationally relevant solutions for students when knowledge and expertise are shared and distributed across intermittent social interactions with IEP team members whose purpose is to identify goals, develop strategies, and monitor student progress (Villeneuve, 2009). Common challenges perceived by occupational therapy practitioners in schools include

- Ambiguity of roles and expectations across IEP team members,
- Personnel shortages,
- Large caseloads,
- Professional isolation,
- Lack of preservice preparation of occupational therapy practitioners and teachers to collaborate, and
- Educational relevance of goals and services provided by occupational therapy (Villeneuve, 2009).

In school practice, it is critical to consider the role and input of various stakeholders, such as parents, students, educators, and administrators. In addition, it is important to account for contextual factors, including cultural responsivity and operational issues, that may affect program performance. Given the dynamic system in which schools operate and students function, consideration of evaluation methods that allow for ongoing changes helps to avoid pitfalls and contributes to evaluation success.

When contemplating a program evaluation, occupational therapy practitioners should consider the following in their discussions with key stakeholders (Newcomer et al., 2015):

- Will the results of the evaluation have the potential to influence decisions about the program?
- Will the evaluation be completed within a reasonable time frame and at a cost that renders it useful?
- Does the program hold enough merit to be evaluated?
- Are there performance concerns or problems associated with the program?
- Where is the program in its stage of development?

Once a commitment has been made to evaluate, practitioners can begin the evaluation planning and design process by focusing on selecting key questions that need to be answered, what information is necessary to answer those questions, methods for data collection, expected outcomes, and potential limitations (Newcomer et al., 2015). The U.S. Government Accountability Office (GAO; 2012) uses a design matrix (see Figure 15.1) as a blueprint for evaluation planning, which is helpful to clarify goals, develop relevant evaluation questions, and identify appropriate data collection methods and analysis procedures to ensure objectivity of the evaluation process.

Logic Model

The *logic model* is a systems model that provides a framework for thinking about planning, implementation, and evaluation. It shows logical relationships among resources that are invested and activities that take place to produce desired outputs and outcomes in a specific context (McLaughlin & Jordan, 2015; U.S. Department of Health and Human Services [DHHS], n.d.). This model provides a visual road map for understanding the elements of a program, assumptions about how they link or work together, and the potential role of context. This information renders the model equally beneficial for planning and designing new programs and for managing existing programs at any point in their life cycle. The logic model also facilitates communication with stakeholders by providing a narrative description of how the program under evaluation operates, like the plot and elements of a story (DHHS, n.d.).

A simple logic model examines inputs (e.g., staff, equipment, materials, time invested), outputs and activities (e.g., what is done, who is reached), and outcomes (e.g., short term, intermediate, long term) to measure impact or performance. This method of evaluation is applicable to single programs (e.g., positive behavioral interventions and supports), single components of a program (e.g., frequency of positive reinforcement per staff member), or a single service (e.g., occupational therapy's impact on behavioral change), and it is helpful for framing a program within a larger organization or context (e.g., school community or classroom; GAO, 2012; see Figure 15.2).

A logic model is meant to be dynamic: It is continually monitored and adjusted accordingly. Standards of quality and usefulness of any logic model design should be examined with input from critical stakeholders before, during, and after the evaluation process.

Assumptions represent values and beliefs, experiences, theories and frames of reference, and research evidence that may influence stakeholders who are engaged in program evaluation (DHHS, n.d.). It is essential to reflect on assumptions throughout the process to avoid bias and yield valid information. Environmental or influential factors, sometimes referred to as *external factors,* are a function of the situational context in which the program exists and may include variables that are driven or restrained by the family; school; or local, state, or federal educational agencies (McLaughlin & Jordan, 2015; GAO, 2012). These factors can have a major influence on the achievement of outcomes.

The logic model can be used to support any of the following 4 major types of program evaluation (Newcomer et al., 2015; Poister, 2015; GAO, 2012; Wholey, 2015):

1. *Exploratory evaluation*—helps establish priorities for further evaluation work
2. *Implementation* or *process evaluation*—examines activities or what happens while a program or service is being carried out

FIGURE 15.1. Sample evaluation design matrix.

Design Matrix Template 2 (GAO version):
Evaluation Name: _____
Evaluation Purpose: _____

RESEARCHABLE QUESTION(S)	INFORMATION REQUIRED AND SOURCE(S)	SCOPE AND METHODOLOGY	LIMITATIONS	WHAT THIS EVALUATION WILL LIKELY ALLOW THE EVALUATOR TO SAY
What questions is the team trying to answer?	What information does the team need to address each evaluation question?	How will the team answer each evaluation question?	What are the design's limitations, and how will it affect the evaluation?	What are the expected results of the work?
Identify specific questions that the team must answer.	Where will they get it?	Describe strategies for collecting the required information or data, such as random sampling, case studies, focus groups, questionnaires, benchmarking to best practices, use of existing databases, etc.	Cite any limitations as a result of the information required or the scope and methodology, such as: —Questionable data quality and/or reliability. —Inability to access certain types of data or obtain data covering a certain time frame. —Security classification or confidentiality restrictions. —Inability to generalize or extrapolate findings to the universe.	Describe what the evaluation team can likely say. Draw on preliminary results for illustrative purposes, if helpful.
Ensure each major evaluation question is specific, objective, neutral, measurable, and doable.	Identify documents or types of information that the team must have.			Ensure that the proposed answer addresses the evaluation question in Column 1.
Ensure key terms are defined.	Identify plans to address internal controls and compliance.			
Each major evaluation question should be addressed in a separate row.	Identify plans to collect documents that establish the "criteria" to be used.	Describe the planned scope of each strategy, including the time frame, locations to visit, and sample sizes.		
	Identify plans to follow up on known significant findings that team found in obtaining background information.	Describe the analytical techniques to be used, such as regression analysis, cost–benefit analysis, sensitivity analysis, modeling, descriptive analysis, content analysis, case study summaries, etc.	Be sure to address how these limitations will affect the evaluation.	
	Identify sources of the required information, such as databases, studies, subject area experts, program officials, models, etc.			

Note. GAO = U.S. Government Accountability Office.
Source. From "The Evaluation Design Matrix: Templates," by Bureau for Policy, Planning and Learning (p. 3), Washington, DC: U.S. Agency for International Development. Copyright © 2015. Available at https://usaidlearninglab.org/sites/default/files/resource/files/evaluation_design_matrix_templates.pdf. In the public domain.

3. *Performance measurement* or *outcome evaluation*—identifies outcomes or results during or after a program or service is completed to determine benefit or improvement
4. *Impact evaluation*—examines effects of the program that are also influenced by external factors to assess net impact.

Target Criteria

IDEA (2004) and other federal laws, state professional regulations, and AOTA practice guidelines and documents outline occupational therapy practices. Occupational therapy practitioners may develop target criteria for their program outcomes from any of these sources.

Procedural outcomes

Occupational therapy practitioners may develop a standard for practice (e.g., district-level evaluation process, documentation requirements, use of assessments) that aligns with state professional regulations or IDEA requirements. AOTA's (2017a) occupational profile template provides a structured format for gathering information and planning an individualized, student-centered approach to intervention.

These types of procedural outcomes may result in the creation of common documentation forms or processes and enhanced communication among IEP team members for assessing and reporting student progress (Frolek Clark & Handley-More, 2017; McKinley-Vargas & Thomas, 2008).

FIGURE 15.2. Sample program logic model.

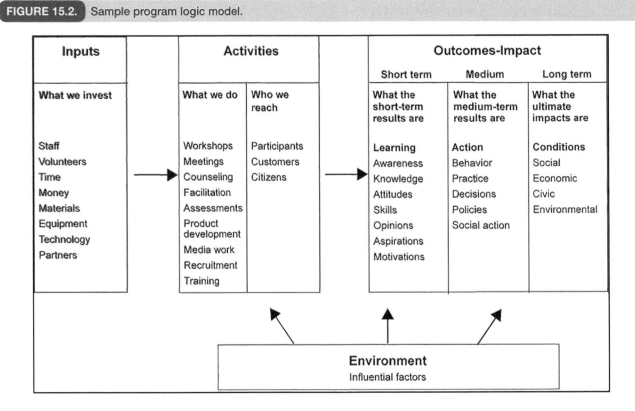

Source. From *Applied Research and Methods: Designing Evaluations*, by U.S. Government Accountability Office, 2012, p. 11. In the public domain.

Improvements in procedural outcomes can be easily planned for and identified through a records review of IEP documents, evaluations, and progress summaries. In addition, productivity concerns can be evaluated with a time study and caseload-to-workload analysis (AOTA, 2014c).

Student outcomes

The role of the occupational therapy practitioner in the educational setting is to provide students with the ability to access and benefit from their educational program. Occupational therapy practitioners support a student's participation and engagement in their education, ADLs, IADLs, social participation, play, leisure, rest and sleep, and work activities in the school environment (AOTA, 2014b, 2016b, 2017b).

Progress monitoring is a scientifically based practice used for ongoing and frequent assessment of students' academic or behavioral performance. This approach may assist practitioners in determining the effectiveness of occupational therapy interventions. Progress monitoring data are collected systematically and frequently during intervention, with adjustments or changes to interventions made on the basis of ongoing analysis and review of the data (Frolek Clark & Handley-More, 2017). When occupational therapy practitioners in schools combine progress monitoring with observation of student performance, work sample reviews, and teacher interviews, they have a variety of methods and tools available for measuring student outcomes.

Substantial and positive student performance gains have been obtained and reported by occupational therapy practitioners in schools in the areas of written communication, fine motor, visual–motor, preacademic and academic, social and behavioral, transition, and work and vocational skills, along with high levels of teacher satisfaction, when a collaborative approach to service provision is used (Dessoye et al., 2017; Ohl et al., 2013; Tomcheck et al., 2016).

Program outcomes

Under ESSA (2015–2016), occupational therapy practitioners are identified as specialized instructional support personnel who should be included in schoolwide planning and the provision of schoolwide intervention programs, including multi-tiered systems of support, under 3 levels of service:
1. *Tier 1 intervention* represents universal programs that are provided to all students with and without disabilities.
2. *Tier 2 intervention* provides targeted group interventions to students who are at risk.
3. *Tier 3 intervention* includes intensive, individualized interventions for students who did not respond to previous interventions and require specialized instruction (AOTA, 2012).

This expansion of services has allowed students with and without disabilities to benefit from occupational therapy practitioners' professional knowledge and skills. Arbesman et al. (2013) found strong evidence for the effectiveness of occupational therapy interventions in all 3 tiers, including schoolwide programs for bullying prevention, after-school performing arts, and stress management; social and life skills programs for at-risk groups of students; and social skills programs for students with autism spectrum disorder, mental illness, and behavior disorders.

Whether they are systemwide or individualized, data-driven interventions should be methodically and systematically measured with specifically defined outcome measures that are identified and reviewed by the IEP team or other appropriate multidisciplinary school teams (Schaaf & Imperatore Blanche, 2012).

BEST PRACTICES

It is important that practitioners use an iterative process of examination and analysis throughout the program evaluation process to facilitate valid, purposeful, meaningful, and applicable information that can support program quality and improvement of services with clients (e.g., students, educational staff, systemwide).

Conducting a Program Evaluation

Occupational therapy practitioners use models or frameworks to plan, implement, and evaluate outcomes or results for their programs. One such model is the logic model described previously. Program evaluation involves the following 8 steps:

1. *Focus:* What will you evaluate (which program or aspect of a program)?
2. *Questions:* What do you want to know?
3. *Indicators or evidence:* How will you know it?
4. *Timing:* When should you collect data?
5. *Data collection:*
   - *Sources*—Who will have the information you need?
   - *Methods*—How will you gather the information?
   - *Sample*—Whom will you question?
   - *Instruments*—What tools will you use?
6. *Analysis*—How will you analyze the data?
7. *Interpretation*—How will you interpret the data?
8. *Communication of results*—How will you communicate the results? To whom? When? Where? How?

EXHIBIT 15.1. Data Inventory Form

Instructions: What evidence do you collect about your program, and at what level? Many programs focus only on the lower levels of evidence (e.g., what the practitioners did, how it went). You can monitor these data using simple record-keeping procedures, but to push further up the hierarchy of evidence, you need to do active assessment. List the data collection tools that you currently use for your program and their data sources. Next, consider other possible data sources for evaluation given your current resources.

LEVELS OF EVIDENCE	DATA COLLECTION TOOLS USED NOW	CURRENT DATA SOURCES	OTHER POTENTIAL DATA COLLECTION TOOLS AND SOURCES
1. *End Results:* Documented increase in students' skills and goal achievement	Achievement-based, standardized, or criterion-based tests	Teacher report	Attendance records, observation- or occupation-based measures of participation and engagement
2. *Practices:* Documented adoption of new behaviors or practices	Observations of teaching or intervention methods	Classrooms	Review of lesson plans and student products and observation of performance in natural settings
3. *Learning:* Documented changes in participants' learning and growth	Preintervention–postintervention comparison of student performance; progress monitoring; performance rubrics	Work samples, clinical observations, assessments	Observation rubrics of staff's or parents' implementation of strategies
4. *Satisfaction:* What participants thought about interventions, their likes and dislikes, their perceptions of quality and utility	Satisfaction survey	General education teachers, special education teachers, teaching assistants	Surveys for students and parents, focus groups
5. *Participation:* Who participated in or was reached by the program, including numbers and descriptive information	Caseload by school	Enrollment reports	Number of students, disability category, hours of teacher planning and collaboration
6. *Interventions:* What was actually done (e.g., direct, indirect, consultation)	Contact reports, intervention plans	Progress reports	Target skill areas, service locations, staff and parent training
7. *Resources:* What it took to develop and deliver the program (e.g., cost, time, staff, resources)	Budget spreadsheet, time tracker, contractual agreements, grant forms	Staff salaries, résumés, work hours, cost estimates for materials and equipment	Support provided by administration, other departments, and community partners and agencies

A data inventory form outlines sample program evaluation levels of evidence (Exhibit 15.1), which may be helpful for planning and documentation. In addition, familiar individual measurement methods and tools currently used in school practice can be considered and included in program evaluation (Frolek Clark & Handley-More, 2017).

Occupational therapists may find that program evaluation of the practitioner's documentation (e.g., are all of the necessary forms being completed in the occupational therapist's working file?) may enhance consistency of services. See Appendix D, "Brief Audit of Occupational Therapy Documentation," and Appendix E, "Full or Partial Audit of Occupational Therapy Documentation," for a template that can be used to identify various forms common to occupational therapy practitioners working in schools.

Program evaluation may also be conducted for student outcomes. The questions asked should reflect information that will be useful in planning or revising occupational therapy services. For example, occupational therapy staff may develop their own questions or pick one of the following questions:

- What percentage of students who receive occupational therapy services are meeting their IEP goals (that are supported by the occupational therapist)?
- How many students being referred are being recommended for services?
- What is the frequency and duration of occupational therapy services for elementary students receiving a particular intervention?
- To what extent is the continuum of occupational therapy services provided to students with disabilities meeting the IDEA LRE requirement?

To collect these data, occupational therapy staff should develop a form for data collection, based on the question. For the first question, codes are developed to indicate the IEP area (e.g., 1 = *dressing*, 2 = *feeding*, 3 = *using materials*, 4 = *play*) and the goal status code (e.g., 5 = *met 95%–100%*, 4 = *not met yet increased 75%–94%*, 3 = *not met yet increased 50%–74%*, 2 = *not met but minimal progress 25%–49%*, 1 = *limited progress under 25%*, 0 = *have not worked on this area*). Staff might want to gather other data as well (e.g., grade, educational disability category, others included on the goal).

At each student's annual review, data should be entered on the form. Initials may be used for confidentiality. If a spreadsheet, such as Excel, is used, the information can be quickly computed and graphed for analysis by the staff or a team of occupational therapy practitioners. If practitioners recognize a pattern across a certain grade, school, or occupation that is not responding to intervention, then they should gather further information (e.g., interviews, observations) to determine whether professional development is needed in that area.

Occupational therapy's contribution to promoting the health and participation of students in the classroom, school context, and greater school community can promote shared discussion and analysis to facilitate efficient achievement of measurable, functional individual and schoolwide outcomes. Given current educational frameworks, occupational therapy practitioners have the opportunity to influence systems-level improvement through the application of practical program evaluation methods and measures.

Occupational therapy practitioners have the opportunity to lead school improvement and performance well beyond the capacity with which the profession was originally envisioned as specialized instructional support personnel. Program evaluation is a critical step in identifying the path for moving occupational therapy practice in schools forward.

SUMMARY

Occupational therapy practitioners strive to achieve continued competence and professional development, to apply research-based interventions, and to provide high-quality services to students in the school setting. Conducting program evaluations can lead to new insights, opportunities to improve programs, measurability of impact, demonstration of accountability, and communication of occupational therapy's distinct value in schools.

REFERENCES

American Occupational Therapy Association. (2012). *AOTA practice advisory on occupational therapy in response to intervention*. Retrieved from http://www.aota.org/~/media/Corporate/Files/Practice/Children/Browse/School/RtI/AOTA%20RtI%20Practice%20Adv%20final%20%20101612.pdf

American Occupational Therapy Association. (2014a). Guidelines for supervision, roles, and responsibilities during the delivery of occupational therapy services. *American Journal of Occupational Therapy, 68*(Suppl. 3), S16–S22. https://doi.org/10.5014/ajot.2014.686S03

American Occupational Therapy Association. (2014b). Occupational therapy practice framework: Domain and process (3rd ed.). *American Journal of Occupational Therapy, 68*(Suppl. 1), S1–S48. https://doi.org/10.5014/ajot.2014.682006

American Occupational Therapy Association. (2014c). *Transforming caseload to workload on school-based occupational therapy services*. Retrieved from https://www.aota.org/~/media/Corporate/Files/Secure/Practice/Children/Workload-fact.pdf

American Occupational Therapy Association. (2016a). *Occupational therapy in school settings*. Retrieved from https://www.aota.org/~/media/Corporate/Files/AboutOT/Professionals/WhatIsOT/CY/Fact-Sheets/School%20Settings%20fact%20sheet.pdf

American Occupational Therapy Association. (2016b). *Occupational therapy's distinct value: Children and youth resource for administrators and policy makers*. Retrieved from https://www.aota.org/~/media/Corporate/Files/Secure/Practice/Children/distinct-value-policy-makers-children-youth.PDF

American Occupational Therapy Association. (2017a). AOTA occupational profile template. *American Journal of Occupational Therapy, 71*(Suppl. 2), 7112420030. https://doi.org/10.5014/ajot.2017.716S12

American Occupational Therapy Association. (2017b). Guidelines for occupational therapy services in early intervention and schools. *American Journal of Occupational Therapy, 71*, 7112410010. https://doi.org/10.5014/ajot.2017.716S01

Arbesman, M., Bazyk, S., & Nochajski, S. M. (2013). Systematic review of occupational therapy and mental health promotion, prevention, and intervention for children and youth. *American Journal of Occupational Therapy, 67*, e120–e130. https://doi.org/10.5014/ajot.2013.008359

Bureau for Policy, Planning and Learning. (2015). *The Evaluation Design Matrix: Templates.* Washington, DC: U.S. Agency for International Development. Retrieved from https://usaidlearninglab.org/sites/default/files/resource/files/evaluation_design_matrix_templates.pdf

Dessoye, J., Davis, L., Mahon, E., Rehrig, S., & Robinson, T. (2017). The effectiveness of a multisensory center-based learning curriculum in prekindergarten students. *American Journal of Occupational Therapy, 71,* 7111520316. https://doi.org/10.5014/ajot.2017.71S1-PO6155

Endrew F. v. Douglas County School District, 15-827 U.S.C. (2017).

Every Student Succeeds Act, Pub. L. 114–195, 129 Stat. 1802 (2015).

Frolek Clark, G. F., & Handley-More, D. (2017). *Best practices for documenting occupational therapy services in schools.* Bethesda, MD: AOTA Press.

Grob, G. F. (2015). Providing recommendations, suggestions, and options for improvement. In K. E. Newcomer, H. P. Hatry, & J. S. Wholey (Eds.), *Handbook of practical program evaluation* (4th ed., pp. 725–738). Hoboken, NJ: Wiley.

Hatry, H. P., Newcomer, K. E., & Wholey, J. S. (2015). Evaluation challenges, issues, and trends. In K. E. Newcomer, H. P. Hatry, & J. S. Wholey (Eds.), *Handbook of practical program evaluation* (4th ed., pp. 816–832). Hoboken, NJ: Wiley.

Individuals With Disabilities Education Improvement Act of 2004, Pub. L. 108–446, 20 U.S.C. §§ 1400–1482.

McKinley-Vargas, J., & Thomas, K. (2008). A framework for change. *OT Practice, 13*(11), 10–15.

McLaughlin, J. A., & Jordan, G. B. (2015). Using logic models. In K. E. Newcomer, H. P. Hatry, & J. S. Wholey (Eds.), *Handbook of practical program evaluation* (4th ed., pp. 62–87). Hoboken, NJ: Wiley.

Newcomer, K. E., Hatry, H. P., & Wholey, J. S. (2015). Planning and designing useful evaluations. In K. E. Newcomer, H. P. Hatry, & J. S. Wholey (Eds.), *Handbook of practical program evaluation* (4th ed., pp. 7–35). Hoboken, NJ: Wiley.

Ohl, A. M., Graze, H., Weber, K., Kenny, S., Salvatore, C., & Wagreich, S. (2013). Effectiveness of a 10-week Tier-1 response to intervention program in improving fine motor and visual–motor skills in general education kindergarten students. *American Journal of Occupational Therapy, 67,* 507–514. https://doi.org/10.5014/ajot.2013.008110

Poister, T. H. (2015). Performance measurement. In K. E. Newcomer, H. P. Hatry, & J. S. Wholey (Eds.), *Handbook of practical program evaluation* (4th ed., pp. 108–136). Hoboken, NJ: Wiley.

Schaaf, R. C., & Imperatore Blanche, E. (2012). Emerging as leaders in autism research and practice: Using the data-driven intervention process. *American Journal of Occupational Therapy, 66,* 503–504. https://doi.org/10.5014/ajot.2012.006114

Tomchek, S., Patten Koenig, K., Arbesman, M., & Lieberman, D. (2016). Occupational therapy interventions for adolescents with autism spectrum disorder. *American Journal of Occupational Therapy, 71,* 7101395010. https://doi.org/10.5014/ajot.2017.711003

U.S. Department of Education. (2016). *Every Student Succeeds Act: Accountability, state plans, and data reporting: Summary of final regulations.* Retrieved from https://www2.ed.gov/policy/elsec/leg/essa/essafactsheet1127.pdf

U.S. Department of Education. (2017). *Questions and answers (Q&A) on U.S. Supreme Court case decision* Endrew F. v. Douglas County School District Re-1. Retrieved from https://www2.ed.gov/policy/speced/guid/idea/memosdcltrs/qa-endrewcase-12-07-2017.pdf

U.S. Department of Health and Human Services, Administration for Children and Families, Office of Planning, Research, and Evaluation (n.d.). *The program manager's guide to evaluation* (2nd ed.). Retrieved from https://www.acf.hhs.gov/sites/default/files/opre/program_managers_guide_to_eval2010.pdf

U.S. Government Accountability Office. (2012). *Applied research and methods: Designing evaluations* (GAO Pub. No. 12-208G). Retrieved from https://www.gao.gov/assets/590/588146.pdf

Villeneuve, M. (2009). A critical examination of school-based occupational therapy collaborative consultation. *Canadian Journal of Occupational Therapy, 76,* 206–218. https://doi.org/10.1177/000841740907600s05

Wholey, J. S. (2015). Exploratory evaluation. In K. E. Newcomer, H. P. Hatry, & J. S. Wholey (Eds.), *Handbook of practical program evaluation* (4th ed., pp. 88–107). Hoboken, NJ: Wiley.

Lauren Holahan, PhD, OTR/L, FAOTA

KEY TERMS AND CONCEPTS

- Children's Health Insurance Program
- Cost settlement process
- Early and Periodic Screening, Diagnostic and Treatment benefit
- Educational relevance
- Fee for service
- Medicaid
- Medical necessity
- Plan of care

OVERVIEW

Depending on the state, estimates suggest that 10%–20% of students with disabilities have occupational therapy as a related service on their individualized education program (IEP). This means that of the 6.5 million students protected under the Individuals With Disabilities Education Improvement Act of 2004 (IDEA; Pub. L. 108–446), between 650,000 and 1.3 million students receive occupational therapy as an essential component of their educational program (U.S. Department of Education, 2016). To meet this service mandate, public schools employ or contract with about 30,000 occupational therapy practitioners[1] nationwide. This results in personnel expenditure that is not supported by general education budgets at the federal, state, or local level.

Fortunately, IDEA (2004) provides funding for special education and related services, such as occupational therapy. Unfortunately, Congress has never allocated the originally promised 40% federal share of the excess cost for educating a student with a disability—historically calculated to be about 2 times greater than the cost of educating a general education student. Most recent data (Dancy, 2016) indicate that federal funding is at 16% (or $1,843 of the $11,534 per student) of the excess cost for educating a student with a disability; the remaining 84% is left to state and local educational agencies (LEAs) to cover, as shown in Figure 16.1.

---

[1]*Occupational therapy practitioner* refers to both the occupational therapist and the occupational therapy assistant. The American Occupational Therapy Association (AOTA; 2014a, p. S18) states, "The occupational therapist is responsible for all aspects of occupational therapy service delivery and is accountable for the safety and effectiveness of the occupational therapy service delivery process" and "must be directly involved in the delivery of services during the initial evaluation and regularly throughout the course of intervention. . . . The occupational therapy assistant delivers safe and effective occupational therapy services under the supervision of and in partnership with the occupational therapist."

In an effort to offset the shortage in federal IDEA funding, in 1988 Congress granted access to Medicaid reimbursement for some health services provided at school with the passage of the Medicare Catastrophic Coverage Act of 1988 (Pub. L. 100–360). As a result, annual Medicaid reimbursement to school services now reduces the $17 billion IDEA burden on states by about $4 billion (McCann, 2013). Although Medicaid fee-for-service reimbursement of some health services provided by schools, including occupational therapy, does not offset the full IDEA funding deficit, it helps significantly.

Moreover, IDEA requires that Medicaid funding precede the financial responsibility of the LEA when it provides services to Medicaid-enrolled students with IEPs (IDEA, 2004, § 300.154). As such, school occupational therapy practitioners and administrators can, in good conscience, participate in compliant school-based Medicaid claiming programs to sustain and strengthen this critical resource.

This chapter provides a brief history of the Medicaid program and describes
- The Medicaid funding mechanisms schools can access;
- Common requirements and challenges for effective school-based claiming; and
- How participation in Medicaid programming affects school occupational therapy practice, including some ethical considerations.

Analysis of future trends and information on where to find additional resources for school-based Medicaid programs are also provided.

ESSENTIAL CONSIDERATIONS

This section provides an overview of the Medicaid program, the history of Medicaid in public education, and key school-based Medicaid program features.

History and Overview of Medicaid

Medicaid, a joint federal–state public health insurance program administered by the Centers for Medicare and Medicaid

---

Copyright © 2019 by the American Occupational Therapy Association. All rights reserved. To reuse this content, contact www.copyright.com.
https://doi.org/10.7139/2019.978-1-56900-591-0.016

FIGURE 16.1. IDEA Part B appropriation vs. full funding estimate.

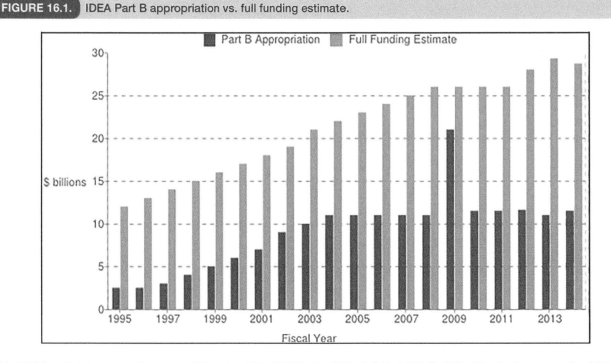

Note. 2009 figure includes American Recovery and Reinvestment Act of 2009 funding. IDEA = Individuals With Disabilities Education Improvement Act of 2004.

Source. From "Fully Funding IDEA: A Democratic Dream or Just an Empty Promise?" [Blog post], by K. Dancy, 2016, March 23. Retrieved from https://www.newamerica.org/education-policy/edcentral/fully-funding-idea/. Open source.

Services (CMS), was established by Congress in 1965 as part of President Lyndon B. Johnson's administration of the Great Society vision. Today, the program serves more than 74 million individuals in low-income working families, older adults, and individuals with disabilities. Children and youth represent 50% of all Medicaid enrollees but account for just 19% of total Medicaid spending, which reached $545.1 billion in 2015 (CMS, 2017). Currently, Medicaid spending represents less than one-fifth of the total national health expenditure in the United States and costs less per enrollee than employer-based insurance (Coughlin et al., 2013).

Two years after the original Medicaid program was established, Congress added the ***Early and Periodic Screening, Diagnostic and Treatment*** (EPSDT) ***benefit*** for children younger than age 21 years who are enrolled in Medicaid. EPSDT supports age-appropriate medically necessary screening, preventive services, and treatment services to address any identified conditions and to ensure that children and youth receive the right care at the right time in the right setting (CMS, 2014).

In 1997, the federal government established the ***Children's Health Insurance Program*** (CHIP) to make possible coverage for children and youth living in families whose income exceeded Medicaid thresholds but who could not afford private coverage. States have considerable flexibility in how they manage their Medicaid, EPSDT, and CHIP programs and leverage the federal share (57% national average) of funding-covered services (Snyder & Rudowitz, 2015). Each state codifies its array of Medicaid services and rules for coverage in a CMS-approved state plan and subsequent amendments.

In terms of the 37 million children enrolled in the program, the Medicaid investment has improved health outcomes, reduced disparities in access to health care, and enhanced academic achievement and greater future earnings of Medicaid-enrolled children (Brown et al., 2015). Children covered by Medicaid during their childhood also experienced fewer hospitalizations and emergency department visits, were more likely to graduate from high school and college, earned higher wages, and paid more in taxes as adults (Wherry et al., 2015). In most states, currently covered services include pediatric primary and specialty care, care for children and youth who are medically fragile to support them living at home rather than in institutional settings, evidence-based therapy services, and transportation support to and from appointments (Cuello et al., 2017).

Medicaid in Schools

As discussed in the introduction, in 1988, state Medicaid entities were required to allow LEAs access to Medicaid-enrolled students' benefits for covered, medically necessary services provided at school, as long as the LEAs met program requirements and before they accessed IDEA funds. To be appropriately educated, many students with disabilities require costly health and therapy services. Medicaid reimbursement for those services reduces special education costs and supports limited education budgets overall, as illustrated in Figure 16.2 (Schubel, 2017).

In 2014, CMS reversed a long-standing position (the "free care" rule) that prohibited reimbursement for school health services provided to any student (e.g., dental, vision, hearing screenings), such that schools may now seek reimbursement for health services named under the Medicaid state plan or EPSDT for all Medicaid-enrolled students, regardless of IDEA eligibility. Funding for Medicaid services provided by schools generally takes the form of fee-for-service payments, as well as support for Medicaid administrative outreach expenditures. ***Fee for service*** is a reimbursement method in which the care provider submits a claim for each discrete, allowable service (e.g., evaluation, intervention, reevaluation) to the payer (e.g., Medicaid) after services have been rendered. The payer then reviews the claim to ensure all program requirements are met and, if so, pays the provider a previously agreed-on fee for the service. Combined reimbursements through the various school-based programs tally less than 1% of the overall federal Medicaid allocation (Pudeleski, 2017). These programs are described in detail.

Fee for service

Although Medicaid fee-for-service policies for school occupational therapy services vary from state to state, all state Medicaid agencies that reimburse schools for services provided to Medicaid-enrolled students include occupational therapy on their lists of covered services. As such, many school occupational therapy practitioners have occasion to interface with the Medicaid program. When occupational therapy is covered, services are typically defined as evaluation, reevaluation, and direct one-on-one intervention. Common requirements for each of these service types are described. Few states reimburse group school occupational therapy interventions or consultation activities, such as time spent in IEP meetings and collaborative planning with parents, teachers, and other team members.

Common requirements for reimbursement of occupational therapy services provided by schools include the following:

- Occupational therapy is a covered Medicaid service, paid at a rate set by an approved methodology.
- Service is provided to a Medicaid-enrolled student.
- The LEA or the occupational therapy practitioner is a recognized Medicaid provider, meeting all federal and state provider qualifications.
- Service is medically necessary.
- Services are not duplicative.
- Providers maintain auditable documentation to support claims.
- The state conducts appropriate financial oversight of provider reimbursement (e.g., audits).
- All other program requirements are met.

Additional program requirements specific to school-based fee-for-service clinical coverage policies may include obtaining physician orders for school occupational therapy services and ensuring that occupational therapy is documented in a formal plan (e.g., IEP, Section 504 plan, behavioral intervention plan, individual health care plan). Moreover, in compliance with the Family Educational Rights and Privacy Act of 1974 (Pub. L. 93–380; 34 C.F.R. Part 99) and IDEA (§ 300.154.d.2.iv), LEAs must obtain one-time parental consent before releasing students'

FIGURE 16.2. How Medicaid reimbursements offset the cost of educating students with disabilities.

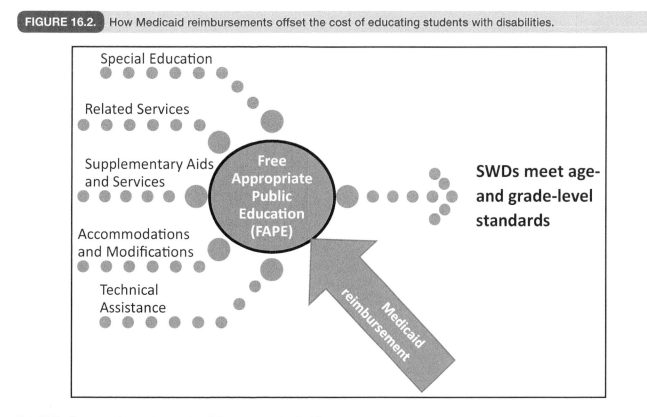

Note. FAPE = free appropriate public education; SWD = students with disabilities.

personally identifiable educational information to the Medicaid agency for the purpose of recovering costs for rendered services. The consent and required annual notification must also ensure that the parent understands that consent is voluntary and does not expire unless the parent revokes it, which they may do at any time. Medicaid-reimbursed services provided at school cannot affect a student's other Medicaid benefits or result in cost to the family.

Medicaid Administrative Claiming Program

An estimated 5% of children younger than age 18 years in the United States are uninsured; most are school-age students, and almost all are eligible for Medicaid (Clarke et al., 2016). Schools are in a unique position to help enroll eligible-but-unenrolled children in Medicaid or CHIP and connect them to other health care services and providers (CMS, 2003). This is both a public health and a public education opportunity: When children are healthy, they perform better on indicators of achievement, including academic performance, attendance, grades, cognitive skills, attitudes, and in-class behavior (Walker et al., 2010). Having health insurance is a primary determinant of overall health.

To that end, federal matching Medicaid funds are available to schools through the Medicaid Administrative Claiming (MAC) program to support the cost of administrative activities aimed at identifying and enrolling eligible children and youth into Medicaid. If school resources are used and employees perform administrative activities that are in support of the state Medicaid plan, federal reimbursement may be available (CMS, 2003). Activities in support of Medicaid might include educating parents and students about Medicaid, assisting with Medicaid applications, and helping families access services both at school and in the community.

In most states, a quarterly random-moment time study identifies the extent to which select employees (occupational therapy practitioners are commonly selected) are engaged in Medicaid-supportive activities. Compliance with MAC program requirements is a prerequisite to accessing fee-for-service reimbursement in many states, given that MAC data are often used to calculate the fee-for-service rates.

Cost settlement

In many states in which Medicaid school-based MAC and fee-for-service programs are aligned, an annual cost-reporting mechanism exists to ensure that LEAs are neither under- nor overpaid for their expenditures for Medicaid-enrolled students. Through the *cost settlement process,* LEAs determine the actual cost of delivering direct medical services (e.g., salaries, materials and supplies, depreciation) to Medicaid beneficiaries. If the LEA's annual expenditures exceed what it received in reimbursement, the state Medicaid agency makes up the difference. If the LEA's annual expenditures are lower than what it received in reimbursement, the state Medicaid agency recoups the overage. Although the technical aspects of cost settlement exceed the scope of this discussion, it is important for school occupational therapy practitioners to understand

that, through processes such as cost reporting, LEAs cannot incur a profit in their Medicaid programs.

Postpayment reviews and audits

All state Medicaid agencies are required to maintain program integrity for each policy covered in the Medicaid state plan, including LEA claiming programs. States have flexibility in how claim validity is monitored, and, as such, considerable variation exists. Many states audit randomly sampled claims by requesting that the LEA produce all relevant documentation connected with the investigated claim. Such documentation can include, for example,

- Evaluation report;
- Plan of care (i.e., occupational therapy intervention plan);
- Progress reports;
- Contact reports;
- IEP, 504, or individual health plan;
- Physician order (if required by the state); and
- Copy of occupational therapy practitioner's license.

In these states, LEA Medicaid program administrators are well served when student records, including occupational therapy reports, are routinely archived. Scheduled internal or self-audits also assist in preparation for a potential Medicaid review. Medicaid agencies may recoup funds when discrepancies or errors are found during review, and in some cases, extrapolation to all claims for a given time period may occur when error rates exceed acceptable standards.

BEST PRACTICES

In this review of best practices for integrating Medicaid claiming requirements with educationally relevant occupational therapy, the occupational therapy process is used as the organizing framework for meeting the mandates of both IDEA and Medicaid standards.

Medicaid and School Occupational Therapy

This section examines how Medicaid claiming programs intersect with the occupational therapy process (AOTA, 2014b) in schools, a common misperception about the incompatibility of the education model, the framework in which school occupational therapy is situated, and the medical model. Before this discussion, however, the framework in which Medicaid is situated bears attention.

To be clear, school occupational therapy practitioners must ensure the *educational relevance* of their services. In simple terms, this means making certain that occupational therapy is required to ensure that a student has access to an appropriate education and experiences educational benefit. Medicaid, conversely, adheres to the standard of *medical necessity* when determining whether a given service will be approved and reimbursed. Medically necessary services generally are

- Essential to prevent, diagnose, or treat medical conditions;
- Essential to enable an individual to attain, maintain, or regain functional capacity;
- Provided within professionally accepted standards of practice and national guidelines;

- Required to meet a person's physical and behavioral health needs;
- Not provided at the convenience of the individual, the provider, or the payer; and
- Reviewed by a physician, who then provides orders for services outlined in the IEP (if required by that state).

Although educational relevance and medical necessity have different parameters, they are not mutually exclusive, particularly when a school team has determined that a health care service (e.g., occupational therapy) is an essential feature of a student's educational program. That is, some educationally relevant occupational therapy services may also be medically necessary and, as such, reimbursable according to a state's school-based Medicaid policy. When services are deemed educationally relevant but not medically necessary, the LEA may be obligated to provide occupational therapy to a student without seeking reimbursement for the service.

Either way, the determination of medical necessity happens well after the decision about the need for educationally relevant occupational therapy. Medical necessity, and Medicaid policy requirements in general, should never influence decisions regarding a student's need for or implementation of (e.g., intensity, duration, location, service focus) occupational therapy at school.

School-Based Medicaid Programs and the Occupational Therapy Process

Best practices for implementing the occupational therapy process in school settings are thoroughly described in other chapters; in this chapter, the analysis focuses primarily on how Medicaid programs affect occupational therapy in schools, with priority given to implications for documentation. As previously indicated, much variability exists among state Medicaid plans and policies for LEA claiming programs.

Although most state Medicaid programs align clinical coverage policies with state licensure rules for occupational therapy (including delineation of responsibilities between occupational therapists and occupational therapy assistants), occupational therapy practitioners and administrators participating in school-based Medicaid programs should carefully review their state's Medicaid policy for LEA claiming requirements. Also, because of the diversity from state to state regarding procedure codes, fee schedules, and the extent to which school occupational therapy practitioners interface with claim creation or submission, that aspect of documentation is not addressed here.

Regardless of state policy variation, Medicaid requires that documentation of school occupational therapy services be auditable at any time to verify both the accuracy of a submitted claim and that services were actually rendered. What follows is an overview of common instances in which Medicaid requirements can be met in concert with special education policies and AOTA's (2018) *Guidelines for Documentation of Occupational Therapy*, such that school occupational therapy documentation is created to meet the needs of a variety of audiences.

Evaluation and reevaluation

Medicaid programs typically require a written evaluation report that includes an occupational profile of the student's participation at school (see Appendix B, "AOTA Occupational Profile Template"), an analysis of occupational performance, and, when appropriate, recommended outcomes to target. The required frequency of evaluation and reevaluation under the LEA Medicaid policies may or may not align with educational evaluation schedules. Practitioners should carefully analyze discrepancies analyzed to determine how program compliance will be reconciled.

The use of standardized assessments is not a Medicaid requirement in most cases, but a suggested list of performance areas to evaluate is often included in a state's school-based Medicaid policy. The Medicaid-suggested areas tend to mirror the language from the *Occupational Therapy Practice Framework: Domain and Process* (3rd ed., or *OTPF–3*; AOTA, 2014b), describing body functions, body structures, and performance skills. Although assessment of student performance at this level may be required to locate evidence-based interventions to match with student need, school occupational therapists are tasked with translating how underlying performance skills and student factors affect participation throughout the school day. Moreover, in the realm of Medicaid, the purposes of an occupational therapy evaluation are to

- Describe a student's disabling condition (if such exists),
- Determine whether the student requires occupational therapy, and, if so,
- Make a case for medical necessity.

For reevaluations, providing evidence for why therapy is recommended to continue or stop is also part of the Medicaid inquiry. Some states' school-based Medicaid policies are so dedicated to this construct that occupational therapy evaluations and reevaluations are only reimbursed when the student's ensuing educational program includes occupational therapy as a direct service.

In contrast, an educationally relevant occupational therapy evaluation provides the school team with a high-definition view of the student's strengths and needs related to the specific occupations a student engages in at school. The educational and Medicaid aims with evaluation are different but not wholly incompatible. School occupational therapists must prioritize the educational relevance mandate and then consider what additional language or rationale could supplement the report to inform a medical necessity determination later, should occupational therapy be part of the student's educational program.

Intervention planning

If a student requires occupational therapy at school to be appropriately educated, then an intervention plan (or, as Medicaid calls it, a **plan of care**) is developed. With the elimination of the free care rule described previously, the number and types of plans accepted by state Medicaid agencies as plans of care—and what constitutes authorization for implementing the plan of care—are rapidly shifting.

In some states, Medicaid allows a team-developed IEP, 504 plan, or individualized health or behavior intervention plan to serve as the authorized, stand-alone plan of care for occupational therapy. In other states, a separate occupational therapy intervention plan is required, in addition to the educational plan. Regardless, the AOTA (2015) *Standards of Practice for Occupational Therapy* require the occupational therapist to complete an intervention plan for any client who is receiving services. The IEP will not meet this requirement.

It is clear across state Medicaid policies that a document describing the student's goals, anticipated skilled interventions, and intensity of services, based on data derived from the evaluation, must exist. It is worth noting that, in terms of intensity of services, Medicaid interprets the prescribed frequency and duration of services as the maximum amount of service that will be reimbursed. In most educational plans, frequency and duration are considered the minimum intensity a student requires to make progress.

Aside from this departure, the Medicaid requirement for a plan of care correlates almost seamlessly with the *OTPF–3*'s description of an intervention plan. It also fits well with the IDEA mandate that IEPs describe specially designed instruction and interventions, which are provided by a specialist (e.g., a licensed school occupational therapy practitioner) to meet a student's unique educational needs.

Intervention

Intervention sessions represent the bulk of school-based Medicaid claims for occupational therapy. Again, each state has its own list of criteria for covered interventions (or procedures), rules for how covered services are documented, the number of intervention sessions that will be reimbursed in a given time period, and who is eligible to provide covered services. As with evaluation and reevaluation, Medicaid's interest in intervention documentation is medical necessity. As a result, the following features of a contact report are commonly highlighted in states' school-based Medicaid claiming policies:

- Description of targeted goals or outcomes;
- Description of skilled or specially designed interventions used;
- Data regarding student's response;
- Plan for continued treatment (intervention);
- Duration of intervention session (usually in minutes);
- Signature and credentials of provider; and
- Clear record of assistant supervision, when relevant.

If occupational therapy assistants are eligible providers under a state's school-based Medicaid policy, practitioners will need to compare licensure standards with the policy to ensure that delegated services are dually compliant.

Progress monitoring and reporting

Most school-based Medicaid policies require a scheduled, data-rich summary of student progress during the authorization period, which often parallels the educational plan dates. As with educational progress monitoring and documentation, the Medicaid interim report provides the following:

- Summary and analysis of student performance data since the last progress report (e.g., every 4.5 or 9 weeks);
- Occupational therapy perspective on the student's progress toward goals;
- Justification for ongoing services and what the student needs to work on next; and
- Opportunity to review or revise the intervention plan.

For Medicaid programs, the interest in progress reporting is to evaluate the medical necessity and effectiveness of recently reimbursed services and to ensure continued student need for medically necessary services. As with evaluation or reevaluation reports, when progress reports are written for a variety of audiences (e.g., parents, educators, education compliance officers, Medicaid claim reviewers or auditors), school occupational therapists may need to deftly embed and define language promoting medical necessity within participation-level descriptions of student occupational performance.

School Occupational Therapy Program Administration and Medicaid

Medicaid programs insert unique management and ethical considerations into oversight of staff and program integrity. As such, this section focuses on administration of school occupational therapy programs and personnel when interfacing with Medicaid claiming occurs.

Employment and contracting

If an LEA has active Medicaid fee-for-service or MAC programs, then participation expectations for employed and contracted occupational therapy practitioners should be clearly defined in open position postings, contracts for services, job descriptions, and performance evaluation instruments. Funding for occupational therapy positions must be carefully examined. If positions are underwritten with federal IDEA dollars, then services provided by those practitioners may not be reimbursable through federal Medicaid dollars.

For independent contractors (e.g., private practitioner, purchased services through agency), best practice in terms of Medicaid programming suggests that the contractor submit service documentation as an agent of or under the LEA Medicaid provider number. The LEA should then pay the contractor their usual and customary rate for services rendered. From there, the LEA can generate Medicaid claims from the contractor data in the same way it produces claims from directly hired staff.

Currently, the United States is experiencing a workforce shortage of allied health service providers, particularly in rural areas (U.S. Department of Health and Human Services, 2013). The shortage includes occupational therapy practitioners (Lin et al., 2015), and schools are particularly affected because they are often unable to compete with salaries for related service providers in health care settings (Bachman & Flanagan, 1999). As such, costs recovered for Medicaid-payable services are critical in supporting recruitment and retention efforts for occupational therapy practitioners in schools.

Workload and logistics

When implemented thoughtfully and efficiently, Medicaid program participation should not increase occupational therapy practitioners' effort, time, or workload. If Medicaid documentation requirements are based on occupational therapy licensure board and national standards of practice—which many states have achieved—then complying with Medicaid policy will not add to a practitioner's workload. Perceived workload increases resulting from Medicaid program participation tend to be rooted in

- Poor alignment among occupational therapy standards of practice, licensure board requirements, and Medicaid policy requirements;
- Occupational therapy practitioners writing multiple or duplicate reports for a single intervention session (e.g., note to parent, handwritten contact report, electronic Medicaid documentation); and
- Lack of accountability or monitoring that results in documentation backlogs, which are experienced as extra work.

Every effort should be made to streamline documentation, such that occupational therapy practitioners compose 1 report per intervention session that is leveraged for communication with a variety of stakeholders, including the agent preparing the Medicaid claim. This streamlining process requires collaborative problem solving among practitioners, LEA administrators, and, when relevant, documentation representatives. When the LEA requires electronic documentation, practitioners need ready access to input devices (e.g., computers, tablets, smartphones) and reliable Internet connections. Medicaid policies for how frequently documentation must be submitted varies across states; in some states, documentation must be completed on the date of service, whereas in other states LEAs have up to 1 year from the date of service to submit a claim.

Ethical Considerations

At no point in the school occupational therapy process should a student's Medicaid enrollment status affect educational decision making. For instance, if a student's IEP team needs performance data from an occupational therapist's professional lens, then an occupational evaluation should be conducted, regardless of anticipated need for service and Medicaid reimbursement of the evaluation. Similarly, during initial placement, annual review, reevaluation, and discontinuation of occupational therapy, the need for therapy, intensity of therapy, and service model should never be influenced by a student's Medicaid eligibility.

To establish equitable and coherent services across the LEA, administrators should avoid assigning all Medicaid-enrolled students to 1 or more select practitioners, including contractors. Given these considerations, it is considered best practice for school occupational therapy practitioners to be blinded to students' Medicaid enrollment whenever possible to limit potential conflicts of interest and help ensure that consistent professional reasoning is used for all students receiving school occupational therapy.

SUMMARY

LEAs optimize financial resources by recovering costs for Medicaid-covered services whenever possible, and these funds help improve education for all students (Pudeleski, 2017). School districts rely on Medicaid to help provide school-based health care, such as vaccinations, vision and hearing screenings, and mental health care. They also use Medicaid funding to help pay for medically necessary special education services under IDEA (2004).

IDEA (2004) requires that LEAs use Medicaid funds before spending federal special education dollars for covered health services that are provided under an IEP (e.g., occupational therapy, audiology, nursing, physical therapy, speech therapy, psychological therapy, social work). In addition, states now have the option to access students' Medicaid benefits for non-IEP services, such as screenings, 504 plan services, and services identified in individual health plan and behavior intervention plans, given that all other Medicaid requirements are met and parental consent is in place.

Future considerations for Medicaid-funded school occupational therapy include growing interest in and advocacy for reimbursement for teletherapy to address staffing shortages and service gaps, particularly in rural and underserved areas. Also, several states have submitted Medicaid state plan amendments to include reimbursement to schools for non-IEP services, which may open opportunities for occupational therapy practitioners to work with general education students and more fully participate in the provision of behavioral and mental health services.

Health care reform deserves attention from school occupational therapy practitioners and administrators as well, given that proposals that include reduction of federal Medicaid allocations to states, block grants, per capita caps, and transitions to managed care will affect schools' ability to provide needed health services such as occupational therapy. One solution to the managed care issue has been to carve out (i.e., exclude) school services from managed care capitation rates and continue with the traditional fee-for-service claiming (Bachman & Flanagan, 1999). Some schools use the Medicaid reimbursements to finance special education or related services. This ensures that students who need the Medicaid-funded services will have access to them in the future.

In all, Medicaid cost recovery in schools is an important resource for the ongoing provision of essential occupational therapy services to students with and, increasingly, without disabilities. School occupational therapy practitioners and administrators are encouraged to continue to educate themselves about the school-based Medicaid program in their state by visiting the state Medicaid agency website, familiarizing themselves with Medicaid policy, and partnering with the state educational agency to advocate for protection and improvement of access to Medicaid funds for school services.

REFERENCES

American Occupational Therapy Association. (2014a). Guidelines for supervision, roles, and responsibilities during the delivery of occupational therapy services. *American Journal of Occupational Therapy, 68*(Suppl. 3), S16–S22. https://doi.org/10.5014/ajot.2014.686S03

American Occupational Therapy Association. (2014b). Occupational therapy practice framework: Domain and process (3rd ed.). *American Journal of Occupational Therapy, 68*(Suppl. 1), S1–S48. https://doi.org/10.5014/ajot.2014.682006

American Occupational Therapy Association. (2015). Standards of practice for occupational therapy. *American Journal of Occupational Therapy, 69*, 6913410057. https://doi.org/10.5014/ajot.2015.696S06

American Occupational Therapy Association. (2018). Guidelines for documentation of occupational therapy. *American Journal of Occupational Therapy, 72*(Suppl. 2), 7212410010. https://doi.org/10.5014/ajot.2018.72S203

American Recovery and Reinvestment Act of 2009, Pub. L. 111–115, 123 Stat. 306.

Bachman, S., & Flanagan, S. (1999). *Medicaid billing for IDEA services: Analysis and policy implications of site visit results.* Washington, DC: U.S. Department of Health and Human Services, Office of the Assistant Secretary for Planning and Evaluation.

Brown, D., Kowalski, A., & Lurie, I. (2015). *Medicaid as an investment: What is the long-term impact on tax receipts?* Suitland, MD: National Bureau of Economic Statistics.

Centers for Medicare & Medicaid Services. (2003). *Medicaid school-based administrative claiming guide.* Baltimore: Author.

Centers for Medicare & Medicaid Services. (2014). *EPSDT—A guide for states: Coverage in the Medicaid benefit for children and adolescents.* Retrieved from https://www.medicaid.gov/medicaid/benefits/downloads/epsdt_coverage_guide.pdf

Centers for Medicare & Medicaid Services. (2017). *Updated November 2017 applications, eligibility, and enrollment data.* Retrieved from https://data.medicaid.gov/Enrollment/2017-11-Updated-applications-eligibility-determina/t8qi-4ycp/data

Clarke, T., Norris, T., & Schiller, J. (2016). *Early release of selected estimates based on data from the 2016 National Health Interview Survey.* Hyattsville, MD: National Center for Health Statistics.

Coughlin, T., Long, S., Clemmons-Cope, L., & Resnick, D. (2013). *What difference does Medicaid make?* San Francisco: Kaiser Family Foundation.

Cuello, L., Reid, D., & Turner W. (2017). *Protect Medicaid funding: Children's health* (Issue 1). Washington, DC: National Health Law Program. Retrieved from https://healthlaw.org/resource/protect-medicaid-funding-childrens-health-issue-1-updated-june-2017/

Dancy, K. (2016, March 23). Fully funding IDEA: A democratic dream or just an empty promise? [Blog post]. Retrieved from https://www.newamerica.org/education-policy/edcentral/fully-funding-idea/

Family Educational Rights and Privacy Act of 1974, Pub. L. 93–380, 20 U.S.C. § 1232g; 34 C.F.R. Part 99.

Individuals With Disabilities Education Improvement Act of 2004, Pub. L. 108–446, 20 U.S.C. §§ 1400–1482.

Lin, V., Zhang, X., & Dixon, P. (2015). Occupational therapy workforce in the United States: Forecasting nationwide shortages. *Physical Medicine and Rehabilitation, 9,* 946–954. https://doi.org/10.1016/j.pmrj.2015.02.012

Medicare Catastrophic Coverage Act of 1988, Pub. L. 100–360, 102 Stat. 68, 42 U.S.C. § 1305.

McCann, S. (2013). *IDEA funding.* Washington, DC: New America.

Pudeleski, S. (2017). *Cutting Medicaid: A prescription to hurt the neediest kids.* Alexandria, VA: School Superintendents Association.

Schubel, J. (2017, April 18). Medicaid helps schools help children [Blog post]. Retrieved from https://www.cbpp.org/research/health/medicaid-helps-schools-help-children

Snyder, L., & Rudowitz, R. (2015). *Medicaid financing: How does it work and what are the implications?* San Francisco: Kaiser Family Foundation.

Walker, S., Kerns, S., Lyon, A., Bruns, E., & Cosgrove, T. (2010). Impact of school-based health center use on academic outcomes. *Journal of Adolescent Health, 46,* 251–257. https://doi.org/10.1016/j.jadohealth.2009.07.002

Wherry, L., Miller, S., Kaestner, R., & Meyer, B. (2015). *Childhood Medicaid coverage and later life health care utilization* (NBER Working Paper No. 20929). Cambridge, MA: National Bureau of Economic Research. Retrieved from https://www.nber.org/papers/w20929

U.S. Department of Education, National Center for Education Statistics. (2016). *Digest of education statistics, 2015* (NCES 2016-014). Washington, DC: Author

U.S. Department of Health and Human Services. (2013). *The U.S. health workforce chartbook.* Rockville, MD: Health Resources and Services Administration, National Center for Health Workforce Analysis.

KEY TERMS AND CONCEPTS

- Alliteration
- Attained curriculum
- Collaborative consultation
- Common Core curriculum
- Conventional literacy
- Coteaching
- Dialogic reading
- Differentiated instruction
- Early literacy
- Emergent literacy
- Engineering design process
- Environmental print
- Family literacy
- Implemented curriculum
- Intended curriculum
- Literacy
- Phonemic awareness
- Phonological awareness
- Preliteracy
- Shared reading
- STEM

OVERVIEW

To be successful in school and the workforce, students need to be proficient readers and writers. The definition of *proficient* is ever changing, however. The constant for proficiency is dependent on the accumulation of experiences and adult–student and student–student interactions in the home, community, and educational settings. In addition, the need for skills in *science, technology, engineering, and mathematics* (STEM)—not just the basics of operation but application in real-world contexts—is necessary in our increasingly complex world (Hwang & Taylor, 2016).

Most recent analysis of reading trends indicates no significant change in reading scores over the past few years (McFarland et al., 2017). A high number of students remain below basic levels of reading (i.e., 31% of 4th graders, 24% of 8th graders, and 28% of 12th graders). In 2014, 43% of 8th graders scored at the proficient level on a new measure that used real-world situations involving technological and engineering problems to assess their knowledge and skills (Nation's Report Card, 2014).

Literacy is embedded in a person's daily life skills and includes reading, writing, speaking, and listening skills (Common Core State Standards Initiative [CCSSI], 2010). It begins in infancy through early literacy and language experiences. In addition, the national movement toward STEM activities brings new learning experiences for students from preschool through high school to prepare them not only for better work-related opportunities but also for an enhanced quality of life. STEM concepts that encompass literacy concepts and have potential for newly embedded language can be found in daily life activities (e.g., calculating tips, using smart devices; Hwang & Taylor, 2016).

In recent years, the number of students interested in STEM careers has declined, whereas the estimated need for workers is projected to grow 14%–62% (U.S. Department of Education, 2018). Unfortunately, the educational field as a whole does not yet know how to support diverse learners in accessing STEM; approximately 5% of students with disabilities have been able to join the STEM workforce (Israel et al., 2013).

Emphasis on and accountability for literacy development are found in federal education laws (Every Student Succeeds Act [ESSA; 2015], Pub. L. 114–195, and Individuals With Disabilities Education Improvement Act of 2004 [IDEA], Pub. L. 108–446). The focus is on

- Teaching to high academic standards that prepare students for college and careers;
- Increasing the number of students participating in the district's statewide assessments;
- Enhancing technology infrastructures at the building level;
- Increasing accessibility to diverse learners; and
- Providing technology training and accessibility for parents to support their children's achievement.

School occupational therapy practitioners[1] have important roles as service providers (IDEA, 2004), specialized instructional support personnel (SISP; ESSA, 2015), and

---

[1]*Occupational therapy practitioner* refers to both the occupational therapist and the occupational therapy assistant. The American Occupational Therapy Association (AOTA; 2014a, p. S18) states, "The occupational therapist is responsible for all aspects of occupational therapy service delivery and is accountable for the safety and effectiveness of the occupational therapy service delivery process" and "must be directly involved in the delivery of services during the initial evaluation and regularly throughout the course of intervention. . . . The occupational therapy assistant delivers safe and effective occupational therapy services under the supervision of and in partnership with the occupational therapist."

Copyright © 2019 by the American Occupational Therapy Association. All rights reserved. To reuse this content, contact www.copyright.com.
https://doi.org/10.7139/2019.978-1-56900-591-0.017

collaborative consultants at the building and district levels. As part of the educational team, occupational therapists can be instrumental in designing and offering interventions that focus on these areas of occupation as well as underlying performance skills (e.g., motor, process, social interaction skills) and the technology to promote literacy and real-world application of STEM activities. Collaborating with other school personnel about connecting learning to everyday life experiences is the true essence of STEM, an interdisciplinary and authentic approach to learning rather than didactic teaching of isolated facts from science and math (Israel et al., 2013).

ESSENTIAL CONSIDERATIONS

Occupational therapy practitioners must understand how literacy skills affect school participation across academic areas, including STEM activities, and the influence of curriculum and instruction on skill development. The movement toward a national core curriculum is also discussed in this chapter.

Occupations

School occupational therapy practitioners are not responsible for the instruction and curriculum of students in a classroom; that is the teacher's role. Occupational therapy practitioners focus on access to, engagement with, and participation in daily life activities (i.e., occupations). When a student is struggling with a meaningful, purposeful activity, such as reading, writing, or a STEM project, an occupational therapist might be asked to evaluate the person, the activity (occupation), or the environment to determine supports and barriers to increase performance. For example, a student with a physical disability might need modifications to access the classroom books for reading or need technology to assist in writing. A student with a mental health condition might require special seating or instruction to focus on the activity, need to avoid areas of the room with too much noise, or need to be closer to the teacher for more frequent positive feedback.

Four Stages of Literacy Development

Occupational therapy practitioners may provide services to students at any of the 4 stages of literacy development outlined by Dunst et al. (2006):
1. *Preliteracy* is the acquisition of the precursors to language, which include the development of nonverbal and social skills, such as acquiring joint attention and reciprocity, making gestures (ranging from body language to pointing), vocalizing, attending to spoken language, looking and recognizing, recognizing pictures, and handling books.
2. *Emergent literacy* is the early use and understanding of language, which includes actual first words, early conventional speech (e.g., requesting, attention getting), language comprehension, symbol and print recognition as meaningful (e.g., understanding a stop sign, recognizing that the word *stop* means to cease what you are doing), and vocabulary acquisition.
3. *Early literacy* includes precursors to reading and writing, such as understanding that words are units of sounds, that words have meaning (both written and

heard words), and the rules of written language (e.g., English is written left to right and top to bottom); inventive spelling; echo reading (i.e., repeating a short chunk of text); and letter and word recognition.
4. *Conventional literacy* includes the actual skills used for reading and writing, such as decoding, reading orally, demonstrating fluency, demonstrating comprehension, generating written sentences or paragraphs, and spelling.

Early Predictors of Literacy Skills

The National Early Literacy Panel (2008) identified the following 6 strong and consistent predictors for the development of literacy skills, even after accounting for IQ and socioeconomic status:
1. Knowing the names of printed letters;
2. Being able to manipulate the sounds of spoken language (breaking words apart, adding or deleting sounds);
3. Being able to rapidly name a sequence of letters, numbers, or objects;
4. Being able to rapidly name a sequence of pictures of objects or colors;
5. Being able to write one's name or even isolated letters; and
6. Being able to remember the content of spoken language for a short time.

Moderate predictors included
- Knowing conventions of English print (e.g., how to use a book);
- Being able to recognize and identify *environmental print*, which consists of the letters, numbers, and shapes found in everyday life (e.g., signs, packages);
- Knowing how to have a conversation with others (e.g., talking, understanding); and
- Being able to see similarities and differences among visual symbols (National Early Literacy Panel, 2008).

Influencing Literacy and School Performance Across Grades

Reading is critical in every aspect of school. When students cannot read and comprehend the curricular materials, they fall behind. Three common difficulties are problems with decoding (e.g., poor sound–letter correspondence to sound out words), poor comprehension (e.g., letter–word recognition, understanding), and speed (e.g., fluency, ability to read quickly by recognizing words by sight rather than having to decode each word).

Lack of quality instruction as well as language-processing disorders (e.g., dyslexia, specific language impairments) can cause struggling learners to feel frustrated and unintelligent compared with their peers (Shapiro et al., 2002). Hernandez (2012) found that 3rd-grade students who did not read at grade level were 4 times more likely to drop out of school later on than students who were proficient readers. In addition, students who were living in poverty were 3 times more likely to drop out or fail to graduate on time, even when they were proficient readers (Hernandez, 2012). Goldston et al. (2007) found that teenagers with reading problems were more likely to have attention deficit hyperactivity disorder, experience anxiety and depression, use drugs, have problems socially, think about harming themselves, and avoid adult responsibilities.

STEM

In contrast to the traditional approach of teaching science, technology, engineering, and mathematics separately, *STEM* is an interdisciplinary instructional method that integrates these concepts into experiences grounded in real-world contexts across the curriculum (Jolly, 2014). The definition of *technology* is broadened to include digital formats and products made by the student to "meet a want or need" (Jolly, 2014, para. 5).

The STEM approach is meant to immerse students, working in teams, to engage in hands-on and open-ended exploration guided by the ***engineering design process.*** This process uses a problem-solving framework by which the problem is identified and continued until a solution is developed, with multiple right answers allowed and generated by the students working together. The STEM approach, like universal design for learning (UDL), considers the different ways people learn and offers diverse learners a chance to use math and science in real situations.

Influence of Curriculum, Instruction, Access to Technology, and Environmental Factors

There are profound differences in knowledge among students across socioeconomic groups as they enter school. Hart and Risley's (1995) study was the first to link vocabulary size with socioeconomic status (i.e., 4-year-olds from families in poverty heard more than 30 million fewer words than children from working-class families). It is important to note that parents who lack strong reading skills can influence their child's learning and later reading success through regular meaningful conversation. Neuman and Wright (2014) indicated that adults who provided quality, quantity, and responsive talk could effectively mediate socioeconomic factors. In turn, this growth in vocabulary skills could predict later reading and literacy performance.

There is now a greater recognition that today's texts (e.g., books, works, documents) are not just accessed through a print medium. More and more information comes from both print and nonprint formats. Educational teams must make use of multimedia, embedding these media into all components of learning and keeping in mind that simply expanding access to technology is not enough on its own. Parents and teachers must help students take advantage of multiple pathways for reading and information seeking (Guernsey et al., 2014).

Having access to an effective curriculum and instruction is critical for learning. IDEA (2004) states that students are not considered to have a disability when the "determinant factor . . . is lack of appropriate instruction in reading [or] math" (§ 1414[b][5]). Therefore, lack of appropriate instruction (e.g., writing) is an exclusionary factor for determining the need for occupational therapy services in schools. A strong evidence-based curriculum that is systematically taught across districts, states, and the nation improves the odds of learning for all students and may enhance the quality of instruction by teachers who are struggling (Marzano, 2003).

Marzano (2003) identified 3 types of curriculum:

1. *Intended curriculum* (i.e., content specified by state, district, or school for a particular grade level),
2. *Implemented curriculum* (i.e., content actually delivered by the teacher), and

3. *Attained curriculum* (i.e., content actually learned by the student).

A discrepancy between the intended curriculum and the implemented curriculum shows that the opportunity to learn is a critical factor that needs to be addressed for student achievement.

Differentiated instruction, or the design of instruction that is individually accessible according to each student's needs, and UDL focus on maximizing each student's potential. Schools accomplish this instructional design by providing learning environments, experiences, and opportunities that are challenging and flexible enough to adjust for each student's interest and preferred way of expression while addressing grade-level content. Occupational therapy practitioners are experts at adapting and modifying activities to challenge students while ensuring successful performance. (For more information on UDL, see Chapter 20, "Best Practices in Universal Design for Learning.")

State Standards and Benchmarks

The ***Common Core curriculum*** is a state-led effort to develop educational standards that outline rigorous knowledge and skills in English language arts and mathematics for students. The standards, developed in collaboration with school administrators, teachers, and national experts, were released initially in 2010 and benchmarked to international standards (CCSSI, 2010). Many individualized education program teams align students' goals with state standards and benchmarks, when applicable. Occupational therapy practitioners should know their state standards and how they are being implemented in the school.

BEST PRACTICES

Occupational therapy practitioners use best practices to support literacy and STEM activities at district (schoolwide), classroom, and student levels. Teachers have the primary role of teaching literacy and STEM skills, whereas occupational therapy practitioners, as related service providers, support the educational team to help students with various learning styles benefit from their educational programs. This role in assisting diverse learners is critical.

Participate in District-Level (Schoolwide) Interventions

Occupational therapy practitioners need to know the focus of district-level, or schoolwide, interventions. Through this understanding, they can position themselves to collaborate and work with school staff to address the needs of the entire student body. This might include curriculum committees, district student improvement teams, professional development, UDL, and family literacy.

Curriculum committees (typically districtwide committees composed of educators) identify, evaluate, select, and make recommendations about curriculum programs. The occupational therapist can assist in determining literacy- and STEM-related curricular criteria and applicability of options on the basis of contextual and environmental factors, child development, and activity demands that influence successful participation in literacy and STEM experiences and instruction.

District student improvement teams, composed of educators and special education providers, usually have a more sustained focus than curriculum committees on explicit and long-term goals for all students' performance. ESSA (2015) includes occupational therapy practitioners as SISP. SISP should be involved in schoolwide planning activities as well as schoolwide interventions and supports. The occupational therapist can assist in analyzing data across age groups while using knowledge of task analysis and context modifications to suggest strategies.

Professional development targets support for literacy skills and participation in STEM activities. Occupational therapy practitioners may present professional development to educational staff on various topics related to these issues, such as using UDL, facilitating handwriting legibility, improving social skills for student teamwork, and enhancing the sensory and physical environments to promote learning. Professional development should emphasize research-based practices and include in-class coaching, teacher mentoring, and demonstration sessions. School occupational therapy practitioners often provide UDL training and implementation ideas for educational staff. Technology offers many potential UDL access options; however, it is important to recognize the differences between access to information and access to curriculum to determine which is a priority for recommendations.

Family literacy, or the promotion of literacy skills at home by the family, can provide the context for establishing and sustaining a child's literacy learning. Students whose parents frequently engage in responsive language and literacy interactions with them and who provide a home environment rich in experiences such as shared book reading, conversations, and reading and writing for real purposes display higher language and cognitive skills into the primary years (Powell & Diamond, 2012). The occupational therapy practitioner can provide support for families by facilitating engagement in early and ongoing literacy experiences while providing information and guidance about environmental characteristics that lead to positive outcomes.

Participate in Classroom-Level Interventions

At the classroom level, interventions allow occupational therapists opportunities to collaborate with educators to enhance classroom environments, curriculum design, and instructional practices for groups of students and individuals, taking into consideration differing personal learning styles and physical needs.

Environmental strategies

AOTA's (2014b) *Occupational Therapy Practice Framework: Domain and Process* (3rd ed.; *OTPF–3*) states that contexts (e.g., cultural, personal, temporal, virtual) and environments (e.g., physical, social) affect access to occupations and can influence the quality of and satisfaction with a person's performance. Although a student might have difficulty in one environment, they could be successful in another environment or in the original environment once it has been modified. Occupational therapy practitioners

are well versed in using environmental strategies and engineering environments where children work and play. They have expertise in analyzing contextual characteristics and making recommendations to structure, modify, or adapt the environment for student participation and success.

Curriculum and instructional strategies

Occupational therapists should be aware of the student's instruction and curriculum and promote evidence-based literacy instruction within the state's or district's core curriculum, keeping in mind that the lack of appropriate instruction is not a reason for identifying a student as a student with a disability (IDEA, 2004, § 1414[b][5][A]).

Individual student's interests

To achieve a higher probability of meaningful engagement and participation, use items that interest the student. The educational team can identify a student's interests, goals to accomplish, struggles that may exist, and strategies already in use. To do so, the team can interview the student, have the student draw pictures or create drawings using technology, and help the student organize and document information according to the student's learning style.

Access to technology

It is important for students to have access to technology as they learn literacy- and STEM-related skills. The use of computer and other digital technologies will continue to grow and has increasingly become a part of literacy instruction. Students need to become users of information-based literacies. Research has found that a high percentage of students at the conventional literacy stage achieved a much higher rate of text production using keyboarding over handwriting, including students who were having specific handwriting difficulties (Preminger et al., 2004; Rogers & Case-Smith, 2002).

Coteaching

Coteaching typically consists of 2 professionals who collaborate in an instructional process. The teachers are responsible for the student's instruction; however, occupational therapists may use their knowledge and skills to plan and provide learning activities with the educator. Coteaching can effectively address literacy, such as handwriting instruction. In this role, the occupational therapist can contribute by adapting the curriculum, modifying materials, and providing specific interventions (Case-Smith et al., 2012).

Professionals participating in coteaching reported increased competence in their colleague's content area (Scruggs et al., 2007). Coteaching has also been shown to contribute to increased handwriting legibility and writing fluency among 1st graders of varying ability (Case-Smith et al., 2012) and an accelerated rate of improvement in emergent literacy and fine-motor development among kindergarten students (Bazyk et al., 2009).

Collaborative consultation

Collaborative consultation is a model of intervention used by occupational therapy practitioners and other professionals since the 1980s to support students in their performance (Dunn, 1988; Individuals With Disabilities Education, 1995; Shasby & Schneck, 2011). In this model, 2 professionals with different backgrounds, perspectives, and expertise work together as equal partners. The teacher has the primary responsibility of instruction; however, the occupational therapy practitioner provides the teacher with skills and resources to assist the student with special needs. The *OTPF–3* (AOTA, 2014b) states that the collaborative approach involves mutual participation between the occupational therapy practitioner and the client.

Shared or dialogic reading

Shared or *dialogic reading* is an effective, interactive reading practice that encourages the student to respond to questions and engage in telling the story. Shared reading engages students in reading experiences that emphasize social interaction among the teacher, the family member, and the student, which makes books meaningful and interesting. A student in the preliteracy or emergent stage of literacy development should not be expected to sit and listen to a story without actively participating, which is the primary purpose of shared reading. The emphasis of shared reading for the adult is to respond to the student's general intentions, such as eye gaze, vocalizations, pointing, and questions, while, most important, engaging the student in a conversation about the reading material at a level that is a good fit for the student's development (Simsek & Erdogan, 2013).

Authentic learning processes for literacy and STEM

When students are presented with authentic or real-life problems, particularly those that involve flexible, hands-on, project-based learning, they become engaged. Students begin to generate solutions and assume different roles in the group learning process. In this capacity, a student may require added support and expertise from the education team. For all students to truly engage in STEM learning, collaboration among the educational team is vital.

The following example illustrates the role of an occupational therapist: The elementary building–level team held a meeting to plan for upcoming science lessons, including kindergarten, 1st-grade, and 2nd-grade teachers; the district curriculum specialist; the speech–language pathologist; and the occupational therapist serving the district. The team decided to use the lesson plan for the water cycle as a means of discussing and planning for the collaboration necessary to include all students.

The teachers explained that the idea was to use sealable plastic bags, water, and food coloring, then hang the bags in a sunny window to help students see and learn how water evaporates in warmth, condenses in cool, and becomes precipitation. The teachers then asked, "How can we ensure that students with individual learning differences can actively participate in this activity?"

The occupational therapist applied her knowledge of material adaptation to suggest other containers and ways to modify the food coloring application. The occupational therapist and speech–language pathologist brainstormed with the teachers about how to set up small groups of students

for making the water cycle together; talking about it afterward; and practicing social skills such as self-regulating, taking turns, and making eye contact. They also provided suggestions on the use of drawing, technology, and pictures to represent the cycle for those students unable to write.

Books and other reading materials

To develop literacy, children must be actively engaged with books and other reading materials in multiple ways. Research has suggested that students learn alphabet knowledge and phonological awareness more effectively when they are presented together as part of everyday activities rather than taught in isolation. For example, practitioners can use letters that are interesting to the student because they are part of the student's name or familiar words rather than teach the alphabet only in sequence (Puranik & Lonigan, 2011).

Environmental print can be found on cereal boxes, snack packages, and signs in restaurants and stores. Familiar sources of environmental print should be used as an integral part of not only the reading curriculum but also other learning activities for students who are in the preliteracy, emergent literacy, and early literacy stages. The use of environmental print to facilitate the introduction to letters as symbols is well documented in the literature as a teaching tool.

More recent research represents how print from the environment encourages not just early reading but also experimenting with early writing by virtue of the student copying what they see (McMahon Giles & Wellhousen Tunks, 2010). Grajo and Candler (2016) suggested that occupational therapy practitioners support children with reading challenges by using a framework grounded in occupation and participation (e.g., having students set outcomes based on their life events). Results of their study indicated significant increases in perceived performance and reading participation despite nonsignificant increases in reading scores after an 8-week intervention. In addition, parents and children reported greater reading confidence and reading time spent at home.

Writing and art

In the emergent and early stages of literacy, writing experiences should emphasize the function of print, not the form. Students in these stages do not distinguish marks, scribbles, or drawings from writing, so all forms and attempts should be regarded as intentional. Adults can highlight and reinforce all representations by adding a written label of what the student intended or says. Familiar words, names, and letters should be available for a student to copy (e.g., names of the child, family members, friends), as well as props such as recipes and cards.

Puranik and Lonigan's (2011) research indicated that by age 3 or 4 years, students demonstrated universal characteristics common to all languages, such as working linearly and separating the units (distinct marks and forms). The language-specific features came later (e.g., letters of the alphabet, their name, inventive spelling), depending on the components of the writing systems to which the student was exposed.

Older students at these literacy stages need meaningful activities, such as writing a card or note to a friend, writing in a journal, or making a list. The focus is to make writing uniquely meaningful for a particular student. Practitioners can include writing adaptations, such as different pencil sizes and shapes, paint brushes of all sizes, adapted tool holders, and slant boards and easels, to accommodate the abilities of all learners.

Music, rhythm, and movement activities

Music, rhythm, and movement activities can help children learn about sound and how it relates to reading. Before students learn to read print, they must be aware that words are made up of small units of sound (i.e., **phonemic awareness**) and of how the sounds in words "work" (i.e., **phonological awareness**). Students in the early literacy stage need multiple opportunities to develop phonemic and phonological awareness by hearing, playing with, and manipulating sounds. Research-based practices include

- Recognizing and using words that start or end with the same sound, playing with sounds (e.g., "Willoughby Wallaby Woo");
- Clapping and performing other rhythmical body movements;
- Reading books that have predictable and repeating phrases or that highlight **alliteration,** which consists of words or phrases that all include the same letter in the same place (e.g., "Silly Sally sells seashells"); and
- Rhyming (e.g., poetry, nursery rhymes, chants; Pierce et al., 2008).

Key to using music, rhythm, or movement activities is integrating everyday activities that are interesting and engaging to the student rather than teaching sounds in isolation (Pierce et al., 2008). Development of these sound-related skills happens simultaneously rather than in sequence, particularly when they are practiced in context, so providing opportunities across literacy stages is preferred.

SUMMARY

Literacy and STEM evolve from many underlying aspects of development and experiences. Occupational therapy practitioners have a critical role in the development of student's literacy and STEM skills. After the evaluation, occupational therapists design interventions that focus on underlying skills that affect performance, and providing professional development for teaching staff. Incorporating literacy materials in occupational therapy interventions is essential to reading and writing development for students, especially those who are at risk for or have been identified as having developmental delays.

REFERENCES

American Occupational Therapy Association. (2014a). Guidelines for supervision, roles, and responsibilities during the delivery of occupational therapy services. *American Journal of Occupational Therapy, 68*(Suppl. 3), S16–S22. https://doi.org/10.5014/ajot.2014.686S03

American Occupational Therapy Association. (2014b). Occupational therapy practice framework: Domain and process (3rd ed.).

American Journal of Occupational Therapy, 68(Suppl. 1), S1–S48. https://doi.org/10.5014/ajot.2014.682006

Bazyk, S., Michaud, P., Goodman, G., Hawkins, E., & Welch, M. (2009). Integrating occupational therapy services in a kindergarten curriculum: A look at the outcomes. *American Journal of Occupational Therapy, 63,* 160–171. https://doi.org/10.5014/ajot.63.2.160

Case-Smith, J., Holland, T., Lane, A., & White, S. (2012). Effect of a coteaching handwriting program for first graders. *American Journal of Occupational Therapy, 66,* 396–405. https://doi.org/10.5014/ajot.2012.004333

Common Core State Standards Initiative. (2010). *Common Core State Standards for English language arts and literacy in history/social studies, science, and technical subjects.* Retrieved from http://www.corestandards.org/ELA-Literacy/

Dunn, W. (1988). Models of occupational therapy service provision in the school system. *American Journal of Occupational Therapy, 42,* 718–723. https://doi.org/10.5014/ajot.42.11.718

Dunst, C., Trivette, C., Masiello, T., Roper, N., & Robyak, A. (2006). Framework for developing evidence-based early literacy learning practices. *CELL Papers, 1*(1). Retrieved from http://www.early literacylearning.org/cellpapers/cellpapers_v1_n1.pdf

Every Student Succeeds Act, Pub. L. 114–195, 129 Stat. 1802. (2015–2016).

Goldston, D. B., Walsh, A., Arnold, E. M., Reboussin, B., Daniel, S. S., Erkanli, A., . . . Wood, F. B. (2007). Reading problems, psychiatric disorders, and functional impairment from mid-to-late adolescence. *Journal of the American Academy of Child and Adolescent Psychiatry, 46,* 25–32. https://doi.org/10.1097/01.chi.0000242241.77302.f4

Grajo, L., & Candler, C. (2016). An occupation and participation approach to reading intervention (OPARI) Part II: Pilot clinical application. *Journal of Occupational Therapy, Schools, and Early Intervention, 9,* 86–98. https://doi.org/10.1080/19411243.2016.1141082

Guernsey, L., Levine, M., Chiong, C., & Severns, M. (2014). *Pioneering literacy in the digital Wild West: Empowering parents and educators.* Retrieved from http://joanganzcooneycenter.org/publication/pioneering-literacy/

Hart, B., & Risley, T. R. (1995). *Meaningful differences in the everyday experience of young American children.* Baltimore: Brookes.

Hernandez, D. (2012). *Double jeopardy: How third-grade reading skills and poverty influence high school graduation.* Retrieved from https://www.aecf.org/m/resourcedoc/AECF-DoubleJeopardy-2012-Full.pdf

Hwang, J., & Taylor, J. (2016). Stemming on STEM: A STEM education framework for students with disabilities. *Journal of Science Education for Students With Disabilities, 19*(1), 39–49.

Individuals With Disabilities Education: Hearings before the Subcommittee on Early Childhood, Youth, and Families, of the Committee on Economic and Educational Opportunities, 104th Cong. D795 (1995) (testimony of Gloria Frolek Clark).

Individuals With Disabilities Education Improvement Act of 2004, Pub. L. 108–446, 20 U.S.C. §§ 1400–1482.

Israel, M., Maynard, K., & Williamson, P. (2013). Promoting literacy-embedded, authentic STEM instruction for students with disabilities and other struggling learners. *Teaching Exceptional Children, 45*(4), 18–25. https://doi.org/10.1177/004005991304500402

Jolly, A. (2014). Six characteristics of a great STEM lesson. *Education Week Teacher.* Retrieved from https://www.edweek.org/tm/articles/2014/06/17/ctq_jolly_stem.html

Marzano, R. (2003). *What works in schools: Translating research into action.* Alexandria, VA: Association for Supervision and Curriculum Development.

McFarland, J., Hussar, W., Brey, C., Snyder, T., Wang, X., Wilkenson-Flicker, S., . . . Hinz, S. (2017). *The condition of education 2017* (NCES 2017-144). Washington, DC: U.S. Government Printing Office.

McMahon Giles, R., & Wellhousen Tunks, K. (2010). Children write their world: Environmental print as a teaching tool. *Dimensions of Early Childhood, 38*(3), 23–30. Retrieved from http://southernearlychildhood.org/upload/pdf/Children_Write_Their_World.pdf

National Early Literacy Panel. (2008). *Developing early literacy: A scientific synthesis of early literacy development and implications for intervention.* Jessup, MD: National Institute for Literacy.

Nation's Report Card. (2014). *Technology and engineering literacy (TEL).* Retrieved from https://www.nationsreportcard.gov/tel_2014/#

Neuman, S., & Wright, T. (2014). The magic words: Teaching vocabulary in the early childhood classroom. *American Educator, 38*(2), 4–13. Retrieved from https://www.aft.org/sites/default/files/periodicals/neuman.pdf

Pierce, P., Abraham, L., Rosenkoetter, S., Knapp-Philo, J., & Summer, G. (2008). Literacy development. In P. Winton, J. McCollum, & C. Catlett (Eds.), *Practical approaches to early childhood professional development: Evidence, strategies, and resources* (pp. 187–206). Washington, DC: Zero to Three.

Powell, D., & Diamond, K. (2012). Promoting early literacy and language development. In R. C. Pianta, L. Justice, C. Blair, S. Barnett, & S. Sheridan (Eds.), *Handbook of early education* (pp. 124–156). New York: Guilford Press.

Preminger, F., Weiss, P., & Weintraub, N. (2004). Predicting occupational performance: Handwriting versus keyboarding. *American Journal of Occupational Therapy, 58*, 193–201. https://doi.org/10.5014/ajot.58.2.193

Puranik, C., & Lonigan, C. (2011). From scribbles to Scrabble: Preschool children's development of written language. *Reading and Writing, 24*, 567–589. https://doi.org/10.1007/s11145-009-9220-8

Rogers, J., & Case-Smith, J. (2002). Relationships between handwriting and keyboarding performance of sixth-grade students. *American Journal of Occupational Therapy, 56*, 34–39. https://doi.org/10.5014/ajot.56.1.34

Scruggs, T., Mastropieri, M., & McDuffie, K. (2007). Coteaching in inclusive classrooms: A metasynthesis of qualitative research. *Exceptional Children, 73*, 392–416. https://doi.org/10.1177/001440290707300401

Shapiro, B. K., Church, R. P., & Lewis, M. E. B. (2002). Specific learning disabilities. In M. L. Batshaw (Ed.), *Children with disabilities* (5th ed., pp. 417–442). Baltimore: Brookes.

Shasby, S., & Schneck, C. (2011). Commentary on collaboration in school-based practice: Positives and pitfalls. *Journal of Occupational Therapy, Schools, and Early Intervention, 4*, 22–33. https://doi.org/10.1080/19411243.2011.573243

Simsek, Z., & Erdogan, N. (2013). Effects of the dialogic and traditional reading techniques on children's language development. *Science Direct, 197*, 754–758. https://doi.org/10.1016/j.sbspro.2015.07.172

U.S. Department of Education. (2018). *Science, technology, engineering and math: Education for global leadership.* Retrieved from https://www.ed.gov/stem

Catherine Candler, OTR, PhD, BCP

KEY TERMS AND CONCEPTS

- Community involvement
- Counseling, psychological, and social services
- Employee wellness
- Family engagement
- Health education
- Health literacy

- Health promotion
- Health services
- Lifestyle choices
- Nutrition environment
- Physical education and physical activity
- Physical environment

- Primary level
- Secondary level
- Social and emotional school climate
- Tertiary level
- Whole School, Whole Community, Whole Child

OVERVIEW

In 1986, the World Health Organization (WHO) defined *health promotion* as the process of enabling people to increase control over and improve their health. A healthy life includes an effective array of functional abilities that allow persons to work, play, and enter fulfilling relationships. Health promotion goes beyond individual behavior and includes a wide range of social and environmental actions, including global initiatives for healthy schools (WHO, 2018).

Health issues directly affect children and often disparately affect children with disabilities. For example, although childhood obesity is a national point of concern (American Occupational Therapy Association [AOTA], 2013b), adolescents with physical and cognitive disabilities have a significantly higher rate of obesity (17.5%) than those without (13.0%; Rimmer et al., 2011). In a 12-year longitudinal study, more extensive histories of respiratory illness, diabetes, and injury-related hospitalizations were present among children with disabilities (Shooshtari et al., 2017).

Reducing health disparities and investing in the provision of health promotion and prevention of disease or disability are a focus of occupational therapy (AOTA, 2013b, 2013c). This investment is in line with the Healthy People 2020 initiative (https://www.healthypeople.gov/), which was launched in 1979 and has since been reaffirmed and updated each decade. Healthy People 2020's goals are to
- Attain high-quality, longer lives free of preventable afflictions;
- Eliminate disparities and achieve health equity;
- Create social and physical environments that promote health; and
- Promote healthy behaviors across all life stages, including childhood.

These goals are consistent with the goals of occupational therapy practitioners[1] to facilitate quality of life through participation and engagement in life activities, support nondiscrimination and inclusion for persons with occupational deprivation, promote the match between persons and environments for optimum function, and help individuals use their adaptive power to master occupational challenges (AOTA, 2014b).

School occupational therapy practitioners have multiple opportunities to positively influence the health of students. According to the National Center for Education Statistics (2013), students in the United States are in school for 30 hours or more each week. Thus, schools have emerged as a focal point for many federal, state, and local mandates; regulations; initiatives; and funding streams related to health.

Varied disciplines operate in this arena, including occupational therapy, education, nursing, social work, psychology, nutrition, and school administration. Collaboration among professionals from different disciplines and organizations is best practice for achieving health promotion goals (Langford et al., 2015). Mechanisms for achieving this collaboration are readily available. Whole School, Whole Community, Whole Child (WSCC) is a strategy developed under the guidance of the Centers for Disease Control and Prevention (CDC;

---

[1]*Occupational therapy practitioner* refers to both the occupational therapist and the occupational therapy assistant. AOTA (2014a, p. S18) states, "The occupational therapist is responsible for all aspects of occupational therapy service delivery and is accountable for the safety and effectiveness of the occupational therapy service delivery process" and "must be directly involved in the delivery of services during the initial evaluation and regularly throughout the course of intervention. . . . The occupational therapy assistant delivers safe and effective occupational therapy services under the supervision of and in partnership with the occupational therapist."

Copyright © 2019 by the American Occupational Therapy Association. All rights reserved. To reuse this content, contact www.copyright.com.
https://doi.org/10.7139/2019.978-1-56900-591-0.018

2017c) and the Association for Supervision and Curriculum Development. *WSCC* includes step-by-step instructions on how to achieve an integrated approach to health and create programs to meet specific health objectives.

School occupational therapy practitioners benefit from participating in school health programs and initiatives. Becoming part of or leading a combined health promotion effort allows occupational therapy practitioners to

- Demonstrate a shared investment in school community concerns,
- Network with the school community, and
- Positively affect the visibility of and respect for the profession among others who are actively involved in the school.

In addition, initiatives to improve the health of all children have the potential to specifically address the goals of occupational therapy and increase the impact and effectiveness of intervention. This benefit is close to the occupational therapy practitioner's primary concerns in day-to-day practice because health issues may complicate the already difficult issues students face because of their disability.

Bullying, obesity, drug use, and other preventable health concerns can be pervasive undoers of the occupational therapy practitioner's efforts. Examples include the student with obesity who cannot independently transfer to a desk because of their body weight, the 7th-grade student with autism whose first experiences with inclusion are fraught with bullying from the peer group, and the student who is homeless and facing numerous challenges. Efforts in health promotion have the potential to directly address individualized education program (IEP) student goals as well as improve collaboration on those goals.

ESSENTIAL CONSIDERATIONS

In the United States, there are differences between the provision of services to treat disease—a task primarily addressed by medicine and the health care industry—and efforts for healthy living, which have been addressed more prominently by public entities and organizations. Although diseases caused by pathology have been reduced (Institute for Health Metrics and Evaluation, 2017), the majority of threats to health in the United States and the world are related to *lifestyle choices,* which are an individual's habits and customs related to daily living (e.g., foods chosen, exercise routines, level of stress, high-risk behaviors).

For example, recent results from a 25-year ongoing global burden of disease study showed high body mass index as the 4th largest contributor to the loss of healthy life, after high blood pressure, smoking, and high blood sugar (Global Burden of Disease Neurological Disorders Collaborator Group, 2017). This knowledge has created shifts in perspective. Engagement in health promotion is now an important part of what health care professionals do.

Continuum of Health Promotion and Wellness

Traditionally, health promotion and wellness efforts are categorized on a continuum made up of primary, secondary, and tertiary levels, which reflects risk for health concerns

and whether an intervention is directed toward an individual or a population (Goldston, 1987). Understanding these levels of health promotion and wellness intervention assists occupational therapy practitioners in selecting the most effective approach for addressing the specific health and wellness concerns of their school setting and clients (AOTA, 2013a). These levels of health promotion intervention mirror concepts used in disease progression.

Primary level

At the *primary level,* health promotion interventions are purely preventive and are aimed at healthy populations and individuals. Although this demographic is often envisioned as consisting of typically abled individuals, in truth, people at all levels of ability are beneficiaries of primary-level health promotion interventions (Rimmer et al., 2014). Primary health promotion interventions are familiar parts of day-to-day life in schools. Examples include removal of sugar-laden snack and beverage vending machines from the school cafeteria (American Academy of Pediatrics, 2004) and participation in

- Programs for drug awareness (National Family Partnership; http://redribbon.org/),
- Jump Rope for Heart and Hoops for Heart (Shape America; https://www.shapeamerica.org/),
- Peaceful Playgrounds (Peaceful Playgrounds Foundation, 2018), and
- National School Backpack Awareness Day (AOTA, 2018; Jacobs et al., 2011).

Secondary level

At the *secondary level,* health promotion interventions are directed toward persons or populations who are at risk for a disease or health concern but have not demonstrated symptoms or are in early stages that can be slowed or arrested. Secondary health promotion interventions can occur in schools. Free school breakfast and lunch programs are a good example, targeting the health risks of students from low-income families.

Students with disabilities form a definite at-risk population, because they disparately experience health issues. One example of a secondary health promotion intervention in schools directly relevant to occupational therapy is establishing a walking club for students with Down syndrome who are at risk for obesity.

Tertiary level

At the *tertiary level,* health promotion interventions address the health concerns of persons with established disease. Tertiary health promotion interventions seek to restore the person to highest function, prevent disease-related complications, and ultimately minimize the effects of the disorder. Direct occupational therapy intervention occurs at the tertiary level, with activities customized to the needs of the affected population. Examples of tertiary health promotion interventions in schools include occupational therapy goals for medication management for an adolescent with juvenile arthritis or development of an anger management program for a student or group of students with behavioral disorders.

WSCC

Public education is a state, not a federal, responsibility, which accounts for the many differences in public education across the nation, such as student–teacher ratios, how kindergarten education is provided, and specific learning outcomes for each grade level. Other than the federal government's responsibility to ensure that whatever education designed by the states is equally applied, the federal government's influence is primarily in its spending power through acts linked to federal funding, such as the Individuals With Disabilities Education Improvement Act of 2004 (Pub. L. 108–446).

The U.S. public schools have long been a meeting ground for divergent health promotion interests, such as nutrition (U.S. Department of Agriculture, 2017a), drug use (National Family Partnership, 2017), and physical activity (Shape America, 2018). Because health promotion in schools has been a complex patchwork of policies and organizations, the federal CDC and the Association for Supervision and Curriculum Development established the WSCC program (Lewallen et al., 2015).

This model integrates the principles of a coordinated school health program with a whole-child approach to education. The child is at the center of the model (see Figure 18.1), surrounded by the tenets of the whole-child approach to education, which seek to shift the concept of child education from a narrow focus on academics to a more global one of development. This approach aims to ensure that each child (student) is

- Healthy,
- Physically and emotionally safe,
- Actively engaged in learning and the community,
- Supported by caring adults, and
- Academically challenged.

Bracketed by the community, the WSCC model works through 10 school health components that form a unified approach to health promotion in the schools:

1. Health education;
2. Nutrition environment and services;
3. Employee wellness;
4. Social and emotional school climate;
5. Physical environment;
6. Health services;
7. Counseling, psychological, and social services;
8. Community involvement;
9. Family engagement; and
10. Physical education and physical activity.

Schools and school districts are encouraged to use this model to draw resources and influences from the whole community to serve the whole child. Occupational therapy

---

FIGURE 18.1.   Whole School, Whole Community, Whole Child.

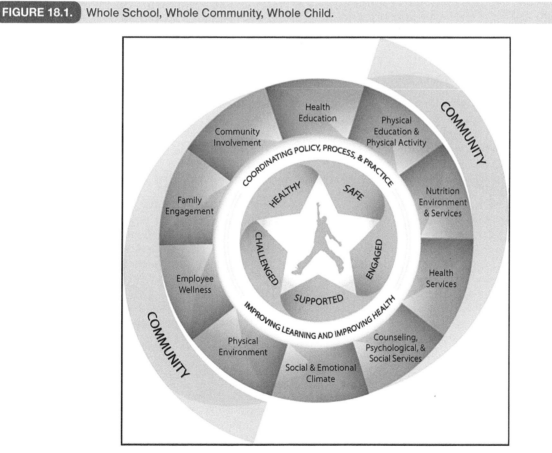

Source. From *Whole School, Whole Community, Whole Child,* by Centers for Disease Control and Prevention, 2017c. Retrieved from https://www.cdc.gov/healthy-schools/wscc/index.htm. In the public domain.

practitioners will find the best fit and connections for their ideas related to school health by connecting with these components at their school or in their school district.

Health education

Health education includes any formal learning experiences that facilitate skills people need to make quality health decisions. A defined sequential kindergarten through 12th-grade curriculum that addresses the physical, mental, emotional, and social dimensions of health is an optimal approach. In the United States, 81.7% of school districts have directed schools to follow established health standards (CDC, 2017b). Most health topics are addressed in high schools, the most common being violence prevention.

Occupational therapists have a primary interest in health education that includes making health-promoting decisions and adopting health-enhancing behaviors. According to Ratzan and Parker (2000), *health literacy* is "the degree to which individuals have the capacity to obtain, process, and understand basic health information and services needed to make appropriate health care decisions" (p. 1). Occupational therapists are responsible for providing information and education that promote self-management for optimum health and participation (AOTA, 2017). Questions to ask are
- How is health education being addressed in my schools?
- What topics are being taught?
- Are these topics inclusive for students with special needs?
- How could an occupation-based approach, incorporating daily life activities, enhance the educational value of what is being offered?

Nutrition environment and services

Nutrition environment refers to providing children opportunities to learn about healthy eating. Nutrition services include the availability of healthy meals and snacks. Two well-known federal programs are National School Lunch and School Breakfast, both sponsored by the U.S. Department of Agriculture (2017a, 2017b).

Nutrition has received much attention in recent years because of the prevalence of obesity among children across the nation. It is estimated that approximately 20% of students are obese (Ogden et al., 2016). Healthy eating habits and access to healthy foods are key health promotion initiatives related to nutrition. In 2013, AOTA (2013b) reissued a position paper on obesity stating the commitment of the profession to use everyday life activities therapeutically in the management of obesity. An example of this commitment is Comfortable Cafeterias, an occupational approach to lunchtime that was developed by and is currently in use by occupational therapists (Bazyk et al., 2014).

Employee wellness

Employee wellness supports students' health and academic success. A healthy work environment is beneficial to all, and school staff members engaged in healthy living provide models for students. Occupational therapy practitioners contribute to this component when they
- Provide training to school staff in safe positioning and handling techniques for students with disabilities,

- Offer in-services related to desk ergonomics for staff, and
- Assist with office arrangement for efficiency to reduce stress on joints.

Social and emotional school climate

Social and emotional school climate directly supports healthy student engagement in school. Good relationships with others support academic performance. Healthy learning environments are safe and supportive. Features of such environments promote a sense of community and welcome, facilitate positive behaviors, and emphasize safety and drug-free lifestyles.

Incorporating activity-based interventions for mental health in schools is good practice for occupational therapy. Strong evidence exists for the effectiveness of programs that focus on social–emotional learning, schoolwide bullying prevention, after-school programs, performing arts offerings, and stress management activities (Arbesman et al., 2013). Opportunity to affect the social and emotional school climate exists throughout the school day, and this strategy is the basis of an occupational therapy–based initiative called Every Moment Counts (Bazyk, 2014). Every Moment Counts presents mental health promotion strategies throughout the school day, including during lunchtime, during class, after school, and at recess.

Recess and the playground have also been the focus of other programs that address social and emotional safety. Playworks (https://www.playworks.org/) is a national non-profit organization that provides training to school staff to transform recess and play into a positive social and physically active experience. Peaceful Playgrounds (Peaceful Playgrounds Foundation, 2018) is another. Playgrounds that promote play unstructured by adults are also important for childhood socialization, an issue that has been addressed by occupational therapy practitioners (Bundy et al., 2008).

Physical environment

Physical environment concerns the school building and its surroundings and the effect of these on the well-being of students and staff at school. Some features of the physical environment of healthy and safe schools that occupational therapy practitioners need to consider are as follows:
- A healthy and safe school building, including the surrounding area;
- Adequate lighting, heating, and ventilation;
- Safe drinking water, air quality, and acoustics;
- Physical security, free from hazards and biological or chemical agents;
- Policies to prevent unintentional injuries and a crisis management plan; and
- School bus and pedestrian safety.

Occupational therapy practitioners are well versed in how the environment affects healthy occupation (AOTA, 2015). The Collaborative for High Performance Schools (2018) sponsors criteria for high-performance schools. These criteria include benchmarks for indoor environment quality, energy, water, school site, materials, and waste management. Occupational therapy practitioners can contribute to healthy and safe school environments by adding their expertise on building modifications or universal design for access.

Another program relevant to a safe and healthy school environment is Safe Routes (http://www.saferoutesinfo.org/). Aimed at students in kindergarten through 8th grade, this program's purpose is to provide surrounding environments that encourage students, including those with disabilities, to walk and bicycle to school, making this option safer and more appealing.

Health services

Health services are a connection between schools and health care providers that facilitate access to and appropriate use of primary health care. Health services include steps to control communicable diseases and intervention with actual health problems, such as first aid, emergency care, and management of chronic conditions. Data from the 2016 School Health Policies and Practices Study have indicated that the management of chronic conditions in schools has risen in the past few years. The American Academy of Pediatrics Council on School Health (2016) has recommended that each school building house a full-time school nurse.

All states authorize the provision of school health services and mandate some basic health prerequisites for school attendance. Occupational therapy practitioners are licensed as health care professionals and listed as potential health service providers. This is an area central to occupational therapy practice. The CDC (2017a) has recommended on-site care coordination that occupational therapy practitioners can contribute to in collaboration with the school nurse.

Counseling, psychological, and social services

Counseling, psychological, and social services address the mental, behavioral, and social–emotional health of students. Services often consist of assessment, intervention, and referral. Since 2012, approximately 10% more school districts have designated a coordinator of these services, but the scope and content of the services vary considerably for students in general education (School Health Policies and Practices Study, 2016). In contrast, special education students must receive these services if indicated on their IEP.

Occupational therapy practitioners are involved in the provision of mental health and social services (Arbesman et al., 2013). Schools have some discretion in how services are provided, and multiple approaches have evolved, ranging from in-school services delivered by school staff to collaborative arrangements with community providers. A public example of an innovative approach is the Occupational Therapy Training Program (OTTP; http://www.ottp .org/) in California.

OTTP originated as functional life skills training for youth in foster and probation programs (Bream, 2010; Hayworth & Cyrs, 2017). Today, the organization operates from 3 sites across the state and uses the occupational therapy principle of engagement in meaningful and purposeful activity to facilitate problem solving, stress management, self-confidence, money management, and job behaviors. OTTP provides school mental health services in

several alternative education settings. In addition, OTTP runs a youth center that provides a safe haven for youth after school, in the evenings, and on the weekends.

Community involvement

Community involvement refers to partnerships between schools and organizations in the community for mutual benefit and the overall goal of a healthy community. Schools, community groups, institutions, and businesses can share health goals and resources. The desire to better integrate health promotion efforts was the impetus for the creation of the WSCC model with strong community involvement (Kolbe et al., 2015). The adoption of this model requires school occupational therapy practitioners to envision themselves as active collaborative members of the local community.

Family engagement

Family engagement is a responsibility for schools and for family. The school should be a welcome place for family, providing opportunities for collaborative efforts to improve the learning, development, and health of students. Families should be engaged in meaningful ways to support involvement across each child's life into young adulthood. Family-centered care has long been a foundational philosophy in pediatric occupational therapy practice (Schaaf & Mulrooney, 1989). Its tenets of family involvement have application for healthy schools.

Physical education and physical activity

Physical education and physical activity refers to a school environment that offers opportunities for activity throughout the school day. Sixty minutes of movement daily is the target amount for healthy schools (Basset et al., 2013). The means to achieve this target amount are encompassed in a comprehensive school physical activity program (Shape America, 2018). Multipronged approaches demonstrate the best results.

A systematic review conducted by the Cochrane Collaboration identified physical activity as a successful outcome for programs based on WHO's Health Promoting Schools framework (Langford et al., 2015). This framework incorporates health education into the curriculum, makes changes to the school environment (i.e., social, physical, or both), and involves families and the community (Langford et al., 2015). Currently in the United States, schools continue to perform poorly in providing opportunities for physical activity. Although 89% of districts support and require formal physical education, only 15% of school districts require someone to oversee a comprehensive school physical activity program at each school.

Recess has emerged as a prime focus for strategies to increase physical activity as well as social–emotional school climate, with positive evidence to support it (Ickes et al., 2013; Playworks, 2018). Other examples of successful programs include Jump Rope for Heart and Hoops for Heart (American Heart Association, 2018), JUMP-in (de Meij et al., 2011), and Movin' Afterschool (Huberty et al., 2013). Occupational therapists engage in the promotion of healthy physical activity and have contributed to health programs in the areas of obesity (Pizzi, 2016), children with assistive mobility devices (Jirikowic & Kerfeld, 2016), autism (Mische Lawson & Foster, 2016), and culturally diverse populations (Kuo et al., 2016; Suarez-Balcazar et al., 2016), to name a few examples.

BEST PRACTICES

The promotion of health is a human concern that spans all people and, as such, involves a broad array of fields of study and professionals. AOTA (2013c) identified the occupational therapy practitioner's role in health promotion to include emphasis on healthy lifestyles with occupation as an essential element and on interventions for persons, groups, and populations. The most basic way occupational therapists can promote health is to routinely address health issues in daily practice. In this capacity, occupational therapists can

- Perform assessments for health risks,
- Teach strategies to incorporate healthy lifestyles,
- Identify solutions to personal and environmental barriers to healthy activities, and
- Educate and provide skills training in healthy occupational engagement.

For example, the CAGE Questionnaire (Ewing, 1984) is a simple yet validated 4-question screening tool to detect problems with alcohol. Occupational therapists can incorporate this type of screening into the occupational profile when working with adolescents.

When occupational therapy practitioners address components of health literacy, they teach strategies and identify solutions to personal and environmental health risks while facilitating client access to care. In addition, work with the issues of time management and occupational balance promotes health. Occupational therapists perform a key role in identifying solutions to barriers to healthy activities. Community access, ADLs that promote healthy lifestyles, and skills training in healthy occupational engagement are the core of the profession.

Health-Promoting Schools

Beyond contributing to health promotion at the person level, occupational therapy practitioners have contributed and should continue to contribute to broader health promotion efforts (Bazyk et al., 2015; Suarez-Balcazar et al., 2016). Health promotion programs incorporating the 3 attributes of WHO's Health Promoting Schools framework have resulted in positive outcomes for body mass, physical activity, healthy eating, tobacco usage, and bullying (Langford et al., 2015). These programs include a formal curricular approach combined with attention to an informal supportive school climate with outreach for community involvement.

Guidelines, Recommendations, and Adaptations That Include Disability

Occupational therapy practitioners can adapt existing and successful health promotion programs to address the needs of individuals with disabilities. Rimmer et al. (2014) proposed a framework to close the gap between available health promotion programs and disability interventions. Piloted on programs that address issues of obesity, Guidelines, Recommendations, and Adaptations That Include Disability has been developed for 11 of 24 CDC obesity programs thus far (Rimmer et al., 2014).

Community Health Implementation Package

Another powerful resource for ensuring inclusion of students with disabilities in healthy school programs meant to be open for all is the Inclusive Community Health Implementation Package. Sponsored by the National Center on Health, Physical Activity and Disability (https://www.nchpad.org/), this online resource has interactive tools that address, among other topics, how to create inclusive policy, communication, and assessment as well as specific training information.

MAP–IT

Healthy People 2020 provides a step-by-step framework to guide the development of or improve existing school health programs. This framework is called *MAP–IT* (Mobilize, Assess, Plan, Implement, and Track; Office of Disease Prevention and Health Promotion, 2018). Understanding the MAP–IT process provides insight for practitioners who wish to initiate or join in with a developing project.

M: Mobilize

The MAP–IT method begins with mobilization, which means finding key partners who share interest in and are willing to contribute to a healthy school initiative or program. Mobilization expands the sphere of influence from one individual to many or, as described in the WSCC model, from one school to an entire community.

Healthy school initiatives started by occupational therapy practitioners typically arise out of a concern realized in daily practice. For example, while addressing the seating needs of a student, a practitioner noticed postural concerns across the general education class and sought support from others to promote healthier seating so students would have the right fit and flexible seating options in classrooms. The practitioner communicated this idea to others and recruited others to meet this goal.

A: Assess

The second step in launching a health promotion initiative is to assess who is affected and how. It is important to determine what resources are available and what resources need to be found. In this process, 2 types of data should be gathered:

1. Numbers and facts to provide an objective picture of the situation and
2. Varied perspectives from those affected by the initiative.

These data provide a deeper understanding of the health promotion concern and any unexplored options. Factual information can be obtained through national, state, and local sources. Nationally, the Data Resource Center for Child and Adolescent Health (http://www.childhealthdata.org/) and the KIDS COUNT Data Center (https://datacenter.kidscount

.org) have statistics about children's health, which may provide guidance in answering questions and assessing the concern.

When collecting data to understand the varied perspectives of those involved, the occupational therapy practitioner and team may draw on different models for assessment. Brunner et al. (2012) applied key concepts from the *Occupational Therapy Practice Framework: Domain and Process* (3rd ed.; AOTA, 2014b) along with ecological models in occupational therapy to identify how people, context, and occupations intersect in a community. Smallfield and Anderson (2009) applied a logic model development guide to create a community profile and understand different perspectives.

P: Plan

Targeting the outcome rather than a specific solution gives the team flexibility when developing the plan. Alternative and potentially more effective approaches can be explored. Healthy school intervention plans should

- Identify key intervention points, on the basis of evidence, where changes can be made;
- Include clear objectives and steps; and
- Include meaningful measures of progress.

Identifying key intervention points involves seeking research evidence for considered approaches and noting opportunities for implementation. For example, data were used to provide evidence for stretching and posture awareness education to improve learning-ready posture. Meaningful measureable outcomes were planned around the effect of the intervention, such as increased time on task.

I: Implement

Successful implementation requires the commitment of involved individuals and ownership of the healthy school intervention. Occupational therapists can accomplish this by designating specific individuals to implement concrete steps as well as naming an individual to oversee the intervention and pull the multiple efforts together.

Communication among team members keeps the project alive. It is important to provide opportunities for support and encouragement as well as to inform others of the progress toward outcomes. Communicating in this way rewards those implementing the health promotion intervention and verifies to participants that they are part of something worthwhile.

T: Track

As the plan is implemented, it is critical to continue to track progress, collecting data about the outcomes of the health promotion intervention. Ongoing data collection informs the implementers of the progressive successes and failures of the intervention, allows for needed changes, and creates efficiency. Outcomes should be a routine part of the communication during implementation and ultimately feed into plans that may proceed beyond the original project.

SUMMARY

Health and school settings have been paired globally (WHO, 2018) and nationally (i.e., WSCC; CDC, 2017c) and are pervasively intertwined at the individual school level. Lifestyle choices are recognized as highly influential to health; thus, health promotion has become an integral part of all health care. Occupational therapy practitioners are calling for a reorientation of the profession toward health, well-being, and quality of life (Pizzi & Richards, 2017). School practitioners can bring the distinct perspective and value of occupation in facilitating life changes in healthy school efforts. In addition, they are well positioned to serve as advocates for all students and staff, including populations at risk for health concerns.

REFERENCES

American Academy of Pediatrics. (2004). Policy Statement: Soft drinks in schools. *Pediatrics, 113*(1), 152–154. Retrieved from http://pediatrics.aappublications.org/content/pediatrics/113/1/152.full.pdf

American Academy of Pediatrics, Council on School Health. (2016). Role of the school nurse in providing school health services. *Pediatrics, 137*(6), 1–7. https://doi.org/10.1542/peds.2016-0852

American Heart Association. (2018). *Kids Heart Challenge.* Retrieved from http://american.heart.org/jump-hoops/

American Occupational Therapy Association. (2013a). AOTA's societal statement on health disparities. *American Journal of Occupational Therapy, 67*(6, Suppl.), S7–S8. https://doi.org/10.5014/ajot.2013.67S7

American Occupational Therapy Association. (2013b). Obesity and occupational therapy. *American Journal of Occupational Therapy, 67*(6, Suppl.), S39–S46. https://doi.org/10.5014/ajot.2013.67S39

American Occupational Therapy Association. (2013c). Occupational therapy in the promotion of health and well-being. *American Journal of Occupational Therapy, 67*(6, Suppl.), S47–S59. https://doi.org/10.5014/ajot.2013.67S47

American Occupational Therapy Association. (2014a). Guidelines for supervision, roles, and responsibilities during the delivery of occupational therapy services. *American Journal of Occupational Therapy, 68*(Suppl. 3), S16–S22. https://doi.org/10.5014/ajot.2014.686S03

American Occupational Therapy Association. (2014b). Occupational therapy practice framework: Domain and process (3rd ed.). *American Journal of Occupational Therapy, 68*(Suppl. 1), S1–S48. https://doi.org/10.5014/ajot.2014.682006

American Occupational Therapy Association. (2015). Occupational therapy's perspective on the use of environments and contexts to facilitate health, well-being, and participation in occupations. *American Journal of Occupational Therapy, 69*(Suppl. 3), 6913410050. https://doi.org/10.5014/ajot.2015.696S05

American Occupational Therapy Association. (2017). AOTA's societal statement on health literacy. *American Journal of Occupational Therapy, 71*(Suppl. 2), 7112410065. https://doi.org/10.5014/ajot.2017.716S14

American Occupational Therapy Association. (2018). *AOTA's National School Backpack Awareness Day: September 18, 2019.* Retrieved from https://www.aota.org/Conference-Events/Backpack-Safety-Awareness-Day.aspx

Arbesman, M., Bazyk, S., & Nochajski, S. M. (2013). Systematic review of occupational therapy and mental health promotion, prevention, and intervention for children and youth. *American Journal of Occupational Therapy, 67*, e120–e130. https://doi.org/10.5014/ajot.2013.008359

Basset, D. R., Fitzhugh, E. C., Heath, G. W., Erwin, P. C., Frederick, G. M., Wolff, D. L., . . . Stout, A. B. (2013). Estimated energy expenditures for school-based policies and active living. *American Journal of Preventive Medicine, 44,* 108–113. https://doi .org/10.1016/j.amepre.2012.10.017

Bazyk, S. (2014). *Every moment counts: Promoting mental health throughout the day.* Retrieved from http://www.everymoment-counts.org/up_doc/EMC_Info_Brief.pdf

Bazyk, S., Demirjian, L., & Horvath, F. (2014). *Creating a comfortable cafeteria program.* Retrieved from http://www .everymomentcounts.org/up_doc/Cafeteria_Info_Brief_7-15 -14.pdf

Bazyk, S., Demirjian, L., LaGuardia, T., Thompson-Repas, K., Conway, C., & Michaud, P. (2015). Building capacity of occupational therapy practitioners to address the mental health needs of children and youth: A mixed-methods study of knowledge translation. *American Journal of Occupational Therapy, 69,* 6906180060. https://doi.org/10.5014/ajot.2015.019182

Bream, S. (2010). Meeting the mental health needs of adolescents. *OT Practice, 15*(11), 15–18.

Brunner, J., Valvano, D., & Lopez, A. (2012). Empowering communities to help at-risk youth engage in healthy occupations. *OT Practice, 17*(13), 10–13, 20.

Bundy, A., Luckett, T., Naughton, G. A., Tranter, P. J., Wyver, S. R., Ragen, J., . . . Spies, G. (2008). Playful interaction: Occupational therapy for all children on the school playground. *American Journal of Occupational Therapy, 62,* 522–527. https://doi .org/10.5014/ajot.62.5.522

Centers for Disease Control and Prevention. (2017a). *Research brief: Addressing the needs of students with chronic health conditions: Strategies for schools.* Retrieved from https://www.cdc .gov/healthyschools/chronic_conditions/pdfs/2017_02_15 -How-Schools-Can-Students-with-CHC_Final_508.pdf

Centers for Disease Control and Prevention. (2017b). *Results from the School Health Policies and Practices Study 2016.* Retrieved from https://www.cdc.gov/healthyyouth/data/shpps/pdf/shpps -results_2016.pdf

Centers for Disease Control and Prevention. (2017c). *Whole school, whole community, whole child.* Retrieved from https:// www.cdc.gov/healthyschools/wscc/index.htm

Collaborative for High Performance Schools. (2018). *Best practices manual.* Retrieved from https://chps.net/best-practices-manual

de Meij, J. S., Chinapaw, M. J., van Stralen, M. M., van der Wal, M. F., van Dieren, L., & van Mechelen, W. (2011). Effectiveness of JUMP-in, a Dutch primary school-based community intervention aimed at the promotion of physical activity. *British Journal of Sports Medicine, 45,* 1052–1057. https://doi.org/10.1136 /bjsm.2010.075531

Ewing, J. A. (1984). Detecting alcoholism: The CAGE Questionnaire. *JAMA, 252,* 1905–1907. https://doi.org/10.1001/jama.1984 .03350140051025

Global Burden of Disease Neurological Disorders Collaborator Group. (2017). Global, regional, and national burden of neurological disorders during 1990–2015: A systematic analysis for the Global Burden of Disease Study 2015. *Lancet Neurology, 16,* P877–P897. https://doi.org/10.1016/S1474-4422(17)30299-5

Goldston, S. E. (Ed.). (1987). *Concepts of primary prevention: A framework for program development.* Sacramento: California Department of Mental Health.

Hayworth, C., & Cyrs, G. (2017). Supporting transitions to the workforce for at-risk youth. *OT Practice, 22*(15), 21–24.

Huberty, J., Beets, M., & Beighle, A. (2013). Effects of a policy-level intervention on children's pedometer-determined physical activity: Preliminary findings from Movin' Afterschool. *Journal of Public Health Management and Practice, 19,* 525–528. https:// doi.org/10.1097/PHH.0b013e31829465fa

Ickes, M. J., Erwin, H., & Beighle, A. (2013). Systematic review of recess interventions to increase physical activity. *Journal of Physical Activity and Health, 10,* 910–926. https://doi .org/10.1123/jpah.10.6.910

Individuals With Disabilities Education Improvement Act of 2004, Pub. L. No. 108–446, 20 U.S.C. §§ 1400–1482.

Institute for Health Metrics and Evaluation. (2017). *IHME releases second annual report on the Sustainable Development Goal indicators.* Retrieved from http://www.healthdata.org/news-release /ihme-releases-second-annual-report-sustainable-development -goal-indicators

Jacobs, K., Wuest, E., Markowitz, J., & Hellman, M. (2011). Planning your own National School Backpack Awareness Day event. *OT Practice, 16*(13), 11–14.

Jirikowic, T. L., & Kerfeld, C. I. (2016). Health-promoting physical activity of children who use assistive mobility devices: A scoping review. *American Journal of Occupational Therapy, 70,* 7005180050. https://doi.org/10.5014/ajot.2016.021543

Kolbe, L. J., Allensworth, D. D., Potts-Datema, W., & White, D. (2015). What have we learned from collaborative partnerships to concomitantly improve both education and health? *Journal of School Health, 85,* 776–774. https://doi.org/10.1111/josh.12312

Kuo, F., Pizzi, M. A., Change, W., Koning, S. J., & Fredrick, A. S. (2016). Exploratory study of the clinical utility of the Pizzi Healthy Weight Management Assessment (PHWMA) among Burmese high school students. *American Journal of Occupational Therapy, 70,* 7005180040. https://doi.org/10.5014/ajot.2016.021659

Langford, R., Bonell, C., Jones, H., Pouliou, T., Murphy, S., Waters, E., . . . Campbell, R. (2015). The World Health Organization's Health Promoting Schools framework: A Cochrane systematic review and meta-analysis. *BioMed Central Public Health, 15*(130). https://doi.org/10.1186/s12889-015-1360-y

Lewallen, T. C., Hunt, H., Potts-Datema, W., Zaza, S., & Giles, W. (2015). The Whole School, Whole Community, Whole Child model: A new approach for improving educational attainment and health development for students. *Journal of School Health, 85,* 729–739. https://doi.org/10.1111/josh.12310

Mische Lawson, L., & Foster, L. (2016). Sensory patterns, obesity, and physical activity participation of children with autism spectrum disorder. *American Journal of Occupational Therapy, 70,* 7005180070. https://doi.org/10.5014/ajot.2016.021535

National Center for Education Statistics. (2013). *Characteristics of private schools in the United States: Results from the 2001–2002 Private School Universe Study.* Retrieved from https://nces.ed .gov/pubs2005/2005305.pdf

National Family Partnership. (2017). *Red ribbon campaign.* Retrieved from http://redribbon.org/

Office of Disease Prevention and Health Promotion. (2018). *Program planning: MAP–IT: A guide for using Healthy People 2020 in your community.* Retrieved from https://www.healthypeople .gov/2020/tools-and-resources/Program-Planning

Ogden, C. L., Carroll, M. D., Lawman, H. G., Fryar, C. D., Kruszon-Moran, D., Kit, B. K., & Flegal, K. M. (2016). Trends in obesity prevalence among children and adolescents in the United States, 1988–1994 through 2013–2014. *JAMA, 315,* 2292–2299. https://doi.org/10.1001/jama.2016.6361

Peaceful Playgrounds Foundation. (2018). *Peaceful Playgrounds Recess Program kit: The recess program that works!* Retrieved from https://peacefulplaygrounds.com/peaceful-playgrounds-recess-program/

Pizzi, M. (2016). Promoting health, well-being, and quality of life for children who are overweight or obese and their families. *American Journal of Occupational Therapy, 70,* 7005170010. https://doi.org/10.5014/ajot.2016.705001

Pizzi, M. A., & Richards, L. G. (2017). Guest Editorial—Promoting health, well-being, and quality of life in occupational therapy: A commitment to a paradigm shift for the next 100 years. *American Journal of Occupational Therapy, 71,* 7104170010. https://doi.org/10.5014/ajot.2017.028456

Playworks. (2018). *What a better recess does.* Retrieved from https://www.playworks.org/

Ratzan, S. C., & Parker, R. M. (2000). Introduction. In C. R. Selden, M. Zorn, S. C. Ratzan, & R. M. Parker (Eds.), *National Library of Medicine current bibliographies in medicine: Health literacy* (NLM Pub. No. CBM 2000-1, pp. v–vii). Bethesda, MD: National Institutes of Health.

Rimmer, J. H., Vanderbom, K. A., Bandini, L. G., Drum, C. E., Luken, K., Suarez-Balcazar, Y., & Graham, I. D. (2014). GRAIDS: A framework for closing the gap in the availability of health promotion programs and interventions for people with disabilities. *Implementation Science, 9*(100). https://doi.org/10.1186/s13012-014-0100-5

Rimmer, J. H., Yamaki, K., Davis, B. M., Wang, E., & Vogel, L. C. (2011). Obesity and overweight prevalence among adolescents with disabilities. *Preventing Chronic Disease, 8,* A41.

Schaaf, R. C., & Mulrooney, L. L. (1989). Occupational therapy in early intervention: A family-centered approach. *American Journal of Occupational Therapy, 43,* 745–754. https://doi.org/10.5014/ajot.43.11.745

School Health Policies and Practices Study. (2016). *Results from the School Health Policies and Practices Study.* Retrieved from https://www.cdc.gov/healthyyouth/data/shpps/pdf/shpps-results_2016.pdf

Shape America. (2018). *Shape America: Society of Health and Physical Educators.* Retrieved from https://www.shapeamerica.org/

Shooshtari, S., Brownell, M., Mills, R. S. L., Dik, N., Yu, D. C. T., Chateau, D., Burchill, C. A., & Wetzel, M. (2017). Comparing health status, health trajectories and use of health and social services between children with and without developmental disabilities: A population-based longitudinal study in Manitoba. *Journal of Applied Research in Intellectual Disabilities, 30,* 584–601. https://doi.org/10.1111/jar.12253

Smallfield, S., & Anderson, A. J. (2009, September). Using after-school programming to support health and wellness: A physical activity engagement program description. *Early Intervention and School System Special Interest Quarterly, 16*(3), 1–4.

Suarez-Balcazar, Y., Hoisington, M., Agudelo Orozco, A., Arias, D., Garcia, C., Smith, K., & Bonner, B. (2016). Benefits of a culturally tailored health promotion program for Latino youth with disabilities and their families. *American Journal of Occupational Therapy, 70,* 7005180080. https://doi.org/10.5014/ajot.2016.021949

U.S. Department of Agriculture. (2017a). *National School Lunch Program (NSLP).* Retrieved from http://www.fns.usda.gov/slp

U.S. Department of Agriculture. (2017b). *School Breakfast Program (SBP).* Retrieved from http://www.fns.usda.gov/sbp

World Health Organization. (1986). *The Ottawa Charter for Health Promotion.* Retrieved from http://www.who.int/healthpromotion/conferences/previous/ottawa/en/

World Health Organization. (2018). *School health and youth health promotion.* Retrieved from http://www.who.int/school_youth_health/en/

Best Practices in School Mental Health

19

Susan Bazyk, PhD, OTR/L, FAOTA

KEY TERMS AND CONCEPTS

- Embedded strategies
- Mental health
- Mental health continuum
- Mental health literacy
- Mental health promotion services
- Mindfulness, yoga, and relaxation approaches
- Positive behavioral interventions and supports
- School mental health
- Social and emotional learning
- Tier 1 services
- Tier 2 services
- Tier 3 services
- Universal services

OVERVIEW

Occupational therapy has a rich history of promoting mental health in all areas of practice through the use of meaningful and enjoyable occupations (Meyer, 1922). This chapter focuses on occupational therapy's role in applying a public health framework for addressing mental health needs of children and youth in schools, including promotion, prevention, and individualized interventions. The chapter also shares practical occupation-based strategies for implementing universal, targeted, and intensive services throughout the school day.

Over the past 2 decades, school mental health programs and services have seen steady growth (Kutash et al., 2006). This growth has been motivated by several factors, including the high prevalence of mental health conditions among children and youth, an awareness that more students can be reached in schools, and important federal initiatives.

The Education for All Handicapped Children Act of 1975 (Pub. L. 94–142), later reauthorized as the Individuals With Disabilities Education Improvement Act of 2004 (Pub. L. 108–446), was the first federal initiative that required schools to meet the mental health needs of students with emotional challenges. Section 504 of the Rehabilitation Act of 1973, as amended (2008; Pub. L. 93–112; 34 C.F.R. Part 104.4), also provides accommodations for students with mental health diagnoses. In 2001, the *World Health Report* called for schools to prevent suicide and help students develop positive mental health (World Health Organization [WHO], 2001). In addition, the health-promoting school model advanced by WHO provides an organizing framework for comprehensive health promotion to create school environments that support students' mental and physical health and family involvement (Jané-Llopis & Mittelmark, 2015).

ESSENTIAL CONSIDERATIONS

School mental health has evolved to become a framework of approaches that expand on traditional mental health services to emphasize promotion, prevention, positive youth development, and schoolwide approaches (National Center for School Mental Health, n.d.). This framework promotes interdisciplinary collaboration among mental health providers, related service providers, school administrators, teachers, and families to meet the mental health needs of all students.

Mental Health Continuum

To address the mental health needs of all children and youth within a promotion, prevention, and intervention framework, it is important to understand the *mental health continuum.* This continuum can be viewed as ranging from complete mental health and flourishing at one end to moderate mental health and becoming unwell in the middle and mental illness at the other end (Keyes, 2007). Research findings suggest that mental health is more than the absence of mental illness—it reflects a positive state of functioning (Keyes, 2007).

Children and youth who experience positive mental health and well-being function better during academic and nonacademic times of the school day (Dix et al., 2012). As such, it is important for occupational therapy practitioners[1] to be aware of this distinction and help school personnel, students, and families understand how to recognize and promote positive mental health as well as identify early indicators of mental illness (Bazyk, 2011).

---

[1] *Occupational therapy practitioner* refers to both the occupational therapist and the occupational therapy assistant. The American Occupational Therapy Association (AOTA; 2014a, p. S18) states, "The occupational therapist is responsible for all aspects of occupational therapy service delivery and is accountable for the safety and effectiveness of the occupational therapy service delivery process" and "must be directly involved in the delivery of services during the initial evaluation and regularly throughout the course of intervention. . . . The occupational therapy assistant delivers safe and effective occupational therapy services under the supervision of and in partnership with the occupational therapist."

Copyright © 2019 by the American Occupational Therapy Association. All rights reserved. To reuse this content, contact www.copyright.com.
https://doi.org/10.7139/2019.978-1-56900-591-0.019

Positive mental health is considered fundamental to overall health and quality of life and contributes to the functioning of individuals, families, communities, and societies (Barry & Jenkins, 2007). In 1999, *mental health* was defined by David Satcher, the U.S. Surgeon General at the time, as "a state of successful performance of mental function, resulting in productive activities, fulfilling relationships with people, and the ability to adapt to change and cope with adversity" (U.S. Department of Health and Human Services, 1999, p. 4). The following cluster of characteristics are associated with the presence of mental health (Bazyk, 2011; Miles et al., 2010):

- Positive affect (e.g., smiling, feeling happy or content);
- Positive psychological and social functioning (e.g., enjoying fulfilling relationships, having friends, feeling positive about oneself);
- Engaging in productive activities (e.g., being able to complete everyday tasks at school and home, such as attending in class); and
- Coping with life stressors and demonstrating resilience when challenged (e.g., bouncing back after a challenge, learning how to regulate emotions).

In terms of mental health disorders, approximately 1 in every 5 children and adolescents ages 9 to 17 years has a diagnosable emotional or behavioral disorder, with about half having mild impairment and the other half having significant impairment (National Research Council & Institute of Medicine, 2009). In a recent national study of lifelong prevalence of mental health disorders among adolescents (13–18 years), prevalence rates were found to be higher, with anxiety disorders being the most common (31.9%), followed by behavioral disorders (19.1%), mood disorders (14.3%), and substance use disorders (11.4%; Merikangas et al., 2010).

Although children with disabilities are 2.5–5 times more likely to develop mental health challenges than their non-disabled peers, attention to their mental health tends to be overshadowed by an emphasis on the remediation of physical limitations (Petrenchik et al., 2011). Increased rates of anxiety, depression, bipolar disorder, obsessive–compulsive disorder, and attention deficit hyperactivity disorder have been identified among children with autism spectrum disorder (Crabtree & Delaney, 2011). Approximately 90%–95% of these children have one or more comorbid psychiatric disorders (Salazar et al., 2015).

Mental health must be perceived as a dynamic state of functioning that can vary throughout a person's life course on the basis of many biological (e.g., genetics), environmental (e.g., poverty), situational (e.g., death of a parent), and developmental factors (Barry & Jenkins, 2007). Research indicates that initial symptoms generally appear 2–4 years before the onset of a full-blown disorder, which suggests the importance of early screening and intervention (Auther et al., 2008).

Accurate identification may take time and relies on information obtained from multiple sources, including the child, family, school personnel, and physicians. For this reason and to promote early intervention, all school personnel must be vigilant for any marked changes in a student's affect, social functioning, and ability to adapt to daily challenges (Bazyk, 2011). Without intervention, mental health issues tend to become more severe over time, causing further emotional pain, school difficulties, and social challenges.

Role of Occupational Therapy

Although many approaches specific to mental health promotion are important to know about and apply, all occupational therapy services share a common emphasis on the use of meaningful occupation to promote participation in needed and desired occupations relevant to school life and routines (education, play, leisure, work, social participation, ADLs, IADLs, sleep and rest) in a variety of contexts (AOTA, 2014b). Occupational therapy practitioners are distinctly qualified to provide occupation-based practice because of their expertise in activity design, task analysis, child development, and group process (Bazyk, 2011).

When interacting with other mental health providers (e.g., psychologists, social workers, school counselors), it is vital that occupational therapy practitioners articulate the distinct value of their services as the use of evidence-based, meaningful activities to promote participation. The findings of an evidence-based review, for example, indicated that activity-based interventions such as arts and crafts, play, and games help improve children's peer interactions, task-focused behaviors, and conformity to social norms (Bazyk & Arbesman, 2013). The authors of that review also recommended

- The use of peer models to foster the practice of new skills,
- Supportive adults to provide coaching, and
- An intervention program long enough to allow ample opportunity for practice of emergent skills.

The use of small groups tends to be the most powerful form of intervention for promoting social competence.

BEST PRACTICES

Understanding multi-tiered systems of support (MTSS) is important for providing services to students at the schoolwide, small group, and individual levels. Examples of application to practice are provided, with an emphasis on schoolwide approaches.

Provide MTSS for School Mental Health

A public health approach to children's mental health has been advocated for internationally (WHO, 2001) and in the United States (Atkins & Frazier, 2011; Miles et al., 2010). Recent occupational therapy publications (Bazyk, 2011) and evidence-based reviews (Bazyk & Arbesman, 2013) have applied this framework to addressing the mental health needs of children and youth in occupational therapy practice. Reflected in MTSS, a public health approach requires a change in thinking from the traditional, individually focused, deficit-driven model of mental health intervention to a schoolwide, strength-based model focusing on promotion, prevention, early intervention, and integration of services for all students.

In a public health model, 3 major levels of service can be provided:

1. *Tier 1 services:* Universal mental health promotion;
2. *Tier 2 services:* Targeted mental health prevention for those at risk of mental health challenges; and
3. *Tier 3 services:* Intensive mental health interventions for those with identified mental health disorders (Bazyk & Downing, 2017; see Figure 19.1).

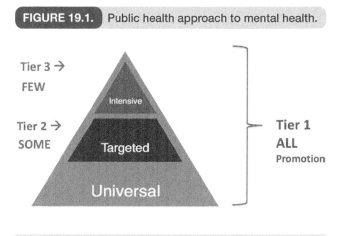

FIGURE 19.1. Public health approach to mental health.

Tier 3 →
FEW

Tier 2 →
SOME

Tier 1
ALL
Promotion

Intensive

Targeted

Universal

Mental health promotion services emphasize teaching competencies associated with mental health, such as social and emotional learning skills and coping strategies (Barry & Jenkins, 2007). Such efforts include creating supportive school environments, reducing stigma, and educating children on mental health literacy—that is, how to develop and maintain positive mental health (Jorm, 2012). Mental health prevention efforts focus on reducing both the incidence of and the seriousness of mental health challenges.

Early prevention programs focus on reducing risk factors (e.g., bullying) and enhancing protective factors (e.g., social and emotional competencies, clear standards for behavior; Bazyk & Downing, 2017). Practitioners provide intensive individualized interventions with a student to reduce symptoms associated with the mental health disorder and help the student participate successfully in school. In addition to diminishing challenges at this level, it is critical to focus on promoting positive mental health (Bazyk, 2011).

Apply a Public Health Approach to Mental Health in Schools

As Atkins et al. (2010) noted, "An important component of integrating mental health efforts into the ongoing routines of schools is the identification and support of indigenous persons and resources within schools as agents of change" (p. 42). Occupational therapy practitioners are among the few team members in schools who have specialized knowledge and skills in addressing the mental health needs of individuals. As such, they are indigenous resources for integrating mental health efforts in schools (Bazyk & Cahill, 2015). Practitioners have an important role in building capacity of the educational team and families to become mental health promoters when interacting with children and youth.

Although school occupational therapy practitioners are well equipped to provide services to promote mental health at the targeted and schoolwide levels, deliberate efforts are needed to shift service provision to an integrated model. Such services give occupational therapy practitioners access to all students, not just those on their caseload, which maximizes their ability to reach students who are at risk of developing mental health challenges.

Even though many school practitioners work within the constraints of a traditional caseload model, they can still provide Tier 1 and 2 services that address the mental health needs of students who are not on their caseload. A good way to accomplish this is by embedding mental health strategies while integrating services in natural contexts (Conway et al., 2015). *Embedded strategies* refers to interactions and activities aimed at promoting positive mental health placed firmly into all aspects of the school day.

In a 3-tiered public health model, occupational therapy practitioners provide a continuum of services geared toward mental health promotion, prevention, early identification, and intervention (Bazyk, 2011). Integrated services can be embedded in several natural contexts throughout the day, including the classroom, cafeteria (e.g., lunch groups), recess (e.g., game clubs), art, music, and physical education.

Use a Variety of Direct and Indirect Service Options

The Individuals With Disabilities Education Improvement Act of 2004 does not mandate any one service model and allows for a range of services, including those provided directly with the student (direct), on behalf of the student (indirect), and as program supports or modifications for teachers and other staff working with the student (indirect; Bazyk & Cahill, 2015). A wide range of direct and indirect service options can be used to address mental health.

For example, occupational therapy practitioners can provide whole-classroom or school programs that focus on helping students be mentally healthy by

- Learning coping and self-regulation skills (e.g., the Zones of Regulation™ program; Kuypers, 2011);
- Engaging in activities focusing on prosocial skills and health behaviors (e.g., the Comfortable Cafeteria and Refreshing Recess programs; Demirjian et al., 2014; Mohler et al., 2014); or
- Participating in relaxation strategies (e.g., the Drive Thru Menus or Calm Moments Cards programs; Bowen-Irish, 2010; Deininger et al., 2014).

Another helpful approach is to conduct occupation-based small-group interventions focusing on

- Prosocial skills (e.g., how to be a good friend),
- Mental health literacy (e.g., learning about positive mental health), and
- Mental health promotion (e.g., engaging in enjoyable activities, talking about feelings).

Such groups can be embedded in cafeteria time (e.g., lunch bunch), at recess (e.g., game group), in the classroom, or after school.

Occupational therapy practitioners can also focus on mental health during individual services. Even when addressing handwriting, for example, practitioners can embed mental health promotion strategies in their sessions (e.g., writing about feelings, identifying character strengths). Another approach is to evaluate and modify school environments to foster student participation and enjoyment. This approach might involve creating sensory-friendly spaces, modifying the physical environment to foster social participation, and helping children and adults interact in prosocial ways.

Finally, occupational therapy practitioners can build the capacity of school personnel and families to be mental health promoters. They can use a variety of creative strategies to help adults learn about positive mental health and how to promote it or give in-services, share newsletters or information sheets, put up posters, hold informal "café" meetings, and share website resources (e.g., the "Moments for Mental Health" tab on the Every Moment Counts website, https://bit.ly/2UK8LzN).

Provide Tier 1: Universal Mental Health Promotion and Prevention Services

Universal services are geared toward the entire school population, including the majority of students who do not demonstrate mental health or behavioral challenges. At this level, it is critical for occupational therapy practitioners to work collaboratively with a wide variety of individuals, including administrators, teachers, health educators, cafeteria and recess supervisors, and families. Services focus on

- Contributing to schoolwide approaches developed outside of the profession,
- Leading occupational therapy–developed universal programs, and
- Embedding mental health promotion and prevention strategies at an individual or small-group level.

Each is described here.

Contribute to universal approaches developed outside of the profession

Occupational therapy practitioners need to learn about and contribute to prominent schoolwide approaches that focus on mental health promotion and prevention, such as

- Social and emotional learning (SEL);
- Positive behavioral interventions and supports (PBIS);

- Mindfulness, yoga, and relaxation strategies; and
- Mental health literacy (Exhibit 19.1).

In a systematic review of universal approaches to mental health, positive evidence of effectiveness was obtained for programs that implemented whole-school approaches for more than a year and emphasized mental health, as opposed to prevention of mental illness (Wells et al., 2003).

Implement universal programs developed by occupational therapy practitioners

Since 2010, several programs developed by occupational therapy practitioners have added to schoolwide mental health promotion and prevention efforts. These programs represent distinct ways in which the occupational therapy profession can contribute to the mental well-being of all students and help create positive school environments that enable participation for children and adults. When they implement the following programs, occupational therapy practitioners use their knowledge of and skills in

- Developing and adapting meaningful activities,
- Using sensory-based strategies,
- Analyzing the environment, and
- Fostering social and emotional development.

This makes occupational therapy practitioners the ideal team members to take the lead in implementation.

The Zones of Regulation (Kuypers, 2011) is a widely used curriculum developed by an occupational therapist that provides a systematic, cognitive–behavioral approach to teach children about their emotional and sensory needs so they can self-regulate, control their emotions and impulses, manage their sensory needs, and improve their ability to problem solve conflicts. The Zones of Regulation combines Social Thinking® concepts and visual supports to help students identify feelings, understand how their behaviors affect

---

EXHIBIT 19.1.   Prominent and Emerging Schoolwide Approaches Emphasizing Mental Health Promotion and Prevention

Social and emotional learning (**SEL**) is a framework used to guide the process of helping children and youth develop critical skills for life—how to get along with others, handle challenges, and behave ethically. Programs that foster SEL help children to recognize and manage emotions, think about their feelings and how they should act, regulate behavior through thoughtful decision making, and acquire important social skills for developing healthy relationships in life. Evidence-based reviews have provided strong support for the use of SEL programming at the universal level to improve social–emotional functioning and reduce problem behaviors (Durlak et al., 2011). For more information, refer to the Collaborative for Academic, Social and Emotional Learning (https://casel.org).

Positive behavioral interventions and supports (**PBIS**) is a framework for promoting positive behavior by creating school environments that proactively encourage appropriate behavior and prevent problem behaviors. PBIS approaches are based on evidence-based behavioral interventions and recognize that a number of relevant factors can influence a student's behavior, including those existing within the student and those reflected in the interaction between the student and the environment. Schoolwide PBIS systems support all students along a continuum of need based on the 3-tiered prevention model (Bradshaw et al., 2010). For more information, refer to http://www.pbis.org.

Mindfulness, yoga, and relaxation approaches have been found to be promising practices in school settings for improving coping abilities and reducing anxiety (Rempel, 2012). Such practices help students step back from stressful situations by teaching them how to purposefully and non-judgmentally be in the moment. Learning how to cope with stressful situations and everyday challenges is an important life skill for all children and youth. Feeling stressed and anxious can negatively affect students' learning (e.g., difficulty concentrating) and everyday functioning (e.g., sleeping, eating, socializing).

Mental health literacy involves helping all children and youth gain a working knowledge of positive mental health and proactive strategies for maintaining mental health (Barry & Jenkins, 2007). It also includes educating students about how to prevent mental health disorders, recognize signs of becoming unwell, engage in self-help strategies, and obtain help when feeling mentally unwell (Jorm, 2012). Youth Mental Health First Aid training courses educate adults on how to provide support to a young person experiencing emotional challenges or distress. These courses have been found to increase adults' confidence in and ability to comfort a young person in emotional distress or crisis (Aakre et al., 2016).

others, and learn tools that they can use to move to a more acceptable state.

The Drive-Thru Menus Relaxation and Attention program (Bowen-Irish, 2010) provides classroom teachers and other school personnel with a menu of 3- to 5-minute activities that can be embedded in the classroom to help students manage stress and relax or to enhance alertness for attending.

Every Moment Counts is an occupational therapy–led, multipronged mental health promotion initiative originally funded by the Ohio Department of Education (Bazyk et al., 2015). A public health approach to mental health is applied in the development and implementation of model programs that make up the initiative (e.g., Comfortable Cafeteria, Refreshing Recess, Calm Moments Cards, Leisure Matters). Every Moment Counts also includes embedded strategies designed to promote inclusive student participation and positive mental health throughout the day (Exhibit 19.2). This initiative also focuses on building the capacity of occupational therapy practitioners to be leaders and collaborators in addressing the mental health needs of all students. Results of a mixed-methods design found that the 6-month building capacity process resulted in statistically significant improvements in occupational therapists' knowledge, beliefs, and actions in applying a public health approach to address the mental health needs of children and youth in schools (Bazyk et al., 2015).

Embed mental health promotion strategies

There are numerous ways in which occupational therapy practitioners can promote positive mental health during individual and group interventions (even if the primary individualized education program goal does not specifically focus on mental health) and build the capacity of school personnel to be mental health promoters.

Informally observe all students. Tune into signs of positive mental health. Look for behaviors that might suggest mental health concerns, and communicate observations to the educational team.

Promote mental health literacy. Make mental health part of everyday conversation. Embed creative strategies for teaching students about positive mental health and how to recognize and cope with mental health challenges during handwriting practice, language arts, and lunch bunch groups. Some effective tools are coloring sheets, mental health apps, books, and posters that focus on mental health. Use downloadable materials from the Mental Health Literacy page on the Every Moment Counts website (http://www.everymomentcounts.org/view.php?nav_id=197).

Clearly articulate the scope of occupational therapy practice. Articulate the scope of occupational therapy as including social participation, social–emotional function, and mental health.

Implement Tier 2: Targeted Mental Health Services

Targeted interventions are designed to support students who have learning, emotional, or life experiences that place them at risk for developing mental health challenges or engaging in problematic behavior. For example, students with physical or developmental disabilities might struggle with low self-esteem, issues related to feeling different, or the stress associated with frequent hospitalizations. In addition, students with and without disabilities are likely at some point in their life to struggle with situational stressors such as friendship issues, bullying, parental divorce, the death of a family member, poverty, or academic challenges.

| **EXHIBIT 19.2.** | Every Moment Counts Model Programs |

Comfortable Cafeteria: This 6-week program (developed by Demirjian et al., 2014), held 1 day per week, is embedded during lunchtime with the purpose of creating a positive cafeteria environment so that all students can enjoy their meal and socialize with friends. The program's goal is to provide the cafeteria staff and students with the necessary knowledge, skills, and resources needed to create and sustain a comfortable cafeteria environment. Some of the weekly themes include how to be a good friend, have a mealtime conversation, and include others. Results of a mixed-methods design found statistically significant improvements in pretest–posttest ratings of participation in and enjoyment for students with low and midrange scores at the outset (Bazyk et al., 2018).

Refreshing Recess: This 6-week program (developed by Mohler et al., 2014), held 1 day each week, is embedded during recess with the purpose of creating a positive recess experience so that all students can enjoy active play and socialization with friends. The ultimate goal is to provide the recess supervisors and students with the necessary knowledge, skills, and resources needed to create and sustain a positive recess environment. Weekly themes include learning how to be a good friend, engaging in active play, including others, and interacting as a team.

Calm Moments Cards: This program was developed to build the capacity of occupational therapists and diverse school personnel (e.g., teachers, paraeducators) to recognize signs of stress and anxiety among students during 17 typical situational stressors (e.g., taking a test, completing a writing assignment). It also teaches them to apply evidence-based embedded strategies (cognitive–behavioral, mindfulness, and sensory) to help them reduce stress and enhance emotional well-being to improve school function (developed by Deininger et al., 2014).

Leisure Matters: The focus of Leisure Matters is to help all children and youth explore, select, and participate in extracurricular leisure activities to develop enjoyable and healthy hobbies and interests. Occupational therapy leisure coaching is the process, used either individually or in a small-group context, of educating youth and families about the health benefits of participation in enjoyable hobbies and interests. This approach also encourages them to explore and participate in community-based leisure activities, and it advocates for inclusive leisure participation in integrated school and community-sponsored extracurricular activities.

Note. See http://www.everymomentcounts.org for free and downloadable information and materials.

During such times, character strengths, coping strategies, participation in enjoyable occupations, and environmental supports can serve as important buffers in the prevention of mental ill health (Bazyk, 2011). When interacting with and observing students, occupational therapy practitioners should remain vigilant to the presence of possible stressors and advocate for and help develop services to counteract stressors and build competencies (e.g., grief support training for school personnel, participation in after-school clubs).

Students at risk of mental health challenges are generally not identified as needing services, but they often begin to display subtle changes in performance. Prevention services help students develop competencies to offset early symptoms (e.g., time management, relaxation strategies) and involve a more direct role in evaluation and intervention compared with Tier 1 services. At this level, occupational therapy practitioners might collaborate with teachers, social workers, or other mental health providers to develop and cofacilitate targeted interventions.

Examples of Tier 2 services include the following:

- Learn about early signs of a variety of mental health disorders and how symptoms might affect school functioning.
- Evaluate social participation with peers during all school activities, especially recess and lunch.
- Consult with teachers to modify learning demands and academic routines to foster successful participation and promote positive psychological functioning (e.g., breaking down school assignments to minimize anxiety, teaching relaxation strategies).
- Develop and run occupation-based small-group programs to foster social participation for students struggling with peer interaction.

Implement Tier 3: Individualized Intensive Mental Health Interventions

Tier 3 services are provided for students with identified mental, emotional, or behavioral disorders that limit participation in needed and desired areas of occupational functioning. Occupational therapy practitioners need to maintain an in-depth knowledge of

- A range of mental health and behavioral disorders,
- How the disorders influence the person's functioning in a variety of occupational areas (e.g., education, leisure, ADLs, social participation),
- Current psychosocial interventions, and
- School and community services (Bazyk, 2011).

Specific Tier 3 services for students with identified mental health challenges include the following:

- Collaborate with the other school mental health providers, teachers, and administrators to ensure a coordinated system of care for students needing intensive interventions.
- Provide ways to modify or enhance school routines to reduce stress and enhance feelings of emotional well-being.
- Offer individual or group interventions for students with serious emotional disturbance, either through special education or Section 504 accommodations or through modifications to enhance participation in education, social participation, play and leisure, and ADLs.
- Analyze the student's unique sensory needs, and develop intervention strategies to promote sensory processing

and successful function in multiple school contexts (e.g., classroom, cafeteria).

- Provide tips to promote successful functioning throughout the school day, including transitioning to classes, organizing work spaces (e.g., a desk, locker), handling stress, and developing strategies for time management.

SUMMARY

Children and youth who experience positive mental health and well-being function better during academic and nonacademic times of the school day. Occupational therapy practitioners are among the few team members in schools with specialized knowledge and skills to address mental health and, as such, serve as indigenous resources for integrating mental health programs and strategies throughout the day.

Ideally, it is possible to address the mental health needs of all students within a multi-tiered public health framework of mental health promotion, prevention, and individualized interventions. Best practice in schools emphasizes the integration of occupational therapy services in the general education classroom and nonacademic settings (e.g., lunch and recess) when possible, offering opportunities to contribute to mental health promotion and prevention efforts for all students.

RESOURCES FOR CHILDREN'S MENTAL HEALTH

AOTA School Mental Health Toolkit (https://bit.ly/1T9XPs0): Free, downloadable information sheets on a variety of topics, including depression, grieving, anxiety, and obesity

Every Moment Counts: Promoting Mental Health Throughout the Day (http://www.everymomentcounts.org): Free, downloadable information and material on how to apply a public health approach to mental health and implement occupation-based embedded strategies and model programs

Children's Mental Health Fact Sheets (Minnesota Children's Mental Health Association; https://bit.ly/2GraDKy): Free, downloadable fact sheets on mental health conditions, the impact on function, and strategies to foster successful participation in schools

Action for Happiness (http://www.actionforhappiness.org): Practical strategies, research, and resources committed to helping people build a happier and more caring society in their homes and communities; provides 10 keys for happier living that are backed by research

Bully Prevention: Office of Special Education Programs Technical Assistance Center on Positive Behavioral Interventions and Supports (free downloadable manuals):

- *Bully Prevention Manual: Elementary School Level* (https://www.pbis.org/resource/785)
- *Bully Prevention Manual: Middle School Level* (https://www.pbis.org/resource/786)
- *Steps to Respect:* Focuses on bully prevention and friendship development; developed by the Committee for Children (https://bit.ly/2BmvSaI)
- *Eyes on Bullying: What Can You Do?* Free, downloadable (https://bit.ly/2EtZjeZ).

REFERENCES

Aakre, J. M., Lucksted, A., & Browning-McNee, L. (2016). Evaluation of Youth Mental Health First Aid USA: A program to assist young people in psychological distress. *Psychological Services, 13,* 121–126. https://doi.org/10.1037/ser0000063

American Occupational Therapy Association. (2014a). Guidelines for supervision, roles, and responsibilities during the delivery of occupational therapy services. *American Journal of Occupational Therapy, 68*(Suppl. 3), S16–S22. https://doi.org/10.5014/ajot.2014.686S03

American Occupational Therapy Association. (2014b). Occupational therapy practice framework: Domain and process (3rd ed.). *American Journal of Occupational Therapy, 68*(Suppl. 1), S1–S48. https://doi.org/10.5014/ajot.2014.682006

Atkins, M. S., & Frazier, S. L. (2011). Expanding the toolkit or changing the paradigm: Are we ready for a public health approach to mental health? *Perspectives on Psychological Science, 6,* 483–487. https://doi.org/10.1177/1745691611416996

Atkins, M. S., Hoagwood, K. E., Kutash, K., & Seidman, E. (2010). Toward the integration of education and mental health in schools. *Administration and Policy in Mental Health, 37,* 40–47. https://doi.org/10.1007/s10488-010-0299-7

Auther, A. M., Gillett, D. A., & Cornblatt, B. A. (2008). Expanding the boundaries of early intervention for psychosis: Intervening during the prodrome. *Psychiatric Annals, 38,* 528–537. https://doi.org/10.3928/00485713-20080801-02

Barry, M. M., & Jenkins, R. (2007). *Implementing mental health promotion.* London: Churchill Livingstone/Elsevier.

Bazyk, S. (Ed.). (2011). *Mental health promotion, prevention, and intervention with children and youth: A guiding framework for occupational therapy.* Bethesda, MD: AOTA Press.

Bazyk, S., & Arbesman, M. (2013). *Occupational therapy practice guidelines for mental health promotion, prevention, and intervention for children and youth.* Bethesda, MD: AOTA Press.

Bazyk, S., & Cahill, S. (2015). School based practice. In J. Case-Smith & J. O'Brien (Eds.), *Occupational therapy for children* (7th ed., pp. 664–703). St. Louis: Elsevier/Mosby.

Bazyk, S., Demirjian, L., Horvath, F., & Dosxey, L. (2018). The Comfortable Cafeteria program for promoting student participation and enjoyment: An outcome study. *American Journal of Occupational Therapy, 72,* 7203205050. https://doi.org/10.5014/ajot.2018.025379

Bazyk, S., Demirjian, L., LaGuardia, T., Thompson-Repas, K., Conway, C., & Michaud, P. (2015). Building capacity of occupational therapy practitioners to address the mental health needs of children and youth: A mixed-methods study of knowledge translation. *American Journal of Occupational Therapy, 69,* 6906180060. https://doi.org/10.5014/ajot.2015.019182

Bazyk, S., & Downing, D. (2017). *Frequently asked questions (FAQ): School mental health for school-based occupational therapy practitioners.* Retrieved from http://www.aota.org/~/media/Corporate/Files/Secure/Practice/Children/School%20Mental%20Health%20FAQ%20Webfin.pdf

Bowen-Irish, T. (2010). *The Drive Thru Menus for relaxation and stress busters.* Framingham, MA: Therapro.

Bradshaw, C. P., Mitchell, M. M., & Leaf, P. J. (2010). Examining the effects of schoolwide positive behavioral interventions and supports on student outcomes: Results from a randomized controlled effectiveness trial in elementary schools. *Journal of Positive Behavioral Interventions, 12,* 161–179. https://doi.org/10.1177/1098300709334798

Conway, C., Kanics, I., Mohler, R., Guidici, M. S., & Wagenfield, A. (2015). *Occupational therapy's role in mental health promotion, prevention and intervention: Inclusion of children with disabilities.* Retrieved from https://www.aota.org/~/media/Corporate/Files/Practice/Children/Inclusion-of-Children-With-Disabilities-20150128.PDF

Crabtree, L., & Delaney, J. V. (2011). Autism: Promoting social participation and mental health. In S. Bazyk (Ed.), *Mental health promotion, prevention, and intervention with children and youth: A guiding framework for occupational therapy* (pp. 163–187). Bethesda, MD: AOTA Press.

Deininger, A., Kolic, S., & Young, D. (2014). *Calm Moments Cards (CMC).* Retrieved from http://www.everymomentcounts.org/view.php?nav_id=213

Demirjian, L., Horvath, F., & Bazyk, S. (2014). *Comfortable Cafeteria.* Retrieved from http://www.everymomentcounts.org/view.php?nav_id=1

Dix, K. L., Slee, P. T., Lawson, M. J., & Keeves, J. P. (2012). Implementation quality of whole-school mental health promotion and students' academic performance. *Child and Adolescent Mental Health, 17,* 45–51. https://doi.org/10.1111/j.1475-3588.2011.00608.x

Durlak, J. A., Weissberg, R. P., Dymnicki, A. B., Taylor, R. D., & Schellinger, K. B. (2011). The impact of enhancing students' social and emotional learning: A meta-analysis of school-based universal interventions. *Child Development, 82,* 405–432. https://doi.org/10.1111/j.1467-8624.2010.01564.x

Education for All Handicapped Children Act of 1975, Pub. L. 94–142, renamed the Individuals With Disabilities Education Improvement Act, codified at 20 U.S.C. §§ 1400–1482.

Individuals With Disabilities Education Improvement Act of 2004, Pub. L. 108–446, 20 U.S.C. §§ 1400–1482.

Jané-Llopis, E., & Mittelmark, M. B. (2015). No health without mental health. *Promotion and Education Supplement, 2,* 4–5. https://doi.org/10.1177/10253823050120020101x

Jorm, A. F. (2012). Mental health literacy: Empowering the community to take action for better mental health. *American Psychologist, 67,* 231–243. https://doi.org/10.1037/a0025957

Keyes, C. L. M. (2007). Promoting and protecting mental health as flourishing: A complementary strategy for improving national mental health. *American Psychologist, 62,* 95–108. https://doi.org/10.1037/0003-066X.62.2.95

Kutash, K., Duchnowski, A. J., & Lynn, N. (2006). *School-based mental health: An empirical guide for decision-makers.* Tampa: University of South Florida, Louis de la Parte Florida Mental Health Institute, Department of Child & Family Studies, Research and Training Center for Children's Mental Health.

Kuypers, L. (2011). *The zones of regulation.* Minneapolis: Social Thinking.

Merikangas, K. R., He, J. P., Burstein, M., Swanson, S. A., Avenevoli, S., Cui, L., . . . Swendsen, J. (2010). Lifetime prevalence of mental health disorders in US adolescents: Results from the National Comorbidity Study–Adolescent Supplement (NCS–A). *Journal of the American Academy of Child and Adolescent Psychiatry, 49,* 980–989. https://doi.org/10.1016/j.jaac.2010.05.017

Meyer, A. (1922). The philosophy of occupational therapy. *Archives of Occupational Therapy, 1,* 1–10.

Miles, J., Espiritu, R. C., Horen, N., Sebian, J., & Waetzig, E. (2010). *A public health approach to children's mental health: A conceptual framework.* Washington, DC: Georgetown University Center for Child and Human Development, National Technical Assistance, Center for Children's Mental Health.

Mohler, R., Kerns, S., & Bazyk, S. (2014). *Refreshing Recess.* Retrieved from http://www.everymomentcounts.org/view.php?nav_id=62

National Center for School Mental Health. (n.d.). *What is (expanded) school mental health?* Retrieved from http://www.schoolmentalhealth.org/Resources/ESMH/DefESMH.html

National Research Council & Institute of Medicine. (2009). *Preventing mental, emotional, and behavioral disorders among young people: Progress and possibilities.* Washington, DC: National Academies Press.

Petrenchik, T. M., King, G. A., & Batoriwicz, B. (2011). Children and youth with disabilities: Enhancing mental health through positive experiences of doing and belonging. In S. Bazyk (Eds.), *Mental health promotion, prevention and intervention in children and youth: A guiding framework for occupational therapy* (pp. 189–205). Bethesda, MD: AOTA Press.

Rehabilitation Act of 1973, Pub. L. 93–112, 29 U.S.C. §§ 701–7961.

Rempel, K. D. (2012). Mindfulness for children and youth: A review of the literature with an argument for school-based implementation. *Canadian Journal of Counseling and Psychotherapy, 46,* 201–220.

Salazar, F., Baird, G., Chandler, S., Tseng, E., O'Sullivan, T., Howlin, P., . . . Simonoff, E. (2015). Co-occurring psychiatric disorders in preschool and elementary school-aged children with ASD. *Journal of Autism and Developmental Disorders, 45,* 2283–2294. https://doi.org/10.1007/s10803-015-2361-5

Section 504 of the Rehabilitation Act of 1973, as amended, 29 U. S. C. § 794 (2008).

U.S. Department of Health and Human Services. (1999). *Mental health: A report of the Surgeon General.* Rockville, MD: U.S. Department of Health and Human Services, Substance Abuse and Mental Health Services Administration, Center for Mental Health, National Institutes of Health, and National Institute of Mental Health.

Wells, J., Barlow, J., & Stewart-Brown, A. (2003). A systematic review of universal approaches to mental health promotion in schools. *Health Education, 103,* 197–220. https://doi.org/10.1108/09654280310485546

World Health Organization. (2001). *The world health report: Mental health—New understanding, new hope.* Geneva: Author.

20

Best Practices in Universal Design for Learning

Judith Schoonover, MEd, OTR/L, ATP, FAOTA

KEY TERMS AND CONCEPTS

- Equitable use
- Flexibility in use
- Interdisciplinary collaboration
- Low physical effort
- Multiple means of action and expression
- Multiple means of engagement
- Multiple means of representation
- Multi-tiered systems of support
- Perceptible information
- Scaffolding
- Simple and intuitive use
- Size and space for approach and use
- Speech recognition
- Text to speech
- Tolerance for error
- Universal design
- Universal design for learning

OVERVIEW

Forcing [all] children to master the same curriculum essentially discriminates against talents that are not consistent with the prescribed knowledge and skills. Students who are otherwise talented but do not do well in the prescribed subjects are often sent to spend more time on the core subjects, retained for another grade, or deprived of the opportunity to develop their talents in other ways.—Zhao (2012, p. 45)

Today's diverse classrooms include an ever-increasing number of students with differing learning styles. Classrooms may be brick and mortar or virtual (i.e., online), and they draw students from great distances with varying cultures, languages, socioeconomic backgrounds, abilities, and needs. Educators are required to accommodate students' unique learning needs and to plan for and create optimal learning opportunities and supports throughout the school day and across subject areas. Educators are being asked to shift from traditional instructional and text-based practice to helping students integrate what they have learned and apply it in real-world settings. Current teaching methodologies include learning experiences that encompass a range of technology in the learning process to increase access to and engagement in the classroom and facilitate learning.

Aided by technology, the 2017 National Educational Technology Plan challenges students to become active learners and contributors in a 21st-century society (U.S. Department of Education, Office of Educational Technology, 2017). It is vital that students be prepared to function in diverse populations, economic conditions, and cultures. The key to stimulating such growth includes student engagement, participation, collaborative learning, personalized learning, project-based learning, and real-world contexts (Luna Scott, 2015).

Changing along with the face of today's learners are the roles of related services providers. New federal requirements have placed increased emphasis on collaboration in the classroom. The Individuals With Disabilities Education Improvement Act of 2004 (IDEA; Pub. L. 108–446) encourages early intervening services and supports initiatives, such as universal design for learning and *multi-tiered systems of support* (MTSS). MTSS is an integrated framework that focuses on data-driven instruction, differentiated learning, student-centered learning, support for individual student needs, and alignment of systems necessary for all students' academic, behavioral, and social success.

The passage of the Americans With Disabilities Act of 1990 (Pub. L. 101–336) required public buildings, including schools, to make architectural changes to provide physical access. Before the *universal design* (UD) movement, the mobility and communication needs of people with disabilities were not always considered, which resulted in buildings that were inaccessible to many. UD originated in the field of architecture and is based on proactively designing physical space from the outset with built-in accessibility (e.g., curb cuts, ramps, automatic doors, low thresholds, motion-sensor paper towel dispensers) rather than reactively retrofitting buildings with ramps, elevators, talking signs, and other access devices. Generally, retrofitting is expensive, is not always adequate, and may not be aesthetically pleasing.

Section 3002, Item (19), of the Assistive Technology Act of 2004 (Pub. L. 108–364) states,

The term "universal design" means a concept or philosophy for designing and delivering products and services that are usable by people with the widest possible range of functional capabilities, which include products and services that are directly accessible (without requiring assistive technologies) and products and services that are interoperable with assistive technologies.

Copyright © 2019 by the American Occupational Therapy Association. All rights reserved. To reuse this content, contact www.copyright.com.
https://doi.org/10.7139/2019.978-1-56900-591-0.020

UD became a framework for reform of the built environment and commercial products. It is based on the principles of

- *Equitable use:* The design is useful and marketable to people with diverse abilities.
- *Flexibility in use:* The design accommodates a wide range of individual preferences and abilities.
- *Simple and intuitive use:* Use of the design is easy to understand, regardless of the user's experience, knowledge, language skills, or concentration level.
- *Perceptible information:* The design communicates necessary information effectively to the user, regardless of ambient conditions or the user's sensory abilities.
- *Tolerance for error:* The design minimizes hazards and the adverse consequences of accidental or unintended actions.
- *Low physical effort:* The design can be used efficiently and comfortably and with a minimum of fatigue.
- *Size and space for approach and use:* Appropriate size and space are provided for approach, reach, manipulation, and use, regardless of the user's body size, posture, or mobility.

UD principles have extended to information and computer technologies. Embedded accessibility features are available on most computer and tablet operating systems. Examples include

- *Text to speech,* which refers to the ability of computers, tablets, and handheld devices to read text aloud;
- Speech to text, or *speech recognition,* which refers to the transcription of spoken words to text;
- Screen magnification;
- Word prediction; and
- On-screen keyboards.

These off-the-shelf tools allow users to customize their device on the basis of their preferences or individual needs. All students, their teachers, and their parents can facilitate learning by taking advantage of features in web browsers and embedded assistive technology (AT) components in the form of Microsoft and Apple operating systems available on current desktops, laptops, tablets, or phones (Koch, 2017).

Just as UD principles are used to inform and guide the design of physical space and products so that all users can have access to and benefit from them, *universal design for learning* (UDL) is an educational initiative for the reform of the learning environment. UDL was expanded from the UD movement in architecture. The Center for Applied Special Technology (Ralabate, 2011) referenced the concept of UD's flexibility and accessibility as a framework to change how students are taught. UDL focuses on providing curricula to support the diversity of students in today's schools.

Applying UD principles to the educational environment, UDL assumes that students with diverse skills and needs will be participants in learning and that the goals, curriculum, instructional materials, and assessments need to anticipate and address this diversity through alternatives, options, and adaptations. UDL is defined in the Higher Education Opportunity Act (2008; Pub. L. 110–315) as

> a scientifically valid framework for guiding educational practice that—(A) provides flexibility in the ways information is presented, in the ways students respond or demonstrate knowledge and skills, and in the ways students are engaged; and (B) reduces barriers in instruction, provides appropriate accommodations, supports, and challenges, and maintains high achievement expectations for all students, including students with disabilities and students who are limited English proficient. (§ 103[a][24])

In 2015, the Every Student Succeeds Act (ESSA; 2015; Pub. L. 114–195) retained the definition of UDL used in the Higher Education Opportunity Act and endorsed it as a tool to use with all students. ESSA included an increased focus on technology as a means of providing accessibility and improving instruction, opportunities, and outcomes for all students. Moreover, it is the first federal education law governing general kindergarten through 12th-grade education, including both a definition and an endorsement of UDL. It also references AT as a means of providing accessible assessments.

UDL applies the UD principles of equitable use, flexibility, simplicity, perceptibility, and efficiency to both the educational environment and the process of teaching and learning. It embraces the concept that "disability results from the interaction between persons with impairments and attitudinal and environmental barriers that hinder their full and effective participation in society on an equal basis with others" (United Nations Programme on Disability, 2006). The Center for Applied Special Technology (CAST) believes that "barriers to learning are not, in fact, inherent in the capacities of learners, but instead arise in learners' interactions with inflexible educational goals, materials, methods, and assessments" (Rose & Meyer, 2002).

A research-based set of principles is used to guide the design of educational materials and methods that are accessible to and effective for students with differing abilities to ensure meaningful participation in the curriculum. The design of instructional goals, assessments, methods, and materials is customized and adjusted to meet diverse needs. This design follows several principles:

- *Multiple means of engagement* (e.g., choices of content and tools, adjustable levels of challenge, choices of rewards, choices of learning context)—the "why" of learning
- *Multiple means of representation* (e.g., more than 1 example, critical features highlighted, use of media and formats, use of background context)—the "what" of learning
- *Multiple means of action and expression* (e.g., flexible models of skilled performance; opportunities to practice with supports; ongoing, relevant feedback; flexible opportunities for demonstrating skill)—the "how" of learning.

Evidence-based strategies for enlisting students' engagement and participation in learning include

- *Scaffolding,* which explicitly ties new information to what a student already knows;
- Providing options for individual choice and autonomy; and
- Giving students tools for managing frustration.

The analogy of training wheels on a bicycle has been used to define *scaffolding* as a form of temporary assistance designed to let the learner progress. UDL recognizes the need to make the student's environment accessible and to promote different modes of engagement. Engagement is a necessary component of the perception and strategic action required for learning (CAST, 2018).

ESSENTIAL CONSIDERATIONS

Although the term *universal* appears to suggest that one size fits all, the true essence of UDL is the belief that the process of designing the academic environment should be proactive rather than reactive. Moreover, it should be flexible in nature, with multiple ways to address variations in learner strengths, needs, styles, and preferences (CAST, 2018). Donna Palley, a special education coordinator, described UDL as "the intersection where all our initiatives—multisensory teaching, multiple intelligences, differentiated instruction, use of computers in schools, performance-based assessment, and others—come together" (Rose & Meyer, 2002, p. 7).

Occupational therapy practitioners[1] can play a vital role in supporting implementation of UDL principles in schools through their knowledge base, skills in activity analysis, and ability to adapt tools and environments. They are able to recommend, model, and provide training in the use of technology and other methods to facilitate learning and performance in the context of classrooms (AOTA, 2015). Occupational therapy practitioners focus on meaningful participation in daily occupations, activities, and tasks.

Models of occupational therapy in schools continue to evolve in response to the changing and complex needs of students (Bissell & Cermak, 2015). School occupational therapy practitioners provide direct services and consultative services to students with disabilities. In addition, there is a role for practitioners to support all students, staff, and administrators—with or without disabilities—in the school climate.

Interdisciplinary collaborations and cooperative sharing of information from various perspectives and professions have the potential to change the way students learn and become productive participants in the educational environment and well beyond the classroom doors. *Interdisciplinary collaboration,* as defined by the World Health Organization (2010), involves collaborative efforts of varied professionals in the delivery of high-quality care.

Ogletree (2017) suggested that "the continuous, reflective, and purposeful collaboration, described as Interprofessional Collaborative Practice (IPCP), is relatively new and likely stems from another more recent concept, Interprofessional Education (IPE)" (p. 158). Interprofessional teams collaboratively design and advocate for physical,

social, and academic environments that promote participation and skill development for all students (Missiuna et al., 2015).

UDL Does Not Eliminate the Need for AT

UDL and AT are related and may coexist. The same strategy or tool can be considered UDL for some students and AT for others. Implementation of UDL does not imply that AT is no longer necessary. Students may require specific and individually selected AT devices (e.g., communication devices, visual aids, mobility supports, specific applications, adapted toys and tools) to meaningfully participate in their role as learner.

Specific AT paired with a learning environment embracing UDL assessments, methods, and materials maximizes learning opportunities for students with disabilities. A key tool in the provision of flexibility prescribed by a UDL approach is achieved through use of technology, including

- Digital books,
- Word prediction software,
- Text-to-speech software,
- Graphic organizers, and
- Word-processing programs.

Provisions in IDEA require state and local educational agencies to ensure that textbooks and related core instructional materials are provided in a timely manner to students with print disabilities (i.e., difficulty accessing instructional material in nonspecialized formats) in specialized formats (§ 300.172). Providing accessible educational materials to eligible students and teaching them to use technology such as text to speech, speech to text, and word prediction software can enhance their learning experiences.

Educators and service providers should be aware that providing access to the educational environment through AT and UDL does not eliminate the need for instruction in educational, vocational, social, and recreational skills pertinent to the tasks of learning and living (Zabala, 2010). A barrier to the use of accessibility features is the issue of students not wanting to appear different from their peers. Although the use of technology might increase a student's autonomy and independence, they may choose not to use an accommodation that calls attention to the manner in which work is being completed (Cook, 2009).

School staff may also need to be educated so that they do not view the use of such features as providing selected students with an unfair advantage. Therefore, incorporating use of technologies into the classroom, modeling, and providing options to all students while objectively analyzing the benefits of those options may increase acceptance of needed features.

Cultural Considerations

The principles of UDL give students and education teams a new lens through which to view multiple means of seeing, hearing, thinking, and knowing (Wilson, 2017). Providing a variety of ways to engage and sustain engagement, presenting information in more than one format, and enabling students to express their knowledge in different ways can result in positive outcomes for learning, self-efficacy, and sense of community (Collins, 2014).

---

[1]*Occupational therapy practitioner* refers to both the occupational therapist and the occupational therapy assistant. The American Occupational Therapy Association (AOTA; 2014, p. S18) states, "The occupational therapist is responsible for all aspects of occupational therapy service delivery and is accountable for the safety and effectiveness of the occupational therapy service delivery process" and "must be directly involved in the delivery of services during the initial evaluation and regularly throughout the course of intervention. . . . The occupational therapy assistant delivers safe and effective occupational therapy services under the supervision of and in partnership with the occupational therapist."

These inclusive practices go beyond accommodations for students with disabilities. They provide options for all students to interact with and respond to information. For example, the use of videos for instruction may provide additional or alternative visual information to students with reading difficulties or those who are English-language learners. Videos might also maintain the attention of students who are easily distracted. In addition to supporting English-language learners, adding closed captioning can support learners who are deaf or hard of hearing. The UDL framework could be used to create a learning environment that recognizes and celebrates cultural diversity by reducing barriers for culturally diverse learners and assisting them in the development of a broader range of expressive, critical, and cognitive styles (Chita-Tegmark et al., 2012).

Edyburn (2010) proposed a blueprint for diversity as a launching point for designing accessible curricula, suggesting that without a blueprint recognizing the full array of diversity, it would be difficult to design curricula that meet the needs of all students. A UD analogy illustrates this well: The provision of "cognitive curb cuts" reduces barriers that might be temporary, situational, or permanent so that no student stands out by using them. Occupational therapy practitioners could advance UDL by providing expertise, knowledge, and theory about occupational roles to promote inclusive practices rather than just accommodations, which some students find stigmatizing.

BEST PRACTICES

Occupational therapists working in schools are challenged to keep current and work within the mandates of school system legislation and initiatives such as MTSS. The first tier of MTSS requires proactive and specific instructional materials supporting the academic achievement and behavioral needs of all students. Consistent with Tier 1, UDL proposes that curricula should be designed to be accessible by all students (Rose & Meyer, 2002). Person-centered, occupation-based practice is the hallmark of occupational therapy. Strategies and tools focused on functional outcomes can open doors and bridge the gap from potential to performance. By supporting all students, school occupational therapy practitioners determine solutions to barriers in the physical, academic, and social environments that benefit everyone. UDL requires a proactive approach and embraces the tools and technology of educational practices.

Be Competent in Choosing Technology

Occupational therapy practitioners need to keep up to date with educational technologies and environmental interventions. AOTA's (2016) official document *Assistive Technology and Occupational Performance* outlines the skills occupational therapy practitioners need to provide ethical, competent services related to technology and environmental interventions. Technology competencies should not be limited to teaching keyboarding as an alternative to handwriting; rather, they should encompass

- The accessibility features of web browsers, computer operating systems, and networked software;

- Use of digital resources to differentiate instruction, such as computer activities and online materials suited to different reading abilities or learning preferences;
- An awareness of the attributes available in instructional tools, such as overhead projectors, interactive whiteboards, digital cameras, and tablet computing; and
- An ability to use online communication tools, connect with others electronically, and more.

Occupational therapy practitioners support literacy, including written language production, in schools and need to educate others that written language expression is more complex than simply picking up a pencil. Most off-the-shelf computers and handheld devices have practical UD applications and embedded accessibility features that can benefit students with sensory, physical, learning, and attention disabilities.

For example, in addition to traditional keyboards, most operating systems offer an on-screen keyboard that can be controlled by a touchpad, traditional mouse, or joystick. When students use the traditional keyboard, adjustments in computer settings can be made for those students who tend to repeat keystrokes ("filter keys" in Microsoft or "slow keys" in Apple) or who cannot hold down multiple keys at once ("sticky keys" feature in Apple and Microsoft). In addition, students can use spoken commands to operate computers or speech-to-text options to compose documents, write emails, and access the Internet. Using the text-to-speech option can also help students focus on the screen versus the keyboard.

Microsoft Word offers a readability feature that identifies the grade level of text. If the reading level is too difficult, then practitioners can edit the text by reducing the length of the sentence, substituting words, and adjusting vocabulary. The same text can be scaffolded to meet a variety of reading levels in the same classroom. Several free and for-fee curricular websites offer the same options. Extensions (Chrome web browser options) can also be added to eliminate unneeded animation and desktop background images so that only text shows on web pages or to add sound, graphics, and videos for those who need to interact with the material in a multisensory manner.

For students who have difficulty with executive function, calendars with color-coding options, reminders, easily programmable alarms, and alerts can help with organization and memory. Calendar reminders can be dictated and read back to students who have writing or reading challenges. The use of visual images (e.g., photos, emojis) in calendar entries can also help guide students.

The use of videos can benefit all students, including English-language learners, students with language-processing disabilities, and students who are hard of hearing. Videos can provide a platform for modeling complex concepts or socially appropriate behaviors. A wide variety of apps for video modeling and scheduling are also available. To ensure accessibility, videos should be closed captioned.

Practitioners should develop a familiarity and comfort level with the use of multimedia applications that allow the combination of text, pictures, movies, and sounds to represent, engage, or express. This familiarity will prepare practitioners to model and promote best practices while creating engaging environments for learners to tap into their multiple intelligences.

Occupational therapy practitioners can apply their expertise in task analysis and sensory processing to make recommendations regarding breaking up assignments into smaller increments, using visuals and graphic organizers to explain concepts, and providing movement breaks and positioning options so that students are alert and engaged. As a means of supporting self-advocacy and self-determination, students can also be taught to alter the amount, cognitive challenge, and appearance of digital text (Norton-Darr & Schoonover, 2012).

Be Collaborative

Occupational therapy practitioners have an active and visible role in the school climate and culture, collaborating with staff and administrators to ensure meaningful student occupations. Occupational therapy practitioners are well positioned to work as members of collaborative teams in schools, using their expertise in applying a top-down, strengths-based approach. When collaborating as a part of an interdisciplinary team designing and providing inclusive services, occupational therapy practitioners should understand the roles and responsibilities of other team members and the curriculum goals of the classroom. They should articulate the role of occupational therapy in supporting educational outcomes as a foundation for successful collaboration among stakeholders, including parents.

As members of a school team, occupational therapy practitioners have the opportunity to address the needs and strengths of all students. For example, rather than concentrating exclusively on handwriting remediation, occupational therapy practitioners could apply UDL principles and recommend modifications to the classroom environment (e.g., seating options, lighting, sound), assist in curriculum development for writing, and suggest writing supports or alternatives that help all students participate (Missiuna et al., 2015).

Answer Questions About Students' Strengths and Needs

Teams ask key evaluation questions in each area (e.g., "What does the student need to do?" "What are the student's special needs?" "What are the student's current abilities?") to gather data and information to support the consideration and implementation of appropriate interventions. These questions provide a framework for the team to communicate, collaborate, and form a consensus on how to proceed.

As part of a team, occupational therapists can exemplify a holistic approach by using the student–environments–tasks–tools (SETT) framework to evaluate and design interventions (i.e., this framework considers the student, the environments, the tasks expected of them, and the best tools for the job). The SETT framework, developed by Joy Zabala (2005), is a 4-part model initially designed for collaborative teams to use in making AT decisions that are student centered, environmentally useful, and task focused to facilitate educational success. The SETT framework guides teams to consider each of the 4 sections when discussing and implementing AT for students in schools. Zabala (2010) proposed that the same framework can be used to guide collaborative teams in designing UDL environments.

Plan and Implement Interventions

Occupational therapy practitioners have traditionally empowered clients by removing barriers and maximizing clients' abilities using a flexible approach to intervention. By providing services within the customary educational environment, occupational therapy practitioners model strategies for educators while giving students the opportunity to practice skills in context (not isolation), scaffolding only when necessary, and removing the scaffolds if and when they are no longer required. As suggested by Press (2016), occupational therapists in schools can follow the guidelines to support, advise, and model the principles of UDL.

Multiple means of engagement

Occupational therapy practitioners can provide guidance on how to gain and sustain students' interest in learning. This guidance might include educating team members about proper positioning for optimal learning, adapting activities to engage students with different academic levels, and understanding sensory processing needs and how to meet these various needs in a classroom environment in socially acceptable ways.

Multiple means of representation

Occupational therapy practitioners can help determine how to make materials available to the widest group of learners. Occupational therapy practitioners are well versed in activity analysis and often scaffold materials and make accommodations to meet individual needs when providing services. Applying these skills on a larger scale, occupational therapy practitioners can work with educational teams to use these same methods on curricular materials.

For example, if a student is assigned to read a book and write a book report, providing multiple means of representation might include options in addition to traditional print. If the text is available digitally, the practitioner can manipulate it by widening margins to reduce the amount of visual tracking required. Other manipulations might include changing the size, color, and spacing of the font; applying a colored background to the text; and taking advantage of text to speech on operating systems.

Practitioners can reduce the amount of text by summarizing, paraphrasing, or using online summarization tools (e.g., https://www.textcompactor.com, http://www.rewordify.com). They can simplify text by substituting words and shortening sentences, using thesaurus and dictionary tools embedded in software, and so on. Reading accommodations might range from low tech (e.g., reading windows or masks, picture symbols) to high tech (e.g., watching a video; using digital tools, websites, and apps) to customize the appearance, content, and modality in which the information is presented.

Multiple means of action and expression

It is a given that all learners do not relate to information in the same way; therefore, provide them with options to reflect on what they learned. If a student is assigned to read a book and write a report yet would be reliant on others, then having the student "show what they know" is an alternative means. Alternatives to writing could include giving an oral report, creating a posterboard display, drawing a picture, making a diorama, acting out the information, or creating a slide presentation. Students who are reluctant to speak in front of an audience could narrate information ahead of time, create a video, or produce digital text that could be presented with text to speech.

SUMMARY

Occupational therapy practitioners have much to offer as members of teams planning and implementing UDL. As collaborators with administrators and educational staff, occupational therapy practitioners can assist with the identification of accommodations and modifications necessary to ensure access to the physical, social, and academic aspects of school environments (e.g., classrooms, hallways, cafeterias, playgrounds) and to build the capacity of the adults in student programming.

Building capacity involves coaching the educational staff to develop the tools and strategies needed for students to fulfill their roles as learners and contributors. It also entails understanding the impact of learning, sensory, and motor difficulties on students' ability to complete these tasks.

Occupational therapy practitioners must use their knowledge and advocate for instructional and environmental designs that provide alternatives to traditional instructional or assessment approaches while supporting student engagement. Edyburn (2010) suggested an action plan for implementing UDL:

- Evaluate current practice methodologies, materials, and environment;
- List 1 immediate change to move toward UDL; and
- Work with others to make long-range improvement plans in your school.

Occupational therapy practitioners embracing UDL principles immerse themselves in the educational process to determine current needs for all students. In doing so, they consider the daily occupational roles of students and the impact of the physical, social, and educational environment on performance.

Technology is empowering. Occupational therapists can coach educators and students in the use of computer operating systems and applications to enhance academic and social performance as well as suggest specialized hardware and software. Because the educational environment includes a wide variety of technology tools that are continually updated, it is imperative that occupational therapy practitioners be competent users of technology. They must also be able to articulate the impact of the use of the right (or wrong) tool for the job, so appropriate scaffolds and supports can be selected and implemented. Occupational therapy practitioners possess the expertise in activity and environmental analysis, tool and environmental modification, low- to high-tech AT, sensory processing, cognitive skills, and strategies to improve or compensate for variances in motor performance to support meaningful participation.

RESOURCES

A Parent's Guide to Universal Design for Learning (https://bit.ly/2UL2y6Q): This article by the National Center for Learning Disabilities describes UDL for parents.

Access Through Universal Design for Learning (http://accessproject.colostate.edu): Hosted by Colorado State University, this website includes UDL, self-advocacy, and disability modules.

Center for Applied Special Technology (CAST; www.cast.org): CAST works to improve opportunities and outcomes for all individuals through UDL. The book *Universal Design for Learning: Theory and Practice* by A. Meyer and colleagues was published in 2014 by CAST (https://bit.ly/2LhQsO6).

Center for Universal Design (https://projects.ncsu.edu/ncsu/design/cud/): The Center for Universal Design promotes accessible and universal design in housing, commercial and public facilities, outdoor environments, and products. Publications include posters of UD principles, which are available for download.

DO–IT Center (https://www.washington.edu/doit/): DO–IT Center promotes the success of individuals with disabilities in postsecondary education and careers by using technology as an empowering tool. Resources include *Equal Access: Universal Design of Instruction* (https://bit.ly/2Bv9ji7).

Early Childhood Technical Assistance Center (https://bit.ly/2UJBnZU): The Early Childhood Technical Assistance Center has a webpage, *Universal Design for Learning*, that contains links to online toolkits, articles, and books.

Fact Sheet: Occupational Therapy and Universal Design for Learning (https://bit.ly/2Emxft2f): AOTA developed this fact sheet on the role of occupational therapy in the implementation of universal design.

IRIS Center's Star Legacy Modules (https://bit.ly/2GhkJ0P): A module called *Universal Design for Learning: Creating a Learning Environment That Challenges and Engages All Students* assists users in creating a UDL environment.

Loudoun County Public Schools (http://lcps.org/at): Loudon County, Virginia, public schools host a multiresource AT website that includes UDL.

Montgomery County Public Schools' High Incidence Accessible Technology (HIAT) pages (https://bit.ly/2PHP3RK): These pages include the **UDL Tool Finder** (https://bit.ly/2rAp0lN).

National Center on Universal Design for Learning (https://medium.com/udl-center): This is a multiresource site on UDL implementation, advocacy, research, community, and resources. For UDL guidelines, see http://udlguidelines.cast.org/

Universal Design for Learning: Policy Challenges and Recommendations (https://bit.ly/2U1tkGP): Published by the Project Forum at the National Association of State Directors of Special Education, this document summarizes panel presentations from higher education and local-, state-, and national-level perspectives.

REFERENCES

American Occupational Therapy Association. (2014). Guidelines for supervision, roles, and responsibilities during the delivery of occupational therapy services. *American Journal of Occupational Therapy, 68*(Suppl. 3), S16–S22. https://doi.org/10.5014/ajot.2014.686S03

American Occupational Therapy Association. (2015). *Occupational therapy and universal design for learning.* Retrieved from https://www.aota.org/-/media/Corporate/Files/AboutOT/Professionals/WhatIsOT/CY/Fact-Sheets/UDL%20fact%20sheet.pdf

American Occupational Therapy Association. (2016). Assistive technology and occupational performance. *American Journal of Occupational Therapy, 70,* 7012410030. https://doi.org/10.5014/ajot.2016.706S02

Americans With Disabilities Act of 1990, Pub. L. No. 101–336, 42 U.S.C. §§ 12101–12213 (2000).

Assistive Technology Act of 2004, Pub. L. 108–364, 118 Stat. 1707.

Bissell, J., & Cermak, S. (2015). Frameworks, models and trends in school-based occupational therapy in the United States. *Israeli Journal of Occupational Therapy, 24,* E49–E69.

Center for Applied Special Technology. (2018). *CAST timeline.* Retrieved from http://www.cast.org/about/timeline.html#.W0ggDdJKhPY

Chita-Tegmark, M., Gravel, J. W., Serpa, M. L. B., Domings, Y., & Rose, D. H. (2012). Using the universal design for learning framework to support culturally diverse learners. *Journal of Education, 192*(1), 17–22.

Collins, B. (2014). Universal design for learning: What occupational therapy can contribute. *Occupational Therapy Now, 16*(6), 22–23. Retrieved from http://eprints.bournemouth.ac.uk/21426/1/Collins.pdf

Cook, A. (2009). Ethical issues related to the use/non-use of assistive technology. *Developmental Disabilities Bulletin, 37*(12), 127–152.

Edyburn, D. L. (2010). Would you recognize universal design for learning if you saw it? Ten propositions for new directions for the second decade of UDL. *Learning Disability Quarterly, 33*(1), 33–41. https://doi.org/10.1177/073194871003300103

Every Student Succeeds Act, Pub. L. No. 114–95, 129 Stat. 1802 (2015).

Higher Education Opportunity Act, Pub. L. No. 110–315, 122 Stat. 3078 (2008).

Individuals With Disabilities Education Improvement Act of 2004, Pub. L. 108–446, 20 U.S.C. §§ 1400–1482.

Koch, K. (2017). Stay in the box! Embedded assistive technology improves access for students with disabilities. *Education Sciences, 7*(4), 82. https://doi.org/10.3390/educsci7040082

Luna Scott, C. (2015). *The futures of learning 3: What kind of pedagogies for the 21st century?* Paris: UNESCO Education Research and Foresight.

Missiuna, C., Pollock, N., Campbell, W., Dix, L., Sahagian Whalen, S., & Stewart, D. (2015). Partnering for change: Embedding universal design for learning into school-based occupational therapy. *Occupational Therapy Now, 17*(3), 13–15.

Ogletree, B. T. (2017). Addressing the communication and other needs of persons with severe disabilities through engaged interprofessional teams: Introduction to a clinical forum. *American Journal of Speech-Language Pathology, 26,* 157–161. https://doi.org/10.1044/2017_AJSLP-15-0064

Norton-Darr, S., & Schoonover, J. (2012, August/September). Spreading "the word" about cognitive rescaling as a tool for inclusion. *Solutions,* 7–13.

Press, M. (2016). Technology and school system practice: A practitioner's guide to success. *SIS Quarterly Practice Connections, 1*(4), 9–10.

Ralabate, P. K. (2011, August 30). Universal design for learning: Meeting the needs of all students. *ASHA Leader.* Retrieved from http://www.readingrockets.org/article/universal-design-learning-meeting-needs-all-students

Rose, D., & Meyer, A. (2002). *Teaching every student in the digital age.* Alexandria, VA: Association for Supervision and Curriculum Development. Retrieved from http://www.ascd.org/publications/books/101042.aspx

United Nations Programme on Disability. (2006). *Convention on the Rights of Persons With Disabilities (CRPD).* Retrieved from https://www.un.org/development/desa/disabilities/convention-on-the-rights-of-persons-with-disabilities.html

U.S. Department of Education, Office of Educational Technology. (2017). *Reimagining the role of technology in education: 2017 National Education Technology Plan update.* Retrieved from https://tech.ed.gov/files/2017/01/NETP17.pdf

Wilson, J. D. (2017). Resisting diagnosis: Reimagining disability and inclusive education through Universal Design for Learning. *Disability Studies Quarterly, 37*(2). Retrieved from http://dsq-sds.org/article/view/5417/4650

World Health Organization. (2010). *Framework for action on interprofessional education and collaborative practice.* Retrieved from http://www.who.int/hrh/resources/framework_action/en/

Zabala, J. (2005). *Using the SETT framework to level the learning field for students with disabilities.* Retrieved from http://www.joyzabala.com/uploads/Zabala_SETT_Leveling_the_Learning_Field.pdf

Zabala, J. (2010). *The SETT framework: Straight from the horse's mouth.* Retrieved from www.joyzabala.com/uploads/CA_Kananaskis__SETT_Horses_Mouth.pdf

Zhao, Y. (2012). *World class learners: Educating creative and entrepreneurial students.* Thousand Oaks, CA: Corwin.

Best Practices in the Use of Assistive Technology to Enhance Participation

21

Judith Schoonover, MEd, OTR/L, ATP, FAOTA, and Matthew Press, MHS, OTR/L, ATP

KEY TERMS AND CONCEPTS

- Assistive
- Assistive technology
- AT device
- AT service
- Interprofessionalism
- Literacy
- Operational competence
- Strategic competence
- Universal design
- Universal design for learning

The direct connection between occupational therapy and [assistive technology] makes it possible to optimize student performance through the promotion of participation in activities that are personally meaningful, relevant, and life sustaining. (Schoonover & Argabrite Grove, 2015, p. 556)

OVERVIEW

Technology is woven into the fabric of everyday life in the United States, with increasingly rapid shifts in the tools used to learn, communicate, work, and play. Whether that technology is the seemingly ubiquitous smartphone, a tablet for punching in sandwich topping preferences at the local convenience store, or a voice-activated environmental control, it is becoming more ever-present in daily routines and key to participation at school, at home, and in the community.

In schools, technology plays a significant role in the instructional process to help individualize learning as well as to provide equal access to the curriculum for all students. Initiatives such as the National Education Technology Plan (U.S. Department of Education, 2017) emphasize the role technology plays in the way educators present information and the ways students are expected to respond. For many students, technology is merely a convenience or one of many options to complete a task. For students with learning or physical differences, technology may be a necessity. In these circumstances, it is thought of as *assistive.*

All students have strengths, weaknesses, and preferred learning styles. In 1984, the Center for Applied Special Technology (2018) began researching the use of computer technologies to provide better educational experiences to students with disabilities. The research resulted in a new approach to improving education with flexible methods and materials, which became known as *universal design for learning* (UDL).

UDL applies *universal design* principles of equitable use, flexibility, simplicity, perceptibility, and efficiency to the educational environment and the process of teaching and learning. It provides the opportunity for all students to access, participate in, and progress in the general education curriculum by reducing barriers to instruction. UDL's principles are multiple means of engagement, representation, and action and expression, which are also embedded in occupational therapy.

Part of the purpose of UDL is to identify systematic variability so that instruction is designed that recognizes and takes advantage of these variables. For example, tasks can be created with attention to social, emotional, and behavioral learning to engage students in ways that are compatible with their affective state (Daley, 2014). When a student with a disability requires individualized and specific interventions to access educational opportunities, those interventions might be considered *assistive technology* (AT). For more information on UDL, see Chapter 20, "Best Practices in Universal Design for Learning."

Occupational therapy practitioners[1] have traditionally used tools—or, given a broader definition of *tools,* technology—in their practice. These tools or technologies promote participation and decrease instances of exclusion brought about by barriers in the physical, academic, or social environment. Occupational therapy practitioners working in schools are in a unique position to serve the needs of the entire district by embracing and applying UDL principles

---

[1]*Occupational therapy practitioner* refers to both the occupational therapist and the occupational therapy assistant. The American Occupational Therapy Association (AOTA; 2014, p. S18) states, "The occupational therapist is responsible for all aspects of occupational therapy service delivery and is accountable for the safety and effectiveness of the occupational therapy service delivery process" and "must be directly involved in the delivery of services during the initial evaluation and regularly throughout the course of intervention. . . . The occupational therapy assistant delivers safe and effective occupational therapy services under the supervision of and in partnership with the occupational therapist."

Copyright © 2019 by the American Occupational Therapy Association. All rights reserved. To reuse this content, contact www.copyright.com.
https://doi.org/10.7139/2019.978-1-56900-591-0.021

and helping to select and implement specific AT. They are equipped to analyze the roles and occupations of learning and identify interventions, inclusive of simple to complex tools, that can support students with identified disabilities as well as struggling learners with difficulties yet to be labeled.

AT can reduce the impact of disabilities and learning differences and provide alternatives for participation in learning opportunities. Occupational therapists working in educational settings are ideally suited to evaluate and determine an appropriate match of AT tools to student needs. The responsibility of those who implement AT intervention is to provide a health-promoting balance between occupational roles and activities consistent with the individualized education program (IEP).

Occupational therapy practitioners need to become familiar with the continuum of AT options available. Continual advances in AT allow many devices to grow and expand with the student through adolescence and into adulthood as they transition into college, career, and community. Therefore, determining the right tool for the job is crucial.

Definitions of AT in Occupational Therapy Literature

Even before a legal definition of AT was established, occupational therapy practitioners incorporated the use of AT in the provision of client-centered intervention to improve or make possible participation (AOTA, 2016). AOTA (2010) defined *technology* as "the combination of assistive, basic, complex, electronic and information, and rehabilitative and educational technologies" (p. S47). Stoller (1998) described AT as

> special devices or structural changes that promote a sense of self-competence, the further acquisition of developmental skills into occupational behaviors, and/or an improved balance of time spent between the occupational roles in an individual's life as determined by the individual's goals and interests and the external demands of the environment. (p. 6)

Relevant AT Legislation

An **AT device** is defined by the Assistive Technology Act of 2004 (Pub. L. 108–364) as "any item, piece of equipment or product system whether acquired commercially off the shelf, modified, or customized that is used to increase, maintain or improve functional capabilities of individuals with disabilities." However, without accompanying support, the device will not necessarily produce the desired results.

Accompanying support, or **AT service,** is defined in the Assistive Technology Act of 2004 as any service that directly assists an individual with a disability in the selection, acquisition, or use of an AT device. Such services include
- Evaluating needs and skills for AT;
- Acquiring AT;
- Selecting, designing, repairing, and fabricating AT;
- Coordinating services with other therapies; and
- Training both individuals with disabilities and the people working with these individuals to use the technologies effectively.

The Individuals With Disabilities Education Improvement Act of 2004 (IDEA; Pub. L. 108–446) requires that AT devices and services be considered for all students receiving special education services as part of the IEP process as a means of providing a free appropriate public education. The Every Student Succeeds Act (ESSA; 2015; Pub. L. 114–195) includes an increased focus on technology as a means to provide accessibility and improve instruction, opportunities, and outcomes for all students. It dictates that states and districts include AT in educational planning.

Education laws do not specify who should assume the role of AT providers in schools. In most schools, those who assess the need for or provide AT services might include general education teachers, special education teachers, occupational therapy practitioners, and speech–language pathologists.

ESSENTIAL CONSIDERATIONS

> Learning experiences enabled by technology should be accessible for all learners, including those with special needs. (U.S. Department of Education, 2016, p. 21)

With this quote in mind, occupational therapy practitioners need to understand the changing landscape in education and be prepared to plan for every student. This requires an understanding of AT, how to best collaborate with team members, and how environmental modifications and specialized tools can optimize a student's participation in school occupations.

Impact on Occupations and Participation in School

Participation can be made possible through environmental modifications and specialized tools. A wide range of considerations can address the functional capabilities of students with disabilities, including
- Seating and positioning,
- Mobility,
- Augmentative communication,
- Aids for daily living,
- Computer access,
- Assistive listening devices,
- Visual aids,
- Academic supports,
- Recreation and leisure, and
- Prevocational aids.

In the school setting, these supports are meant to circumvent barriers, as opposed to being curative.

Best practices start with considering the least restrictive no-tech or low-tech solutions, then proceeding along a continuum of tools to best match the student's needs, abilities, and activity requirements (see Table 21.1). No-tech solutions should also be considered and typically involve accommodations, modifications, and services rather than devices or equipment (e.g., preferential seating, social scripts, incentive charts, schedule changes to support the student's availability for instruction).

The provision of AT services takes time and coordination of staff and services. Barriers such as lack of appropriate staff training and support, negative staff attitudes, inadequate assessment and planning processes, and time

TABLE 21.1.   Examples of AT Categories Along a Continuum

CATEGORIES	LOW TECH	MID-TECH	HIGH TECH
Seating and positioning	Seat cushions, footrests, TheraBand	Specialized seating and positioning equipment	Motorized lifts
Mobility	Walker	Manual wheelchair	Power wheelchair
Augmentative communication	Paper-based communication books, eye gaze boards	Static-screen voice output device	Tablet with communication app
Aids for daily living	Nonslip materials, universal cuff, adapted utensils	Mobile arm support	Electronic feeder
Computer access	Pointing and positioning aids for keyboard stickers, "mouse house"	Built-in accessibility features (e.g., "sticky" keys, magnifier), alternative keyboard, mouse	Voice recognition, switch scanning
Listening devices	Print copies of lecture notes	Personal amplification systems, vibrating alerting systems	Classroom amplification systems, closed captioning
Visual aids	Handheld magnifier	Enlarged print (paper or digital)	Digital access to content, Braille note-taking devices
Academic supports			
Reading	Access tools (page fluffers, slant boards, color overlays, reading windows), adapted books	Audiobooks, content adaptations to digital text (scaffolded reading levels)	Digital text with voice output
Writing	Pencil grips, slant boards, editing checklists	Portable word processors, word prediction software	Word processors, spelling and grammar check features, speech to text
Math	Adapted manipulatives	Calculators, talking timers and watches	Electronic worksheets; apps for calculation, graphing, time, and money skills
Executive function	Number stamps, charts for computation	Timers, digital highlighters, and sticky notes	Wearable technology (smart watches, fitness trackers), apps
	Visual schedules, organizational supports (sticky notes, labels, highlighters), rubrics		
Recreation and leisure	Adapted toys, games, art tools, musical instruments, sporting equipment	Video games, battery-operated spin art and pottery wheel	Online virtual
Prevocational aids	Picture-based task analysis sheets	Video modeling, battery-operated timers	Tablet with apps pertaining to work activities

Note. AT = assistive technology.

constraints can negatively affect outcomes (Alharbi, 2016; Copley & Zivani, 2004). A team model for AT assessment and planning is ideal but might not be feasible for face-to-face coordination. Use of online collaboration tools, such as polls, surveys, shared documents, and video conferencing, can provide teams with opportunities to meet and share perspectives, data, and concerns.

Special Training Needed for Occupational Therapy Practitioners Working With AT

On the basis of their training, occupational therapists are skilled in the analyses of client factors (body structures and functions), performance skills, demands of a task or activity, performance of that task or activity, and environmental and contextual barriers to performance, which are basic prerequisites to determining effective AT interventions (AOTA, 2016). Studies have revealed that many professionals who provide AT services do not have adequate competencies to recommend and deliver AT in school settings (Burgos, 2015). Because of the constant evolution of specifically designed AT devices as well as the accessibility features built into standard tools, software, operating systems, and web browsers, occupational therapy practitioners are challenged to keep up with technology.

Choosing the right tool begins with a feature match (i.e., describing what the tool needs to do). Occupational therapy practice with AT encompasses a broad range of knowledge and skills, including evaluating needs, developing and implementing intervention, training in the use of AT, and coordinating resources as part of an interdisciplinary team (AOTA, 2016).

Interprofessional Collaborative Practice

Occupational therapy practitioners in schools should work toward collaborating effectively with education partners, including families, and connect that collaboration to mandates such as IDEA and ESSA to promote student participation in the general education curriculum (Hanft & Shepherd, 2016). The Interprofessional Education Collaborative, which represents 20 organizations for health professionals, including AOTA, defined *interprofessionalism* as the "consistent demonstration of core values evidenced by professionals working together . . . and wisely applying principles of altruism, excellence, caring, ethics, respect, communication, and accountability to achieve optimal health and wellness in individuals and communities" (Stern, 2006, p. 19). Interprofessional teams collaboratively design and advocate for physical, social, and academic environments that promote participation and skill development for all students (Missiuna et al., 2015).

Cultural Considerations

There is little research about the intersection of AT and culture (Ripat & Woodgate, 2011). The culture of the classroom, the classroom teacher, and social acceptance or participation can greatly affect use of AT in the educational setting. Research suggests that school staff might not feel adequately prepared to implement AT interventions (Bruinsma, 2011; Estrada-Hernandez & Stachowiack, 2015).

Determining new uses for familiar tools may help school staff overcome reluctance to implement tools. Taking advantage of features in a web browser and embedded AT components (e.g., Microsoft and Apple operating systems available on current desktops, laptops, tablets, or phones) can enable students with disabilities, their teachers, and their parents to facilitate learning (Koch, 2017). Educators, related service providers, students, and parents require ongoing support and opportunities to practice AT use (Karlsson et al., 2017).

BEST PRACTICES

The goal of occupational therapy has always been to empower individuals, enhancing or enabling meaningful participation in their occupational roles through tools and strategies. Occupational therapy practitioners have expertise in considering interaction among person, environment, and occupation (Law et al., 1996). In collaboration with school teams, occupational therapy practitioners can affect the selection of appropriate tools that match the physical, cognitive, and sensory capabilities of students. Because technology and AT are imperative to accessing and responding to information in schools, occupational therapy practitioners have a responsibility to keep abreast of current educational practices and available technologies to support all students.

Evaluate Students' Needs for AT

The student–environments–tasks–tools (SETT) framework is one of the best-known interprofessional collaborative tools used for considering a student's need for AT in schools (Zabala, 2005, 2010). The SETT framework provides a road map to help occupational therapy practitioners recognize barriers to student performance and identify the specific features or tools they can use to overcome those barriers.

Designed as a conversation starter to be used collaboratively, the SETT framework provides teams with a lens through which to view the interplay of the student's skills, environmental factors, and the tasks the student needs to accomplish. Teams choose to respond to the relevant questions, depending on the student's needs. Many of the questions are consistent with the type of information that occupational therapy practitioners gather as part of an occupational profile and occupational performance analysis and are applicable to a variety of settings.

When conducting an AT evaluation, best practices include gathering information about the student's customary environments and routines. SETT promotes collaboration, communication, sharing of knowledge and perspectives, flexibility, and ongoing processes that result in student-centered, environmentally specific, and task-focused tool systems to support a student's participation in curricular and extracurricular activities throughout the school day. Once the student, environmental, and task components are considered, the IEP team can focus on determining tools that meet those identified needs.

The Wisconsin Assistive Technology Initiative (WATI; 2004) developed the WATI Assessment on the basis of the SETT framework. The WATI Assessment, updated in 2017, includes model forms, suggested procedures, resource materials, and access to AT for trial use. (For additional information, see WATI, n.d.)

This tool begins with a place for users to record the student's sensory, motor, and cognitive abilities and their environmental considerations and then allows for a breakdown of the component tasks that are difficult for the student. Next, the team narrows the focus to where technology intervention should be considered. Last, the team works together to brainstorm ideas, prioritize tools to be trialed, and develop an intervention and follow-up plan to be implemented.

Provide No-Technology to High-Technology Intervention

AT interventions range from no technology to high technology on the basis of the practicality, complexity, or electrical power required (Edyburn, 2009). In the school environment, a continuum of AT may be provided to facilitate participation and academic achievement, depending on
- The environment;
- The context;

- The student's cognitive, mobility, and sensory needs; and
- The purpose of the tool (e.g., communication system, text to speech).

Several AT tools could be indicated, depending on the task and the environment in which the task is performed. For example, a student experiencing difficulty editing written work might use pencil and paper and an editing checklist for brief responses. For lengthier written assignments, the same student might also require access to word processing with built-in spell and grammar check features. The student might also benefit from digital supports, including text to speech to hear what they have written and check for omissions and other grammatical errors.

AT for access

To benefit from educational opportunities, students must have access to information, materials, and school tools. At the most basic level, this access might center on ensuring proper seating and desk sizing. At a more complex level, it might require equal access to computers and communication. Low-tech interventions for positioning can be as simple as foot rests, slant boards, and adapted chairs.

For students who need high-tech interventions, a range of computer operating system adjustments exist, such as settings that allow easier and more flexible access to the standard keyboard and mouse. (For Windows operating system features, see https://www.microsoft.com/en-us/accessibility/windows. For iOS features, see https://www.apple.com/accessibility/.)

In addition to built-in features, external hardware, such as adapted keyboards and mice, provide input. Switches are alternative "buttons" or input–output devices that users can access physically through minimal motor movement. Once a switch is selected, interfacing it with the device allows the user to control multiple settings on a toy, computer, or communication device. Positioning of the switch and the device being accessed is a complex endeavor and may require the use of mounts to put each object in the optimal position for access. Other options include eye (gaze) control and voice recognition of the entire computer or communication device.

AT for literacy

Literacy is reading, writing, listening, and speaking. According to the International Reading Association and National Association for the Education of Young Children (1998), "One of the best predictors of whether a child will function competently in school and go on to contribute actively in an increasingly literate society is the level to which the child progresses in reading and writing" (p. 30). This position statement frames the importance of access to literacy and thus furthers the importance of AT supports for students who struggle with traditional methods of accessing the reading and writing process.

Reading can be broken down into 5 main instructional areas:

1. Phonemic awareness,
2. Phonics,
3. Fluency,
4. Vocabulary, and
5. Text comprehension.

The expectation of instruction through the 6th-grade level is that individuals can read accurately out loud at a rate of at least 150 words per minute. Another expectation of that instruction is the comprehension of the content being read. Although practitioners may continue to explore strategies through traditional instructional methods, technology-based interventions may support a variety of learning styles and needs. Low-tech interventions include using

- Colored overlays to change the tint or glare of the printed page,
- Reading guides to isolate small chunks of passages, and
- Highlighters to draw attention to important details.

From a UDL perspective, digital text provides flexibility that print text does not. For students with physical impairments, digital text removes the barriers of holding and transporting books as well as turning pages. Digital text also supports accommodations such as increasing the font size, spacing, and color contrast for students with the need for visual accommodations. For students who have good listening comprehension skills, adding text to speech can accommodate for the decoding process or delays in fluency. Electronic dictionaries with or without speech support can be used as a cognitive scaffold to increase comprehension.

Text that can be accessed electronically opens the door to instructional resources, such as Rewordify.com (www.rewordify.com), which takes complex vocabulary out of a passage and substitutes simpler wording, or Text Compactor (www.textcompactor.com), which allows the user to select a smaller percentage of the passage to be shown rather than the entire passage. Coupling these websites together allows a struggling reader to have access to shorter passages at a lower reading level.

Eligible students with visual, physical, or specific cognitive disabilities can access digital content through the National Instructional Materials Accessibility Center, run by Bookshare Organization (https://bit.ly/17hLICu). For students who are not eligible, digital content is available on the Internet and through commercial products. When digital text is not readily available, those who have access to smart devices, such as iPads or Droids, can use free or inexpensive apps to take a photograph of typed text and then use optical character recognition to convert the image to digital text. The user can then "read" this text through text-to-speech interfaces.

For writing, low-tech tools such as magnetic letters, alphabet stickers, and ink-based stamps allow students to engage in the academic aspect of writing without the demands of holding a traditional writing tool. Further strategies include adapting writing utensils with different types of grips and using alternative pens or pencils or adapted paper. When low-tech strategies are not effective, occupational therapy practitioners should explore alternatives, such as a word processor or speech to text.

Keyboarding can be accomplished through devices as simple as dedicated portable word processors that have no functions beyond word processing. Alternatively, students can use laptops or tablets that have word processing capabilities coupled with software that may enhance the rate of typing or provide access to other features, such as word prediction, that the student needs for the academic aspects of written language expression. Speech to text can be accessed through built-in accessibility tools found in Windows, Droid, Chrome, and iOS device operating systems.

Although universally accessible options work for most students, some may require more specific voice-typing software with added features, such as complete control of the entire computer or voice recognition that is trained to the user. It should be noted that multimodal tools that incorporate both handwriting and technology should be considered, depending on the tasks the students are completing. According to Berninger (2013), it is important to "teach strategies for composing using both modes. For example, handwriting is useful for graphic organizers during planning or generating a rough first draft, but technology-supported word processing programs are useful for creating multiple drafts during the revision process" (p. 3).

Steps for written language composition include prewriting, drafting, revising, editing, and publishing. Low-tech tools that are common to the composition process include the use of index cards or sticky notes to capture quick ideas and then placing them on a print-based graphic organizer. Graphic organizer software can be used to accomplish the same tasks in a digital manner.

One benefit to moving to the digital platform is the use of tools that can provide immediate feedback to the student as they complete the task. Using auditory feedback, a student can hear the information generated as it is typed. Real-time feedback on spelling, grammar, and word choice provided through word processing software offers the student independent opportunities to begin the self-editing process to improve the accuracy of their final work product. Regardless of the tools being used, "accommodations alone are not sufficient for students with persisting writing disabilities" (Thompson et al., 2017, p. 138).

AT for math

Learning basic concepts in math is a foundational skill that has profound effects across the life course. From managing money, to measuring during cooking, to showing up on time, math is ever present in daily life. Low-tech strategies that can increase access to functional activities involving math include adapted manipulatives and rulers as well as talking calculators. These items can help with concepts related to basic math calculations and number sense.

In some cases, students need accommodations for the writing process during math activities. AT resources can help students increase legible completion without assisting with the calculation process. For example, specialized graph paper can be made online (https://incompetech .com/graphpaper/), and digital math paper can be found on tablet apps, such as ModMath (http://www.modmath .com/).

As math reasoning concepts are taught, digital tools can take over to help build the necessary visual mental models for learning. A mental model coupled with strong visualization and spatial reasoning skills allows students to be more successful in math and science classes (Matheson & Hutchinson, 2014). Tools (e.g., free ones posted at http:// www.conceptuamath.com/math-tools/) can be used to build a strong mental model of concepts related to fractions, multiplication, and division.

Apps such as PhotoMath (iOS and Droid) allow students to take a picture of math problems and see them solved, step by step, and graphed if needed. Students who struggle with memory, such as retaining steps for completion of math problems, can use this app to reinforce instruction provided by the teacher.

AT for executive functioning

Low-tech tools such as visual strategies for a classroom schedule, steps to a routine or task, or reminders of behavioral expectations can be used to enhance students' ability to meaningfully participate in classroom activities. For younger students, visual supports might appear as a graphic or pictorial representation of concepts. As students increase their literacy skills, the visuals might move to a text-based format. In either representation, both paper and digital options are available.

Mid-tech options include digital personal reminders, such as watches that have programmable features, and organizational tools that are readily available on the typical smartphone. Such features include the clock for setting alarms and the calendar for showing up at appointments and turning in assignments on time. The increasing presence of smart technologies provides an opportunity to enhance independent participation in life's daily routines, with the support of technology rather than dependence on people for those prompts.

AT for art, music, and physical education

Low-tech tools for positioning instruments, art activities that use adapted art utensils, and sports activities that use adapted equipment all increase students' engagement, well-being, and social participation. Flexible time lines for projects, individual or collaborative activities, and assignments that are highly participatory and interactive can facilitate success.

Occupational therapy practitioners can create basic tools from easily found materials or purchase more complex ones to assist students with viewing, understanding, holding on to, and manipulating materials, which can result in meaningful participation for all (Coleman & Cramer, 2015; Schoonover & Schwind, 2017). Specialized equipment can be modified from existing equipment or purchased and used independently of or in conjunction with computer-facilitated and computer-based activities or online experiences.

Document AT Services and Outcomes

School occupational therapy practitioners should give careful consideration to documenting the AT implementation process on the IEP, including the time needed to teach students and their support team as well as successful use of the needed technologies. Light and McNaughton (2014) defined competencies for augmentative communication, some of which can be generalized to a broader range of AT—in particular, *operational competence* (i.e., knowing how to use the technology) and *strategic competence* (i.e., knowing when to use the technology). Without adequate supports to reach competence, students are more likely to abandon the technology. Documenting services, tracking progress, identifying outcomes, and adjusting intervention plans are critical to students' success with AT and access to learning and school activities.

Stay Current With AT

AT providers should maintain their competence in AT through ongoing professional development and reflection. Referring to the Quality Indicators of AT Matrices (QIAT Community, 2015), they should review their own performance and reflect on ways to improve the quality of AT service in their district.

In addition, occupational therapy practitioners may access professional development modules through Assistive Technology Internet Modules (in partnership with WATI; https://atinternetmodules.org/user_mod.php). This online learning environment contains AT topics from assessment and funding to content areas such as

- Access to mobile devices,
- Communication,
- Seating and positioning, and
- AT for students with complex needs.

Developed with partnering universities and nationally renowned experts in the field, the modules are available at no cost and designed to provide high-quality information and professional development on AT for educators, professionals, families, and persons with disabilities. The self-paced modules guide the user through case studies, instructional videos, pre- and postassessments, and a glossary. Additional resources can be found at http://www.atinternetmodules.org/.

SUMMARY

The right AT devices and services can remove barriers in the physical and academic environment and provide students with options to increase participation. Occupational therapy practitioners working in schools can influence how educators teach and how students learn. Occupational therapy practitioners are ideally suited to serve on interprofessional collaborative teams to evaluate students who are experiencing difficulty accessing the learning environment and determine an appropriate match of AT tools. It is essential that occupational therapy practitioners in schools become familiar with the continuum of AT options available. Many mainstream devices offer accessibility features that can be customized and adjusted to meet individual needs and preferences.

Occupational therapy practitioners have a responsibility to educate themselves and others about the possibilities offered by new technologies. Ongoing assessment of the effectiveness of AT interventions is necessary to ensure that students are equipped with the tools they need as they transition to college, career, or community. In addition, shifting from an expert model to a coaching model will help school teams build capacity in the delivery of AT services, ensuring that AT will be used throughout the day in all school environments (DeCoste, 2013).

AT changes and reshapes attitudes about what people do and can do (Schoonover & Argabrite Grove, 2015).

Ongoing communication, collaboration, and professional development are necessary practice components of AT that require both time and commitment. The direct connection between occupational therapy and AT has always existed; it allows participation in activities that are personally meaningful, relevant, and life sustaining. The challenge is to increase collaborative practices, insist on opportunities for professional development, advocate for the provision of appropriate AT, and continue to define the role of occupational therapy in the provision of AT devices and services.

REFERENCES

Alharbi, S. (2016). Benefits and barriers: Incorporating assistive technology in an inclusive setting for primary school students with learning disabilities in language arts. *American Research Journal of Humanities and Social Sciences, 2,* 1–11. Retrieved from https://www.arjonline.org/papers/arjhss/v2-i1/16.pdf

American Occupational Therapy Association. (2010). Specialized knowledge and skills in technology and environmental interventions for occupational therapy practice. *American Journal of Occupational Therapy, 64*(6, Suppl.), S44–S56. https://doi.org/10.5014/ajot.2010.64S44

American Occupational Therapy Association. (2014). Guidelines for supervision, roles, and responsibilities during the delivery of occupational therapy services. *American Journal of Occupational Therapy, 68*(Suppl. 3), S16–S22. https://doi.org/10.5014/ajot.2014.686S03

American Occupational Therapy Association. (2016). Assistive technology and occupational performance. *American Journal of Occupational Therapy, 70,* 7012410030. https://doi.org/10.5014/ajot.2016.706S02

Assistive Technology Act of 2004, Pub. L. 108–364, 118 Stat. 1707.

Berninger, V. (2013, March). Educating students in the computer age to be multilingual by hand. *Commentaries: A Continuing Dialogue on Critical Education Policy Issues, 19*(1). Retrieved from https://www.schools.utah.gov/file/3affb2e5-74ce-4d94-a31e-bbd39b9a22b1

Bruinsma, A. M. (2011). *Implementation of assistive technology in the classroom* (Unpublished master's thesis). St. John Fisher College, Rochester, NY. Retrieved from https://fisherpub.sjfc.edu/cgi/viewcontent.cgi?article=1064&context=education_ETD_masters

Burgos, B. B. (2015). *A study of assistive technology competencies of specialists in public schools* (Unpublished doctoral dissertation). Nova Southeastern University, Fort Lauderdale, FL. Retrieved from https://nsuworks.nova.edu/cgi/viewcontent.cgi?article=1059&context=gscis_etd

Center for Applied Special Technology. (2018). *CAST timeline.* Retrieved from http://www.cast.org/about/timeline.html#.W0diCtJKhPY

Coleman, M. B., & Cramer, S. (2015). Creating meaningful art experiences with assistive technology for students with physical, visual, severe, and multiple disabilities. *Art Education, 68*(2), 6–13. https://doi.org/10.1080/00043125.2015.11519308

Copley, J., & Ziviani, J. (2004). Barriers to the use of assistive technology for children with multiple disabilities. *Occupational Therapy International, 11,* 229–243. https://doi.org/10.1002/oti.213

Daley, S. (2014, May 16). *Universal design for learning: Variability in emotion and learning* [video file]. TU Office of Academic

Innovation. Retrieved from https://www.youtube.com/watch?v=LDaP-THd-9c

DeCoste, D. (2013). The changing roles of assistive technology teams in public school settings. *Perspectives on Language and Literacy, 39*(4), 19–23.

Edyburn, D. L. (2009). Hindsight, understanding what we got wrong, and changing directions. *Journal of Special Education Technology, 24*(1), 61–64.

Estrada-Hernandez, N., & Stachowiack, J. R. (2016). Factors that affect the successful implementation of assistive technology. *Eastern Education Journal, 45*(1), 2–22.

Every Student Succeeds Act, Pub. L. No. 114–95, 129 Stat. 1802 (2015).

Hanft, B., & Shepherd, J. (Eds.). (2016). *Collaborating for student success: A guide for school-based occupational therapy* (2nd ed.). Bethesda, MD: AOTA Press.

Individuals With Disabilities Education Improvement Act of 2004, Pub. L. 108–446, 20 U.S.C. §§ 1400–1482.

International Reading Association & National Association for the Education of Young Children. (1998). Learning to read and write: Developmentally appropriate practices for young children. *Young Children, 53*(4), 30–46. Retrieved from https://www.naeyc.org/sites/default/files/globally-shared/downloads/PDFs/resources/position-statements/PSREAD98.PDF

Karlsson, P., Johnston, C., & Barker, K. (2017). Influences on students' assistive technology use at school: The views of classroom teachers, allied health professionals, students with cerebral palsy and their parents. *Disability and Rehabilitation: Assistive Technology, 13,* 763–771. https://doi.org/10.1080/17483107.2017.1373307

Koch, K. (2017). Stay in the box! Embedded assistive technology improves access for students with disabilities. *Education Sciences, 7*(4), 82. https://doi.org/10.3390/educsci7040082

Law, M., Cooper, B., Strong, S., Stewart, D., Rigby, P., & Letts, L. (1996). The Person–Environment–Occupational Model: A transactive approach to occupational performance. *Canadian Journal of Occupational Therapy, 63,* 9–23. https://doi.org/10.1177/000841749606300103

Light, J., & McNaughton, D. (2014). Communicative competence for individuals who require augmentative and alternative communication: A new definition for a new era of communication? *Augmentative and Alternative Communication, 30,* 1–18. https://doi.org/10.3109/07434618.2014.885080

Matheson, I., & Hutchinson, N. (2014). *Visual representation in mathematics.* Retrieved from http://www.ldatschool.ca/numeracy/visual-representation/

Missiuna, C., Pollock, N., Campbell, W., Dix, L., Sahagian Whalen, S., & Stewart, D. (2015). Partnering for change: Embedding universal design for learning into school-based occupational therapy. *Occupation Therapy Now, 17*(3), 13–15.

QIAT Community. (2015). *Quality indicators for assistive technology services.* Retrieved from http://qiat.org/indicators.html

Ripat, J., & Woodgate, R. (2011). The intersection of culture, disability and assistive technology. *Disability and Rehabilitation: Assistive Technology, 6*(2), 87–96. https://doi.org/10.3109/17483107.2010.507859

Schoonover, J. W., & Argabrite Grove, R. E. (2015). Influencing participation through assistive technology. In J. Case-Smith & J. O'Brien (Eds.), *Occupational therapy for children and adolescents* (7th ed., pp. 525–559). St. Louis: Mosby.

Schoonover, J., & Schwind, D. B. (2017). Grant's ART toolbox: Adapted repurposed tools. *OT Practice, 22*(9), 8–10, 12–13.

Stern, D. T. (2006). *Measuring medical professionalism.* New York: Oxford University Press.

Stoller, L. C. (1998). *Low-tech assistive devices: A handbook for the school setting.* Framingham, MA: Therapro.

Thompson, R., Tanimoto, S., Abbott, R., Nielsen, K., Lyman, R. D., Geselowitz, K., . . . Berninger, V. (2017). Relationships between language input and letter output modes in writing notes and summaries for students in Grades 4 to 9 with persisting writing disabilities. *Assistive Technology, 29,* 131–139. https://doi.org/10.1080/10400435.2016.1199066

U.S. Department of Education, Office of Educational Technology. (2016). *Reimagining the role of technology in education: 2017 National Education Technology Plan update.* Washington, DC: Author. Retrieved from http://tech.ed.gov/netp/

U.S. Department of Education, Office of Educational Technology. (2017). *Reimagining the role of technology in education: 2017 National Education Technology Plan update.* Washington, DC: Author.

Wisconsin Assistive Technology Initiative. (2004). *The W.A.T.I. Assessment package.* Retrieved from https://dpi.wi.gov/sites/default/files/imce/sped/pdf/at-wati-assessment.pdf

Wisconsin Assistive Technology Initiative. (n.d.). *Assistive technology consideration to assessment.* Retrieved from http://www.wati.org/free-publications/assistive-technology-consideration-to-assessment/

Zabala, J. (2005). *Using the SETT framework to level the learning field for students with disabilities.* Retrieved from http://www.joyzabala.com/uploads/Zabala_SETT_Leveling_the_Learning_Field.pdf

Zabala, J. (2010). *The SETT framework: Straight from the horse's mouth.* Retrieved from www.joyzabala.com/uploads/CA_Kananaskis__SETT_Horses_Mouth.pdf

Best Practices in Safe Transportation

22

Susan Englert Shutrump, OTR/L

KEY TERMS AND CONCEPTS

- Cam wrap
- Child safety restraint system
- Compartmentalization
- Individualized transportation plan
- Integrated child safety seat
- School-bus–specific CSRS
- School-bus–specific lap belt add-on CSRS
- Seat bight
- Tether strap
- Transportation

OVERVIEW

Transportation, as defined in Part B of the Individuals With Disabilities Education Improvement Act of 2004 (IDEA; Pub. L. 108–446), includes "travel to and from school and between schools . . . travel in and around school buildings" and provision of "specialized equipment (such as special or adapted buses, lifts, and ramps), if required to provide special transportation for a child with a disability" (§ 300.34[c][16]). Under IDEA, the transportation of students with disabilities is a related service. Section 504 of the Rehabilitation Act of 1973 (as amended, 2008; Pub. L. 93–112) and the ADA Amendments Act of 2008 (Pub. L. 110–325) require students with disabilities to have equal opportunities to participate in school district activities (e.g., transportation).

The occupational therapist works with the team to determine the need for specialized equipment on the school vehicle (an educational environment). This equipment may include necessary supports for the student, including

- Assistive technology and equipment,
- Modified procedures and accommodations, and
- Supervision and assistance provided by transportation staff trained to meet individualized student needs.

Decisions should be determined at the individualized education program (IEP) meeting and documented in the IEP.

School bus drivers and monitors work with students who have a variety of medical conditions while operating in a remote location mired with risks and few supports. However, transportation personnel are not typically included in the IEP meeting. School occupational therapy practitioners[1] should advocate for the inclusion of transportation personnel in the IEP and other formal planning meetings. All team members, including the student and their family, need to understand that full educational access and independence are often vehicle dependent.

Students with special needs should be safe and comfortable on all school transportation vehicles that access educational activities (e.g., field trips, community sites for community mobility). Occupational therapy practitioners must understand the basic construction of a school bus as built or with modifications to transport students with special needs. They must also be familiar with the equipment that is most commonly used to secure a student with special needs on a school bus or other transport vehicle used by the educational system.

ESSENTIAL CONSIDERATIONS

Occupational therapists' expertise in positioning seating and modifying the environment for safe use of adaptive equipment, while supporting students in self-advocacy,

---

[1]*Occupational therapy practitioner* refers to both the occupational therapist and the occupational therapy assistant. The American Occupational Therapy Association (2014, p. S18) states, "The occupational therapist is responsible for all aspects of occupational therapy service delivery and is accountable for the safety and effectiveness of the occupational therapy service delivery process" and "must be directly involved in the delivery of services during the initial evaluation and regularly throughout the course of intervention. . . . The occupational therapy assistant delivers safe and effective occupational therapy services under the supervision of and in partnership with the occupational therapist."

Copyright © 2019 by the American Occupational Therapy Association. All rights reserved. To reuse this content, contact www.copyright.com. https://doi.org/10.7139/2019.978-1-56900-591-0.022

makes them obvious leaders in establishing an individualized transportation plan (ITP) for students. Working as an interdisciplinary team and documenting important decisions regarding transportation is essential to ensure transportation safety and independence on a daily basis.

Individualized Transportation Plan

The development of an *ITP* (University of Michigan Transportation Research Institute, 2015) as part of the student's IEP provides additional information about all aspects of the ride, from entering to disembarking the vehicle. ITPs are necessary for students who require specialized transportation equipment or support, and they should include concerns for daily travel and emergencies. Section 504 plans may also include an ITP for general education students.

Formation of the ITP involves a team analysis of a variety of factors, including the student's

- Age,
- Size,
- Sensory reactions,
- Physical development,
- Health impairments,
- Cognition, and
- Behavioral status.

The occupational therapist provides information about the

- Need for and type of seating and occupant restraint;
- Seating location;
- Type and proximity of supervision;
- Emergency evacuation procedures;
- Access to and egress from the bus, including use of the lift; and
- Opportunities for socialization.

A copy of each student's ITP should be carried on the vehicle whenever they are riding, which allows prompt reference to it in case of an emergency or question. Transportation personnel are responsible for full and accurate implementation. For passengers with a wheelchair, it is recommended that the team document securement locations for proper follow-through on a daily basis. An easy way to do this is to take a digital picture of the student wearing the shoulder lap belt in the secured chair, print it, and include it in the ITP. Bullet points highlighting any special needs or concerns can be included with these pictures, which can be of great assistance to substitute bus drivers or monitors.

Specialized Equipment

This section does not provide an exhaustive list. In addition, examples of vendors are used, but this is not an endorsement of their product. Rather, vendors are listed to provide an understanding of the availability of products on the market. When using specialized equipment, team members need to follow the manufacturer's guidelines and state safety standards with best practice in mind.

School-bus–specific child safety restraint systems

A *child safety restraint system* (CSRS) is a crash-tested device that is designed to provide crash protection (National Highway Traffic Safety Administration [NHTSA], 2015). Some manufacturers have designed CSRSs specifically to be used on school buses for students who need occupant restraint or support in addition to that afforded through the traditional school bus occupant protection system of compartmentalization. *Compartmentalization* keeps bus passengers safe through closely spaced, densely padded, high-backed bus seats. Occupants bounce within the compartment, which is designed to reduce crash forces by spreading them across a large portion of the body.

School-bus–specific CSRSs attach to the school bus seat through a portable seat mount, often referred to as a *cam wrap*. These systems can be used on traditional bus seats because they do not use a lap belt in their installation. These systems meet the needs of preschool children and can also accommodate heavier and taller school-age children.

Some examples of these bus-specific add-on CSRSs are

- Safeguard Student Transportation Add-On Restraints (IMMI, Westfield, IN),
- Pro-Tech II or III (BESI, Hamilton, OH), and
- Portable Child Restraint (HSM Transportation Solutions, Hickory, NC).

These systems seat the student closer to the *seat bight* (i.e., the space where the seat back and bottom meet), thus allowing for more leg room than allowed for by a conventional car seat. In addition, the larger, flattened seat pans allow for students with bulky casts or lower extremity or pelvic bracing to be more comfortably secured. The systems are very easily installed and therefore can quickly be moved for a route change or for a field trip.

For safety, when a student uses any system that attaches to the seat through a portable seat mount or cam wrap, the seat behind the secured student must remain empty, or its occupants must be secured in CSRSs. For the safety of the student in the bus-specific add-on CSRS, the occupational therapy practitioner must ensure that the student seated directly behind the student will not be relying solely on compartmentalization in a crash because their impact to the seat back will cause a double-loading effect. An unrestrained student thrown into the seat back causes it to deflect by design, sending the student secured in the CSRS forward, with potentially injury-producing force to the head and neck.

School-bus–specific lap belt add-on CSRSs

Some state laws require lap belts to be installed on school buses. In states without regulations, some districts have opted to install lap belts on buses used to transport students with special needs. *School-bus–specific lap belt add-on CSRSs* are an option for students riding on buses with lap belts who need additional upper torso restraint.

These systems are 5-point harness systems that include crotch straps and shoulder straps through which lap belts are threaded. They attach to the bus seat through a portable seat mount or cam wrap. Some examples of these CSRSs include

- KidCam for School Buses (E-Z-ON, Jupiter, FL),
- CamHarness for School Buses (E-Z-ON, Jupiter, FL), and
- Over the Shoulder Securement (BESI, Hamilton, OH).

Students secured in these systems sit directly on the bus seat, which allows for more leg room. They accommodate larger and taller students and are often used for students who grow out of school-bus–specific or traditional CSRSs. This is especially true for students with longer torso height.

Safety vests

Zippers on 2-piece safety vests used on school buses are always positioned on the student's back. Although extra-small- and small-sized safety vests have a crotch strap to ensure that the vest is in a low position on the student's trunk (e.g., to prevent the horizontal straps from slipping onto the child's neck), practitioners should advocate that crotch straps be used on all safety vests to prevent the student from slipping under the vest, which poses a risk for strangulation.

It is difficult for the student to get out of a well-fitted safety vest, so it is often the restraint of choice for students with interfering behaviors. When the safety vest is used primarily for behavioral reasons, the team's rationale should be clearly documented in the ITP and IEP, along with a plan to support the student to learn appropriate behavior for eventual discontinuation of the safety vest. Support through the use of

- Lightweight toys,
- Headsets,
- Social Stories, and
- Visual supports or schedules.

Other items to improve compliance with bus safety rules should be instituted before use of a safety vest. Seating-plan modifications to prompt improved behavior (e.g., window seating with a peer in the aisle to cue staying in the seat) should be attempted.

Occupational therapists should advise transportation staff to order safety vests with as many options as possible to ease fit and allow for better customization. Safety vests are easily installed on traditional bus seats because most do not use a lap belt. They come with the options of adjustable shoulder straps on the vest and portable seat mounts as well as zipper inserts to adjust torso girth size and allow for seasonal clothing changes.

With this adjustability comes responsibility to ensure proper follow-through on a daily basis. Those who will assist the student into and out of the safety vest need to be trained in fit and use. An advantage of using 2-part safety vests is that parents and school staff can put them on the student before the student boards the bus. The safety vest can be worn under a coat as long as transportation staff can access the metal fasteners at the shoulders and hips to attach all 4 buckles of the portable seat mount. Once an adjustable safety vest and cam wrap are fitted to meet the needs of a student, the equipment and method of use are documented on the ITP and IEP to ensure consistency.

Special considerations need to be made for students with shunts. Given that the large metal buckles of a 2-part safety vest are often placed close to the student's head or neck, the shunt site might be affected by the buckle, which poses a risk for damage or malfunction. The team should choose another type of occupant restraint for these students. The seating plan should also be modified to position these students away from the window, with their shunt site facing the aisle.

Integrated child safety seats

The *integrated child safety seat* (CSS) is a restraint system built into the bus seat. The seat cushion can be flipped up when not in use to allow the bus seat to be used for larger passengers. These seats are similar to those available for use in private vehicles.

Students With Specific Physical Needs

School teams must consider transportation safety for students with specific physical needs, such as poor head control, poor trunk control, need for leg support, particular orthopedic concerns, small stature, and wheelchair use.

Poor head control

Because none of the bus-specific CSRSs offer the ability to provide any support to the head or neck, a traditional rear-facing car seat, installed semireclined, may be a better option for a smaller passenger with poor head control. When students have outgrown the rear-facing seat, a forward-facing seat that allows for some recline should be considered. Students with severe head control problems may require a car seat designed for students with special needs that allows for more recline, with support to align the head.

Occupational therapists should advise teams about the least restrictive options to meet the student's needs. CSRSs for students with disabilities are costly, and they tend to be large and difficult, if not impossible, to secure to a bus seat. Also, to date, only 1 has been designed for specific use on a school bus with cam wrap technology (STAR Special Needs, IMMI, Westfield, IN).

A *tether strap* is typically required to manage the additional loads or forces that these CSRSs generate. The tether is a strap attached to the top of the restraint system that secures to a vehicle anchor point (usually on the floor or back dashboard of a private vehicle) to prevent excessive forward movement in the event of a sudden stop or force. Many manufacturers allow an alternative method of tether attachment on a school bus (e.g., buckled onto a lap belt in the seat behind); however, tether use still results in reduced occupancy and a more difficult, restrictive, and time-consuming installation. For the student's safety, the occupational therapist might suggest the need for specialized restraint systems in private vehicles.

Modifications to CSRSs must not alter their effectiveness. For example, firm towels or sheets can be rolled and used to better align the student, or they can be put just behind the crotch strap of the CSS to position the student's hips farther into the seat (e.g., to maintain flexed hips to break up full-body extension or increased tone, which may prevent a comfortable, stable sitting posture). No compressible material should be used, nor should any padding be put under or behind the student because these modifications could introduce slack into the fit of the harness, making it ineffective in case of an accident.

The webbing of the CSRS harness stretches in a crash, allowing the torso to move forward considerably to ride down the crash (i.e., extending the time over which the occupant feels the forces to reduce injury potential).

If the head is secured against the back of the CSRS as the torso moves forward, a serious cervical injury could occur. For this reason, no strapping system should be used, and any neck collar advised should be free floating and in no way attached to the seat. It should also be the lightest and smallest collar to meet the student's needs.

Poor trunk control

CSSs that allow for recline to reduce the effects of gravity may be used with students with limited trunk control. More restrictive options also are available in CSSs designed for students with special needs. These CSSs include those allowing for significant recline in a forward-facing position as well as a modified safety vest that secures a student lying in a bus seat. To use the Modified E-Z-ON vest (E-Z-ON Products, Jupiter, FL), the student must fit entirely on the bus seat with the head positioned toward the aisle. This option also can work for students in body or hip spica casts who are unable to sit.

Small stature

Practitioners must work with school staff to ensure that no student is carried onto or off of the bus. This is a safety concern for both the student and adults and is a discriminating and inappropriately restrictive practice. Students with small stature may need a step stool with a nonslip surface to allow for independent access. Bus steps are typically deep and difficult to access, with the lowest step being the most challenging.

Need for lower extremity support

Students with paralysis, heavy legs, pelvic casting, or bracing may experience discomfort when riding in a CSRS with their feet unsupported. Pressure on the femoral artery on an already compromised circulatory system can often be alleviated through use of an integrated CSS or bus-specific add-on CSRS. In contrast with traditional CSSs, these systems, with reduced seat-back bulk, position the student farther into the seat bight while providing greater support and increased foot and leg room. Moreover, seating the student over a wheel well can provide additional support to the feet.

If the school district is using traditional CSSs, then more lower extremity room can be gained through a change from a CSS designed to secure smaller students with a full harness to a combination CSS (i.e., the seat can be used with a harness system and can be used as a booster seat in a private vehicle with the child secured with a lap shoulder belt). Because they are designed to secure larger passengers (albeit in a private vehicle), these combination CSSs tend to have larger and flatter seat pans and position the passenger more erect; therefore, they provide more leg and hip room. Because booster seats cannot be used on a school bus, combination CSS use is limited to those children who meet the harness weight and height restrictions.

Other orthopedic concerns

Students who have brittle bones, spinal rods, or other orthopedic concerns may not be able to tolerate a rough ride and should be positioned at the front of the bus, away from wheel-well positions. The team can also achieve a smoother ride by equipping the bus with air ride, which is offered as an option during the purchase of a new vehicle. Even with special seating, the team should discuss and plan for additional padding or careful positioning and fit of CSRS harnesses. The IEP or 504 team should discuss modifications needed to ensure a safe evacuation and document them on the ITP. Drivers and other adults on the bus should be trained in use of the evacuation drag blanket and a protected lift out of the rear door.

Wheelchair use

Wheelchairs, which were designed for mobility rather than stability, have long been identified by their manufacturers as not suitable as seats in a motor vehicle. This safety warning is clearly stated in wheelchair owner's manuals and is often reiterated on literature and labels on the chair's frame. The recommendation is for the passenger to transfer into a seat designed for transportation, with the empty wheelchair tied down.

It is important that students and their families understand these safety precautions, learn how to advocate for them, and learn the skills necessary to travel as safely as possible. If it is determined that it is safe and appropriate for the student to transfer, practitioners should assist in determining and training for the most efficient and safe transfer procedures. If support on the school bus seat is necessary, therapists should use their knowledge of positioning and seating to suggest a proper CSRS.

If it is not reasonable for a student to transfer from their wheelchair, the IEP team must work together to identify a safe transportation plan based on best practice transportation safety principles. In doing so, the team needs to contemplate supporting research and follow safety standards in their decision making. Leaders in conducting research and establishing standards for safe transportation in the United States include the University of Michigan Transportation Research Institute, the Rehabilitation Engineering Society of North America (RESNA) Committee on Wheelchairs and Transportation, and the American National Standards Institute (ANSI).

If the student will continue to need to use the wheelchair as a seat in a motor vehicle, then the wheelchair should be designed and ordered with transportation safety in mind. Many wheelchairs are now available with transit technology that meets voluntary industry standards. One voluntary standard is the WC 19 standard (ANSI & RESNA, 2012a). A wheelchair compliant with this standard comes with 4 easily identifiable and accessible securement points to which the school bus's wheelchair tie-down straps can be attached. These securement points have been proven to withstand crash tests at 30 miles per hour with 20-g-force impacts. This is the level of testing required of CSRSs and other vehicle safety equipment.

Compliant chairs are required to achieve an acceptable rating for ease in proper placement and fit of the shoulder lap belt, which must be used in conjunction with the wheelchair tie-downs to properly secure the passenger. Standards also require an optional crash-tested, wheelchair-anchored pelvic safety belt with a standard interface to allow for the bus-mounted shoulder belt to connect to it. This decreases the amount of intrusion into the personal space of the student by transporters positioning a lap belt.

Wheelchairs designed for children who weigh 50 pounds or less are required to provide the option of a crashworthy, wheelchair-anchored 5-point harness to allow for occupant protection similar to that offered by regulated CSRSs. WC 19–compliant wheelchairs are best pursued at the time of purchase, because retrofitting options are limited. For these reasons, it is important to work with and educate students, family members, school staff, and transportation staff as to the importance of these options for safe community mobility.

The WC 20 standard (ANSI & RESNA, 2012b) is a voluntary standard that allows for seating systems and their attachment hardware to be crash tested on surrogate wheelchair frames under the same impact conditions. This is an important advancement for those who need highly customized seating and are unable to transfer out of their wheelchair for transport.

The IEP or 504 plan team must develop individualized emergency evacuation plans that do not rely on use of the wheelchair or mobility equipment to get the student out of the bus as quickly as possible in an emergency. The plan should include

- What kind of assistance is necessary to get the student out of the wheelchair (e.g., 1- or 2-person lift or drag),
- What kind of equipment is needed,
- How much physical involvement in evacuation drills is appropriate, and
- What kind of training is necessary to implement the plan.

Other issues that teams should address include ensuring that

- The wheelchair is in good working order and structurally sound, with the seating system securely attached to the base, securement sites on the chair frame, and anchor points on the vehicle floor to meet tie-down manufacturers' guidelines for effectiveness;
- Proper fit of the shoulder lap belt will safely secure the passenger;
- Safe use of the lift is followed; and
- The role and fit of postural supports and securement of accessory equipment (e.g., lap trays, crutches, canes, book bags, laptop computers, augmentative communication systems) are in place.

Students With Specific Health Concerns and Needs

Students with specific health concerns and needs, such as respiratory problems, tracheotomies, allergies, seizure disorders, feeding concerns, or ostomy bags, have specific issues related to safe transportation.

Emergency medical procedures

Well-designed emergency medical procedures specific to the school bus environment must be detailed in the ITP. Proper training in implementation must be provided for students with respiratory conditions, severe allergies (especially to bee stings and latex), seizures, and swallowing

problems. IEP and 504 building teams need to carefully analyze the bus environment, making plans that

- Decrease exposure to triggers (e.g., seating the student away from rear windows and across from the lift to reduce exposure to temperature changes, fumes, or dust by students with respiratory conditions; requiring a mouth sweep before boarding for students with swallowing concerns; replacing latex gloves with nonlatex gloves in bus cleanup kits);
- Ensure transportation staff's ability to follow CPR protocol (e.g., transfer students to a firm surface for effective chest compressions or abdominal thrusts);
- Allow for necessary adult supervision and assistance; and
- Ensure proper seating and support during and after a medical emergency (e.g., stroller, CSRS).

In case of an emergency, the plan should document a student's ability to use their rescue medications (e.g., EpiPen, rescue inhalers) or their need for assistance. High-backed, padded bus seats make it especially difficult for students to communicate an immediate need for help. Therefore, teaching students to advocate for and be involved in the development of a crisis plan is vital to their safe transport on both the school bus and community transit vehicles.

Occupant protection concerns

Proper fit of the occupant restraint for passengers with tracheotomies is vital. Harness systems of CSRSs or the shoulder belt should lie over the clavicle, avoiding the neck and tube site to allow for unrestricted forward movement of the head and neck during impact. Families concerned that the shoulder belt could dislodge the tube must learn the importance of consistent use and that the shoulder belt should never be worn under the arm, where it could contribute to rib injury in a crash.

Students with tracheotomies often have significant weakness of their trunk and neck muscles, which puts them at greater risk of injury during daily stops and starts without a well-fitted shoulder lap belt. A properly adjusted postural harness cannot be relied on for occupant protection; however, it can be beneficial in aligning the student with better posture to enhance the effectiveness of the shoulder lap belt.

School-bus–specific systems with hip and waist straps that are fitted and adjusted daily typically work better for students with ostomy bags or feeding tubes or buttons because they offer more adjustment at the waist to account for the bag's content or tube placement. Two-part safety vests, which are fitted by waist size, are usually not a good choice.

Students With Cognitive Impairments or Behavioral Challenges

A CSRS may be necessary to keep the student with intellectual disabilities or unsafe behaviors within the compartment and available for effective supervision. A clear rationale should be documented for any system of restraint not needed for a medical or physical concern, especially for use with students identified with severe behavior disorders. Restraint use is highly regulated, controversial, and debated for these students, and least restrictive options need to be tried, deemed ineffective by the team, and documented. These options include

- Presentation of bus safety rules and expectations in alternative ways,
- Carryover of classroom behavior intervention plans and reinforcement schedules,
- Environmental modifications to reduce the impact of unsafe behavior triggers, and
- Use of toys and visual or sensory supports to aid compliance.

Students who are a flight risk often attempt to get out of CSRSs. It is vital for the team to try less restrictive strategies (e.g., zipping the student's coat to cover the harness buckle, refitting the CSRS with adjustment features inherent to the system) before progressing to a more restrictive CSRS. It is also imperative that adjustment features are only those allowed by the manufacturer and proven to be compliant with related motor vehicle safety standards. After-market buckle guards, arm and leg restraints, or homemade fabricated restraints should not be used. The team should also weigh potential benefits of the CSRS assisting in safe containment during evacuation when the tendency to flee can present great safety concerns.

As with all other IEP-driven service provision, goals and objectives should support teaching the student expected behaviors to allow for discontinuation of the CSRS and to move toward a more traditional bus ride. Additional support may also be necessary for boarding and leaving the bus on a daily basis and during evacuation, given that it is more difficult to predict how the student might react under stress. Documentation on ITPs and IEPs of who will receive the student at both destinations is necessary as well as what backup plans will be followed with emergency contacts.

Students With Sensory Processing Issues

The nonobvious nature of a sensory processing disorder often leads transportation staff to conclude that disruptive or inappropriate responses of their passengers with sensory regulation challenges are the result of behavior problems. Occupational therapists should lead the team in careful analysis of the student's performance during the entire transportation experience to uncover sensory triggers. They can then implement strategies to help students cope in the stimulating and unpredictable environment of the school bus.

Student interaction strategies

For students who are hypersensitive to light touch or movement, drivers and monitors should be educated that firm, sustained touch will go a long way in establishing rapport. This is particularly true when they supplement the touch by talking the student through the experience and, whenever possible, initiating contact from within the student's line of sight.

Students with auditory sensitivity may struggle to filter ambient or background sounds to hear voices and may have difficulty responding to instructions or commands. They may use noises to drown out irritating ambient sounds or self-stimulate (e.g., hum, yell, repeat phrases). Transporters should

- Speak to these students in simple, short phrases with a moderate tone and volume;
- Give multistep directions 1 step at a time to prompt understanding; and
- Provide touch cues to the student before beginning to speak to ensure that they have gained attention.

Gestures, signs, visual cues, and pictures can also help communication.

When conveying important safety information to students with visual processing concerns and reduced eye contact, transporters can greatly enhance communication through the use of gestures, pictures, or physical cues positioned in the student's visual field. It is important that transporters understand that decreased eye contact does not reflect a student's lack of caring and that some students are more comfortable looking out of the corners of their eyes.

Seating, positioning, and securement strategies

Movement of the bus, coupled with densely padded seating, often results in sliding and brushing of the skin or dangling body parts. The team can reduce this light touch source by providing a CSRS or by seating the student over a wheel well for support to the feet. Firmly fitting the harness system of the CSRS can provide sensory input similar to that of a weighted or pressure vest. Loose straps of the CSRS harness must be secured, and collars and clothing should be adjusted around the CSRS to avoid irritation. Transportation staff should be taught to remove scarves, mittens, or hats when they present a problem for a student who is touch sensitive.

Many students who are properly supported in a CSRS actually benefit from the bouncing movement of the bus (which can be enhanced when the student sits over the wheel well or in the back of the bus). Students may benefit from having equipment initially fitted in a familiar environment (e.g., classroom, home). The occupational therapy practitioner could also make a sensory storybook with pictures of the student being secured in the CSRS, which could be read in the classroom and at home to prepare the student.

Whenever possible, students should assist in getting themselves into and out of the CSRS harness, with transportation staff checking the end fit. Sitting near the window avoids inadvertent touch of students in the aisle. Leaning into the side wall of the bus can also provide firm pressure. Students bothered by visual busyness and bright light, including those for whom blinking light might trigger a seizure (light filtering between buildings can be a source of blinking light), are often most comfortable sitting in the aisle.

Strategies to enhance an understanding of personal space and seat boundaries can improve student interaction and behavior. For example, the team could reinforce the concept of a student's own space with tape or a square of nonstick shelving matting put on the bus seat. An initial seating plan might allow for the student to sit alone, with gradual reintroduction into sitting with others. Seat placement of fragile students should avoid physical contact with passengers who cannot grade movement. Students should be taught to use their words to get a peer's attention rather than touch.

Students who are insecure with movement often benefit from being seated next to the window with a peer in the aisle, with their feet firmly planted on a wheel well and with their body properly supported (secured in a CSRS, if necessary). Transporters must realize that students with movement difficulties often have difficulty positioning their body in getting into CSRSs and require additional assistance. For the impulsive mover, a peer in the aisle provides a natural cue to stay within the compartment.

Students with auditory filtering difficulty should be seated away from loud noises (e.g., pressurized door opener) as well as persistent ambient sound, such as that emanating from the heating vent and motor. Sensitivity to sounds in the confines of a bus's compartmentalized seating may make it necessary to seat the student alone initially, with a plan in place for reintroducing seating with a peer. Peer modeling can help appropriate follow-through of commands, especially those to prompt timely evacuation.

Self-regulation strategies

Students who need firm pressure may benefit from weighted blankets, toys, or comfort items. However, anything that could become a harmful missile in the event of a crash must be avoided. It may also be useful for these students to do seat push-ups while parked, have a chewy or crunchy snack, or rub on hand lotion before boarding. Proper clothing choices can benefit the student who engages in self-injurious or self-stimulating behaviors to cope with touch processing deficits.

A desensitization program to assist the student in coping with auditory sensitivity on the bus may include transitioning from wearing earplugs to earphones, then earmuffs, and then a hat with earflaps. Students may be allowed to use headphones to decrease sound or listen to music, although they should be taught to periodically look to the transporters or monitors for cues or instructions.

Students who are overly sensitive to visual stimuli may benefit from wearing sunglasses or a hat with a brim. Mounting a cling sunscreen window gel to control light may be another option. A picture landmark map may help some students to navigate the route.

Boarding strategies

Often, students with touch processing challenges display poor body awareness and coordination. This can present a problem for the student whose touch-sensitive fight-or-flight response may be to lash out at the student who brushes against them (Kuhaneck et al., 2007). A poorly graded reflexive swat can be construed as a conscious physical assault. Allowing students with touch processing challenges to board early or late to avoid having to stand in line can reduce opportunities for inadvertent light touch. This is also beneficial for those who have difficulty safely negotiating the stairs because of poor body awareness and coordination.

The process of negotiating steps (or even slightly raised surfaces) for a student with poor balance and body awareness or one who fears heights may need to be modified to

enhance independence and safety during boarding. Transporters need to be taught to recognize that students who have a death grip on the handrail, who are resistant or slow to board, or who appear stiff or ill-coordinated in their movement may be fearful and need added assistance. They might benefit from turning sideways to hold the rail with 2 hands.

Students who have difficulty processing movement sensation can also struggle in understanding spatial terminology (e.g., *up, behind*). Transporters need to know that true conceptualization of spatial terminology is learned through movement, so the student's understanding may be limited, and use of gestures and tactile cues may be necessary to support the verbal commands.

For students with vestibular challenges who need to ride the lift, allowing them a familiar adult and the use of a comfort item in the process may be beneficial. Allowing the student to cue or direct transportation staff to initiate movement of the lift can give them a better feeling of control. For students who are underresponsive to movement sensation, safety risks can be even greater because they may seek more intense movement experiences with little regard for safety. Their impulsive responses make it difficult for them to stay still and in their seat until the bus stops. It is imperative that these students receive hands-on supervision during the boarding process to prevent impulsive darting into traffic and to cue careful and slowed movement on the steps.

Use of the concept of moving in slow motion may help students who are underresponsive to movement to adjust their pace. Implementing a sensory program with heavy work activities before boarding may enhance body awareness and facilitate improved impulse control.

Students who have difficulty processing visual input and coordinating their eyes to work together to accurately perceive depth require extra supervision, especially when boarding and leaving the bus. These students may not notice critical visual details or judge traffic distance. This can make it very difficult for the driver alone to keep the student safe in the dangerous zone immediately surrounding the bus. In addition, transportation staff need to be aware that the student's visual abilities may significantly change during the day, especially when muscles that coordinate eye teaming become tired. Impaired depth perception can make it difficult for the student to find their bus in the parking lot. Use signage (e.g., color, size) to increase the student's independence in locating their assigned seat.

General instructions for all students as they line up to board the bus might consist of keeping 1 arm's length from the person in front of them. This can help reduce problem behaviors as well as cue position in space for the student with visual challenges. If the height of bus steps and curbs poses a problem, then consider textured or colored striping on the stair or curb edge. If the sun's glare disrupts students from seeing and using the handrail, then wrap the rail with reflective or brightly colored tape or teach students to turn toward the rail to hold it with 2 hands as they negotiate the stairs. Teaching students to drag their foot against the stair back can also cue body awareness.

Evacuation strategies

Environmental fears, such as walking through high grass or negotiating various terrains, must be considered with students who are touch sensitive. Unexpected touch sensation involved in an unplanned evacuation may require more supervision or hands-on assistance, such as full lifting or carrying when the student freezes in their tracks, hides, or returns to the bus.

During evacuation, the team must not assume that a student with auditory sensitivity will understand even simple commands in times of stress. The team should practice use of visual cues, gestures, and signs daily with the student to support understanding of instructions needed during an actual evacuation. A rear-door evacuation must take into account the extra support and assistance that may be necessary due to fear of the alarm.

Rear door or window exit evacuation for students with impaired depth perception may also require more adult assistance. Difficulty visually scanning the area and locating and judging the distance to the evacuation destination may further slow efficient evacuation without support. Students who could be a flight risk because of sensory sensitivities may need to be evacuated last to ensure appropriate supervision outside the bus.

BEST PRACTICES

Good teamwork, communication, and coordinated interdisciplinary training are necessary when an IEP or 504 plan team is designing an ITP and ensuring its daily implementation.

Advocate for Transportation Staff to Assist in Developing ITP

In accordance with IDEA (2004), "when a child requires specialized equipment their need should be determined at the IEP meeting and documented on the IEP" (§ 300.5). Therefore, whenever specialized equipment and related procedures are necessary, transportation staff should be present at the IEP meeting. If that is not possible, information should be fully communicated. Occupational therapists should participate in the development of the ITP and provide strategies to the transportation staff.

Document a Plan and Train Transportation Staff

The complexity of transportation-related programming requires additional forms that detail the decision-making process as well as the training required for implementation. Therapists' expertise can be beneficial in helping to design forms that guide the team to first consider least restrictive accommodations or supports allowed for on traditional bus routes so the student can ride with neighborhood peers. Should these prove insufficient, the therapist can then suggest more restrictive options that require more specialized equipment or procedures.

Documentation must detail supports needed for safe daily transport as well as those necessary in an emergency. Conducting a test ride with fast stops, starts, and turns to ensure that the ITP translates well into practice can be especially beneficial. The final ITP should be considered an addendum to the IEP. All team members, including family members, should be informed of their responsibility to notify the district of any changes that could necessitate modifications.

The plan should identify training needs along with who is responsible for providing the instruction. Interdisciplinary training is most effective, and occupational therapy practitioners' varied expertise makes them the natural choice in many areas to provide this instruction. With safety being paramount, ITPs should ensure that the level of support through equipment, staff, and procedural modifications is comparable to that given in other educational environments.

Advocate for Safety on All Vehicles

Occupational therapists must advise the student's educational team to incorporate the self-advocacy goals the student will need for lifetime educational pursuits and safe community access. These goals might aim to increase the student's understanding of their own needs, ability to access available resources, and communication with others around transportation safety. Increased self-sufficiency

---

EXHIBIT 22.1. Online Resources Related to Safe Transportation of Children

- **17th National Congress on School Transportation** (http://ncstonline.org): This website provides national school transportation specification and procedures available for download or purchase.
- **Automotive Safety Program** (http://www.preventinjury.org): This program at Indiana University School of Medicine, affiliated with Riley Hospital for Children, provides literature, training, and resources dedicated to child passenger safety, with a focus on children with special needs.
- **Challenging Behavior and Autism—A Guide for Transportation Personnel** (http://faptflorida.org/wp-content/uploads/2015/10/THE-BUS-1 -Ideas-for-Challenging-Behavior-and-Autism.pdf): Jocelyn Taylor, MS, CCC-SLP, an autism specialist, outlines strategies for dealing with challenging behavior on the bus.
- **National Highway Traffic Safety Administration** (https://www.nhtsa.gov/): This website contains extensive training literature, programs, and videos specific to school bus safety and use of child safety restraint systems, and driver training related to transportation of students with special needs.
- **Safe Ride News Publications** (https://www.saferidenews.com): This independent press publishes a bimonthly newsletter (*Safe Ride News*) and other educational materials related to child passenger safety, such as the *School Bus Safety Handbook: Choosing and Using Child Safety Restraint Systems and Wheelchairs* (Stewart & Donaldson, 2013).
- **Wheelchair Transportation Safety** (http://wc-transportation-safety.umtri.umich.edu): This arm of the University of Michigan's Transportation Research Institute provides information on crash tests and related research to support best practice principles regarding safe transportation of people who use wheelchairs. It also lists wheelchairs and seating systems that are compliant with WC 19 and WC 20.

in transportation subskills (e.g., boarding, using a bus stop, seating in the compartment), combined with reduced need for support equipment, may be a focus leading to independence in use of public transportation or the pursuit of driver training.

SUMMARY

Transportation safety and independence can be greatly enhanced through occupational therapy practitioners' leadership and work with students on this important IADL. Practitioners must consider many constraints and procedural guidelines when making decisions about effective seating and positioning. These concerns are outlined in a chart titled "Effective School Bus Occupant Restraints for Students With Special Needs" included in the appendix of NHTSA's (2015) 8-hour training course. Occupational therapy practitioners who want to further educate themselves in meeting the needs of students with special needs are directed to the list of online resources in Exhibit 22.1.

REFERENCES

ADA Amendments Act of 2008, Pub. L. 110–325, 122 Stat. 3553.

American National Standards Institute & Rehabilitation Engineering Society of North America. (2012a). *ANSI/RESNA WC19: Wheelchairs used as seats in motor vehicles* [Wheelchair standard]. Arlington, VA: Rehabilitation Engineering Society of North America.

American National Standards Institute & Rehabilitation Engineering Society of North America. (2012b). *ANSI/RESNA WC20: Wheelchairs and transportation.* Arlington, VA: Rehabilitation Engineering Society of North America.

American Occupational Therapy Association. (2014). Guidelines for supervision, roles, and responsibilities during the delivery of occupational therapy services. *American Journal of Occupational Therapy, 68*(Suppl. 3), S16–S22. https://doi.org/10.5014/ajot.2014.686S03

Individuals With Disabilities Education Improvement Act of 2004, Pub. L. 108–446, 20 U.S.C. §§ 1400–1482.

Kuhaneck, H. M., Henry, D., & Glennon, T. (2007). *Sensory Processing Measure (SPM).* Los Angeles: Western Psychological Services.

National Highway Traffic Safety Administration. (2015). *Child passenger safety restraint systems on school buses national training instructor manual.* Washington, DC: Author.

Rehabilitation Act of 1973, Pub. L. 93–112, 29 U.S.C. §§ 701–796l.

Section 504 of the Rehabilitation Act of 1973, as amended, 29 U.S.C. § 794 (2008).

Stewart, D., & Donaldson, D. (2013). *School bus safety handbook* (2nd ed.). Greenbank, WA: Safe Ride News.

University of Michigan Transportation Research Institute. (2015). *Transportation review checklist.* Retrieved from http://wc-transportation-safety.umtri.umich.edu/consumers/transportation-review-checklist-rev-02-07

Best Practices in Transition Planning for Preschoolers

23

Christine Teeters Myers, PhD, OTR/L, and Mara C. Podvey, PhD, OTR

KEY TERMS AND CONCEPTS

- Adjustment to school
- Annual performance report
- Head Start
- School readiness
- State-identified measurable result

OVERVIEW

Transition is a hallmark of life, and the transition to school is one of the first experiences a young child will remember. In 2015, more than 300,000 children receiving special education services transitioned to kindergarten (U.S. Department of Education, Office of Special Education Programs, 2018a). Changes in environment and in family and child routines and roles as well as new expectations, policies, and people shape the transition process. A positive initial school experience is important because early school transitions may provide the foundation for future school experiences of children and families (Schulting et al., 2005; Wildengar & McIntyre, 2012).

As children transition from preschool to kindergarten, the personnel working with them should provide guidance and support to the child and family as well as address school readiness and form relationships with community agencies (e.g., Head Start, public school districts). An overarching goal of the transition to school is to support school success through child and family preparation and positive early school experiences (Kang et al., 2017; Rous, Hallam, et al., 2007).

Occupational therapy practitioners[1] have much to offer in the transition from one program and environment to the next (Myers, 2006; Podvey & Hinojosa, 2009). This chapter focuses on the role of the school occupational therapy practitioner in preschool to kindergarten transitions under Part B

---

[1]*Occupational therapy practitioner* refers to both the occupational therapist and the occupational therapy assistant. The American Occupational Therapy Association (AOTA; 2014a, p. S18) states, "The occupational therapist is responsible for all aspects of occupational therapy service delivery and is accountable for the safety and effectiveness of the occupational therapy service delivery process" and "must be directly involved in the delivery of services during the initial evaluation and regularly throughout the course of intervention. . . . The occupational therapy assistant delivers safe and effective occupational therapy services under the supervision of and in partnership with the occupational therapist."

of the Individuals With Disabilities Education Improvement Act of 2004 (IDEA; Pub. L. 108–446). The chapter also suggests practices and strategies that occupational therapy practitioners may use to support children and families throughout the transition process.

ESSENTIAL CONSIDERATIONS

This section presents an overview of various aspects of the transition process related to occupational therapy services, such as understanding laws and regulations, working with community agencies, measuring outcomes for accountability, and learning about transition processes and procedures.

Transition From Preschool Into Kindergarten

Schools have high expectations for kindergartners, both academically and socially. The transition into kindergarten should be focused on a successful *adjustment to school* (i.e., adaptation to the student role and school environment) with an emphasis on school readiness during preschool (Rous, Hallam, et al., 2007). The transition process may be supported by occupational therapy practitioners, who act as important team members for students with disabilities or developmental delays.

IDEA (2004) and regulations provide very little guidance pertaining to the transition practices for children in this age group. However, students who meet state eligibility for special education and related services or who are eligible under Section 504 of the Rehabilitation Act of 1973, as amended (2008; Pub. L. 93–112) may need assistance in transitioning to kindergarten programming. The Improving Head Start for School Readiness Act of 2007 (Pub. L. 110–134) mandates continuity of services into kindergarten.

Head Start is a program that provides school readiness services for children from families with low income. Staff must provide guidance for families and children entering elementary school by coordinating with educational and social agencies, which may include meetings with parents

Copyright © 2019 by the American Occupational Therapy Association. All rights reserved. To reuse this content, contact www.copyright.com.
https://doi.org/10.7139/2019.978-1-56900-591-0.023

and kindergarten teachers. Under the Every Student Succeeds Act (ESSA; 2015; Pub. L. 114–195), related service providers, such as occupational therapy practitioners, are considered specialized instructional support personnel and may provide support to transition teams.

Although IDEA (2004) lacks specific guidelines for the transition to kindergarten, the student's educational team should discuss and consider the transition when developing the initial individualized education program (IEP) and in subsequent IEP meetings during preschool years. In particular, team members should emphasize the importance of school readiness in preparation for kindergarten transition. *School readiness* should encompass more than academic competence, emphasizing social–emotional competence as well. Occupational therapy practitioners should attend transition planning meetings for students on their workload (Myers, 2008).

Office of Special Education Programs Indicators and Outcomes

IDEA (2004; § 1416[b][1]) requires each state to have a state performance plan that evaluates Part B implementation in the state and describes how implementation improvements will occur. The Office of Special Education Programs (OSEP) requires that state performance plans be reported annually through the *annual performance report,* which describes the goals and intended outcomes of U.S. Department of Education programs and initiatives. Indicator B-11 relates to early childhood transition: "*B–11 (timely evaluation):* Percentage of children with parental consent to evaluate who were evaluated and eligibility determined within 60 days (or state-established timeframe; § 1416[a][3][B])" (U.S. Department of Education, Office of Special Education Programs, 2018b). School occupational therapists working under Part B services are involved in helping to meet these requirements by conducting evaluations within established time frames and assisting in implementing a child's IEP.

OSEP also collects outcome data on children from birth to age 5 years, which includes students transitioning to kindergarten who are receiving Part B services. Two Part B indicators measure outcomes that relate to early childhood transitions:

> *B–7 (Preschool outcomes):* Percentage of preschool children with IEPs who demonstrate improved
> - Positive social–emotional skills (including social relationships)
> - Acquisition and use of knowledge and skills (including early language or communication and early literacy)
> - Use of appropriate behaviors to meet their needs (§ 1416[a][3][A])
>
> *B–8 (Parental involvement):* Percentage of parents with a child receiving special education services who report that schools facilitated parent involvement as a means of improving services and results for children with disabilities (§ 1416[a][3][A]). (U.S. Department of Education, Office of Special Education Programs, 2018b)

As part of the transition team, the occupational therapist may find this information beneficial when considering a student's needs. A student who begins kindergarten with the ability to communicate effectively and who has developed early literacy skills may adjust more quickly. Significant associations have been found between cognitive and social–emotional readiness at kindergarten entry and reading fluency and social–emotional well-being in Grade 5 (Quirk et al., 2017). Likewise, executive functioning (EF) skills, such as delay of gratification, are associated with social–emotional readiness for school (Mann et al., 2016).

Occupational therapy practitioners who engage parents to become more involved in their child's transition to kindergarten help to support school adjustment and potentially influence school experiences (this is a B-8 indicator). Occupational therapy practitioners can also support school readiness by understanding family routines, because engagement in more family routines predicts better reading scores, math scores, and physical health and is associated with fewer teacher-reported conduct problems and better social skills (Ferretti & Bub, 2017). Research suggests that a positive teacher–student relationship can decrease the negative impacts of a student's EF limitations on their readiness for school (Graziano et al., 2016). For this reason, occupational therapy strategies should include ways to support the teacher–student relationship.

Occupational therapy practitioners working in transition may also have a role in addressing the *state-identified measurable result* (SIMR) from each state's systemic improvement plan. The SIMR is based on one of these indicators. For instance, in Florida, the SIMR is the percentage of youth with an IEP graduating from high school with a standard diploma. The occupational therapy practitioner working with a kindergarten student may assist in the transition process to improve school readiness and therefore improve the likelihood of the student's graduation many years later.

Understand Transition Processes and Procedures

Confusion and complexity are characteristics of the transition process for both service providers and families (Starr et al., 2016). Ongoing training in transition processes (e.g., from preschool to kindergarten) in the agency should be provided, with the goal of an efficient and trained staff (Branson & Bingham, 2009). More experienced staff members and novice ones can share strategies. See Exhibit 23.1 for a list of online resources related to understanding and improving preschooler transition.

BEST PRACTICES

Best practices in early childhood transitions are those that include child and family preparation, parent and family involvement in planning and transitions, and support for interprofessional collaboration and communication regarding the transition process (Rosenkoetter et al., 2009; Rous, 2008; Rous, Myers, et al., 2007). Some occupational therapists are already participating in early childhood transition activities that are considered best practices, including
- Evaluating the child,
- Attending transition meetings,

EXHIBIT 23.1. Online Resources for Preschool Transitions

- **CONNECT: The Center to Mobilize Early Childhood Knowledge** (http://community.fpg.unc.edu/): CONNECT is a series of 8 self-paced and self-guided courses for professionals working in inclusive learning environments such as child care centers, preschools, and Head Start programs.
- **Early Childhood Technical Assistance Center** (ECTA Center; http://ectacenter.org): The ECTA Center is funded by OSEP to offer technical assistance to state early intervention and early childhood special education service programs while supporting efforts to implement effective early childhood practices and improve outcomes of services provided to children and families. The National Early Childhood Technical Assistance Center, the Center for Early Literacy Learning, Technical Assistance Center on Social Emotional Intervention for Young Children, and Early Childhood Outcomes Center are now at the ECTA Center. The ECTA Center website has information on all aspects of early childhood transitions, state resources (e.g., transition guides, forms), transition-related research, and parent resources (e.g., tip sheets, parent guides to transition). Information on the transition from preschool to kindergarten is found at http://ectacenter.org/topics/transition/transtoK.asp
- **Head Start Early Childhood Learning and Knowledge Center–Transitions** (https://eclkc.ohs.acf.hhs.gov/transitions): Head Start's Early Childhood Learning and Knowledge Center website has information for early childhood professionals on ways to help support Head Start students and families during transitions. Strategies for collaboration with other professionals, helping students and families transition to kindergarten, and in-class transition strategies are provided.
- **National Early Childhood Transition Center** (NECTC; http://www.hdi.uky.edu/nectc/NECTC/Home.aspx): NECTC was funded by OSEP to conduct research related to factors that support successful early childhood transitions. NECTC's website provides many products for occupational therapy practitioners interested in learning more about transitions, including research briefs, presentations, references to publications, a database of transition literature, a webinar series, and a transition toolkit.

Note. OSEP = Office of Special Education Programs.

- Helping to develop the student's IEP,
- Working with families, and
- Referring children and families to additional services as needed (Myers, 2008).

These practices are critical for those who are at risk for developing difficulties down the road (National Institute of Mental Health, 2002). To offer the highest quality services, occupational therapists must be aware of these best practices and implement them as a routine part of service provision. The Early Childhood Technical Assistance (ECTA) Center has developed transition practice guidelines for practitioners (ECTA Center, 2017b) and transition checklists (ECTA Center, 2017a) to assist in the implementation of best practices.

Address the Needs of the Student in the Next Environment

Contextual changes are a hallmark of early childhood transitions from preschool to kindergarten. As students move to a new physical context (e.g., from home-based to community- or classroom-based care), they also see additional changes to the cultural (e.g., routines, daily activities), social (e.g., peer-to-peer relationships, engagement with personnel), and philosophical (e.g., developmental vs. academic) contexts. Given that the ultimate goal of successful transitions is to support the student's engagement in kindergarten occupations, occupational therapy practitioners must develop a deep understanding of the contextual demands as well as the student's strengths and challenges.

Evaluate the student

Under Part B of IDEA (2004), teams must complete the full and individual initial evaluations, determine eligibility, and complete the IEP meeting within 60 days (some states may require less than 60 days) of receipt of parental consent. If the parent has requested it or if the team feels it is necessary,

an occupational therapy evaluation may be conducted. This evaluation must be completed within the timelines as well.

Continuity between programs is important during early childhood transitions (Rosenkoetter et al., 2009), and completing the initial evaluation, eligibility determination, and IEP in a timely manner can facilitate this continuity.

The occupational therapist should be aware of both the curriculum and expectations in the new environment. The evaluation process can help identify necessary modifications to the school environment, adaptations to materials, and intervention strategies that can improve a student's participation in the school program.

Lack of sufficient qualified personnel to perform those evaluations (Kasprzak et al., 2012) is not acceptable. If these evaluations are not conducted within the required timelines stipulated under Indicator Part B-11, as previously discussed, the state must report this lack of compliance to OSEP in its annual state report.

Help the student learn skills needed for the next environment

All parents, regardless of their children's abilities, report concerns about kindergarten readiness (McIntyre et al., 2010). Rosenkoetter et al. (2009) reported that teaching skills needed in the next environment lead to successful transition and successful outcomes. The occupational therapy evaluation can help the team identify the student's present level of performance and needs for the next environment.

To create an appropriate occupational therapy intervention plan, an occupational therapist must understand the expectations for performance in each environment where the student will participate. Development of environment-specific skills (e.g., hanging a coat on a hook, washing hands, following simple directions) and adaptation or modification of environments support participation in the school setting and should be accounted for in such a plan.

Adjustment to school may be predicted by social and behavioral competencies (Welchons & McIntyre, 2017), which are supported by the development of EF skills (Moreno et al., 2017). Self-regulation, choice making, and engagement in school routines are skills developed in early childhood that determine success in earlier grades. They also foster development of the self-determination skills (Erwin et al., 2016) that are the basis of later transitions, including the transition to adulthood. Engagement in common classroom activities as well as interaction with peers and teachers provide the foundation for skill development in social and behavioral competencies (Welchons & McIntyre, 2017).

There is limited evidence in the literature that students with motor deficits, including poor kinesthesia, muscle tone, and visual–motor integration, have greater difficulty than peers in adjusting to kindergarten (Bart et al., 2007). However, addressing the motor skill needs of preschool children with delays can positively affect their transition outcomes by improving the skills they need for early learning (McClelland & Cameron, in press).

Support Families

One of the most crucial indicators of success in transitions to inclusive environments is a positive relationship between service providers and families. Supporting families throughout transitions is a way to reduce families' stress levels (Rosenkoetter et al., 2009) and is associated with better child outcomes (Kemp, 2003; Mantzicopoulos, 2005; Peisner-Feinberg et al., 2001).

Family studies underscore the importance of the IEP team in identifying and selecting program options for students, sharing information about the environment that the child will enter, and discussing the expectations and needs of that environment (Campbell, 1997; Hanline & Halvorsen, 1989; Hanson et al., 2000; Kemp, 2003; Lovett & Haring, 2003; Pianta & Kraft-Sayre, 1999). Most parents want more information about their child's skill levels and the expectations in the new environment (Wildengar & McIntyre, 2011), which should be shared so parents can be included in the evaluation, planning, and intervention processes at all levels.

Occupational therapy practitioners use a client-centered approach to understand what is important and meaningful to the client (e.g., child, family, school staff; AOTA, 2014b). When practitioners view the client as both the student and their family, it becomes clear that practitioners' role includes empowering families to be active participants in and advocates for their child's education (Lovett & Haring, 2003).

Explain procedural safeguards and due process procedures

Procedural safeguards and due process procedures for parents of children with disabilities are included in IDEA (§300.500–§300.536) to offer parents options for fairly resolving disagreements that might arise surrounding their child's special education program. Included in the safeguards are parental rights related to evaluation, such as to consent to perform full and individual initial evaluations, as well as the right to refuse such evaluations. In addition, parents have the right to notification before changes are made to their children's special education programs by the local educational agency.

Explain various programs' eligibility processes

IDEA requires a 60-day timeline for conducting a full and individual initial evaluation of a child and for developing an IEP. The law provides each district the latitude to develop its own procedures for completing the process within the given time frame. These procedures should be shared with all members of the evaluation team. Occupational therapists participating in the evaluation process should contact the family to request specific information about their child (e.g., medical history, parental concerns). Once the evaluation process has been completed, the occupational therapist should contact the family again to discuss the findings of that process.

Encourage families and staff to participate in site visits

Visiting potential programs that the child may enter is one way to reduce the anxiety associated with transition (Rous et al., 2010). Equally important in a site visit is the participation of school-based personnel. Site-visit participation by all stakeholders allows for more universal identification of the student's strengths, needs, and any preparations necessary (e.g., ordering new equipment) for the student's ultimate entrance into the program.

Provide regular communication

A critical factor in school success for children is parental involvement (Mantzicopoulos, 2003), so including parents in the transition process is critical. The transition process includes an adjustment period after the move to the new environment (Rimm-Kaufman & Pianta, 2000; Starr et al., 2016). This process can be made easier and more comfortable with regular communication between families and personnel throughout the transition period, including after arrival at the new program (Kemp, 2003; Podvey et al., 2013).

Any method of communication (e.g., email, written notes, telephone calls) used by the occupational therapy practitioner should be based on parent preference. All team members should be aware of and abide by this preference whenever possible. Practitioners should document and securely store original notes related to family contact.

Communicate and Collaborate With Other Programs and Providers

Effective communication is identified in the literature as a best practice (Branson & Bingham, 2009; Rosenkoetter et al., 2009). Interprofessional communication is facilitated when team members participate in transition meetings. These exchanges provide the opportunity for a universal understanding of team member roles within and between programs. Occupational therapy practitioners can improve the perceived value of their field to the team by participating in meetings and contributing valuable information to the individualized family service plan's family outcomes and IEP goals (Myers, 2008).

SUMMARY

The transition from preschool to kindergarten is important, and federal law offers guidance (IDEA, 2004). Practices that promote collaboration and communication between families and professionals have the best potential to support early school transitions (Myers et al., 2011; Rosenkoetter et al., 2009).

Communication and collaboration should not be limited to families but should include personnel involved in the programs as well as professionals working with the student outside of early intervention or preschool programs. With the contribution of all team members, including occupational therapy practitioners, working with families and students before, during, and after the transition and using best practices, the process can be positive.

REFERENCES

American Occupational Therapy Association. (2014a). Guidelines for supervision, roles, and responsibilities during the delivery of occupational therapy services. *American Journal of Occupational Therapy, 68*(Suppl. 3), S16–S22. https://doi.org/10.5014/ajot.2014.686S03

American Occupational Therapy Association. (2014b). Occupational therapy practice framework: Domain and process (3rd ed.). *American Journal of Occupational Therapy, 68*(Suppl. 1), S1–S48. https://doi.org/10.5014/ajot.2014.682006

Bart, O., Hajami, D., & Bar-Haim, Y. (2007). Predicting school adjustment from motor abilities in kindergarten. *Infant and Child Development, 16,* 597–615. https://doi.org/10.1002/icd.514

Branson, D. M., & Bingham, A. (2009). Using interagency collaboration to support family-centered transition practices. *Young Exceptional Children, 12*(3), 15–31. https://doi.org/10.1177/1096250609332306

Campbell, J. (1997). The next step: Parent perspectives of transition to preschool of children with disabilities. *Australian Journal of Early Childhood, 22,* 30–34.

Early Childhood Technical Assistance Center. (2017a). *Transition from early intervention services to Part B preschool special education checklist.* Retrieved from http://ectacenter.org/~pdfs/decrp/TR-2_EI_to_Preschool_2017.pdf

Early Childhood Technical Assistance Center. (2017b). *Transition from early intervention to preschool special education services* [Practitioner practice guide]. Retrieved from http://ectacenter.org/~pdfs/decrp/PG_Trn_EItoPreschool_prac_print_2017.pdf

Erwin, E. J., Maude, S. P., Palmer, S. B., Summers, J. A., Brotherson, M. J., Haines, S. J., . . . Peck, N. F. (2016). Fostering the foundations of self-determination in early childhood: A process for enhancing child outcomes across home and school. *Early Childhood Education Journal, 44,* 325–333. https://doi.org/10.1007/s10643-015-0710-9

Every Student Succeeds Act, Pub. L. No. 114–95, 129 Stat. 1802 (2015).

Ferretti, L. K., & Bub, K. L. (2017). Family routines and school readiness during the transition to kindergarten. *Early Education and Development, 28,* 59–77. https://doi.org/10.1080/10409289.2016.1195671

Graziano, P. A., Garb, L. R., Ros, R., Hart, K., & Garcia, A. (2016). Executive functioning and school readiness among preschoolers with externalizing problems: The moderating role of the student–teacher relationship. *Early Education and Development, 27,* 573–589. https://doi.org/10.1080/10409289.2016.1102019

Hanline, M. F., & Halvorsen, A. (1989). Parent perceptions of the integration transition process: Overcoming artificial barriers. *Exceptional Children, 55,* 487–492. https://doi.org/10.1177/001440298905500601

Hanson, M. J., Beckman, P. J., Horn, E., Marquart, J., Sandall, S. R., Greig, D., . . . Brennan, E. (2000). Entering preschool: Family and professional experiences in this transition process. *Journal of Early Intervention, 23,* 279–293. https://doi.org/10.1177/105381510002300407 01

Improving Head Start for School Readiness Act of 2007, Pub. L. 110–134, 42 U.S.C. § 9801 *et seq.*

Individuals With Disabilities Education Improvement Act of 2004, Pub. L. No 108–446, 20 U.S.C. §§ 1400–1482.

Kang, J., Horn, E. M., & Palmer, S. (2017). Influences of family involvement in kindergarten transition activities on children's early school adjustment. *Early Childhood Education Journal, 45,* 789–800. https://doi.org/10.1007/s10643-016-0828-4

Kasprzak, C., Hurth, J., Rooney, R., Goode, S. E., Danaher, J. C., Whaley, K. T., . . . Cate, D. (2012). States' accountability and progress in serving young children with disabilities. *Topics in Early Childhood Special Education, 32,* 151–163. https://doi.org/10.1177/0271121411408119

Kemp, C. (2003). Investigating the transition of young children with intellectual disabilities to mainstream classes: An Australian perspective. *International Journal of Disability, Development, and Education, 50,* 403–433. https://doi.org/10.1080/1034912032000155194

Lovett, D. L., & Haring, K. A. (2003). Family perceptions of transitions in early intervention. *Education and Training in Developmental Disabilities, 38,* 370–377. https://www.jstor.org/stable/23879913

Mann, T. D., Hund, A. M., Hesson-McInnis, M. S., & Roman, Z. J. (2016). Pathways to school readiness: Executive functioning predicts academic and social–emotional aspects of school readiness. *Mind, Brain and Education, 11*(1), 21–31. https://doi.org/10.1111/mbe.12134

Mantzicopoulos, P. (2003). Flunking kindergarten after Head Start: An inquiry into the contribution of contextual and individual variables. *Journal of Educational Psychology, 95,* 268–278. https://doi.org/10.1037/0022-0663.95.2.268

Mantzicopoulos, P. (2005). Conflictual relationships between kindergarten children and their teachers: Associations with child and classroom context variables. *Journal of Social Psychology, 43,* 425–442.

McClelland, M. M., & Cameron, C. E. (in press). Developing together: The role of executive function and motor skills in children's early academic lives. *Early Childhood Research Quarterly.* https://doi.org/10.1016/j.ecresq.2018.03.014

McIntyre, L. L., Eckert, T. L., Fiese, B. H., Reed, F. D. D., & Wildenger, L. K. (2010). Family concerns surrounding kindergarten transition: A comparison of students in special and general education. *Early Childhood Education Journal, 38,* 259–263. https://doi.org/10.1007/s10643-010-0416-y

Moreno, A. J., Schwayder, I., & Friedman, I. D. (2017). The function of executive function: Everyday manifestations of regulated thinking in preschool settings. *Early Childhood Education Journal, 45,* 143–153. https://doi.org/10.1007/s10643-016-0777-y

Myers, C. T. (2006). Exploring occupational therapy and transitions for young children with special needs. *Physical and Occupational Therapy in Pediatrics, 26,* 73–88. https://doi.org/10.1080/J006v26n03_06

Myers, C. T. (2008). Descriptive study of occupational therapists' participation in early childhood transitions. *American Journal of Occupational Therapy, 62,* 212–220. https://doi.org/10.5014/ajot.62.2.212

Myers, C. T., Schneck, C. M., Effgen, S. K., McCormick, K. M., & Shasby, S. B. (2011). Factors associated with therapists' involvement in children's transition to preschool. *American Journal of Occupational Therapy, 65,* 86–94. https://doi.org/10.5014/ajot.2011.09060

National Institute of Mental Health. (2002). *A good beginning: Sending America's children to school with the social and emotional competence they need to succeed.* Bethesda, MD: Author.

Peisner-Feinberg, E., Burchinal, M. R., Clifford, R. M., Culkin, M. L., Howes, C., Kagan, S. L., & Yazejian, N. (2001). The relation of preschool child-care quality to children's cognitive and social developmental trajectories through second grade. *Child Development, 72,* 1534–1553. https://doi.org/10.1111/1467-8624.00364

Pianta, R. C., & Kraft-Sayre, M. (1999). Parents' observations about their children's transitions to kindergarten. *Young Children, 54,* 47–52.

Podvey, M. C., & Hinojosa, J. (2009). Transition from early intervention to preschool special education services: Family-centered practice that promotes positive outcomes. *Journal of Occupational Therapy, Schools, and Early Intervention, 2,* 73–83. https://doi.org/10.1080/19411240903146111

Podvey, M. C., Hinojosa, J., & Koenig, K. P. (2013). Reconsidering insider status for families during the transition from early intervention to preschool special education. *Journal of Special Education, 46,* 211–222. https://doi.org/10.1177/0022466911407074

Quirk, M., Dowdy, E., Goldstien, A., & Carnazzo, K. (2017). School readiness as a longitudinal predictor of social–emotional and reading performance across the elementary grades. *Assessment for Effective Instruction, 42,* 248–253. https://doi.org/10.1177/1534508417719680

Rehabilitation Act of 1973, Pub. L. 93–112, 29 U.S.C. §§ 701–7961.

Rimm-Kaufman, S. E., & Pianta, R. C. (2000). An ecological perspective on the transition to kindergarten: A theoretical perspective to guide empirical research. *Applied Developmental Psychology, 21,* 491–501. https://doi.org/10.1016/S0193-3973(00)00051-4

Rosenkoetter, S., Schroeder, C., Rous, B., Hains, A., Shaw, J., & McCormick, K. (2009). *A review of research in early childhood transition: Child and family studies* (Technical Report No. 5).

Lexington: University of Kentucky, Human Development Institute, National Early Childhood Transition Center.

Rous, B. (2008). *Recommended transition practices for young children and families: Results from a national validation survey* (Technical Report No. 3). Lexington: University of Kentucky, Human Development Institute, National Early Childhood Transition Center. Retrieved from http://www.hdi.uky.edu/nectc/Libraries/NECTC_Papers_and_Reports/Technical_Report_3.sflb.ashx

Rous, B., Hallam, R., Harbin, G., McCormick, K., & Jung, L. A. (2007). The transition process for young children with disabilities: A conceptual framework. *Infants and Young Children, 20,* 135–148. https://doi.org/10.1097/01.IYC.0000264481.27947.5f

Rous, B., Hallam, R., McCormick, K., & Cox, M. (2010). Practices that support the transition to public preschool programs: Results from a national survey. *Early Childhood Research Quarterly, 25,* 17–32. https://doi.org/10.1016/j.ecresq.2009.09.001

Rous, B., Myers, C., & Stricklin, S. (2007). Strategies for supporting transitions of young children with special needs and their families. *Journal of Early Intervention, 30,* 1–18. https://doi.org/10.1177/105381510703000102

Schulting, A. B., Malone, P. S., & Dodge, K. A. (2005). The effect of school-based kindergarten transition policies and practices on child academic outcomes. *Developmental Psychology, 41,* 860–871. https://doi.org/10.1037/0012-1649.41.6.860

Section 504 of the Rehabilitation Act of 1973, as amended, 29 U.S.C. § 794 (2008).

Starr, E. M., Martini, T. S., & Kuo, B. H. (2016). Transition to kindergarten for children with autism spectrum disorder. *Focus on Autism and Other Developmental Disabilities, 31,* 115–128. https://doi.org/10.1177/1088357614532497

U.S. Department of Education, Office of Special Education Programs. (2018a). *IDEA Section 618 data products: State level data files: 2015 child count and educational environments.* Retrieved from https://www2.ed.gov/programs/osepidea/618-data/state-level-data-files/index.html#bcc

U.S. Department of Education, Office of Special Education Programs. (2018b). *Part B state performance plan/annual performance report 2018 indicator analyses.* Retrieved from https://osep.grads360.org/#communities/pdc/documents/17333

Welchons, L. W., & McIntyre, L. L. (2017). The transition to kindergarten: Predicting socio-behavioral outcomes for children with and without disabilities. *Early Childhood Education Journal, 45,* 83–93. https://doi.org/10.1007/s10643-015-0757-7

Wildengar, L. M., & McIntyre, L. L. (2011). Family concerns and involvement during kindergarten transition. *Journal of Child and Family Studies, 20,* 387–396. https://doi.org/10.1007/s10643-010-0416-y

Wildengar, L. M., & McIntyre, L. L. (2012). Investigating the relation between kindergarten preparation and child socio-behavioral outcomes. *Early Childhood Education Journal, 40,* 169–176.

Best Practices in Transition Planning for Independent Living and Workplace Readiness

24

Meira L. Orentlicher, PhD, OTR/L, FAOTA

KEY TERMS AND CONCEPTS

- Client-centered practice
- Community-based instruction
- Discovery
- Ecological inventories
- Employment preparation program
- Functional assessment
- Guardianship
- Inclusion
- Interagency collaboration
- Peer-focused strategy
- Person-centered planning
- Self-determination
- Social competence
- Social model of disability
- Supported decision making
- Support-focused strategy

OVERVIEW

The goal of education is to prepare all students to be adults who are as independent as possible, and the Individuals With Disabilities Education Improvement Act of 2004 (IDEA; Pub. L. 108–446) stipulates that students who receive special education and related services should be prepared for "further education, employment, and independent living" (§ 1401[d]). This explicit statement clarifies that school personnel, parents, and students must consider adult outcomes as they plan each student's school experiences and individualized education programs (IEPs). To improve adult outcomes for students with disabilities, schools are mandated to provide transition services beginning no later than age 16 years.

Occupational therapy practitioners[1] are particularly well placed to provide supports for students with disabilities who are seeking opportunities for an independent and fulfilling life in the community. The occupational therapy practitioner's distinct focus on human engagement in meaningful occupations in a variety of natural contexts is critical for students seeking an independent life in the community. The practitioner's expertise in activity analysis, task

[1]*Occupational therapy practitioner* refers to both the occupational therapist and the occupational therapy assistant. The American Occupational Therapy Association (AOTA; 2014a, p. S18) states, "The occupational therapist is responsible for all aspects of occupational therapy service delivery and is accountable for the safety and effectiveness of the occupational therapy service delivery process" and "must be directly involved in the delivery of services during the initial evaluation and regularly throughout the course of intervention. . . . The occupational therapy assistant delivers safe and effective occupational therapy services under the supervision of and in partnership with the occupational therapist."

adaptations, and environmental modifications is essential as well.

ESSENTIAL CONSIDERATIONS

The focus of this chapter is on the transition from school to meaningful employment, independent living, and community participation. For the transition to postsecondary education, see Chapter 25, "Best Practices in Preparing Students and Families for Postsecondary Education."

Laws That Shape Practice

IDEA (2004) requires that each IEP must include "appropriate measurable post-secondary goals based upon age-appropriate transition assessments related to training, education, employment, and, where appropriate, independent living skills" (§ 1414[d][1][A][VIII]). Services must be provided to assist each student in meeting these goals. These services may be provided by the local educational agency or by agencies outside of the school.

Although IDEA requires transition planning to begin no later than age 16 years, research suggests that planning should begin earlier (Cimera et al., 2013) to increase employment after high school and help the student earn higher wages. In fact, many states now mandate that transition services begin at age 14 (e.g., Iowa, North Carolina, Nevada, Mississippi) or 15 (e.g., New York). Occupational therapy researchers also proposed preemployment and other transition preparation programs for students in middle school (Hollenbeck et al., 2015).

In addition to IDEA, other laws stipulate various resources (e.g., vocational counseling training assistance, job placement); promote equal access to education, employment, and daily activities; and provide funding for insurance or benefits for qualified persons. Examples include the

Copyright © 2019 by the American Occupational Therapy Association. All rights reserved. To reuse this content, contact www.copyright.com.
https://doi.org/10.7139/2019.978-1-56900-591-0.024

- Rehabilitation Act of 1973 (Pub. L. 93–112),
- ADA Amendments Act of 2008 (Pub. L. 110–325), and
- Social Security Disability Insurance and Supplemental Security Income (Social Security, 2017).

Staying current on regulations and resources at the federal and state levels is wise.

State vocational rehabilitation services offer a range of employment and independent living services, with a goal of promoting a greater level of independence in work and living environments. Medicaid's Home and Community-Based Services waiver programs offer benefits for individuals with intellectual and developmental disabilities (IDDs) on a long-term basis so they can remain in the community. Networking to understand these offerings benefits the student, family, and educational team.

Transition Outcomes

Predictors of transition outcomes for young adults with disabilities include race, gender, and disability. According to the secondary analysis of the Second National Longitudinal Transition Study (Wagner et al., 2003), 67% of young adults with disabilities who had paid work were White. Erickson et al. (2013) documented that 31.1% of women with disabilities between ages 21 and 64 years were employed compared with 35.9% of men. Young adults with emotional disturbances (Wagner et al., 2017), autism spectrum disorder (Alverson & Yamamoto, 2017), and mild IDDs (Bouck, 2017) had the poorest transition outcomes.

Evidence suggests that academic achievement in high school and social skills are predictors of postsecondary success (Hein et al., 2013; National Technical Assistance Center on Transition, 2016b). Students with better social skills demonstrated greater persistence and ability to navigate the demands of postsecondary education than with students with lesser social skills (Dymnicki et al., 2013).

On another positive note, transition programs that provide vocational skills instruction and work experiences helped young adults with IDDs secure long-term employment and independent living (Southward & Kyzar, 2017). Family participation and young adults' self-determination and career awareness were found to be linked to increased graduation rates, employment, and achievement of positive postschool outcomes.

Self-determination is a predictor of employment, independent living, and community access for students with disabilities (Shogren et al., 2015). It is defined as having the skills to

- Make choices and decisions,
- Solve problems,
- Set and attain goals,
- Advocate and be a leader, and
- Self-regulate and control oneself (Wehmeyer, 2015).

In 1 study (Nonnemacher & Bambara, 2011), youth expressed that it was important for them to

- Have the support of others,
- Receive good medical care,
- Know how to obtain accommodations,
- Know about their rights,

- Have reliable transportation, and
- Have involvement in community agencies.

Individuals with disabilities also listed choosing what to do during free time, how to spend personal money, and where to live or work as ways in which they can express their independence. These promising findings provide empirical support for transition planning and service approaches that are considered best practice.

Research on transition practices (Landmark et al., 2010) indicated that they can be ranked from most to least substantiated as follows:

- Paid and unpaid work experiences,
- Employment preparation emphasizing job-searching skills and vocational training,
- Family involvement,
- Inclusion in general education classrooms,
- Social skills and independent living skills training,
- Self-determination,
- Community integration, and
- Interagency collaboration.

Occupational therapy practitioners should advocate for these transition practices to enhance student outcomes.

Role of Occupational Therapy Practitioners in Transition

Best practices in transition focus on providing opportunities for students with disabilities to identify preferences, make choices in everyday life, and participate in meaningful current and future activities. This is consistent with occupational therapy's specific focus on occupational engagement in meaningful activities in natural environments. Orentlicher and Gibson (2015) identified 3 philosophical approaches that underline the occupational therapy role in transition:

- Inclusion,
- Social model of disability, and
- Client-centered practice.

Inclusion means "everyone is treated fairly and equitably but also that all individuals have the same opportunities to participate in naturally occurring activities of society" (AOTA, 2014c, p. S23). These activities include education, social events, and school sports. The *social model of disability* proposes that people with disabilities have difficulty participating in activities and community settings because of society's failure to provide appropriate accommodations and services (Oliver, 1996). Therefore, the focus of intervention should be on changing and accommodating the environment, tools, and tasks rather than trying to "fix" the individual. *Client-centered practice* is an approach to evaluation and intervention that requires the student and family to take an active role in program decisions (e.g., identifying desired occupations, transition goals, and performance gaps; setting priorities for intervention).

BEST PRACTICES

This section outlines strategies for providing best practices for occupational therapy evaluation and intervention in transition.

Conduct Evaluation to Determine Student's Transition Needs

An essential element in high-quality transition evaluation is the integration of the perspectives of individuals who know the student well and are familiar with the current or future environments in which the student will participate, such as parents and teachers (Carter et al., 2014). Occupational therapists can contribute to the transition evaluation in the following areas:

- Interests and student and family preferences,
- Sensory and motor skills,
- Cognitive performance (e.g., attention, executive functioning),
- Daily living and community living skills,
- Vocational skills,
- Socialization skills, and
- Skills in self-determination and self-advocacy (Orentlicher, 2007).

Transition assessment measures for occupational therapy include but are not limited to

- Assessment of Work Performance (Version 1.0; Sandqvist et al., 2010),
- Children's Assessment of Participation and Enjoyment and Preferences for Activities of Children (King et al., 2004),
- Kohlman Evaluation of Living Skills (Kohlman Thomson & Robnett, 2016), and
- Transition Planning Inventory–Updated Version (Clark & Patton, 2009).

Additional measures (or tools) can be found in the *Age Appropriate Transition Assessment Toolkit* of the National Secondary Transition Technical Assistance Center (2016a).

In addition to formal measures, occupational therapists should use informal approaches during observations, such as

- *Functional assessments* (i.e., the measurement of purposeful activities in interaction with the environment),
- *Ecological inventories* (i.e., environmental assessments), and
- Task and activity analyses.

Wehman and Brooke (2013) introduced an informal method for getting to know the student known as ***discovery.*** The discovery process means learning about the student and creating a profile of their interests and strengths, their ideal employment conditions, and available employment opportunities in their community. Once the profile is created, the young adult can then pursue internships, competitive or supported employment, or customized employment.

Another commonly used informal method for learning about the student is ***person-centered planning,*** which is an alternative process for transition evaluation that is frequently suggested as a best practice approach that can empower students' self-determination and increase their involvement in transition planning (Orentlicher, 2011). Commonly used person-centered planning tools include

- Personal Futures Planning (Mount, 2000),
- Making Action Plans (O'Brien et al., 2010), and
- Promoting Alternative Tomorrows With Hope (O'Brien et al., 2010).

Each of these tools outlines specific steps that the team must follow throughout the planning process.

For example, Promoting Alternative Tomorrows With Hope (known as PATH) emphasizes goal development, starting with long-term goals based on the student's vision and dreams for the future and ending with short-term objectives and a specific plan to achieve the goals. The short-term objectives are broken further into steps that can be taken immediately. Person-centered planning is commonly used to design the individual service plan for people with disabilities when they are applying for Medicaid self-directed Home and Community-Based Services waivers. Thus, many states now offer a variety of free workshops on person-centered planning.

Use Evidence-Based Intervention Strategies in Transition

The occupational therapist analyzes the evaluation results along with other sources of information. The IEP team prioritizes performance gaps, giving priority to skills used in many environments. Occupational therapy practitioners provide support to school personnel and offer direct interventions to enhance the outcomes for students by being involved in the following research-supported interventions.

Employment preparation

Employment preparation programs, which are classroom- and curriculum-based programs that teach students how to prepare for the workforce and find a job, emphasize job-search skills and participation in career education. They also offer work–study programs and have been linked to more positive employment outcomes after graduation (Baer et al., 2011).

Family involvement

Widely recognized as important to successful transition, family involvement has been substantiated as a best practice (Landmark et al., 2010). Research indicates that young adults with disabilities often rely on their parents for support when making important decisions or facing problems, use their parents' contacts to secure employment and other community-based opportunities, and participate in community activities in which their parents engage (Eisenman et al., 2009). In terms of transition outcomes, students with disabilities work more hours, earn higher wages, live more independently, and have an overall higher quality of life when their parents are involved in the transition process (Landmark et al., 2010).

Planning for the long term. One of the main concerns parents have is what will happen to their adult son or daughter after their death or when they lose the ability to care for their child (Orentlicher, 2018). Occupational therapy practitioners can help parents plan for the long term by identifying relatives, friends, or service organizations that will help support the young adult in the future. They can also refer families to local disability lawyers, who can assist the family in putting together long-term financial plans and disability trusts to support their child with disabilities.

Planning for guardianship. **Guardianship** is when an adult (guardian) is authorized by a judge to make decisions for another adult (ward), when the court determines that the ward is totally or partially unable to make decisions or care for their own person or property. Depending on the judge's order, all or some of the ward's civil and legal rights are removed and given to the guardian (Millar, 2014). This means that a guardian is authorized to decide, without input from the ward, where the ward will reside or work, what health care they will receive, and how their money will be spent.

Millar (2014) argued that families should consider alternatives to guardianship, so that young adults with disabilities do not lose civil and legal rights unnecessarily and can maintain their self-determination and choice. Other, less restrictive options are available, including **supported decision making,** which allows the individual with a disability to get help from trusted friends, family members, or professionals in making decisions but retain control over who provides that help and what the ultimate decisions are (Jameson et al., 2015). Occupational therapy practitioners can assist families when they begin to consider guardianship options by providing information on the student's level of independence and the type of supports needed for the student to manage their own ADLs and IADLs as well as the student's cognitive skills and decision-making abilities.

Inclusion in general education

IDEA (2004) supports the inclusion of students with disabilities in schools and communities to the maximum extent possible, with the appropriate individualized supports necessary for successful experiences. Researchers have determined that students with disabilities who are included in and have access to the general education curriculum have better postschool outcomes (Griffin et al., 2014). Moreover, a high school diploma and strong academic skills have been identified as predictors of employment (McDonnall, 2011).

Typical students in inclusive classrooms in high school can provide a wealth of opportunities for students with disabilities to develop interpersonal relationships and effective work habits (Agran et al., 2017). By participating in the full range of activities offered in a typical high school, students with disabilities become better prepared with skills, experiences, and relationships to lead an integrated adult life.

Inclusion translates into full participation in community life, including multiple and equal opportunities, in a manner consistent with how people without disabilities typically participate. Occupational therapy supports nondiscrimination and inclusion (AOTA, 2009). Occupational therapy practitioners can use their understanding of reasonable accommodations to broaden the focus of their services to influence opportunities for full inclusion in education and other community settings.

Occupational therapists should collaborate with teachers to include functional academic skills, such as reading (e.g., read street signs) or math (e.g., counting change), as necessary. Literature on best practices in inclusive education includes **community-based instruction** (i.e., teaching instructional objectives and performing meaningful activities in natural contexts) to help students retain and generalize information (Cavkaytar et al., 2017).

Transition preparation in elementary and middle school

Best practices in transition recommend beginning to teach young students transition-related skills appropriate for their development stage, such as IADLs, organization, direction following, social skills, and self-determination (Hollenbeck et al., 2015; Wehmeyer, 2015). Occupational therapy practitioners may coteach IADLs and social and work readiness skills with students in elementary and middle school. These skills can be taught to entire classrooms or groups of selected students (e.g., baking and cooking groups, supplies and recycling programs for the school).

Social skills training

Social skills are important for the achievement of postschool success. Carter and Hughes (2013) recommended the use of **peer-focused strategies** (i.e., teach peers and coworkers how to interact with the student with disabilities) and **support-focused strategies** (i.e., create supportive environments for peer interactions and social skills development).

When working with students, occupational therapy practitioners should focus on enhancing the student's **social competence,** a multidimensional construct that includes sociocognitive skills such as social problem solving and perspective taking (Fraser et al., 2005), as well as skills for emotional regulation (Spinrad et al., 2006). It also includes the ability to independently choose friends, network, and initiate social activities. Appropriate expressions of sexuality and participation in recreational activities are also components of social competence.

Occupational therapy practitioners can help students learn how to modulate their emotional states by teaching them to use their emotions as cues and guides in social interactions. For example, anger can be a cue that one's rights are not being recognized and that a social situation is not fair. The student should also learn how to identify signs of impending emotional stress and explore strategies to proactively regulate their own emotions in everyday environments (Orentlicher & Olson, 2010). Occupational therapy practitioners can teach or coteach social skills in group settings. In these groups, students can learn how to accurately read social cues or how to interpret the perspectives of others while interacting in a variety of social situations.

Independent living skills training

Independent living skills (i.e., basic and instrumental) should be taught to students while they are in high school. For young adults with disabilities, having functional daily living skills has been linked to better postschool outcomes in employment, friendships, social participation, and independent living (Gray et al., 2014).

In addition to ADLs and IADLs, which are described in detail in AOTA's (2014b) *Occupational Therapy Practice Framework: Domain and Process* (3rd ed.), evidence shows support for teaching students personal responsibility, including habits and patterns such as self-control, the ability to save money, punctuality, and the ability to accept criticism (Wehman, 2013). The teaching of these habits should be infused into the curriculum geared toward students with disabilities, and individual goals, such as financial management goals, should be included in the student's transition plan. In addition to basic budgeting, topics taught should include more complex subjects, such as using credit or managing one's disability benefits.

Health and health care transitions

Young adults with disabilities often have complex health needs, which may include physical and mental health conditions (Croen et al., 2015). They rely heavily on their medical providers and may struggle through required transitions and changes in care. Health care transitions should be addressed with the student and family.

Occupational therapy practitioners can help students and families explain their disability and health conditions to new providers. They can also teach students to carry out the skills and tasks necessary to manage their own health care—for example, teaching them to keep track of and take their own medication and order new prescriptions as needed.

Self-determination

Self-determination is considered the most important practice for successful transition (McDougall et al., 2010). Wehmeyer (2015) argued that the emergence from adolescence into adulthood is characterized as a quest for self-determination, whereas Halloran (1993) identified self-determination as the "ultimate goal of education" (p. 214). Self-determination has been linked to increased quality of life and feelings of personal development and self-fulfillment (Shogren et al., 2015).

Students with disabilities should be provided with the knowledge, competency, and opportunities to exercise valuable choices (Agran & Hughes, 2008). Skills taught should include choice making, decision making, problem solving, goal setting, risk taking, self-evaluation, and self-advocacy (Wehmeyer, 2015). Students should be encouraged to evaluate their own performance toward achieving their goals.

Community participation

Adolescents with disabilities may have fewer opportunities to participate in social and leisure activities. It is important to promote the participation of young adults in activities outside of work, in particular those that provide opportunities for socialization and for the young adult to demonstrate special interests and talents (Orentlicher & Olson, 2010).

In a study exploring the transition experiences of young adults with severe disabilities, Orentlicher (2008) found that promoting socialization and securing recreational options were especially important for young adults who worked in integrated settings but who did not make friends or become socially involved with coworkers. These young adults reported being socially isolated. Leisure activities can be typical community-based options,

such as swimming in the local pool, working out in a local gym, or joining a book club or a bowling team. Specialized options for young adults with disabilities include Special Olympics and programs offered by disability service organizations. Social media also offer opportunities for socialization, but Internet safety training should be provided.

Another important aspect of community integration is transportation. Consideration of any program option should include how the young adult will get to it. Driving instruction or travel training for students who plan to use public transportation should be provided. Specialized transportation services tend to be costly but may be covered by the young adult's disability benefit program.

Interagency collaboration

Interagency collaboration is a predictor of postschool success in employment and education (Flowers et al., 2018). Researchers have emphasized the importance of *interagency collaboration,* which involves community agencies, including federal, state, and local representatives, and incorporates information from local businesses to create relevant employment preparation courses for students with disabilities (Trainor et al., 2012).

Seamless transition that includes additional services in school, such as follow-up support from community adult agencies, leads to more successful employment (Wehman, 2013). Trainor et al. (2012) recommended building relationships with community stakeholders by holding regular meetings with community and agency representatives throughout the school year to

- Introduce students to community representatives and businesses;
- Provide opportunities for networking that can lead to internships or employment; or
- Brainstorm solutions to common problems, such as transportation.

Occupational therapy practitioners should become familiar with the resources in and outside of school and target community agencies and organizations that can provide support for students with disabilities who are transitioning to adult life in the community. It is important to build relationships with these agencies by touring their offices or inviting their representatives to the school, so all stakeholders can better coordinate transition services.

SUMMARY

Best practices advocate that successful transition can only be achieved by engaging students with disabilities in meaningful community-based activities and by addressing performance skills, performance patterns, client factors, activity demands, and contexts in ways that are directly aligned with students' dreams, strengths, and desires.

Students should determine the course of their own transition process. Evaluation should use informal approaches and person-centered planning. Service provision should include student training and environmental and task adaptations in employment, higher education, and independent living. While in school, students should make connections with adult disability services in their community.

REFERENCES

ADA Amendments Act of 2008, Pub. L. 110–325, 122 Stat. 3553.

Agran, M., & Hughes, C. (2008). Students' opinions regarding their individualized education program involvement. *Career Development and Transition for Exceptional Individuals, 31,* 69–76. https://doi.org/10.1177/0885728808317657

Agran, M., Wojcik, A., Cain, I., Thoma, C., Achola, E., Austin, K. M., . . . Tamura, R. B. (2017). Participation of students with intellectual and developmental disabilities in extra-curricular activities: Does inclusion end at 3:00? *Education and Training in Autism and Developmental Disabilities, 52*(1), 3–12.

Alverson, C. Y., & Yamamoto, S. H. (2017). Employment outcomes of vocational rehabilitation clients with autism spectrum disorders. *Career Development and Transition for Exceptional Individuals, 40,* 144–155. https://doi.org/10.1177/2165143416629366

American Occupational Therapy Association. (2014a). Guidelines for supervision, roles, and responsibilities during the delivery of occupational therapy services. *American Journal of Occupational Therapy, 68*(Suppl. 3), S16–S22. https://doi.org/10.5014/ajot.2014.686S03

American Ocupational Therapy Association. (2014b). Occupational therapy practice framework: Domain and process (3rd ed.). *American Journal of Occupational Therapy, 68*(Suppl. 1), S1–S48. https://doi.org/10.5014/ajot.2014.682006

American Occupational Therapy Association. (2014c). Occupational therapy's commitment to nondiscrimination and inclusion. *American Journal of Occupational Therapy, 68*(Suppl. 3), S23–S24. https://doi.org/10.5014/ajot.2014.686S05

Baer, R. M., Daviso, A. W., Flexor, R. W., McMahan, Q. R., & Meindl, R. (2011). Students with intellectual disabilities: Predictors of transition outcomes. *Career Development and Transition for Exceptional Individuals, 33,* 132–141. https://doi.org/10.1177/0885728811399090

Bouck, E. C. (2017). Educational outcomes for secondary students with mild intellectual disability. *Education and Training in Autism and Developmental Disabilities, 52,* 369–382.

Carter, E. W., Brock, M. E., & Trainor, A. A. (2014). Transition assessment and planning for youth with severe intellectual and developmental disabilities. *Journal of Special Education, 47,* 245–255. https://doi.org/10.1177/0022466912456241

Carter, E. W., & Hughes, C. (2013). Teaching social skills and promoting supportive relationships. In P. Wehman (Ed.), *Life beyond the classroom: Transition strategies for young people with disabilities* (5th ed., pp. 261–281). Baltimore: Brookes.

Cavkaytar, A., Acungil, A. T., & Tonris, G. (2017). Effectiveness of teaching cafe waitering to adults with intellectual disability through audio-visual technologies. *Education and Training in Autism and Developmental Disabilities, 52*(1), 77–90.

Cimera, R. E., Burgess, S., & Wiley, A. (2013). Does providing transition services early enable students with ASD to achieve better vocational outcomes as adults? *Research and Practice for Persons With Severe Disabilities, 38,* 88–93. https://doi.org/10.2511/027494813807714474

Clark, G. M., & Patton, J. R. (2009). *Transition Planning Inventory: Updated version.* Austin, TX: ProEd.

Croen, L. A., Zerbo, O., Qian, Y., Massolo, M. L., Rich, S., Sidney, S., & Kripke, C. (2015). The health status of adults on the autism spectrum. *Autism: The International Journal of Research and Practice, 19,* 814–823. https://doi.org/10.1177/1362361315577517

Dymnicki, A., Sambolt, M., & Kidron, Y. (2013). *Improving college and career readiness by incorporating social and emotional learning.* Retrieved from https://ccrscenter.org/sites/default/files/Improving%20College%20and%20Career%20Readiness%20by%20Incorporating%20Social%20and%20Emotional%20Learning_0.pdf

Eisenman, L. T., Tanverdi, A., Perrington, C., & Geiman, A. (2009). Secondary and postsecondary community activities of youth with significant intellectual disabilities. *Education and Training in Developmental Disabilities, 44,* 168–176.

Erickson, W., Lee, C., & von Schrader, S. (2013). *Disability statistics from the 2011 American Community Survey (ACS).* Ithaca, NY: Cornell University Employment and Disability Institute.

Flowers, C., Test, D. W., Povenmire-Kirk, T. C., Diegelmann, K. M., Bunch-Crump, K. R., Kemp-Inman, A., & Goodnight, C. I. (2018). A demonstration model of interagency collaboration for students with disabilities: A multilevel approach *Journal of Special Education, 51,* 211–221. https://doi.org/10.1177/0022466917720764

Fraser, M. W., Galinsky, M. J., Smokowski, P. R., Day, S. H., Terzian, M. A., Rose, R. A., & Guo, S. (2005). Social information-processing skills training to promote social competence and prevent aggression behavior in the third grades. *Journal of Consulting and Clinical Psychology, 73,* 1045–1055. https://doi.org/10.1037/0022-006X.73.6.1045

Gray, K. M., Keating, C. M., Taffe, J. R., Brereton, A. V., Einfeld, S. L., Reardon, T. C., & Tonge, B. J. (2014). Adult outcomes in autism: Community inclusion and living skills. *Journal of Autism and Developmental Disorders, 44,* 3006–3015. https://doi.org/10.1007/s10803-014-2159-x

Griffin, M. M., Taylor, J. L., Urbano, R. C., & Hodapp, R. M. (2014). Involvement in transition planning meetings among high school students with autism spectrum disorders. *Journal of Special Education, 47,* 256–264. https://doi.org/10.1177/0022466913475668

Halloran, W. D. (1993). Transition services requirement: Issues, implications, challenge. In R. C. Eaves & P. J. McLaughlin (Eds.), *Recent advances in special education and rehabilitation* (pp. 210–224). Boston: Andover Medical.

Hein, V., Smerdon, B., & Sambolt, M. (2013). *Predictors of postsecondary success.* Retrieved from https://ccrscenter.org/sites/default/files/CCRS%20Center_Predictors%20of%20Postsecondary%20Success_final_0.pdf

Hollenbeck, J., Orentlicher, M. L., & Handley-More, D. (2015). Expanding roles, expanding impact: Supporting work readiness in middle school. *Early Intervention and School Special Interest Section Quarterly, 22*(3), 1–4.

Individuals With Disabilities Education Improvement Act of 2004, Pub. L. 108–446, 20 U.S.C. §§ 1400–1482.

Jameson, J. M., Riesen, T., Polychronis, S., Trader, B., Mizner, S., Martinis, J., & Hoyle, D. (2015). Guardianship and the potential of supported decision making with individuals with disabilities. *Research and Practice for Persons With Severe Disabilities, 40,* 1–16. https://doi.org/10.1177/1540796915586189

King, G., Law, M., King, S., Hurley, P., Hanna, S., Kertoy, M., . . . Young, N. (2004). *Children's Assessment of Participation and Enjoyment (CAPE) and Preferences for Activities of Children (PAC).* San Antonio: Harcourt Assessment.

Kohlman Thomson, L., & Robnett, R. (2016). *Kohlman Evaluation of Living Skills (KELS)* (4th ed.). Bethesda, MD: AOTA Press.

Landmark, L. J., Ju, S., & Zhang, D. (2010). Substantiated best practices in transition: Fifteen plus years later. *Career Development for Exceptional Individuals, 33,* 165–176. https://doi.org/10.1177/0885728810376410

McDonnall, M. C. (2011). Predictors of employment for youth with visual impairments: Findings from the second National Longitudinal Transition Study. *Journal of Visual Impairment and Blindness, 105,* 453–466.

McDougall, J., Evans, J., & Baldwin, P. (2010). The importance of self-determination to perceived quality of life for youth and young adults with chronic conditions and disabilities. *Remedial and Special Education, 31,* 252–260. https://doi.org/10.1177/0741932509355989

Millar, D. S. (2014). Extending transition to address guardianship alternatives: An issue concerning students who have intellectual disability. *Education and Training in Autism and Developmental Disabilities, 49,* 449–463.

Mount, B. (2000). *Person-centered planning: Finding directions for change using personal futures planning.* New York: Graphic Futures.

National Secondary Transition Technical Assistance Center. (2016a). *Age Appropriate Transition Assessment Toolkit* (4th ed.). Retrieved from https://transitionta.org/system/files/toolkitassessment/AgeAppropriateTransitionAssessmentToolkit2016_COMPLETE_11_21_16.pdf

National Technical Assistance Center on Transition. (2016b). *Evidence-based practices and predictors in secondary transition: What we know and what we still need to know.* Retrieved from https://transitionta.org/system/files/effectivepractices/EBPP_Exec_Summary_2016_12_13_16.pdf

Nonnemacher, S. L., & Bambara, L. M. (2011). "I'm supposed to be in charge": Self-advocates' perspectives on their self-determination support needs. *Intellectual and Developmental Disabilities, 49,* 327–340. https://doi.org/10.1352/1934-9556-49.5.327

O'Brien, J., Pearpoint, J., & Kahn, L. (2010). *The PATH and MAPS handbook: Person-centered ways to build community.* Toronto: Inclusion Press.

Oliver, M. (1996). *Understanding disability: From theory to practice.* New York: St. Martin's Press.

Orentlicher, M. L. (2007). Transition from school to adult life. In L. Jackson (Ed.), *Occupational therapy services in schools and early childhood settings* (pp. 143–167). Bethesda, MD: AOTA Press.

Orentlicher, M. L. (2008). *Striving for typical: Collective experiences of person-centered planning for young adults with disabilities during transition* (Unpublished doctoral dissertation). New York University, New York.

Orentlicher, M. L. (2011). Person-centered planning: An innovative approach for transition planning. *OT Practice, 16*(1), CE-1–CE-8.

Orentlicher, M. L. (2018). *Participatory action research on the experiences and perceptions of people who receive disability funding through consumer-directed funding models.* Manuscript submitted for publication.

Orentlicher, M. L., & Gibson, R. W. (2015). Foundations of transition. In M. L. Orentlicher, S. Schefkind, & R. W. Gibson (Eds.), *Transitions across the lifespan: An occupational therapy approach* (pp. 21–30). Bethesda, MD: AOTA Press.

Orentlicher, M. L., & Olson, L. J. (2010). Transition from school to adult life for students with an autism spectrum disorder. In H. Miller-Kuhaneck & R. Watling (Eds.), *Autism: A comprehensive occupational therapy approach* (3rd ed., pp. 665–700). Bethesda, MD: AOTA Press.

Rehabilitation Act of 1973, Pub. L. 93–112, 29 U.S.C. §§ 701–7961.

Sandqvist, J., Lee, J., & Kielhofner, G. (2010). *Assessment of Work Performance (AWP): Version 1.0.* Chicago: Model of Human Occupation Clearinghouse.

Shogren, K., Wehmeyer, M., Palmer, S., Rifenbark, G., & Little, T. (2015). Relationships between self-determination and postschool outcomes for youth with disabilities. *Journal of Special Education, 48,* 256–267. https://doi.org/10.1177/0022466913489733

Social Security. (2017). *Overview of our disability programs.* Retrieved from https://www.ssa.gov/redbook/eng/overview-disability.htm

Southward, J. D., & Kyzar, K. (2017). Predictors of competitive employment for students with intellectual and/or developmental disabilities. *Education and Training in Autism and Developmental Disabilities, 52*(1), 26–37.

Spinrad, T. L., Eisenberg, N., Cumberland, A., Fabes, R. A., Valiente, C., Shepard, S. A., . . . Guthrie, I. K. (2006). Relation of emotion-related regulation to children's social competence: A longitudinal study. *Emotion, 6,* 498–510. https://doi.org/10.1037/1528-3542.6.3.498

Trainor, A. A., Carter, E. W., Swedeen, B., & Pickett, K. (2012). Community conversations: An approach for expanding and connecting opportunities for employment for adolescents with disabilities. *Career Development for Exceptional Individuals, 35,* 50–60. https://doi.org/10.1177/0885728811419166

Wagner, M., Cameto, R., & Newman, L. (2003). *Youth with disabilities: A changing population.* Menlo Park, CA: SRI International.

Wagner, M., Newman, L. A., & Javitz, H. S. (2017). Vocational education course taking and post-high school employment of youth with emotional disturbances. *Career Development and Transition for Exceptional Individuals, 40,* 132–143. https://doi.org/10.1177/2165143415626399

Wehman, P. (2013). Transition: New horizons and challenges. In P. Wehman (Ed.), *Life beyond the classroom: Transition strategies for young people with disabilities* (5th ed., pp. 3–39). Baltimore: Brookes.

Wehman, P., & Brooke, V. (2013). Securing meaningful work in the community. In P. Wehman (Ed.), *Life beyond the classroom: Transition strategies for young people with disabilities* (5th ed., pp. 309–337). Baltimore: Brookes.

Wehmeyer, M. (2015). Framing the future: Self determination. *Remedial and Special Education, 36,* 20–23. https://doi.org/10.1177/0741932514551281

KEY TERMS AND CONCEPTS

- Academic persistence
- Alternative diploma
- ARC framework
- Inclusive individual support model
- Mixed or hybrid model
- Occupational performance coaching
- Open admissions
- Professional or vocational diploma
- Selective admissions
- Self-determination
- Standard diploma
- Substantially separate model
- Summary of performance
- Vocational education

OVERVIEW

Education is an occupation that literally has the power to transform lives. Students with disabilities have more opportunities than ever to receive education (i.e., primary, secondary, postsecondary) along with services and supports to access that education. Understanding variations across educational environments, preparing students for the next steps in their education, and framing what "successfully completing one's education" means is important.

In the United States, more students are pursuing postsecondary education than ever before. This may be due to the job market, given that the entry point for many jobs now requires postsecondary education or training (Getzel & Wehman, 2005). According to the 2011 National Longitudinal Transition Study–2, 60% of students with disabilities identified that they intended to continue to a postsecondary education within 8 years of leaving high school (Newman et al., 2011); however, their postsecondary completion rate (i.e., 34% at 4-year universities, 22% at 2-year colleges, 57% at career and technical schools) lagged behind that of students in the general population (i.e., 51% at 4-year universities, 41% at 2-year colleges, 66% at career and technical schools).

Various factors have been implicated as contributing to poor postsecondary completion, many of which can be addressed before high school graduation. Occupational therapy practitioners[1] are instrumental in assisting students with disabilities as they prepare for postsecondary environments, although roughly 7.5% of students with disabilities receive occupational therapy services during their transition to adult years (Eismann et al., 2017).

ESSENTIAL CONSIDERATIONS

This section contrasts laws that govern postsecondary environments with those that regulate the kindergarten through 12th-grade system. Factors that contribute to students' *academic persistence,* or their ability to remain enrolled, at the postsecondary level are identified, and strategies that occupational therapy practitioners can implement to more effectively prepare students for this major life transition are shared.

High School Graduation and Postsecondary Options

According to 2013–2014 data collected by the National Center for Education Statistics (2015), 63.1% of students with disabilities in the United States graduated from high school. Despite this figure, graduation rates for students with disabilities varied significantly across states. Some states reported graduation rates surpassing 80%, whereas 7 reported rates less than 50%, and 2 reported rates of less than 30%.

---

[1]*Occupational therapy practitioner* refers to both the occupational therapist and the occupational therapy assistant. The American Occupational Therapy Association (AOTA; 2014a, p. S18) states, "The occupational therapist is responsible for all aspects of occupational therapy service delivery and is accountable for the safety and effectiveness of the occupational therapy service delivery process" and "must be directly involved in the delivery of services during the initial evaluation and regularly throughout the course of intervention. . . . The occupational therapy assistant delivers safe and effective occupational therapy services under the supervision of and in partnership with the occupational therapist."

Copyright © 2019 by the American Occupational Therapy Association. All rights reserved. To reuse this content, contact www.copyright.com.
https://doi.org/10.7139/2019.978-1-56900-591-0.025

With respect to interpreting graduation data, understanding diploma and exiting options provides insight into the variability across states. Even more critical is understanding how different options affect students' future prospects (U.S. Department of Education, Office of Special Education and Rehabilitative Services [U.S. DOE OSERS], 2017).

Distinguished diploma programs offer a college preparatory track and certify completion of a rigorous program of study. ***Standard diplomas*** confirm that students completed credit requirements for graduation. ***Professional or vocational diplomas*** endorse students' knowledge and skills related to a particular field of work. ***Alternative diplomas,*** including certificates of completion, indicate that students completed high school courses yet did not meet grade-level academic achievement. Although alternative diplomas acknowledge students' efforts and may boost graduation rates, they do not prepare students adequately for postsecondary opportunities (Getzel & Wehman, 2005).

Postsecondary options include education specifically designed for students with disabilities, career and technical education, and academic degree programs. The Rehabilitation Services Administration offers services designed to assist students with disabilities in their transition to postsecondary education in preparation for competitive employment (U.S. DOE OSERS, 2017).

Individual support, substantially separate, and mixed or hybrid models

Three models of postsecondary education have been designed specifically for students with disabilities (Hart et al., 2006). The first is an ***inclusive individual support model,*** which involves multiple agencies collaborating to enable students to establish and enact a vision for their individualized career goals. Costs are distributed among multiple agencies.

The second model, the ***substantially separate model,*** involves life skills or transition programs. Classes are composed exclusively of students with disabilities; however, students have opportunities to participate in general social activities on campus. The third model is the ***mixed or hybrid model*** in which students with disabilities participate in social activities and classes (either for credit or audit) with students without disabilities. These programs may include additional opportunities for students with disabilities, such as specialized life skills classes as well as opportunities to engage in campus employment.

Postsecondary career and technical education

Postsecondary career and technical education programs (U.S. Department of Education, International Affairs Office [U.S. DOE IAO], 2008c), also known as ***vocational education,*** may be offered as short-term programs within degree-granting institutions or as stand-alone entities. Students who complete training in an organized program of study can earn an award, certificate, or diploma, as opposed to an academic degree. Program structure varies; some are brick-and-mortar programs offering on-site opportunities, but many are online.

Both for-profit and nonprofit agencies offer programs, and this distinction affects costs significantly. Although many career and technical education programs are available for everyone, state vocational rehabilitation programs offer services designed for people with disabilities who meet the agency's criteria (U.S. DOE OSERS, 2017).

Academic degree programs

Academic programs include associate degree programs, which require the student to complete an organized 2- to 4-year program of full-time study consisting of 60–120 semester credit hours (U.S. DOE IAO, 2008a). Approximately 23% of students with learning disabilities pursue this type of degree (Wagner et al., 2005).

Students can also enroll in baccalaureate or bachelor's degree programs, which take 4–5 years of full-time study (U.S. DOE IAO, 2008b). Approximately 11% of students with learning disabilities pursue this credential.

Postsecondary Enrollment Rates

In a 2008–2009 study, students with disabilities composed approximately 11% of the total student population in higher education (Raue et al., 2011). Of this group, 31% self-identified as having learning disabilities, 18% as having attention deficit disorder with or without hyperactivity, 15% as having a mental illness, 11% as having other types of health impairment, and 2% as having autism spectrum disorder.

Laws: Entitlement vs. Eligibility

During elementary and secondary education, students with a disability, in accordance with the Individuals With Disabilities Education Improvement Act of 2004 (IDEA; Pub. L. 108–446), are entitled to receive special education services to access a free appropriate public education (FAPE). For elementary and secondary students with medical disabilities that substantially limit their participation in accessing their education, protections are available under Section 504 of the Rehabilitation Act of 1973, as amended (2008; Pub. L. 93–112), and schools must provide them with FAPE.

Once students with a disability exit high school, they bear the burden of proof for self-disclosing their disability, presenting documentation of that disability, and seeking eligibility for services and supports (e.g., reasonable and necessary accommodations to access their postsecondary education; U.S. Department of Education, Office of Civil Rights [U.S. DOE OCR], 2011). IDEA (2004) and FAPE no longer apply, yet protections remain under Section 504 of the Rehabilitation Act of 1973 and the ADA Amendments Act of 2008 (Pub. L. 110–325). For a brief snapshot of how these laws and others differ across kindergarten to graduation and postsecondary environments, see Table 25.1.

Admissions Process

Some higher education institutions have ***open admissions,*** whereby everyone holding a high school diploma who applies is admitted until the student body is filled. Other institutions may have ***selective admissions,*** whereby

TABLE 25.1.   Laws Across Kindergarten Through Graduation and Postsecondary Environments

LAWS	KINDERGARTEN–GRADUATION	POSTSECONDARY
IDEA (Pub. L. 108–446)	Students who fall in an IDEA disability category and need special education are entitled to specially designed instruction and related services as needed in the least restrictive environment.	Not applicable
Section 504 of the Rehabilitation Act of 1973, as amended (2008; Pub. L. 93–112)	Requires LEAs to "provide a free appropriate public education to each qualified" (34 C.F.R. Subpart D 104.33) student with a disability that substantially limits a major life activity (e.g., access to education and extracurricular activities). LEAs must identify the student's educational needs and provide necessary services and related aids	To be eligible for accommodations, students need to voluntarily disclose and provide supporting documentation of their disability to the federally funded academic institution. The academic institution is then required to maintain confidentiality and provide reasonable and appropriate academic adjustments to ensure equal access to education similar to that of peers in the general population. The student needs to self-advocate to obtain accommodations in each instance in which they are required. This includes housing and nonacademic services (e.g., physical education, counseling and placement, social organizations) when applicable.
ADA Amendments Act of 2008 (Pub. L. 110–325)	Provides students with disabilities protection to access places used by the public (e.g., field trips, work sites, community outings).	Same standards apply as in kindergarten through graduation and for Section 504 in postsecondary education. Broadens to include postsecondary institutions that do not receive federal dollars.
FERPA (Pub. L. 93–380)	Protects the confidentiality of students' educational records in schools that receive federal funds. Requires parent's written permission to share information. Rights transfer to the student at age 18 years.	Rights transfer to the student no matter the age. Protects the confidentiality of students' educational records in schools that receive federal funds. Requires student's written permission to share information (even with parents).
Assistive Technology Act of 2004 (Pub. L. 108–364)	Funds state projects aimed at awareness and access to AT devices and services.	Same
Higher Education Opportunity Act (Pub. L. No. 110–315)	Not applicable.	Financial assistance available to students who meet requirements. Encourages organizations to collaborate with postsecondary institutions to enhance accessibility for students with disabilities.

Note. AT = assistive technology; FERPA = Family Educational Rights and Privacy Act of 1974; IDEA = Individuals With Disabilities Education Improvement Act of 2004; LEA = local educational agency.

admission is competitive and offered on a limited basis. Entrance requirements for selective admissions may pose barriers for students with disabilities (e.g., admissions tests with sensory, manual, or speaking components). To receive reasonable accommodations, students must voluntarily disclose their disability.

The literature suggests that only 35% of eligible students self-disclose information about disabilities to postsecondary environments (Newman & Madaus, 2015; Raue et al., 2011). The low rate has been attributed to students'

- Beliefs that they will be perceived or treated differently,
- Incomplete awareness of their needs, and
- Uncertainty about where to obtain assistance (Hong, 2015).

When students do request accommodations, more than 90% of postsecondary settings require supporting documentation to verify the presence of a disability and adverse impact on performance (Newman & Madaus, 2015; U.S. DOE OCR, 2011).

Documentation accepted varies significantly. Only 44% of schools will accept a copy of the student's individualized education program (IEP), and 40% will accept a 504 plan (Raue et al., 2011). Many institutions deny accommodations on the basis of documentation that is incomplete, old, or unclear in describing the impact that the health condition has on the student's performance (Hamblet, 2014).

Postsecondary Transition Planning

Special education laws mandate postsecondary transition planning to prepare students for life after high school. However, critics suggest that schools may fall short in preparing students (Harrison et al., 2017; Lombardi et al., 2017). Test and Cease-Cook (2012) conducted a review of evidence-based practices that support aligning students' transition goals with their program of study and diploma track. Lombardi et al. (2017) further emphasized the inclusion of transition goals that prepare students for meeting future academic and social demands (e.g., building social networks and supports).

In addition, aligning transition goals with the skills outlined by the College and Career Readiness Movement (Achieve, 2018) enhances postsecondary success. These skills are demanded by postsecondary institutions and include the ability to

- Engage academically;
- Analyze information and solve problems;
- Persist; and
- Communicate, collaborate, and present information.

Other skills include transition competencies, such as early planning, awareness of college cultures, and an understanding of adult roles and responsibilities (Connor, 2012; Hamblet, 2014; Lombardi et al., 2017; Test & Cease-Cook, 2012).

BEST PRACTICES

Many students with disabilities experience difficulties transitioning from high school to postsecondary education; however, planning makes a difference (Barnard-Brak et al., 2009; Cobb et al., 2013). Multiple factors that contribute to these difficulties fall within occupational therapy's domain of practice. This section provides guidance for practitioners who support high school students' preparation for postsecondary transitions.

Conduct a Needs Assessment at the Program Level

Completing a needs assessment may be a useful opportunity for occupational therapists to explore with others the postsecondary transition needs of students with disabilities. The process may also help the occupational therapist ascertain how the postsecondary transition process functions in the district. Finlayson et al. (2002) delineated a 3-phase process for completing a needs assessment to guide practitioners as they create new initiatives. These phases align with the *Occupational Therapy Practice Framework: Domain and Process* (3rd ed.; AOTA, 2014b) evaluation process that outlines gathering data about the student's needs and barriers and supports to occupations (occupational profile), analyzing the information, and synthesizing data to make recommendations and develop the occupational therapy intervention plan.

The first phase starts with obtaining background information and gaining an understanding of the needs and strengths of clients (in this case, students) and the needs and strengths of the specific setting (e.g., the local educational agency [LEA], high school, classroom). Identifying important stakeholders is essential to this phase because therapists understand the student's needs most fully and accurately when they understand the issues from multiple perspectives. Potential stakeholders could include students, families, teachers, and school administrators as well as personnel from postsecondary institutions. Occupational therapists must analyze their own role as well (e.g., will they function as a direct service provider, a consultant, or a program developer?). Understanding what services exist as well as any gaps can also be useful.

The second phase requires data collection and analysis. Data might be collected through a thorough literature review, artifact examination (e.g., current curriculum, trends in the program, student's IEP), interviews, observations, and student journaling. Once data are collected, the occupational therapist can begin analysis to determine a formal plan that includes evidence-based interventions. The third phase involves implementing the plan and collecting data on its effectiveness, with ongoing adjustments as needed.

Several resources can guide school practitioners regarding best postsecondary transition practices. AOTA's Postsecondary Transition Community of Practice made several recommendations (Orentlicher et al., 2017) that mirror domains identified by the College and Career Readiness Movement (Lombardi et al., 2017). Orentlicher et al. (2014) recommended that practitioners reconsider the practice of discontinuing students at earlier ages and instead "consider students' needs in a broader sense. . . . Related services should ebb and flow during an individual's academic program and beyond" (p. 3). Practitioners should analyze their own recommendations for discontinuation of services and explore mechanisms with educational teams to reevaluate students' needs or resume involvement at future points when students may benefit from additional skilled occupational therapy services.

Know Available Resources

School occupational therapy practitioners need to explore their knowledge about current environments and postsecondary environments. Practitioners should be aware of existing options in their districts. Knowing what programs of study are offered after high school may help practitioners educate students and their families about options.

Likewise, practitioners need to know about external agencies that support students' postsecondary transitions. Each state has a designated vocational rehabilitation program that offers services for students and supports postsecondary transitions. Each state also has a designated AT center that offers resources (https://www.ataporg.org/).

Prepare Students for Postsecondary Transitions

In preparation for postsecondary transitions, students with disabilities need to

- Understand their strengths as well as their disability,
- Receive support for setting their own goals and making decisions,
- Learn to advocate for reasonable accommodations,
- Get ready for curriculum demands, and
- Develop their time management, networking, and technical skills.

Promote self-determination and self-advocacy

Occupational therapy interventions support "empower[ing] clients to seek and obtain resources to fully participate in daily life occupations" (AOTA, 2014b, p. S30). Students with disabilities can be empowered through *self-determination* and by having the knowledge, skills, and beliefs that they can participate in goal-directed, self-regulated, and autonomous behavior (Wehmeyer, 2005). Understanding and acknowledging one's disability as well as one's strengths and limitations, learning to succeed, solving one's own problems, and managing oneself are fundamental to self-determined behaviors. These must be cultivated over time across different contexts and environments.

Students who volunteer to self-disclose information about their disability are more likely to complete postsecondary education (Newman & Madaus, 2015). Lombardi et al. (2017) stressed the importance of assisting students to establish a growth-oriented mindset. Cognitive–behavioral approaches may promote the student's ability to think in graded ways. Literature on resilience emphasizes the importance of engagement, graded thinking, and connection to something or someone outside of the self. This literature seems to align with factors supporting students' academic persistence.

Empower students to envision the future through goals

For students seeking postsecondary education, evidence suggests that having measurable goals toward that education supports positive outcomes (Karpur et al., 2013). In addition, Karpur et al. (2013) advocated that students establish goals related to the development of their independent living skills. Unfortunately, studies have suggested that students with disabilities are often not fully included in the creation of postsecondary goals, and many of these goals are written too broadly and too vaguely to be actionable (Harrison et al., 2017).

Occupational therapists can use Goal Attainment Scaling to personalize goals and measure a student's progress (Wallen & Stewart, 2015). They can also use the Canadian Occupational Performance Measure (COPM; Law et al., 2014) as an outcome measure to provide the student with insight into their self-perceptions of abilities and difficulties, satisfaction with performance, and priorities. When administering the COPM, occupational therapists can intentionally structure questions about the student's performance in different contexts to strengthen self-knowledge of their own strengths and challenges. In addition, the COPM can be paired with some of the cognitive approaches described later to support the student's self-awareness and critical thinking skills.

Occupational therapy practitioners need to ask students about their goals and dig deeper with further questions. Poulsen et al. (2015) discussed the importance of considering the dimensions of autonomy, relatedness, and competence (ARC) when setting goals. They detailed a process for creating feasible goals using the *ARC framework.*

Following the ARC framework process, the practitioner asks questions about how each ARC component affects the stage. The first stage is goal setting; it occurs before the student formulates goals. The practitioner asks, "How important is this goal?" and provides additional clarification for the student when needed. Poulsen et al. (2015) stressed that the student must feel supported in creating goals versus coerced to create a specific goal. Students must feel safe to consider and relay their performance with the practitioner.

The second stage involves goal planning. Any obstacles and supports are identified, and a plan is created regarding committing to and pursuing the goal. The last stage is

goal progress, during which work toward the goal is initiated, progress is monitored, and the student engages in self-reflection to determine next steps.

Educate students on postsecondary educational environments and resources

Although IDEA mandates starting transition planning when students turn age 16 years, Hamblet (2014) recommended beginning this process during 8th grade, when students make decisions about educational tracks. When they are young, students should know their health conditions, the impact on performance in various environments, and strategies for self-advocacy. This knowledge assists them in identifying their strengths and needs in activities and environments. This allows students to self-advocate when meeting with staff in the postsecondary environment.

During elementary and secondary education, occupational therapy practitioners facilitate students' ability to access classroom and school activities by reducing physical and social barriers and providing technology or adaptations to activities or environments (AOTA, 2017). Although this often supports students' success, it is prudent to consider whether students are aware of the adaptations and whether they will be available after the student transitions. Environmental factors can become normalized and easily overlooked. It is essential to unpack these elements to increase the student's self-knowledge, identify existing needs, and explore strategies to effectively meet those needs in postsecondary environments.

Assistive technology. AT can make a significant difference for students with disabilities; however, these needs may not be fully addressed in anticipation of postsecondary education (Asselin, 2014; Hamblet, 2014). School occupational therapy practitioners have an important role in addressing these needs and continuing to support students during middle and high school (Orentlicher et al., 2014). Asselin (2014) recommended asking students with disabilities who are college bound several questions when addressing their AT needs:

- Will devices transfer with the student or remain at the school?
- Will the user's manual transfer with the device?
- Does the student have a plan for maintenance of the device?
- Is the student aware of funding sources for new or replacement devices when needed?

Many postsecondary settings have AT and student resources on campus, so students should ask what they are and how to access them. Although Hamblet (2014) advocated the use of AT, she also recommended paring down supports because they may not available or deemed appropriate in postsecondary settings. Educating students to think explicitly about how supports such as AT contribute to their performance may strengthen their self-knowledge and ability to effectively advocate for themselves.

Personal strategies. The Cognitive Orientation to daily Occupational Performance (CO–OP) is a client-centered, evidence-based intervention designed to enable people who experience difficulties performing activities that are important to them (Dawson et al., 2017; Polatajko & Manditch, 2004). Through a process of discovery that allows students to identify strategies to support their performance, monitor their performance, and self-evaluate outcomes, CO–OP enables them to

- Acquire skills,
- Develop cognitive strategies,
- Generalize skills and strategies to everyday life, and
- Transfer learning to perform new skills in new contexts.

Using CO–OP, the practitioner assists the student in applying a global problem-solving approach: Goal, Plan, Do, Check. First the student selects a target goal and makes decisions regarding how to address the goal, with support from the occupational therapy practitioner as needed (Ziviani et al., 2015). Next, the therapist asks questions to assist the student in formulating a plan to achieve the goal. Then the student implements the plan. Last, the student and practitioner review the outcome to determine whether the plan resulted in the intended outcome or whether adjustments to the plan are required. This process actively involves the student in goal setting, develops the student's metacognitive skills, and promotes problem solving (Polatajko & Manditch, 2004; Rodger & Vishram, 2010).

Parents as a support system. Many interventions focus on students; however, parents are important to consider. Gibbs and Breen-Franklin (2016) detailed a need to support parents during the transition process. ***Occupational performance coaching*** (Graham et al., 2009, 2010, 2012) is a structured, goal-directed intervention designed to support youth development by supporting caregivers' competence in solving problems and understanding what motivates their children. This approach can be useful in nurturing self-determination behaviors.

Social support networks. The literature discusses social support as a significant contributor to academic completion. Students with disabilities experience challenges creating social support networks in postsecondary settings, and many spend increased time involved in academic pursuits and have less time for socialization. Skills training can assist students in the development of skills related to effective communication, assertiveness, organization, and living (e.g., ADLs, IADLs).

Provide Input on Student's Summary of Performance

IDEA (2004) requires LEAs to create a ***summary of performance,*** which reviews the functional performance and academic achievements of students who are exiting special education services (Shaw et al., 2012). Practitioners can ask how their districts create a summary of performance and who is involved in this process. Morgan et al. (2017) advocated for guiding the student to create a self-directed summary of performance. In this process, students create a portfolio summary. This provides them with opportunities to learn self-advocacy skills, become more in tune with their own strengths and challenges, and communicate their goals and visions for future education.

The occupational therapist can provide documentation for the summary of performance by describing how the student's health condition could affect the student's functioning in the postsecondary environment. Documentation should include academic performance and performance in other areas, such as self-care and social participation. Practitioners can describe how assistive technologies and environmental adaptations support the student.

SUMMARY

First, best practices in transitioning students to postsecondary education are collaborative. They begin early, extend over time, and empower students to act as agents on their own behalf. Students and families are provided with accurate information and scaffolding to support choice making along the way. During high school, students build their self-awareness, understand their rights, advocate for their needs, access resources, and grow their support system.

RESOURCES

1. **American Occupational Therapy Association (AOTA):**
- *Frequently Asked Questions (FAQ): What Is Occupational Therapy's Role in Transition Services and Planning?* (https://bit.ly/2VstgBm)
- *Transitions Across Contexts: Checklist for Occupational Therapy Practitioners* (https://bit.ly/2IatZnI)
- *Transitions for Children and Youth: How Occupational Therapy Can Help* (https://bit.ly/2VtTPWN)
2. **College Internship Program** (https://cipworldwide.org/)
3. **Disabilities, Opportunities, Internetworking, and Technology (DO-IT) Center** (https://www.washington.edu/doit/)
4. **I'm Determined** (https://www.imdetermined.org/)
5. **National Center for Learning Disabilities** (https://www.ncld.org/transitioning-to-life-after-high-school)
6. **National Technical Assistance Center on Transition** (https://www.transitionta.org/)

REFERENCES

Achieve. (2018). *College and career readiness.* Retrieved from https://www.achieve.org/college-and-career-readiness

ADA Amendments Act of 2008, Pub. L. 110–325, 122 Stat. 3553.

American Occupational Therapy Association. (2014a). Guidelines for supervision, roles, and responsibilities during the delivery of occupational therapy services. *American Journal of Occupational Therapy, 68*(Suppl. 3), S16–S22. https://doi.org/10.5014/ajot.2014.686S03

American Occupational Therapy Association. (2014b). Occupational therapy practice framework: Domain and process (3rd ed.). *American Journal of Occupational Therapy, 68*(Suppl. 1), S1–S48. https://doi.org/10.5014/ajot.2014.682006

American Occupational Therapy Association. (2017). Guidelines for occupational therapy services in early childhood and schools. *American Journal of Occupational Therapy, 71*(Suppl. 2), 7112410010. https://doi.org/10.5014/ajot.2017.716S01

Asselin, S. B. (2014). Learning and assistive technologies for college transition. *Journal of Vocational Rehabilitation, 40,* 223–230. https://doi.org/10.3233/JVR-140687

Assistive Technology Act of 2004, Pub. L. 108–364, 118 Stat. 1707.

Barnard-Brak, L., Davis, T., Tate, A., & Sulak, T. (2009). Attitudes as a predictor of college students requesting accommodations. *Journal of Vocational Rehabilitation, 31,* 189–198. https://doi.org/10.3233/JVR-2009-0488

Cobb, R., Lipscomb, S., Wolgemuth, J., Schulte, T., Veliquette, A., Alwell, M., . . . Weinberg, A. (2013). *Improving post-high school outcomes for transition-age students with disabilities: An evidence review* (NCEE 2013-4011). Washington, DC: National Center for Education Evaluation and Regional Assistance, Institute of Education Sciences.

Connor. D. J. (2012). Helping students with disabilities transition to college: 21 tips for students with LD and/or ADHD. *TEACHING Exceptional Children, 44*(5), 16–25. https://doi.org/10.1177/004005991204400502

Dawson, D., McEwen, S. E., & Polatajko, H. J. (2017). *Cognitive Orientation to daily Occupational Performance in Occupational Therapy: Using the CO–OP Approach™ to enable participation across the lifespan.* Bethesda, MD: AOTA Press.

Eismann, M. M., Weisshaar, R., Capretta, C., Cleary, D. S., Kirby, A. V., & Persch, A. C. (2017). Centennial Topics—Characteristics of students receiving occupational therapy services in transition and factors related to postsecondary success. *American Journal of Occupational Therapy, 71,* 7103100010. https://doi.org/10.5014/ajot.2017.024927

Family Educational Rights and Privacy Act of 1974, Pub. L. 93–380, 20 U.S.C. § 1232g, 34 C.F.R. Part 99.

Finlayson, M., Baker, M., Rodman, L., & Herzberg, G. (2002). The process and outcomes of a multimethod needs assessment at a homeless shelter. *American Journal of Occupational Therapy, 56,* 313–321. https://doi.org/10.5014/ajot.56.3.313

Getzel, E. E., & Wehman, P. (2005). *Going to college: Expanding opportunities for people with disabilities.* Baltimore: Brookes.

Gibbs, V. D., & Breen-Franklin, A. (2016). When an adult child with a developmental disability goes to college: A transition for parents. *SIS Quarterly Practice Connections, 1*(2), 8–10.

Graham, F., Rodger, S., & Ziviani, J. (2009). Coaching parents to enable children's participation: An approach for working with parents and their children. *Australian Occupational Therapy Journal, 56*(3), 16–33. https://doi.org/10.1111/j.1440-1630.2008.00736.x

Graham, F., Rodger, S., & Ziviani, J. (2010). Enabling occupational performance of children through coaching parents: Three case reports. *Physical and Occupational Therapy in Pediatrics, 30*(1), 4–15. https://doi.org/10.3109/01942630903337536

Graham, F., Rodger, S., & Ziviani, J. (2012). Effectiveness of occupational performance coaching in improving children's and mothers' performance and mothers' self-competence. *American Journal of Occupational Therapy, 67,* 10–18. https://doi.org/10.5014/ajot.2013.004648

Hamblet, E. C. (2014). Nine strategies to improve college transition planning for students with disabilities. *TEACHING Exceptional Children, 46*(3), 53–59. https://doi.org/10.1177/004005991404600306

Harrison, J. R., State, T. M., Wills, H. P., Custer, B. A., & Miller, E. (2017). Transition goals for youth with social, emotional, and behavioral problems: Parent and student knowledge. *Preventing School Failure: Alternative Education for Children and Youth, 61,* 248–257. https://doi.org/10.1080/1045988X.2016.1266596

Hart, D., Grigal, M., Sax, C., Martinez, D., & Will, M. (2006). *Postsecondary options for students with intellectual disabilities* (Research to Practice Brief 46). Boston: Institute for Community Inclusion, University of Massachusetts.

Higher Education Opportunity Act, Pub. L. No. 110–315, 122 Stat. 3078 (2008).

Hong, B. S. S. (2015). Qualitative analysis of the barriers college students with disabilities experience in higher education. *Journal of College Student Development, 56,* 209–226. https://doi.org/10.1353/csd.2015.0032

Individuals With Disabilities Education Improvement Act of 2004, Pub. L. 108–446, 20 U.S.C. §§ 1400–1482.

Karpur, A., Brewer, D., & Golden, T. (2013). Critical program elements in transition to adulthood: Comparative analysis of New York State and the NLTS2. *Career Development and Transition for Exceptional Individuals, 37,* 119–130. https://doi.org/10.1177/2165143413476880

Law, M., Baptiste, S., Carswell, A., McColl, M. A., Polatajko, H., & Pollock, N. (2014). *Canadian Occupational Performance Measure* (5th ed.). Ottawa: CAOT Publications.

Lombardi, A., Kern, L., Flannery, K. B., & Doren, B. (2017). Is college and career readiness adequately addressed in annual and postsecondary goals? *Journal of Disability Policy Studies, 28,* 150–161. https://doi.org/10.1177/1044207317716147

Morgan, R. L., Kupferman, S., Jex, E., Preece, H., & Williams, S. (2017). Promoting student transition planning by using a self-directed summary of performance. *TEACHING Exceptional Children, 50*(2), 66–73. https://doi.org/10.1177/0040059917734383

National Center for Education Statistics. (2015). *Table 1. Public high school 4-year adjusted cohort graduation rate (ACGR), by race/ethnicity and selected demographics for the United States, the 50 states, and the District of Columbia: School year 2013–14.* Retrieved from https://nces.ed.gov/ccd/tables/ACGR_RE_and_characteristics_2013-14.asp

Newman, L. A., & Madaus, J. W. (2015). An analysis of factors related to receipt of accommodations and services by postsecondary students with disabilities. *Remedial and Special Education, 36,* 208–219. https://doi.org/10.1177/0741932515572912

Newman, L., Wagner, M., Knokey, A., Marder, C., Nagle, K., Shaver, D., & Wei, X. (2011). *The post-high school outcomes of young adults with disabilities up to 8 years after high school: A report from the National Longitudinal Transition Study–2* (NCSER 2011-3005). Menlo Park, CA: SRI International.

Orentlicher, M. L., Case, D., Podvey, M. C., Myers, C. T., Rudd, L. Q., & Schoonover, J. (2017). *Frequently asked questions (FAQ): What is occupational therapy's role in transition services and planning?* Bethesda, MD: American Occupational Therapy Association. Retrieved from https://www.aota.org/~/media/Corporate/Files/Secure/Practice/Children/FAQ-What-is-OTs-Role-in-Transition-Services-and-Planning-20170530.pdf

Orentlicher, M. L., Demchick, B. B., Gibson, R. W., Case, D., Jackson-Pena, H., & Schoonover, J. (2014). Secrets from the field: Secondary transition resources and tips. *Early Intervention and School Special Interest Quarterly, 21*(3), 1–3.

Polatajko, H., & Manditch, A. D. (2004). *Enabling occupation in children: Cognitive Orientation to daily Occupational Performance (CO–OP) approach.* Ottawa: CAOT Publications.

Poulsen, A. A., Ziviani, J., & Cuskelly, M. (2015). *Goal setting and motivation in therapy: Engaging children and parents.* Philadelphia: Jessica Kingsley.

Raue, K., Lewis, L., & Coppersmith, J. (2011). *Students with disabilities at degree-granting postsecondary institutions* (NCES

2011-018). Washington, DC: U.S. Department of Education, National Center for Education Statistics.

Rodger, S., & Vishram, A. (2010). Mastering social and organization goals: Strategy use by two children with Asperger syndrome during Cognitive Orientation to daily Occupational Performance. *Physical and Occupational Therapy in Pediatrics, 30,* 264–276. https://doi.org/10.3109/01942638.2010.500893.

Section 504 of the Rehabilitation Act of 1973, as amended, 29 U.S.C. § 794 (2008).

Shaw, D. F., Dukes, L. L., & Madaus, J. W. (2012). Beyond compliance: Using the summary of performance to enhance transition planning. *TEACHING Exceptional Children, 44*(5), 6–12. https://doi.org/10.1177/004005991204400501

Test, D. W., & Cease-Cook, J. (2012). Evidence-based secondary transition practices for rehabilitation counselors. *Journal of Rehabilitation, 78*(2), 30–38.

U.S. Department of Education, International Affairs Office. (2008a). *Structure of the U.S. education system: Associate degrees.* Retrieved from https://www2.ed.gov/about/offices/list/ous/international/usnei/us/associate.doc

U.S. Department of Education, International Affairs Office. (2008b). *Structure of the U.S. education system: Bachelor's degrees.* Retrieved from https://www2.ed.gov/about/offices/list/ous/international/usnei/us/bachelor.doc

U.S. Department of Education, International Affairs Office. (2008c). *Structure of the U.S. education system: Career and technical qualifications.* Retrieved from https://www2.ed.gov/about/offices/list/ous/international/usnei/us/cte.doc

U.S. Department of Education, Office of Civil Rights. (2011). *Students with disabilities preparing for postsecondary education: Know your rights and responsibilities.* Retrieved from https://www2.ed.gov/about/offices/list/ocr/transition.html

U.S. Department of Education, Office of Special Education and Rehabilitative Services. (2017). *A transition guide to postsecondary education and employment for students and youth with disabilities.* Retrieved from https://www2.ed.gov/about/offices/list/osers/transition/products/postsecondary-transition-guide-may-2017.pdf

Wagner, M., Newman, L., Cameto, R., Garza, N., & Levine, P. (2005). *After high school: A first look at the post-school experiences of youth with disabilities. A report from the National Longitudinal Transition Study–2 (NLTS2).* Washington, DC: U.S. Department of Education, Office of Special Education Programs. Retrieved from https://eric.ed.gov/?id=ED494935

Wallen, M., & Stewart, K. (2015). The GAS approach: Scaling tailored goals. In A. A. Poulsen, J. Ziviani, & M. Cuskelly (Eds.), *Goal setting and motivation in therapy: Engaging children and parents* (pp. 153–162). Philadelphia: Kingsley.

Wehmeyer, M. (2005). Self-determination and individuals with severe disabilities: Re-examining meanings and misinterpretations. *Research and Practice for Persons With Severe Disabilities, 30,* 113–120. https://doi.org/10.2511/rpsd.30.3.113

Ziviani, J., Polatajko, H., & Rodger, S. (2015). Embedding goal setting in practice: The CO-OP approach. In A. A. Poulsen, J. Ziviani, & M. Cuskelly (Eds.), *Goal setting and motivation in therapy: Engaging children and parents* (pp. 80–88). Philadelphia: Jessica Kingsley.

SECTION III.

Evidence-Guided Practices: Population-Level Considerations to Support Participation

Best Practices in Multi-Tiered Systems of Support

Susan M. Cahill, PhD, OTR/L, FAOTA

KEY TERMS AND CONCEPTS

- Common Core Standards
- Early intervening services
- Educational standards
- Every Student Succeeds Act
- General education
- General education curriculum
- Individuals With Disabilities Education Improvement Act of 2004
- Positive behavioral interventions and supports
- Problem-solving teams
- Response to intervention
- Specialized instructional support personnel
- Universal screening

OVERVIEW

The majority of the more than 55 million students attending elementary and secondary schools in the United States receive general education (McFarland et al., 2017; U.S. Department of Education, 2016). *General education* refers to the common curriculum, expectations, and instructional practices that are thought to be beneficial to the majority of students in a school or district. Some students receiving general education are at risk for academic failure because of learning or social–emotional difficulties (National Center on Response to Intervention, 2010). Occupational therapy practitioners[1] collaborate with teachers and other service providers to support students receiving general education within the context of multi-tiered systems of support (MTSS; Cahill et al., 2014; Frolek Clark, 2016; Frolek Clark & Miller, 1996).

Occupational therapy practitioners add value to general education teams by designing supportive learning environments and making recommendations to maximize students' learning, social participation, and mental health (AOTA, 2012). To truly collaborate with general education teams, occupational therapy practitioners must understand the influence of educational standards, legislation, and models of service provision.

---

[1] *Occupational therapy practitioner* refers to both the occupational therapist and the occupational therapy assistant. The American Occupational Therapy Association (AOTA; 2014a, p. S18) states, "The occupational therapist is responsible for all aspects of occupational therapy service delivery and is accountable for the safety and effectiveness of the occupational therapy service delivery process" and "must be directly involved in the delivery of services during the initial evaluation and regularly throughout the course of intervention. . . . The occupational therapy assistant delivers safe and effective occupational therapy services under the supervision of and in partnership with the occupational therapist."

Curriculum in General Education and the Common Core

The *general education curriculum* is the course of study that is offered to students in a school or a school district. The curriculum includes the *scope,* or the breadth and depth, of the material that will be covered as well as the *sequence,* or the order, in which it will be presented. Decisions about what knowledge and skills are included in the curriculum are often made by a curriculum committee and school administrators. Many schools and districts adopt educational standards to guide the scope and sequence of their curricula.

Educational standards are the goals and grade-level expectations that students are projected to meet, usually by the completion of the academic year. Standards-based education began in the late 1980s and gained increasing popularity in the 2000s (Coburn et al., 2016). Critics of standards-based education argue that educational standards result in the narrowing of the curricular scope as well as a tendency on the part of teachers to prepare students to perform well on high-stakes tests, which inadvertently results in the deemphasis of authentic learning (Coburn et al., 2016). However, many educators and policymakers favor the increased accountability provided by standards-based education (Coburn et al., 2016).

The *Common Core Standards,* which provide schools and districts with common educational expectations for students in kindergarten through Grade 12 in the subject areas of English and math, were introduced in 2010 (Porter et al., 2011). They were developed in response to the need to prepare students for life after high school and steered by the National Governors Association Center for Best Practices and the Council of Chief State School Officers (Porter et al., 2011). The development of the Common Core Standards included a review of evidence associated with the knowledge and skills that are needed to prepare students

---

Copyright © 2019 by the American Occupational Therapy Association. All rights reserved. To reuse this content, contact www.copyright.com.
https://doi.org/10.7139/2019.978-1-56900-591-0.026

for college and career readiness and current state educational standards and feedback from teachers, parents, and administrators (Common Core Standards Initiative, n.d.).

The Common Core Standards provide an opportunity and a framework for schools and districts in the United States to develop a national curriculum (Porter et al., 2011). This shared framework allows for increased consistency and equity in educational content and expectations across schools, districts, and states (Porter et al., 2011). These standards can serve as a point of reference when making decisions about curriculum, resources, faculty, and support services. The Common Core Standards have been voluntarily adopted by most states (Common Core Standards Initiative, n.d.), and practitioners should be aware of them (see https://bit.ly/PiGYUF).

Legislation That Supports the Role of Occupational Therapy in General Education

Federal legislation provides the framework for public education in the United States and the supports and services that are provided to children in public schools. Two important pieces of legislation, the *Every Student Succeeds Act* (ESSA; 2015; Pub. L. 114–95) and the *Individuals With Disabilities Education Improvement Act of 2004* (IDEA; Pub. L. 108–446), include provisions associated with the delivery of occupational therapy in general education and with students not receiving special education.

ESSA

ESSA is the most recent iteration of the Elementary and Secondary Education Act of 1965 (ESEA; Pub. L. 89–313). The implementation of the ESEA was the first time that the federal government attempted to equalize the distribution of education funding to offset the needs experienced by persons living in disadvantaged regions of the country (Kantor, 1991).

ESSA includes provisions for school districts to establish their own goals and monitoring systems for accountability. The ESSA legislation identifies related services (e.g., occupational therapy) as *specialized instructional support personnel* (SISP). SISP also includes other professionals such as social workers, speech–language pathologists, and school counselors (National Alliance of Specialized Instructional Support Personnel, n.d.). Under ESSA, SISP consult with other professionals to support students' academic achievement and engage in the provision of MTSS. The SISP recognition, in effect, sanctions the involvement of occupational therapy practitioners to provide supports in general education.

IDEA

IDEA (2004) provides some important provisions associated with the work of occupational therapy practitioners in general education as well as in special education. IDEA is a reauthorization of the Education for All Handicapped Children Act of 1975 (Pub. L. 94–142) and the primary legislation associated with the education of students with disabilities. In 2004, IDEA's focus on the evaluation of students

at risk or suspected of having disabilities was expanded to emphasize prevention. Prevention was addressed in IDEA by enabling local educational agencies to provide early intervening services (EIS).

School districts are permitted to spend up to 15% of their special education funds for *EIS,* including "scientifically based academic instruction and behavioral interventions, including scientifically based literacy instruction, and, where appropriate, instruction on the use of adaptive and instructional software; and providing educational and behavioral evaluations, services, and supports" (34 C.F.R. § 300.224). School districts in which a disproportionate number of students from racial/ethnic minority backgrounds are receiving special education services are required to spend 15% of their funds on EIS (IDEA, 2004). Related services (e.g., occupational therapy) are included in IDEA 2004 (§ 300.208) as possible EIS.

Because of IDEA and ESSA, general education practices now emphasize prevention and support a proactive (vs. a wait-and-see) approach, and school personnel, including occupational therapy practitioners, have expanded their roles in public schools.

ESSENTIAL CONSIDERATIONS

Many school districts provide EIS through MTSS. However, not all states have adopted this approach, and requirements for providing occupational therapy services within MTSS may vary (AOTA, 2012). Before engaging in MTSS, occupational therapy practitioners should review their state practice act and licensure laws to determine the types of services that they may provide to students without an individualized education program (AOTA, 2012).

The primary aims of an MTSS framework are to identify students who are struggling, to provide students with the supports they need to address learning and behavioral needs, and to promote student success in general education. To address these aims, school districts implementing MTSS use several common practices, which include

- High-quality general education instruction based on scientific evidence,
- Continuous progress monitoring of student performance,
- Universal screening of academics and behavior, and
- The use of multiple tiers of instruction that are progressively more intense, based on the student's response to intervention (RtI; Jimerson et al., 2015).

MTSS

MTSS are used to address learning as well as social and behavioral needs of students in general education. Because RtI and positive behavioral interventions and supports (PBIS) follow a similar tiered structure, they can easily be used by school teams in combination under the MTSS umbrella.

RtI is a system of implementing EIS based on students' progress within the context of high-quality instruction and intervention matched to student needs, followed by the systematic evaluation of their responses to education and interventions (National Association of State Directors of Special Education, 2006). *PBIS* is an MTSS framework that uses the systematic implementation of tiered interventions targeting prosocial behavior and social–emotional development (Benner et al., 2013).

Many MTSS models are composed of 3 levels: Tier 1 (universal or core instruction), Tier 2 (targeted intervention plus Tier 1), and Tier 3 (intensive intervention plus Tier 1 and Tier 2). The tiers used in MTSS refer to the levels of intensity associated with the academic or behavioral intervention. Some MTSS frameworks include 4 or 5 tiers. In some cases, the final tier or tiers of MTSS may lead to referral for special education services. Table 26.1 includes the components that are commonly found in a 3-tier MTSS framework.

Generally, in a 3-tiered model of support, the first tier includes high-quality instructional, behavioral, and social support provided through school- or classroom-wide interventions (RTI Action Network, 2014). Whole-class screening and peer-to-peer comparison are often used to assess whether academic and behavioral performance is appropriate for the student's age and grade. When students are struggling despite Tier 1 supports, Tier 2–targeted interventions may be considered. Tier 2 interventions are often designed and sometimes implemented by the school's problem-solving team (PST), sometimes referred to as the *student support team* or the *instructional support team*. Interventions and supports provided at Tier 2 are more intensive and might include small group interventions or more intensive academic instruction (RTI Action Network, 2014). The third tier usually comprises the most intensive interventions, often provided on a one-to-one basis (RTI Action Network, 2014).

Within an MTSS framework, occupational therapy practitioners can work with educational teams to provide a continuum of services to students in general education to support promotion, prevention, early identification, and intervention associated with occupational performance needs. MTSS allows occupational therapy practitioners to expand their role in school systems practice by providing services to students who are at risk and may not traditionally

be part of their caseloads (Cahill, 2007). Depending on the state's licensure law, occupational therapy practitioners can work with educational teams to participate at every level of MTSS.

SISP

As SISP, occupational therapy practitioners share their specialized knowledge and skills to enhance the learning and participation of students in general education environments. Occupational therapists and occupational therapy assistants, under the occupational therapist's supervision, perform critical tasks associated with this role. According to the National Alliance of Specialized Instructional Support Personnel (n.d.), some of these critical tasks for SISP are

- Consulting with teachers and families to promote effective teaching and assessment practices that support student learning,
- Developing a safe and positive school climate,
- Designing behavioral supports and interventions to support classroom management and promote students' positive mental health,
- Designing programs and activities that enhance student learning and behavioral outcomes,
- Providing a continuum of services for all students,
- Engaging in collaborative professional development to promote student outcomes, and
- Supporting the integration of general education and special education programming.

Problem Solving With Educational Teams

Many schools use PSTs to integrate and sustain implementation of MTSS. Often, the PST is responsible for the coordination of all activities associated with the implementation of RtI and PBIS (Florida's Positive Behavior Support Project, 2011). The *PST* is composed of educators, administrators, and SISP who are all committed to engaging in a collaborative problem-solving process. In many instances, the PST analyzes data from universal screening measures and interprets other progress-monitoring data to make decisions about whether specific students would benefit from more intensive intervention at a higher tier (Cahill, 2007).

The PST also works to discern the reason why a student is having difficulty and develop an intervention and method for monitoring the student's progress. The process used by the PST to make such decisions is outlined in Table 26.2. Although this process is described in 7 discrete steps, it is cyclical. If the PST finds that an intervention is not effective or needs to be modified for intensity, the problem-solving process may start again at the beginning.

Working with educational teams to implement the problem-solving process, occupational therapy practitioners able to work in the general education through an MTSS framework must provide services associated with MTSS in the student's natural learning environment (Conway et al., 2015). Providing services in the student's classroom or in the cafeteria or gymnasium, for example, allows the occupational therapy practitioner to understand how the student's occupational performance compares with that of same-age

TABLE 26.1. Components Commonly Found in Each Tier of Multi-Tiered Systems of Support

TIER	COMPONENTS
Tier 1	Research-based core curriculum
	Evidence-based instructional practices
	Problem-solving team
	Universal screening
	Professional development
	Regular progress monitoring
Tier 2	Small group instruction or more intensive interventions
	Differentiated instruction
	Plus Tier 1 components
Tier 3	Individual or small group instruction and the most intensive interventions
	Wraparound services and connections to community agencies
	Plus Tier 1 and Tier 2 components

Source. Positive Behavioral Intervention & Support, OSEP Technical Assistance Center (2018).

TABLE 26.2.   Sample Process Used by Problem-Solving Teams to Make Decisions in Multi-Tiered Systems of Support

STEP	PROCESS
1	Identify and describe a student's academic or behavioral concern. Identification is often based on comparing the student's performance with that of peers and use of multiple sources of information (e.g., universal screenings, data collection tools).
2	Examine the data and formulate a hypothesis to explain the student's performance concern.
3	Formulate an academic performance or behavior target for measuring progress.
4	Develop an intervention plan based on evidence and a progress monitoring system (e.g., who will collect data, what type of data will be collected, the frequency with which the data will be collected, when the data will be reviewed).
5	Execute the intervention plan and monitor progress at regular intervals.
6	Evaluate the student's progress using progress monitoring data.
7	Determine whether the intervention plan should be discontinued, modified for increased intensity, or continued as is.

Source. Florida's Positive Behavior Support Project (2011).

peers. This comparison may help the PST to identify why the student is having performance difficulties and select the most appropriate intervention. Integrating services into the student's routine also provides the occupational therapy practitioner with an opportunity to educate and consult with other team members in real time using concrete examples (Bazyk & Cahill, 2015).

Services in the Educational Environment and Routine

The success of SISP and ultimately of the supports and services with students and educators in general education are dependent on the integration of their services into daily routines. High levels of integration are based on successful collaboration and communication (Benson et al., 2016). Collaboration in school systems is based on classroom teachers and SISP having a mutual understanding of the common goal they are working toward and how this goal benefits students (Friend & Cook, 2000).

Occupational therapy practitioners should be present in the natural school environments in which students typically perform their daily routines and carry out their student role. Because occupational therapy practitioners are skilled in supporting outcomes associated with students' achievement in academics, social participation (e.g., playing at recess), and essential student role behaviors (e.g., organization of learning materials), the contexts in which occupational therapy practitioners can provide services are varied and include classrooms, restrooms, playgrounds, cafeterias, hallways, buses, and gymnasiums (Bazyk & Cahill, 2015). Interventions integrated into natural environments more readily lead to lasting functional changes in performance (AOTA, 2017).

Removing students from natural environments to provide interventions in isolation is ineffective for students unless an intensive instruction associated with learning a new skill is required (Bazyk & Cahill, 2015; Frolek Clark, 2016). When this is the case, the occupational therapy practitioner should have a plan for moving services into the natural environment as soon as is practical.

Occupational therapy practitioners may provide services with students for a number of reasons (Frolek Clark & Polichino, 2010), including to address self-regulation (e.g., attention, self-management of behavior, transitioning between activities), use of school materials, handwriting (Cahill, 2010), reading (Grajo et al., 2016), and positive mental health (Bazyk & Cahill, 2015).

BEST PRACTICES

Occupational therapy practitioners working in general education may provide professional development to school staff, serve as MTSS case managers, develop universal screenings to be used by teachers (and assist in the screenings if allowed by state licensure and school district policy), and assist in data collection through progress monitoring.

Provide Professional Development to School Staff

Professional development is included as an EIS under IDEA (34 C.F.R. 300.226) and is an important part of working in an MTSS framework. Occupational therapy practitioners may provide professional development to teachers and other school staff to support their use of evidence-based academic and behavioral interventions and advocate for the needs of students in general education. Professional development may be informal, such as conversations during a meeting or in the classroom, or formal, such as in-services or trainings.

Whether informal or formal, professional development opportunities are one way in which occupational therapy practitioners may convey their knowledge of different intrinsic and environmental factors that affect student role performance and the interventions that optimize performance and participation.

Occupational therapy practitioners providing professional development trainings should carefully consider the knowledge and skills that are the focus of the training as well as the method that will be used to assess learning (Castillo et al., 2016). Professional development trainings are most effective when they are scheduled at regular intervals, based on the most current and up-to-date evidence, include demonstrations and modeling, and allow for reflection. In addition, context-embedded practice and coaching are also effective in helping teachers and other school staff implement strategies and interventions in the classroom and other learning environments.

Serve as Case Manager

Some SISPs, such as occupational therapists, are responsible for MTSS case management (American Institute for Research, 2014). Case management in an MTSS framework involves coordinating MTSS supports and services, monitoring the provision of services, overseeing data collection and progress monitoring, and leading the problem-solving process (American Institute for Research, 2014).

In addition, an SISP serving in a case management role may be responsible for communicating with students' families, connecting with outside community agencies, and maintaining MTSS documentation. Case managers in MTSS frameworks may also provide some direct services to students by using coaching strategies to address self-management, organization, or increasing participation in academic and social contexts (U.S. Department of Education, Office of Planning, Evaluation, and Policy Development, 2017).

Develop Classroom-Level Programs

Occupational therapists may engage in systems-level practice by developing programs for general education students (AOTA, 2014b). Program development is generally a collaborative endeavor that involves the participation of multiple stakeholders. The program development process includes a needs assessment, program planning, implementation, evaluation, and the development of a sustainability plan (Scaffa & Brownson, 2014).

Occupational therapists are well suited for program development because they are able to apply the systematic approach used in the occupational therapy process with groups and populations (AOTA, 2014b). This process includes an examination of how client factors, contexts, occupations, activities, and performance patterns interact to support or limit participation. Examples of school programs developed by occupational therapists and used in MTSS include Comfortable Cafeteria (Bazyk et al., 2014a), Refreshing Recess (Bazyk et al., 2014b), and Write Start (Case-Smith et al., 2012).

Assist With Universal Screening

Universal screening (i.e., screening groups of students at the whole class or grade level) is often used to ensure that students are making the expected progress on grade-level academic and behavioral indicators. If allowed by licensure in that state, occupational therapy practitioners may participate in universal screenings associated with academic performance and behavior to assist in the identification of students who are at risk for learning and social–emotional difficulties. A universal screening in MTSS is proactive rather than reactive and avoids the implementation of a "wait-to-fail" approach (Turse & Albrecht, 2015, p. 83) to monitoring students' concerns. This proactive approach helps to ensure that students receive interventions and support as they need it, ideally in time for them to catch up to their peers (Turse & Albrecht, 2015).

Universal screenings, sometimes called *probes,* are generally easily repeatable and often low-cost methods of assessing age- or grade-appropriate academic skills or behaviors (Hughes & Dexter, n.d.). The most common screening tools used in MTSS are curriculum-based measures associated with reading and math (Hughes & Dexter, n.d.).

There is a lack of consensus on how to use screening data to make decisions about which students receive higher intensity tiered interventions and which do not (Hughes & Dexter, n.d.). Many schools and PSTs choose to use a normative approach based on percentile ranks associated with standardized screening measures (Hughes & Dexter, n.d.) or the discrepancy model. When the discrepancy model is used during screening, the student's performance is often compared with that of a local group of same-age peers on the screening measure or probe to determine whether the student's performance is comparable or not. When a student demonstrates a difference in performance, intervention or further assessment may be warranted.

Use Progress Monitoring and Data-Informed Decision Making

Progress monitoring is used in an MTSS framework to assess students' performance related to learning or behavior (Frolek Clark, 2010). Information gained through progress monitoring is used to make data-informed decisions about whether or not a student would benefit from more intensive interventions and supports (Frolek Clark et al., 2015). Students receiving Tier 2 and Tier 3 interventions are monitored at 2- to 8-week intervals, depending on their needs and the level of intensity of the intervention (Brown-Chidsey & Steege, 2010). The schedule for monitoring is often based on the severity of the student's needs; it is expected that as the severity of the student's needs increases, so too does the frequency of progress monitoring (Frolek Clark & Handley-More, 2017; Harlacher et al., 2014).

Teams should collect progress monitoring data frequently enough that they are able to make decisions (e.g., weekly minimum for Tier 3). Generally, most teams collect data at least 8 times before making a decision about the efficacy of an intervention with a particular student (Harlacher et al., 2014). The frequency, type, and amount of progress monitoring data collected may also be dictated by local policy or the variability of the student's performance (Harlacher et al., 2014). The data collected through progress monitoring may be plotted against baseline data to determine the student's progress and compare it with desired outcomes.

SUMMARY

Federal legislation such as the ESSA (2015) and IDEA (2004) provides occupational therapy practitioners with an expanded role in general education. Working in general education requires that occupational therapy practitioners understand the influence of educational standards, legislation, and models of service provision. Occupational therapy practitioners working in general education collaborate with teachers and

PSTs to provide multi-tiered interventions to promote students' learning, behavior, and participation at school.

REFERENCES

American Institute for Research. (2014). *Evaluating specialized instructional support personnel.* Retrieved from https://files.eric.ed.gov/fulltext/ED555666.pdf

American Occupational Therapy Association. (2004). Occupational therapy services in early intervention and school-based programs. *American Journal of Occupational Therapy, 59,* 681–685. https://doi.org/10.5014/ajot.58.6.681

American Occupational Therapy Association. (2014a). Guidelines for supervision, roles, and responsibilities during the delivery of occupational therapy services. *American Journal of Occupational Therapy, 68*(Suppl. 3), S16–S22. https://doi.org/10.5014/ajot.2014.686S03

American Occupational Therapy Association. (2014b). Occupational therapy practice framework: Domain and process (3rd ed.). *American Journal of Occupational Therapy, 68*(Suppl. 1), S1–S48. https://doi.org/10.5014/ajot.2014.682006

American Occupational Therapy Association. (2017). Guidelines for occupational therapy services in early intervention and schools. *American Journal of Occupational Therapy, 71*(Suppl. 2), 7112410010. https://doi.org/10.5014/ajot.2017.716S01

Bazyk, S., & Cahill, S. (2015). School-based occupational therapy. In J. Case-Smith & J. O'Brien (Eds.), *Occupational therapy for children* (7th ed.; pp. 664–703). St. Louis: Elsevier.

Bazyk, S., Mohler, R., & Kerns, S. (2014a). *Creating a Comfortable Cafeteria program information brief.* Retrieved from http://www.everymomentcounts.org/up_doc/Cafeteria_Info_Brief_7-15-14.pdf

Bazyk, S., Mohler, R., & Kerns, S. (2014b). *Refreshing Recess program.* Retrieved from http://www.everymomentcounts.org/up_doc/Recess_Info_Brief.pdf

Benner, G. J., Kutash, K., Nelson, J. R., & Fisher, M. B. (2013). Closing the achievement gap of youth with emotional and behavioral disorders through multi-tiered systems of support. *Education and Treatment of Children, 36,* 15–29. https://doi.org/10.1353/etc.2013.0018

Benson, J., Szucs, K., & Mejasic, J. (2016). Teachers' perceptions of the role of occupational therapist in schools. *Journal of Occupational Therapy, Schools, and Early Intervention, 9,* 290–230. https://doi.org/10.1080/19411243.2016.1183158

Brown-Chidsey, R., & Steege, M. W. (2010). *Response to intervention: Principles and strategies for effective practice.* New York: Guilford Press.

Cahill, S. (2007). A perspective on response to intervention. *School System Special Interest Section Quarterly, 14*(3), 1–4.

Cahill, S. (2010). The contributions made by occupational therapists in RtI: A pilot study. *Journal of Occupational Therapy, Schools, and Early Intervention, 3,* 3–10. https://doi.org/10.1080/19411241003683771

Cahill, S. M., McGuire, B., Krumdick, N. D., & Lee, M. M. (2014). National survey of occupational therapy practitioners' involvement in response to intervention. *American Journal of Occupational Therapy, 68,* e234–e240. https://doi.org/10.5014/ajot.2014.010116

Case-Smith, J., Holland, T., Lane, A., & White, S. (2012). Effect of a co-teaching handwriting program for first graders: One group pretest–posttest design. *American Journal of Occupational Therapy, 66,* 396–405. https://doi.org/10.5014/ajot.2012.004333

Castillo, J. M., March, A. L., Tan, S. Y., Stockslager, K. M., Brundage, A., Mccullough, M., & Sabnis, S. (2016). Relationships between ongoing professional development and educators' perceived skills relative to RtI. *Psychology in the Schools, 53,* 893–910. https://doi.org/10.1002/pits.21954

Coburn, C. E., Hill, H. C., & Spillane, J. P. (2016). Alignment and accountability in policy design and implementation: The Common Core State Standards and implementation research. *Educational Researcher, 45,* 243–251. https://doi.org/10.3102/0013189X16651080

Common Core Standards Initiative. (n.d.). *Development process.* Retrieved from http://www.corestandards.org/about-the-standards/development-process/

Conway, C. S., Kanics, I. M., Mohler, R., & Giudici, M. (2015). *Inclusion of children with disabilities: Occupational therapy's role in mental health promotion, prevention, and intervention with children and youth.* Retrieved from https://www.aota.org/~/media/Corporate/Files/Practice/Children/Inclusion-of-Children-With-Disabilities-20150128.PDF

Education for All Handicapped Children Act of 1975, Pub. L. 94–142, renamed the Individuals With Disabilities Education Improvement Act, codified at 20 U.S.C. §§ 1400–1482.

Elementary and Secondary Education Act of 1965, Pub. L. 89–313, 20 U.S.C. §§ 2701–3386.

Every Student Succeeds Act, Pub. L. 114–95, 129 Stat. 1802 (2015).

Florida's Positive Behavior Support Project. (2011). *Implementing a multi-tiered system of support for behavior: A practical guide.* Retrieved from https://www.pbis.org/common/cms/files/pbisresources/RTIB_Guide_101811_final.pdf

Friend, M., & Cook, L. (2000). *Interactions: Collaboration skills for school professionals.* New York: Addison Wesley Longman.

Frolek Clark, G. (2010). Using data to guide your designs. In H. Miller Kuhaneck & R. Watling (Eds.), *Autism: A comprehensive occupational therapy approach* (3rd ed.; pp. 743–776). Bethesda, MD: AOTA Press.

Frolek Clark, G. (2016). Collaboration within the *Paces:* Structures and routines. In B. Hanft & J. Shepherd (Eds.), *Collaborating for student success: A guide for school-based occupational therapy* (pp. 177–207). Bethesda, MD: AOTA Press.

Frolek Clark, G., Cahill, S. M., & Ivey, C. (2015). School practice documentation: Documenting and organizing quantitative data. *OT Practice, 20*(15), 12–15.

Frolek Clark, G., & Handley-More, D. (2017). *Best practices for documenting occupational therapy services in schools.* Bethesda, MD: AOTA Press.

Frolek Clark, G., & Miller, L. (1996). Providing effective occupational therapy services: Data-based decision making in school-based practice. *American Journal of Occupational Therapy, 50,* 701–708. https://doi.org/10.5014/ajot.50.9.701

Frolek Clark, G., & Polichino, J. (2010). Response to intervention and early intervening services: Occupational therapy roles in general education. *OT Practice, 15*(1), 1–7.

Grajo, L. C., Candler, C., Bowyer, P., Schultz, S., Thomson, J., & Fong, K. (2016). Determining the internal validity of the Inventory of Reading Occupations: An assessment tool of children's reading participation. *American Journal of Occupational Therapy, 70,* 7003220010. https://doi.org/10.5014/ajot.2016.017582

Harlacher, J. E., Sanford, A., & Nelson Walker, N. (2014, May 15). Distinguishing between Tier 2 and Tier 3 instruction in order to support implementation of RTI. *RTI Action Network Monthly Newsletter*. Retrieved from http://www.rtinetwork.org/essential /tieredinstruction/tier3/distinguishing-between-tier-2-and -tier-3-instruction-in-order-to-support-implementation-of-rti

Hughes, C., & Dexter, D. (n.d.). *Universal screening within a response-to-intervention model*. Retrieved from http://www .rtinetwork.org/learn/research/universal-screening-within -a-rti-model?tmpl=component&print=1

Individuals With Disabilities Education Improvement Act of 2004, Pub. L. 108–446, 20 U.S.C. §§ 1400–1482.

Jimerson, S., Burns, M., & VanDerHeyden, A. (2015). From RtI to MTSS: Advances in the science and practice of assessment and intervention. In S. Jimerson, M. Burns, & A. VanDerHeyden (Eds.), *Handbook of RtI: The science and practice of multi-tiered systems of support* (pp. 1–8). New York: Springer.

Kantor, H. (1991). Education, social reform, and the state: ESEA and federal education policy in the 1960s. *American Journal of Education, 100(1)*, 47–83. https://doi.org/10.1086/444004

McFarland, J., Hussar, B., de Brey, C., Snyder, T., Wang, X., Wilkinson-Flicker, S., . . . Hinz, S. (2017). *The condition of education 2017* (NCES 2017-144). Retrieved from https://nces.ed .gov/pubsearch/pubsinfo.asp?pubid=2017144

National Alliance of Specialized Instructional Support Personnel. (n.d.). *Fact Sheet: Specialized instructional support personnel*. Retrieved from http://nasisp.org/uploads/NASISP_SISP_Fact _Sheet.pdf

National Association of State Directors of Special Education. (2006). *Response to intervention: Policy considerations and implementation*. Alexandria, VA: Author.

National Center on Response to Intervention. (2010). *Essential components of RTI: A closer look at response to intervention*. Washington, DC: U.S. Department of Education, Office of Special Education Programs, Author.

Porter, A., McMaken, J., Hwang, J., & Yang, R. (2011). Common Core Standards: The new U.S. intended curriculum. *Educational Researcher, 40*, 103–116. https://doi.org/10.3102 /0013189X11405038

Positive Behavioral Interventions and Supports, OSEP Technical Assistance Center. (2018). *Multi-tiered system of support (MTSS) and PBIS*. Retrieved from https://www.pbis.org /school/mtss

RTI Action Network. (2014). *What is RTI?* Retrieved from www .rtinetwork.org/learn/what/whatisrti

Scaffa, M. E., & Brownson, C. A. (2014). Program planning and needs assessment. In M. E. Scaffa & S. E. Reitz (Eds.), *Occupational therapy in community-based practice settings* (pp. 61–78). Philadelphia: F. A. Davis.

Turse, K. A., & Albrecht, S. F. (2015). The ABCs of RTI: An introduction to the building blocks of response to intervention. *Preventing School Failure: Alternative Education for Children and Youth, 59(2)*, 83–89. https://doi.org/10.1080/10459 88X.2013.837813

U.S. Department of Education, National Center for Education Statistics. (2016). *Digest of education statistics, 2015* (NCES 2016-014). Retrieved from https://nces.ed.gov/pubsearch/pubs -info.asp?pubid=2016014

U.S. Department of Education, Office of Planning, Evaluation, and Policy Development. (2017). *Issue Brief: Case management in high schools*. Retrieved from https://www2.ed.gov/rschstat /eval/high-school/case-management.pdf

Leslie L. Jackson, DrOT, MEd, OT/L, FAOTA

KEY TERMS AND CONCEPTS

- Accommodation
- ADA Amendments Act of 2008
- Americans With Disabilities Act of 1990
- Every Student Succeeds Act
- Free appropriate public education
- Individuals With Disabilities Education Improvement Act of 2004
- Modification
- Section 504

OVERVIEW

Education reform efforts continue to evolve, with an increasing focus on all students, including those with disabilities in general education or receiving special education (Thurlow et al., 2016). National data from the 2016–2017 school year indicate that more than 62% of all students with disabilities ages 3–21 years received a major portion of their education in the general education classroom (U.S. Department of Education [U.S. DOE], 2017a). Despite the rising number of students with disabilities in general education classrooms, many general educators do not feel prepared to appropriately plan for and teach these students in their classrooms (Holmes, 2018; Jerome, 2017; LeMay, 2017). School occupational therapy practitioners[1] work with students with and without disabilities in general and special education environments and provide supports to educational staff to support student engagement and participation in daily living activities (AOTA, 2017).

Occupational therapy in schools is designed to facilitate students' learning, development, and behavior that enable them to organize, manage, and perform their daily life occupations and activities (AOTA, 2017). In most instances,

school services are provided under the auspices of the *Individuals With Disabilities Education Improvement Act of 2004* (IDEA; Pub. L. 108–446), which requires schools to provide a *free appropriate public education* (FAPE) that includes special education and related services for students with disabilities.

The *Every Student Succeeds Act* (ESSA; 2015; Pub. L. 114–195), which replaced the No Child Left Behind Act of 2001 (Pub. L. 107–110), identifies related services as "specialized instructional support personnel" who can provide supports for students in grades K–12. For students with eligible disabilities who do not need specialized instruction under IDEA, supports and accommodations may be available under Section 504 of the Rehabilitation Act of 1973, as amended (2008), and the *ADA Amendments Act of 2008* (ADAAA; Pub. L. 110–325).

Section 504 is a civil rights law that prohibits any organization that receives any federal funding from discriminating against people with disabilities. It refers to a specific section of the Rehabilitation Act of 1973 (as amended in 2008) that provides funding to states for vocational rehabilitation services, supported employment, independent living, and client assistance programs (U.S. DOE, 2017b). The law also includes provisions that address rights and advocacy for persons with disabilities.

Section 504 applies to all organizations that receive financial assistance from any federal department or agency (U.S. Department of Health and Human Services [U.S. DHHS], Office for Civil Rights, 2017), including public schools, charter schools, and magnet schools (U.S. DOE, Office for Civil Rights, 2016). Under Section 504, no additional funding is provided to school districts to provide supports and services for eligible students, as is required under other federal education laws. School districts must consider whether a student with a disability needs support to access and succeed in the learning environment (AOTA,

---

[1]*Occupational therapy practitioner* refers to both the occupational therapist and the occupational therapy assistant. The American Occupational Therapy Association (AOTA; 2014, p. S18) states, "The occupational therapist is responsible for all aspects of occupational therapy service delivery and is accountable for the safety and effectiveness of the occupational therapy service delivery process" and "must be directly involved in the delivery of services during the initial evaluation and regularly throughout the course of intervention. . . . The occupational therapy assistant delivers safe and effective occupational therapy services under the supervision of and in partnership with the occupational therapist."

Copyright © 2019 by the American Occupational Therapy Association. All rights reserved. To reuse this content, contact www.copyright.com.
https://doi.org/10.7139/2019.978-1-56900-591-0.027

2017). As recipients of federal funds, school systems cannot deny

- Qualified individuals the opportunity to participate in or benefit from federally funded programs, services, or other benefits;
- Access to program, services, benefits, or opportunities to participate as a result of physical barriers; or
- Employment opportunities, including hiring, promotion, training, and fringe benefits for which they are otherwise entitled or qualified ("Nondiscrimination on the Basis of Handicap in Programs or Activities Receiving Federal Financial Assistance," 1977).

Compliance is not optional (Wrightslaw, 2008). Lack of compliance can result in loss of all federal funds received by the school district.

The focus of this chapter is school systems' obligations to all students with disabilities served by the district to ensure those students in elementary, middle, and high school academic, nonacademic, and extracurricular programs are identified and provided appropriate and effective occupational therapy services.

ESSENTIAL CONSIDERATIONS

Occupational therapy practitioners should understand the various federal laws that allow for occupational therapy services in schools and how they protect students with disabilities. Since the 1960s, Congress has passed federal education laws (such as ESSA, IDEA, and Section 504) aimed at ensuring equal opportunity and access for different classes of students (i.e., students with disabilities, racial and ethnic minorities, English-language learners, disadvantaged students). According to Thurlow et al. (2016), these efforts to include all students come at the same time as new and more rigorous, internationally competitive standards are being implemented and greater accountability is required of school administrators and educators, of special education systems (through results-based accountability), and of students themselves. Education systems are considering how to make education accessible to all students, including students with disabilities who may be served under IDEA or Section 504 as well as those who do not have identified disabilities (National Center on Educational Outcomes, 2015).

Impact on Student Participation in School and Learning

Section 504 and the IDEA work in tandem to ensure that school districts do not discriminate against students identified with disabilities while also ensuring each student's right to special education services, if appropriate (Martín, 2010). Section 504 emphasizes equal access to education rather than educational benefit (e.g., need for specialized education instruction), as under IDEA. Services may include modifications to the general education program, such as adjustments in test-taking procedures and adjustments to attendance rules when a student's absences are due to a disability (U.S. DOE, 2012). Even when the condition is considered temporary (episodic) or controlled by medication (mitigated), a student may be covered under Section 504

(Martín, 2010; U.S. DOE, 2016). If occupational therapy services are provided under Section 504, it is reasonable to expect the goal would be to support student engagement in learning, skill development, and participation in school activities.

The ***Americans With Disabilities Act of 1990*** (ADA; Pub. L. 101–336) and the ***ADAAA*** (Pub. L. 110–325) also provide protections for students with disabilities. The ADA and its amendments prohibit discrimination based on disability in public entities, including state and local governments and school districts (ADAAA, 2008). The language of ADA is similar to that in Section 504 and explains that the remedies, procedures, and rights are the same as those under Section 504 (Wrightslaw, 2012). Title II of the ADA sets out requirements for public educational entities (U.S. DOE, 2016); regulations can be found in the *Code of Federal Regulations* at 28 C.F.R. Part 35 ("Nondiscrimination on the Basis of Disability in State and Local Government Services," 1991).

Public and charter schools are public entities and recipients of federal funds. As such, they are covered by Section 504 and the ADAAA (U.S. DOE, 2016), in addition to IDEA and other federal education requirements. Under Section 504 and the ADAAA, schools cannot

- Exclude students with disabilities from a program or activity;
- Deny students with disabilities the benefits of a program or activity;
- Provide students with disabilities opportunities to participate in or benefit from a benefit or service that is not equal to what is provided to others;
- Provide a benefit or service to students with disabilities that is not as effective as what is provided to others;
- Provide different or separate benefits or services to students with disabilities, unless necessary to provide benefits or services that are as effective as what are provided to others; or
- Apply eligibility criteria that tend to screen out students with disabilities unless necessary for the provision of the service, program, or activity (U.S. DHHS, 2017).

In other words, students with disabilities must have equal opportunity to "obtain the same result, gain the same benefit, or reach the same level of achievement as other students" (PEER Project, 2008, "Key Concepts Under Section 504 and the ADA," para. 2) for benefits and services to be considered equally effective.

Comparing IDEA, Section 504, and the ADAAA

All students with disabilities who receive IDEA supports are also covered by Section 504 and the ADAAA. However, the converse is not true. Therefore, it is critical that school occupational therapy practitioners understand the similarities and differences between the laws. Table 27.1 provides a comparison of selected areas of the IDEA with Section 504 and the ADAAA.

Generally speaking, IDEA provides more specialized services and safeguards for students with disabilities and their parents than Section 504 (Wrightslaw, 2012). Students with disabilities must be determined to need special

TABLE 27.1. Key Differences Between IDEA and Section 504 and the ADAAA

TOPIC	IDEA	SECTION 504 AND ADAAA
Purpose	• Ensures that eligible students receive FAPE that includes special education and related services.	• Protects individuals with disabilities from discrimination because of their disabilities.
Eligibility	• Students with a disability that adversely affects their educational performance and who therefore require special education and related services to receive FAPE. • Requires a multidisciplinary evaluation that gathers information from a variety of sources.	• Students with a physical or mental impairment that substantially limits at least one major life activity (e.g., walking, seeing, hearing, speaking, learning, reading, writing, working, caring for oneself, performing manual tasks). • Expanded list of major life activities. • Requires an evaluation that draws information from a variety of sources.
Benefits and rights	• Students who receive special education and related services have an array of rights and protections. • Protections do not follow students after they leave school.	• Fewer protections than provided under IDEA. • Protections follow students after they leave public school system. (Also apply to charter schools; elementary and secondary schools; higher education; employment practices; accessibility; and health, welfare, and social services.)
Protection against discrimination	• Students who receive special education and related services are also covered under Section 504 and the ADAAA.	• Students with disabilities are protected from discrimination because of their disabilities.
Accommodations or modifications	• Students may receive accommodations and modifications to receive educational benefit. Must be included in the IEP.	• Students may receive accommodations and modifications to receive equal access to education. Should be included in a 504 plan.
Access vs. educational benefit	• Guarantees that students with disabilities receive an IEP designed to meet their unique needs and provide educational benefit so that the students are prepared for "further education, employment and independent living" (IDEA, § 602[d]).	• Provides access to the same FAPE that is available to students without disabilities. *FAPE* is defined in Section 504 regulations as "the provision of regular or special education and related aids and services that . . . are designed to meet individual educational needs of persons with disabilities as adequately as the needs of persons without disabilities are met and . . . are based upon adherence to specified procedures" ("Nondiscrimination on the Basis of Handicap in Programs or Activities Receiving Federal Financial Assistance," 1977; 34 C.F.R. § 104.33[b][1]). • Related services can be provided alone or in combination with general or special education services.
Written plans	• Schools must provide each eligible student with a written IEP that outlines specific services, accommodations, and modifications; the degree to which the student will or will not be educated with students with disabilities; and more. • Parents must be involved in developing the IEP. • IEPs must be reviewed at least annually.	• Requires schools to develop a plan that is a written document. • Schools are not required to invite parents to the meeting when the plan is developed, but they do have to notify the parent that a plan was developed. • No formal requirement for schools to review the plan after it is developed.
Procedural safeguards	• Provides an elaborate system of procedural safeguards designed to protect students and their parents, including written notice before any change of placement and the right to an independent educational evaluation at public expense.	• Requires schools to develop a system of safeguards that includes notice, an opportunity for parents to review records, and an impartial hearing and review procedure.
Impartial hearings	• Requires school districts to conduct impartial hearings for parents who disagree with the identification, evaluation, or placement of their child.	• Requires school districts to conduct impartial hearings for parents. Parents have the opportunity to participate and obtain counsel, but other details are left to the discretion of the district.

Note. ADAA = ADA Amendments Act of 2008; FAPE = free appropriate public education; IDEA = Individuals With Disabilities Education Improvement Act of 2004; IEP = individualized education program; Section 504 = Section 504 of the Rehabilitation Act of 1973.
Sources. Howey (2012); Jackson (2013); U.S. DOE (2016); Wright and Wright (2012).

education and related services (U.S. DOE, 2012). The key factor is whether the disability is such that the student requires special education and related services so that the student can receive an appropriate educational (FAPE).

In IDEA, *special education* is defined as specially designed instruction that can be provided in an array of locations, including general education classrooms, physical education, and a student's home. In other words, special education is not a specific place or classroom that students go to in school but rather a combination of supports and services (Jackson, 2013; Wrightslaw, 2012). As a related service, occupational therapy is a support to the specially designed instruction and also can be provided anywhere within the educational environment (Jackson, 2013).

If students have a disability but do not need special education services, then they may receive protections under Section 504 and the ADAAA. Unlike IDEA, *disability* has a broader meaning under both Section 504 and the ADAAA. Both statutes define *disability* as "(1) A physical or mental impairment that substantially limits a major life activity; (2) a record of such an impairment; or (3) being regarded as having such an impairment" (U.S. DOE, 2012, "How Does the Amendments Act Alter Coverage Under Section 504 and Title II?" para. 2).

If a student is indeed found to have a disability that substantially limits their major life activities "in a way that impacts their functioning in the school setting" (Martín, 2010, p. 3), then the district must provide an individualized and systematic plan for accommodations and services so that the student can access the same education that is provided to students without disabilities. Even when students do not need an accommodation plan, they are still entitled to other 504 protections, including the right to be free from actions that discriminate on the basis of disability, the right to protection from accumulations of short-term disciplinary removals that result in a pattern of exclusion, the right to 504 due process hearings, and equal right to access extracurricular activities and nonacademic services (Martín, 2010).

Eligibility for Section 504

Disability determination and eligibility for Section 504 is specific (i.e., individualized) to each student but not disability specific. The process is based on whether the student's disability significantly affects a major life activity, including learning, reading, and thinking and concentration (U.S. DOE, 2016). There are no per se disabilities in Section 504 (U.S. DOE, 2012) as in IDEA. For that reason, both Section 504 and the ADAAA broadly define *disability* (see 29 U.S.C. §705[9][B] and 42 U.S.C. §12101[1]). The need for special education in order to benefit from educational programming is essential for IDEA eligibility. A student with a disability who does not need special education (specialized instruction) is not eligible for IDEA services but may be protected from discrimination under Section 504 (U.S. DOE, 2016).

The ADAAA significantly changed how the term *disability* is to be interpreted. According to U.S. DOE (2012, para. 10), Congress directed that the definition of disability "shall be construed broadly and that the determination of whether an individual has a disability should not demand extensive analysis." In other words, school districts should focus their attention on how to ensure equal educational opportunities rather than spending a great deal of time deciding whether or not a student has a disability under Section 504 or ADAAA (U.S. DOE, 2012). To that end, the ADAAA expanded the list of major life activities to include "major bodily functions . . . and to include sleeping, standing, lifting, bending, reading, concentrating, thinking, communicating and working" (Martín, 2010, p. 7).

Another factor in determining eligibility for Section 504 is whether the student utilizes any mitigating measures. According to U.S. DOE (2016), the school has to consider whether the impairment would substantially limit a major life activity if the condition were not ameliorated with medication or other measures. For example, a student with a nut allergy may have problems in the major life areas of breathing and respiratory function when the allergy is active, even if the student receives medication to combat the allergy. In another example, a student with low vision who is able to read with a computer reader that enlarges the print is still considered to have an impairment that affects a major life activity (reading). Moreover, even when an impairment occurs only periodically or is in remission, it is still considered a disability if it would substantially limit a major life activity when in an active phase (U.S. DOE, 2016). For example, a student with epilepsy is a student with a disability if, during a seizure, the student is substantially limited in a major life activity, such as thinking, breathing, or neurological function.

Occupational Therapy Code of Ethics

Section 504 and the ADAAA prohibit schools from discriminating against students with disabilities; compliance is not optional (Weber, 2011). Some school personnel may mistakenly believe they are not obligated to provide 504 services and supports because, unlike IDEA or the ESSA, there is no additional funding. In fact, nothing can be further from the truth. Public education is not a federal responsibility. Each state operates public schools, although there is a federal role (Fryer, 2009). As such, it is rational for parents to expect schools to provide an appropriate education to their children. Federal education law and related court findings serve only to further clarify and codify this expectation.

School occupational therapy practitioners, faced with the dilemma of schools that do not recognize their responsibility under Section 504 or ADAAA, have an obligation to seek ethical action under the *Occupational Therapy Code of Ethics (2015)* (AOTA, 2015a). In particular, practitioners have a responsibility to advocate for students to receive the services to which they are entitled, whether they are under IDEA, Section 504, ADAAA, or ESSA. The ethical values of Nonmaleficence (refraining from actions that cause students harm), Social Justice (ensuring fair and equitable treatment for all students in school), and Procedural Justice (compliance with local, state, and federal laws) apply in this instance (AOTA, 2015a). School personnel are misinformed if they say the district does not "do 504." School occupational therapy practitioners should bring this issue to the attention of the proper administrators to comply with federal laws.

BEST PRACTICES

School occupational therapy practitioners are actively involved in supporting learning and school success. They promote student health and wellness and address the needs of those who are at risk of developing activity limitations and restrictions in participation as a result of disability, illness, injury, or other conditions (AOTA, 2015b).

Conduct the Evaluation

Decisions about who has a disability and is, therefore, eligible under Section 504 should be made on a case-by-case basis by a group of people, including school occupational therapists, who are knowledgeable about the student (Durheim, 2017; Martín, 2010; U.S. DOE, 2016). Although anyone can refer a student for evaluation under Section 504, schools must also have a reason to believe the student is in need of services under Section 504 (Durheim, 2017). Although Section 504 does not require formalized testing, the team needs to consider a variety of information sources, for example, occupational therapy evaluations, student grades, teacher reports, information from parents, health records, observations, and state assessment scores (Durheim, 2017).

Occupational therapists assist schools in appropriately identifying students who may be protected by Section 504. When conducting the evaluation, the occupational therapist should use multiple data sources to clearly "identify the child's performance in his or her occupations, the affordances and barriers to successful engagement, and expectations for the child's development and participation and synthesize information to develop a working hypothesis" (AOTA, 2017, p. 4). In these instances, the therapist has a responsibility to collaborate with the district to identify student skills, the demands of the environment, and appropriate solutions for interventions.

For students who already have a diagnosed condition, such as cerebral palsy, autism, Down syndrome, HIV/AIDS, arthritis, asthma, or epilepsy, the district can focus on identifying what specific accommodations or modifications these students may need to fully access the curriculum, learning environment, and other school activities or programs rather than on disability determination. For example, the school might need to adapt the physical education curriculum with different activity levels so a middle school student with asthma can physically participate along with classmates. This accommodation would be outlined in the student's 504 plan.

Develop the 504 Plan

School occupational therapists often assist the school district in developing the 504 plan, which outlines the individualized accommodations, modifications, or services that will be provided to the student by the school district. Identifying the accommodations (e.g., no changes in learning expectations) and modifications (e.g., reduction in learning expectations) needed by each student requires knowledge of the student's disability and expectations in the school environment.

When a student is found to be eligible for Section 504, the school should develop an individualized plan (i.e., 504 plan) to make sure the student, the student's parents, and school personnel understand their responsibilities in providing the student with the same access to education as other students. Section 504 does not mandate a timeline for 504 meetings or for implementing the plan, although the district may have developed specific procedures for doing so. On a related note, Section 504 also does not require parent participation in the development of the plan; however, the school must notify parents that a plan has been developed.

The format of the plan can vary from district to district or from school to school. Each plan should be adapted to the specific needs, abilities, and medical condition or disability of the individual child. The Council of Chief State School Officers (CCSSO; 2005) identified a list of questions that can help guide the 504 plan committee in selecting appropriate accommodations (see Exhibit 27.1). The committee should also identify how and when the student will learn to use each accommodation (e.g., make sure there is ample time for the student to learn how to use assessment accommodations before an assessment occurs) and plan for ongoing evaluation and improvement of the use of accommodations. Depending on the specific condition or disability, such as diabetes, the 504 plan also may include information targeted to the condition, such as medications needed, disability-specific procedures, training for staff to ensure they know what to do and how to do it, and what to do and whom to contact in an emergency.

An *accommodation* allows the student to complete the same assignment or test as other students but with a change in the timing, formatting, setting, scheduling, response, or presentation. The accommodation does not alter in any significant way what the test or assignment measures (Families and Advocates Partnership for Education, 2001). According to the CCSSO (2005), accommodations are intended to reduce or eliminate the effects of the disability but do not

EXHIBIT 27.1.	Questions to Guide Selecting Accommodations

- What are the student's learning strengths and areas of further development?
- How do the student's learning needs affect their achievement of grade-level standards?
- What specialized instruction(s) does the student need to achieve grade-level standards?
- What accommodations will increase the student's access to instruction and assessment?
- What accommodations, if any, are regularly used by the student during instruction and assessments?
- What are the results for assignments and assessments when accommodations were used and not used?
- What is the student's perception of how well an accommodation worked?
- Are there effective combinations of accommodations?
- What difficulties did the student experience when using accommodations?
- What are the perceptions of parents, teachers, and specialists about how the accommodation worked?
- Should the student continue to use an accommodation, are changes needed, or should its use be discontinued?

Source. Council of Chief State School Officers (2005).

EXHIBIT 27.2. Examples of Accommodations and Modifications for Students

Changes to Presentation
- Using a marker to highlight important sections of books/readings
- Extra set of textbooks for home
- List of discussion questions before reading the material
- Books and other written materials in alternative formats
- Computer-aided instruction
- Individualized rules for the student
- Recorded lectures
- Reduction of visual distractions
- Oral and printed directions
- Visual aids
- Using sticky notes to mark assignments in textbooks
- Handing out worksheets one at a time
- Provide study guides and questions that directly relate to tests
- Peer tutors
- Positive reinforcements
- Drawing arrows on worksheets, chalkboard, or overheads to show how ideas are related, or use other graphic organizers

Changes to Setting or Location
- Keeping the classroom quiet during intense learning times
- Using a study carrel
- Preferred seating assignments
- Providing separate location for testing with fewer distractions

Alternate Ways to Respond
- Audio versions of books to have the student follow text while listening
- Alternatives to long written reports (e.g., oral reports, audiovisual presentations, short written reviews)
- Designated note taker or a copy of other students' notes
- Dictating answers on assignments that require copying
- Reading test materials and allow the student to respond orally
- Additional time to complete a test
- Allowing take-home or open-book tests
- Arranging a "check-in" time to organize the day
- Enlarged graph paper to help the student keep numbers in columns

Changes to Timing or Scheduling
- Shortening assignments to focus on mastery of key concepts
- Minimizing the number and sequence of steps
- Fewer math problems on a worksheet page
- Frequent feedback
- Alerting student several minutes before a transition is planned; giving several reminders
- Standing near the student when giving directions or presenting a lesson

Sources. Council of Chief State School Officers (2005); Durheim (2017); Families and Advocates Partnership for Education (2001).

---

reduce learning expectations. Accommodations provided to a student must be the same for classroom instruction, classroom assessments, and district and state assessments (CCSSO, 2005).

Modification, however, is adjustment to a test or assignment that changes, lowers, or reduces what is measured or learned (CCSSO, 2005; Families and Advocates Partnership for Education, 2001), such as having a student complete part of an assignment or an alternative assignment, or revising assignments to make them easier. Decisions about any needed accommodation or modification should be based on the student's individual needs. All accommodations or modifications that will be provided must be included in this 504 plan. Many state departments of education have developed a list of accommodations that have been approved for use by local school districts. Exhibit 27.2 provides examples of accommodations and modifications that schools might provide for students.

Some schools may not allow related service providers to participate in Section 504 activities because their position is funded solely by IDEA funds. This is an administrative issue that can be adjusted within the district and should not be used as a means to exclude a student from benefiting from the expertise of an occupational therapist in developing an appropriate 504 plan.

Provide Interventions: Accommodations and Modifications

When determining occupational therapy interventions, school practitioners should consider accommodations before modifications. Interventions may also include services to teach students how to use the accommodation and to support them in gaining access. A best practice is to involve students in identifying the accommodations they will need. Staff training and education is another intervention school practitioners might use to ensure that staff know when and how to use a given accommodation appropriately.

When providing occupational therapy services, the occupational therapist is responsible for developing and documenting the occupational therapy intervention plan (e.g., occupation-based goals, intervention approach, methods of service delivery) that provides a framework for the implementation of the student's 504 plan (AOTA, 2017). Occupational therapy assistants may provide input for the plan, under the supervision of the occupational therapist.

Identify Outcomes

Unlike the individualized education program, which must be reviewed at least annually (and more frequently when needed), the 504 plan has no such requirements. Given the interest of most school districts in appropriately educating students, however, it is reasonable to expect school personnel to be willing to regularly discuss the effectiveness of a given student's 504 plan and to determine what adjustments, if any, might be needed to support success. Christensen et al. (2009) indicated the importance of monitoring as an important component of improving outcomes for students with disabilities. When the provision of accommodations is systematically attended to, students with disabilities are best able to show what they know and can do.

In a survey of general and special educators, Thurlow et al. (2017) found that most educators agreed that accommodations and other accessibility features have a positive impact on students who use them. This finding is supported by Troccoli (2017), who looked at the attitudes of college students with disabilities toward the use of accommodations. Accommodations were identified in this study as critical to the academic success of students with disabilities. Moreover, students with more positive attitudes about accommodations were more likely to use them (Troccoli, 2017).

SUMMARY

School occupational therapy is an important support for students with disabilities who are protected under Section 504 and the ADAAA. School practitioners need to position themselves within their schools to help administrators, teachers, and parents to understand the full breadth of occupational therapy expertise in identifying the underlying factors that both support and interfere with learning and school success.

Occupational therapy practitioners' deep understanding of student participation and engagement in learning-related occupations, activities, and routines makes them a natural fit to help schools provide equal educational opportunities for students with disabilities that will allow them to both access and benefit from the general education environment. The ultimate outcome of school occupational therapy services is to enable students to successfully participate in their learning and functional aspects of school and to support the school system in providing an appropriate public education for all students with and without disabilities.

REFERENCES

ADA Amendments Act of 2008, Pub. L. 110–325, 122 Stat. 3553.

American Occupational Therapy Association. (2014). Guidelines for supervision, roles, and responsibilities during the delivery of occupational therapy services. *American Journal of Occupational Therapy, 68*(Suppl. 3), S16–S22. https://doi.org/10.5014/ajot.2014.686S03

American Occupational Therapy Association. (2015a). Occupational therapy code of ethics (2015). *American Journal of Occupational Therapy, 69*(Suppl. 3), 6913410030. https://doi.org/10.5014/ajot.2015.696S03

American Occupational Therapy Association. (2015b). Standards of practice for occupational therapy. *American Journal of Occupational Therapy, 69*(Suppl. 3), 6913410057. https://doi.org/10.5014/ajot.2015.696S06

American Occupational Therapy Association. (2017). Guidelines for occupational therapy services in early intervention and schools. *American Journal of Occupational Therapy, 71*(Suppl. 2), 7112410010. https://doi. org/10.5014/ajot.2017.716S01

Americans With Disabilities Act of 1990, Pub. L. 101–336, 42 U.S.C. §§ 12101–12213.

Christensen, L. L., Thurlow, M. L., & Wang, T. (2009). *Improving accommodations outcomes: Monitoring instructional and assessment accommodations for students with disabilities.* Minneapolis: University of Minnesota, National Center on Educational Outcomes. Retrieved from https://nceo.umn.edu/docs/OnlinePubs/AccommodationsMonitoring.pdf

Council of Chief State School Officers. (2005). *Accommodations manual: How to select, administer, and evaluate use of accommodations for instruction and assessment of students with disabilities.* Retrieved from https://nceo.umn.edu/docs/OnlinePubs/AccommodationsManual.pdf

Durheim, M. (2017). *A parent's guide to Section 504 in public schools.* Retrieved from https://www.greatschools.org/gk/articles/section-504-2/

Every Student Succeeds Act, Pub. L. 114–195, 129 Stat. 1802 (2015).

Families and Advocates Partnership for Education. (2001). *School accommodations and modifications.* Retrieved from http://www.wrightslaw.com/info/sec504.accoms.mods.pdf

Fryer, W. (2009). *Federal or state responsibility for education and inequitable education funding formulas.* Retrieved from http://www.speedofcreativity.org/2009/01/14/federal-or-state-responsibility-for-education-and-inequitable-education-funding-formulas

Holmes, K. E. (2018). *Educators' attitudes towards implementation of inclusive education* (Master's thesis). Retrieved from http://scholarworks.lib.csusb.edu/etd/613

Howey, P. (2012). *Key differences between Section 504 and IDEA.* Retrieved from http://www.wrightslaw.com/howey/504.idea.htm

Individuals With Disabilities Education Improvement Act of 2004, Pub. L. 108–446, 20 U.S.C. §§ 1400–1482.

Jackson, L. (2013). Best practices in supporting students with a 504 plan. In G. F. Clark & B. E. Chandler (Eds.), *Best practices for occupational therapy in schools* (pp. 263–272). Bethesda, MD: AOTA Press.

Jerome, S. K. (2017). *An analysis of inclusion in the field of special education* (Honors thesis). Retrieved from http://firescholars.seu.edu/honors/65

LeMay, H. N. (2017). *Administrator and teacher attitudes toward inclusion* (Doctoral dissertation). Retrieved from http://dc.etsu.edu/etd/3278

Martín, J. L. (2010). *Determining eligibility under Section 504: Fundamentals and new challenge areas.* Retrieved from http://www.504idea.org/Council_Of_Educators/Resources_files/Modern%20504%20Eligibility.pdf

National Center on Educational Outcomes. (2015). *Making accessibility decisions for ALL students* (NCEO Brief No. 11). Minneapolis: University of Minnesota, National Center on Educational Outcomes. Retrieved from https://nceo.info/Resources/publications/OnlinePubs/briefs/brief11/brief11.html

No Child Left Behind Act of 2001, Pub. L. 107–110, 20 U.S.C. §§ 6301–8962.

Nondiscrimination on the basis of disability in state and local government services, 28 C.F.R. Part 35, §§ 35.101, 35.191–35.999. (1991).

Nondiscrimination on the basis of handicap in programs or activities receiving federal financial assistance, 45 C.F.R. Part 84, §§ 84.1–84.61. (1977).

Nondiscrimination on the basis of handicap in programs or activities receiving federal financial assistance, 34 C.F.R. Part 104, §§ 104.1–104.61. (1980).

PEER Project. (2008). *Section 504, the Americans with Disabilities Act, and education reform.* Retrieved from http://www.wrightslaw.com/info/section504.ada.peer.htm

Rehabilitation Act of 1973, Pub. L. 93–112, 29 U.S.C. §§ 701–796l.

Section 504 of the Rehabilitation Act of 1973, as amended, 29 U.S.C. § 794 (2008).

Thurlow, M. L., Larson, E. D., Lazarus, S. S., Shyyan, V. V., & Christensen, L. L. (2017). *Educators' experiences with and attitudes toward accessibility features and accommodations.* Minneapolis: University of Minnesota, Data Informed Accessibility—Making Optimal Needs-based Decisions (DIAMOND).

Thurlow, M. L., Lazarus, S. S., Christensen, L. L., & Shyyan, V. (2016). *Principles and characteristics of inclusive assessment systems in a changing assessment landscape* (NCEO Report 400). Minneapolis: University of Minnesota, National Center on Educational Outcomes. Retrieved from https://nceo.info/Resources/publications/OnlinePubs/Report400/default.html

Troccoli, A. E. (2017). *Attitudes toward accommodations and academic well-being of college students with disabilities* (Master's thesis). Retrieved from http://rdw.rowan.edu/etd/2408

U.S. Department of Education. (2012). *Questions and answers on the ADA Amendments Act of 2008 for students with disabilities attending public elementary and secondary schools.* Retrieved from http://www2.ed.gov/about/offices/list/ocr/docs/dcl-504faq-201109.html

U.S. Department of Education. (2016). *Disability discrimination.* Retrieved from https://www2.ed.gov/about/offices/list/ocr/front-page/faq/disability.html

U.S. Department of Education. (2017a). *IDEA Part B child count and educational environments for school year 2016–2017.* Retrieved from https://www2.ed.gov/programs/osepidea/618-data/collection-documentation/index.html

U.S. Department of Education. (2017b). *The Rehabilitation Act of 1973.* Retrieved from www2.ed.gov/policy/speced/reg/narrative.html

U.S. Department of Education, Office for Civil Rights. (2016). *Frequently asked questions about the rights of students with disabilities in public charter schools under Section 504 of the Rehabilitation Act of 1973.* Retrieved from https://www2.ed.gov/about/offices/list/ocr/docs/dcl-faq-201612-504-charter-school.pdf

U.S. Department of Health and Human Services, Office for Civil Rights. (2017). *Discrimination on the basis of disability.* Retrieved from https://www.hhs.gov/civil-rights/for-individuals/disability/index.html

Weber, M. C. (2011). *A new look at Section 504 and the ADA in special education cases.* Retrieved from https://apps.americanbar.org/litigation/committees/childrights/content/articles/summer2011-section-504-ada-idea.html

Wright, P., & Wright, P. (2012). *Key differences between Section 504, the IDEA, and the ADA.* Retrieved from http://www.wrightslaw.com/info/sec504.summ.rights.htm

Wrightslaw. (2008). My school district doesn't do 504s. Will a child study plan work? [Blog post]. Retrieved from http://www.wrightslaw.com/blog/my-district-doesnt-do-504s-will-a-child-study-plan-work/

Wrightslaw. (2012). What is the timeline for developing a Section 504 plan? [Blog post]. Retrieved from http://www.wright-slaw.com/blog/?p=7085

Best Practices in Supporting Students With Attention Deficit Hyperactivity Disorder

Gloria Frolek Clark, PhD, OTR/L, BCP, SCSS, FAOTA

28

KEY TERMS AND CONCEPTS

- Attention deficit hyperactivity disorder
- Executive function
- Multi-tiered systems of support
- Occupational profile
- Self-regulation

OVERVIEW

Attention deficit hyperactivity disorder (ADHD) is a childhood-onset neuropsychiatric disorder characterized by persistent and maladaptive symptoms of inattention, hyperactivity, and impulsivity (American Psychiatric Association [APA], 2013). As the most common neurobehavioral disorder of children, ADHD affects academic performance, well-being, and social interactions and is the top reason for referral for mental health treatment (American Academy of Pediatrics [AAP], 2011; APA, 2013).

On the basis of data from the National Health Interview Survey, a national, population-based, cross-sectional survey, approximately 10.2% of children in the United States in 2016 were diagnosed with ADHD (Xu et al., 2018)—an increase from 6.1% in 1997–1998. Several factors appear to be related to this increase, including expanded medical education for physicians that increased diagnosis in girls, public awareness, improved access to health care, and increased referral from primary health care providers to specialty mental health services.

There is no medical test to diagnose ADHD. The AAP (2011) recommends that the primary care clinician rule out other possible causes, determine that *Diagnostic and Statistical Manual of Mental Disorders* (5th ed., or *DSM–5*; APA, 2013) criteria have been met, and obtain information from parents and teachers (when applicable). Comorbid conditions (e.g., physical, developmental, mental health) should be assessed as well. Behavior rating scales and parent self-report measures are often used for a diagnostic evaluation.

The *DSM–5* criteria for the diagnosis of ADHD (APA, 2013) include

- A pattern (at least 6 months with negative impact on social and academic or occupational activities) of inattention or hyperactivity–impulsive behaviors that interfere with functioning or development (see Table 28.1);
- Several symptoms present before age 12 years;
- Symptoms present in 2 or more settings;
- Clear evidence that symptoms interfere with or reduce quality of academic, social, or occupational functioning; and
- Symptoms that are not better explained by another mental disorder.

Severity is determined by the number of symptoms present and their impact on functional performance (APA, 2013):

- *Mild*—few symptoms in excess of those needed for diagnosis; symptoms result in minor functional impairments
- *Moderate*—symptoms between the mild and severe categories
- *Severe*—many symptoms in excess of those needed for diagnosis; symptoms may be severe or present with marked impairment in social or occupational functioning.

Etiology is a complex mixture of genetic and environmental factors. Estimated heritability of ADHD is 70%–80% (Adams et al., 2013). Environmental factors are as follows:

- Prenatal (e.g., prenatal alcohol exposure, smoking),
- Perinatal (e.g., very low birthweight, increased pregnancy and birth complications), and
- Postnatal (e.g., malnutrition and dietary deficiency, iron deficiency, early social deprivation; National Institute of Mental Health, 2012).

Reduced volumes of white matter, midsagittal corpus callosum areas, and cortical thickening were also found in persons with ADHD compared with study control groups (Curatolo et al., 2010). Neurotransmitters, especially dopamine, have received much study related to ADHD because insufficient levels of dopamine can interfere with cognitive and executive functions (Antshel et al., 2011).

Studies by Neuman et al. (2007) found that joint effects of gene variants (of DRD4 and DAT1) along with prenatal exposure to substances such as cigarette smoke were associated with combined ADHD in children who were genetically susceptible. For example, maternal smoking increased the risk of ADHD 2.7 times (Milberger et al., 1996), and a direct relationship was found between maternal smoking during pregnancy and hyperactivity (Kotimaa et al., 2003). Very low birthweight and increased complications

Copyright © 2019 by the American Occupational Therapy Association. All rights reserved. To reuse this content, contact www.copyright.com.
https://doi.org/10.7139/2019.978-1-56900-591-0.028

TABLE 28.1. Inattentive and Hyperactivity–Impulsive Symptoms

INATTENTIVE SYMPTOMS	HYPERACTIVE–IMPULSIVE SYMPTOMS
▪ Does not give close attention to details	▪ Fidgets with hands or feet; squirms in seat
▪ Has difficulty sustaining attention	▪ Leaves seat when being seated is expected
▪ Does not listen when spoken to directly	▪ Runs or climbs when it is inappropriate (restless)
▪ Does not follow through or finish tasks	▪ Has difficulty playing quietly
▪ Has difficulty organizing tasks and activities	▪ Is often "on the go"
▪ Avoids tasks that require sustained mental effort	▪ Often talks excessively
▪ Loses things often	▪ Blurts out answers frequently
▪ Is easily distracted	▪ Has difficulty waiting turn
▪ Is forgetful in daily activities	▪ Interrupts or intrudes on others

Note. In each category, there must be 6 or more of the symptoms that lasted 6 months or more with a negative impact on social and academic–occupational activities (see the *Diagnostic and Statistical Manual of Mental Disorders* [5th ed.] for a complete description and examples). *Combined attention deficit hyperactivity disorder* is used when a person exhibits both inattention and hyperactive–impulsive symptoms.
Source. American Psychiatric Association (2013).

in pregnancy and birth produced a twofold increase in ADHD (Taylor & Rogers, 2005).

Shaw et al. (2012) conducted a systematic review of long-term outcomes of persons with ADHD that indicated that persons without treatment had poorer long-term outcomes in all categories (academic, antisocial behavior, driving, nonmedicinal drug use or addictive behavior, obesity, occupation, services use, self-esteem, and social function outcomes). Driving and obesity outcomes appeared the most responsive to treatment (72% of outcomes); drug use and addictive behavior (67%), antisocial behavior (50%), services use (50%), and occupation (33%) were less responsive. Comorbid conditions may have affected these outcomes.

Students with ADHD may require support to access, participate in, and progress in their educational program. ADHD affects *executive function* (EF), a set of cognitive processes such as working memory, attention, inhibitory control, and self-regulation (e.g., self-management, emotional, cognitive, behavioral regulation). In addition, motor and sensory deficits have been reported in children with ADHD.

Occupational therapy practitioners[1] address the needs of students with ADHD through general education, multi-tiered systems of support (MTSS), Section 504 plans, and special education and related services. The role of the occupational therapy practitioner is discussed further in the "Best Practices" section.

ESSENTIAL CONSIDERATIONS

Occupational therapy practitioners working with students with ADHD must be aware of comorbid conditions,

---

[1]*Occupational therapy practitioner* refers to both the occupational therapist and the occupational therapy assistant. The American Occupational Therapy Association (2014, p. S18) states, "The occupational therapist is responsible for all aspects of occupational therapy service delivery and is accountable for the safety and effectiveness of the occupational therapy service delivery process" and "must be directly involved in the delivery of services during the initial evaluation and regularly throughout the course of intervention. . . . The occupational therapy assistant delivers safe and effective occupational therapy services under the supervision of and in partnership with the occupational therapist."

medications, and impact on occupational performance. Students with ADHD have many strengths that should be identified and used when designing services.

Comorbid Conditions

Children with ADHD have an 80% chance of having at least 1 other condition (Kaplan et al., 2001). Comorbid conditions may include emotional (e.g., mood and anxiety disorders, depression, conduct disorders, oppositional defiant disorder), developmental (e.g., learning disabilities, language and motor delays), physical (e.g., sleep apnea, tics), and neurogenetic disorders (e.g., neurofibromatosis I, Fragile X syndrome; AAP, 2011; Biederman & Faraone, 2005).

Fifty percent of children with ADHD have developmental coordination disorder, a marked impairment in motor coordination that interferes with academic achievement and ADLs (Kadesjo & Gillberg, 1999; Pitcher et al., 2003). Compared with neurotypical children, children with ADHD are more likely to exhibit sensory processing challenges in all areas (Pfeiffer et al., 2015).

Mental health disorders such as depression, anxiety, and disruptive behavior disorders are common in children with ADHD. Halmoy et al. (2010) found that approximately 20% of adults with ADHD also have bipolar disorder, so it is important to enhance the mental health of students of all ages.

With age, hyperactivity and impulsivity tend to decrease, but attention and disorganization continue. Sometimes the hyperactivity may become more inward (e.g., restlessness, difficulty sleeping, impatient), but few longitudinal studies exist.

Medical and Behavioral Interventions

The Centers for Disease Control and Prevention (2018) reported that only 6 out of 10 children received some type of psychosocial treatment during their lives to deal with this condition (4 out of 10 received social skills training). The AAP (2011) has recommended cognitive–behavioral therapy and medication for children who are ages 6 years or older. A parent survey indicated that 43% of children were treated with medication alone, and fewer than 1 in 3 children received both.

Children receiving combined treatment (e.g., intensive behavioral intervention and medication) demonstrated better outcomes than children receiving medication alone or behavioral interventions only (Swanson et al., 2001); however, at the 8-year follow-up, no difference was found between the groups (Molina et al., 2009).

Occupational therapy practitioners must be aware of the medications prescribed by primary care providers, understand common side effects, and report observable data. Evidence is strong for stimulant medications and sufficient but not as strong for atomoxetine (e.g., Strattera), extended-release guanfacine (Intuniv ER), and extended-release clonidine (Kapvay). Stimulant medication includes short-acting (e.g., Adderall, Dexedrine, Focalin, Ritalin), intermediate-acting (e.g., Evekeo, Ritalin SR), and long-acting (e.g., Adzenys XR-ODT, Focalin XR, Adderall XR, Vyvanse, Concerta, Daytrana, Ritalin LA). Stimulants are not habit forming in doses that are used for children and teens with ADHD.

People with ADHD who use medication have a lower rate of substance abuse than people with ADHD who are not treated. People should not take stimulants when they have severe anxiety, glaucoma, tics, Tourette's syndrome, or a history of psychosis or if they have taken a monoamine oxidase inhibitor within 14 days of starting a stimulant. Common side effects of stimulants (e.g., headache, upset stomach, higher blood pressure) usually go away after a few weeks as the person's body adjusts to the medication.

Positive Attributes of ADHD

Although ADHD is considered a chronic condition and has many negative connotations, people with ADHD see the positive aspects of their condition. Some traits of persons with ADHD include humor, drive, passion, ability to channel attention into work (e.g., artists, scientists), brightness, creativity, a commitment to helping others who need different things to succeed (e.g., compassion), willingness to take a risk, spontaneity, and high energy (ADDitude, 2018). Applying a strengths-based approach, occupational therapy practitioners can identify and frame students' strengths during team discussions and planning.

Impact on Occupations

Any area of occupation may be challenging. The ability to attend, concentrate, plan, and organize can impair occupations (e.g., ADLs, IADLs, education, work, play, leisure, rest and sleep, social participation). Self-care skills such as dressing, grooming, and eating may be affected. Social play and interactions are often affected. Research indicates that students with ADHD have lower grades, higher dropout rates, and higher absenteeism (DuPaul et al., 2011). Goldston et al. (2007) found that teenagers with reading problems were more likely to have ADHD, experience anxiety and depression, use drugs, have problems socially, think about harming themselves, or avoid adult responsibilities. Executive dysfunction may affect occupations such as self-care, academics, leisure, and social participation (Antshel et al., 2014; Tseng & Gau, 2013).

Increased risk behaviors are common in people with ADHD, including substance use, risky driving, and risky sexual behavior. The leading cause of death and disability among adolescents is car accidents (Koisaari et al., 2015). Compared with adolescents with ADHD who were taking methylphenidate (MPH; Ritalin), adolescents with ADHD who are not taking MPH have an increased risk for center-line crossings, road-edge excursions, and driving faster while driving a simulator (Ratzon et al., 2017). Although school occupational therapy practitioners may not be responsible for teaching driving instruction, they may educate parents and teachers about activities to enhance skills needed for driving.

A study comparing teenagers with ADHD and autism spectrum disorder with peers indicated significant errors in visual acuity, selective attention, cognition, visual–motor integration, and motor performance (Classen et al., 2013). Classen et al. (2013) found errors using a driving stimulator that included difficulty with visual scanning, speed regulation, lane maintenance, adjustment to stimuli, and total driving errors. They also found moderate correlations between impaired functioning on visual–motor integration and motor performance and driving errors.

Motor performance issues are reported in 30%–50% of children with ADHD (Fliers et al., 2009). These issues may include fine motor control, dexterity, bilateral coordination, balance, gross motor coordination, and postural control. These performance skills affect ADLs, academic skills, play, and leisure skills, resulting in a negative impact on participation, self-esteem, and self-concept.

Davies and Tucker (2010) found multiple studies indicating sensory modulation difficulties such as increased sensory seeking, sensory sensitivity, and avoiding in children with ADHD compared with peers. One study found increased cortical brain activity to somatosensory stimulation and significantly more tactile defensiveness compared with peers (Parush et al., 1997). Other studies have suggested adolescents with ADHD have more difficulty in sustaining eye tracking on moving objects, especially when extended visual attention is required. Despite these barriers, most people with ADHD engage in happy and productive lives.

BEST PRACTICES

Students with ADHD may have minor or severe symptoms affecting access, participation, and performance. Occupational therapy practitioners should screen all areas to determine which support or impede occupational performance. This section reviews evidence-based research in evaluation and intervention for students with ADHD.

Educate and Collaborate With Family as a Team Member

Educating parents with information about the condition, impact of occupational performance, and effective methods of discipline (e.g., modification of the environment or student's pattern of thinking or interactions) is necessary. Research indicates that positive interaction and support from parents allows children to achieve better long-term outcomes (Harrison & Sofronoff, 2002; Hinojosa et al., 2002).

Consider MTSS

When a student in general education indicates difficulty with occupations (e.g., coloring, writing, social interactions, toileting and hygiene skills), the occupational therapist may be asked to provide professional development for the teaching staff or screen the student to determine strategies to enhance general education performance. *MTSS* is an umbrella term for tiered intervention supports, such as positive behavioral interventions and supports (PBIS), response to intervention, and school mental health. (For more information, see Chapter 26, "Best Practices in Multi-Tiered Systems of Support.") Students with ADHD can often benefit from a varying intensity of support throughout their school years.

Evaluate Students' Strengths and Needs

The purpose of an occupational therapy evaluation under the Individuals With Disabilities Education Improvement Act of 2004 (IDEA; Pub. L. 108–446) is to contribute information to the team for decision making to determine whether the student has a disability (one of the IDEA categorical labels) and identify educational needs to decide whether special education and related services are necessary. If the student does not present with educational needs, eligibility for a Section 504 plan should be considered (see Chapter 27, "Best Practices in Supporting Students With a 504 Plan").

The evaluation process should include an *occupational profile* (summary of the student's current concerns and ability to access and participate in occupations). Data should be collected using multiple methods of data collection (e.g., record review, interview, observation, various tools) across multiple settings (e.g., classroom, outdoors, hallways, lunchroom, bathrooms, locker room) to formulate a hypothesis regarding the student's performance strengths and limitations.

Conduct Evidence-Based Intervention to Facilitate Performance and Participation

Interventions should focus on educating the family and teacher in classroom interventions to enhance participation in occupations. Using a person–occupation or activity–environment model allows the practitioner to observe and enhance interactions between these components.

Consider student, occupation, and environment

Chu and Reynolds (2007) presented a model of practice for children with ADHD that considers the child, task, and environment. Results of the family-centered program showed statistically significant changes in scores on at least 1 of the subscales, and 11 children showed statistically significant changes in scores in either 1 or both of the total scales of the whole ADHD Rating Scales. Intervention included education of parents and teachers about ADHD; sensory modulation techniques; adaptation of home or classroom environments and routines; integrated educational management strategies, behavioral management strategies, and sensory modulation techniques to promote the student's engagement in different tasks; and remediation of any developmental or functional challenges that interfere (e.g., self-care, handwriting, visual–motor).

Although this program was used in community-based settings, school occupational therapy practitioners may be able to apply most of this information to their practice.

Consider academic needs

Students who are interested and motivated are more likely to endure when challenges in learning occur. Modifications to the environment may be necessary to decrease visual and auditory distractions (e.g., quiet, free of distractions). DuPaul et al. (2011) found that specific training in study and organizational skills, note taking, social skills, and self-regulation were effective. In addition, on-task behavior and performance may be enhanced by computer programs for academic areas such as math, reading, and writing. Last, incorporating peers as tutors or during interventions has a positive impact on school performance as well as social skills (Daley & Birchwood, 2010).

The classroom environment should be relatively calm with clear expectations. A teacher who is structured and uses PBIS increases the chance of appropriate performance. Using concepts in universal design for learning (see Chapter 20, "Best Practices in Universal Design for Learning") and providing multiple methods of instruction and representation of learning should be encouraged. Many students with ADHD need to move, so classes that are primarily auditory lecture may result in increased negative behaviors.

Add movement to student routine

Aerobic exercise has a moderate to large effect on the core symptoms of ADHD (e.g., attention, hyperactivity, impulsivity, EF, related conditions such as social disorders and anxiety), and short-term exercise has the best outcome (e.g., 50 minutes/day, 2–3 times per week, for 5 weeks at 50%–75% maximum heart rate; Archer & Kostrzewa, 2012; Cerrillo-Urbina et al., 2015; Gapin et al., 2011). Active participation in physical education and activities improves EF in children with ADHD (Grassmann et al., 2017).

Enhance EF

Occupational therapy practitioners use various cognitive programs to enhance EF and participation in children with ADHD. The Cognitive–Functional (Cog–Fun) intervention was based on cognitive rehabilitation models in occupational therapy (Maeir et al., 2012) and addresses cognitive, emotional, and environmental barriers to participation in their context. The aim of Cog–Fun is to promote acquisition of executive strategies and self-efficacy in occupational performance (Hahn-Markowitz et al., 2017). Cog–Fun improves EF and participation among children with ADHD (Hahn-Markowitz et al., 2017; Rosenberg et al., 2015).

Another cognitive intervention is the Cognitive Orientation to daily Occupational Performance (CO–OP; Dawson et al., 2017; Miller et al., 2001). CO–OP is a problem-solving approach initially used for children with developmental coordination disorder, and it is an effective intervention for children with ADHD. Increases in motor performance and improvements in self-goals (e.g., handwriting, cutting, washing hands, dressing, reading, catching, soccer) were observed in children with ADHD (Gharebaghy et al., 2015).

Address self-regulation and build coping skills

Children with ADHD have sensory deficits across all modalities (Dunn & Bennet, 2002). Programs to enhance *self-regulation* (e.g., ability to regulate sensation, behavior, emotions) can be used with students who have ADHD. The development of self-regulation requires coregulation, which is provided by caregiving adults (e.g., parents, teachers) through warm and responsive interaction that can model and support the student to express thoughts and behavior in an appropriate and excepted manner (Murray et al., 2016). A student must be motivated to self-regulate through external sources (e.g., rewards, consequences) or intrinsic motivation (e.g., internal values, goals).

Curricula have been developed by occupational therapists for self-regulation and are typically run by or with the input of occupational therapy practitioners. These curricula include the Alert Program (Williams & Shellenberger, 1996) and the Zones of Regulation (Kuypers, 2011). Both programs are easy to use, provide terminology to explain various factors, use visual examples and multiple practice opportunities, and link the information to natural routines. For example, the Alert Program discusses engines that run too fast, too slow, or just right. This program was developed to address EF skills in children. The Zones of Regulation provides a colored chart with various facial expressions that can be used to provide the student with input regarding the "zone" the student is currently in.

The evidence for weighted vests and stability balls is limited and insufficient for children with ADHD. Studies are usually small in number and have not been conducted in natural settings. For example, Lin et al. (2014) found immediate effects on attention and behavioral performance when children wore a weighted vest loaded at 10% of the child's body weight, but this study was conducted in a controlled laboratory area, not during functional performance in a classroom.

Occupational therapy practitioners should always use the best evidence available when developing interventions. When the only evidence for an intervention is low, practitioners may implement a short trial of the intervention and systematically collect ongoing data to determine the effectiveness of the intervention. The intervention should be terminated if there are adverse reactions or if progress (beyond typical growth) is not noted.

SUMMARY

Approximately 1 in 10 (5.4 million) children in the United States has ADHD that may affect participation in academic, behavior, and occupational functioning. Students with ADHD often display problems with sensory, learning, motor, or mental health conditions. School occupational therapy practitioners have the knowledge to modify the task and environment, educate staff and parents, and provide interventions to students so that they can benefit from their educational program.

REFERENCES

Adams, P. F., Kirzinger, W. K., & Martinez, M. (2013). Summary health statistics for the US population: National Health Interview Survey, 2012. *Vital and Health Statistics, 10*(259), 1–95.

ADDitude. (2018). *17 things to love about ADHD.* Retrieved from https://www.additudemag.com/slideshows/benefits-of-adhd-to-love/

American Academy of Pediatrics. (2011). ADHD: Clinical practice guidelines for the diagnosis, evaluation, and treatment of attention-deficit/hyperactivity disorder in children and adolescents. *Pediatrics, 128,* 1–16. https://doi.org/10.1542/peds.2011-2654

American Occupational Therapy Association. (2014). Guidelines for supervision, roles, and responsibilities during the delivery of occupational therapy services. *American Journal of Occupational Therapy, 68*(Suppl. 3), S16–S22. https://doi.org/10.5014/ajot.2014.686S03

American Psychiatric Association. (2013). *Diagnostic and statistical manual of mental disorders* (5th ed.). Arlington, VA: American Psychiatric Publishing.

Antshel, K. M., Hargrave, T., Simonescu, M., Kaul, P., Hendricks, K., & Faraone, S. V. (2011). Advances in understanding and treating ADHD. *BMC Medicine, 9,* 72. https://doi.org/10.1186/1741-7015-9-72

Antshel, K. M., Hier, B. O., & Barkley, R. (2014). Executive functioning theory and ADHD. In S. Goldstein & J. Naglieri (Eds.), *Handbook of executive functioning* (pp. 107–120). New York: Springer.

Archer, T., & Kostrzewa, R. M. (2012). Physical exercise alleviates ADHD symptoms: Regional deficits and developmental trajectory. *Neurotoxicity Research, 21,* 195–209. https://doi.org/10.1007/s12640-011-9260-0

Biederman, J., & Faraone, S. V. (2005). Attention-deficit hyperactivity disorder. *Lancet, 366,* 237–248. https://doi.org/10.1016/S0140-6736(05)66915-2

Centers for Disease Control and Prevention. (2018). *Attention-deficit/hyperactivity disorder (ADHD): Data and statistics.* Retrieved from https://www.cdc.gov/ncbddd/adhd/data.html

Cerrillo-Urbina, A. J., Garcia-Hermoso, A., Sanchez-Lopex, M., Pardo-Guijarro, J. J., Santos Gomex, J. L., & Martinex-Vizcaino, V. (2015). The effect of physical exercise in children with attention deficit hyperactivity disorder: A systematic review and meta-analysis of randomized control trials. *Child: Care, Health and Development, 41,* 779–788. https://doi.org/10.1111/cch.12255

Chu, S., & Reynolds, F. (2007). Occupational therapy for children with attention deficit hyperactivity disorder (ADHD), Part 1: A delineation model of practice. *British Journal of Occupational Therapy, 70,* 372–383. https://doi.org/10.1177/030802260707000902

Classen, S., Monahan, M., & Wang, Y. (2013). Driving characteristics of teens with attention deficit hyperactivity and autism spectrum disorder. *American Journal of Occupational Therapy, 67,* 664–673. http://dx.doi.org/10.5014/ajot.2013.008821

Curatolo, P., D'Agati, E., & Moavero, R. (2010). The neurobiological basis of ADHD. *Italian Journal of Pediatrics, 36*(79), 1–7. https://doi.org/10.1186/1824-7288-36-79

Daley, D., & Birchwood, J. (2010). ADHD and academic performance: Why does ADHD impact on academic performance and what can be done to support ADHD children in the classroom? *Child Care Health Development, 36,* 455–464. https://doi.org/10.1111/j.1365-2214.2009.01046.x

Davies, P. L., & Tucker, R. (2010). Evidence review to investigate the support for subtypes of children with difficulty processing and integrating sensory information. *American Journal of Occupational Therapy, 64,* 391–402. https://doi.org/10.5014/ajot.2010.09070

Dawson, D., McEwen, S. E., & Polatajko, H. J. (2017). *Cognitive Orientation to daily Occupational Performance in Occupational Therapy: Using the CO–OP Approach™ to enable participation across the lifespan.* Bethesda, MD: AOTA Press.

Dunn, W., & Bennett, D. (2002). Patterns of sensory processing in children with attention deficit hyperactivity disorder. *OTJR: Occupation, Participation and Health, 22,* 4–15. https://doi.org/10.1177/153944920202200102

DuPaul, G. J., Weyant, L., & Janusis, G. (2011). ADHD in the classroom: Effective intervention strategies. *Theory Into Practice, 50*(1), 35–42. https://doi.org/10.1080/00405841.2011.534935

Fliers, E. A., Franke, B., Lambregts-Rommelse, N. N., Altink, M. E., Buschgens, C. J., Nijhuis-van der Sanden, M. W., . . . Buitelaar, J. K. (2009). Undertreatment of motor problems in children with ADHD. *Child and Adolescent Mental Health, 15,* 85–90. https://doi.org/10.1111/j.1475-3588.2009.00538.x

Gapin, J. I., Labban, J. D., & Etnier, J. L. (2011). The effects of physical activity on attention deficit hyperactivity disorder symptoms: The evidence. *Preventive Medicine, 52*(Suppl. 1), S70–S74. https://doi.org/10.1016/j.ypmed.2011.01.022

Gharebaghy, S., Rassafiani, M., & Cameron, D. (2015). Effect of cognitive intervention on children with ADHD. *Physical and Occupational Therapy in Pediatrics, 35*(1), 13–23. https://doi.org/10.3109/01942638.2014.957428

Goldston, D., Walsh, A., Arnold, E., Reboussin, B., Daniel, S., Erkanli, A., . . . Wood, F., (2007). Reading problems, psychiatric disorders, and functional impairment from mid- to late adolescence. *Journal of the American Academy of Child and Adolescent Psychiatry, 46,* 25–32. https://doi.org/10.1097/01.chi.0000242241.77302.f4

Grassman, V., Alves, M. V., Santos-Galduroz, R. F., & Galduroz, J. C. (2017). Possible cognitive benefits of acute physical exercise in children with ADHD: A systematic review. *Journal of Attention Disorders, 21,* 367–371. https://doi.org/10.1177/1087054714526041

Hahn-Markowitz, J., Berger, I., Manor, I., & Maeir, A. (2017). Impact of the Cognitive–Functional (Cog–Fun) intervention on executive functions and participation among children with attention deficit hyperactivity disorder: A randomized controlled trial. *American Journal of Occupational Therapy, 71,* 7105220010. https://doi.org/10.5014/ajot.2017.022053

Halmoy, A., Halleland, H., Dramsdahl, M., Bergsholm, P., Fasmer, O. B., & Haavik, J. (2010). Bipolar symptoms in adult attention-deficit/hyperactivity disorder: A cross-sectional study of 510 clinically diagnosed patients and 417 population-based controls. *Journal of Clinical Psychiatry, 71*(1), 48–57. https://doi.org/10.4088/JCP.08m04722ora

Harrison, C., & Sofronoff, K. (2002). ADHD and parental psychological distress: Role of demographics, child behavioural characteristics, and parental cognitions. *Journal of the American Academy of Child and Adolescent Psychiatry, 41,* 703–711. https://doi.org/10.1097/00004583-200206000-00010

Hinojosa, J., Sproat, C. T., Mankhetwit, S., & Anderson, J. (2002). Shifts in parent–therapist partnerships: Twelve years of change.

American Journal of Occupational Therapy, 56, 556–563. https://doi.org/10.5014/ajot.56.5.556

Individuals With Disabilities Education Improvement Act of 2004, Pub. L. 108–446, 20 U.S.C. §§ 1400–1482.

Kadesjo, B., & Gillberg, C. (1999). Developmental coordination disorder in Swedish 7-year-old children. *Journal of the American Academy of Child and Adolescent Psychiatry, 38,* 820–828. https://doi.org/10.1097/00004583-199907000-00011

Kaplan, B. J., Dewey, D. M., Crawford, S. G., & Wilson, B. N. (2001). The term comorbidity is of questionable value in reference to developmental disorders: Data and theory. *Journal of Learning Disabilities, 34,* 555–565. https://doi.org/10.1177/002221940103400608

Koisaari, T., Michelsson, K., Holopainen, J. M., Maksimainen, R., Päivänsalo, J., Rantala, K., & Tervo, T. (2015). Traffic and criminal behavior of adults with attention deficit–hyperactivity with a prospective follow-up from birth to the age of 40 years. *Traffic Injury Prevention, 16,* 824–830. https://doi.org/10.1080/15389588.2015.1029068

Kotimaa, A. J., Moilanen, I., Taanila, A., Ebeling, H., Smalley, S. L., McGough, J. J., . . . Jarvelin, M. R. (2003). Maternal smoking and hyperactivity in 8-year-old children. *Journal of the American Academy of Child and Adolescent Psychiatry, 42,* 826–883. https://doi.org/10.1097/01.CHI.0000046866.56865.A2

Kuypers, L. (2011). *The Zones of Regulation.* San Jose, CA: Think Social.

Lin, H.-Y., Lee, P., Chang, W.-D., & Hong, F.-Y. (2014). Effects of weighted vests on attention, impulse control, and on-task behavior in children with attention deficit hyperactivity disorder. *American Journal of Occupational Therapy, 68,* 149–158. https://doi.org/10.5014/ajot.2014.009365

Maeir, A., Hahn-Markowitz, J., Fisher, O., & Traub Bar-Ilan, R. (2012). *Cognitive–Functional (Cog–Fun) intervention in occupational therapy for children aged 5–10 with ADHD: Treatment manual.* Jerusalem: Hadassah and Hebrew University, Faculty of Medicine, School of Occupational Therapy.

Milberger, S., Biederman, J., Faraone, S. V., Chen, L., & Jones, J. (1996). Is maternal smoking during pregnancy a risk factor for attention deficit hyperactivity disorder in children? *American Journal of Psychiatry, 153,* 1138–1142. https://doi.org/10.1176/ajp.153.9.1138

Miller, L., Polatajko, H., Missiuna, C., Mandich, A., & Macnab, J. (2001). A pilot trial of a cognitive treatment for children with developmental coordination disorder. *Human Movement Science, 20,* 183–210. https://doi.org/10.1016/S0167-9457(01)00034-3

Molina, B. S., Hinshaw, S. P., Swanson, J. M., Arnold, L. E., Vitiello, B., Jensen, P. S., . . . Houck, P. R.; MTA Cooperative Group. (2009). The MTA at 8 years: Prospective follow-up of children treated for combined-type ADHD in a multisite study. *Journal of the American Academy of Child and Adolescent Psychiatry, 48,* 484–500. https://doi.org/10.1097/CHI.0b013e31819c23d0

Murray, D. W., Rosanbalm, K., & Christopoulos, C. (2016). *Self regulation and toxic stress: Seven key principles of self regulation in context* (OPRE Report No. 2016-39). Washington, DC: U.S. Department of Health and Human Services.

National Institute of Mental Health. (2012). *Attention-deficit/hyperactivity disorder (ADHD).* Retrieved from https://www.nimh.nih.gov/health/statistics/attention-deficit-hyperactivity-disorder-adhd.shtml

Neuman, R. J., Lobos, E., Reich, W., Henderson, C. A., Sun, L. W., & Todd, R. D. (2007). Prenatal smoking exposure and dopaminergic genotypes interact to cause a severe ADHD subtype. *Biological Psychiatry, 61,* 1320–1328. https://doi.org/10.1016/j.biopsych.2006.08.049

Parush, S., Sohmer, H., Steinberg, A., & Kaitz, M. (1997). Somatosensory functioning in children with attention deficit hyperactivity disorder. *Developmental Medicine and Child Neurology, 39,* 464–468. https://doi.org/10.1111/j.1469-8749.1997.tb07466.x

Pfeiffer, B., Daly, B. P., Nicholls, E. G., & Gullo, D. F. (2015). Assessing sensory processing problems in children with and without attention deficit hyperactivity disorder. *Physical and Occupational Therapy in Pediatrics, 35*(1), 1–12. https://doi.org/10.3109/01942638.2014.904471

Pitcher, T. M., Piek, J. P., & Hay, D. A. (2003). Fine and gross motor ability in males with ADHD. *Developmental Medicine and Child Neurology, 45,* 525–535. https://doi.org/10.1111/j.1469-8749.2003.tb00952.x

Ratzon, N. Z., Lunievsky, E. K., Ashkenasi, A., Laks, J., & Cohen, H. A. (2017). Simulated driving skills evaluation of teenagers with attention deficit hyperactivity disorder before driving lessons. *American Journal of Occupational Therapy, 71,* 7103220010. https://doi.org/10.5014/ajot.2017.020164

Rosenberg, L., Maeir, A., Yochman, A., Dahan, I., & Hirsch, I. (2015). Effectiveness of a cognitive–functional group intervention among preschoolers with attention deficit hyperactivity disorder: A pilot study. *American Journal of Occupational Therapy, 69,* 6903220040. http://dx.doi.org/10.5014/ajot.2015.014795

Shaw, M., Hodgkins, P., Caci, H., Young, S., Kahle, J., Woods, A., & Arnold, L. E. (2012). A systematic review and analysis of long-term outcomes in attention deficit hyperactivity disorder: Effects of treatment and non-treatment. *BMC Medicine, 10,* 99. https://doi.org/10.1186/1741-7015-10-99

Swanson, J. M., Kraemer, H. C., Hinshaw, S. P., Arnold, L. E., Conners, C. K., Abikoff, H. B., . . . Wu, M. (2001). Clinical relevance of the primary findings of the MTA: Success rates based on severity of ADHD and ODD symptoms at the end of treatment. *Journal of the American Academy of Child and Adolescent Psychiatry, 40,* 168–179. https://doi.org/10.1097/00004583-200102000-00011

Taylor, E., & Rogers, J. W. (2005). Practitioner review: Early adversity and developmental disorders. *Journal of Child Psychology and Psychiatry, 46,* 451–467. https://doi.org/10.1111/j.1469-7610.2004.00402.x

Tseng, W.-L., & Gau, S. S. (2013). Executive function as a mediator in the link between attention-deficit/hyperactivity disorder and social problems. *Journal of Child Psychology and Psychiatry, 54,* 996–1004. https://doi.org/10.1111/jcpp.12072

Williams, M. S., & Shellenberger, S. (1996). *"How does your engine run?" A leader's guide to the Alert Program for self-regulation.* Albuquerque, NM: Therapy Works.

Xu, G., Strathearn, L., Liu, B., Yang, B., & Bao, W. (2018). Twenty-year trends in diagnosed attention-deficit/hyperactivity disorder among US children and adolescents, 1997–2016. *JAMA Network Open, 1*(4), e181471. https://doi.org/10.100/jamanetworkopen.2018.1471

Best Practices in Supporting Students With Autism

29

Heather Kuhaneck, PhD, OTR/L, FAOTA, and Renee Watling, PhD, OTR/L, FAOTA

KEY TERMS AND CONCEPTS

- Antecedent approaches
- Autism
- Ayres Sensory Integration®
- Positive reinforcement
- Socially significant behaviors
- Strengths-based approach
- Universal design for learning

OVERVIEW

In the United States, it is currently estimated that 1 in 59 children is diagnosed with autism spectrum disorder (ASD; Baio et al., 2018) and that access to diagnosis and treatment services remains disparate across geographic and socioeconomic factors (Boswell et al., 2014; Durkin et al., 2017). In schools, the student with autism may have a medical diagnosis, educational diagnosis, or both.

Medical and educational diagnoses are not synonymous. The *Diagnostic and Statistical Manual of Mental Disorders* (5th ed.; *DSM–5;* American Psychiatric Association [APA], 2013) is used by medical and psychiatric professionals to diagnose mental health conditions. A medical diagnosis is typically provided by a medical professional, usually a doctor or psychiatrist, in order to obtain necessary medical and health-related services in the community. When given as an educational diagnosis, the term used is **autism,** which is defined by the Individuals With Disabilities Education Improvement Act of 2004 (IDEA; Pub. L. 108–446) as

> a developmental disability significantly affecting verbal and nonverbal communication and social interaction, generally evident before age three, that adversely affects a child's educational performance. Other characteristics associated with autism are engagement in repetitive activities and stereotyped movements, resistance to environmental change or change in daily routines, and unusual responses to sensory experiences. (34 C.F.R. § 300.8 [c][1][i-iii])

An educational diagnosis is documented via a thorough multidisciplinary assessment from a variety of professionals on the educational team and is meant to assist the team in developing and delivering an appropriate educational program.

Key features of ASD indicated in the diagnostic criteria of the *DSM–5* (APA, 2013) include difficulties with social communication and behavior, limited interests, repetitive movements or behaviors, need for routine and sameness, and atypical sensory reactivity. The term *ASD,* as opposed to *autism,* was chosen for *DSM–5* to reflect the significant variation in profiles of persons with the disorder in terms of both strengths and difficulties (APA, 2013).

Occupational therapy practitioners[1] may function as specialized instructional support personnel for a student with ASD in general education (Every Student Succeeds Act [ESSA], 2015; Pub. L. 114–95) as a related service provider to assist a special education teacher in improving the educational performance of a student with ASD (IDEA, 2004) or as a building team member to determine modifications for a student with ASD in general education (Section 504 of the Rehabilitation Act of 1973, as amended [2008]; Pub. L. 93–112). Occupational therapy practitioners promote access and participation of students in all aspects of classroom and school routine, including academic performance; social interaction; play with peers; and engagement in extracurricular, afterschool, and sports activities. Occupational therapy practitioners are important team members because of their ability to consider the student, the educational environment, and the specific educational activity to enhance and optimize student performance.

ESSENTIAL CONSIDERATIONS

Students with ASD present with complex patterns of strengths and challenges that, combined with the tasks required of

---

[1]*Occupational therapy practitioner* refers to both the occupational therapist and the occupational therapy assistant. The American Occupational Therapy Association (AOTA; 2014, p. S18) states, "The occupational therapist is responsible for all aspects of occupational therapy service delivery and is accountable for the safety and effectiveness of the occupational therapy service delivery process" and "must be directly involved in the delivery of services during the initial evaluation and regularly throughout the course of intervention. . . . The occupational therapy assistant delivers safe and effective occupational therapy services under the supervision of and in partnership with the occupational therapist."

Copyright © 2019 by the American Occupational Therapy Association. All rights reserved. To reuse this content, contact www.copyright.com.
https://doi.org/10.7139/2019.978-1-56900-591-0.029

them in the classroom and the sensory and social aspects of the environment, may lead to a multitude of performance difficulties and limited participation.

Common Educational Strengths

Recent research documents unique strengths or *special skills* of persons with ASD; the most common is a special skill in memory, reported in 52% of participants with ASD (Meilleur et al., 2015). Other special skills include visuospatial, reading, drawing, music, and computation skills. Special skills were most commonly noted in older children with ASD and those with higher scores on measures of intelligence (Meilleur et al., 2015). Special interests such as machines and technology, numerical systems, sports and games, particular objects, sensory experiences, factual information, sorting and organizing, food and drink, animals, and sciences such as chemistry or meteorology are also commonly reported in persons with ASD (Caldwell-Harris & Jordan, 2014).

Common Educational Difficulties

Academic performance in persons with ASD is highly variable. Multiple studies have reported discrepancies between academic achievement and intellectual ability, but predictors of academic performance include verbal and nonverbal IQ, social behavior, and sensory responsiveness (Keen et al., 2016).

Challenging behaviors

Behavior problems reported among school-age persons with ASD include both active and passive behaviors. Active behaviors include verbal or physical aggression directed toward self, environment, or others; sexualized behavior; and elopement (Jang et al., 2011). Passive behaviors include poor initiation in response to instructional cues; poor attention to task; uncooperativeness; and lack of engagement in classroom, playground, or other specialist activities. Behavior challenges may be due to poor understanding of expectations, mismatch between performance demands and student capabilities, poor self-regulation, ineffective communication skills, poor sensory processing, or a learned behavior pattern and can vary with student age and relevant social norms.

Because managing change can be difficult for youth with ASD, the transitions that occur while attending school may create particular barriers to successful performance. Within each school day, there are multiple transitions between activities that may become stressful for the person with ASD. Each of these transitions may prompt anxiety or behavioral difficulties. Managing behaviors during transitions can be an important intervention area for the educational team.

Sensory processing

Atypical sensory processing, including poor praxis, is a common feature of ASD (Marco et al., 2011). Classrooms are sensory-intense environments, increasing the potential for mismatch between students' sensory needs and their daily sensory experiences at school (Kuhaneck & Kelleher, 2015; Miller Kuhaneck & Kelleher, 2018). Students with sensory difficulties may be unable to tolerate the noises and visual stimuli in the classroom, the smells of the cafeteria, or the frequent touching and bumping of other students, resulting in avoidant or explosive behaviors. Uncomfortable sensory experiences, particularly with noise, may increase a student's repetitive behaviors (Kanakri et al., 2017). Students may also have difficulties with classroom self-care such as shoe tying or challenges with playground equipment or physical education activities because of problems with motor skills resulting from poor sensory integration and dyspraxia (Kaur et al., 2018; Smith Roley et al., 2015).

Social skills difficulties

Consistent with the diagnostic criteria for ASD (APA, 2013), poor social skills development is frequently noted, but social function varies widely, with each student displaying a unique profile of strengths and challenges. Social difficulties can stem from challenges with development and social use of communication skills; poor understanding of social pragmatics; anxiety related to social engagement; and limitations in cognition, executive function (EF), or awareness of and conformation with social norms for appearance or behavior.

The social challenges that occur as a result of the symptoms of ASD often leave youth with ASD open to social isolation, loneliness, and bullying from their peers (Deckers et al., 2017). Risk factors for bullying include age, behavioral difficulties, attending a public school, and being in an inclusive classroom (Hebron et al., 2017). Bullying can lead to loneliness and increased awareness of differentness as students with ASD age, putting them at high risk for depression and anxiety, which further hinders their performance.

Some studies suggest that 35% to almost 40% of students with ASD have comorbid anxiety disorders, whereas 30% of those with ASD have comorbid depression (Strang et al., 2012; van Steensel et al., 2011). As youth with ASD experience puberty, challenges with sexuality and dating may emerge, and remain as a result of lack of experience or education, difficulties with communication, or sensory dysregulation (Barnett & Maticka-Tyndale, 2015).

BEST PRACTICES

Occupational therapy practitioners who work with students with ASD must be aware of the students' limitations and challenges as well as their unique strengths and interests in order to best serve them and assist their teachers. There has been an explosion of research on ASD, providing practitioners with many evidence-based practices to choose from for evaluation and intervention.

Support Team Collaboration for Participation in Least Restrictive Environment

Collaboration between the professionals working with an individual student has extensive support as best practice. Students with ASD frequently receive services from a multitude of professionals in school as well as outside of the school context. Given the multiple professionals involved in providing care, it is possible to discover overlap in areas of expertise. School teams should discuss the primary concerns for the student, identify the merits of the philosophical approaches being recommended, and assess the goodness of fit between each approach and the student's needs. Any inaccuracies in the understanding of occupational therapy should be clarified, including the role of the occupational therapy practitioner and the potential benefit of the various evidence-based interventions that practitioners can provide.

Behavior analytic services often overlap with occupational therapy in providing services for students with ASD. Behavior analysts intervene using applied behavior analysis principles such as reinforcement and manipulation of environmental stimuli or consequences to improve the student's socially significant behaviors (Association of Professional Behavior Analysts [APBA], 2017). *Socially significant behaviors* are defined as any behavior the person needs or wants to use throughout their day (APBA, 2017). This focus directly overlaps with the domain of occupational therapy, which, in school practice, addresses person-, context-, and occupation-based factors to enhance or enable participation in the myriad environments, activities, and situations that the student encounters throughout the school day (AOTA, 2014).

The structured, systematic intervention practices used by behavior analysts to change or modify students' behavior (APBA, 2017) contrast with the broad range of occupation-based methods and frames of reference that occupational therapy practitioners use to address the health, wellness, performance, participation, and quality of life of their clients (AOTA, 2014). For example, both occupational therapists and behavior analysts provide intervention to improve a student's ADLs; play; and social, motor, and adaptive skills; however, the philosophical approaches to service provision and theories that guide intervention approaches vary widely between these professions. To promote the collaboration that characterizes best practice and maximizes therapeutic benefit for the student, practitioners can use the following strategies:

- Build rapport by respecting peer knowledge and contributions—even when disagreements occur;
- Learn about the other professions;
- Educate others about occupational therapy;
- Gain trust by understanding and articulating the evidence for interventions; and
- Take a proactive approach to solving any conflicts that occur (Watling & Jones, 2018).

Remain Immersed in Evidence for Continual Professional Development

To remain up to date, a continual and comprehensive strategy must be used. Methods of tracking and notification about research articles of interest exist through PubMed and Google Scholar. Continual education may require a significant but critical investment in time and attention. One important place to begin is with large-scale, thorough, and methodologically sound evidence-based reviews (e.g., Wong et al., 2015). See Appendix H, "Evidence-Based Practice and Occupational Therapy," for further information about evidence-based practice.

Conduct Strengths-Based Evaluation of Students

Occupational therapy evaluation is meant to provide both documentation of a need for therapy services and the information necessary to guide goal development and intervention planning.

Strengths-based evaluation and report

A strengths-based focus in evaluation suits the occupational therapy philosophy of supporting optimal performance and enhancing well-being. One strengths-based assessment model, called the *Resources, Opportunities, Possibilities, Exceptions,* and *Solutions* (ROPES) Model (Graybeal, 2001), can be helpful in guiding the process. The therapist should include questions during the evaluation that ask about specific strengths and resources (see Exhibit 29.1). Although a strengths-based focus is ideal, therapists must understand and balance this approach with the reality of the setting and the legal requirements and restraints that guide practice in schools. The ultimate goal is to complete an evaluation that documents needs, measures discrepancies in performance as required by federal or state law, and provides information about a student's strengths and capacities.

The occupational therapy practitioner recognizes the family is the expert on their child. During the evaluation process, the therapist should include the family's concerns as well as the educational expectations. Parents prefer a strengths-based approach (Klein et al., 2011). In the form of an evaluation report, a *strengths-based approach* would explain how the student's relative strengths and special interests can be used to enhance their educational performance.

Multiple methods of assessment

The occupational therapist in the school evaluates the student to identify areas of strengths or needs. Therapists may use interviews, questionnaires, and observation to determine the strengths and barriers in the student's access

EXHIBIT 29.1.	Strengths-Based Assessment: Sample Questions for Students, Parents, or Teachers

- What do you do when you have a problem? How do you handle it?
- What is working now? What are you doing that you think you should keep doing?
- What options have you tried already to address this ___ (specific problem identified)?
- How much can you count on family and friends?
- Do you feel there are people who care about you?
- What do you do when you're stressed?
- How have you been able to thrive even with this ___ (specific problem identified)?
- When is ___ (specific problem identified) not happening or when is it different? Why do you think that is?

Sources. Resources, Opportunities, Possibilities, Exceptions, and Solutions Model (Graybeal, 2001; Tedeschi & Kilmer, 2005).

and academic and social functioning to assist the team in determining eligibility and need for special education and related services. Multiple methods of assessment in multiple settings are preferred because students with ASD may not perform to the best of their ability on norm-referenced assessments, different raters may perceive student performance differently, and performance may vary substantially in different contexts.

Implement Evidence-Based Interventions

Occupational therapy practitioners use client-centered, contextual, and evidence-based interventions. The best available evidence for students with ASD that can be incorporated into occupational therapy interventions is listed next.

Strengths- and interests-based intervention

In a review of 20 articles examining the use of special interests in the classroom, all reported enhanced learning, enhanced behavior, or both (Gunn & Delafield-Butt, 2016); in 3 instances, there were also reports of increased perseverative or inappropriate behaviors. Special interests and skills can create unparalleled opportunities for engagement in the classroom and may open doors to social interaction with peers or opportunities for leadership in the classroom for the student with ASD.

Evidence-based student interventions for behavior

Antecedent approaches to intervention aim to prevent difficult behaviors or to elicit desired behaviors that may not be readily performed by the student. Occupational therapy practitioners must identify and then reduce or remove the triggers for a problem behavior so that it becomes less frequent, or they must increase stimuli that elicit positive behavior at times when the behavior is desired. One approach, functional communication training, teaches the person productive strategies for communication that result in the same outcome as is typically acquired through an undesired behavior. For example, if screeching and falling to the floor allow the student to avoid doing math, the student could be taught to express his disinterest in completing the task another way. Just as human behavior is individualized, so are the antecedents that trigger behaviors. Some common categories of antecedents include a particular person, room, visual stimulus, or sound or cognitive, motor, or communicative performance demands.

The most common consequence intervention is *positive reinforcement.* Positive reinforcement is any response to student behavior that results in that behavior occurring again. Because positive reinforcement strengthens a behavior, therapists must be cognizant of inadvertently reinforcing undesired behaviors by allowing a student with ASD to escape from or avoid a demand as a result of the undesired behavior. Using antecedent and consequent strategies together can help support student compliance with classroom expectations and shape functional behaviors for classroom success.

Exercise is one method of improving behavior that may be overlooked in schools. Multiple studies document the efficacy of exercise in ASD for reducing aggressive

behaviors, stereotypies, and elopement while increasing on-task behavior, although many studies have methodological flaws (Dillon et al., 2017; Lang et al., 2010). Moreover, physical activity and exercise have significant sensory properties and affect physiological functions that support regulatory abilities and social–emotional functioning among people with ASD (Sowa & Meulenbroek, 2012). Occupational therapy practitioners can customize exercise interventions to match student strengths, interests, and capabilities and support behavioral and social–emotional needs of students with ASD across school environments.

Coaching methods allow an occupational therapist to collaborate with parents or teachers with the goal of enabling their success, competence, and efficacy in managing the child's behaviors. Studies to date on coaching methods with parents have been positive (e.g., Graham et al., 2017). Less is known about the effectiveness of these methods with teachers; however, in Canada, a model based on collaborative coaching has been successfully implemented with students with developmental coordination disorder (Dancza et al., 2017).

Evidence-based student interventions for social–emotional and psychosocial needs

Incorporating individual strengths and interests into interventions validates the student's personal interests, values, and abilities, leading to improved self-efficacy, volition, and social–emotional health (Tomchek & Koenig, 2016). For example, a student's interest in technology could be incorporated into a coping plan by using stress management apps to help the student increase follow-through. Providing opportunities for participation in hobbies and interests that elicit a student's positive emotions, creativity, and the right level of challenge may promote mental health and resilience.

Occupational therapy practitioners can teach students with ASD individualized mindfulness strategies to support coping and stress management. Spek et al. (2013) found positive results from a protocol that emphasized the experience of mindfulness by excluding metaphors and ambiguous language, including acceptance of the present moment in a nonjudgmental way, viewing thoughts and feelings as temporary mental phenomena, and increasing time spent on breathing. This approach, referred to as *mindfulness-based therapy for individuals on the autism spectrum,* reduced rumination, depression, and anxiety in adults with ASD and could be graded and customized for application with middle school or high school students.

Evidence-based student interventions for improving social skills

Although inclusion has increased for students with ASD, and inclusion promotes peer interaction, inclusion alone is insufficient to create peer engagement (Locke et al., 2015). Group-based social skills training programs are strongly supported for their ability to increase social skills acquisition, decrease problem behaviors, and affect participants' social–emotional development (Olsson et al., 2017; Tanner et al., 2015). Social skills groups typically include the explicit teaching of social skills, role playing to practice skills within the group, and performing activities outside the group to promote transfer and generalization.

Peer-mediated interventions are also supported for social skills development (Zhang & Wheeler, 2011); however, evidence suggests that these interventions are most effective when implemented in the home with a sibling serving as the peer (Zhang & Wheeler, 2011). Activity-based interventions in which students with ASD participate in a goal-directed activity have moderate evidence for effectiveness in promoting social skills (Tanner et al., 2015). Evidence also supports group activity, such as building with LEGOs, completing a cooking project, or working together with others to solve a problem.

Other evidence-based interventions for improving social skills include video modeling, reinforcement of specific social skills, Social Stories, and peer modeling (Watkins et al., 2015; Wong et al., 2015). Specific peer modeling strategies include peer initiation, prompting and reinforcement, and proximity, with and without additional strategies such as using visual supports or preferred interests (Watkins et al., 2015). Successful implementation of peer modeling strategies appears to require the selection of appropriate peers as well as adequate peer training. For all social interaction methods, however, school policies, staffing shortages, limited staff training in working with students with ASD, competing demands for time, varying levels of support by administration, and limited resource availability may be barriers to implementation in schools (Locke et al., 2015).

Evidence-based student interventions for altering the environment

Multiple studies have reported the sensory issues of students with ASD and the impact of these issues on participation (Marco et al., 2011; Pfeiffer et al., 2017; Reynolds et al., 2011; Schaaf et al., 2011). Recent studies have documented the intense sensory environments of classrooms and school buildings (Kuhaneck & Kelleher, 2015) as well as the behavioral impact of exposure to these environments, particularly in regard to noise (Kanakri et al., 2017). The most commonly reported outcome for classroom sensory experiences of adolescents with ASD and atypical sensory processing is a reduction in their ability to concentrate (Howe & Stagg, 2016). Teachers have similarly reported distraction in relation to the elementary classroom sensory environment (Miller Kuhaneck & Kelleher, 2018). Therefore, occupational therapy practitioners can fill an important role by collaborating with teachers to find ways to reduce noise, limit distractions, and improve the match between a student's sensory needs and the classroom sensory environment.

The literature base for the effectiveness of certain specific sensory techniques and environmental modifications based on *Ayres Sensory Integration*® is currently limited (Bodison & Parham, 2018; Case-Smith et al., 2015). Kinnealey et al. (2012) demonstrated that modifying the environment to address sensory processing differences reduced distractions and student stress, leading to improved student-perceived performance and emotional well-being. Literature reviews suggest possible physical adaptations to classroom environments for students with ASD (Martin, 2016; see Exhibit 29.2), but these should be used cautiously and with thorough data collection to ensure efficacy

EXHIBIT 29.2.	Samples of Classroom Adaptations to Support Students With ASD

- Provide clear visual boundaries for different types of learning
- Provide a visually quiet space with limited visual stimulation
- Use visual supports, such as labeling items in the classroom and photo schedules
- Use physical objects to block sight and reduce visual distractions
- Allow for additional personal space by leaving more open spaces in the classroom
- Eliminate clutter
- Reduce visual distractions on wall and floor surfaces, including colors and patterns
- Use natural lighting or avoid lighting that hums or flickers
- Cover windows to reduce glare and outdoor distractions
- Increase lighting in areas in which table work occurs
- Minimize noise through carpeting, acoustical tiles, and in-floor heat
- Provide flexible options to allow teachers to provide appropriate environments for a variety of students who may have differing needs
- Provide routine and predictability for uncomfortable sensory experiences
- Allow students as much control as possible regarding exposure to sensory experiences
- Maximize safety by eliminating sharp edges and opportunities for unsafe climbing or flight
- Provide sensory options for sensory seekers (e.g., ball chairs, fidget toys)
- Provide a space for withdrawal for sensory avoiders

Note. ASD = autism spectrum disorder.
Sources. Martin (2016); Pfeiffer et al. (2017).

for specific students (see Chapter 45, "Best Practices in School Occupational Therapy Documentation and Data Collection").

Universally designed curricula provide learners with varied ways to acquire knowledge, demonstrate what they have learned, and engage with learning by using their individual interests to increase motivation (CAST, 2011). *Universal design for learning* (UDL) is a method of education that creates learning environments that are flexible enough to accommodate learning differences. For these reasons, UDL is a good match for students with ASD. In addition, assistive technology interventions provide options for improved communication, peer interaction and social skills, play, life skills, and behaviors and may also promote motivation for learning. In particular, tablet use and apps have been documented as effective options for enhancing communication and social interaction that can motivate children with ASD (Kagohara et al., 2013).

A list of helpful apps is maintained by Autism Speaks (https://www.autismspeaks.org/autism-apps). Similarly, personal digital assistants have been used with adolescents with ASD to promote their EF and cognitive performance (Gentry et al., 2010). However, the evidence to support computer-aided instruction for academic skills is limited (Knight et al., 2013).

Measure Outcomes

With any chosen intervention, it is imperative that the practitioner implement some method of data collection to document the efficacy of the intervention for the particular student with ASD. Even with intervention practices strongly supported by evidence, there will be some persons for whom the intervention does not work. Methods of data-based decision making and outcome assessment must be put in place (see Chapter 45).

SUMMARY

Best practices for occupational therapy in supporting students with ASD in school settings are comprehensive and individualized, addressing behavior, sensory, social, emotional, and participation needs. Occupational therapy practitioners use occupation-based approaches that incorporate student strengths and interests while providing direct and indirect services, addressing family priorities, partnering with teachers, and collaborating with the educational team. Skilled evaluation and intervention services informed by both research evidence and student data-driven decision making result in effective occupational therapy services for students with ASD.

REFERENCES

American Occupational Therapy Association. (2014). Occupational therapy practice framework: Domain and process (3rd ed.). *American Journal of Occupational Therapy, 68*(Suppl. 1), S1–S48. https://doi.org/10.5014/ajot.2014.686S03

American Psychiatric Association. (2013). *Diagnostic and statistical manual of mental disorders* (5th ed.). Arlington, VA: American Psychiatric Publishing.

Association of Professional Behavior Analysts. (2017). *Identifying applied behavior analysis interventions.* Retrieved from https://www.bacb.com/wp-content/uploads/APBA-2017-White-Paper-Identifying-ABA-Interventions1.pdf

Baio, J., Wiggins, L., Christensen, D. L., Maenner, M. J., Daniels, J., Warren, Z., . . . Dowling, N. F. (2018). Prevalence of autism spectrum disorder among children aged 8 years—Autism and Developmental Disabilities Monitoring Network, 11 sites, United States, 2014. *Morbidity and Mortality Weekly Report Surveillance Summary, 67*(SS-6), 1–23. http://dx.doi.org/10.15585/mmwr.ss6706a1

Barnett, J. P., & Maticka-Tyndale, E. (2015). Qualitative exploration of sexual experiences among adults on the autism spectrum: Implications for sex education. *Perspectives on Sexual and Reproductive Health, 47,* 171–179. https://doi.org/10.1363/47e5715

Bodison, S. C., & Parham, L. D. (2018). Specific sensory techniques and sensory environmental modifications for children and youth with sensory integration difficulties: A systematic review. *American Journal of Occupational Therapy, 72,* 7201190040. https://doi.org/10.5014/ajot.2018.029413

Boswell, K., Zablotsky, B., & Smith, C. (2014). Predictors of autism enrollment in public school systems. *Exceptional Children, 81,* 96–106. https://doi.org/10.1177/0014402914532230

Caldwell-Harris, C. L., & Jordan, C. J. (2014). Systemizing and special interests: Characterizing the continuum from neurotypical to autism spectrum disorder. *Learning and Individual Differences, 29,* 98–105. https://doi.org/10.1016/j.lindif.2013.10.005

Case-Smith, J., Weaver, L. L., & Fristad, M. A. (2015). A systematic review of sensory processing interventions for children with autism spectrum disorders. *Autism, 19,* 133–148. https://doi.org/10.1177/1362361313517762

CAST. (2011). *Universal design for learning guidelines* (Version 2.0). Retrieved from http://www.udlcenter.org/aboutudl/udlguidelines

Dancza, K., Missiuna, C., & Pollock, N. (2017). Occupation-centred practice: When the classroom is your client. In S. Rodger & A. Kennedy-Behr (Eds.), *Occupation-centred practice with children: A practical guide for occupational therapists* (2nd ed., pp. 257–288). Chichester, England: Wiley-Blackwell.

Deckers, A., Muris, P., & Roelofs, J. (2017). Being on your own or feeling lonely? Loneliness and other social variables in youths with autism spectrum disorders. *Child Psychiatry and Human Development, 48,* 828–839. https://doi.org/10.1007/s10578-016-0707-7

Dillon, S. R., Adams, D., Goudy, L., Bittner, M., & McNamara, S. (2017). Evaluating exercise as evidence-based practice for individuals with autism spectrum disorder. *Frontiers in Public Health, 4,* 290. https://doi.org/10.3389/fpubh.2016.00290.

Durkin, M. S., Maenner, M. J., Baio, J., Christensen, D., Daniels, J., Fitzgerald, R., . . . Wingate, M. S. (2017). Autism spectrum disorder among US children (2002–2010): Socioeconomic, racial, and ethnic disparities. *American Journal of Public Health, 107,* 1818–1826. https://doi.org/10.2105/AJPH.2017.304032.

Every Student Succeeds Act, Pub. L. No. 114–95, § 129 Stat. 1802 (2015).

Gentry, T., Wallace, J., Kvarfordt, C., & Lynch, K. B. (2010). Personal digital assistants as cognitive aids for high school students with autism: Results of a community-based trial. *Journal of Vocational Rehabilitation, 32,* 101–107. https://doi.org/10.3233/JVR-2010-0499

Graham, F., Rodger, S., & Kennedy-Behr, A. (2017). Occupational performance coaching (OPC): Enabling caregivers' and children's occupational performance. In S. Rodger & A. Kennedy-Behr (Eds.), *Occupation-centred practice with children: A practical guide for occupational therapists* (2nd ed., pp. 209–232). Chichester, England: Wiley-Blackwell.

Graybeal, C. (2001). Strengths-based social work assessment: Transforming the dominant paradigm. *Families in Society, 82,* 233–242. https://doi.org/10.1606/1044-3894.236

Gunn, K. C., & Delafield-Butt, J. T. (2016). Teaching children with autism spectrum disorder with restricted interests: A review of evidence for best practice. *Review of Educational Research, 86,* 408–430. https://doi.org/10.3102/0034654315604027

Hebron, J., Oldfield, J., & Humphrey, N. (2017). Cumulative risk effects in the bullying of children and young people with autism spectrum conditions. *Autism, 21,* 291–300. https://doi.org/10.1177/1362361316636761

Howe, F. E., & Stagg, S. D. (2016). How sensory experiences affect adolescents with an autistic spectrum condition within the classroom. *Journal of Autism and Developmental Disorders, 46,* 1656–1668. https://doi.org/10.1007/s10803-015-2693-1

Individuals With Disabilities Education Improvement Act of 2004, Pub. L. 108–446, 20 U.S.C. §§ 1400–1482.

Jang, J., Dixon, D. R., Tarbox, J., & Granpeesheh, D. (2011). Symptom severity and challenging behavior in children with ASD. *Research in Autism Spectrum Disorders, 5,* 1028–1032. https://doi.org/10.1016/j.rasd.2010.11.008

Kagohara, D. M., van der Meer, L., Ramdoss, S., O'Reilly, M. F., Lancioni, G. E., Davis, T. N., . . . Green, V. (2013). Using iPods and iPads in teaching programs for individuals with developmental disabilities: A systematic review. *Research in Developmental Disabilities, 34,* 147–156. https://doi.org/10.1016/j.ridd.2012.07.027

Kanakri, S. M., Shepley, M., Tassinary, L. G., Varni, J. W., & Fawaz, H. M. (2017). An observational study of classroom acoustical design and repetitive behaviors in children with autism. *Environment and Behavior, 49,* 847–873. https://doi.org/10.1177/0013916516669389

Kaur, M., Srinivasan, S. M., & Bhat, A. N. (2018). Comparing motor performance, praxis, coordination, and interpersonal synchrony between children with and without ASD. *Research in Developmental Disabilities, 72,* 79–95. https://doi.org/10.1016/j.ridd.2017.10.025

Keen, D., Webster, A., & Ridley, G. (2016). How well are children with autism spectrum disorder doing academically at school? An overview of the literature. *Autism, 20,* 276–294. https://doi.org/10.1177/1362361315580962

Kinnealey, M., Pfeiffer, B., Miller, J., Roan, C., Shoener, R., & Ellner, M. L. (2012). Effect of classroom modification on attention and engagement of students with autism or dyspraxia. *American Journal of Occupational Therapy, 66,* 511–519. https://doi.org/10.5014/ajot.2012.004010

Klein, S., Wynn, K., Ray, L., Demeriez, L., LaBerge, P., Pei, J., & Pierre, C. S. (2011). Information sharing during diagnostic assessments: What is relevant for parents? *Physical and Occupational Therapy in Pediatrics, 31,* 120–132. https://doi.org/10.3109/01942638.2010.523450

Knight, V., McKissick, B. R., & Saunders, A. (2013). A review of technology-based interventions to teach academic skills to students with autism spectrum disorder. *Journal of Autism and Developmental Disorders, 43,* 2628–2648. https://doi.org/10.1007/s10803-013-1814-y

Kuhaneck, H. M., & Kelleher, J. (2015). Development of the Classroom Sensory Environment Assessment (CSEA). *American Journal of Occupational Therapy, 69,* 6906180040. https://doi.org/10.5014/ajot.2015.019430

Lang, R., Koegel, L. K., Ashbaugh, K., Regester, A., Ence, W., & Smith, W. (2010). Physical exercise and individuals with autism spectrum disorders: A systematic review. *Research in Autism Spectrum Disorders, 4,* 565–576. https://doi.org/10.1016/j.rasd.2010.01.006

Locke, J., Olsen, A., Wideman, R., Downey, M. M., Kretzmann, M., Kasari, C., & Mandell, D. S. (2015). A tangled web: The challenges of implementing an evidence-based social engagement intervention for children with autism in urban public school settings. *Behavior Therapy, 46,* 54–67. https://doi.org/10.1016/j.beth.2014.05.001

Marco, E. J., Hinkley, L. B., Hill, S. S., & Nagarajan, S. S. (2011). Sensory processing in autism: A review of neurophysiologic findings. *Pediatric Research, 69*(5, Pt. 2), 48R–54R. https://doi.org/10.1203/PDR.0b013e3182130c54

Martin, C. S. (2016). Exploring the impact of the design of the physical classroom environment on young children with autism spectrum disorder (ASD). *Journal of Research in Special Educational Needs, 16,* 280–298. https://doi.org/10.1111/1471-3802.12092

Meilleur, A. A. S., Jelenic, P., & Mottron, L. (2015). Prevalence of clinically and empirically defined talents and strengths in autism. *Journal of Autism and Developmental Disorders, 45,* 1354–1367. https://doi.org/10.1007/s10803-014-2296-2.

Miller Kuhaneck, H., & Kelleher, J. (2018). The Classroom Sensory Environment Assessment as an educational tool for teachers. *Journal of Occupational Therapy, Schools, and Early Intervention, 11,* 161–171. https://doi.org/10.1080/19411243.2018.1432442

Olsson, N. C., Flygare, O., Coco, C., Gorling, A., Rade, A., Lindstedt, K., . . . Bolte, S. (2017). Social skills training for children and adolescents with autism spectrum disorder: A randomized controlled trial. *Journal of the American Academy of Child and Adolescent Psychiatry, 56,* 585–692. https://doi.org/10.1016/j.jaac.2017.05.001

Pfeiffer, B., Coster, W., Snethen, G., Derstine, M., Piller, A., & Tucker, C. (2017). Caregivers' perspectives on the sensory environment and participation in daily activities of children with autism spectrum disorder. *American Journal of Occupational Therapy, 71,* 7104220020. https://doi.org/10.5014/ajot.2017.021360

Rehabilitation Act of 1973, Pub. L. 93–112, 29 U.S.C. §§ 701–796l.

Reynolds, S., Bendixen, R. M., Lawrence, T., & Lane, S. J. (2011). A pilot study examining activity participation, sensory responsiveness, and competence in children with high functioning autism spectrum disorder. *Journal of Autism and Developmental Disorders, 41,* 1496–1506. https://doi.org/10.1007/s10803-010-1173-x

Schaaf, R. C., Toth-Cohen, S., Johnson, S. L., Outten, G., & Benevides, T. W. (2011). The everyday routines of families of children with autism: Examining the impact of sensory processing difficulties on the family. *Autism, 15,* 373–389. https://doi.org/10.1177/1362361310386505

Section 504 of the Rehabilitation Act of 1973, as amended, 29 U.S.C. § 794 (2008).

Smith Roley, S., Mailloux, Z., Parham, L. D., Schaaf, R. C., Lane, C. J., & Cermak, S. (2015). Sensory integration and praxis patterns in children with autism. *American Journal of Occupational Therapy, 69,* 6901220010. https://doi.org/10.5014/ajot.2015.012476

Sowa, M., & Meulenbroek, R. (2012). Effects of physical exercise on autism spectrum disorders: A meta-analysis. *Research in Autism Spectrum Disorders, 6,* 46–57. https://doi.org/10.1016/j.rasd.2011.09.001

Spek, A. A., van Ham, N. C., & Nyklíček, I. (2013). Mindfulness-based therapy in adults with an autism spectrum disorder: A randomized controlled trial. *Research in Developmental Disabilities, 34,* 246–253. https://doi.org/10.1016/j.ridd.2012.08.009

Strang, J. F., Kenworthy, L., Daniolos, P., Case, L., Wills, M. C., Martin, A., & Wallace, G. L. (2012). Depression and anxiety symptoms in children and adolescents with autism spectrum disorders without intellectual disability. *Research in Autism Spectrum Disorders, 6,* 406–412. https://doi.org/10.1016/j.rasd.2011.06.015

Tanner, K., Hand, B. N., O'Toole, G., & Lane, A. E. (2015). Effectiveness of interventions to improve social participation, play, leisure, and restricted and repetitive behaviors in people with autism spectrum disorder: A systematic review. *American Journal of Occupational Therapy, 69,* 6905180010. https://doi.org/10.5014/ajot.2015.017806

Tedeschi, R. G., & Kilmer, R. P. (2005). Assessing strengths, resilience, and growth to guide clinical interventions. *Professional Psychology: Research and Practice, 36,* 230–237. https://doi.org/10.1037/0735-7028.36.3.230

Tomchek, S. D., & Koenig, K. P. (2016). *Occupational therapy practice guidelines for individuals with autism spectrum disorder.* Bethesda, MD: AOTA Press.

van Steensel, F. J., Bögels, S. M., & Perrin, S. (2011). Anxiety disorders in children and adolescents with autistic spectrum disorders: A meta-analysis. *Clinical Child and Family Psychology Review, 14,* 302–317. https://doi.org/10.1007/s10567-011-0097-0

Watkins, L., O'Reilly, M., Kuhn, M., Gevarter, C., Lancioni, G. E., Sigafoos, J., & Lang, R. (2015). A review of peer-mediated social interaction interventions for students with autism in inclusive settings. *Journal of Autism and Developmental Disorders, 45,* 1070–1083. https://doi.org/10.1007/s10803-014-2264-x

Watling, R., & Jones, C. J. (2018). *Managing challenging behavior in pediatric clients: Occupational therapy–behavior analyst collaboration* [Online continuing education course]. Seattle: Medbridge. Retrieved from https://www.medbridgeeducation.com/

Wong, C., Odom, S. L., Hume, K. A., Cox, A. W., Fettig, A., Kucharczyk, S., . . . Schultz, T. R. (2015). Evidence-based practices for children, youth, and young adults with autism spectrum disorder: A comprehensive review. *Journal of Autism and Developmental Disorders, 45,* 1951–1966. https://doi.org/10.1007/s10803-014-2351-z

Zhang, J., & Wheeler, J. J. (2011). A meta-analysis of peer-mediated interventions for young children with autism spectrum disorders. *Education and Training in Autism and Developmental Disabilities, 46,* 62–77.

Best Practices in Supporting Students With Childhood Trauma

Rachel Ashcraft, OTR/L, TBRI® Practitioner; Amy K. Lynch, PhD, TBRI® Educator, OTR/L, SCFES; and Lisa Tekell, OTD, OTR/L

30

KEY TERMS AND CONCEPTS

- Adverse childhood experiences
- Compassion fatigue
- Co-regulation
- Developmental trauma
- Homeschooling
- Insecure attachment
- Secondary (vicarious) trauma
- Self-regulation

OVERVIEW

Each year, more than 7 million children experience early adversity (Child Welfare Information Gateway, n.d.; U.S. Department of Health and Human Services, 2016). Childhood trauma results from psychologically chronic or acute stress experiences, which involve actual or serious threat of injury, violence, or death (American Occupational Therapy Association [AOTA], 2015). Childhood trauma transcends all levels of economic status, ethnicities, and geographic regions.

A large number of children in the United States are not equipped with the internal and external resources to overcome traumatic events (see Table 30.1). Moreover, the cumulative impact of "exposure to actual or threatened death, serious injury, or sexual violence" (American Psychiatric Association, 2013, p. 261) negatively affects occupational performance and occupational satisfaction across the life course (Anda et al., 2006).

Understanding the Terms *Adverse Childhood Experiences* and *Developmental Trauma*

Occupational therapy practitioners[1] who work in schools will most likely encounter students who have experienced or are actively experiencing adversity. Therefore, it

is imperative for all practitioners to recognize and understand adverse childhood experiences (ACEs) and how adversity affects a student's participation and performance in school.

ACEs are a set of defined, negative life experiences known to affect the emergence of childhood development and to significantly alter the trajectory of a child's life course (Anda et al., 2006; Van der Kolk et al., 2005). ACEs include abuse (physical, verbal, sexual), neglect (physical, emotional), and distress related to an immediate family member in the home (e.g., mental illness, substance abuse, incarceration, sudden loss of a primary parent as a result of divorce or death). The extent of early adversity experienced by a person can be reflected in an ACE score, with each identified adversity equal to 1 point (i.e., a summative higher ACE score indicates greater risk for physical health problems such as obesity, hypertension, and cardiac problems, as well as mental health issues such as addiction, anxiety, and depression; Felitti et al., 1998). ACE experiences correlate with reduced quality of life and occupational engagement into adulthood, including a higher risk of unemployment (Liu et al., 2013).

The term *developmental trauma* (Van der Kolk, 2017) was coined after extensive research evaluating the impact of adverse childhood experiences. Students with early adversity and complex developmental trauma do not experience typical physical and emotional nurturing, which is important in building attachment, trust, self-regulation, self-efficacy, and self-worth (Van der Kolk, 2017). Moreover, developmental trauma means a lack of scaffolding of learning and instrumental enrichment by a trusted caregiver, both of which are vital to a child's development of cognitive, motor, language, and social–emotional skills. Occupational therapy practitioners recognize how the impact of cumulative trauma in early development constrains a student's performance in daily activities (AOTA, 2017). Unfortunately, neither identification nor removal from trauma will, in isolation, shift the student's life trajectory back on course.

---

[1]*Occupational therapy practitioner* refers to both the occupational therapist and the occupational therapy assistant. AOTA (2014, p. S18) states, "The occupational therapist is responsible for all aspects of occupational therapy service delivery and is accountable for the safety and effectiveness of the occupational therapy service delivery process" and "must be directly involved in the delivery of services during the initial evaluation and regularly throughout the course of intervention. . . . The occupational therapy assistant delivers safe and effective occupational therapy services under the supervision of and in partnership with the occupational therapist."

Copyright © 2019 by the American Occupational Therapy Association. All rights reserved. To reuse this content, contact www.copyright.com.
https://doi.org/10.7139/2019.978-1-56900-591-0.030

TABLE 30.1. Examples of Internal and External Resources for a Child

RESOURCES	TYPICAL RESILIENCE FACTORS
Internal	▪ Good coping ▪ Self-regulation skills ▪ Communication skills ▪ Positive self-image ▪ Adequate problem solving ▪ Adequate physical growth ▪ Medical stability
External	▪ Safe and supportive family or extended community ▪ Safe housing ▪ Consistent access to nutrition and hydration, education, health care

Research on Trauma and Academic Performance

Trauma changes the typical development of the brain at chemical, cellular, and cortical levels. Changes can begin prenatally with exposure to prenatal stress, such as exposure to toxins. One study suggested that 90% of children with posttraumatic stress disorder in the foster care system had documented prenatal toxin exposure (Charil et al., 2012; Nadeem, 2017).

After birth, the developing central nervous system, under stress, establishes atypical patterns of "wiring and firing" that ultimately modify the brain's response to future experiences of stress. At a chemical level, the brain's chemical reward system, the dopaminergic system, is drastically altered by stress, resulting in a negative impact on learning, memory, and motivation. Chronic traumatic stress and maternal deprivation lower production of oxytocin, an important chemical in both mood regulation and social recognition.

Developmental trauma also elicits excess production of cortisol and atypical hypothalamic–pituitary–adrenal activity; excessively elevated cortisol in early childhood damages brain structures, including the hippocampus (Lupien et al., 2009), contributing to vigilance and hyperresponsiveness of fight, flight, and freeze mechanisms driven by the sympathetic nervous system. Unfortunately, the chemical differences perpetuate; children who experience trauma earlier in life also have a greater risk for greater atypical production of diurnal cortisol when experiencing later life trauma (Bevans et al., 2008).

Changes at a cellular level continue to perpetuate because of the atypical excess of hormones. For example, neuronal cell death in the hippocampus occurs with the presence of excessive glucocorticoid, making the hippocampus less capable of accessing and storing memories in their true form. Ultimately, the atypically high presence of hormones disrupts brain circuitry and perpetuates elevated states of the sympathetic nervous system, triggering an increase in fear-based responses (Rodrigues et al., 2009).

At a cortical level, research also finds deficits in the frontostriatal region that is vital to executive functioning (EF), regulation of emotion, insight, and judgment abilities (Gunnar & Quevedo, 2007). Moreover, chronic stress causes differences

in cortical areas of the brain, including the somatosensory cortex and medial temporal lobe, leading to differences and hyperresponsiveness to type of task, expected outcome of task, and reinforcement of decisions in task (Gerin et al., 2017). In summary, the neurobiological damage resulting from trauma establishes a child with significant nervous system instability, contributing to vulnerability of an explosive response system that cannot process the situational details properly and that will have an impact on every aspect of participation in school.

Layered on this identifiable neurobiological damage is the impact of lack of relational trust that is regularly paired with childhood experiences of chronic developmental trauma. As noted in Table 30.1, external resilience factors include the consistent presence of supportive and nurturing caregivers. Emergent development without the guidance of an invested, consistently present adult to ensure a child receives not only basic care and safety but also emotional nurturing leads to attachment difficulties. *Insecure attachment* often occurs in parallel with trauma and exacerbates the neurobiological challenges (Moutsiana et al., 2014). The brain of a student who has experienced early adversity is at risk for being ill equipped to take on typical learning and relational demands and even less capable of responding and coping with the positive and negative stress associated with development.

Research suggests that adverse childhood experiences collectively result in a negative impact on brain development as well as relational understanding. In addition to these findings and those that suggest motor differences, students who have experienced trauma are at risk for difficulties in school performance. Essential considerations for occupational therapy practitioners to address when working with students who have experienced trauma include

- Protecting children and families by identifying signs and symptoms of trauma,
- Promoting child readiness for learning and participation in the classroom,
- Educating and providing support for teachers regarding childhood trauma,
- Educating and providing support for homeschooling parents, and
- Assuring trauma informed care among all school stakeholders.

ESSENTIAL CONSIDERATIONS

It is essential that occupational therapy practitioners practicing in schools not only understand but also be able to identify students who have signs of trauma. Signs and symptoms of trauma include but are not limited to difficulties with occupational engagement reflected in atypical coping responses, regulation (social, emotional, and sensory), cognition, EF, and social participation, especially when not otherwise explained by a medical diagnosis.

Occupational Engagement and Coping Response

Students exhibit different forms of coping mechanisms in light of their own interpersonal trauma experiences. The occupational therapy practitioner understands that fight, flight, or freeze reactions are all neurobiological coping mechanisms that occur as result of trauma (Kinniburgh et al., 2005). Hypervigilance is a protective fear-based response. Students may display this differently.

For example, Student A may hyperfocus on the internal and external visual, auditory, or tactile input in the environment rather than the teacher (e.g., freeze, passive avoidance response); Student B may be highly disruptive in the classroom, with frequent physical altercations with peers or teachers (e.g., fight, active engagement response); Student C may avoid difficult tasks and act as a class clown to get out of an assignment (e.g., flight, active engagement response); and Student D may be extremely compliant yet not retain any of the academic information imparted during the school day (e.g., freeze, passive response). These students are at risk for having neurobiological systems that are attuned more toward negative emotion, so they may show more attention and engagement in whatever their coping mechanism is when they receive negative emotion from others (Lanius et al., 2010; Pollak et al., 2000). It is essential to recognize the individual nature of trauma responses when evaluating a student and determining the need for services.

Occupational Engagement and Self- and Co-Regulation

Self-regulation refers to a person's ability to obtain the adequate arousal level needed for occupational participation on their own. *Co-regulation* refers to the process of achieving a regulated state of adequate arousal for occupation with the external support of another individual guiding and modeling the regulation state (Efklides, 2008). For children of trauma, co-regulation ideally occurs through a process of sharing occupations with the co-regulating, nurturing individual.

Co-regulation is an important component of intervention necessary to build trust with the student and to help the student develop the skills necessary for self-regulation. However, children who have experienced trauma with relational difficulties present a challenge to safe adults who attempt to engage them in co-regulation interactions or activities. Regulation is vital for these students. With gains in regulation and awareness, the student increases the potential for development of interoception awareness, thus empowering internal cognitive and self-regulation skills to increase stability (Warner et al., 2014).

Occupational Engagement, Cognition, and EF in School

Students who have experienced complex trauma often struggle with cognition, maintaining sustained attention, and completing school learning tasks that require EF. Research identifies sequelae of trauma involving impairments in cognition, including working memory and pattern recognition (Gould et al., 2012; Majer et al., 2010). In addition to providing support for students with respect to cognitive impairments, occupational therapists also play a role in assessing EF challenges as barriers to school performance (DePrince et al., 2009).

Occupational Engagement and Social Participation in School

Students who have experienced complex developmental trauma often have difficulty participating in play, engaging in social occupations, and developing close peer relationships at school (Cole et al., 2005). This difficulty stems from the student's having limited social pragmatic skills and a greater tendency toward poor self-efficacy (Benight & Bandura, 2004) and self-concept (Saigh et al., 2008).

Characteristic differences that put a student with a history of trauma at a disadvantage in a social situation include poor self-esteem, impairments in understanding the emotions of others (including facial emotion recognition difficulties and difficulties with understanding tone of voice; Pollak et al., 2000), limitations in expressing own emotions, and compromised EF. The combination of any of these characteristics limits the student's ability to engage in social situations and produce appropriate social responses (e.g., understanding social expectations, identifying social strategies for engagement, generating appropriate social actions).

Establishing and maintaining healthy relationships in the school community is difficult, and students may struggle not only with peer groups or friendship circles but also with transitions in personnel, such as new teachers each year, substitute teachers, or rotating through teachers for different academic subjects. It is an important job of the occupational therapist to identify the differences among teacher style, approach, classroom culture, and environment as influences on the student with trauma in the school setting.

Occupational Engagement in School and Homeschool Settings

In the school setting (K–12), social and academic demands increase yearly, which may challenge students' academic performance and social skills. Sometimes problems may be related to earlier trauma when another medical explanation is not available.

Some district policies allow students who are homeschooled to access special education services through the local school system. *Homeschooling* is an option used by many parents whose child has experienced trauma. A family may feel this choice allows them to promote secure attachments and family involvement, which are important factors in successful learning (Gathercole, 2007); remove the child from an environment that may have frequent turnover in staff, depending on the school, or because the child struggles with new teachers each year; and provide an opportunity to build a predictable environment to ensure that the child feels safe throughout the day.

The occupational therapy practitioner may collaborate with the parent to identify opportunities for social inclusion and healthy friendship development and assist the family with environmental adaptations to create an effective area for learning.

TABLE 30.2. Evidence-Based Models for Trauma-Informed Training	
EVIDENCE-BASED MODEL	**REFERENCE WEBSITE**
Circle of Security	https://www.circleofsecurityinternational.com/
Neurosequential Model (NMT)	http://childtrauma.org/nmt-model/
Parent–Child Interaction Therapy	http://www.pcit.org/
Theraplay®	https://www.theraplay.org/
Trauma-Focused Cognitive Behavioral Therapy (TF–CBT®)	https://tfcbt.org/
Trust-Based Relational Intervention® (TBRI)	https://child.tcu.edu/

Professional Development

Trauma-informed training is important for professional development. Providers should be qualified, and the model should have an evidence base. Several complementary models align well with occupational therapy values and serve to inform the practitioner working with students. Some examples of evidence-based models are provided in Table 30.2.

Collaboration With Teacher and Family

When students have experienced trauma, their belief in a safe, encouraging, happy environment can be lost. This lack of belief alters what the student values; as a result, typical academic behavior programs do not work for children of trauma. Behavioral approaches that shame bad behavior foster self-doubt for the student who has experienced trauma. Instead, collaborative efforts should focus on

- Creating "felt safety" (Purvis et al., 2013), a feeling of being safe (e.g., create routines that are consistent and predictable; embed the school day with activities graded to promote success; modify environments to increase success; ensure consistent and predictable access to food, drink, and sensory activity; Purvis et al., 2013);
- Promoting relationship first, new performance skills second, for students for whom there are "gaps" (e.g., motor, social, emotional, self-regulation);
- Maintaining consistency in student and adult expectations, the student's performance, and goals; and
- Educating school staff on information that is pertinent to the student's current needs. Trauma triggers are especially important for people to be aware of; however, avoid release of confidential information that may be overshared by staff or others and may further breach any potential trust established with the student.

When the occupational therapy practitioner, teacher, guardian, or parent empathizes with the student, it helps to create a feeling of a safe environment and develop stable, predictable relationships. In addition, when a student engages with others in shared meaningful occupations, positive relationships develop that can enhance resiliency. Routines are very important to helping a student learn to trust and predict what will happen in their routine. The routines should be realistic and mindful of occupations or activities that the student may need to complete and should include important meaningful rituals. Engaging in shared meaningful rituals provides an opportunity for the group to form a feeling of community (e.g., reciting the Pledge of Allegiance, lining up for lunch).

Cultural Considerations: Culture of Trauma as a Disability

As more information and research become available regarding the specific needs that occur as a result of childhood trauma, an additional risk arises of defining people in terms of their trauma. No student should be defined by the adverse experiences they have encountered. Trauma, similar to other diagnoses that influence occupational participation, is only one piece of who the student is. Moreover, unlike other diagnoses such as cerebral palsy or autism, a unique aspect of trauma is that other providers around the child may also be victims of trauma. A sustainable approach to trauma-informed practice in the school system must consider the potential of trauma history in other providers as well as sustain consistent personnel able to implement trauma-informed approaches.

Trauma history does not go away with time; it is a hidden disability that flashes its features at expected and unexpected times across the life course. Every person has their own life experiences that contribute to their strengths and needs. This is as true for students as for others. Parents, educators, and service providers may be triggered by the student's expressions of trauma, may develop compassion fatigue, or may experience secondary trauma. Dismissing this reality may cause turnover and burnout in staff and families, which does not contribute to a stable environment for the student.

Compassion fatigue (e.g., becoming mentally and physically depleted as a result of caring for another person) can make it challenging to implement best practices. Professionals may detach from the student, become too depleted to implement trauma-informed approaches, react out of their own trauma triggers, or quit working with the student. Secondary trauma can result for a school provider who is consistently involved in a student's trauma-related behaviors. Childhood trauma behaviors (e.g., an argumentative spirit, physical outbursts, constant behaviors) take a huge toll on providers and contribute to the risk of secondary trauma for providers.

Occupational therapy practitioners in the school community need to address stability across the community for students, educating and supporting the educational team about these potentials. Together with the educational team, occupational therapy practitioners need to consider what proactive approaches are needed to keep providers healthy, because the potential for *secondary (vicarious) trauma* resulting from processing the trauma another person has experienced is significant. The occupational therapy practitioner must enter all interactions and educational planning meetings with great empathy for the parent or primary guardian and educators because they may also be experiencing secondary trauma.

BEST PRACTICES

Occupational therapy evaluations and interventions should address the student's performance and participation within natural routines of the school environment. It is imperative that evaluations and interventions be student centered, grounded in appropriately graded occupation-based approaches, and within a trauma-informed perspective.

Conduct an Evaluation to Determine Strengths and Barriers in Occupations

The occupational therapy evaluation should include an occupational profile and observation of the student in natural routines and environments to determine access, performance, and participation in the student's school day. It is critical to gather data about the curriculum, instruction, environment, and the student. Here are some sample questions to consider:

- *Academic history:* How many schools has the student been in? What is the student's academic and peer history at those schools? Is there a classroom where the student experienced greater success? What was different about that classroom?
- *Family history:* How many homes has the student been in? Does the student have siblings, and does the student live with their siblings? What is the stability of the current home environment (e.g., placement stability, predictable daily routines, regular access to food, consistent sleep)?
- *Social history:* Does the student have at least 1 friend from prior schools or homes? Is there any known social history or issues from prior schools? Does the student have at least 1 adult who values the child and is a consistent presence across school and home placements?
- *Classroom evaluation:* If the student has trauma triggers, then what are they, and when do they typically occur? What training or consultation does the teacher want to appropriately manage the student's needs? What is the structure of the classroom, teacher instruction, level of empathy, and assignments?
- *Communication plans to ensure a team approach:* Is there an established communication plan with the parent or caregiver? What is the preferred communication method between school and family? Among the educational team?
- *Safety plan:* Is there a safety plan in place so that all providers in the educational milieu will respond in the same manner?

Evaluating and addressing the dynamics of the teacher, school culture, and family are beneficial to intervention. Ensure that the establishment of daily communication between parent and teacher does not expose the student to shaming when the report is taken home. Appropriate means of communication should be established during the initial individualized education program (IEP) or Section 504 planning meetings. A team approach helps the student to understand that teachers and parents are working together and will minimize using the student as the communication agent between teacher and parent.

Students who have experienced trauma are more likely to have delays in development, including motor and visual perception (Roebar et al., 2014). Regulation and sensory processing differences occur at a much higher rate for students who have experienced trauma than for the general population, especially (but not only) if that trauma included physical abuse or neglect (Howard et al., 2018; Lynch, 2016; Lynch et al., 2017).

EF and cognition can be adversely affected by childhood trauma. However, because these students may lack physical signs of a disability, they are at further risk of being overlooked in the school or mislabeled as a behavior problem. The school occupational therapist should inquire about the student's participation in all domains of occupational therapy to determine whether these areas are affecting engagement in occupations.

Provide Evidence-Based Interventions

The occupational therapy practitioner's role is to address occupational engagement and barriers to occupation. Building internal and external coping and resiliency factors is key to removal of barriers to occupational performance. It is more important to address the student's needs and verify that the student feels validated and safe than to require completion of a specific task. Every interaction with the student must begin with validation. The school team must be able to provide the necessary assistance throughout the student's day. A dysregulated adult cannot help a student become regulated.

Educate staff to avoid triggers

All educators and service providers should avoid activities that may be triggers for a student. Triggers are extremely

TABLE 30.3.   Activity Alternatives to Avoid Triggers

ACTIVITY	ALTERNATIVES
Write Your Life Story	If the goal is a "get to know classmates" activity, an alternative could be to engage students in a team-building shared occupation at an age-appropriate level (e.g., "I like to fish").
	If the goal is to learn to plot points in a story, an alternative could be to describe a special event day at school or write an imaginative story.
Grandparent Day	Renaming "Grandparent Day" as "Special Guest Day" allows students who may not have grandparents in their life to honor other people important in their lives (e.g., aunts, uncles, a close friend of the family).
Family Tree	Instead of a geneological tree, each branch could represent a category, such as family, friends, teachers, relatives, coaches, or pets.

common in elementary school when family-based and "all about me" activities are used in classrooms. Activities that meet the educational goal and allow for diversity without shaming the student should be used. Table 30.3 includes a few simple examples of activities that may trigger a student unnecessarily, along with alternative ideas.

Minimize student fears

As much as possible, any fears that the student may have should be minimized. As an example, a student in foster care may have a specific fear of police because the police were the ones who initially removed them from the home.

EXHIBIT 30.1.   Occupational Considerations for Students Who Have Experienced Trauma

ELEMENTARY AGE GROUP

Bathroom and Toileting
- Be mindful of regressions with restroom behavior because they may indicate an emerging stress in the student's life.
- Emphasize teaching hygiene skills.

Mealtimes and Feeding
- Eliminate any food insecurity felt at school: Check that the student is eating breakfast at home or school. Does this student need access to the school breakfast program?
- Does the student have access to appropriate snacks during snack time?
- If the student is not eating, evaluate for sensory needs, oral–motor delays, and food saving (i.e., is the student trying to save food for later?).

Sleep
- Educate the family regarding sleep hygiene along with intervention strategies to build co-regulation and self-regulation skills. Be aware of the impact of sleep quality on occupations.

Dressing and Clothing Management for Toileting
- Use interventions to improve motor planning, coordination, and strength as needed to complete ADLs. Directly address ADLs.

Social Participation
- Participate in social skills groups and skill building to make and keep friends.
- Emotional and sensory regulation skills are needed for social participation.

Safety Considerations
- Teach the student healthy body boundaries and establish a safety plan for the student regarding who to tell and what to do if they are unsafe.
- Teach smartphone, Internet, and social media safety if the student has access to these resources.

INTERMEDIATE THROUGH HIGH SCHOOL AGE GROUP

Mealtimes and Feeding
- Continue to eliminate any food insecurity felt at school. Consider social implications of food and mealtimes. Does the student miss social opportunities because they do not have funds for a special snack, or is this student stigmatized for being the only student in the free lunch program?

Sleep
- Educate student on sleep hygiene and continue to build self-regulation skills, building responsibility to manage bedtime and wake-up time.

Dressing
- Address any underlying factors inhibiting ADLs. Include cognitive pieces of dressing, such as planning attire for activity or weather as well as accessing needed clothing for weather conditions.

Access to Sexual Health Information Taught at School (If Applicable)
- Partner with health class curriculums in relation to sexual health being taught at school. Students who have been sexually assaulted may need the content delivered in a safer space, such as with the occupational therapist or school counselor, rather than in a general education environment.

Social Participation
- Address adverse social experiences occurring at school (student may be bullied or engage in bullying behavior).
- Social skills groups and skills to both make and keep friends may be indicated.
- Consider teaching healthy relationships and establishing healthy boundaries.
- Social skills related to anger management as well as positive coping skills may be indicated.

Safety
- Teach healthy body boundaries and establish safety plans.
- Teach social media skills for appropriateness of posts, antibullying, and safety.

IADLs in Context of Transitional Services
- Basic life skills will be important for all students but crucial for the student nearing the end of school who may not have a stable support system into adulthood. These skills include money management; IADLs; interviewing skills; locating and securing housing when needed; and job training, assistance in transition to college, or both.

Leisure
- Development of positive leisure skills and opportunities to access healthy leisure may support a child's transitioning to adulthood in building positive leisure activities as well as positive support systems. Moreover, education and assistance to avoid or cease negative health behaviors, such as substance use, may be indicated.

It may be that the student experiences fear when they see the officer routinely on duty at the school. Developing a plan with the student to decrease the fear may begin with getting to know the school officer.

Establish clear expectations and boundaries

Students need to understand the rules and the consequences if the rules are not followed. Positive behavioral interventions and supports provide clear training for students. If a student needs assistance in calming after escalation when trying to escape a task, then they should redo the task once they are calm. Punishments such as restricting access to meals or hydration, adding extreme physical activity (e.g., pushups, running sprints), threatening physical or verbal abuse, or leaving a student alone in a space that the student perceives as unsafe should not be allowed.

Use self-regulation programs

Curricula that provide information on self-regulation and social thinking are beneficial in intervention planning. Regulation programs such as How Does Your Engine Run? (Williams & Shellenberger, 1996) or the Zones of Regulation (Kuypers, 2011) are excellent options to begin teaching regulation skills (AOTA, 2017). Because of the lack of evidence, sensory diet programs should never be used in isolation from evidence-based interventions. When regulation curricula are used for students who have experienced trauma, students need to know that the adult provider will remain calm and help them regain regulation without loss of relationship (Lynch, 2016).

Foster resilience

The occupational therapy practitioner can have a powerful impact on helping students advocate for themselves, which will help them to develop resilience (Samuels & Pryce, 2008). A sense of hope is important. The practitioner can work with students to overcome irrational thoughts and self-defeating behaviors.

In addition, students can begin to learn what things are within their control and what things are not. The occupational therapy practitioner can work with students to help them with positive communication as well as identification and creating positive social interactions and networks. As students identify their talents and what they need and want, the practitioner can work with them to identify rewards to improve performance as part of their overall IEP goals.

Use an occupation-based approach

Interventions should be guided by occupation-based practice. ADLs, IADLs, and social participation are all critical components of occupational therapy practitioners' intervention for students who have experienced trauma (Atchison, 2007; Tirella et al., 2012). Specific needs will vary, depending on the student's school support, family system, or both, as well as the student's individual strengths and needs. Exhibit 30.1 provides examples of occupational challenges that may arise across childhood.

Measure Outcomes

Outcomes in the school system can be measured at the student and system levels. Outcomes for students who are at risk for academic or behavior concerns are measured by their ability to return to Tier 1 (general education classroom). For the student with a disability, outcomes are measured on the basis of their performance on the IEP goals. Student progress may not be a direct sequence of improvements but may improve and regress at various times, depending on the person.

Systems-level outcomes may relate to reduced dropout rate, reduced use of restraints, decreased frequency of visits to the peace or conflict resolution room, improved staff awareness regarding managing behavior and understanding student needs, and improved community and parent partnerships with the school.

SUMMARY

Best practices of occupational therapy practitioners in the school include supporting the academic performance and social needs of at-risk students or students with disabilities. For many students with exposure to trauma, school may be the most stable and safe environment. Occupational therapy practitioners are ideally suited to implement strength-based strategies that meet students' ability to participate in their educational program.

REFERENCES

American Occupational Therapy Association. (2014). Guidelines for supervision, roles, and responsibilities during the delivery of occupational therapy services. *American Journal of Occupational Therapy, 68*(Suppl. 3), S16–S22. https://doi.org/10.5014/ajot.2014.686S03

American Occupational Therapy Association. (2015). *Occupational therapy's role in mental health promotion, prevention, and intervention with children and youth: Childhood trauma.* Retrieved from https://www.aota.org/~/media/Corporate/Files/Practice/Children/Childhood-Trauma-Info-Sheet-2015.pdf

American Occupational Therapy Association. (2017). *Foster care.* Retrieved from https://www.aota.org/~/media/Corporate/Files/Practice/Children/SchoolMHToolkit/Foster-Care-Info-Sheet-20170320.pdf

American Psychiatric Association. (2013). *Diagnostic and statistical manual of mental disorders* (5th ed.). Arlington, VA: American Psychiatric Publishing.

Anda, R. F., Felitti, V. J., Bremner, J. D., Walker, J. D., Whitfield, C., Perry, B. D., . . . Giles, W. H. (2006). The enduring effects of abuse and related adverse experiences in childhood. *European Archives of Psychiatry and Clinical Neuroscience, 256,* 174–186. https://doi.org/10.1007/s00406-005-0624-4

Atchison, B. (2007). Sensory modulation disorders among children with a history of trauma: A frame of reference for speech–language pathologists. *Language, Speech, and Hearing Services in Schools, 28,* 109–116. https://doi.org/10.1044/0161-1461(2007/011)

Benight, C. C., & Bandura, A. (2004). Social cognitive theory of post-traumatic recovery: The role of perceived self-efficacy. *Behaviour Research and Therapy, 42,* 1129–1148. https://doi.org/10.1016/j.brat.2003.08.008

Bevans, K., Cerbone, A., & Overstreet, S. (2008). Relations between recurrent trauma exposure and recent life stress and salivary cortisol among children. *Development and Psychopathology, 20,* 257–272. https://doi.org/10.1017/S0954579408000126

Charil, A., Laplante, D. P., Vaillancourt, C., & King, S. (2012). Prenatal stress and brain development. *Brain Research Reviews, 65,* 56–79. https://doi.org/10.1016/j.brainresrev.2010.06.002.

Child Welfare Information Gateway. (n.d.). *Extending out-of-home care for youth past age 18.* Retrieved from https://www.child welfare.gov/topics/outofhome/independent/outofhomecare/

Cole, S. F., Greenwald O'Brien, J., Gadd, M. G., Ristuccia, J., Wallace, D. L., & Gregory, M. (2005). *Helping traumatized children learn: Supportive school environments for children traumatized by family violence.* Retrieved from https://trauma sensitiveschools.org/tlpi-publications/download-a-free-copy -of-helping-traumatized-children-learn/

DePrince, A. P., Weinzierl, K. M., & Combs, M. D. (2009). Executive function performance and trauma exposure in a community sample of children. *Child Abuse and Neglect, 33,* 353–361. https://doi.org/10.1016/j.chiabu.2008.08.002

Efklides, A. (2008). Metacognition: Defining its facets and levels of functioning in relation to self-regulation and co-regulation. *European Psychologist, 13,* 277–287. https://doi.org/10.1027/1016 -9040.13.4.277

Felitti, V. J., Anda, R. F., Nordenberg, D., Williamson, D. F., Spitz, A. M., Edwards, V., . . . Marks, J. S. (1998). Relationship of childhood abuse and household dysfunction to many of the leading causes of death in adults: The Adverse Childhood Experiences (ACE) Study. *American Journal of Preventive Medicine, 14,* 245–258. https://doi.org/10.1016/S0749-3797(98)00017-8

Gathercole, R. (2007). *The well adjusted child: The social benefits of homeschooling.* Denver: Mapletree.

Gerin, M. I., Puetz, V. B., Blair, R. J. R., White, S., Sethi, A., Hoffmann, F., . . . McCrory, E. J. (2017). A neurocomputational investigation of reinforcement-based decision making as a candidate latent vulnerability mechanism in maltreated children. *Development and Psychopathology, 29,* 1689–1705. https://doi.org/10.1017/S095457941700133X.

Gould, F., Clarke, J., Heim, C., Harvey, P. D., Majer, M., & Nemeroff, C. B. (2012). The effects of child abuse and neglect on cognitive functioning in adulthood. *Journal of Psychiatric Research, 46,* 500–506. https://doi.org/10.1016/j.jpsychires.2012 .01.005

Gunnar, M. R., & Quevedo, K. M. (2007). Early care experiences and HPA axis regulation in children: A mechanism for later trauma vulnerability. *Progress in Brain Research, 167,* 137–149. https://doi.org/10.1016/S0079-6123(07)67010-1

Howard, A., Lynch, A., Call, C., & Cross, D. (2018). *Sensory processing in children with a history of maltreatment.* Manuscript submitted for publication.

Kinniburgh, J. K., Blaustein, M., Spinazzola, J., & Van der Kolk, B. A. (2005). Attachment, self-regulation, and competency: A comprehensive intervention framework for children with complex trauma. *Psychiatric Annals, 35,* 424–430. https://doi.org /10.3928/00485713-20050501-08

Kuypers, L. (2011). *The Zones of Regulation.* San Jose, CA: Think Social.

Lanius, R., Frewen, P., Vermetten, E., & Yehuda, R. (2010). Fear conditioning and early life vulnerabilities: Two distinct pathways of emotional dysregulation and brain dysfunction in PTSD. *European Journal of Psychotraumatology, 1*(1), 5467. https://doi .org/10.3402/ejpt.v1i0.5467

Liu, Y., Croft, J. B., Chapman, D. P., Perry, G. S., Greenlund, K. J., Zhao, G., & Edwards, V. J. (2013). Relationship between adverse childhood experiences and unemployment among adults from five US states. *Social Psychiatry and Psychiatric Epidemiology, 48,* 357–369. https://doi.org/10.1007/s00127-012-0554-1

Lupien, S. J., McEwen, B. S., Gunnar, M. R., & Heim, C. (2009). Effects of stress throughout the lifespan on the brain, behaviour and cognition. *Nature Reviews Neuroscience, 10,* 434–445. https://doi.org/10.1038/nrn2639

Lynch, A. (2016). *From early adversity to permanency: Implications for occupational and life course health development* [Webinar]. Retrieved from http://www.lcrn.net/from-early -adversity-to-permanency-implications-for-occupational -and-life-course-health-development/

Lynch, A., Ashcraft, R., & March Tekell, L. (2017). Understanding children who have experienced early adversity: Implications for practitioners practicing sensory integration. *SIS Quarterly Practice Connections, 2*(3), 5–7.

Majer, M., Nater, U. M., Lin, J. M. S., Capuron, L., & Reeves, W. C. (2010). Association of childhood trauma with cognitive function in healthy adults: A pilot study. *BMC Neurology, 10*(1), 61. https://doi.org/10.1186/1471-2377-10-61

Moutsiana, C., Fearon, P., Murray, L., Cooper, P., Goodyer, I., Johnstone, T., & Halligan, S. (2014). Making an effort to feel positive: Insecure attachment in infancy predicts the neural underpinnings of emotion regulation in adulthood. *Journal of Child Psychology and Psychiatry, 55,* 999–1008. https://doi. org/10.1111/jcpp.12198

Nadeem, E. (2017). Long-term effects of pre-placement risk factors on children's psychological symptoms and parenting stress among families adopting children from foster care. *Journal of Emotional and Behavioral Disorders, 25*(2), 67–81. https://doi .org/10.1177/1063426615621050

Pollak, S. D., Cicchetti, D., Hornung, K., & Reed, A. (2000). Recognizing emotion in faces: Developmental effects of child abuse and neglect. *Developmental Psychology, 36,* 679–688. https:// doi.org/10.1037/0012-1649.36.5.679

Purvis, K. B., Cross, D. R., Dansereau, D. F., & Parris, S. R. (2013). Trust-based relational intervention (TBRI): A systemic approach to complex developmental trauma. *Child and Youth Services, 34,* 260–368. https://doi.org/10.1080/0145935X.2013.859906

Rodrigues, S. M., LeDoux, J. E., & Sapolsky, R. M. (2009). The influence of stress hormones on fear circuitry. *Annual Review of Neuroscience, 32,* 289–313. https://doi.org/10.1146/annurev .neuro.051508.135620

Roebar, B. J., Gunnar, M. R., & Pollak, S. D. (2014). Early deprivation impairs the development of balance and bilateral coordination. *Developmental Psychobiology, 56,* 1110–1118. https:// doi.org/10.1002/dev.21159.

Saigh, P. A., Yasik, A. E., Oberfield, R., & Halamandaris, P. V. (2008). The self-concept of traumatized children and adolescents with or without PTSD. *Behaviour Research and Therapy, 46,* 1181–1186. https://doi.org/10.1016/j.brat.2008.05.003

Samuels, M., & Pryce, J. (2008). "What doesn't kill you makes you stronger": Survivalist self-reliance as resilience and risk among young adults aging out of foster care. *Children and Youth Services Review, 30,* 1198–1210. https://doi.org/10.1016/j.childyouth. 2008.03.005

Tirella, L. G., Tickle-Degnen, L., Miller, L. C., & Bedwell, G. (2012). Parent strategies for addressing the needs of their newly adopted child. *Physical and Occupational Therapy in Pediatrics, 32*(1), 97–110. https://doi.org/10.3109/01942638.2011.610434

U.S. Department of Health and Human Services. (2016). *Child maltreatment 2016.* Retrieved from https://www.acf.hhs.gov /cb/research-data-technology/statistics-research/child-mal treatment

Van der Kolk, B. A. (2017). Developmental trauma disorder: Toward a rational diagnosis for children with complex trauma histories. *Psychiatric Annals, 35,* 401–408. https://doi.org/10.3928 /00485713-20050501-06

Van der Kolk, B. A., Roth, S., Pelcovitz, D., Sunday, S., & Spinazzola, J. (2005). Disorders of extreme stress: The empirical foundation of a complex adaptation to trauma. *Journal of Traumatic Stress, 18,* 389–399. https://doi.org/10.1002/jts.20047

Warner, E., Spinazzola, J., Westcott, A., Gunn, C., & Hilary, H. (2014). The body can change the score: Empirical support for somatic regulation in the treatment of traumatized adolescents. *Journal of Child and Adolescent Trauma, 7,* 237–246. https:// doi.org/10.1007/s40653-014-0030-z

Williams, M. S., & Shellenberger, S. (1996). *How does your engine run? A leader's guide to the alert program for self regulation.* Albuquerque, NM: TherapyWorks.

31

Best Practices in Supporting Students With Emotional Disturbance

Gretchen Scheibel, MS, OTR/L, BCBA

KEY TERMS AND CONCEPTS

- Behavior intervention plan
- Cognitive Orientation to daily Occupational Performance
- Cognitive–behavioral intervention
- Emotional disturbance
- Functional behavior assessment
- Positive behavioral interventions and supports
- Self-regulation

OVERVIEW

Students eligible for special education under emotional disturbance[1] (ED) make up an increasing percentage of students receiving special education services in public schools. In 2015, 6% of students in public education programs were receiving special education services under this category (National Center for Education Statistics, 2017), yet they are the smallest percentage of students receiving occupational therapy as a related service. For special education eligibility, the Individuals With Disabilities Education Improvement Act of 2004 (IDEA; Pub. L. 108–446) defines **ED** as

a condition exhibiting one or more of the following characteristics over a long period of time and to marked degree that adversely affects a child's educational performance: (A) An inability to learn that cannot be explained by intellectual, sensory, or health factors; (B) An inability to build or maintain satisfactory interpersonal relationships with peers and teachers; (C) Inappropriate types of behaviors or feelings under normal circumstances; (D) A general pervasive mood of unhappiness or depression; (E) A tendency to develop physical symptoms or fears associated with personal or school problems.

(ii) Emotional disturbance includes schizophrenia. The term does not apply to children who are socially maladjusted, unless it is also determined that they have an emotional disturbance under paragraph (c)(4)(i) of this section. (34 CFR §300.8(c)(4)(i-ii))

The term *ED* includes a wide range of psychological diagnoses, such as affective disorders (e.g., depression, bipolar disorder), anxiety disorders (e.g., separation anxiety, generalized anxiety, obsessive–compulsive disorder), disruptive behavior disorders (e.g., oppositional defiant disorder, conduct disorder), pervasive developmental disorders, and psychotic disorders (e.g., schizophrenia).

Role of Occupational Therapy

Occupational therapy practitioners[2] have a role in mental health promotion, prevention, and intervention (AOTA, 2017b). They can apply a public health model to address the range of needs presented by students with ED. Use of this model may look like occupational therapy practitioners working at the systems level to promote (i.e., focus on competency enhancement) a healthy school climate, locate internal and external resources to emphasize students' healthy engagement in school occupations, and identify students' strengths to build on and minimize mental health barriers (AOTA, 2009; Arbesman et al., 2013).

They may target their services toward prevention (i.e., intervention aimed to prevent occurrence of occupational performance barriers) by working with curriculum specialists to design courses that embed cognitive–behavioral interventions, working with students to identify their triggers and develop personalized strategies to reduce or eliminate unhealthy responses, and collaborating with teachers to structure the environment for active learning.

---

[1]In the literature, terms include *emotional and behavioral disorders* and *serious emotional disorders*. For the purposes of this chapter, we use the term *ED* to align with IDEA (2004).

[2]*Occupational therapy practitioner* refers to both the occupational therapist and the occupational therapy assistant. The American Occupational Therapy Association (AOTA; 2014a, p. S18) states, "The occupational therapist is responsible for all aspects of occupational therapy service delivery and is accountable for the safety and effectiveness of the occupational therapy service delivery process" and "must be directly involved in the delivery of services during the initial evaluation and regularly throughout the course of intervention. . . . The occupational therapy assistant delivers safe and effective occupational therapy services under the supervision of and in partnership with the occupational therapist."

Copyright © 2019 by the American Occupational Therapy Association. All rights reserved. To reuse this content, contact www.copyright.com.
https://doi.org/10.7139/2019.978-1-56900-591-0.031

Focusing on evaluation and intervention, occupational therapists may work with or on behalf of individual students, groups, classrooms, and schools to identify strategies to minimize students' stressors, contribute to functional behavior assessments, or build student skills for greater self-determination and social participation.

Occupational Therapy Practitioners' Qualifications as Mental Health Providers

Occupational therapy is well rooted in mental health (AOTA, 2017b). Occupational therapists in their preservice education acquire knowledge and skills in analyzing the effects of mental health disorders on children's participation and engagement in occupation; occupational therapy assistants acquire an understanding of these effects (Accreditation Council for Occupational Therapy Education, 2012). The *Occupational Therapy Practice Framework: Domain and Process* (3rd ed.; OTPF–3; AOTA, 2014b) further describes an overarching professional tenet of "achieving health, well-being, and participation in life through engagement in occupation" (p. S4). Health specifically encompasses mental and social well-being.

In this capacity, occupational therapists can assist in the identification of mental illness; evaluate students to determine their strengths and barriers in the learning environment; and outline interventions to target outcomes for social–emotional learning, self-regulation, and mental functions (Bazyk & Arbesman, 2018). Occupational therapy assistants can implement interventions and contribute to discussions in determining programming needs. Together, their skills in collaboration and maintaining an occupation-based, student-centered focus make them valuable contributors to this population.

ESSENTIAL CONSIDERATIONS

This section explores common circumstances for and characteristics of students meeting the IDEA category of ED and various actions by school teams.

Common Circumstances for Students With ED

Students with ED may present with a multitude of challenges. They are more likely to experience involvement with child protection services, be placed outside of the home, be unsupervised in the home environment, be involved in criminal activities, experience substance abuse or engage in risky behavior or both, and have fewer opportunities to engage in formative childhood experiences (Maggin, Wehby, Farmer, et al., 2016). Occupational therapists' expertise in understanding interrelated conditions (e.g., student's abilities, context, environment) and their effect on engagement in occupation (AOTA, 2014c) is critical to student programming.

Common Characteristics of Students With ED and Effect on Occupational Performance

Students with ED may exhibit a variety of characteristics depending on their intellectual abilities, previous exposure to intervention, and varying symptoms related to psychological diagnoses. A similar pattern of characteristics (e.g., limited self-regulation, cognitive distortions, low self-esteem, vulnerability, relationship challenges, impaired performance) may underlie many students with ED, which can greatly affect their occupational performance in schools.

Limited self-regulation

Self-regulation is the student's ability to observe the environment; identify expectations; and adjust or change their alertness, emotions, and impulses to match the expectations of the situation (Kuypers, 2013). Students with ED may demonstrate disruption in their ability to continually assess and adjust their emotions and actions in educational settings. This inability may be due to their challenges not only with processing and preparing responses to sensory input but also with regulating their emotions and drawing on executive function (EF). Limited self-regulation may further affect their opportunity to engage with peers and experience success, to build tolerance for performance failures essential for skill development and refinement, and to focus attention on relevant environmental stimuli (e.g., speakers, instructional materials; AOTA, 2017b).

Cognitive distortions or misperceptions

Students with ED may display distorted or inaccurate thoughts, meaning they may view the world with a negative perspective, misinterpret others' actions, make inaccurate assumptions about others' intentions, negatively perceive positive social cues (e.g., smiles, kind words), and be resistant to new information or information that challenges their understanding of the world (Maggin, Wehby, Farmer, et al., 2016). These thought patterns can extend beyond their perception of the world to their perception of themselves and can include over- or underestimating their abilities, positive attributions, and acceptance in the community. Cognitive distortions, feelings of vulnerability, and low self-esteem can affect a student's willingness to engage in occupations that foster a sense of accomplishment and relaxation (e.g., participate in group activities that facilitate peer interactions, solve problems, perform ADLs; AOTA, 2017b).

Difficulty developing a clear and positive identity

Students with ED may demonstrate low self-esteem, feelings of insignificance, and lack of control, and have a reduced sense of meaning or purpose (Maggin, Wehby, Farmer, et al., 2016). These feelings can manifest as a distorted perception of one's self or the appearance of arrogance, which is often a compensation to protect themselves from feeling vulnerable and may even be related to distorted thought patterns; a lack of motivation, engagement, or forward thinking; or feeling a lack of control to improve their situation.

When students struggle with the development of a clear and positive identity, they may present with a false arrogance; lash out at others; blame others for mistakes or misunderstandings; or appear unmotivated, apathetic, or pessimistic (Jones et al., 2016). Limited development of a clear and positive identity can affect all areas of occupation, especially leisure pursuits. Students' involvement in structured leisure participation can enhance their personal development as they begin to understand what interests them, develop initiative to persist through challenges, and make a commitment over time (AOTA, 2017b).

Vulnerability

Students with ED may have experienced childhood trauma and, as a result, may feel vulnerable or more vigilant than their peers. These feelings may increase the likelihood of students' using challenging or avoidance behaviors to protect themselves or evade perceived demands. When students experience feelings of vulnerability, they may react impulsively, lash out unexpectedly, miss important directions, or miss social overtures from peers (Jones et al., 2016). (See Chapter 30, "Best Practices in Supporting Students With Childhood Trauma.")

Challenging relationships

Positive and healthy relationships with peers and adults can be a particular challenge for students with ED. Often, these students have been exposed to volatile, dysfunctional, or negative relationships that affect their ability to trust others, manage boundaries, and recognize negative relationships. Students with ED may develop relationships with adults in the educational environment that can range from overly personal or attached to disrespectful or combative. Adults working with this population need to be intentional in their efforts to develop positive relationships that demonstrate clear boundaries and model respectful and genuine interactions (Jones et al., 2016).

Students with ED typically need support in learning how to engage with peers in a healthy and positive manner; recognizing what friendship looks like; and problem solving social challenges such as managing disagreements, bullying, or social isolation. When difficulties persist with forming meaningful peer relationships, students can appear to be withdrawn, isolated, bullish, or standoffish (Jones et al., 2016).

Limited performance skills

Students with ED may present with deficits related to fine motor, visual–motor, and sensory processing skills that can increase the effort required to complete academic tasks or remain engaged in the classroom environment, thereby increasing the response effort of these tasks and furthering the student's disruption in the development of a clear,

positive identity. Occupational therapists can assist in evaluating the environment, conduct activity analyses, and recommend strategies to promote just-right challenges for students who struggle with limited performance (AOTA, 2017b).

Common Education Team Actions for Students With ED

As a member of the special education team, occupational therapists may collaborate with the team to gather data on students who may have challenges that could affect behavior (e.g., social interactions, self-care skills, self-regulation). The team can use these data to complete a functional behavior assessment (FBA) and create an individualized behavior intervention plan (BIP).

Functional behavior assessment

An **FBA** is conducted through a systematic process used to determine the function of the negative behavior (e.g., to gain or avoid something) and what conditions in the environment affect the occurrence of the behavior and the continued use of the behavior (see Exhibit 31.1). FBAs and the use of BIPs are mandated by IDEA (2004) and are considered to be an essential portion of program planning for students with ED (Scott & Alter, 2017).

IDEA requires that FBAs be completed by a qualified professional, meaning a professional who has received comprehensive training in the principles of behavior, essential components, and assessment procedures. Often, psychological and behavior professionals conduct these assessments, yet occupational therapists who have received the appropriate training can rely on their mental health background and unique view of occupation to conduct practical and informative FBAs. Occupational therapists who have not received this training along with occupational therapy assistants remain valuable members of the team and have the opportunity to contribute crucial information regarding the student's occupational performance.

FBAs can be conducted by a single person who gathers information from team members; however, Gable et al. (2014) suggested that students with ED benefit most clearly from a team-based FBA approach, to provide the richest understanding of the student's behavior. In a team-based FBA, all members of an interdisciplinary team contribute throughout the FBA process and work together to identify the function of the behavior.

EXHIBIT 31.1.   Functional Behavior Assessment

Functional behavior assessments (FBAs) use the principles of behaviors to better understand how and why behaviors happen. This includes the basic assumption that behaviors occur as the result of setting events or antecedents that trigger the occurrence of a behavior and that the changes in the environment that occur after a behavior is exhibited (otherwise known as *consequences*) control the future occurrences of behavior. Reponses to a behavior that have a desirable effect are anticipated to increase the future likelihood of the same behavior (otherwise known as *reinforcement*), and responses that have an undesirable effect are anticipated to decrease the future likelihood of the same behavior (otherwise known as *punishment*).

FBAs rely solely on objective information to guide assessment and interpretation of data, meaning that the only information included is information that is observable and measurable by all parties on the special education team. FBAs can target single or multiple behaviors; however, any behavior must be operationally defined to provide an objective and precise description of the behavior that is easily recognized. This precision allows the team to be confident in multiple observers' and data collectors' measurement of a behavioral occurrence (Alberto & Troutman, 2017).

EXHIBIT 31.2.   Functional Behavior Assessment (FBA) Data Collection Tools

The "ABC" data collection sheet is frequently used to determine how often specific environmental events trigger (**A**ntecedent) the **B**ehavior or occur as a result of the behavior (**C**onsequence). This information is analyzed by the team to determine the event's relationship to the behavior. The ABC data collection sheets can also be used outside of the FBA to provide context and objective information regarding a student's performance (see Figure 31.1).

FIGURE 31.1.   ABC data collection.

What was happening before the incident occurred? (Antecedent)	What behaviors occurred during the incident? (Behavior)	What happened after the behavior? (Consequence)
_X_ Sitting next to friend ___ Told to start working ___ Corrected/told to do something different	___Kicking ___ Biting _X_ Calling out (3 times)	_X_ Peer laughed ___ Teacher reminder ___ Left group _X_ Teacher ignored
_X_ Sitting next to friend ___ Told to start working _X_ Corrected/told to do something different	___Kicking ___ Biting _X_ Calling out (5 times)	_X_ Peer laughed ___ Teacher reminder _X_ Left group _X_ Teacher ignored

Scatterplot data sheets allow the team to identify trends or patterns in the behavior because the data collector records when the behavior occurs in the student's schedule over many days. This information can help to identify whether the student struggles more with academic demands vs. unstructured social time or whether behavior occurs on specific days of the week. It can guide the team to look at what makes days or times successful or unsuccessful (see Figure 31.2).

FIGURE 31.2.   Scatterplot of student behavior (highlight behaviors when and where they occur).

	Monday	Tuesday	Wednesday	Thursday	Friday
Arrival	Rude behavior Disruption Aggression	Rude behavior Disruption Aggression	Rude behavior Disruption Aggression	Rude behavior Disruption Aggression	Rude behavior Disruption Aggression
Homeroom	Rude behavior Disruption Aggression	Rude behavior Disruption Aggression	Rude behavior Disruption Aggression	Rude behavior Disruption Aggression	Rude behavior Disruption Aggression
Math	Rude behavior Disruption Aggression	Rude behavior Disruption Aggression	Rude behavior Disruption Aggression	Rude behavior Disruption Aggression	Rude behavior Disruption Aggression

Most FBAs include 2 phases of assessment: indirect and direct. *Indirect assessment* (i.e., descriptive assessment) includes the use of behavior rating scales; record reviews; direct observations; and structured interviews of teachers, paraeducators, related service providers, parents, community supports, and, when possible, the student (Alberto & Troutman, 2017; Gable et al., 2014). This process can look different, depending on the FBA procedure being used by the team.

Regardless of the procedure, the indirect phase presents an opportunity for occupational therapists to provide valuable information regarding specific occupational performance deficits that could affect the student's ability to perform in the educational environment. These challenges should be explored during this phase to determine whether they are contributing to an increase in environmental or task demands that appear to be setting events or antecedents to challenging behaviors. Adaptation or accommodation of these occupations could mitigate the need for further behavioral intervention or allow the team to consider less restrictive behavioral interventions.

Direct assessment of challenging behavior, the second phase, includes the use of data collection to objectively identify the variables that influence behavior (i.e., setting events or environmental conditions that encourage challenging behavior, antecedents, and consequences; see Exhibit 31.2). To complete this phase, a data collection sheet is created to catalog the frequency, duration, or intensity of target behaviors; specific environmental events that occur before and after the behavior; and the times when behaviors are most likely to occur (Alberto & Troutman, 2017).

The direct assessment phase of the FBA presents another opportunity for occupational therapists to contribute expertise, such as identifying objective descriptions of behavioral states (e.g., frustration can look like tensed shoulders and arms, avoidance of eye contact, and a change in tone of voice) and occupational performance barriers occurring in the environment that may influence behavioral performance (e.g., presence of environmental noise, proximity to peers, motor or organizational demands) to streamline data collection. Once the data are collected, they must be analyzed to identify specific variables that influence behavior. Occupational therapists are valuable collaborators in this process, lending their occupational lens to assess the specific challenges associated with antecedent events and determining occupational performance barriers that contribute to the demand of those events.

One potential challenge of conducting FBAs is that all information provided during the FBA process must be objective and grounded in concrete observation of the behavior. To conduct a valid FBA, it is imperative that a strictly objective view is used when participating in the direct assessment phase of an FBA, relying only on concrete observation of observable and measurable performance and avoiding use of jargon or speculation about internal states.

For example, when contributing expertise regarding environmental demands that may affect the student's performance, the occupational therapist reports specific behaviors with clear language (e.g., "When a peer joined circle and sat within 5 inches of the student, he immediately moved his body 1 foot away from the peer. This pattern of behavior was repeated 5 times during the observation whenever a peer or adult was within 6 inches of the student."), not subjective language (e.g., "During circle time, the student demonstrated a heightened response to tactile input as demonstrated by withdrawing from peers in close proximity.").

Although occupational therapists may use their professional expertise to glean performance information from this observation in their own intervention planning, FBAs require that only observable data be presented to ensure precise measurement and analysis of behavior.

Behavior intervention plan

The **BIP** is an individualized written plan based on the FBA to describe the positive behavioral interventions, strategies, and supports needed to implement the student's individualized education program (IEP) goals in the area of social, emotional, and behavioral development. IDEA (2004) mandates that a BIP be developed for any student who exhibits interfering behavior that affects their learning or the learning of others. Most BIPs include the following components: operational definition of behaviors, positive behavior instructional strategies, reinforcement procedure to strengthen positive behaviors, proactive strategies, and responses to negative behaviors.

Occupational therapists provide valuable input during the BIP process to promote student success in the classroom and prevent challenging behaviors. It is important to identify environmental and activity adaptations as well as to recommend exercise routines and movement breaks that can help to regulate the student's energy level and attention to facilitate performance. Occupational therapy practitioners need to be familiar with each student's BIP and be confident in implementing the documented strategies and reinforcement systems when working with students to maintain consistent implementation of the plan.

Evidence-Based Social–Emotional Curriculum

Social–emotional learning is an area of high need for students with ED. To meet this need, the use of an evidence-based curriculum that targets the development of social–emotional learning competencies is an essential component of programming for students with ED (Jones et al., 2016). The Collaborative for Academic, Social, and Emotional Learning (CASEL) is a multidisciplinary research team working to integrate social–emotional learning into elementary and secondary education (AOTA, 2014c; CASEL, 2013). CASEL's research has identified social–emotional learning competencies as self-awareness, self-management, social awareness, relationship skills, and responsible decision making.

Using multi-tiered systems of support found in schoolwide positive behavioral interventions and supports initiatives is important:

- *Tier 1:* Provide a positive learning environment for learning (e.g., explicit group instruction of positive behavioral expectations, frequent acknowledgment of positive behavior, consistent constructive adult responses when problem behaviors occur, a positive school climate)
- *Tier 2:* Skill instruction groups and least restrictive interventions (e.g., check in–check out, organizational and problem-solving supports, academic supports)
- *Tier 3:* Evaluations; begin process for BIP.

Occupational therapy practitioners support social–emotional learning competencies by planning interventions to target specific areas, collaborating with team members to provide social skills interventions, and developing strategies to enable the student to regulate emotions and actions. When assessing performance, occupational therapists should pay careful attention to a student's limitations in social–emotional learning competencies that might affect their ability to participate.

Academic Accommodations

Students with ED often demonstrate academic underachievement in learning environments. This population can present with academic performance similar to students with learning disabilities, despite demonstrating average cognitive profiles (Maggin, Wehby, & Gilmour, 2016). Jones et al. (2016) suggested that a student's academic underachievement could be related to disruption in academic instruction because of problem behaviors as well as limited academic engagement and motivation to learn. To manage these challenges and maximize academic success, students with ED benefit from strategies listed in Exhibit 31.3. Strategies can be incorporated into occupational therapy sessions, as can consulting with education staff to facilitate the use of strategies in the educational environment.

Least Restrictive Environment

IDEA (2004) mandates that all students be placed to learn in the least restrictive environment appropriate to their individual needs. This may pose a challenge for IEP teams because students with ED often possess cognitive skills that allow them to participate in the general education curriculum yet exhibit behaviors that greatly disrupt the learning environment for themselves and others.

When making placement decisions for a student with ED, the team needs to consider any potential harmful effect on the student or quality of services provided. The prevalence of a high frequency and intensity of a student's problem behavior—specifically, physical aggression—is a common consideration for self-contained or alternative school placements (Hoge et al., 2014). Students with ED are more likely to be placed in more restrictive settings (e.g., self-contained classrooms, alternative schools, homebound programming, hospital placements) and are more likely to move between schools and service providers multiple times during their academic careers (Becker et al., 2014).

Some studies have identified that students who enter into more restrictive settings demonstrate higher rates of problem behavior and lower rates of academic achievement (Becker et al., 2014). Also, recent research has suggested that entrance criteria into alternative placements tend to be less strict than the criteria required to exit the placement, suggesting that once students enter an alternative placement, they are less likely to transition back to a less restrictive environment (Hoge et al., 2014).

Occupational therapists can support the IEP team by advocating for early behavioral intervention and social–emotional learning support for students who meet the criteria for ED. Providing students with high-quality intervention to promote positive behaviors and social–emotional learning competencies may decrease the need for more restrictive placement in the future.

Restraint and Seclusion

Some students with ED may exhibit severe and dangerous forms of challenging behavior. At times, this type of behavior can pose an imminent danger to the student, school staff, and peers. IDEA (2004) mandates that positive behavioral interventions and supports (PBIS) be used to manage challenging behaviors for students receiving special education. *PBIS* requires that positive behavior approaches be used to respond to and manage behaviors instead of aversive interventions, such as restraint and seclusion (Gagnon et al., 2017).

Although federal law does not regulate the use of restraint and seclusion in schools, 27 states have adopted guidelines or policies around their use. Most states clearly outline that the emergency use of restraint and seclusion is a last resort to maintain the safety of the student, staff, and peers and is prohibited as a behavioral intervention to reduce the frequency of a behavior. State legislation routinely identifies requirements for the proactive use of PBIS, specifies training for use of restraint or seclusion, and prohibits the use of dangerous restraints and aversive procedures (Jones et al., 2016).

Despite state regulations and limitations on the use of these procedures, concerns regarding their use remain. Gagnon et al. (2017) cited multiple examples of research indicating that the use of restraint and seclusion could result in physical and emotional harm for the student; is generally ineffective for decreasing the problem behavior; and can exacerbate problem behavior by angering the

---

EXHIBIT 31.3.   Strategies to Maximize Academic Success

- Set clear expectations of the learning environment and behaviors associated with learning (e.g., successful learners are well organized, keep eyes focused on the speaker, use time wisely).
- Preteach expected procedures associated with learning (e.g., being prepared for class means that the desk is clear of all materials except a pencil and notebook, glasses are on, and conversations with peers are finished).
- Have strategies in place to facilitate learning (e.g., organizational materials, visually structured materials, limited disruptions in the learning environment).
- Instruct student in goal setting, self-monitoring, and self-assessment (e.g., use Goal–Plan–Do–Check, Self-Determined Learning Model of Instruction, self-monitoring of time on task, self-regulated strategy development).
- Use choice to allow students to exert some amount of control over academic demands.
- Use peer-mediated instruction and intervention to provide tutoring or support.
- Match instructional methods and cultural styles.
- Use experiential learning (e.g., real-world learning, work experience, service learning, place-based education).

Source. Jones et al. (2016).

student, triggering associations of previous traumatic experiences, and damaging student–teacher relationships.

Students who are "chronically restrained or secluded . . . may experience occupational deprivation as a result of being kept from their peers and what most would consider typical school activities" (AOTA, 2015, p. 1). Occupational therapy practitioners can reduce the likelihood of the use of restraint or seclusion by promoting occupational enrichment and supporting meaningful participation in educational and leisure pursuits (e.g., organizing a checkers club, cheering for a sports team, setting up chairs for an assembly).

Positive Student–Teacher Relationships

Students with ED may have experienced dysfunctional familial relationships, adverse childhood experiences, and extreme stress in home and community environments, leading to challenges forming relationships with teachers and educational staff. Research has demonstrated that when positive student–teacher relationships are developed, a correlated reduction is seen in problem behavior, anxiety, and loneliness and an increase in academic achievement, school engagement, and overall student satisfaction (Jones et al., 2016).

Occupational therapy practitioners should engage in an individual connection with the student, communicate openly and honestly, attend and respond to nonverbal communication, use high rates of positive statements and limit negative ones, provide effective feedback regarding performance, and demonstrate respect and unconditional positive regard for the student (Jones et al., 2016).

Collaboration With Family and Community Service Providers

Collaborating with parents and community service providers is essential to working with students with ED. Most students with ED demonstrate similar rates and intensities of behaviors at home and in the community and can be a challenge to manage outside of school. Parents of children with ED are more likely to experience mental health needs (Jones et al., 2016); they benefit from additional time and attention to understand evaluation results and intervention plans and build a positive home–school partnership.

Students with ED are likely to receive mental health services outside of school. In these instances, IEP teams (including the occupational therapist) should gain parent permission to collaborate with community professionals, coordinate intervention practices, and share important student updates.

BEST PRACTICES

Occupational therapy practitioners provide services to students under IDEA, including students with mental health and behavioral challenges. To allow for the most effective and efficient provision of services, occupational therapy practitioners must be prepared to provide evidence-based interventions using data-driven decision making to guide their practice.

Conduct Evaluation to Identify Student Strengths and Needs

Occupational therapists evaluate the student's ability to engage in learning and school activities across the day. Emphasis is often placed on identifying those activities that pose challenges and those that do not. The process begins with the occupational profile (AOTA, 2014c) to gain a perspective on the student and background. Data are gathered about the student's history, experiences, interests, needs, daily living routines, and the supports or barriers during occupations.

Occupational therapy evaluations include a record review (e.g., to provide pertinent background history and educational performance) as well as observation of the student in the settings and routines where concerns are present. If practitioners determine areas that require additional information, assessments, such as the Canadian Occupational Performance Measure (5th ed.; Law et al., 2014), School Function Assessment (Coster et al., 1998), or Child Occupational Self-Assessment (Keller et al., 2005), may provide a structured approach to investigating areas of occupational performance need. For additional resources, see Appendix F, "Selected Assessment Tools for Analysis of Students' Occupational Performance."

Identify Factors Affecting Occupational Performance

When necessary to understand the barriers to participation in common occupations, occupational therapists may use systematic observation to identify environmental factors, performance skills, or performance patterns that contribute to performance deficits. Bellini (2016) differentiated skill deficits into performance deficits and acquisition deficits. Students with acquisition deficits lack the specific skills to complete the task; performance deficits occur when the student possesses all the skills necessary to complete the task yet does not perform the necessary skills.

For example, an occupational therapy practitioner may observe that a student puts on his coat independently and quickly packs his school bag on days he needs to leave school early for community activities; however, on other days, the student needs multiple reminders and supervision to perform these tasks. This reflects that the student presents with performance deficits versus acquisition deficits. Students with acquisition deficits lack specific skills (performance skills or patterns) and may require specific intervention to develop these skills.

Address Educational Performance Deficits

The presence of multiple variables affecting a student's educational outcomes indicates the need for systematic and intensive intervention. Maggin, Wehby, Farmer, et al. (2016) stated that students with ED require individualized interventions that are continually monitored by objective data collection to achieve optimal outcomes. Occupational therapy practitioners are encouraged to access AOTA's systematic reviews, evidence-based practice resources, and practice guidelines series when contemplating which interventions to select (AOTA, 2017a).

Self-management interventions

Common and evidence-based strategies used with students with ED include self-management interventions such as

- Self-monitoring (the ability to continuously monitor own performance)
- Self-instruction (the ability to select and apply strategy or accommodation to change own performance)
- Self-evaluation (the ability to evaluate the change in performance)
- Self-reinforcement (the ability to access a desirable event or activity contingent on positive performance change).

Occupational therapy practitioners can follow a self-management intervention protocol (e.g., the Zones of Regulation; Kuypers, 2011) to assist students in demonstrating on-task behavior; accessing a break appropriately; and accessing strategies to support management of feelings of stress, anxiety, or frustration.

Cognitive–behavioral interventions

Cognitive–behavioral interventions aim to alter behavior by using cognitive strategies to change thoughts and perspectives on a given situation. Most often, cognitive–behavioral interventions address social–emotional learning competencies and EF skills to support student performance in the education environment (Jones et al., 2016).

Strong research supports the use of cognitive–behavioral interventions with students with ED, including self-monitoring, self-instruction or self-talk, social skills development, goal setting, contracts, and accurate and effective interpretation of events (AOTA, 2017a; Jones et al., 2016). Cognitive–behavioral theory is a frame of reference frequently used by occupational therapists in practice, allowing cognitive–behavioral interventions to be applied to occupation-based practice.

Cognitive Orientation to daily Occupational Performance. The ***Cognitive Orientation to daily Occupational Performance*** (CO–OP) is an occupational therapy intervention developed to support occupational performance in children using problem solving, learning and motor learning theories, cognitive strategies, client-centered practice, goal setting, and motivation (Dawson et al., 2017; Missiuna et al., 2001).

CO–OP uses a cognitive–behavioral approach (well known for effectiveness with students with ED) to address goal setting and motivation (specific areas of need for students with ED), suggesting that the intervention contains practice elements and principles of behavior that may be effective with this population. The Goal–Plan–Do–Check framework (Polatajko & Mandich, 2004) may be used for enhancing occupational performance during complex or unstructured tasks. This is a framework that evolved out of occupational therapy practice in mental health.

Organizational and educational strategies. Students with ED may exhibit occupational performance barriers around the completion of academic tasks, often related to EF and motor challenges. They may benefit from the use of organizational strategies such as making instructions very explicit, breaking the assignment into manageable steps or parts, grading or altering the complexity of the task, scaffolding instruction, and developing and using appropriate questions. Use of assistive technology may increase a student's success and decrease frustration associated with organization or handwriting demands. Occupational therapists can incorporate these strategies into collaboration with special education staff to facilitate a student's occupational performance in academic tasks throughout the school day.

Self-determination. Students with ED demonstrate characteristics that adversely affect their perception of their performance, abilities, and ability to advocate effectively for their individual needs. Occupational therapy practitioners can support students in overcoming these barriers using coaching interventions such as Occupational Performance Coaching (OPC) to facilitate students' understanding of unique skills and abilities, how to leverage their strengths, and how to achieve occupational success in the educational environment (Dunn, 2017; Graham et al., 2009).

Coaching interventions can help students learn to monitor, evaluate, and modify their occupational performance, furthering success in the educational environment. Currently, limited evidence exists to support the use of coaching to improve occupational performance for students with ED; however, Detrich et al.'s (2013) framework can be used to determine whether this intervention may be effective for students with ED. OPC uses a strengths-based and cognitive–behavioral approach (both are well known as effective interventions for students with ED) to facilitate goal achievement (a specific area of need for students with ED).

Establish skills and abilities. Occupational therapy intervention may focus on students' acquisition of skills to enhance their participation and engagement in occupations. In this case, occupational therapy practitioners would apply approaches and interventions described in the *OTPF–3* (AOTA, 2014b) while working to develop a positive relationship with the student and providing additional encouragement and praise for effort and task completion.

SUMMARY

Occupational therapy practitioners can have a significant effect on educational programming for students with ED. Their unique understanding of the interrelated conditions that affect students' occupational performance is a valuable contribution to the IEP for students with ED.

RESOURCES

- **AOTA** (https://www.aota.org) provides fact sheets on AOTA's role, evidence-based materials, and information about restraint and seclusion (https://www.aota.org).
- The **National Professional Development Center for Autism Spectrum Disorder** (https://autismpdc.fpg.unc .edu/sites/autismpdc.fpg.unc.edu/files/imce/documents /Self-management-Complete-10-2010.pdf) provides modules on implementing self-management intervention with high fidelity.

REFERENCES

Accreditation Council for Occupational Therapy Education. (2012). *Accreditation Council for Occupational Therapy Education (ACOTE®) standards and interpretive guide.* (<June 2018> Interpretive Guide version). Retrieved from https://www.aota.org/-/media/Corporate/Files/EducationCareers/Accredit/Standards/2011-Standards-and-Interpretive-Guide.pdf

Alberto, P. A., & Troutman, A. C. (2017). *Applied behavior analysis for teachers* (9th ed.). New York: Pearson.

American Occupational Therapy Association. (2009). *Fact Sheet: Occupational therapy and school mental health.* Retrieved from https://www.aota.org/~/media/corporate/files/secure/practice/children/ot%20and%20school%20mental%20health.pdf

American Occupational Therapy Association. (2014a). Guidelines for supervision, roles, and responsibilities during the delivery of occupational therapy services. *American Journal of Occupational Therapy, 68*(Suppl. 3), S16–S22. https://doi.org/10.5014/ajot.686S03

American Occupational Therapy Association. (2014b). Occupational therapy practice framework: Domain and process (3rd ed.). *American Journal of Occupational Therapy, 68*(Suppl. 1), S1–S48. https://doi.org/10.5014/ajot.2014.682006

American Occupational Therapy Association. (2014c). *Occupational therapy's role in mental health promotion, prevention, and intervention: Social and emotional learning.* Retrieved from https://www.aota.org/~/media/Corporate/Files/Practice/Children/SchoolMHToolkit/Social-and-Emotional-Learning-Info-Sheet.pdf

American Occupational Therapy Association. (2015). *Reducing restraint and seclusion: The benefit and role of occupational therapy.* Retrieved from https://www.aota.org/~/media/Corporate/Files/Practice/Children/Reducing-Restraint-and-Seclusion-20150218.PDF

American Occupational Therapy Association. (2017a). *AOTA's evidence-based practice resources.* Retrieved from https://www.aota.org/~/media/Corporate/Files/Practice/Researcher/EBP-Resources.pdf

American Occupational Therapy Association. (2017b). Mental health promotion, prevention, and intervention in occupational therapy practice. *American Journal of Occupational Therapy, 71*(Suppl. 2), 7112410035. https://doi.org/10.5014/ajot.2017.716S03

Arbesman, M., Bazyk, S., & Nochajski, S. M. (2013). Systematic review of occupational therapy and mental health promotion, prevention, and intervention for children and youth. *American Journal of Occupational Therapy, 67*, e120–e130. https://doi.org/10.5014/ajot.2013.008359

Bazyk, S., & Arbesman, M. (2018). *Occupational therapy practice guidelines for mental health promotion, prevention, and intervention for children and youth.* Bethesda, MD: AOTA Press.

Becker, S. P., Paternite, C. E., & Evans, S. W. (2014). Special educators' conceptualizations of emotional disturbance and educational placement decision making for middle and high school students. *School Mental Health, 6*, 163–174. https://doi.org/10.1007/s12310-014-9119-7

Bellini, S. (2016). *Building social relationships 2.* Lenexa, KS: AAPC.

Collaborative for Academic, Social, and Emotional Learning. (2013). *About CASEL.* Retrieved from https://casel.org

Coster, W., Deeney, T., Haltiwanger, J., & Haley, S. (1998). *School Function Assessment.* San Antonio: Psychological Corp.

Dawson, D., McEwen, S. E., & Polatajko, H. J. (2017). *Cognitive Orientation to daily Occupational Performance in Occupational Therapy: Using the CO–OP Approach™ to enable participation across the lifespan.* Bethesda, MD: AOTA Press.

Detrich, R., Slocum, T. A., & Spencer, T. D. (2013). Evidence-based education and best available evidence: Decision-making under conditions of uncertainty. In B. G. Cook, M. Tankersley, & T. J. Landrum (Eds.), *Evidence-based practices* (pp. 21–44). Bingley, England: Emerald Group.

Dunn, W. (2017). Strengths-based approaches: What if even the "bad" things are good things? *British Journal of Occupational Therapy, 80*, 395–396. https://doi.org/10.1177/0308022617702660

Gable, R. A., Park, K. L., & Scott, T. M. (2014). Functional behavioral assessment and students at risk for or with emotional disabilities: Current issues and considerations. *Education and Treatment of Children, 37*, 111–135. https://doi.org/10.1353/etc.2014.0011

Gagnon, D. J., Mattingly, M. J., & Connelly, V. J. (2017). The restraint and seclusion of students with a disability: Examining trends in U.S. school districts and their policy implications. *Journal of Disability Policy Studies, 28*(2), 66–76. https://doi.org/10.1177/1044207317710697

Graham, F., Rodger, S., & Bauer, J. (2009). *Occupational performance coaching: An exploration of a therapist's strategy use.* Paper presented at the University of Queensland School of Health and Rehabilitation Sciences Post-Graduate Conference, Brisbane, Queensland, Australia.

Hoge, M. R., Liaupsin, C. B., Umbreit, J., & Ferro, J. B. (2014). Examining placement considerations for students with emotional disturbance across three alternative schools. *Journal of Disability Policy Studies, 24*, 218–226. https://doi.org/10.1177/1044207312461672

Individuals With Disabilities Education Improvement Act of 2004, Pub. L. 108–446, 20 U.S.C. §§ 1400–1482.

Jones, V., Greenwood, A., & Dunn, C. (2016). *Effective supports for students with emotional and behavioral disorders.* New York: Pearson.

Keller, J., Kafkes, A., Basu, S., Federico, J., & Kielhofner, G. (2005). *A user's guide to Child Occupational Self-Assessment (COSA).* Chicago: University of Illinois.

Kuypers, L. (2011). *The Zones of Regulation.* San Jose, CA: Think Social.

Kuypers, L. (2013). The Zones of Regulation: A framework to foster self-regulation. *Sensory Integration Special Interest Section Quarterly, 36*(4), 1–4.

Law, M., Baptiste, S., Carswell, A., McColl, M., Polatajko, H., & Pollock, N. (2014). *Canadian Occupational Performance Measure* (5th ed.). Ottawa: CAOT Publications.

Maggin, D. M., Wehby, J. H., Farmer, T. W., & Brooks, D. S. (2016). Intensive interventions for students with emotional and behavioral disorders: Issues, theory, and future directions. *Journal of Emotional and Behavioral Disorders, 24*, 127–137. https://doi.org/10.1177/1063426616661498

Maggin, D. M., Wehby, J. H., & Gilmour, A. F. (2016). Intensive academic interventions for students with emotional and behavioral disorders: An experimental framework. *Journal of Emotional and Behavioral Disorders, 24*, 138–147. https://doi.org/10.1177/1063426616649162

Missiuna, C., Mandich, A. D., Polatajko, H. J., & Malloy-Miller, T. (2001). Cognitive Orientation to daily Occupational Performance (CO–OP): Part I. Theoretical foundations. *Physical and Occupational Therapy in Pediatrics, 20*(2/3), 69–81.

National Center for Education Statistics. (2017). *The condition of education.* Retrieved from https://nces.ed.gov/programs/coe/

Polatajko, H., & Mandich, A. (2004). *Enabling occupation in children: The Cognitive Orientation to daily Occupational Performance (CO–OP) approach.* Ottawa: CAOT Publications.

Scott, T. M., & Alter, P. J. (2017). Examining the case for functional behavior assessment as an evidence-based practice for students with emotional and behavioral disorders in general education classrooms. *Preventing School Failure: Alternative Education for Children and Youth, 61*(1), 80–93. https://doi.org/10.1080/1045988X.2016.1196645

Best Practices in Supporting Students With Hearing Impairments or Deafness

32

Elizabeth A. Fain, EdD, OTR/L

KEY TERMS AND CONCEPTS

- American Sign Language
- Assistive technology
- Cultural sensitivity
- Deaf culture
- Deaf Gain
- Eye gaze
- Facial processing
- Fragmented hearing
- Hearing impairment
- Hearing loss
- Lipreading
- Person–Environment–Occupation Model
- Self-advocacy
- Sensory processing disorders

OVERVIEW

For children, **hearing loss** is associated with long-term academic and communication difficulties (Rajendran & Roy, 2011). The World Health Organization (2018) estimates that 5% of the population (i.e., 466 million persons of whom 34 million are children) has a disabling hearing loss. Of every 1,000 children in the United States, 2–3 are born with a congenital hearing loss.

Because there are no obvious signs, the perception may often be that the child has an attention problem or learning disability. Hearing loss, similar to learning disabilities, also affects perception, language processing, processing time, memory, and attention (Anderson, 2014). It is not uncommon for a student with a hearing impairment to miss at least 20% of the information conveyed in the classroom, even with aids and a quiet environment. A student with a mild hearing loss can miss as much as 50% of classroom discussion (Hearing Loss Association of America, 2018). Forty percent of children classified as having hearing loss also have other conditions (Beams, 2007; Jerome et al., 2013).

Children with hearing loss typically demonstrate vestibular dysfunction, clumsiness, incoordination, and balance deficits (Jerome et al., 2013; Rajendran & Roy, 2011). Many children and teenagers who have a **hearing impairment** (HI; including deafness) also have deficits in the functional skills necessary for functional independence (Meinzen-Derr et al., 2013).

The Education for All Handicapped Children Act of 1975 (Pub. L. 94–142) enabled students with HI to attend their local public schools in lieu of environments that were more restrictive. Today, the Individuals With Disabilities Education Improvement Act of 2004 (IDEA; Pub. L. 108–446) recognizes that students with HI may need special accommodations in the least restrictive environment with highly qualified professionals. Specific regulations under IDEA require that a student determined eligible for specialized instruction as a child with an HI receive an individualized education program (IEP). The IEP addresses and documents any adverse effect of the HI on the student's access to and participation in the general education curriculum.

Evidence-based accommodations have been developed to guide best practices for people with HI; however, implementation of accommodations is sparse as specifically related to occupational therapy. See Exhibit 32.1 for general recommendations for communicating with a Deaf person.

Terminology, Communicating, and Awareness

The terminology of hearing loss and deafness is often misunderstood, which contributes to misunderstanding because several terms are often used interchangeably (see Exhibit 32.2 for common definitions).

ESSENTIAL CONSIDERATIONS

Occupational therapy practitioners[1] working with students with HI need to understand cultural considerations, communication styles, effect on participation in an educational program, and common assistive technology (AT). *AT* includes devices or equipment that is used to promote

---

[1]*Occupational therapy practitioner* refers to both the occupational therapist and the occupational therapy assistant. The American Occupational Therapy Association (AOTA; 2014a, p. S18) states, "The occupational therapist is responsible for all aspects of occupational therapy service delivery and is accountable for the safety and effectiveness of the occupational therapy service delivery process" and "must be directly involved in the delivery of services during the initial evaluation and regularly throughout the course of intervention. . . . The occupational therapy assistant delivers safe and effective occupational therapy services under the supervision of and in partnership with the occupational therapist."

Copyright © 2019 by the American Occupational Therapy Association. All rights reserved. To reuse this content, contact www.copyright.com.
https://doi.org/10.7139/2019.978-1-56900-591-0.032

EXHIBIT 32.1.	Recommendations for Communicating With a Deaf Person

- Expect to feel uncomfortable when initiating the communication process.
- Accept being uncomfortable; the comfort level will increase as efforts to be understood are made.
- It is okay to write to a Deaf person. However, be cognizant that literacy and language skills affect their comprehension.
- Efforts will be appreciated more if you use a combination of gestures, facial expressions, body language, and written communication.
- When a Deaf person uses their voice to communicate, it is fine to ask them to write responses to you if you do not understand.
- Recognize that patience is needed during a conversation, and do not fake understanding the communication or trivialize the conversation.
- Deaf people listen with their eyes and cannot look at an object at the same time you are communicating to them.
- Speak directly to a Deaf person instead of to an interpreter.

Source. Greer et al. (2004).

functional skills. Occupational therapy practitioners are valuable team members and are vital for optimal learning and success in the school environment. IDEA (2004) mandates that children and youth between the ages of 3 and 21 years with disabilities be provided a free appropriate public education.

Cultural Sensitivity

Cultural sensitivity entails understanding the culture of the client receiving the therapy services and being responsive to those attitudes, feelings, and circumstances throughout the occupational therapy process. These key components of cultural sensitivity include awareness or knowledge, appropriate skill set, and contextual understanding (AOTA, 2014b). Occupational therapy practitioners need to be aware of cultural components, along with communication techniques, fragmented hearing, increased efforts of listening with resulting increased fatigue, dos and don'ts of working with sign language interpreters, self-advocacy competency, and various types of assistive technology for HI.

Students with HI are influenced by their perspective; family, home, and educational environments; social mores; and cultural components. Most people perceive deafness merely as a medical condition and tend to focus on correcting the perceived problem. However, many Deaf people do not view themselves as disabled—rather, they see themselves as members of *Deaf culture,* a distinct cultural community with its own language, values, and social mores (Deaf Inc., 2017).

There are no specific hearing levels or personal characteristics that determine whether a student will identify with a hearing culture or Deaf culture. Therefore, practitioners need to engage with students with profound hearing loss to know whether they identify themselves as hard of hearing or as deaf. How a person chooses to identify is based on a variety of factors that include hearing status, communication preference, cultural orientation, and use of technology. This will directly affect the approach that the occupational therapy practitioner uses with the student.

Communication Techniques With the Deaf and Hard of Hearing

Communication styles vary according to the culture with which persons who are deaf and hard of hearing identify and with the environmental situation. The most widely used

EXHIBIT 32.2.	Common Definitions of Hearing Loss and Deafness

- **Audiogram:** Responses to sounds that are recorded on a chart for each sound frequency tested.
- **deaf** (lowercase D): Having minimal or no hearing.
- **Deaf** (capital D) **culture:** Generally refers to Deaf people who use ASL as their primary mode of communication and who enjoy socializing with others who are Deaf, creating close-knit communities based on shared beliefs, customs, arts, and history.
- **Decibel** (dB): Unit of measure for intensity or loudness of sound.
- **Hard of hearing:** Having some level of hearing loss but not profound hearing loss.
- **Hearing impairment:** Having reduced hearing sensitivity. Note that people with hearing impairment generally do not consider themselves part of the Deaf culture even when they know sign language. *Hearing impaired* is the term most often used by the media or society; however, the Deaf culture perceives this term as offensive, suggesting that Deaf people are "broken" (Greer et al., 2004).
- **Hertz:** Frequency or pitch of a sound.
- **Hearing loss:**
  - *Acquired hearing loss:* Occurs after birth.
  - *Congenital hearing loss:* Present at birth.
  - *Perilingual hearing loss:* Occurs during the acquisition of spoken language.
  - *Postlingual hearing loss:* Occurs after the acquisition of spoken language.
  - *Prelingual hearing loss:* Occurs before acquisition of spoken language.
  - *Progressive hearing loss:* Occurs over time.
- **Types of hearing loss:**
  - *Conductive hearing loss:* Sound waves are obstructed from traveling to the inner ear by ossified bones or malformed auditory canals.
  - *Sensorineural hearing loss:* Damage to the inner ear or auditory nerve prevents the sound message from being sent to the brain for processing.
  - *Mixed hearing loss:* Having both a conductive hearing loss and a sensorineural hearing loss.
  - *Central auditory processing disorder:* The ear is not damaged, but the neural system involved with processing or understanding language is damaged (Lanfer, 2006).

Note. ASL = American Sign Language.

communication mode in the Deaf culture in the United States is American Sign Language (ASL). *ASL* is a visual language using hand motions and consists of a distinct vocabulary, grammar, and syntax separate from the English language (Deaf Inc., 2017). If the occupational therapy practitioner is not familiar with ASL, then an interpreter is necessary. The process of using an ASL interpreter is much like that of using an interpreter for a foreign language: Face the student when communicating.

Other students may choose to use AT to help them use their residual hearing to communicate orally. AT could be hearing aids, amplifying devices, or note takers to help them read the material at a later time. When working with the students in the classroom environment, get their attention before proceeding with the conversation and be sure to face them so that they can read your lips and use facial expressions for additional contextual meaning. Ask for their preferred communication method and follow through with it.

Forcing use of different communication methods alters the accuracy of information gained. Be aware of the environment for lighting, noise level, and types of activities occurring simultaneously, especially when the intervention is occurring in the classroom. Communicate clearly without raising your voice or speaking quickly. Each student's communication mode is unique and shaped by many factors, including educational experiences, cultural or linguistic identity of family of origin, and peer influences.

Impact on Participation

Fragmented hearing consists of missing pieces or words in the story or educational topic being presented. Envision a completed puzzle with many pieces missing and the visual effect that results. Even with the latest hearing technology, hearing is not restored to the normal hearing ability. For example, a student with an aided hearing threshold of a 20-dB hearing loss will have a 20% listening gap; hearing peers will have a 5% listening gap (Anderson, 2014). The occupational therapy practitioner addresses the fragmented hearing by ensuring optimal fit among person, environment, and occupation and by educating teachers and other team members about the cascading effect of the hearing loss that requires the student to exert extra effort to understand the speech and contextual relevance, and the resulting fatigue (Hornsby et al., 2014; Valente et al., 2012; see Figure 32.1 for common sounds).

According to Hornsby et al. (2014) and Valente et al. (2012), any degree of hearing loss requires greater effort, regardless of amplification. Researchers have investigated this fatigue using the Test of Auditory Processing Skills, which looks at language processing for phonological or phonemic processing, memory, and language comprehension and reasoning. The fatigue that resulted was substantial even when compared with that resulting from other chronic health conditions such as cancer, diabetes, and rheumatoid arthritis (Hornsby et al., 2014; Valente et al., 2012).

The Functional Listening Evaluation may be more relevant for understanding the student's listening skills and performance in the classroom as opposed to audiological assessments in a soundproof booth (Johnson & VonAlmen, 1993). Because hearing loss is invisible, it is easy

to comprehend how effects of fragmented hearing, listening effort fatigue, and contextual components of the environment contribute to the overall disconnect for optimal performance in the learning environment. Therefore, occupational therapy practitioners, along with other team members, must ensure equal and effective access to communication and learning in the classroom.

Sensory Processing: Auditory, Visual, and Vestibular

Students with partial or total HI are vulnerable to *sensory processing disorders* that may affect occupational performance such as self-care skills, functional mobility, and learning when students have difficulty with sensitivity to certain types of clothing, coordination and balance difficulties, or oral sensitivity to various textures. Studies by Tharpe et al. (2008) indicated that visual attention of children with HI was more disorganized than that of children with normal hearing. The rationale was that children with normal hearing were able to achieve and maintain sustained visual attention, whereas those with HI had to use their visual skills to perceive the visual stimulants. However, evidence suggests that this improves with further auditory stimulation (Parasnis et al., 2003).

Lipreading is the visual identification of speech gestures that enhances the intelligibility of speech (Schwartz et al., 2004). Reading the speaker's lips enhances the sensitivity to auditory information (Grant, 2001). Studies support that the brain develops language skills irrespective of visual or auditory stimulus, suggesting the benefits of early sign language even if the goal is spoken language (Hoffmeister, 2000; Mayberry & Lock, 2003). In light of these studies, occupational therapy practitioners need to promote a fit for the Person–Environment–Occupation (PEO) framework.

Students with deafness are at risk for vestibular dysfunction as a result of comorbid conditions such as profound sensorineural hearing loss; acquired deafness as a result of meningitis; damage to the central nervous system; damage to the inner ear extending to the vestibular receptors; and Usher, Waardenburg, and Pendred syndromes, among others (De Kegel et al., 2012; Suarez et al., 2007). Several studies have yielded data supporting that children who have HI demonstrate motor and balance deficits (De Kegel et al., 2012; Hartman et al., 2011; Livingstone & McPhillips, 2011).

Postural stability integrates visual, vestibular, and somatosensory information by the nervous system to produce motor responses that maintain balance. Published reports yield data that vestibular dysfunction is noted in approximately 30%–70% of children with HI (Jacot et al., 2009; Shinjo et al., 2007; Zhou & Stevens, 2009). One implication for occupational therapy practitioners is that functional limitations and learning challenges may be attributed to the vestibular and proprioceptive systems, whereas bilateral integration and sequencing may be attributed to sensory integration dysfunction (Koester et al., 2014).

Technology and AT

Students with HI are unaware of various sounds that occur throughout the day in various functional activities and

FIGURE 32.1. Audiogram of familiar sounds.

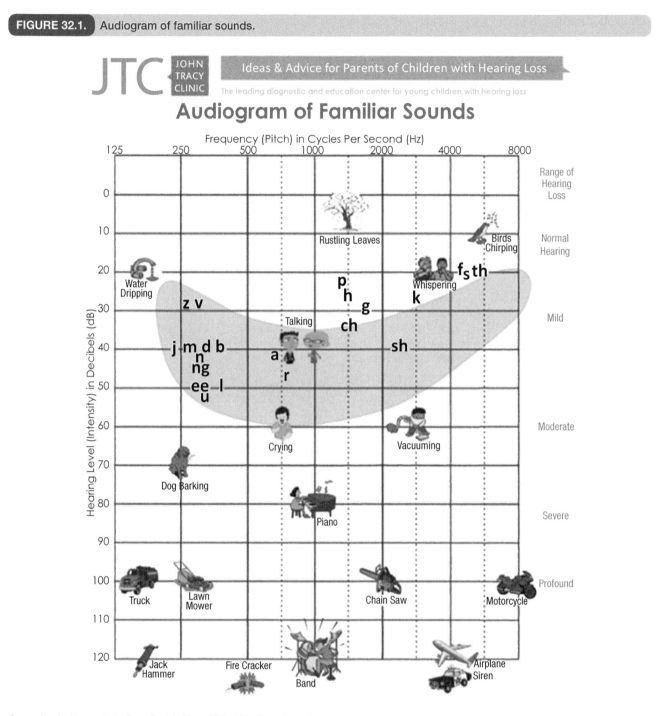

FIGURE 32.1. Audiogram of familiar sounds.

Source. Used with permission from the John Tracy Clinic, 2012, https://www.jtc.org.

contexts, which can adversely affect their security and functional skills. Hearing dogs are trained to alert for sounds such as alarms, school bells ringing, or someone calling the student's name, among other sounds (Mowry et al., 1994). The hearing dog—even with the sole task of lying near the reader during a reading task—can facilitate an increase in a student's reading ability (Pillow-Price et al., 2014).

Assessment and provision of AT is an important strategy to promote a fit between students and their environment to enhance optimal engagement in occupations (Ivanhoff et al., 2006). According to Ivanhoff et al. (2006), AT and physical environmental interventions are important strategies to promote occupational performance.

Several studies have indicated that persons with HI explore and see the world differently because of their adaptation to hearing loss and communication approaches (Dye et al., 2009; Tharpe et al., 2008). *Facial processing* is the ability to recognize expressions, a person's appearance, and social interactions (Watanabe et al., 2011). McCullough and Emmorey (1997) provided data indicating that Americans who are deaf are better at detecting subtle differences in facial differences, which suggests that long-term experience of facial processing with ASL and lipreading may contribute to enhanced detection of facial expression nuances.

Eye gaze is being used in technology and is designed to help steer the acoustics of hearing through a highly directional beamforming microphone. The principle is that such a directed hearing aid will preferentially amplify sounds from one direction as opposed to all the sounds in the environment (Best et al., 2017).

BEST PRACTICES

Occupational therapy practitioners promote maximal independence and participation in occupational performance. The **PEO Model** can be used by occupational therapists to guide the evaluation and intervention process. After a comprehensive evaluation, occupational therapists share information with the team to determine the need for related services, modifications, and accommodations for students with HI.

Using the PEO Model With Students With HI

In the school setting, occupational therapy practitioners support learning through enhancement of students' abilities and by addressing the fit of the PEO frame of reference. Students who are deaf or hard of hearing have unique barriers to occupational performance in the school setting.

Using an occupation-based model, such as the PEO Model (Law et al., 1996), entails promoting optimal occupational performance while ensuring a good fit in the interaction among the person, the occupation, and the environment. Desired activities for students include successful learning, participation in daily routines, academic performance, and social participation (occupations) in their environment (AOTA, 2014b). Students with HI may experience challenges engaging in their occupations in the environment because of fragmented hearing, even with optimal technology usage and environmental circumstances (see Figure 32.2).

Facilitating functional independence entails that occupational therapy practitioners demonstrate awareness of the language and culture surrounding the perception of and terms related to deafness and hearing loss. Dirksen et al. (2014) proposed that *deafness* be defined as a distinct way of interacting with the environment using perceptions, perspectives, and insights that are less commonly shared by the hearing population. Therefore, using the term *Deaf Gain* lines up with the philosophy of occupational therapy to view the condition as abilities.

Deaf Gain refers to the alternate ways of thinking, perceiving sensory information, creative problem solving, and cultural gains manifested through being deaf when interacting in the world (Dirksen et al., 2014). Illustrations of the Deaf Gain concept might include intensified visual–perceptual skills for observation of environmental contexts and awareness of facial and body language such that the person with HI uses their visual sensory skills to offset their hearing limitations. Tactile sensory skills of persons with HI may be enhanced such that they focus on tactile input, including vibrations, to alert them to environmental events (Dirksen et al., 2014).

FIGURE 32.2. Model adapted for people who are Deaf or hard of hearing.

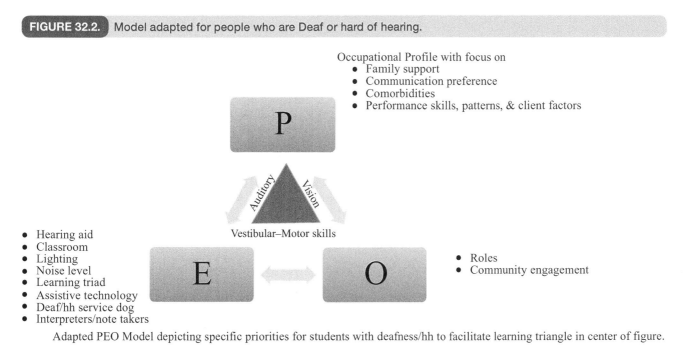

Adapted PEO Model depicting specific priorities for students with deafness/hh to facilitate learning triangle in center of figure.

Note. hh = hard of hearing; PEO = Person–Environment–Occupation.

Conduct a Comprehensive Evaluation

The evaluation follows the process outlined in the *Occupational Therapy Practice Framework: Domain and Process* (3rd ed.; AOTA, 2014b) for examining occupations, client factors, performance skills, performance patterns, and contexts and environment. Special considerations when evaluating students with HI must address the following:

- Understand the culture and use a competent interpreter (when appropriate);
- Consider the PEO fit when assessing the student;
- Assess supports and barriers to occupations (e.g., self-care, social interactions, education); and
- Consider sensory processing skill, especially visual, vestibular, and tactile.

When analyzing a student's occupational performance, there are limited yet applicable assessments standardized for children with HI. In addition, adaptation of standardized instruments may be a consideration for collecting data; however, one needs to be aware of the mode being used and whether the student is culturally and linguistically skilled to determine whether an accurate picture of the student's performance is captured (Dirksen et al., 2014).

Support Plan and Implement Interventions

Best practice for occupational therapists working with students with HI should include addressing vision, communication, learning, environment and context, visual perception for lipreading, sign language, facial recognition, and eye gaze for hearing aid sound localization. It should also include other compensatory strategies that need to be assessed and developed by occupational therapy practitioners to provide optimal occupational performance and to promote self-advocacy.

Promote Self-Advocacy

Self-advocacy is the awareness of one's needs and seeking support for obtaining the right to reasonable needs and accommodations (Pocock et al., 2002). Specifically, self-advocacy for students with HI entails reflecting on strengths and weaknesses as related to performance in the environment, formulating goals, being assertive, and making decisions to achieve the desired outcome. The occupational therapy practitioner can guide students through describing their skills; setting goals; formulating a plan on who, how, and when to ask for assistance; learning how to make decisions; and taking responsibility to deal with the consequences of those decisions.

The occupational therapy practitioner facilitates this process with an intervention approach, as described by Gronski (2012), expanding the school approach to consist of paradigms that promote the development of needed skills for successful engagements in a variety of environments such as school, community, and home. Using the Self-Advocacy Competency Skills Checklist can help assess and guide the intervention addressing self-advocacy skills for students with HI (Pocock et al., 2002). Examples of self-advocacy skills include "I hear better when I can see you talking" or "I can explain to you how my hearing aid works in different environments." Provide feedback to guide students in linking cause and effect so that they can evaluate their own work (Pocock et al., 2002).

Promote Environmental Adaptations

An analogy for capturing the significance of the environment for a student with HI is to imagine being in a sound-proof glass box and relying on vision to capture everything that is occurring in the room. It seems challenging, yet the compensatory strategies required to understand the environment begin to make sense (e.g., using vision, touch, and movement to explore and gather needed information; removing clutter; seeking clarifications). Considerations for adapting the environment include classroom acoustics, lighting, language use, and more.

Classroom acoustics

The occupational therapy practitioner can address challenges with acoustics and environmental accommodations for students with HI. The practitioner should be aware of principles of sound acoustical design and their effect on educational outcomes. After completion of the evaluation, the occupational therapist needs to educate the other team members, disseminate the information, and act as a resource for teachers, parents, and other team members. Include other experts to ensure adequate assessment of the acoustics and equipment needs to promote adequate acoustical design to promote learning (Dockrell & Shield, 2012).

Arranging classroom seating in a U shape provides full visual access to peers during discussions. Be mindful of appliances such as air conditioning units, fans, and computers that may create additional noise and interfere with hearing. Carpet or classroom rugs help to dampen sounds, whereas hardwood floors allow sounds to bounce around (Weber, 2016). Haertl (2015) indicated that compensation strategies for students with deafness or blindness need to include additional sensory cues to complement the traditional pedagogical approaches. These approaches include efforts to enhance fit between the student and learning environment in addition to communication.

Lighting

Fluorescent lights emit a sound that is amplified along with other sounds and interferes with hearing aids and cochlear implants, making it harder to distinguish what is being said. Consider placing the student so these lights are not behind the interpreter or teacher (Weber, 2016).

Language deficiencies

Be aware of the cultural context; the student's first or second language may not be English. Be sure to enlist an appropriate interpretation service that will use the student's primary language (Weber, 2016).

Other considerations

The ultimate goal for occupational therapy practitioners is to promote learning and optimal occupational function for the students who are deaf or hard of hearing in the school setting. Other considerations to weigh when developing the IEP are listed here:

- Research supports that students who are deaf lag behind in learning; emphasis needs to be placed on how to bridge this gap. Being flexible and engaging the PEO framework to promote learning needs to be considered (Weber, 2016).

■ Although students with HI may use lipreading for comprehension of spoken language, only 30%–40% of spoken English is distinguishable on the lips. Therefore, face the student at all times when speaking.

■ Each student's learning needs are unique; therefore, the approach needs to be student centered to promote learning and engagement (Weber, 2016). Consider lists of tasks that outline the agenda and direct the student to upcoming changes in topics or activities.

■ Students with HI often feel isolated because of the differences in communication. Consider smaller groups for these students. Promote a variety of interaction games to increase awareness and socialization among all students.

Collaborate With the Team

All team members need to communicate closely and regularly to ensure the student's academic progress and to adjust the IEP as needed. The student should have copies of class lectures, assignments, and notes. Interactive whiteboards allow teachers to write information on the board and then print it out for the student with HI.

SUMMARY

HI has a unique effect on persons and is the 3rd major public health issue after arthritis and heart disease (Hearing Loss Association of America, 2018). Given its prevalence and significance for occupational performance, occupational therapy practitioners are likely to have students with HI on their caseload.

REFERENCES

American Occupational Therapy Association. (2014a). Guidelines for supervision, roles, and responsibilities during the delivery of occupational therapy services. *American Journal of Occupational Therapy, 68*(Suppl. 3), S16–S22. https://doi.org/10.5014/ajot.2014.686S03

American Occupational Therapy Association. (2014b). Occupational therapy practice framework: Domain and process (3rd ed.). *American Journal of Occupational Therapy, 68*(Suppl. 1), S1–S48. http://dx.doi.org/10.5014/ajot.2014.682006

Anderson, K. (2014). *Supporting success for children with hearing loss.* Retrieved from http://successforkidswithhearingloss.com

Beams, D. (2007). *Communication considerations: Deaf plus.* Retrieved from http://www.handsandvoices.org/comcon/articles/deafplus.htm

Best, V., Keidser, G., Freeston, K., & Buchholz, J. M. (2017). A dynamic speech comprehension test for assessing real-world listening ability. *Journal of the American Academy of Audiology, 27,* 515–526. https://doi.org/10.3766/jaaa.15089

Deaf Inc. (2017). *About deafness and hearing loss.* Retrieved from http://www.deafinconline.org/about-us/deafness/

De Kegel, A., Maes, L., Baetens, T., Dhooge, I., & Waelvelde, H. (2012). The influence of a vestibular dysfunction on the motor development of hearing-impaired children. *Laryngoscope, 122,* 2837–2843. https://doi.org/10.1002/lary.23529

Dirksen, H., Bauman, H., & Murray, J. (2014). *Deaf Gain: Raising the stakes for human diversity.* Minneapolis: University of Minnesota Press.

Dockrell, J., & Shield, B. (2012). The impact of sound-field systems on learning and attention in elementary school classrooms. *American Journal of Speech, Language, and Hearing Research, 55,* 1163–1176. https://doi.org/10.1044/1092-4388(2011/11-0026)

Dye, M., Hauser, P., & Bavalier, D. (2009). Is visual selective attention in deaf individuals enhanced or deficient? The case of useful field of view. *PLoS ONE, 4*(5), e540. https://doi.org/10.1371/journal.pone.0005640

Education for All Handicapped Children Act of 1975, Pub. L. 94–142.

Grant, K. (2001). The effect of speechreading on masked detection thresholds for filtered speech. *Journal of the Acoustical Society of America, 109,* 2272–2275. https://doi.org/10.1121/1.1362687

Greer, L., Holcomb, B., & Siple, L. (2004). *Deaf culture.* Retrieved from https://www.rit.edu/ntid/radscc/sites/rit.edu.ntid.radscc/files/file_attachments/deaf_culture_tip_sheet.pdf

Gronski, M. (2012). Team efforts to serve children who are deaf or hard of hearing. *OT Practice, 17*(17), 15–18.

Haertl, K. (2015). Interdisciplinary sensorimotor approaches to learning: Applications for populations who are deaf blind. *OT Practice, 20*(12), 7–12.

Hartman, E., Houwen, S., & Vischer, C. (2011). Motor skill performance and sports participation in deaf elementary school children. *Adaptive Physical Activity, 28,* 132–145.

Hearing Loss Association of America. (2018). *Basic facts about hearing loss.* Retrieved from https://www.hearingloss.org/hearing-help/hearing-loss-basics/

Hoffmeister, R. (2000). A piece of the puzzle: ASL and reading comprehension in deaf children. In C. Chamberlain, J. Morford, & R. Mayberry (Eds.), *Language acquisition by eye* (pp. 143–163). Mahwah, NJ: Erlbaum.

Hornsby, B., Werfel, K., Camarata, S., & Bess, F. (2014). Subjective fatigue in children with hearing loss: Some preliminary findings. *American Journal of Audiology, 23,* 129–134. https://doi.org/10.1044/1059-0889(2013/13-0017)

Individuals With Disabilities Education Improvement Act of 2004, Pub. L. 108–446, 20 U.S.C. §§ 1400–1482.

Ivanhoff, S., Iwarsson, S., & Sonn, U. (2006). Occupational therapy research on assistive technology and physical environmental issues: A literature review. *Canadian Journal of Occupational Therapy, 2,* 109–119. https://doi.org/10.1177/000841740607300203

Jacot, E., Van Den Abbeele, T., Debre, H., & Wiener-Vascher, S. (2009). Vestibular impairments pre- and post-cochlear implant in children. *International Journal of Pediatric Otorhinolaryngology, 73,* 209–217. https://doi.org/10.1016/j.ijporl.2008.10.024

Jerome, A., Kannan, L., Lakhani, H., & Palekar, T. (2013). Prevalence of vestibular dysfunction in hearing impaired children. *International Journal of Pharmaceutical Science and Health Care, 3*(2), 1–6. https://doi.org/10.1016/j.ijporl.2008.10.024

Johnson, C. D., & VonAlmen, P. (1993). The Functional Listening Evaluation. In C. D. Johnson, P. V. Benson, & J. B. Seaton (Eds.), *Educational audiology handbook* (pp. 336–339). San Diego: Singular.

Koester, A. C., Mailloux, Z., Coleman, G. G., Mori, A. B., Paul, S. M., Blanche, E., & Cermak, S. A. (2014). Sensory integration functions of children with cochlear implants. *American Journal of Occupational Therapy, 68,* 562–569. https://doi.org /ajot.2014.012187

Lanfer, E. (2006). *A resource guide: Mainstreaming a child with a hearing impairment: What teachers need to know* (Capstone paper). Retrieved from http://digitalcommons.wustl.edu/pacs _capstones/92

Law, M., Cooper, B., Strong, S., Stewart, D., Rigby, P., & Letts, L. (1996). The Person–Environment–Occupation Model: A transactive approach to occupational performance. *Canadian Journal of Occupational Therapy, 63,* 9–23. https://doi.org/10 .1177/000841749606300103

Livingstone, N., & McPhillips, M. (2011). Motor skill deficits in children with partial hearing. *Developmental Medicine and Child Neurology, 53,* 836–842. https://doi.org/10.1111/j.1469-8749 .2011.04001.x.

Mayberry, R. I., & Lock, E. (2003). Age constraints on first versus second language acquisition: Evidence for linguistic plasticity and epigenesis. *Brain and Language, 87,* 369–384. https://doi.org /10.1016/S0093-934X(03)00137-8

McCullough, S., & Emmorey, K. (1997). Face processing by deaf ASL signers: Evidence for expertise in distinguishing local features. *Journal of Deaf Studies and Deaf Education, 2,* 212–222.

Meinzen-Derr, J., Wiley, S., Grether, S., & Choo, D. I. (2013). Functional performance among children with cochlear implants and additional disabilities. *Cochlear Implants International, 14,* 181–189. https://doi.org/10.1179/1754762812Y.0000000019

Mowry, R., Carnahan, S., & Watson, D. (1994). *A national study of the training, selection and placement of hearing dogs.* Fayetteville: University of Arkansas, Arkansas Rehabilitation Services.

Parasnis, I., Samar, V., & Berent, G. (2003). Deaf adults without attention deficit hyperactivity disorder display reduced perceptual sensitivity and elevated impulsivity on the Test of Variables of Attention. *Journal of Speech Language and Hearing Research, 46,* 1166–1183. https://doi.org/10.1044/1092 -4388(2003/091)

Pillow-Price, K., Yonts, N., & Stinson, L. (2014). Sit, stay, read: Improving literacy skills using dogs! *Dimensions of Early Childhood, 42*(1), 5–9.

Pocock, A., Lambros, S., Karvonen, M., Test, D., Algozzine, B., Wood, W., & Martin, J. E.; LEAD Group. (2002). Successful strategies for promoting self-advocacy among students with LD. *Intervention in School and Clinic, 37,* 209–216. https://doi .org/10.1177/105345120203700403

Rajendran, V., & Roy, F. (2011). An overview of motor skill performance and balance in hearing impaired children. *Italian Journal of Pediatrics, 37,* 33. https://doi.org/10.1186/1824-7288-37-33

Schwartz, J., Berthommier, F., & Savariaux, C. (2004). Seeing to hear better: Evidence for early audio-visual interactions in speech identification. *Cognition, 93,* B69–B78. https://doi.org /10.1016/j.cognition.2004.01.006

Shinjo, Y., Jin, Y., & Kaga, K. (2007). Assessment of vestibular function of infants and children with congenital and acquired deafness using the ice-water caloric test, rotational chair test and vestibular-evoked myogenic potential recording. *Acta Oto-Laryngologica, 127,* 736–747. https://doi.org/10.1080 /00016480601002039

Suarez, H., Angeli, S., Suarez, A., Rosales, B., Carrera, X., & Alonso, R. (2007). Balance sensory organization in children with profound hearing loss and cochlear implants. *International Journal of Pediatric Otorhinolaryngology, 71,* 629–637. https://doi.org/10.1016/j.ijporl.2006.12.014

Tharpe, A., Ashmead, D., Sladen, D., Ryan, H., & Rothpletz, A. (2008). Visual attention and hearing loss: Past and current perspectives. *Journal of the American Academy of Audiology, 19,* 741–748. https://doi.org/10.3766/jaaa.19.10.2

Valente, D., Plevinsky, H., Franco, J., Heinrichs-Graham, E., & Lewis, D. (2012). Experimental investigation of the effects of the acoustical conditions in a simulated classroom on speech recognition and learning in children. *Journal of the Acoustical Society of America, 131,* 232–246. https://doi.org/10.1121/1.3662059

Watanabe, K., Matsuda, T., Nishioka, T., & Namatame, M. (2011). Eye gaze during observation of static faces in deaf people. *PLoS ONE, 6*(2), e16919. https://doi.org/10.1371/journal.pone.0016919

Weber, M. (2016). *10 challenges deaf students face in the classroom.* Retrieved from http://www.gettingsmart.com/2016/08/10 -challenges-deaf-students-face-in-the-classroom/

World Health Organization. (2018). *Constitution of the World Health Organization* (45th ed.). Retrieved from http://www.who .int/features/factfiles/deafness/en/

Zhou, G., & Stevens, K. (2009). Assessment of saccular function in children with sensorineural hearing loss. *Archives of Otolaryngology Head and Neck Surgery, 135,* 40–44. https://doi.org /10.1001/archoto.2008.508

Best Practices in Supporting Students With Intellectual Disability

Meghan Suman, OTD, OTR/L, BCP, SCSS

33

KEY TERMS AND CONCEPTS

- Adaptive behavior
- Free appropriate public education
- Intellectual disability
- Intellectual functioning
- Least restrictive environment

OVERVIEW

The definition and terminology related to intellectual disability have changed as the understanding of this condition and its effect on persons and stakeholders continues to evolve. *Intellectual disability* refers to a cluster of different conditions caused by genetic or environmental factors (Bertelli et al., 2016) and is sometimes referred to as *mental retardation, disorder of intellectual development, global developmental delay,* or *early developmental impairment* (Bertelli et al., 2016). The way intellectual disability is defined, named, and categorized can have a significant effect on the funding and services that are available to persons with intellectual disability.

In 2013, with the publication of the 5th edition of the *Diagnostic and Statistical Manual of Mental Disorders (DSM–5)*, the American Psychiatric Association (APA) replaced *mental retardation* with two conditions: *intellectual disability* and *intellectual developmental disorder.* The American Association on Intellectual and Developmental Disabilities (AAIDD; n.d.) acknowledges that *intellectual disability* is synonymous with *mental retardation* but identifies *intellectual disability* as the preferred terminology. In 2017, in response to Rosa's Law (2010; Pub. L. 111–256), the U.S. Department of Education amended federal laws by replacing the term *mental retardation* with *intellectual disability* (Rosa's Law Final Regulations, 2017).

The Individuals With Disabilities Education Improvement Act of 2004 (IDEA; Pub. L. 108–446), as amended, defines *intellectual disability* as "significantly subaverage general intellectual functioning, existing concurrently with deficits in adaptive behavior and manifested during the developmental period, that adversely affects a child's educational performance" (34 C.F.R. §300.8[c][6]). Adaptive behavior and age of onset are as important as intelligence when identifying intellectual disability. IDEA's definition for intellectual disability is consistent with the diagnostic criteria in the *DSM–5*, in which intelligence test scores (e.g., IQ) have been deemphasized and clinical assessment of the person's functional abilities has been emphasized. General IQ guidelines (2 standard deviations or more below the mean; i.e., an IQ of 70 or less) are included in the text but are not used as the defining factor for diagnosing intellectual disability (AAIDD, n.d.; APA, 2013).

ESSENTIAL CONSIDERATIONS

Intellectual disability is not one single condition; rather, it is a term that identifies a cluster of conditions characterized by below-average intellectual functioning and adaptive skills (Bertelli et al., 2016). The characteristics of students with intellectual disability vary on the basis of the etiology of their disability, associated health conditions, and environmental factors.

Etiology

In approximately 75% of cases of intellectual disability, no cause is known ("Intellectual Disability," n.d.). Intellectual disability can be caused by factors in the prenatal, antenatal, or childhood environment such as infection, hypoxia, prenatal alcohol exposure, trauma, malnutrition, or lack of stimulation (ARC, 2011; Emerson, 2007; Palusci et al., 2015). Severe intellectual disability is most often caused by genetic factors (Reichenberg et al., 2016). Genetic causes of intellectual disability include Down syndrome, Williams syndrome, Fragile X syndrome, and many others (Karam et al., 2015). Some conditions, such as Rett syndrome, are progressive and associated with ongoing decline in cognition and adaptive function (Rettsyndrome.org, n.d.).

Continued advances in genetic testing are creating increased opportunities to identify the etiology of intellectual disability (Sun et al., 2015; Vissers et al., 2016). Advanced genetic testing holds the promise of greater understanding of intellectual disability, more accurate prognoses, and opportunities to provide condition-specific support to persons and families. However, genetic testing also raises ethical concerns, such as the effect of identifying genetic factors that are unrelated to intellectual disability and balancing the

Copyright © 2019 by the American Occupational Therapy Association. All rights reserved. To reuse this content, contact www.copyright.com.
https://doi.org/10.7139/2019.978-1-56900-591-0.033

cost of genetic testing with potential clinical benefits (Sun et al., 2015).

Conditions With Co-Occurring Intellectual Disability

Students may present with a variety of diagnostic conditions that have co-occurring intellectual disabilities. A study conducted by Van Naarden Barun et al. (2015) that examined 15–20 years of data identified a prevalence of co-occurring intellectual disabilities in children with cerebral palsy, heart defects, autism spectrum disorder, and sensory deficits (e.g., hearing, vision). Other developmental research (Burack et al., 2012) has linked intellectual disabilities in children with Down syndrome and Angelman syndrome. In addition, children and adolescents with intellectual disabilities have been observed to have a higher rate of anxiety disorders (Green et al., 2015; Reardon et al., 2015). Green et al. (2015) found that children with intellectual disabilities may present with separation anxiety that persists until kindergarten age and beyond (i.e., ages 5 years or older).

Intellectual Functioning

Intellectual functioning, also referred to as *intelligence,* is typically measured with tests that assess a variety of factors including comprehension, reasoning, and memory to generate an IQ score (Kazdin, 2000). Students with higher IQ scores are likely to obtain better grades and experience greater school success (Hogan et al., 2010). Intellectual functioning is also a key component of identifying intellectual disability (APA, 2013).

IQ is typically measured by a psychologist using an individually administered standardized general intelligence test, such as the Stanford–Binet Intelligence Scales or the Wechsler Intelligence Scale for Children. This type of testing presents a challenge for clinicians assessing students with intellectual disability because of reduced measurement sensitivity when testing clients in the lower ranges of intelligence (Sansone et al., 2014) and difficulty completing standardized assessments with students with intellectual disability who also have motor or sensory deficits (Gabis et al., 2015).

It is important to consider that these standardized general intelligence tests do not measure social intelligence, life experience, or personal characteristics, such as determination, curiosity, dedication, or kindness. Occupational therapy's holistic focus positions practitioners[1] to help team members draw meaning from and recognize the limitations of intelligence testing. The occupational therapy evaluation

should identify additional strengths of students with intellectual disability.

Adaptive Behavior

Adaptive behavior encompasses a range of skills that enable people to navigate the demands of daily life. *Adaptive behavior* includes personal care, social interaction, community engagement, school participation, and leisure occupations. Students with an intellectual disability often require scaffolded assistance, training, and accommodations to successfully participate in age-appropriate daily tasks. Educational programming should explicitly address adaptive behavior related to daily function at school and in the community. Occupational therapists and occupational therapy assistants, in partnership with their supervising occupational therapist, have specific expertise in adaptive behavior and play an important role in the evaluation and development of these skills.

Accurate Application of Classification Criteria

Accurately identifying a student with an intellectual disability is important for the well-being of the student and family, for educational planning, and for financial reasons. Accurate identification of intellectual disability allows families to more fully comprehend their child's condition and select appropriate supports and interventions. An accurate identification of intellectual disability can also enable school personnel to customize the student's programming, aimed to maximize participation and reduce frustration. Families of persons with intellectual disability often struggle to plan for their children's financial future and express concern about their child's ability to access funding in the future (Hewitt et al., 2010). Identifying and diagnosing intellectual disability may enable students and families to access government financial support, including Supplemental Security Income and Medicaid (Social Security Administration, 2017).

Free Appropriate Public Education and Least Restrictive Environment

The requirement that school districts provide a *free appropriate public education* (FAPE) is one of the most important elements of IDEA (2004) and the most common area of concern leading to litigation in special education (Zirkel & Hetrick, 2017). In 2002, a settlement was approved in a class action lawsuit (*P.J. v. Connecticut Board of Education,* 2013) on behalf of 5 students with intellectual disability and their families, who claimed a denial of FAPE. Students were segregated in special education classrooms rather than being educated along with their nondisabled peers whenever possible. Education provided in an inclusive setting gives students with intellectual disability the opportunity to interact with peers and become familiar with topics addressed in general education classes. Although the number of students with disabilities educated alongside their peers has increased steadily in recent years, students with intellectual disability have not experienced the same rate of change and are one of the groups most likely to have limited or no access to general education settings (McLeskey et al., 2012; Morningstar et al., 2017; Williamson et al., 2006).

---

[1]*Occupational therapy practitioner* refers to both the occupational therapist and the occupational therapy assistant. The American Occupational Therapy Association (AOTA; 2014a, p. S18) states, "The occupational therapist is responsible for all aspects of occupational therapy service delivery and is accountable for the safety and effectiveness of the occupational therapy service delivery process" and "must be directly involved in the delivery of services during the initial evaluation and regularly throughout the course of intervention. . . . The occupational therapy assistant delivers safe and effective occupational therapy services under the supervision of and in partnership with the occupational therapist."

Ensuring that students with intellectual disability are educated in the *least restrictive environment* (LRE) is not only an educational concern but also an issue of civil rights and occupational justice. As experts in maximizing participation in daily life for students with disabilities, occupational therapy practitioners should take a leadership role in helping school teams develop plans to support students with intellectual disability in the LRE.

Social–Emotional Functioning

Although social–emotional functioning can be an area of challenge or strength for students with intellectual disability, it may be overlooked by team members (Lyons et al., 2016). Communication deficits may limit students' ability to express their feelings and connect socially with others. Exclusion of students with intellectual disability from general education classrooms further limits opportunities to learn from age-appropriate peer models and engage in reciprocal social relationships.

Behavior

Persons with intellectual disability often demonstrate delayed emotional development and challenging behaviors (Sappok et al., 2014). Mild behaviors such as task refusal and off-task behavior may be easily managed at school through redirection and behavioral incentives. More severe challenging behaviors, such as self-injurious or aggressive behavior, may require a more comprehensive behavioral intervention program, which may include multidisciplinary behavioral, environmental, or pharmaceutical interventions (Heyvaert et al., 2010). In schools, occupational therapy practitioners can promote positive behavior in students with intellectual disability by adapting tasks and the environment to reduce frustration and create opportunities for independence.

Friendships

Friendships are an important part of school participation for all students. Students with intellectual disability are often less socially engaged with friends outside of school (Shields et al., 2014; Tipton et al., 2013; Tonkin et al., 2014). Students with intellectual disability can benefit from developing friendships with classmates who have disabilities as well as with typically developing peers (Nijs & Maes, 2014; Salmon, 2013). Delays in social skills, functional independence, communication, and problem solving may contribute to challenges in developing and maintaining friendships for students with intellectual disability. Occupational therapy interventions to facilitate social development at school may include social play, music, and recreational groups (Arbesman et al., 2013).

Life Course Considerations

Because of the lifelong nature of intellectual disability, it is important to take a prospective approach that considers the student's current and future needs. Even without significant changes in intellectual functioning, changes in age, health, and environment have a significant effect on the occupational performance of persons with intellectual disability across the life course. Occupational therapy practitioners should take a long-term perspective when planning for students with intellectual disability.

Health

In addition to the commonly co-occurring conditions addressed in this chapter, persons with intellectual disability are at greater risk of chronic health conditions related to lifestyle and environment. Social determinants of health such as socioeconomic status, education, physical environment, social support, and access to health care play a key role in influencing the health and well-being of persons with intellectual disability. Obesity occurs at a higher rate among children with intellectual disability, which may be related to nutritional factors as well as sedentary lifestyle (Segal et al., 2016). As they mature into late adolescence and adulthood, persons with intellectual disability are at greater risk of other chronic health problems such as diabetes, arthritis, gastrointestinal disorders, and cardiovascular disease (Krahn & Fox, 2014). Sleep disorders are also common in children and adults with intellectual disability (Greydanus, 2015).

Occupational therapy practitioners should help the school system (e.g., administration, staff, community members) recognize the importance of developing skills and promoting behaviors that contribute to lifelong health for students with intellectual disability. The emotional, social, and financial effect of having a child with intellectual disability may make it difficult for families to adopt healthy lifestyle practices. Occupational therapy practitioners can improve the lifelong health of students with intellectual disability by collaborating with families to reduce stress, improve daily routines, facilitate access to community resources, and enable participation in health-promoting self-care and leisure occupations.

Sexuality

Generally, adolescents with intellectual disability experience the same sexual maturation, romantic desires, and sexual feelings as their typically developing peers, although parents and teachers may be hesitant to acknowledge or address issues of sexuality. Students with intellectual disability are more likely than their typically developing peers to be excluded from sex education in school (Barnard-Brak et al., 2014). This is especially concerning because this group of students has a greater risk for sexual abuse (Fogden et al., 2016; Spencer et al., 2005) and online sexual victimization (Normand & Sallafranque-St-Louis, 2016).

Whether provided at school or elsewhere, sex education is essential for students with intellectual disability. The confusion of emerging sexual feelings may be compounded because of delays in emotional maturity and communication. A comprehensive approach to sexual education, including discussion of friendships, romantic relationships, and safe sexual practices, can help meet the unique needs of students with intellectual disability (Swango-Wilson, 2011). As with other areas of education, concepts may be best communicated using objects, pictures, video, role play, and simplified materials.

Supports

The effects of intellectual disability cannot be reversed or cured, so people typically require ongoing supports throughout the life course. Although persons with intellectual disability may always need support for successful participation in daily life, occupational therapy practitioners can help students develop skills to reduce the need for one-on-one adult support, increase efficiency of daily routines, and promote self-advocacy. Supports should be individualized to meet the unique needs of each student. The nature of supports should be expected to change as age or maturity lead to new and different occupations. In schools, the primary focus of supports is often on maximizing participation in the LRE, as required by IDEA (2004). Care is needed to develop supports that meet student needs and respect the dignity and age of the student.

BEST PRACTICES

To best meet the needs of students with intellectual disability, occupational therapists should take a holistic, practical, and evidence-based approach to planning evaluations and interventions.

Evaluate Students With Intellectual Disability

Evaluating a student with intellectual disability requires a multifaceted approach that incorporates various sources of information to form a complete picture of the student's occupational performance. There is no single approach to evaluation that will work for all students with intellectual disability. Using a broad battery of standardized sensory–motor assessments may not be helpful to plan interventions because students with intellectual disability may have below-average skills in all areas. The first step of the evaluation process is the creation of an occupational profile in which the occupational therapist identifies the student's "occupational history and experiences, patterns of daily living, interests, values, and needs" (AOTA, 2014b, p. S10). The information from the occupational profile will guide the selection of additional elements of the evaluation (see Chapter 40, "Best Practices in School Occupational Therapy Evaluation and Planning to Support Participation").

Standardized assessments and procedures

Using some norm-referenced assessments with students with intellectual disability may be difficult or improbable for gaining meaningful information (Gabis et al., 2015). Cognition and attention may impair the student's ability to follow instructions for standardized assessments of motor skills. Motor, sensory, and communication deficits may affect the student's ability to complete standardized assessments of process or social skills. When a standardized assessment is needed, practical and informative options may include criterion-referenced measures such as the School Function Assessment (Coster et al., 1998) or those with simple instructions and familiar activities, such as the Goal-Oriented Assessment of Lifeskills™ (Miller & Oakland, 2013).

Interview, observation, and self-report

Often, interview and observation are the most appropriate evaluation methods for gathering meaningful information regarding students with intellectual disability. Occupational therapists should interview multiple persons with knowledge about the student, including parents, teachers, paraeducators, support personnel (e.g., bus drivers, lunchroom workers), peers, and community contacts (e.g., coaches, clinical therapists). Therapists should be aware of and adhere to privacy laws such as the Health Insurance Portability and Accountability Act of 1996 (Pub. L. 104–191) and the Family Educational Rights and Privacy Act of 1974 (Pub. L. 93–380) before contacting stakeholders outside of school. Although interviews alone are not sufficient to evaluate occupational performance, information gathered through the interview process can guide the occupational therapist to select relevant parts of the student's routine to observe or specific skills to assess.

Observation and analysis of the student's performance within the educational environment are an essential component of the occupational therapy evaluation. The occupational therapist should select elements of the students' day to observe on the basis of the occupational profile and the information gathered through the interview process. Ideally, observations should be completed in multiple educational environments (e.g., classroom, hallways, lunchroom), and the occupational therapist should confirm with school personnel that the observation period was representative of the student's typical performance.

The occupational therapist should first attempt to observe the student unobtrusively, without attempting to change the student's performance, to provide an accurate baseline measure. Comparing the student's performance with the expected performance and with peer performance provides insight into strengths and needs. As part of the reasoning process, the therapist may then choose to make changes to the student's environment or routine to evaluate the student's performance under various conditions.

When possible, self-report should be used to determine the student's perceptions, interests, and priorities. Although the student may have difficulty communicating effectively in an unstructured interview, there are formal measures that can be useful. The Pediatric Activity Card Sort (Mandich et al., 2004) allows students to communicate nonverbally by using picture cards depicting common childhood occupations. The Child Occupational Self-Assessment (Keller et al., 2006) allows students with intellectual disability to use simple icons (e.g., smiley faces, stars) to communicate their perspectives on the importance of a variety of daily occupations and their performance on them. Information gathered via self-report can provide valuable insight into the behavior and performance of students with intellectual disability and can be a key factor in creating student-centered goals.

Include families in the evaluation process

Family involvement is an essential element of an occupational therapy evaluation. A student's experiences at home (e.g., social opportunities, behavior management, leisure activities, self-care, nutrition, sleep routines) can have a significant effect on school participation. Information obtained through family interviews can contribute to the development of the occupational profile and help guide the planning of the occupational therapy evaluation. The occupational therapist should take care to explain evaluation results in a clear and compassionate manner, avoiding overly technical language and allowing ample opportunity for families to ask questions.

Implement Interventions for Students With Intellectual Disabilities

Interventions should be developed using occupational therapy theory and the best available evidence. Because intellectual disability affects almost all areas of occupational performance, occupational therapy practitioners should collaborate with the student, family, and school team to determine priority areas for intervention. Occupational therapy interventions that incorporate ongoing collaborative consultation have been found to be more effective than teacher training alone for increasing the classroom participation of students with intellectual disability (Selanikyo et al., 2018).

When choosing an intervention approach, it is important to consider the student's rate of progress and potential for growth. Skill development may be slow for students with intellectual disability, which may make environmental and task adaptations the best options to improve occupational performance and participation. In some circumstances, it is appropriate to use environmental and task adaptations in the short term while also providing opportunities for skill development. Skill development for students with intellectual disability should be incorporated into daily routines whenever possible and may require task simplification and frequent repetition. The frequency and duration of occupational therapy services should increase or decrease on the basis of the student's unique needs. For example, a student may have less need for occupational therapy services in late elementary school when routines and supports have been well established but may require increased services when adjusting to the new self-care routines of adolescence.

Elementary school interventions

Mild or moderate intellectual disability may be identified for the first time at the elementary school level, when students' work involves more academic tasks and a decreased focus on play. Occupational therapy may be needed to address a wide range of skills related to participation in elementary school. Functional occupations such as walking in line with the class, zipping a jacket, accessing playground equipment, eating lunch, and using the restroom may be priorities for students with intellectual disability. Occupational therapy may also address skills directly related to academic participation, such as cutting, coloring, writing, and technology use. Social and play skills for this age group may include expressing feelings, inviting a friend to play, and following classroom rules.

Middle and high school interventions

At the middle and high school levels, expectations for students with intellectual disability often broaden to include an increased focus on workplace readiness and independent living skills. Occupational therapy may address safety and independence in navigating the school building, job site, and local community. Self-care occupations also change significantly at this time. Modifications, accommodations, and skill development may be warranted to enable students with intellectual disability to manage menstruation, shaving, or application of makeup. Occupational therapy may also continue to address skills related to academic participation, such as using technology, following a schedule, and accessing and maintaining a locker. Social and leisure occupations addressed in occupational therapy may include developing and maintaining friendships, dating, leisure exploration, and sports participation.

Transition planning

Occupational therapy practitioners have a distinct knowledge of life course issues that can help students with intellectual disability, their families, and teachers to plan for the transition to adulthood. IDEA requires that individualized education programs for students ages 16 years or older include a discussion of transition needs (some states' laws may require this by the student's 14th birthday). For many students with intellectual disability, however, it may be appropriate to begin transition planning at a younger age. Factors to consider in a transition plan include family and social connections, community access, support for ADLs and IADLs, employment, and financial resources.

Employment is a significant challenge for young adults with intellectual disability. Adequate social–emotional skills have been found to be more important than IQ in supporting employment for this population (Sappok et al., 2014). Occupational therapy practitioners can participate in transition planning by helping students and their families explore community resources, thoroughly documenting student needs and supports, and identifying supports that reduce the student's need for assistance. For more information, see Chapter 24, "Best Practices in Transition Planning for Independent Living and Workplace Readiness."

Establish Outcomes

Outcomes for students with intellectual disability can vary significantly as a result of differences in the underlying cause of the student's disability, other health conditions, and environmental factors. Because of the lifelong effects of intellectual disability, effective occupational therapy interventions are often focused on identifying supports that affect occupational participation and quality of life.

SUMMARY

Although all students with intellectual disability have below-average intellectual and adaptive functioning, each student has unique needs and requires individualized evaluation and programming. Occupational therapists should take a holistic approach to evaluating and contributing to educational planning for students with intellectual disability. School teams should consider the student's strengths, prognosis, health conditions, family situation, future plans, and individual interests. Supports are especially important to ensuring long-term access to the LRE for students with intellectual disability.

It is important to consider that students with intellectual disability will likely need supports throughout life. Occupational therapy practitioners can meet the needs of students with intellectual disability through targeted skill development and by identifying supports that contribute to participation, well-being, and quality of life.

REFERENCES

American Association on Intellectual and Developmental Disabilities. (n.d.). *Frequently asked questions on intellectual disability.* Retrieved from https://aaidd.org/intellectual-disability /definition/faqs-on-intellectual-disability#.WjlJDTdMGUk

American Occupational Therapy Association. (2014a). Guidelines for supervision, roles, and responsibilities during the delivery of occupational therapy services. *American Journal of Occupational Therapy, 68*(Suppl. 3), S16–S22. https://doi.org/10.5014 /ajot.2014.686S03

American Occupational Therapy Association. (2014b). Occupational therapy practice framework: Domain and process (3rd ed.). *American Journal of Occupational Therapy, 68*(Suppl. 1), S1–S48. https://doi.org/10.5014/ajot.2014.682006

American Psychiatric Association. (2013). *Diagnostic and statistical manual of mental disorders* (5th ed.). Arlington, VA: American Psychiatric Publishing.

Arbesman, M., Bazyk, S., & Nochajski, S. M. (2013). Systematic review of occupational therapy and mental health promotion, prevention, and intervention for children and youth. *American Journal of Occupational Therapy, 67,* e120–e130. https://doi.org /10.5014/ajot.2013.008359

ARC. (2011). *Causes and prevention of intellectual disabilities.* Retrieved from https://www.thearc.org/what-we-do/resources /fact-sheets/causes-and-prevention

Barnard-Brak, L., Schmidt, M., Chesnut, S., Wei, T., & Richman, D. (2014). Predictors of access to sex education for children with intellectual disabilities in public schools. *Intellectual and Developmental Disabilities, 52,* 85–97. https://doi.org/10.1352 /1934-9556-52.2.85

Bertelli, M. O., Munir, K., Harris, J., & Salvador-Carulla, L. (2016). "Intellectual developmental disorders": Reflections on the international consensus document for redefining "mental retardation-intellectual disability" in *ICD–11. Advances in Mental Health and Intellectual Disabilities, 10,* 36–58. https:// doi.org/10.1108%2FAMHID-10-2015-0050

Burack, J. A., Hodapp, R. M., Iarocci, G., & Zigler, E. (Eds.). (2012). *The Oxford handbook of intellectual disability and development.* New York: Oxford University Press.

Coster, W., Deeney, T., Haltiwanger, J., & Haley, S. (1998). *School Function Assessment.* San Antonio: Therapy Skill Builders.

Emerson, E. (2007). Poverty and people with intellectual disabilities. *Developmental Disabilities Research Reviews, 13,* 107–113. https://doi.org/10.1002/mrdd.20144

Family Educational Rights and Privacy Act of 1974, Pub. L. 93–380, 20 U.S.C. § 1232g, 34 C.F.R. Part 99.

Fogden, B. C., Thomas, S. D. M., Daffern, M., & Ogloff, J. R. P. (2016). Crime and victimisation in people with intellectual disability: A case linkage study. *BMC Psychiatry, 16,* 170. https:// doi.org/10.1186/s12888-016-0869-7

Gabis, L. V., Tsubary, N. M., Leon, O., Ashkenasi, A., & Shefer, S. (2015). Assessment of abilities and comorbidities in children with cerebral palsy. *Journal of Child Neurology, 30,* 1640–1645. https://doi.org/10.1177/0883073815576792

Green, S. A., Berkovits, L. D., & Baker, B. L. (2015). Symptoms and development of anxiety in children with or without intellectual disability. *Journal of Clinical Child and Adolescent Psychology, 44,* 137–144. https://doi.org/10.1080/15374416.2013.873979

Greydanus, D. (2015). Intellectual disability: Sleep disorders. *Journal of Alternative Medicine Research, 7,* 287–304.

Health Insurance Portability and Accountability Act of 1996, Pub. L. 104–191, 42 U.S.C. § 300gg, 29 U.S.C. §§ 1181–1183, and 42 U.S.C. §§ 1320d–1320d9.

Hewitt, A., Lightfoot, E., Bogenschutz, M., McCormick, K., Sedlezky, L., & Doljanac, R. (2010). Parental caregivers' desires for lifetime assistance planning for future supports for their children with intellectual and developmental disabilities. *Journal of Family Social Work, 13,* 420–434. https://doi.org/10.1080 /10522158.2010.514678

Heyvaert, M., Maes, B., & Onghena, P. (2010). A meta-analysis of intervention effects on challenging behaviour among persons with intellectual disabilities. *Journal of Intellectual Disability Research, 54,* 634–649. https://doi.org/10.1111/j.1365-2788.2010.01291.x

Hogan, M. J., Parker, J. A., Wiener, J., Watters, C., Wood, L. M., & Oke, A. (2010). Academic success in adolescence: Relationships among verbal IQ, social support and emotional intelligence. *Australian Journal of Psychology, 62,* 30–41. https://doi.org /10.1080/00049530903312881

Individuals With Disabilities Education Improvement Act of 2004, Pub. L. 108–446, 20 U.S.C. §§ 1400–1482.

Intellectual disability. (n.d.). In *MedlinePlus.* Retrieved from https://medlineplus.gov/ency/article/001523.htm

Karam, S. M., Riegel, M., Segal, S. L., Félix, T. M., Barros, A. J. D., Santos, I. S., . . . Black, M. (2015). Genetic causes of intellectual disability in a birth cohort: A population-based study. *American Journal of Medical Genetics: Part A, 167,* 1204–1214. https:// doi.org/10.1002/ajmg.a.37011

Kazdin, A. E. (2000). *Encyclopedia of psychology.* Washington, DC: American Psychological Association.

Keller, J., Kafkes, A., Basu, S., Federico, J., & Kielhofner, G. (2006). *Child Occupational Self-Assessment.* Chicago: University of Illinois at Chicago.

Krahn, G. L., & Fox, M. H. (2014). Health disparities of adults with intellectual disabilities: What do we know? What do we do? *Journal of Applied Research in Intellectual Disabilities, 27,* 431–446. https://doi.org/10.1111/jar.12067

Lyons, G. L., Huber, H. B., Carter, E. W., Chen, R., & Asmus, J. M. (2016). Assessing the social skills and problem behaviors of adolescents with severe disabilities enrolled in general education classes. *American Journal on Intellectual and Developmental Disabilities, 121,* 327–345. https://doi.org/10.1352/1944-7558 -121.4.327

Mandich, A., Polatajko, H., Miller, L., & Baum, C. (2004). *The Pediatric Activity Card Sort.* Ottawa: CAOT Publications.

McLeskey, J., Landers, E., Williamson, P., & Hoppey, D. (2012). Are we moving toward educating students with disabilities in less restrictive settings? *Journal of Special Education, 46,* 131–140. https://doi.org/10.1177/0022466910376670

Miller, L. J., & Oakland, T. (2013). *Goal-Oriented Assessment of Lifeskills.* Torrance, CA: Western Psychological Services.

Morningstar, M. E., Kurth, J. A., & Johnson, P. E. (2017). Examining national trends in educational placements for students with significant disabilities. *Remedial and Special Education, 38*(1), 3–12. https://doi.org/10.1177%2F0741932516678327

Nijs, S., & Maes, B. (2014). Social peer interactions in persons with profound intellectual and multiple disabilities: A literature review. *Education and Training in Autism and Developmental Disabilities, 49,* 153–165.

Normand, C. L., & Sallafranque-St-Louis, F. (2016). Cybervictimization of young people with an intellectual or developmental disability: Risks specific to sexual solicitation. *Journal of Applied Research in Intellectual Disabilities, 29,* 99–110. https://doi.org/10.1111/jar.12163

Palusci, V. J., Datner, E., & Wilkins, C. (2015). Developmental disabilities: Abuse and neglect in children and adults. *International Journal of Child Health and Human Development, 8,* 407.

P.J. v. Connecticut Board of Education, 10-3586-cv (2d Cir. 2013).

Reardon, T. C., Gray, K. M., & Melvin, G. A. (2015). Anxiety disorders in children and adolescents with intellectual disability: Prevalence and assessment. *Research in Developmental Disabilities, 36,* 175–190. https://doi.org/10.1016/j.ridd.2014.10.007

Reichenberg, A., Cederlöf, M., McMillan, A., Trzaskowski, M., Kapara, O., Fruchter, E., . . . Plomin, R. (2016). Discontinuity in the genetic and environmental causes of the intellectual disability spectrum. *Proceedings of the National Academy of Sciences, 113,* 1098–1103. https://doi.org/10.1073/pnas.1508093112

Rettsyndrome.org. (n.d.). *What is Rett syndrome?* Retrieved from https://www.rettsyndrome.org/about-rett-syndrome/what-is-Rettsyndrome

Rosa's Law, Pub. L. 111–256, 124 Stat. 2643 (2010).

Rosa's Law Final Regulations, 82 Fed. Reg. 31910 (proposed July 11, 2017) (to be codified at 34 C.F.R. pts. 103, 105, 222, 300, 361, 373, 385, 668, & 674).

Salmon, N. (2013). "We just stick together": How disabled teens negotiate stigma to create lasting friendship. *Journal of Intellectual Disability Research, 57,* 347–358. https://doi.org/10.1111/j.1365-2788.2012.01541.x

Sansone, S. M., Schneider, A., Bickel, E., Berry-Kravis, E., Prescott, C., & Hessl, D. (2014). Improving IQ measurement in intellectual disabilities using true deviation from population norms. *Journal of Neurodevelopmental Disorders, 6,* 16. https://doi.org/10.1186/1866-1955-6-16

Sappok, T., Budczies, J., Dziobek, I., Bolte, S., Dosen, A., & Diefenbacher, A. (2014). The missing link: Delayed emotional development predicts challenging behavior in adults with intellectual disability. *Journal of Autism and Developmental Disorders, 44,* 786–800. https://doi.org/10.1007/s10803-013-1933-5

Segal, M., Eliasziw, M., Phillips, S., Bandini, L., Curtin, C., Kral, T., . . . Must, A. (2016). Intellectual disability is associated with increased risk for obesity in a nationally representative sample of U.S. children. *Disability and Health Journal, 9,* 392–398. https://doi.org/10.1016/j.dhjo.2015.12.003

Selanikyo, E., Weintraub, N., & Yalon-Chamovitz, S. (2018). Effectiveness of the Co-PID for students with moderate intellectual disability. *American Journal of Occupational Therapy, 72,* 7202205090. https://doi.org/10.5014/ajot.2018.024109

Shields, N., King, M., Corbett, M., & Imms, C. (2014). Is participation among children with intellectual disabilities in outside school activities similar to their typically developing peers? A systematic review. *Developmental Neurorehabilitation, 17,* 64–71. https://doi.org/10.3109/17518423.2013.836256

Social Security Administration. (2017). *Benefits for children with disabilities.* Retrieved from https://www.ssa.gov/pubs/EN-05-10026.pdf

Spencer, N., Devereux, E., Wallace, A., Sundrum, R., Shenoy, M., Bacchus, C., & Logan, S. (2005). Disabling conditions and registration for child abuse and neglect: A population-based study. *Pediatrics, 116,* 609–613. https://doi.org/10.1542/peds.2004-1882

Sun, F., Oristaglio, J., Levy, S. E., Hakonarson, H., Sullivan, N., Fontanarosa, J., & Schoelles, K. M. (2015). *Genetic testing for developmental disabilities, intellectual disability, and autism spectrum disorder* (Technical Brief No. 23). Rockville, MD: Agency for Healthcare Research and Quality.

Swango-Wilson, A. (2011). Meaningful sex education programs for individuals with intellectual/developmental disabilities. *Sexuality and Disability, 29,* 113–118. https://doi.org/10.1007/s11195-010-9168-2

Tipton, L. A., Christensen, L., & Blacher, J. (2013). Friendship quality in adolescents with and without an intellectual disability. *Journal of Applied Research in Intellectual Disabilities, 26,* 522–532. https://doi.org/10.1111/jar.12051

Tonkin, B. L., Ogilvie, B. D., Greenwood, S. A., Law, M. C., & Anaby, D. R. (2014). The participation of children and youth with disabilities in activities outside of school: A scoping review. *Canadian Journal of Occupational Therapy, 81,* 226–236. https://doi.org/10.1177%2F0008417414550998

Van Naarden Braun, K., Christensen, D., Doernberg, N., Schieve, L., Rice, C., Wiggins, L., . . . Yeargin-Allsopp, M. (2015). Trends in the prevalence of autism spectrum disorder, cerebral palsy, hearing loss, intellectual disability, and vision impairment, metropolitan Atlanta, 1991–2010. *PLos ONE, 10*(4), e0124120. https://doi.org/10.1371/journal.pone.0124120

Vissers, L. E., Gilissen, C. F., & Veltman, J. A. (2016). Genetic studies in intellectual disability and related disorders. *Nature Reviews Genetics, 17,* 9–18. http://dx.doi.org/10.1038/nrg3999

Williamson, P., McLeskey, J., Hoppey, D., & Rentz, T. (2006). Educating students with mental retardation in general education classrooms. *Exceptional Children, 72,* 347–361. https://doi.org/10.1177%2F001440290607200306

Zirkel, P. A., & Hetrick, A. (2017). Which procedural parts of the IEP process are the most judicially vulnerable? *Exceptional Children, 83,* 219–235. https://doi.org/10.1177%2F0014402916651849

Best Practices in Supporting Students With Low-Incidence Disabilities

34

Yvonne Swinth, PhD, OTR/L, FAOTA

KEY TERMS AND CONCEPTS

- Deaf–blindness
- Ecological approach
- Individualized transportation plan
- Low-incidence disabilities
- Multiple disabilities
- Peer-mediated instruction
- Role release

OVERVIEW

Fewer than 10% of students in schools have low-incidence disabilities. These students have complex and varied needs that include medical conditions or physical limitations that affect movement, vision, communication, or hearing. The Individuals With Disabilities Education Improvement Act of 2004 (IDEA; Pub. L. 108–446, § 1401[3][i]) does not define *low-incidence disabilities* as an eligibility category for a "child with a disability"; however, ***low-incidence disabilities*** are specifically defined in IDEA:

- A visual or hearing impairment, or simultaneous visual and hearing impairments;
- A significant cognitive impairment; or
- Any impairment for which a small number of personnel with highly specialized skills and knowledge are needed in order for children with that impairment to receive . . . a free appropriate public education. (IDEA, 2004, § 1462[c][3])

Specific low-incidence disabilities such as deaf–blindness and multiple disabilities are also defined in the regulations. IDEA (2004) defines ***deaf–blindness*** as hearing and vision impairments, "the combination of which causes . . . severe communication and other developmental and educational needs" (§ 300.8[a][2]). ***Multiple disabilities*** are defined as

concomitant impairments (such as intellectual disability–blindness or intellectual disability–orthopedic impairments), the combination of which causes such severe educational needs that they cannot be accommodated in special education programs solely for one of the impairments. Multiple disabilities does not include deaf–blindness. (IDEA, 2004, § 300.8[c][7])

Although students with low-incidence disabilities are eligible for special education under categories such as multiple disabilities, other health impairment, or visual impairment, including blindness, this chapter focuses on students with deaf–blindness and multiple disabilities and includes persons with severe disabilities (a "low-incidence" population). Information about students with hearing, intellectual, and visual disabilities can be found in Chapter 32, "Best Practices in Supporting Students With Hearing Impairments or Deafness"; Chapter 33, "Best Practices in Supporting Students With Intellectual Disability"; and Chapter 39, "Best Practices in Supporting Students With Visual Impairments."

According to the National Consortium on Deaf–Blindness (2017), in 2016 approximately 9,635 children in the United States had a diagnosis of deaf–blindness, a majority of whom (91.6%) lived at home. Many of these students (61%) received at least part of their education in general education settings for a portion of the day. These children may have had 1 or more medical conditions, including CHARGE syndrome, Hunter syndrome, Down syndrome, fetal alcohol syndrome, congenital rubella, encephalitis, and others. Cognitive or motor impairments may or may not have been present. However, most had some level of cognitive impairment and typically had delays in adaptive, motor, and communication skills as well as sensory functioning. Of note, the National Consortium on Deaf–Blindness stated,

The apparent under-identification and referral to state and multi-state deaf–blind programs of very young infants and children remains an important issue. Infants and toddlers benefit greatly from having access to expertise in deaf–blindness. They require appropriate services that address the impacts of dual sensory impairments. . . . Without such early identification and referral to state and multi-state deaf–blind programs, access to needed services and supports is compromised. (pp. 7–8)

These students may come to school having received few appropriate services in their earlier years.

Copyright © 2019 by the American Occupational Therapy Association. All rights reserved. To reuse this content, contact www.copyright.com.
https://doi.org/10.7139/2019.978-1-56900-591-0.034

The key principles of IDEA (2004), specific to service provision, hold true for students with low-incidence disabilities: These students should be educated in the context of general education (Browder et al., 2014; TASH, 2017). However, many of these students will require a network of services and supports to be able to participate in the least restrictive environment (LRE) as well as careful planning to prepare them for life after school (see Chapter 24, "Best Practices in Transition Planning for Independent Living and Workplace Readiness").

These services include related service providers, varied accommodations and adaptations, assistive technology (AT), peer supports, and personal assistant support services in the LRE. Related services should be provided in the general education setting with more restrictive settings used only when the LRE has been shown to be ineffective or disruptive. School occupational therapy practitioners[1] working with this population need to consider transition and future planning as part of their initial evaluation and ongoing intervention.

Some of these students and families may come to the educational setting with specific expectations about the type and intensity of services needed because of the medical services they have received since they were very young. The complexity of their needs often affects school performance, family interactions, community access, and future planning. The role of the occupational therapist with this population is broad and varied. It should include ongoing evaluation and a broad range of interventions, including services with the student and services on behalf of the student.

ESSENTIAL CONSIDERATIONS

The educational team, which includes the family, determines what a student needs in order to access and participate in their educational program, with the expectation that every student can and does learn. Research has shown that coordination between service providers and family members leads to better outcomes for this population (Browder et al., 2014), including improved participation, improved family functioning, increased quality of life, and less stress.

Health Needs for Students With Low-Incidence Disabilities

All stakeholders (e.g., family, educational staff, related services, medical community, community agencies) involved with students with low-incidence disabilities must communicate and cooperate in a collaborative manner in order to provide services that maximize learning and functional activities. The health needs of these students are often complex and varied, and some students may be medically fragile. Many have more than one health concern that may be a characteristic of the disability or may be secondary to the disability. Conditions experienced by these students may include eating and swallowing disorders, lung function and breathing control issues, movement limitations, skeletal deformities, and medical and other equipment needs and medications, as well as heart defects, seizures, the tendency to become sick easily, failure to thrive, and skin integrity problems (which may be related to positioning of the body).

These students often require more hospitalizations than others; therefore, they miss more school per year (Browder et al., 2014). To prevent students from falling behind in school, teams should plan for how educational services, including related services such as occupational therapy, will be provided during extended absences. School occupational therapy practitioners and school nurses may work closely with the family regarding the student's complex health needs and help to gather and interpret medical information and implement relevant recommendations.

Eating, feeding, and swallowing

School practitioners collaborate with other team members to support mealtime occupations and oral hygiene. Students with low-incidence disabilities may have dysphagia, poor oral–motor control, and other specific eating and feeding disorders. Moreover, limitations in movement, poor motor control, or muscle tone issues may make independent feeding difficult or unsafe (e.g., an aspiration risk). To receive proper nutrition, they may be reliant on feeding tubes (e.g., nasogastric, gastrostomy).

Students may also have dietary limitations as a result of allergies or the ability to eat only specific types of food, or they may require special food preparation such as blending. In addition, they may have few or no teeth or may be unable to fully attend to oral hygiene needs without the help of caregivers (for more information, see Chapter 47, "Best Practices in School Mealtimes to Enhance Participation").

Lung function and breathing control

Students with low-incidence disabilities may have limitations in lung function and breathing control, leading to a restriction in activities, the need for oxygen, or ongoing respiration support. Occupational therapy practitioners must always consider positioning of the body when working with a student with a compromised respiratory system. Basic knowledge about respiration support equipment should be acquired by any occupational therapy practitioner working with students who use such equipment.

Movement

Many students with low-incidence disabilities have conditions affecting performance skills (e.g., moves, stabilizes), body functions (e.g., range of motion [ROM], muscle strength), and limitations imposed by equipment needed for medical support. The severity of conditions and the effect on participation and performance varies across students, even among those with the same condition.

---

[1]*Occupational therapy practitioner* refers to both the occupational therapist and the occupational therapy assistant. The American Occupational Therapy Association (AOTA; 2014a, p. S18) states, "The occupational therapist is responsible for all aspects of occupational therapy service delivery and is accountable for the safety and effectiveness of the occupational therapy service delivery process" and "must be directly involved in the delivery of services during the initial evaluation and regularly throughout the course of intervention. . . . The occupational therapy assistant delivers safe and effective occupational therapy services under the supervision of and in partnership with the occupational therapist."

Skeletal conditions

Skeletal conditions may be a result of ongoing muscle tightness or limitations in ROM (e.g., students with severe scoliosis). *Fixed* (normal movement is not possible) or *flexible* (some movement is possible) skeletal conditions may affect students with low-incidence disabilities. These conditions may require ongoing intervention to prevent further deterioration. These deformities may also occur or increase when students with limitations in movement are not afforded consistent opportunities to be assisted with movement and ROM. Attention to positioning and the type of equipment used across school contexts is critical with this population.

Equipment

A variety of equipment, such as wheelchairs, standers, IV poles, respirators, and various kinds of AT (see Chapter 21, "Best Practices in the Use of Assistive Technology to Enhance Participation"), to support physical and medical needs can be used by many students with low-incidence disabilities. Equipment may require additional space, ramps for access to the house and school, and other accommodations and adaptations to a student's environments. Equipment may need to be transported to and from school and should be part of the **individualized transportation plan.** This plan, which details all aspects of the student's transportation needs, such as equipment and getting on or off the vehicle, is developed by the individualized education program (IEP) team, which consists of teachers, parents, student, related service providers, and other persons significant to the student's education (see Chapter 22, "Best Practices in Safe Transportation").

Educational Planning to Support Positive Student Outcomes

The needs of this population are usually complex, requiring more time for planning and coordination and sustained input from the IEP team. Potential or anticipated short-term (1–5 years) and long-term (7–10 years) needs in relation to transition planning should be discussed early in the process. An expanded core curriculum should use universal design for learning and AT as well as functional academics, life skills training (e.g., ADLs, IADLs, leisure activities), community access, and vocational training (Figure 34.1). Minimal to full-time paraeducator support may be required, and alternative assessments may be needed (Jackson, 2010). For more information, see Chapter 20, "Best Practices in Universal Design for Learning."

Services may also need to be provided across a variety of contexts, including but not limited to the classroom, the gym, the playground, and the cafeteria, to evaluate whether equipment is implemented appropriately and that skills are generalized. School occupational therapy practitioners may also need to work at the systems level to ensure that all appropriate school environments are accessible and able to support the complex needs of these students (Hanft et al., 2016).

Homebound instruction

Some students with low-incidence disabilities may live at home with caregiver support, including respite or nursing services (sometimes up to 24 hours a day). Some live in residential facilities, even though the number of such facilities continues to decrease (Rosenau, 2000).

Home environments can present challenges in service provision considerations for the family and service providers. Because of their medical needs, students who are unable to ever leave their home, or those who must remain home during high illness periods (e.g., October–March), must participate in their educational program in the home when other students are receiving services at school. A written statement from the physician may be required to verify that the student is unable to attend school and that homebound instruction will not affect their health or recovery. IEP teams may need to modify the student's IEP for homebound instruction—for example, shortening the school day to accommodate medical and health concerns. A highly qualified teacher is responsible for the student's homebound instruction; however, the school occupational therapy practitioner may provide services in the home and may support collaboration between service providers if a community-based occupational therapist is addressing medical needs.

Importance of the team approach

The need for effective collaboration across all school environments and all populations by all team members has been receiving increased attention (Hanft & Shepherd, 2016) with positive results (Shasby & Schneck, 2011). Given the multifaceted and complex needs of these students, effective collaborative teaming throughout decision making and service provision is critical and leads to a more cohesive and comprehensive program. More than 20 years ago, Giangreco (1996) discussed the importance of professionals in the school working together to establish and implement effective programs for these students. He recommended that teams use consensual decision making related to shared student goals to avoid gaps, contradictions, or overloads in services.

Teams should consider **role release** (transferring or sharing an intervention practice with another qualified member of the team) as appropriate. When role release is appropriate, an occupational therapy practitioner may provide information and training to another person (e.g., teacher, paraeducator, speech–language pathologist [SLP]), who then provides these supports with the student (e.g., providing instruction to the classroom paraeducator on positioning and safe feeding techniques).

In the LRE, methods of teaching and learning that are the most socially acceptable, least intrusive, and least stigmatizing should be implemented. In addition, these methods should lead to access to and participation in individualized education and achievement of learning outcomes. These recommendations continue to be highlighted as evidence-based practices for students with severe disabilities (Browder et al., 2014).

Unique issues

Issues unique to this population can take considerable time to address and require not only strong professional reasoning by the school occupational therapy practitioner but also creative and ongoing problem solving. Methodical instruction that includes clearly defined outcomes and systematic

FIGURE 34.1. Students with severe disabilities: General program considerations.

Preschool	Elementary	Middle	High School	18–21 Program
3–5 years	6–11 years	11–14 years	14–18 years	18–21 years

Communication --→

Social–Emotional --Social–Emotional,----------------------→
Self-Determination,
Self-Management

Preacademics, -----------------Academics, ------------------------------Functional Academics, ---------Consumer--------------------------→
Early Literacy   Functional   Academics   Skills
Academics
(independent living)

Self-Help, Safety ---Independent Living---→
(focuses on basic functional
skills needed on a daily/frequent
basis—self-help, personal care, safety,
home living, community living)

Motor Skills----------------------PE,---→ ←------------------------Recreation–leisure----------------------------→
Gross Motor   adaptive PE,
Developmental   recreation–leisure
Fine Motor
Developmental------------------Use of Classroom Tools,-------------------------→ ←---------------------Fine Motor Skills for Functional Tasks/Work---------→
written communication,
AT access

←-----------------------Community Access -------------→ Community Access -------------------------------→
(on a limited basis—   (transportation & mobility focused)
orientation/mobility focus)

←-------------------------School Based---------------→ ←---School &-------------------------------------→
community-based
vocational experience
& training
(job sampling; career path)

Note. AT = assistive technology; PE = physical education.
Source. From 6.28.05 (PROD.SEV.GeneralCurriculumFlow). Based on work with the DI Program of the Spokane Public Schools. Valerie Lynch, EdD, Puget Sound Educational Service Districts, Special Services, Seattle, WA 98116. Adapted with permission.

data collection to measure progress must occur (Browder et al., 2014). In addition, the necessary adaptive equipment and AT must consistently be available.

BEST PRACTICES

Research specific to occupational therapy for students with low-incidence disabilities is scarce. However, within general education, research has established that high teacher quality leads to better outcomes for students (Howell & Gengel, 2005). Howell and Gengel (2005) identified 5 characteristics of effective teachers of students with low-incidence disabilities:

1. Holding high expectations and helping others (e.g., families, paraeducators, general education teachers) to do the same;
2. Engaging in effective communication with other team members and the student;
3. Maintaining respect for the student and all other team members, including intentionally getting to know the student's interests, values, and needs;
4. Fostering professionalism, including participating in ongoing professional development, especially given the rapid changes in technology and instructional practices that may work for this population; and
5. Developing positive partnerships among team members, especially general education teachers.

These findings are consistent with the work of Browder et al.'s (2014) summary of evidence-based practices for this population. These characteristics would be invaluable for the school occupational therapy practitioner working with these students to embrace as well.

Evaluate the Student's Strengths and Needs

Services start with a comprehensive evaluation that identifies a student's strengths and needs for school performance and participation. A team-based ecological approach would collect the most meaningful information when evaluating students with low-incidence disabilities. Through an *ecological approach,* the team considers the student across all contexts to identify academic and functional needs, including present and future environments and expectations. On the basis of a survey of occupational therapists, Clark-Boll (2002) concluded that evaluation practices for this population should focus on addressing students' skills, roles, and tasks in the environment and then directly link the evaluation data to goals and services. Although the focus of their article is on teachers, Browder et al. (2014) confirmed these findings when describing evidence-based practices with this population.

Ecological approach

IDEA (2004, § 1414[b][2][A]) states that "a variety of assessment tools and strategies to gather relevant functional, developmental, and academic information" should be used. Occupational therapists gather these data to determine personal (e.g., roles, routines, response to transitions) and environmental (e.g., physical space, social groups, occupational demands) factors that facilitate or impede the student's participation in learning and school activities across educational contexts.

Strategies include reviewing existing evaluations and information about the student, conducting observations (e.g., during physical education, recess, lunch, other school activities), and conducting interviews. Tools such as the Canadian Occupational Performance Measure (Law et al., 2014), Pediatric Evaluation of Disability Inventory (Haley, 1992), and Short Child Occupational Profile (Bowyer et al., 2008) that are ecologically based and address occupation may be more effective for these students than developmental or norm-referenced assessments.

Team-based assessments are commonly used with this population and can be organized around curriculum, person-centered planning, or functional skill areas. One curriculum-based measure is the Assessment, Evaluation and Programming System for Infants and Children (Bricker et al., 2002). Two examples of person-centered planning tools are Choosing Options and Accommodations for Children (Giangreco et al., 1998) and Making Action Plans (Pearpoint et al., 1996). Every Move Counts is an assessment designed around understanding a specific functional skill area (Korsten et al., 1993). This assessment uses a sensory-based approach to communication and AT that provides both assessment and program information. Last, the SETT Framework (Zabala, 1995) can be helpful in guiding AT determination.

Client factors

During the ecological evaluation process, school occupational therapists may identify concerns in specific client factors that need to be explored further. This evaluation may include gathering specific ROM measurements and manual muscle testing. Other client factors to consider during the evaluation process include body functions such as mental functions; pain and sensory functions (e.g., hearing, vision); neuromusculoskeletal and movement-related functions; cardiovascular, immunological, and respiratory system functions; and voice and skin integrity (AOTA, 2014b).

Provide Effective Interventions to Enhance Participation

Education research has suggested that systematic instruction should be used to teach students academic, daily living, work, and community skills in general education, when possible, with appropriate adaptations and supports (Delano et al., 2008; Spooner et al., 2011). Sufficient evidence is lacking to fully determine which occupational therapy practices and interventions are most effective, yet intervention considerations should consider the needs of the student and family, the student's program and placement, and the educational context.

Given occupational therapy practitioners' skills in activity analysis, they can bring vital knowledge to the team to promote increased opportunities for student engagement and participation across contexts and environments. When working with this population, services on behalf of the student (e.g., collaboration with teachers, paraeducators, team members) and program supports may require more time from school occupational therapy practitioners. Effective use of services on behalf of the child in addition to services with the student is more likely to result in the student having an increased ability to access and participate across all educational environments (Mu & Royeen, 2004).

The school occupational therapist should consider a range of interventions as defined in the *Occupational Therapy Practice Framework: Domain and Process* (3rd ed.; AOTA, 2014b). Regardless of the complexity of the student's disability, emphasis should be on engagement and participation in occupations and activities. However, this may require increased attention to preparatory methods and tasks (e.g., positioning), education and training (e.g., teaching the paraeducator to transfer the student safely), advocacy, and group interventions.

Use developmentally or chronologically appropriate practices

There is an ongoing discussion regarding the use of developmentally appropriate versus chronologically appropriate interventions with students with low-incidence disabilities. Some authors feel that instruction too far beyond a student's developmental level may result in increased stress, decreased motivation, and nonfunctional skills (Carta et al., 1991), as well as rote learning of nonfunctional information across contexts (National Association for the Education of Young Children, 2009). However, others have stated that using activities that are developmentally appropriate but not age appropriate can reduce the quality of life and well-being of persons with disabilities (Reinders, 2002).

Brollier et al. (1994) discussed the importance of focusing on chronologically appropriate as well as environmentally based functional activities as a way of contributing to community living and the development of life skills. Forster (2010) stated that the use of age-appropriate activities and tools might be a way to gain community acceptance. The school occupational therapy practitioner should be aware of this ongoing discussion and choose the best intervention that provides opportunities for participation and performance across contexts. What follow are some intervention considerations for occupational therapy practitioners working with this population.

Support academic performance. The occupation of the student is a primary focus when working with this population in the schools. The literature supports the importance of access and participation in traditional academics (e.g., literacy, math, science) for students with low-incidence disabilities (Browder et al., 2012; Spooner et al., 2011).

The school occupational therapy practitioner can support access and participation in academics in a variety of ways. For example, there is a growing evidence base for occupational therapy services that support literacy development through interventions that support the use of adaptive equipment, AT, or both; positioning; and the development of fine motor, executive functioning, processing, and visual–perceptual skills. The occupational therapist may also support the teaching and learning of math by adapting math manipulatives so that the student can easily access them.

Enhance social participation. Social participation can be difficult for students with low-incidence disabilities because

of several factors, including communication challenges, difficulty accessing social environments, poor social skills, and sensory–motor impairments as well as health concerns that may limit interaction with other students. However, social skills are a daily requirement for any student and can be a necessity for successful postschool outcomes (AOTA, 2010).

Although the teacher may have the primary responsibility for addressing social skills with this population, the occupational therapy practitioner should consider providing input to the team, especially when issues such as sensory-processing difficulties, limitations in movement, or the need for adaptive equipment make social participation difficult. Social skills programs should incorporate sensory processing, movement, and communication skills (Baltazar-Mori & Piantanida, 2007; Kuypers, 2011) and preferred interests (Koegel et al., 2013). The practitioner may incorporate general education peers into social skills instructional programs (Hughes et al., 2011; Rossetti, 2011) or friendship groups for students with low-incidence disabilities. Training for general education students may include learning about a particular disability, learning how to use a piece of adaptive equipment for communication, or learning how to model interaction strategies.

Address mealtime needs. Eating, feeding, and swallowing can be particularly challenging for students with low-incidence disabilities. When a student has a challenge with this skill area, it is important that the school occupational therapist work closely with the medical community and educational team to ensure safe swallowing and proper nutrition. Delegation should be done only after the therapist is sure that the person providing the service is competent in a particular skill and student safety is not compromised.

Documenting the program is important for consistent follow-through. If the student is tube fed, the therapist needs to be aware of any licensure limitations. For example, in Washington State, only the school nurse can reinsert a gastrostomy tube if it happens to come out. The occupational therapist may also be involved in addressing the type and consistency of food (e.g., blended) and should include this information in the student's IEP and health care plan.

According to the U.S. Department of Agriculture (2001) and Section 504 of the Rehabilitation Act of 1973, as amended (2008; Pub. L. 93–112), schools receiving federal funds cannot discriminate against a student who has special dietary needs for school meals (e.g., food substitutions, food modifications). For more information, see Chapter 47.

Use AT to support participation. Many students with low-incidence disabilities use a variety of AT to access and participate in the learning environment. This equipment may include low-tech aids, such as a universal cuff, or high technology, such as an eye-gaze or complex computer system. For students requiring a functional communication system, the school occupational therapy practitioner should collaborate with the SLP and teacher to help set up and establish strategies (low or high tech) that work best for the student (Tiger et al., 2008).

Active learning can be facilitated with the use of toys, tools, or switches that have sound (including amplified sound) or texture and that emphasize foundation skills for learning, engagement, and play (Dunnett, 1997). Dr. Lilli Nielsen, a Danish researcher, introduced the theory of active learning, which is based on the belief that all students can learn when environments and opportunities promote free and active exploration (LilliWorks Active Learning Foundation, n.d.). To promote this concept, she created active learning materials and environments such as the Little Room; the Resonance Board; the Support Bench; and the Scratch, Pull, and Grab Board. The Little Room is a 3-walled container in which the student can actively explore and interact with suspended or mounted toys or textures; it can be used to support learning, access the curriculum, and to demonstrate what the student knows.

Address positioning needs. Because of the complexity of the student's physical needs, proper positioning is a critical part of their programs (Browder et al., 2014). Adaptive equipment for positioning can be as simple as a foam wedge or as complex as a power wheelchair. School occupational therapy practitioners should work closely with other team members in the selection, procurement, setup, and use of this equipment. The input from the practitioner regarding the proper positioning of a student can significantly affect engagement in school tasks and activities. Proper positioning and the change of position over time are also important in preventing skin breakdown, contractures, and other body function and body structure issues.

Provide professional development and training for staff. A primary role of school occupational therapy practitioners with students with low-incidence disabilities is to provide initial training; monitor continued competence after the initial training; and contribute to professional development for teachers, paraeducators, other team members, and peer tutors.

For example, occupational therapists may train paraeducators in proper body mechanics when lifting, transferring, and positioning a specific student; educate peer tutors to optimize interactions and exchange with the student who uses AT; or collaborate with the SLP and school nurse to design a student's mealtime support plan. In addition, practitioners are often part of the AT team or are the primary service providers in this area. Training in the setup, use, and ongoing maintenance of AT or other adaptive equipment may be needed. With proper training and supervision, paraeducators can implement the practitioner's suggestions into the student's daily program, as documented in the student's IEP.

Use peer-mediated instruction to support participation. A strong body of literature supports the use of **peer-mediated instruction** to support participation across school contexts, specifically to support literacy (Brady & Honsberger, 2016), math skills (Davis, 2016), and social skills (Simpson & Bui, 2016). School occupational therapy practitioners can help support peer-mediated instruction through activities such as training, program development, and monitoring the peer-mediated activities that are within the domain of occupational therapy.

Participate in transition planning. School occupational therapy practitioners should anticipate future environments

for this student population, given that some students may take longer to learn functional skills and develop habits and routines. Practitioners should work closely with the family and other team members to identify any splinter skills (ability to do a specific task or activity without foundational skills, out of a developmental sequence, and that does not generalize to other tasks or activity) that should be taught to support engagement and participation and to advocate for any needed supports. Discussion of expectations and needs for future environments should be ongoing throughout the student's educational career and should include the entire team (Wells et al., 2012).

Outcomes

When working with this population, data-based decision making should be used as part of systematic instruction throughout the intervention process to ensure that students are meeting their goals. The school occupational therapy practitioner should record data that not only document strengths and needs in areas of client factors but also enable evaluation of the student's participation and performance in the curriculum and across school contexts.

Thus, data should reflect the student's improvement in client factors such as ROM or positioning, as well as the student's ability to access the curriculum or participate in school activities (e.g., physical education, art, field trips). When the student is having difficulty participating across school contexts or meeting goals, the occupational therapist, in collaboration with the school team, can make adjustments to the student's program (see Chapter 45, "Best Practices in School Occupational Therapy Documentation and Data Collection").

SUMMARY

Through comprehensive, occupation-based evaluations that emphasize an ecological and team-based approach, occupational therapy practitioners become key team members for students with low-incidence disabilities. Interventions are varied and should include services required by the student and on behalf of the student to implement research-based best practices that meet the student's complex and varied needs, and that support access and participation in current environments. Needs for future environments should also be considered.

REFERENCES

American Occupational Therapy Association. (2010). Occupational therapy services in the promotion of psychological and social aspects of mental health. *American Journal of Occupational Therapy, 64,* 578–591. https://doi.org/10.5014/ajot.2010.64S78

American Occupational Therapy Association. (2014a). Guidelines for supervision, roles, and responsibilities during the delivery of occupational therapy services. *American Journal of Occupational Therapy, 68*(Suppl. 3), S16–S22. https://doi.org/10.5014/ajot.2014.686S03

American Occupational Therapy Association. (2014b). Occupational therapy practice framework: Domain and process (3rd ed.). *American Journal of Occupational Therapy, 68*(Suppl. 1), S1–S48. https://doi.org/10.5014/ajot.2014.682006

Baltazar-Mori, A., & Piantanida, D. B. (2007). *Every child wants to play: Simple and effective strategies for teaching social skills.* Torrance, CA: Pediatric Therapy Network.

Bowyer, P. L., Kramer, J., Ploszaj, A., Ross, M., Schwartz, O., Kielhofner, G., & Kramer, K. (2008). *The Short Child Occupational Profile (SCOPE), Version 2.2.* Chicago: University of Illinois at Chicago.

Brady, M., & Honsberger, T. (2016). Effects of a peer-mediated literacy based behavioral intervention on the acquisition and maintenance of daily living skills in adolescents with autism. *Education and Training in Autism and Developmental Disabilities, 51,* 122–131. Retrieved from http://daddcec.org/Publications/ETADDJournal/ETADDArchives.aspx

Bricker, D., Pretti-Frontczak, K., Johnson, J., & Straka, E. (2002). *AEPS: Assessment, Evaluation, and Programming System for Infants and Children* (2nd ed.). Baltimore: Brookes.

Brollier, C., Shepherd, J., & Markley, K. F. (1994). Transition from school to community living. *American Journal of Occupational Therapy, 48,* 346–353. https://doi.org/10.5014/ajot.48.4.346

Browder, D. M., Trela, K., Courtade, G. R., Jimenez, B. A., Knight, V., & Flowers, C. (2012). Teaching mathematics and science standards to students with moderate and severe developmental disabilities. *Journal of Special Education, 46,* 26–35. https://doi.org/10.1177/0022466910369942

Browder, D. M., Wood, L., Thompson, J., & Ribuffo, C. (2014). *Evidence-based practices for students with severe disabilities* (Document No. IC-3). Retrieved from http://ceedar.education.ufl.edu/tools/innovation-configurations/

Carta, J., Schwartz, I., Atwater, J., & McConnell, S. (1991). Developmentally appropriate practice: Appraising its usefulness for young children with disabilities. *Topics in Early Childhood Special Education, 11,* 1–20. https://doi.org/10.1177%2F027112149101100104

Clark-Boll, R. (2002). *School-based occupational therapists' reported frames of reference, therapeutic approaches, assessment practices, and goals for students with moderate to severe disabilities* (Doctoral dissertation). Albany: State University of New York.

Davis, L. L. (2016). *Effects of peer-mediated instruction on mathematical problem solving for students with moderate/severe intellectual disability* (Doctoral dissertation). Available from ProQuest Dissertations and Theses database. (UMI No. 10111913)

Delano, M. E., Keefe, L., & Perner, D. (2008). Personnel preparation: Recurring challenges and the need for action to ensure access to general education. *Research and Practice for Persons With Severe Disabilities, 34,* 232–240. https://doi.org/10.2511/rpsd.33.4.232

Dunnett, J. (1997). Nielsen's little room: Its use with a young blind and physically disabled girl. *Journal of Visual Impairment and Blindness, 91,* 145–150.

Forster, S. (2010). Age-appropriateness: Enabler or barrier to a good life for people with profound intellectual and multiple disabilities? *Journal of Intellectual and Developmental Disability, 35,* 129–131. https://doi.org/10.3109/13668251003694606

Giangreco, M. F. (1996). *Vermont interdependent services team approach: A guide to coordinating educational support services.* Baltimore: Brookes.

Giangreco, M. F., Cloninger, C. J., & Iverson, V. S. (1998). *Choosing Options and Accommodations for Children (COACH): A guide to educational planning for students with disabilities* (2nd ed.). Baltimore: Brookes.

Haley, S. M. (1992). *Pediatric Evaluation of Disability Inventory (PEDI): Development, standardization and administration manual.* Boston: New England Medical Center Hospital.

Hanft, B., & Shepherd, J. (Eds.). (2016). *Collaborating for student success: A guide for school-based occupational therapy* (2nd ed.). Bethesda, MD: AOTA Press.

Hanft, B., Swinth, Y., & Shepherd, J. (2016). Initiating and sustaining system supports. In B. Hanft & J. Shepherd (Eds.), *Collaborating for student success: A guide for school-based occupational therapy* (2nd ed., pp. 243–281). Bethesda, MD: AOTA Press.

Howell, J. J., & Gengel, S. (2005). Perspectives of effective teachers of students with low-incidence disabilities. *TEACHING Exceptional Children Plus, 1*(4), Article 6. Retrieved from https://files.eric.ed.gov/fulltext/EJ966520.pdf

Hughes, C., Golas, M., Cosgriff, J., Brigham, N., Edwards, C., & Cashen, K. (2011). Effects of a social skills intervention among high school students with intellectual disabilities and autism and their general education peers. *Research and Practice for Persons With Severe Disabilities, 36*(1–2), 46–61. https://doi.org/10.2511%2Frpsd.36.1-2.46

Individuals With Disabilities Education Improvement Act of 2004, Pub. L. 108–446, 20 U.S.C. §§ 1400–1482.

Jackson, R. (2010). *Curriculum access for students with low-incidence disabilities: The promise of universal design for learning.* Wakefield, MA: National Center on Accessing the General Curriculum. Retrieved from http://aem.cast.org/about/publications/2005/ncac-curriculum-access-low-incidence-udl.html#.W8YPEPZRfyQ

Koegel, R., Kim, S., Koegel, L., & Schwartzman, B. (2013). Improving socialization for high school students with ASD by using their preferred interests. *Journal of Autism and Development Disorders, 43,* 2121–2134. https://doi.org/10.1007/s10803-013-1765-3

Korsten, J. E., Dunn, D. K., Foss, T. V., & Francke, M. K. (1993). *Every Move Counts: Sensory-based communication techniques.* Austin, TX: Pro-Ed.

Kuypers, L. (2011). *The Zones of Regulation.* San Jose, CA: Think Social.

Law, M., Baptiste, S., Carswell, A., McColl, M., Polatajko, H., & Pollock, N. (2014). *Canadian Occupational Performance Measure manual* (5th ed.). Ottawa: CAOT Publications.

LilliWorks Active Learning Foundation. (n.d.). *About active learning.* Retrieved from http://www.lilliworks.org/?page_id=2

Mu, K., & Royeen, C. (2004). Facilitating participation of students with severe disabilities: Aligning school-based occupational therapy practice with best practices in severe disabilities. *Physical and Occupational Therapy in Pediatrics, 24*(3), 5–21. https://doi.org/10.1300/J006v24n03_02

National Association for the Education of Young Children. (2009). *Developmentally appropriate practice in early childhood programs serving children from birth through age 8.* Retrieved from http://www.naeyc.org/DAP

National Consortium on Deaf–Blindness. (2017). *The 2016 national child count of children and youth who are deaf-blind.* Retrieved from http://www.nationaldb.org/reports/national-child-count-2016

Pearpoint, J., Forest, M., & O'Brien, J. (1996). MAPS, Circle of Friends, and PATH: Powerful tools to help build caring communities. In S. Stainback & W. Stainback (Eds.), *Inclusion: A guide for educators* (pp. 67–86). Baltimore: Brookes.

Rehabilitation Act of 1973, Pub. L. 93–112, 29 U.S.C. §§ 701–796l.

Reinders, J. S. (2002). The good life of citizens with intellectual disability. *Journal of Intellectual Disability Research, 46,* 1–5. https://doi.org/10.1046/j.1365-2788.2002.00386.x

Rosenau, N. (2000). Do we really mean families for *all* children? Permanency planning for children with developmental disabilities. *Policy Research Brief, 11*(2), 1–12. Retrieved from https://ici.umn.edu/products/prb/112/default.html

Rossetti, Z. S. (2011). "That's how we do it": Friendship work between high school students with and without autism or developmental disability. *Research and Practice for Persons With Severe Disabilities, 36*(1–2), 23–33. https://doi.org/10.2511%2Frpsd.36.1-2.23

Section 504 of the Rehabilitation Act of 1973, as amended, 29 U.S.C. § 794 (2008).

Shasby, S., & Schneck, C. (2011). Commentary on collaboration in school-based practice: Positives and pitfalls. *Journal of Occupational Therapy, Schools, and Early Intervention, 4,* 22–33. https://doi.org/10.1080/19411243.2011.573243

Simpson, L., & Bui, Y. (2016). Effects of a peer-mediated intervention on social interactions of students with low-functioning autism and perceptions of typical peers. *Education and Training in Autism and Developmental Disabilities, 51,* 162–178. Retrieved from http://daddcec.org/Publications/ETADDJournal/ETADD Archives.aspx

Spooner, F., Knight, V., Browder, D. M., Jimenez, B., & DiBiase, W. (2011). Evaluating evidence-based practice in teaching science in context to students with severe developmental disabilities. *Research and Practice in Severe Disabilities, 36,* 62–75. https://doi.org/10.2511/rpsd.36.1-2.62

TASH. (2017). *About TASH.* Retrieved from http://tash.org/about/

Tiger, J. H., Hanley, G. P., & Bruzek, J. (2008). Functional communication training: A review and practical guide. *Behavior Analysis in Practice, 1,* 16–23. https://doi.org/10.1007/BF03391716

U.S. Department of Agriculture. (2001). *Accommodating children with special dietary needs in the school nutrition programs: Guidance for school food service staff.* Washington, DC: Author.

Wells, J., Sheehey, P., & Moore, A. (2012). Postsecondary expectations for a student in a rural middle school: Impact of person-centered planning on team member agreement. *Rural Special Education Quarterly, 31,* 25–33. https://doi.org/10.1177%2F875687051203100305

Zabala, J. S. (1995). *The SETT framework: Critical areas to consider when making informed assistive technology decisions.* Retrieved from https://eric.ed.gov/?id=ED381962

Best Practices in Supporting Students With Other Health Impairments

35

Janice Harman Flegle, MA, OTR/L, BCP, and Christina M. Edelbrock, MA, OTR/L, BCP, SCSS

KEY TERMS AND CONCEPTS

- Acute condition
- Chronic care model
- Chronic condition
- Collaborative consultation
- Healthy learner
- Medical home
- Other health impairment
- Students with special health care needs

OVERVIEW

Young people with health impairments are commonly referred to as *children and youth with special health care needs*. These persons experience at least 1 type of ongoing health condition that results in a greater-than-routine need for health and related services. **Students with special health care needs** are those who "have or are at increased risk for chronic physical, developmental, behavioral, or emotional condition and who also require health and related services of a type or amount beyond that required by children generally" (McPherson et al., 1998, as cited in Maternal and Child Health Bureau, 2018, para. 1).

A national survey conducted by the Maternal and Child Health Bureau (Data Resource Center for Child and Adolescent Health, 2016), more than 1 in 5 households reported having at least 1 child with special health care needs. More than 25% of the respondents to the 2016 National Survey of Children With Special Health Care Needs described functional difficulties that affect day-to-day life, and 10% described difficulty concentrating, remembering, or making decisions because of a physical, mental, or emotional condition. In the households surveyed, nearly 40% of the students did not meet the criteria for school success: being always or usually engaged in school, participating in extracurricular activities, and feeling safe at school (Blumberg et al., 2007).

Persons with special health care needs may have functional limitations or behavioral health problems that require additional accommodations and support for them to succeed in school and learn to manage their chronic condition effectively (Forrest et al., 2011). When a student has a health condition that affects access to and participation in their educational program, the verification category of other health impairment (OHI) should be considered.

According to the Individuals With Disabilities Education Improvement Act of 2004 (IDEA; Pub. L. 108–446), **OHI** means

> having limited strength, vitality, or alertness, including a heightened alertness to environmental stimuli, that results in limited alertness with respect to the educational environment, that—
>
> (i) is due to chronic or acute health problems such as asthma, attention deficit disorder or attention deficit hyperactivity disorder, diabetes, epilepsy, a heart condition, hemophilia, lead poisoning, leukemia, nephritis, rheumatic fever, sickle cell anemia, and Tourette syndrome; and
>
> (ii) adversely affects a child's educational performance. (§ 300.8[c][9])

The phrase *such as* indicates that there are other chronic health conditions that might support a student's eligibility under this category when considered by a team of qualified professionals and the family. The multidisciplinary team's responsibility is to determine whether the student's health problem adversely affects the student's educational performance. A medical diagnosis is not required by IDEA, but some state rules may require a medical condition for this category. Best practices in school occupational therapy evaluation and intervention to improve student outcomes are discussed later.

ESSENTIAL CONSIDERATIONS

This section presents current evidence describing the characteristics of students with OHI or special health care needs and some of the educational participation risks documented for this population of students.

Copyright © 2019 by the American Occupational Therapy Association. All rights reserved. To reuse this content, contact www.copyright.com.
https://doi.org/10.7139/2019.978-1-56900-591-0.035

EXHIBIT 35.1.	Online Resources Related to OHI

- **American Diabetes Association** (http://www.diabetes.org): Advocacy efforts, research, and resources for living with and managing diabetes
- **American Lung Association** (https://www.lung.org/lung-disease/asthma/): Information about lung disease and asthma for health professionals and volunteers
- **Asthma and Allergy Foundation of America** (http://www.aafa.org/): Education, advocacy, and research pertaining to asthma and allergies
- **Center for Parent Information and Resources** (http://www.parentcenterhub.org/disability-landing/): Information and connections on a full spectrum of disabilities in children, including developmental delays and rare disorders
- **Children and Adults With Attention Deficit/Hyperactivity Disorder** (http://www.chadd.org/): Education, advocacy, and support for persons with ADHD
- **American Heart Association** (https://www.aha.org/): Information about impact, risk factors, symptoms and treatment for CHDs
- **Environmental Protection Agency** (http://www.epa.gov/lead): Information about lead poisoning symptoms and prevention, laws, regulations, and research spanning many environmental and human health protection topics
- **Epilepsy Foundation** (http://www.epilepsy.org): Information, resources, and research activities about epilepsy
- **Juvenile Diabetes Research Foundation** (http://www.jdrf.org/): Information on juvenile diabetes advocacy and research
- **Leukemia and Lymphoma Society** (http://www.lls.org): Information about research, services, and public policy concerning blood cancer
- **National Association of Special Education Teachers** (http://www.naset.org/2278.0.html): Information for teachers and families about various chronic health conditions considered under the OHI category
- **Cystic Fibrosis Foundation** (http://www.cff.org/): Information, resources, and treatment of this progressive condition
- **National Institute of Mental Health** (https://www.nimh.nih.gov/health/topics/anxiety-disorders/index.shtml): Information about a variety of mental health issues, including risk factors, signs and symptoms, treatments and therapies
- **National Organization for Rare Disorders** (http://www.rarediseases.org/): Information, resources, advocacy efforts, and research pertaining to rare disorders
- **Tourette Association of America** (https://www.tourette.org/): Information, advocacy efforts, and professional resources about the diagnosis and treatment of Tourette syndrome

Note. ADHD = attention deficit hyperactivity disorder; CHD = congenital heart defect; OHI = other health impairment.

OHI and Comorbidities

According to the National Center for Education Statistics (2013), approximately 11% of students were found eligible for special education under OHI. These rates are increasing. One possible reason for this increase could be the rise in the number of students diagnosed with attention deficit hyperactivity disorder (ADHD), one of the most common chronic health conditions encountered in the educational setting. Exhibit 35.1 lists various online resources related to OHI.

The literature is unequivocal about the increased risks for emotional and behavioral difficulties in children with chronic health conditions (Forrest et al., 2011; Shaw & McCabe, 2008; Wodrich, Hasan, & Parent, 2011). Mental health disorders in children and youth are on the rise, and students with special health care needs have a disproportionately higher incidence of mental, emotional, and behavioral disorders than the general population (Green et al., 2017). Overall, 30% of students with health care needs have a mental, emotional, or behavioral disorder or condition requiring medical treatment (Glassgow & Voorhees, 2017). Consideration for students' mental health in the context of the educational setting is essential, because educators may not be aware of the signs and symptoms of various mental health conditions, and the signs of half of all mental health disorders are seen before age 14 years (American Occupational Therapy Association [AOTA], 2010).

Students living in poverty and those at risk for or with disabilities also have a higher rate of health issues and encounter more barriers to accessing appropriate health care than their peers (Sanetti, 2017). Guerrero et al. (2017) found that Latino families were less likely to have a ***medical home*** (a partnership between medical and community settings; American Academy of Pediatrics, 2004); Latino children with health care needs (ages 6–17 years) missed 11 or more school days a year in comparison with children with special health care needs who were White or Black, and they were more likely to have unmet medical needs than the same counterparts. School occupational therapy practitioners[1] working with ethnically diverse student populations should be aware of the cultural values and practices of their students' families regarding health and medical care.

Establishing communication between clinical and educational teams is essential for students with special health care needs. Limited communication between the clinical and educational systems was identified as a primary concern during standardized, open-ended, 1-on-1 interviews with 10 mothers of children with health care needs (Anderson, 2009). A majority of those interviewed felt that they were the sole liaison between the health care and educational settings and found limited system supports for effective transfer of information between the 2 settings. It is extremely important that all on-site school staff members understand the implications and utility of the OHI verification and be familiar with the school district's special education referral process.

---

[1]*Occupational therapy practitioner* refers to both the occupational therapist and the occupational therapy assistant. AOTA (2014a, p. S18) states, "The occupational therapist is responsible for all aspects of occupational therapy service delivery and is accountable for the safety and effectiveness of the occupational therapy service delivery process" and "must be directly involved in the delivery of services during the initial evaluation and regularly throughout the course of intervention. . . . The occupational therapy assistant delivers safe and effective occupational therapy services under the supervision of and in partnership with the occupational therapist."

Identifying Students Under OHI

Health and school performance are interdependent. Good health is required for learning, and students with good health are more successful in school (Forrest et al., 2011). Research has shown that academic outcomes can be adversely affected when health conditions impose limits on a student's activity (Bethell et al., 2012). Although not all students with health impairments struggle in the educational setting, identifying students with chronic health conditions that affect educational performance and participation is essential.

The OHI verification should only be considered for students with acute or chronic special health care needs that interfere with educational participation. When a student with special health care needs requires accommodations to access learning and school activities in a general education environment, a 504 plan should be considered. Section 504 of the Rehabilitation Act of 1973, as amended (2008; Pub. L. 93–112), requires schools that receive federal funds to provide supports and accommodations for students who are eligible (see Chapter 27, "Best Practices in Supporting Students With a 504 Plan").

The process to determine eligibility for special education varies by state and school district (e.g., a local educational agency may have a worksheet to determine eligibility; some may require a diagnosis from a medical professional). Documentation that the condition is either *acute* (i.e., expected to last for more than 60 calendar days) or *chronic* (i.e., permanent) may be required by the school district. Evaluations to determine the impact of the health impairment on educational performance (for students kindergarten–graduation) must be completed. A comprehensive evaluation of intellectual ability and developmental history should also be obtained when that information will provide important insight for educational programming (American Academy of Special Education Professionals [AASEP], 2012).

Management of a Student's Chronic Health Conditions

It is extremely important for all members of the school staff who support students with special health care needs to be well informed about the students' condition and related needs (Shaw & McCabe, 2008). The management of some chronic health conditions is quite routine, whereas others require constant monitoring and dynamic management strategies to support optimal educational participation. For example, students with diabetes need to be diligent about monitoring blood glucose levels to determine their insulin needs (Cooke & Plotnick, 2008). Students with asthma or severe allergies may experience seasonal or activity-related exacerbations of their condition (Bray et al., 2008); students with cancer may struggle with unpredictable side effects related to the disease or their treatment regimen (Shaw & McCabe, 2008).

Most students with chronic conditions will require life-long medical and psychological support. Those who are young, are newly diagnosed, or have complex health care needs require more dedicated oversight and direct support from their family and educational team to maintain an optimal level of health and educational participation.

Responsibility for the management of aspects of their health care needs can be shifted gradually from the family (or responsible adult) to students when they begin to show interest and readiness to take responsibility. However, premature shifting of responsibility may result in deterioration of (e.g., metabolic) control and management of the condition (Cooke & Plotnick, 2008).

Students with special health care needs may miss instructional time as a result of their condition. These students may have increased absences as a result of illness, injury, or required medical appointments. Students with complex medical needs will leave the classroom to manage personal needs related to their condition such as tube feedings, suctioning, tracheostomy management, intermittent catheterization, and administration of prescribed medications (National Dissemination Center for Children With Disabilities, 2012).

Although students with health care needs might recognize that their health and well-being are dependent on this support, they might also feel self-conscious about their need for equipment and procedural support that sets them apart from their peers. The potential for embarrassment after an emergency triggered by their condition might also exacerbate anxiety for a student with a volatile health condition (Wodrich et al., 2008). Moreover, school days missed due to illness can undermine students' confidence, affect their motivation to learn, and hinder their ability to sustain positive peer relationships (Shaw & McCabe, 2008).

Challenges in the Educational Setting

The unique challenges faced by students with health care needs include but are not limited to mobility issues, coordination difficulties, muscle weakness, poor school attendance, excessive tardiness, poor stamina, and problems maintaining focused attention (AASEP, 2012). In a study of students in Grades 4–6, students with special health care needs participated less in classroom activities, were less motivated to do well in school, missed more school days, and were more likely to exhibit disruptive behaviors in school than their peers without health conditions (Forrest et al., 2011). In addition, students with disabilities were either the victim of bullying or the perpetrator at a rate twice the national average, according to an extensive review of foundational studies examining bullying in schools (Rose et al., 2011).

Unfortunately, a student's health condition may even have an impact on their education after graduation. One study examined how or whether certain personal characteristics of transition-age youth served by a Midwest state vocational rehabilitation agency predicted successful employment postgraduation. Oswald et al. (2016) found that an OHI verification was negatively predictive of employment. School occupational therapy practitioners need to partner with school transition coordinators and vocational rehabilitation counselors to develop or expand programs that encourage students with OHI to explore job and career options and supported work experiences before graduation to improve outcomes for this population. Students with special health care needs appear to be at greater risk for underemployment or unemployment than their peers.

Role of Occupational Therapy Practitioners

The school occupational therapy practitioner has a unique understanding of how the relationship among student factors, occupations, performance skills, and performance patterns in all pertinent contexts can affect a student's health, well-being, and participation in life (AOTA, 2014b). The school occupational therapy practitioner must be able to articulate this professional perspective clearly to the student, family, and multidisciplinary educational team.

BEST PRACTICES

It is important for occupational therapists to know and use evidence-based strategies when evaluating and supporting students with OHI or health care needs in the educational setting.

Evaluate Students With Health Care Needs to Identify Strengths and Needs

A critical element of the school occupational therapist's evaluation process is to learn as much about a student's health condition as necessary to understand how their health condition might affect their access to and participation in education.

First, a thorough review of medical history and medications should be gathered through record review, family interviews, and medical reports from any medical provider with whom the family authorizes an information exchange. Understanding characteristics of the student's condition or diagnosis before the evaluation is important. When a student is likely to experience exacerbation and remission cycles related to a health condition, the evaluator should include information about factors known to prevent or trigger variance. In addition, the evaluation should describe how performance skills might be adversely affected during exacerbation cycles. Observable performance patterns that might be attributed to side effects of medication should be documented in the report and communicated to the parents and health care team when applicable.

Standardized assessments are not always possible because of the student's special health care needs and lack of normative data for the population of people with such needs. Ecological assessment and structured observation of the student's participation in all aspects of their school routine and environment with comparison with peer performances, school standards, and classroom or teacher expectations may be used to identify how the student's condition affects educational participation, performance, or both. Throughout the evaluation process, school occupational therapy practitioners should be aware of behaviors that may predispose students with disabilities to victimization or perpetration of bullying, and an intervention plan to address such behaviors should be considered.

The School Function Assessment (Coster et al., 1998) is a criterion-referenced measure that can be used to provide information pertaining to the student's participation and performance across school settings. Mancini and Coster (2004) found that some aspects of function are context specific, meaning a student's participation in any given setting may be associated with the ability to meet the physical, cognitive, and behavioral requirements common in that environment or context. School occupational therapy practitioners should consider the full extent of functional skills that each context demands and the barriers that may impede successful participation.

When the student possesses the maturity and insight to participate in a self-assessment process, the Canadian Occupational Performance Measure (COPM; Law et al., 2014) can be used to identify and prioritize everyday issues that restrict or affect the student's performance in the school setting. The COPM can also be used to structure an interview with the student's family and members of the student's educational team.

Implement Evidence-Based Interventions

After a thorough evaluation, school occupational therapy practitioners provide interventions on the basis of research and professional judgment. Collaboration with the student and significant adults in the student's life is critical for ongoing monitoring of the health condition and educational performance. Addressing social and emotional skills is necessary because of increased risk for problems in these areas.

Build collaborative consultation

For many years, school occupational therapy practitioners have embraced **collaborative consultation,** which is an "interactive problem-solving process that enables people with diverse expertise to generate creative solutions to mutually defined problems" (Villenueve, 2009, p. 207). Strategies for building collaborative relationships in schools involve listening to families, other team members, and community partners; observing students' activities in contextual settings (e.g., classroom, lunchroom, playground); educating administrators and key stakeholders about the unique contributions of occupational therapy; and establishing effective communication among team members (Hanft & Shepherd, 2016).

Missiuna et al. (2012) described a model for occupational therapy service delivery in the schools that emphasizes the partnership of occupational therapy practitioners, educators, and parents of children with a chronic condition. The Partnering for Change model shifts the focus from direct service (or fixing impairments) to collaboration and coaching in the student's educational context (Campbell et al., 2012). Team members are encouraged to support early identification of students with a chronic health condition and build the capacity of school professionals and others to manage each student's condition (Missiuna et al., 2012).

School occupational therapists might support students by working with the school nurse and principal to find resources for a student in need of eyeglass repair or replacement, communicating with a student's family and health care providers when a student presents with symptoms of depression, or collaborating with a student's family and a wheelchair vendor to order and fit the student for a new wheelchair.

Members of the educational team (e.g., nurses, psychologists, occupational therapy practitioners) may work with many students in different school buildings. Each member must be equally dedicated to building relationships with one another and with family members to support collaborative communication to benefit students with health care needs—even more so when a student's health care needs fluctuate.

Occupational therapy practitioners may also provide consultation to educational teams to support students with health care needs even when these students do not receive special education services. Using multi-tiered systems of support (MTSS), a range of interventions based on the needs of individual students can be provided (Office of Special Education Programs, 2017). Although MTSS is focused primarily on academic and behavior concerns, it reflects a new way to think about both disability identification and early intervention for at-risk students, including those with health care needs. MTSS focus on collaborative, team-based approaches to the development, implementation, and evaluation of research-based interventions. Occupational therapy practitioners in schools are members of the interdisciplinary team whose unique skills may be called on to support all students, including students with health care needs in educational settings.

Provide transition planning between medical and educational settings

Episodic hospitalization or an acute exacerbation of symptoms associated with a chronic health problem can isolate students with health care needs from their peers and disrupt school attendance. Proactive communication and planning among the student's family, medical providers, and educational personnel are imperative, whether the transition is from hospital to home, home to school, school to school, or hospital to school (National Dissemination Center for Children With Disabilities, 2012).

The American Academy of Pediatrics (2004) stated that management of children and young adults with special health care needs should follow the principles of the **chronic care model,** which fosters collaborative participation of persons with chronic health problems and their care providers. Ongoing communication among community programs, medical providers, and educational teams is the hallmark of the medical home wherein everyone works together to ensure that the special needs of these students and families are addressed.

Support student participation

School occupational therapy practitioners working with students with health care needs are ultimately partners in a team effort to promote the student's active participation in learning activities that support academic progress, positive peer relationships, and sustained wellness. Erickson et al. (2006) described the **healthy learner** as one who attends school, whose chronic condition is well managed, and who is an active participant in the educational process. Occupational therapy interventions might focus on the establishment of routines or skills that support optimal participation throughout the school day or identify adaptations or accommodations that will modify either the current context or activity demands to support the student's performance in their natural learning environment.

The Partnering for Change model shifts the focus from direct service to collaboration and coaching within the student's educational context (Campbell et al., 2012). Working at the building or classroom level rather than the individual level allows school occupational therapy practitioners to enable early identification of students with a chronic health condition and build the capacity of school professionals and others to manage this condition (Missiuna et al., 2012). When families and educators have more knowledge about chronic health conditions, students who may be in need of supports can be identified earlier, and accommodations can be put in place sooner to maximize educational participation and performance (Campbell et al., 2012; Missiuna et al., 2012).

The Centers for Disease Control and Prevention has developed a model that integrates educational and medical outcomes. The Whole School, Whole Community, Whole Child (WSCC) model focuses on student outcomes related to health and education, with an emphasis on collaboration between medical and educational providers to ensure that all students feel safe and healthy at school (Lewallen et al., 2015). The WSCC model provides a framework for building a health-focused school community to promote the safety and well-being of all students.

Anticipate and support student social and emotional needs

Emotional strength is a byproduct of successful participation. School occupational therapy practitioners can listen and watch for participation opportunities for which the student may lack confidence to pursue without support. Through the use of everyday activities, occupational therapy practitioners promote mental health and support functioning in people with or at risk of experiencing a range of mental health disorders (AOTA, 2010). When designing interventions for students with OHI, as well as for students with health care needs who are not receiving special education services, consideration of the student's mental health in the context of the educational setting is essential.

Students with health care needs who experience symptoms of anxiety and depression in the educational setting may receive accommodations or modifications to increase their school success. One study found that 82% of students with anxiety who had an individualized education program or 504 plan reported receiving at least 1 anxiety-related accommodation (Green et al., 2017). Occupational therapy practitioners provide a unique perspective to educational teams because "occupational therapy practitioners recognize that mental well-being is an integral part of the ability of people to engage in desired and necessary life occupations regardless of physical and social situation or context" (AOTA, 2016, p. 2).

The focus of occupational therapy practitioners in schools is on student participation. Well-intentioned family members might suggest that a student with anxiety should be accommodated by allowing them to leave the classroom when the student's anxiety escalates (e.g., during a group classroom activity). However, it is important for educational teams to understand that providing accommodations that allow avoidance in the short term may limit the student's ability to manage their anxiety in the long term (Green et al., 2017). Occupational therapy providers should advocate for accommodations that facilitate participation and engagement rather than avoidance of anxiety-producing activities.

Extracurricular and community activities provide opportunities for participation in areas of interest for students of all ages. School occupational therapy practitioners may help students navigate the application process to become a library aide, timekeeper at junior varsity games, or crossing guard. When needed, occupational therapy practitioners can advocate for late transportation services for the student who is interested in after-school extracurricular activities. Sharing information about sports teams in the community that are more inclusive than competitive would be most helpful. Occupational therapy practitioners could also share information with families about community resources and scholarships or stipends.

Finally, school occupational therapy practitioners can encourage transition-age students to consider work–study or supported employment opportunities that complement the personal strengths and interests they have demonstrated throughout their school career.

SUMMARY

Students with OHI or health care needs face significant barriers to positive school experiences. School occupational therapy practitioners provide a unique, holistic perspective on the dynamic relationship between a student's health and participation. Students eligible for special education services under the OHI category must meet the state's criteria and demonstrate performance skill deficits or problems that can be attributed to their underlying medical condition.

During the evaluation, the school occupational therapist should integrate information about the student's medical history and health condition in addition to structured observations of their current level of participation in all aspects of their natural school environment. Occupational therapy providers should consider the social–emotional needs of students with health care needs in the educational setting and proactively identify and reinforce the unique strengths and interests of students whose social, cultural, and personal contexts might make it difficult for them to access community resources.

Peer performance, school standards, and classroom and teacher expectations can provide a baseline when determining the educational effect of a student's health condition. Current evidence supports a collaborative consultation model for intervention in which the school occupational therapy practitioner partners with parents, other school personnel, and medical professionals to identify, understand, and accommodate students with health care needs as early as possible.

REFERENCES

American Academy of Pediatrics. (2004). Medical Home Initiatives for Children with Special Needs Project Advisory Committee: The medical home. *Pediatrics, 113,* 1545–1547. https://doi.org/10.1542/peds.110.1.184

American Academy of Special Education Professionals. (2012). *Other health impairments.* Retrieved from http://aasep.org/professional-resources/exceptionalstudents/otherimpairments/index.html

American Occupational Therapy Association. (2010). Occupational therapy services in the promotion of psychological and social aspects of mental health. *American Journal of Occupational Therapy, 64*(6, Suppl.), S78–S91. https://doi.org/10.5014/ajot.2010.64S78

American Occupational Therapy Association. (2014a). Guidelines for supervision, roles, and responsibilities during the delivery of occupational therapy services. *American Journal of Occupational Therapy, 68*(Suppl. 3), S16–S22. https://doi.org/10.5014/ajot.2014.686S03

American Occupational Therapy Association. (2014b). Occupational therapy practice framework: Domain and process (3rd ed.). *American Journal of Occupational Therapy, 68*(Suppl. 1), S1–S48. https://doi.org/10.5014/ajot.2014.682006

American Occupational Therapy Association. (2016). Occupational therapy services in the promotion of mental health and well-being. *American Journal of Occupational Therapy, 70*(Suppl. 2), 7012410070. https://doi.org/10.5014/ajot.2016.706S05

Anderson, L. S. (2009). Mothers of children with special health care needs: Documenting the experience of their children's care in the school setting. *Journal of School Nursing, 25,* 342–351. https://doi.org/10.1177/1059840509334146

Bethell, C., Forrest, C. B., Stumbo, S., Gombojav, N., Carle, A., & Irwin, C. E. (2012). Factors promoting or potentially impeding school success: Disparities and state variations for children with special health care needs. *Maternal and Child Health Journal, 16*(Suppl. 1), S35–S43. https://doi.org/10.1007/s10995-012-0993-z

Blumberg, S. J., Foster, E. B., Frasier, A. M., Satorius, J., Skalland, B. J., Nysse-Carris, K. L., & O'Connor, K. S. (2007). *Design and operation of the National Survey of Children's Health.* Hyattsville, MD: U.S. Department of Health and Human Services, Centers for Disease Control and Prevention, National Center for Health Statistics.

Bray, M. A., Kehle, T. J., Grigerick, S. E., Loftus, S., & Nicholson, H. (2008). Children with asthma: Assessment and treatment in school settings. *Psychology in the Schools, 45,* 63–73. https://doi.org/10.1002/pits.20279

Campbell, W. N., Missiuna, C. A., Rivard, L. M., & Pollock, N. A. (2012). "Support for everyone": Experiences of occupational therapists delivering a new model of school-based service. *Canadian Journal of Occupational Therapy, 79,* 51–59. https://doi.org/10.2182%2Fcjot.2012.79.1.7

Cooke, D. W., & Plotnick, L. (2008). Type 1 diabetes mellitus in pediatrics. *Pediatrics in Review, 29,* 374–384. https://doi.org/10.1542/pir.29-11-374

Coster, W. J., Deeney, T. A., Haltiwanger, J. T., & Haley, S. M. (1998). *School Function Assessment.* San Antonio: Psychological Corporation.

Data Resource Center for Child and Adolescent Health. (2016). *2016 and 2016–2017 Combined National Survey of Children's Health.* Retrieved from http://childhealthdata.org/browse/survey

Erickson, C. D., Splett, P. L., Mullett, S. S., & Heiman, M. B. (2006). The healthy learner model for student chronic condition management: Part I. *Journal of School Nursing, 22,* 310–318. https://doi.org/10.1177%2F1059840506022006020

Forrest, C. B., Bevans, K. B., Riley, A. W., Crespo, R., & Louis, T. A. (2011). School outcomes of children with special health care needs. *Pediatrics, 128,* 303–312. https://doi.org/10.1542/peds.2010-3347

Glassgow, A. E., & Voorhees, B. V. (2017). Behavioral health disparities among children and youth with special health care needs. *Pediatric Annals, 46,* e382–e386. https://doi.org/10.3928/19382359-20170920-02

Green, J. G., Comer, J. S., Donaldson, A. R., Elkins, R. M., Nadeau, M. S., Reid, G., & Pincus, D. B. (2017). School functioning and use of school-based accommodations by treatment-seeking anxious children. *Journal of Emotional and Behavioral Disorders, 25,* 220–232. https://doi.org/10.1177%2F1063426616664328

Guerrero, A. D., Zhou, X., & Chung, P. J. (2017). How well is the medical home working for Latino and Black children? *Maternal Child Health Journal, 22,* 175–183. https://doi.org/10.1007/s10995-017-2389-6

Hanft, B., & Shepherd, J. (2016). Initiating and sustaining support systems. In B. Hanft & J. Shepherd (Eds.), *Collaborating for student success: A guide for school-based occupational therapy* (2nd ed., pp. 243–281). Bethesda, MD: AOTA Press.

Individuals With Disabilities Education Improvement Act of 2004, Pub. L. 108–446, 20 U.S.C. §§ 1400–1482.

Law, M., Baptiste, S., Carswell, A., McColl, M. A., Polatajko, H. J., & Pollock, N. (2014). *Canadian Occupational Performance Measure* (5th ed.). Ottawa: CAOT Publications.

Lewallen, T. C., Hunt, H., Potts-Datema, W., Zaza, S., & Giles, W. (2015). The Whole School, Whole Community, Whole Child model: A new approach for improving educational attainment and healthy development for students. *Journal of School Health, 85,* 729–739. https://doi.org/10.1111/josh.12310

Mancini, M. C., & Coster, W. J. (2004). Functional predictors of school participation by children with disabilities. *Occupational Therapy International, 11,* 12–25. https://doi.org/10.1002/oti.194

Maternal and Child Health Bureau. (2018). *Children with special health care needs.* Retrieved from https://mchb.hrsa.gov/maternal-child-health-topics/children-and-youth-special-health-needs#ref1

McPherson, M., Arango, P., Fox, H., Lauver, C., McManus, M., Newacheck, P. W., & Strickland, B. (1998). A new definition of children with special health care needs. *Pediatrics, 102,* 137–140. https://doi.org/10.1542/peds.102.1.137

Missiuna, C., Pollock, N. A., Levac, D. E., Campbell, W. N., Sahagian Walen, S. D., Bennett, S. M., . . . Russell, D. J. (2012). Partnering for change: An innovative school-based occupational therapy service delivery model for children with developmental coordination disorder. *Canadian Journal of Occupational Therapy, 79,* 41–50. https://doi.org/10.2182/cjot.2012.79.1.6

National Center for Education Statistics. (2013). *Children and youth with disabilities.* Retrieved from https://nces.ed.gov/programs/coe/indicator_cgg.asp

National Dissemination Center for Children With Disabilities. (2012). *Other health impairment.* Retrieved from https://www.parentcenterhub.org/ohi/

Office of Special Education Programs Technical Assistance Center. (2017). *Positive behavioral interventions and supports.* Retrieved from http://www.pbis.org/

Oswald, G., Flexer, R., Alderman, L. A., & Huber, M. (2016). Predictive value of personal characteristics and the employment of transition-aged youth in vocational rehabilitation. *Journal of Rehabilitation, 82,* 60–66.

Rehabilitation Act of 1973, Pub. L. 93–112, 29 U.S.C. §§ 701–796l.

Rose, C. A., Monda-Amaya, L. E., & Espelage, D. L. (2011). Bullying perpetration and victimization in special education: A review of the literature. *Remedial and Special Education, 32,* 114–130. https://doi.org/10.1177%2F0741932510361247

Sanetti, L. M. H. (2017). Increasing equitable care for youth through coordinated school health. *Psychology in the Schools, 54,* 1312–1318. https://doi.org/10.1002/pits.22081

Section 504 of the, Rehabilitation Act of 1973, as amended, 29 U.S.C. § 794 (2008).

Shaw, S. R., & McCabe, P. C. (2008). Hospital-to-school transition for children with chronic illness: Meeting the new challenges of an evolving health care system. *Psychology in the Schools, 45,* 74–87. https://doi.org/10.1002/pits

Villenueve, M. (2009). A critical examination of school-based occupational therapy collaborative consultation. *Canadian Journal of Occupational Therapy, 76,* 206–218. https://doi.org/10.1177%2F000841740907600s05

Wodrich, D. L., Hasan, K., & Parent, K. B. (2011). Type 1 diabetes mellitus and school: A review. *Pediatric Diabetes, 12,* 63–70. https://doi.org/10.1111/j.1399-5448.2010.00654.x

Best Practices in Supporting Students With Physical Disabilities

36

Cheryl Colangelo, MS, OT/L, and Laurette Olson, PhD, OTR/L, FAOTA

KEY TERMS AND CONCEPTS

- Executive functioning
- Positioning
- Regular interruptions
- Self-determination
- Self-efficacy

OVERVIEW

As students with physical disabilities enter school, their access to academic tasks, classroom participation, and school mobility may pose pressing concerns for students, their parents, school administrators, and teachers. The expertise of occupational therapy practitioners[1] is often immediately sought because they understand the nature of physical disabilities and medical conditions at the level of body functions and structures.

Occupational therapists assess and recommend ways to meet the participation and performance needs of a student with a physical disability within the contextual demands of the school setting and academic program. In the process, the student's goals and preferences are identified to promote and strengthen the student's *self-efficacy* (the belief that they can competently accomplish particular tasks) and *self-determination* ("a combination of skills, knowledge, and beliefs that enable an individual to take responsibility and advocate for personal life goals"; Palisano et al., 2012, p. 1041). Concerns related to the student's medical disorder or disability must not overshadow the student's mental health and social needs and their developing sense of self.

To be covered under the Individuals With Disabilities Education Improvement Act of 2004 (IDEA; Pub. L. 108–446), a student must be identified as a child with a disability (i.e., meet one of the eligibility categories) and need special education, related services, or both (§ 300.8). Some students with physical disabilities do not require specially designed instruction to benefit from their education, yet they need equal access to education because of their disability. These students may be eligible for services under Section 504 of the Rehabilitation Act of 1973, as amended (2008, Pub. L. 93–112; see Chapter 27, "Best Practices in Supporting Students With a 504 Plan").

ESSENTIAL CONSIDERATIONS

Occupational therapy practitioners need to understand the individual needs of students with physical disabilities, not only in terms of their physical health, age, family supports, and education but also in terms of participation.

Performance and Participation in School

With good intentions, educators and staff may unnecessarily limit activities or complete tasks for students with physical disabilities. Studies describing the perspectives of youth with disabilities have reported that on one hand, their participation was positively influenced by adults and peers who provided an appropriate level of cognitive, emotional, and physical support at the right time (Kramer et al., 2012). On the other hand, their participation was negatively affected when adults over- or underestimated their needs. Students also reported that when adults made decisions about what the students' needs were without collaborating with them, it resulted in misunderstandings and ineffective accommodations.

Occupational therapy practitioners address students' movement limitations that interfere with school and academic participation. These limitations may include students' limited use of upper or lower extremities, decreased endurance and strength for participation in activities, need for adaptive equipment, and training in the use of mobility devices, including wheelchairs and walkers. Occupational therapy practitioners also provide interventions to address

---

[1] *Occupational therapy practitioner* refers to both the occupational therapist and the occupational therapy assistant. The American Occupational Therapy Association (AOTA; 2014a, p. S18) states, "The occupational therapist is responsible for all aspects of occupational therapy service delivery and is accountable for the safety and effectiveness of the occupational therapy service delivery process" and "must be directly involved in the delivery of services during the initial evaluation and regularly throughout the course of intervention. . . . The occupational therapy assistant delivers safe and effective occupational therapy services under the supervision of and in partnership with the occupational therapist."

Copyright © 2019 by the American Occupational Therapy Association. All rights reserved. To reuse this content, contact www.copyright.com.
https://doi.org/10.7139/2019.978-1-56900-591-0.036

less observable sequelae of physical disabilities such as pain, fatigue, impaired sensation and perception, and executive function (EF) deficits (Wicksell et al., 2004).

Types and Frequency of Physical Disabilities

Cerebral palsy (CP), a nonprogressive neuromotor disorder, is the most common motor impairment in children, with an estimated prevalence of 2–3 per 1,000 live births (Lindsay, 2016). Arthritis or other rheumatic conditions affect an estimated 294,000 children, as reported by the Centers for Disease Control and Prevention (CDC; 2009). The CDC has further reported that 30–40 students per million have a spinal cord injury. Children with traumatic brain injury may also have orthopedic impairments. Table 36.1 summarizes key features of the most common physical disabilities seen in children.

Challenges of Students' Physical Disabilities at Different Developmental Stages

How a student's physical disability affects school learning and participation varies with grade level and developmental demands. In schools, academic learning is the emphasis

of education. Therefore, addressing barriers to academic participation often takes precedence over acquiring motor, self-care, or play skills. When the student and family identify these last areas as important, the occupational therapist can help determine the school's role and appropriate educational goals and intervention strategies to support students' skill development.

Like typically developing teens, adolescents with physical disabilities seek greater autonomy and increased engagement in peer activities of their own choosing. Unfortunately, barriers in the environment and insufficient task adaptations may interfere. Ensuring social supports and opportunities to participate is important (Lindsay, 2014). Occupational therapy practitioners need to keep this in mind as they address students' occupation-based needs.

Conditions Related to the Primary Diagnosis

The nature of a physical disability often disrupts gross motor capacities (e.g., postural stability, motor coordination, mobility) and fine motor capacities (e.g., manipulating tools and materials for academic, social, and self-care activities). Often, participation of students with physical disabilities is also affected by secondary conditions, including fatigue, pain,

TABLE 36.1.   **Key Features of Common Physical Disabilities in Children**

DIAGNOSIS	CHARACTERISTICS	RELATED CONDITIONS
Cerebral palsy	Static encephalopathy resulting in problems with movement, posture, and coordination. The most common symptom is abnormal muscle tone. There is a wide range of levels of motor impairment and the presence of related conditions (CDC, 2018a).	• Seizures, contractures, and pain • Problems with vision, hearing, or speaking • Feeding, nutritional, and gastrointestinal problems • Pulmonary complications • Intellectual disability (Goldstein & Morewitz, 2011) • EF impairment (Pirila et al., 2011)
Muscular dystrophy	Hereditary, progressive group of disorders that result in muscle weakness and a decrease in muscle mass over time. The most frequent is Duchenne's muscular dystrophy (CDC, 2009). Academic performance is frequently affected by associated conditions.	• Nonprogressive cognitive deficits, including memory, information processing, and EF (Hinton et al., 2004; Wicksell et al., 2004) • Fatigue related to respiratory and heart health and muscle weakness • Affected emotional health
Juvenile rheumatoid arthritis	At least 3 clinical classification schemes exist—juvenile rheumatoid arthritis (the most common form), juvenile chronic arthritis, and juvenile idiopathic arthritis. Juvenile rheumatoid arthritis causes at least 6 weeks of persistent arthritis in a child younger than age 16 years.	• Joint pain and destruction • Fatigue • Adverse effects of medication (e.g., obesity, growth retardation, osteoporosis) • Increased risk for anxious and depressive symptoms (Rapoff & Lindsley, 2009)
Spina bifida	Neural tube defects resulting in leg (and possibly trunk) weakness and paralysis, orthopedic abnormalities (e.g., club foot, hip dislocation, scoliosis), incontinence and urinary tract infections, pressure sores and skin irritations, and abnormal eye movements (CDC, 2018b).	• EF and visual planning difficulties (Snow, 1999) • Social immaturity (Holmbeck et al., 2003) • Pain associated with pressure sores and tethered spinal cord (cord may be attached to the spinal canal)
Spinal cord injury	Motor, sensory, and visceral (e.g., bowel, bladder, sexual) functions impaired or lost below level of lesion.	• Chronic pain • Greater vulnerability to respiratory and heart difficulties • Growth problems and potential scoliosis • Reduced overall psychological well-being, including feelings of grief and loss or adjustment difficulties related to self-identity, sexual health, and self-control (Lindwall et al., 2012)

Note. CDC = Centers for Disease Control and Prevention; EF = executive function.

decreased physical activity, and learning disabilities. Over the course of students' development, they need to learn how to manage their own health conditions in the interest of their quality of life across their lifetime. Outcomes of studies that focused on children and adolescents' development of self-management behaviors reported increased health knowledge, decreased pain, and decreased family stress (Lindsay et al., 2014).

Pain and fatigue

Pain experienced by children with disabilities often goes unrecognized or is trivialized. Children may not share the extent and frequency of their pain unless adults facilitate an open discussion about it. Children and adolescents who live with pain are at high risk for decreased participation, mental health problems, and anxiety (Sienko, 2018; Westbom et al., 2017). In a systematic review, Lindsay (2016) reported that in 14 studies, youth with CP reported experiencing constant pain, which contributed to feelings of frustration and social isolation. Their hips, back, bladder, and upper limbs were often the locations of pain.

Interventions that are designed to support function may also cause pain, including range of motion (ROM), functional mobility training, and use of splints or other devices (Britton & Moore, 2002a, 2002b; McKearnan et al., 2004). Children with juvenile rheumatoid arthritis reported intense episodic pain that disrupted their ability to participate in activities like their peers and feeling "tired, powerless, and incapacitated" (Tong et al., 2012, p. 1395).

Pain is a significant condition that contributes to sleep problems of children with physical disabilities. Inadequate sleep (e.g., poor sleep quality and quantity, inconsistent routines) has been associated with decreased capacity for learning and participation, including EF deficits, and negative academic outcomes (Wright et al., 2006).

Mental health

Youth with CP reported anxiety, stress, and depressive symptoms related to being bullied by peers, being socially isolated, longing to be normal, or being frustrated by their differences (Lindsay, 2016). Likewise, children living with juvenile idiopathic arthritis reported despair and feeling misunderstood and stigmatized (Tong et al., 2012). In a qualitative study examining the perspectives of 15 youth with CP on how to increase their peer inclusion and decrease bullying of youth like them, they reported wanting the opportunity to raise the disability awareness of their peers, increase inclusion opportunities, and decrease teachers pointing out their differences (Lindsay & McPherson, 2011).

Decreased physical activity

When children with physical disabilities engage in physical activity, they can prevent fatigue and functional decline and improve their quality of life and psychological well-being (Bloeman et al., 2017). Unfortunately, this population is at high risk for developing an inactive lifestyle and prolonged periods of sedentary behavior. This pattern can be reasonably altered in the context of the school day by addressing behavioral, motivational, and environmental

barriers (Verschuren et al., 2016). In addition, listening to the viewpoints of youth about their experiences and what accommodations and adaptations they believe they need is important. Youth reported that they are often relegated to "fringe participation" in peer activities, referring to inadequate accommodations or adaptations to facilitate authentic participation (Kramer et al., 2012).

Learning disabilities

As a result of cerebral damage associated with neurological conditions, students with physical disabilities may have concomitant learning disabilities. In particular, students with spina bifida and those with CP may have deficits in spatial cognition (Jansen-Osmann et al., 2008; Van Rooijen et al., 2011). These deficits increase students' challenges in learning arithmetic and mastering related academics (Jenks et al., 2009).

Interactional Impact of Environmental and Personal Factors

To competently and actively participate in tasks with motor components, students with physical disabilities may require task or environmental modifications and adaptations. Although teachers are able to adjust cognitive or behavioral demands of academic tasks, adapting the physical demands of those tasks may be more difficult. Without individualized accommodations or modifications, students are reliant on others and may not have an opportunity to improve their self-efficacy and mastery motivation (Majnemer et al., 2010).

Aspects of the physical environment—particularly when there are barriers related to space, movement, manipulation, or speed (e.g., physical education, recess)—may interfere with participation and motivation. Students with neuromotor impairments exhibit lower levels of motivation than their peers and experience more failure and less sense of control (Majnemer et al., 2010), as well as disengagement and boredom (Egilson & Traustadottir, 2009b).

Without the physical skill capacities to participate on par with peers, students with physical disabilities may spend recess on the periphery of the physical space and group activity. Without considering how environmental barriers affect students' emotional state and ability to participate, adults may inaccurately view students' behaviors as an indication of poor social skills or low motivation. Hemmingsson and Borell (2002) found that students with disabilities between ages 10 and 19 years reported barriers to their participation in physical and social environments. A majority of barriers centered on how school activities were organized or carried out—all things that can be adjusted.

Paraeducators

Students with physical disabilities may need support from a paraeducator to access and participate in their school day. Before justifying the need for support, the educational team needs to consider the setup of a classroom, the teacher's perspective, paraeducators' training in providing help, and the student's own priorities and needs. Egilson and Traustadottir (2009a) reported that students with disabilities may receive excessive support or may underuse available paraeducators. Lack of curriculum modification, differentiated instruction, and accessible educational activities unnecessarily increase the need for paraeducators as well as the student's dependency and social isolation.

Routine experiences of shared management and decision making with school personnel about strategies for reducing social, academic, and environmental barriers, as well as for managing their health conditions in school, are essential for the health and well-being of students with physical disabilities—not only in their present school environment but also in preparing and motivating them to take charge of their own health and participation needs in adulthood. Students with considerable physical disabilities must learn how to be independent throughout their lives by defining when they require physical assistance and their preferred methods of receiving that assistance.

Parents as Members of the Educational Team

Parents of students with physical disabilities reported a desire for joint decision making, including having active, manageable roles on the educational team without significant time and energy burdens when planning interventions (Egilson, 2011). Parents need support in understanding their children's abilities and needs, knowing their rights and how to advocate for them, gaining access to community resources and support systems, and helping their children to develop and learn (Bailey et al., 2006). Chiarello et al. (2010) reported that parents' priorities varied with their child's chronological age and developmental expectations; however, the first priority of all parents was their children's participation in daily activities, including dressing, self-feeding, and nutrition. For older children, parents were concerned with productivity; for adolescents, parents focused on socialization and leisure.

Participation Barriers

The World Health Organization (2007) has defined *participation* as being actively involved and taking part in a life situation. Adair et al. (2015) reported that as children with physical disabilities age, their participation decreases in diversity and intensity. In a study of 472 students with disabilities, Almqvist and Granlund (2005) found that the severity of disability did not predict a student's pattern of participation. Instead, the student's high scores in autonomy, internal locus of control, and perceived interaction with peers and teachers were predictors.

Hemmingsson and Borell (2000) identified key concerns expressed by parents and students with disabilities as students' physical access to space, materials, and peers for participation. Although many school systems identify only goals for academic improvement, from a human rights perspective, "students with disabilities should have the same opportunity to participate in all aspects of the educational experience as students without disabilities" (Coster et al., 2013, p. 535).

BEST PRACTICES

Understanding a student's strengths, limitations, and ability to navigate the school and access facilities where academic and social events (curricular and extracurricular) occur is

critical. The evaluation methods used should inform how the student's disability affects their participation in the general education curriculum and access to the learning environment. A focus on how the environment and psychosocial factors support or constrain the student's participation allows the individualized education program (IEP) team to identify goals and services that promote inclusive participation academically and socially. The roles of self-efficacy and self-determination as supports for participation should be considered in developing interventions. The student's experience, from their perspective, should be a primary focus in this process.

Use Various Evaluation Methods to Identify the Student's Strengths and Needs

Although a top-down approach to evaluation is best practice, occupational therapists should also use various evaluation methods to identify the student's performance skills and patterns related to the particular physical disability. The occupational therapy evaluation should use multiple measures for decision making, addressing activity and participation, contextual and personal factors (e.g., self-efficacy, self-determination), and body structures and function (AOTA, 2014b).

A review of available records (e.g., academic, behavioral, medical) may provide a history of performance patterns and previous interventions. A positive alliance with teachers and parents supports productive interviews that may yield critical data regarding the student's performance and the adult's perception of it. Observation during classroom routines, transitions, and academic instruction provides an opportunity for the occupational therapist to analyze the student's interaction with the task, environment, and possibly teacher and other children. When assessment measures (see Appendix F, "Selected Assessment Tools for Analysis of Students' Occupational Performance") are required, they should be selected to best understand the student's educational needs. When appropriate, methods used should include self- and family reporting.

An occupational therapist, singly or as part of a team, may conduct an assistive technology (AT) evaluation to identify the needs of the student. This technology evaluation may relate to participation, including positioning and seating, as well as accessing tools, materials, and curricula. Most important, the evaluation should include observation of students' ability to use the equipment within their natural routine. Ongoing evaluation of the effectiveness of the device in school is also important (see Chapter 21, "Best Practices in the Use of Assistive Technology to Enhance Participation").

Provide Effective Interventions

In schools, the focus of effective intervention centers on access to and participation in the student's role, academic success, and school activities. Intervention should be client centered, with the student participating in establishing goals and judging improvement. To increase the quality of student participation, the student's perspective must be included along with the perspectives of educators and parents. Rather than focusing on the right way to accomplish a task, intervention should address the effectiveness of task outcomes on an individual basis.

Provide collaboration, education, and training

Occupational therapy practitioners must have strong collaborative skills and competency in education and training strategies with educational staff, parents, and students to relay how to adapt or modify activities or environments to support the student. Information needs to be shared in ways that are compelling to the student's team so that they understand the importance of strategies, including use of equipment (Brentnall & Bundy, 2012; Szlut, 2012).

Support proactive prevention of pain

Many students with physical disabilities have constant or intermittent pain. An occupational therapy practitioner should explore sources of pain relative to students' particular physical disabilities, learn how to recognize signs of pain, and understand how to talk to students about experiences that may be painful. The practitioner should share this information with other educational staff so that students' pain is recognized and respected throughout their day and they are supported while engaged in necessary activities that cause pain. Adaptations for optimal postural support in all classroom activities and opportunities for movement in students' daily routines can lessen pain. When possible, expectations should be altered and activities redesigned to lessen pain.

Strategies to decrease sedentary behavior can contribute to decreased pain. These may include *regular interruptions* of inactivity through repositioning (e.g., sitting to supported standing; sitting with, then without back support), light-intensity activity, and counseling to decrease patterns of screen time. Individualized plans for repositioning are ideally developed collaboratively with educators and other related service providers.

Address dignity, competence, and social inclusion during self-care

The student's dignity, competence, and social inclusion must be considered when performing self-care. Physical support and adaptations during self-care such as eating, dressing, and toileting may be needed. Accommodations must be provided, and the student's potential for independence (or lessened dependence) must be evaluated. The occupational therapist may act as the lead decision maker for the team (e.g., student, educational staff, speech–language pathologist, nurse) regarding optimal time, place, and appropriateness for direct intervention.

Self-care is a sensitive issue. What may seem efficient and helpful from an adult's perspective may be experienced as intrusive, infantilizing, or embarrassing for the student. Some students may prefer or benefit from a private setting, rather than the natural environment, to address skill development, or they may opt for maximal adult assistance (e.g., eating in the cafeteria, putting on a jacket before recess). A student with physical disabilities may require much more time than peers to complete self-care tasks. This time may take away from classroom activities and from social engagement (especially at snack or mealtimes), particularly when the student is expected to practice skill development in context.

The occupational therapist should provide input to the team regarding necessary adaptations, equipment, and, in the case of eating, food modifications for students with self-care needs. Modifications and supports should be outlined in the student's IEP. When the student is making measurable progress toward functional independence, the therapist should develop a plan with the team that includes time and place for direct intervention and training designed for adults to foster physical independence, support student choices, and minimize learned helplessness.

Promote the student's sense of self-efficacy

Personal factors that are not always apparent—including learned helplessness, social isolation, and a poorly developed sense of self-efficacy—impede not only the student's ability to participate fully but also the student's ability to feel like a participant. In an effort to physically help students, adults or peers may inadvertently disempower them by making decisions for them.

Ylvisaker and Feeney (2002) noted that adults need to support students in developing self-awareness of their strengths and needs, capacity to determine what makes an activity easy or hard for them, skills for predicting their degree of success with an activity, and skills for monitoring their own performance. The critical aspect is that adults facilitate children's development of *executive functioning* capacities (e.g., self-awareness, initiating, goal setting, planning, problem solving) that support self-determination in students with disabilities. In this process, adults also become aware of how they might unwittingly be interfering with children's development of self-determination.

Embed occupational therapy services in natural environments and activities

To increase opportunities for students to meaningfully participate in school activities, services need to be offered in natural environments and embedded in everyday activities (as appropriate and feasible). Occupational therapists working in general education classrooms can better determine where universal design and curricular adaptations will benefit students with disabilities.

Occupational therapists need to support teachers in conceptualizing curricular adaptations differently. Guiding teachers to understand how a student's physical disabilities may pose difficulties for participation in particular learning activities or understand certain concepts is important in the collaborative process.

Students with severe motor impairments may also have difficulties understanding spatial concepts because of their limited opportunities to independently move through space. They may need alternative experiences to strengthen spatial cognition in either real or virtual space. Virtual reality activities can make exploration of space accessible (Harris & Reid, 2005), offer variability, challenge and provide competition, and promote volition in students with CP, and they may be useful in improving spatial functioning (Akhutina et al., 2003).

Although students with physical disabilities may still require adult assistance for managing classroom materials and self-care, carefully reorganizing physical space and using adaptations can allow for optimal independence. In addition, the occupational therapy practitioner can guide teachers and staff to address special safety issues related to a student's physical disability without placing unnecessary limitations on the student.

In addition to considering the physical environment, occupational therapy practitioners have special knowledge and skill in adapting the social environment in ways that promote students' self-efficacy and social inclusion. Occupational therapy practitioners can also provide training to students in the use of the Internet for social networking, which has been shown to have a positive impact on social participation (Raghavendra, 2013). Last, practitioners may consider alternative roles or adaptations for students with disabilities during group activities so they can experience leadership and personal control.

Use AT

AT may be used to position the student's body to facilitate ROM and postural symmetry, improve circulation and respiration, maintain musculoskeletal integrity, and decrease skin breakdown. It also enables the student to move through space, maintain alertness, manipulate objects, communicate, and engage in academic learning. When a student requires a device, the school district is the payer of last resort. If a student requires a wheelchair at school and the parents have not purchased one, the school may need to provide one for use in school. In addition, when a student requires AT to complete assigned homework, the school may be required to lend technology, such as an adapted keyboard or speech-to-text software, for use in the home.

A general principle of AT is to address ***positioning*** to provide a stable base of support (Colangelo & Shea, 2010) from which the student can better control movement. In the general education classroom, wheelchairs, adapted classroom chairs, and equipment to support a standing position commonly provide proper positioning. The school occupational therapy practitioner, often in collaboration with the school physical therapist, addresses how to use equipment and consults with staff regarding furniture and activity placement to optimize participation.

Positioning equipment may signify disability. Respecting the perceptions of the student, peers, school staff, and parents when considering equipment is important. Students should be encouraged to use their most efficient motor strategies when completing a task or playfully engaging with friends. Professionals' intentions to fix anatomical positioning so that a student's posture always approximates the norm, despite social and participatory consequences, may be interpreted by the student to mean that they are of lesser value or broken (Cramm, 2011).

For students with physical disabilities, optimal positioning in seating and standing contributes to arm and hand control and use of augmentative communication (Colangelo & Shea, 2010; Costigan & Light, 2010). Adaptive positioning is associated with improved cognitive test scores for

students with CP (Miedaner & Finuf, 1993). The demands of maintaining postural stability divides attentional resources and decreases cognitive performance in typical children and those with CP (Reilly et al., 2008).

SUMMARY

Occupational therapy practitioners need to focus on students' participation as opposed to being guided by the typical developmental profile, which is not achievable for most students with physical disabilities. The occupational therapy practitioner addresses motor impairments in the context of students' global well-being as they engage in academic activities and interactions that make up the school day.

It is important that school occupational therapy practitioners support students in developing the capacity for participation in their present and future activities and roles. Practitioners recognize the barriers in activities, tasks, and environments for each student and determine when and where physical remediation may be a realistic and meaningful component of intervention. Students' development of self-sufficiency, mastery, academic competence, and belonging are at the core of every intervention.

REFERENCES

Adair, B., Ullenhag, A., Keen, D., Granlund, M., & Imms, C. (2015). The effect of interventions aimed at improving participation outcomes for children with disabilities: A systematic review. *Developmental Medicine and Child Neurology, 57,* 1093–1104. https://doi.org/10.1111/dmcn.12809

Akhutina, T., Foreman, N., Krichevets, A., Matikka, L., Narhi, V., Pylaeva, N., & Vahakuopus, J. (2003). Improving spatial functioning in children with cerebral palsy using computerized and traditional game tasks. *Disability and Rehabilitation, 25,* 1361–1371. https://doi.org/10.1080/09638280310001616358

Almqvist, L., & Granlund, M. (2005). Participation in school environment of children and youth with disabilities: A person-oriented approach. *Scandinavian Journal of Psychology, 46,* 305–314. https://doi.org/10.1111/j.1467-9450.2005.00460.x

American Occupational Therapy Association. (2014a). Guidelines for supervision, roles, and responsibilities during the delivery of occupational therapy services. *American Journal of Occupational Therapy, 68*(Suppl. 3), S16–S22. https://doi.org/10.5014/ajot.2014.686S03

American Occupational Therapy Association. (2014b). Occupational therapy practice framework: Domain and process (3rd ed.). *American Journal of Occupational Therapy, 68*(Suppl. 1), S1–S48. https://doi.org/10.5014/ajot.2014.682006

Bailey, D. B., Bruder, M. B., Hebbeler, K., Carta, J., DeFosset, M., Greenwood, C., . . . Barton, L. (2006). Recommended outcomes for young children with disabilities. *Journal of Early Intervention, 28,* 227–251. https://doi.org/10.1177%2F105381510602800401

Bloeman, M., Van Wely, L., Mollema, J., Dallmeijer, A., & deGroot, J. (2017). Evidence for increasing physical activity in children with physical disabilities: A systematic review. *Developmental Medicine and Child Neurology, 59,* 1004–1010. https://doi.org/10.1111/dmcn.13422

Brentnall, J., & Bundy, A. C. (2012). Consultation: Can I talk to you a minute? In S. J. Lane & A. C. Bundy (Eds.), *Kids can be kids:*

A childhood occupations approach (pp. 396–411). Philadelphia: F. A. Davis.

Britton, C., & Moore, A. (2002a). Views from the inside: Part 2. What children with arthritis said and the experiences of siblings, mothers, fathers, and grandparents. *British Journal of Occupational Therapy, 65,* 413–419. https://doi.org/10.1177%2F030802260206500904

Britton, C., & Moore, A. (2002b). Views from the inside: Part 3: How and why families undertake prescribed exercise and splinting programmes and a new model of the families' experience of living with juvenile arthritis. *British Journal of Occupational Therapy, 65,* 453–460. https://doi.org/10.1177%2F030802260206501004

Centers for Disease Control and Prevention. (2009). Prevalence of Duchenne/Becker muscular dystrophy among males aged 5–24 years—Four states, 2007. *MMWR Morbidity and Mortality Weekly Report, 58,* 1119–1122.

Centers for Disease Control and Prevention. (2018a). *Basics about cerebral palsy.* Retrieved from http://www.cdc.gov/ncbddd/cp/facts.html

Centers for Disease Control and Prevention. (2018b). *What is spina bifida?* Retrieved from http://www.cdc.gov/ncbddd/spinabifida/facts.html

Chiarello, L. A., Palisano, R. J., Maggs, J. M., Orlin, M. N., Almasri, N., Kang, L.-J., & Change, H.-J. (2010). Family priorities for activity and participation of children and youth with cerebral palsy. *Physical Therapy, 90,* 1254–1263. https://doi.org/10.2522/ptj.20090388

Colangelo, C. A., & Shea, M. (2010). A biomechanical frame of reference for positioning children for functioning. In P. Kramer & J. Hinojosa (Eds.), *Frames of reference for pediatric occupational therapy* (3rd ed., pp. 489–567). Philadelphia: Lippincott Williams & Wilkins.

Coster, W., Law, M., Bedell, G., Liljenquist, K., Kao, Y.-C., Khetani, M., & Teplicky, R. (2013). School participation, supports and barriers of students with and without disabilities. *Child: Care, Health and Development, 39,* 535–543. https://doi.org/10.1111/cch.12046

Costigan, F. A., & Light, J. (2010). Effect of seated position on upper-extremity access to augmentative communication for children with cerebral palsy: A preliminary investigation. *American Journal of Occupational Therapy, 64,* 596–604. https://doi.org/10.5014/ajot.2010.09013

Cramm, H. (2011). Can interventions have negative impacts? The importance of seeing the bigger picture. *Physical and Occupational Therapy in Pediatrics, 31,* 217–221. https://doi.org/10.3109/01942638.2011.589716

Egilson, S. T. (2011). Parent perspectives of therapy services for their children with physical disabilities. *Scandinavian Journal of Caring Sciences, 25,* 277–284. https://doi.org/10.3109/01942638.2011.565865

Egilson, S. T., & Traustadottir, R. (2009a). Assistance to pupils with physical disabilities in regular schools: Promoting inclusion or promoting dependency. *Educational Psychology, 24*(1), 21–36. https://doi.org/10.1080/08856250802596766

Egilson, S. T., & Traustadottir, R. (2009b). Participation of students with physical disabilities in the school environment. *American Journal of Occupational Therapy, 63,* 264–272. https://doi.org/10.5014/ajot.63.3.264

Goldstein, M., & Morewitz, S. (2011). *Chronic disorders in children and adolescents.* New York: Springer.

Harris, K., & Reid, D. (2005). The influence of virtual reality play on children's motivation. *Canadian Journal of Occupational Therapy, 72,* 21–29. https://doi.org/10.1177%2F000841740507200107

Hemmingsson, H., & Borell, L. (2000). Accommodation needs and student–environment fit in upper secondary schools for students with severe physical disabilities. *Canadian Journal of Occupational Therapy, 67,* 162–172. https://doi.org/10.1177%2F000841740006700311

Hemmingsson, H., & Borell, L. (2002). Environmental barriers in mainstream schools. *Child: Care, Health and Development, 28,* 57–63. https://doi.org/10.1046/j.1365-2214.2002.00240.x

Hinton, V., De Vivo, D., Fee, R., Goldstein, E., & Stern, Y. (2004). Investigation of poor academic achievement in children with Duchenne muscular dystrophy. *Learning Disabilities Research and Practice, 19,* 146–154. https://doi.org/10.1111/j.1540-5826.2004.00098.x

Holmbeck, G. W., Westhoven, V. C., Shapera, W., Bowers, R., Gruse, C., Nicolopoulos, T., & Davidson, K. (2003). A multi-method, multi-informant, and multi-dimensional perspective on psychosocial adjustment in pre-adolescents with spina bifida. *Journal of Consulting and Clinical Psychology, 71,* 82–796. http://psycnet.apa.org/doi/10.1037/0022-006X.71.4.782

Individuals With Disabilities Education Improvement Act of 2004, Pub. L. 108–446, 20 U.S.C. §§ 1400–1482.

Jansen-Osmann, P., Wiedenbauer, G., & Heil, M. (2008). Spatial cognition and motor development: A study of children with spina bifida. *Perceptual and Motor Skills, 106,* 436–446. https://doi.org/10.2466%2Fpms.106.2.436-446

Jenks, K. M., van Lieshout, E. C. D. M., & de Moor, J. (2009). Arithmetic achievement in children with cerebral palsy or spina bifida meningomyelocele. *Remedial and Special Education, 30,* 323–329. https://doi.org/10.1177%2F0741932508321009

Kramer, J. M., Olsen, S., Mermelstein, M., Balcells, A., & Liljenquist, K. (2012). Youth with disabilities' perspectives of the environment and participation: A qualitative meta-synthesis. *Child: Care, Health and Development, 38,* 763–777. https://doi.org/10.1111/j.1365-2214.2012.01365.x

Lindsay, S. (2014). A qualitative synthesis of adolescents' experiences of living with spina bifida. *Qualitative Health Research, 24,* 1298–1309. https://doi.org/10.1177%2F1049732314546558

Lindsay, S. (2016). Child and youth experiences and perspectives of cerebral palsy: A qualitative systematic review. *Child: Care, Health and Development, 42,* 153–175. https://doi.org/10.1111/cch.12309

Lindsay, S., Kingsnorth, S., Mcdougall, C., & Keating, H. (2014). A systematic review of self-management interventions for children and youth with physical disabilities. *Disability and Rehabilitation, 36,* 276–288. https://doi.org/10.3109/09638288.2013.785605

Lindsay, S., & McPherson, A. C. (2011). Strategies for improving disability awareness and social inclusion of children and young people with cerebral palsy. *Child: Care, Health and Development, 38,* 809–816. https://doi.org/10.1111/j.1365-2214.2011.01308.x

Lindwall, J., Russell, H., Kelly, E., Klaas, S., Mulcahey, M., Betz, R., & Vogel, L. (2012). Coping and participation in youth with spinal cord injury. *Topics in Spinal Cord Injury Rehabilitation, 18,* 220–231. https://doi.org/10.1310/sci1803-220

Majnemer, A., Shevell, M., Law, M., Poulin, C., & Rosenbaum, P. (2010). Level of motivation in mastering challenging tasks in children with cerebral palsy. *Developmental Medicine and Child Neurology, 52,* 1120–1126. https://doi.org/10.1111/j.1469-8749.2010.03732.x

McKearnan, K. A., Kieckhefer, G. M., Engel, J. M., Jensen, M. P., & Labyak, S. (2004). Pain in children with cerebral palsy: A review. *Journal of Neuroscience Nursing, 36,* 252–259.

Miedaner, J., & Finuf, I. (1993). Effects of adaptive positioning on psychological test scores for preschool children with cerebral palsy. *Pediatric Physical Therapy, 5,* 177–182.

Palisano, R. J., Chiarello, L. A., King, G. A., Novak, I., Stoner, T., & Fiss, A. (2012). Participation-based therapy for children with physical disabilities. *Disability and Rehabilitation, 34,* 1041–1052. https://doi.org/10.3109/09638288.2011.628740

Pirila, S., van der Meere, J. J., Rantanen, K., Jokiluoma, M., & Eriksson, K. (2011). Executive functions in youth with spastic cerebral palsy. *Journal of Child Neurology, 26,* 817–821. https://doi.org/10.1177/0883073810392584

Raghavendra, P. (2013). Participation of children with disabilities: Measuring subjective and objective outcomes. *Child: Care, Health and Development, 39,* 461–465. https://doi.org/10.1111/cch.12084

Rapoff, M., & Lindsley, C. (2009). Juvenile rheumatoid arthritis. In W. O'Donohue (Ed.), *Behavioral approaches to chronic disease in adolescence: A guide to integrative care* (pp. 129–142). New York: Springer Science+Business Media.

Rehabilitation Act of 1973, Pub. L. 93–112, 29 U.S.C. §§ 701–796l.

Reilly, D., Woollacott, M., Donkelaar, P., & Saavedra, S. (2008). The interaction between executive attention and postural control in dual-task conditions: Children with cerebral palsy. *Archives of Physical Medicine and Rehabilitation, 89,* 834–842. https://doi.org/10.1016/j.apmr.2007.10.023

Section 504 of the Rehabilitation Act of 1973, as amended, 29 U.S.C. §794 (2008).

Sienko, S. (2018). An exploratory study investigating the multidimensional factors impacting the health and well-being of young adults with cerebral palsy. *Disability and Rehabilitation, 40,* 660–666. https://doi.org/10.1080/09638288.2016.1274340

Snow, J. H. (1999). Executive processes for children with spina bifida. *Children's Health Care, 28,* 241–253. https://doi.org/10.1207/s15326888chc2803_3

Szlut, S. E. (2012). Indirect intervention: Teaching therapeutic techniques. In S. J. Lane & A. C. Bundy (Eds.), *Kids can be kids: A childhood occupations approach* (pp. 384–395). Philadelphia: F. A. Davis.

Tong, A., Jones, J., Craig, J. C., & Singh-Grewal, D. (2012). Children's experiences of living with juvenile idiopathic arthritis: A thematic synthesis of qualitative studies. *Arthritis Care and Research, 64,* 1392–1404. https://doi.org/10.1002/acr.21695

Van Rooijen, M., Verhoeven, L., & Steenbergen, B. (2011). Early numeracy in cerebral palsy: Review and future research. *Developmental Medicine and Child Neurology, 53,* 202–209. https://doi.org/10.1111/j.1469-8749.2010.03834.x

Verschuren, O., Peterson, M. D., Balemans, A. C. J., & Hurvitz, E. A. (2016). Exercise and physical activity recommendations for people with cerebral palsy. *Developmental Medicine and Child Neurology, 58,* 798–808. https://doi.org/10.1111/dmcn.13053

Westbom, L., Rimstedt, A., & Nordmark, E. (2017). Assessments of pain in children and adolescents with cerebral palsy: A retrospective population-based registry study. *Developmental Medicine and Child Neurology, 59,* 858–863. https://doi.org/10.1111/dmcn.13459

Wicksell, R., Kihlgren, M., Melin, L., & Eeg-Olofsson, O. (2004). Specific cognitive deficits are common in children with Duchenne muscular dystrophy. *Developmental Medicine and Child Neurology, 46,* 154–159. https://doi.org/10.1111/j.1469-8749.2004.tb00466.x

World Health Organization. (2007). *International classification of functioning, disability and health: Children and youth version.* Geneva: Author.

Wright, M., Tancredi, A., Yundt, B., & Larin, H. (2006). Sleep issues in children with physical disabilities and their families. *Physical and Occupational Therapy in Pediatrics, 26,* 55–72. https://doi.org/10.1080/J006v26n03_05

Ylvisaker, M., & Feeney, T. (2002). Executive functions, self-regulation, and learned optimism in paediatric rehabilitation: A review and implications for intervention. *Pediatric Rehabilitation, 5,* 51–70. https://doi.org/10.1080/1363849021000041891

Best Practices in Supporting Students With Specific Learning Disabilities

Dottie Handley-More, MS, OTR/L, FAOTA

37

KEY TERMS AND CONCEPTS

- Differentiated instruction
- Disability of written expression
- Dyscalculia
- Dysgraphia
- Dyslexia
- Mathematics disability
- Nonverbal learning disability
- Reading disability
- Self-determination
- Specific learning disability
- Strategy instruction
- Strengths-based approach
- Universal design for learning

OVERVIEW

More than 8% of children and adolescents in the United States are estimated to have a learning disability (Pullen, 2016). In schools, these children may be eligible for special education under the disability category of specific learning disability in accordance with the Individuals With Disabilities Education Improvement Act of 2004 (IDEA; Pub L. 108–446). During the 2015–2016 school year, more than 2.2 million students received special education under this category (National Center for Education Statistics, 2017). This number represented 34.4% of all students identified under IDEA and 4.6% of all students enrolled in public schools.

Learning disabilities are generally considered to be "a neurological disorder that affects the brain's ability to receive, process, store, and respond to information" (Pullen et al., 2017, p. 286). The term *learning disabilities* was first used by Samuel Kirk in the early 1960s and, with the passage of the Education for All Handicapped Children Act of 1975 (Pub. L. 94–142), public schools were required to provide a free appropriate public education to students with learning disabilities (Hallahan et al., 2013).

Since 1975, there have been differing opinions on how to define learning disabilities. IDEA (2004) defines a *specific learning disability* as

> a disorder in one or more of the basic psychological processes involved in understanding or in using language, spoken or written, that may manifest itself in the imperfect ability to listen, think, speak, read, write, spell, or to do mathematical calculations, including conditions such as perceptual disabilities, brain injury, minimal brain dysfunction, dyslexia, and developmental aphasia. (34 C.F.R. 300.8[a][10][i])

IDEA (2004) also clarifies that the criteria for a specific learning disability are not met if the learning difficulties result primarily from vision or hearing impairments; motor disabilities; intellectual disabilities; emotional difficulties; or environmental, cultural, or economic factors (34 CFR 300.8[a][10][ii]).

Despite having average or above-average intelligence, persons with a learning disability demonstrate difficulties with development of basic academic and functional skills (Pullen et al., 2017). Learning disabilities last throughout a person's life and can affect organization, attention, memory, auditory and visual processing, and social and emotional well-being in addition to reading, writing, spelling, and math (Berninger & Wolf, 2016; Cortiella & Horowitz, 2014). Individual differences are common, including the levels of severity and the area or areas of learning affected (National Center for Learning Disabilities [NCLD], 2013).

Although the causes are unknown, learning disabilities are assumed to have a neurological basis. Studies have indicated hereditary factors; prenatal factors such as exposure to drugs or alcohol; complications at birth (e.g., prematurity, lack of oxygen, low birthweight); and postnatal factors such as exposure to toxins, poor nutrition, head injuries, or serious illness as possible causes for learning disabilities (NCLD, 2013).

ESSENTIAL CONSIDERATIONS

This section presents criteria used to identify or diagnose learning disabilities, identifies the types of learning disabilities, and discusses general education initiatives that support diverse learners.

Multi-Tiered Systems of Support to Identify a Specific Learning Disability

Historically, the presence of a learning disability was determined by testing a struggling student to identify the existence of a severe discrepancy between the student's academic

Copyright © 2019 by the American Occupational Therapy Association. All rights reserved. To reuse this content, contact www.copyright.com.
https://doi.org/10.7139/2019.978-1-56900-591-0.037

achievement and the expected level of performance on the basis of age, grade, and intellectual ability. Since the passage of IDEA (2004, § 300.307[a][1]), states are not allowed to "require the use of a severe discrepancy between intellectual ability and achievement" to determine the presence of a learning disability. States must now "permit the use of a process based on the child's response to scientific research-based intervention" (IDEA, 2004, § 300.307[a][2]). The use of other research-based procedures is also allowed (IDEA, 2004, § 300.307[a][3]).

Multi-tiered systems of support (MTSS) is an education initiative for struggling learners in general education. Under this initiative, research-based instructional practices are used in the general education environment. Progress data are regularly collected and analyzed. Students who do not make adequate progress receive supplemental or intensive instructional interventions. A student who receives intensive instructional interventions but continues to struggle is suspected of having a disability, and data regarding the lack of progress are used to identify the presence of a learning disability.

The MTSS model ensures that all students receive high-quality instruction. Regular progress monitoring is used in general education classrooms to support early identification of students who struggle academically and give them access to preventive interventions so that inappropriate special education referrals are less likely to occur (see Chapter 26, "Best Practices in Multi-Tiered Systems of Support").

Medically Diagnosed Specific Learning Disorder

The term *specific learning disorder* is used when problems with learning are medically diagnosed by a physician or other professional on the basis of specific criteria described in the *Diagnostic and Statistical Manual of Mental Disorders* (5th ed.; *DSM–5*; American Psychiatric Association [APA], 2013). The *DSM–5* considers the person's history and response to intervention in addition to intelligence test scores (IQ) and academic testing. The *DSM–5* designates 3 types of disorder:
1. Reading disorder,
2. Mathematics disorder, and
3. Disorder of written expression.

Secondary Conditions Associated With Specific Learning Disabilities

According to the *DSM–5* (APA, 2013), learning disorders (disabilities) often co-occur with other neurodevelopmental conditions. About one-third of people with learning disabilities also have attention deficit hyperactivity disorder (Cortiella & Horowitz, 2014), and about 30% of students with learning disabilities have emotional and behavioral problems (Sahoo et al., 2015). Anxiety disorders and problems with social skills are also common.

A meta-analysis completed by Nelson and Harwood (2011) found that about 70% of students with learning disabilities had higher anxiety symptoms than students without disabilities. Estimates have reported the incidence of social problems among students with learning disabilities as 35%–75% (Bryan, 2005). Poor motor skills may also co-occur,

especially in students with learning disabilities in mathematics (Pieters et al., 2015). These students may also experience difficulties with working memory, visual and auditory processing, and executive function (EF; Chen et al., 2017; Cortiella & Horowitz, 2014).

Types and Characteristics of Specific Learning Disabilities

Under IDEA (2004), state and local educational agencies may consider learning disabilities in the areas of oral expression, listening comprehension, written expression, reading (i.e., basic reading, fluency and comprehension), and mathematics (i.e., calculation and problem solving). Emerging research suggests the existence of subtypes within the learning disability categories on the basis of patterns of strengths and weaknesses (Compton et al., 2012), and neuroimaging studies have indicated brain-based differences between the subtypes (Berninger et al., 2015).

A *reading disability* is described as difficulty with reading comprehension or with speed, accuracy, and fluency of reading (APA, 2013). This difficulty could include problems with phonemic awareness and phonological processing, as well as difficulties with decoding words, spelling, and vocabulary (Cortiella & Horowitz, 2014). The term *dyslexia* is often used interchangeably with *reading disability,* but some researchers define *dyslexia* more narrowly, using it to refer to students who struggle with decoding, spelling, and reading words. The *DSM–5* (APA, 2013) cautioned that any additional learning difficulties (e.g., reading comprehension or math reasoning) should be specified when the term *dyslexia* is used. Berninger and Wolf (2016) also used this narrower definition of dyslexia and referred to students who have difficulty with listening comprehension, reading comprehension, oral expression, and written expression as having an *oral written language disability.*

A *mathematics disability* includes difficulty with number sense, memorizing math facts, doing calculations accurately or fluently, and demonstrating accurate math reasoning (APA, 2013). This difficulty could include problems with counting, solving math problems, doing mental math, counting money, telling time, and estimating quantities (Cortiella & Horowitz, 2014). The term *dyscalculia* is often used interchangeably with mathematics disability, although the *DSM–5* (APA, 2013) describes dyscalculia as a term that does not include math reasoning. Berninger and Wolf (2016) defined *dyscalculia* as an impairment of calculation. Persons with dyscalculia "may or may not be impaired in all quantitative skills or the visual–spatial skills involved in math learning" (Berninger & Wolf, 2016, p. 22).

A *disability of written expression* affects spelling, grammar, and punctuation as well as clarity or organization of written expression (APA, 2013). Common characteristics include fatiguing quickly when writing, avoiding writing or drawing tasks, difficulty forming letters and spacing between and within words, difficulty organizing thoughts on paper, and difficulty with sentence structure and grammar (Cortiella & Horowitz, 2014).

The term *dysgraphia* is sometimes used broadly to refer to a specific learning disability that affects written language (e.g., Cortiella & Horowitz, 2014). It has also been used more narrowly to refer to difficulties with producing legible writing automatically and consistently, a skill that involves both the motor aspects of handwriting (e.g., sequencing strokes) and the language skills of finding, retrieving, and producing letters (Berninger & Wolf, 2016). Difficulties with these language skills may also affect spelling by students with dysgraphia (Berninger & Wolf, 2016).

Nonverbal learning disabilities (NLDs) have been identified in the literature but are not officially recognized in the *DSM–5* or IDEA as a specific disorder or disability. An **NLD** is "a neuropsychological disorder composed of a specific pattern of assets and deficits related to right hemispheric dysfunction" (Ellis, 2013, p. 1850). Students with NLD may demonstrate difficulties with EF; visual attention and visual memory; academic delays in writing, reading comprehension, and math; and difficulties with social skills (Ellis, 2013). Consistent diagnostic criteria for NLD have not yet been established. However, on the basis of a review of the literature, Mammarella and Cornoldi (2014) proposed 5 criteria for a diagnosis of NLD:

1. Good verbal intelligence and poor visual–spatial or perceptual intelligence, with a substantial discrepancy between the 2 scores
2. Difficulties with fine motor and visual–motor skills
3. Poor achievement in math (showing visual–spatial type errors) with good reading or decoding
4. Difficulties with spatial working memory
5. Difficulties with social and emotional skills.

For students with an NLD, Ellis (2013, p. 1850) recommended multidisciplinary and individualized interventions, including "academic accommodations as necessary, language therapy, occupational therapy, social skills training, psychotherapy to assist with emotional difficulties, organizational skills, behavioral difficulties, and adaptive skills."

General Education Approaches That Support Students With Specific Learning Disabilities

Two instructional approaches that are effective in supporting students with specific learning disabilities in general education are differentiated instruction and universal design for learning. *Differentiated instruction* provides strategies for teaching learners of differing abilities in the same classroom. Tomlinson (2014) described the following ways to differentiate instruction:

- Teachers vary the content—that is, they vary the input by scaffolding the instruction on the basis of students' prior knowledge of the subject (e.g., some students receive additional learning activities to have a solid base to learn from; others receive additional learning activities to extend their learning).
- Teachers may also alter the process for teaching the material. Alterations might include introducing content in different ways, providing different learning activities (e.g., having some children do a hands-on activity and other children listen to a story), or assigning students to different groups.
- Teachers vary the ways students demonstrate learning (e.g., allowing students to choose among doing an oral

report, writing an essay, or creating a poster) and the ways they are evaluated (e.g., using different criteria to measure learner progress).
- Teachers provide an environment that supports student learning.

In a classroom using differentiated instruction, decisions are made on the basis of the student's readiness to learn the content, personal interests related to the content, and how the student learns.

Universal design for learning (UDL) supports students with specific learning disabilities in general education by offering learning options (including tools and materials) that all students can use, unlike differentiated instruction, which provides individualized supports for specific students (for more information, see Chapter 20, "Best Practices in Universal Design for Learning"). **UDL** is "a research-based framework for teachers to incorporate flexible materials, techniques, and strategies for delivering instruction and for students to demonstrate their knowledge in a variety of ways" (Council for Exceptional Children [CEC], 2017, p. 129). UDL principles eliminate barriers for students with learning disabilities and, when applied to instructional technology, common assistive technology (AT) tools can be embedded in curricula to support access to needed AT for students with learning disabilities.

BEST PRACTICES

Best practices for students with learning disabilities involve evaluating the student's ability to participate at school and providing interventions that support the student's daily school activities and routines.

Evaluate Students With Specific Learning Disabilities

An occupational therapy evaluation begins with gathering data through record reviews, interviews, and observations to develop an occupational profile that identifies the student's strengths, limitations, and needs (American Occupational Therapy Association [AOTA], 2014b). For students with learning disabilities, it is important to use a strengths-based perspective.

A *strengths-based approach* focuses on identifying a student's abilities and preferences as well as the supports that are available in the school context (Morris & Hollenbeck, 2016). Using this approach helps to identify strategies that support student success (Climie & Henley, 2016). Important considerations include identifying the student's interests and the activities in which the student feels successful, noting how the student approaches activities and responds to expectations, and comparing their performance with that of other students.

Analysis of educational activities, curricula, and teacher and grade-level expectations will provide information regarding aspects of the school environment that support participation and potential needs for curricula adaptations and AT. Additional data, when needed, can be gathered through the administration of standardized assessments. These data can be combined with other sources of information to complete the analysis of occupational performance.

The literature has identified several performance skills, patterns, and client factors that can present challenges for students with learning disabilities, including behavior, memory, motor and visual–motor skills, attention and hyperactivity, visual processing, self-regulation, and social and emotional well-being (e.g., low self-esteem, low motivation; Berninger & Wolf, 2016; Cortiella & Horowitz, 2014; Pullen et al., 2017). The effect of these areas on occupational performance would be relevant to address in an occupational therapy evaluation along with skills, interests, and supports that can help to foster improved participation.

Implement Evidence-Based Interventions

Occupational therapy practitioners[1] focus on facilitating participation in school. For students with learning disabilities, that may include supporting handwriting and writing quality, addressing AT needs, teaching learning strategies and social skills, and making curricular adaptations and environmental modifications. However, research that is directly related to occupational therapy with students with specific learning disabilities is limited. Therefore, occupational therapy practitioners may want to examine and keep abreast of the extensive research from the field of education. Drawing on this research will be critical when developing evidence-based intervention plans.

An education-related meta-analysis of 272 intervention studies across all types of specific learning disabilities identified the strongest effect sizes for interventions that combined direct instruction of content and instruction in specific learning strategies (Swanson, 2013). Elements of the interventions included "attention to sequencing, drill–repetition–practice, segmentation of information, control of task difficulty, technology (e.g., use of diagrams), teacher's systematic modeling of problem-solving steps, making use of small interactive groups, and cuing (prompting) students to use taught strategies" (Swanson, 2013, p. 630). Similar intervention components were identified in a synthesis of writing interventions for students with specific learning disabilities (Kaldenberg et al., 2016).

Strategy instruction

Strategy instruction involves explicitly teaching "cognitive and metacognitive processing strategies to support memory, attention, and self-regulation of learning" (CEC, 2017, p. 76). Research studies support strategy instruction as an effective intervention for students with specific learning disabilities (CEC, 2017; Reid et al., 2013). Cognitive strategies "must be taught explicitly with teacher demonstration

using a think-aloud procedure followed by guided practice with feedback" (Wendling & Mather, 2009, p. 231). Ongoing instruction and practice are needed for the strategies to become automatic. Common cognitive strategies followed by self-regulation strategies include the following examples.

Mnemonics. A *mnemonic* is a memory aid that helps students store and retrieve information from long-term memory. Mnemonics include acronyms that use the first letter of each word to be remembered, visual representations of information (e.g., the student might draw a picture to illustrate the meaning of a word), keywords that use a familiar word to link new information to a mental image, pegwords (words that rhyme with numbers) to help with remembering a numbered sequence, and acrostics or word cues that form a sentence (Reid et al., 2013). Mnemonic devices can be used to remember a variety of strategies, such as the sequence of operations in a math problem or the story elements in a personal narrative. They should be carefully chosen so that they connect the student to the content in ways that are meaningful to the student.

Chunking strategies. Chunking strategies group individual pieces of information together into units to make them easier to remember, such as putting a series of 4 separate digits into one 4-digit number (3, 6, 9, and 8 become the single number 3698; Reid et al., 2013).

Self-monitoring. Self-monitoring involves the student observing their own behavior and then recording that behavior (Bruhn et al., 2015). This strategy has been used successfully to address academic and behavior problems in students with learning disabilities (Bruhn et al., 2015). Specifically, it can be used to measure productivity, accuracy, and strategy use during academic tasks and to monitor behaviors such as whether the student is paying attention when cued (Reid et al., 2013). The process for setting up a self-monitoring program involves identifying the target behavior, collecting baseline data, gaining student buy-in, and training the student (Reid et al., 2013). A more complete description of the process is provided in Table 37.1. Once the program is implemented, ongoing evaluation should occur to check for accuracy and to assess the program's effectiveness.

Self-evaluation. Students are asked to compare their performance with an external standard, and reinforcement is provided on the basis of their accuracy (Reid et al., 2013). Initially, the teacher performs the ratings and shares the ratings with the student until the behavior is consistently acceptable. Next, both the student and the teacher rate the behavior and compare their ratings. Finally, the comparisons are gradually faded (Reid et al., 2013).

Self-instruction. Students use self-talk to guide themselves through a task (Reid et al., 2013). Self-instruction can be task specific or more general and applicable to multiple activities.

Goal setting. Students select a goal, identify a timeline, monitor progress, and develop skills and strategies to support goal achievement (Reid et al., 2013).

---

[1]*Occupational therapy practitioner* refers to both the occupational therapist and the occupational therapy assistant. AOTA (2014a, p. S18) states, "The occupational therapist is responsible for all aspects of occupational therapy service delivery and is accountable for the safety and effectiveness of the occupational therapy service delivery process" and "must be directly involved in the delivery of services during the initial evaluation and regularly throughout the course of intervention. . . . The occupational therapy assistant delivers safe and effective occupational therapy services under the supervision of and in partnership with the occupational therapist."

TABLE 37.1. Steps for Setting Up a Self-Monitoring Intervention

STEP	DESCRIPTION
1. Identify target behavior	▪ Choose a discrete, observable behavior. ▪ Ensure the behavior is one that the student can perform but not to the desired level (e.g., frequency, quality, or quantity). ▪ Ensure the behavior is one the student can control and occurs regularly.
2. Collect baseline data	▪ Determine when and where the self-monitoring will occur and how the intervals will be prompted (e.g., auditory cue, visual cue). ▪ Choose a quick and easy method to collect and record data. ▪ Analyze baseline data and adjust the plan if needed.
3. Gain student buy-in	▪ Discuss the target areas with the student and explain the benefits of self-monitoring. ▪ Set up a trial period with a reinforcer if needed.
4. Provide training	▪ Provide a clear description of the target behavior. ▪ Provide examples and nonexamples of the target behavior. ▪ Provide specific step-by-step directions, modeling and naming each step, then having the student model and name each step. ▪ Check for accuracy and provide feedback. ▪ Allow time for structured practice and initiate the program when the desired level of accuracy is achieved.

Source. Reid et al. (2013).

Additional examples of strategy instruction can be found in interventions developed by occupational therapists. The Alert Program (Williams & Shellenberger, 1996) teaches self-regulation through sensory strategies. Another example is Cognitive Orientation to daily Occupational Performance (CO–OP), a problem-solving approach that uses cognitive strategies and goal setting to support successful achievement of client-centered goals (Dawson et al., 2017; Polatajko & Mandich, 2004). Originally developed for children with developmental coordination disorder, the CO–OP approach has also been used to support self-generation of strategies for struggling readers as part of the Occupation and Participation Approach to Reading Intervention (Grajo & Candler, 2016).

Occupational therapy practitioners could teach strategies that support implementation of a cognitive or sensory strategy to support attention. Once the student successfully uses the strategy, they could learn to self-monitor their strategy use, and the self-monitoring data could be used to determine the effectiveness of the strategy. Checklists for self-monitoring record keeping could be developed on the basis of a task analysis of relevant school routines, such as work completion, transitions, or organizational skills. Similarly, rubrics could be developed and implemented to help students evaluate the quality of their classwork (Handley-More, 2008).

Occupational therapy practitioners can also work with teachers to develop or adapt strategies to meet individual needs, such as pairing mnemonics with actions. (For additional information, see Chapter 54, "Best Practices in Cognition and Executive Functioning to Enhance Participation.")

Self-determination

Self-determination is the ability of an individual to "cause things to happen in her or his own life" (Wehmeyer et al., 2017, p. 295). It has been connected with positive engagement in school, better postsecondary outcomes, and

academic achievement for students with learning disabilities (Zheng et al., 2014). Using self-directed learning strategies such as self-monitoring, self-evaluation, self-instruction, and goal setting, discussed earlier in this chapter, is one way to promote self-determination (Wehmeyer et al., 2017). Instruction in making choices, solving problems, making decisions, and self-advocacy skills can also support self-determination (Wehmeyer et al., 2017). These strategies can be embedded within occupational therapy interventions related to the student's area of need (e.g., reading, writing, social participation).

Social skills

A systematic review found that universal social skills programs (e.g., social–emotional learning, social skills training, bullying prevention programs) and play, recreation, or leisure programs (e.g., drama and after-school recreation that emphasize cooperation and teamwork) are effective in supporting social skills development and reducing problem behaviors (Bazyk & Arbesman, 2013). Both of these areas can be difficult for students with learning disabilities (Pullen et al., 2017), and emerging evidence has shown that universal interventions are effective for these students.

In a study that included 11- and 12-year-old students with disabilities (47% with learning disabilities), participation in a social–emotional learning program resulted in decreased bullying behaviors, and students reported an increased willingness to intervene in situations when bullying occurs (Espelage et al., 2016). Students also showed improved grades on their report cards. In another study, greater time spent participating in unstructured extracurricular activities (e.g., activities that included elements of free play) was associated with greater social competence for 8- to 11-year-olds with specific learning disabilities and intellectual disabilities than time spent in structured, competitive activities (Brooks et al., 2015). A follow-up interview indicated that parents of children with learning and intellectual disabilities monitored the unstructured play activities to support successful play experiences (e.g., carefully matching playmates and activities with their child's strengths).

Targeted interventions that provide social skills training have also been effective in improving social skills and reducing problem behaviors in students with learning disabilities (Bazyk & Arbesman, 2013; Milligan et al., 2016). Ruegg (2006) recommended supporting social skills in the classroom by demonstrating appropriate skills and behaviors through

- Role-playing, video modeling, and peer modeling in the natural environment;
- Practicing skills in a structured setting;
- Helping students recognize challenging social interactions, develop possible solutions, and think critically about the consequences of their actions; and
- Providing positive feedback for prosocial behaviors.

Occupational therapy practitioners are well suited to use occupation-based strategies to support mental health at school through universal and targeted interventions (Bazyk & Arbesman, 2013). Examples of occupational therapy interventions include advocating for universal social skills programs and ensuring that students with learning disabilities are included in these programs, partnering with coaches and teachers to include students with learning disabilities in after-school arts and leisure programs that foster cooperation and teamwork, providing activity-based social skills groups for students with learning disabilities, ensuring that appropriate recess options are available for students with learning disabilities, and supporting social participation during free play at recess. (For more information, see Chapter 53, "Best Practices in Enhancing Social Participation.")

Curricular adaptations and environmental modifications

> There is logical support for teachers to adapt instructional materials and tasks to support specific learning goals. By substituting, simplifying, and highlighting important instructional content, teachers increase the likelihood that students, including those with disabilities, will meet these learning goals. (CEC, 2017, p. 76)

Occupational therapy practitioners can apply their skills in activity analysis and environmental modifications to analyze and adapt the curricula and school environment. Curricular adaptations may be needed to simplify cognitive demands, promote self-assessment and monitoring, teach or develop specific skills, support intrinsic motivation, support increased independence, and encourage social participation. Research has demonstrated the positive effect of a few specific adaptations, including graphic organizers and guided notes (CEC, 2017). Environmental modifications such as seating arrangements, alternative seating devices, and desk organizers may support organization and attention, whereas pencil grips, modified paper, and modified textbooks can support engagement in classroom activities.

AT

A meta-analysis conducted by Perelmutter et al. (2017) found that, for secondary and postsecondary students with specific learning disabilities, AT can support access to instructional materials and work completion. Large effect sizes were found for word processing–based tools (e.g., spell check, word prediction) and small effect sizes for text-to-speech and smart pens. Speech recognition and multimedia presentation also showed positive effects overall, but the studies were too diverse for meta-analysis.

A critical review of AT to address written work of students with learning disabilities identified some improvements in transcription, revision, quality, and organization of written work using word processing, word prediction, speech recognition, and mind-mapping tools paired with instruction (Batorowicz et al., 2012, p. 222). The review also noted a positive effect on student motivation and behavior. For study skills, students may benefit from digital note-taking tools such as an electronic pen paired with structured note-taking strategies (Belson et al., 2013). As with any AT device, it must be selected on the basis of the individual needs of the student.

Student involvement in the decision-making process may also be important. Perelmutter et al. (2017, p. 159) noted that "many students who reported success with AT used systems they had set up at their own time and cost." (For more information, see Chapter 21, "Best Practices in the Use of Assistive Technology to Enhance Participation.")

Handwriting and writing interventions

Many students with specific learning disabilities struggle with writing. Graham et al. (2013) identified 4 factors that affect struggling writers:
1. Inefficient strategies for planning and revising,
2. Skills needed for evaluating and transcribing text (e.g., spelling, fluent handwriting),
3. Knowledge about writing (e.g., genres, literary devices, conventions), and
4. Cognitive resources for sustaining effort and motivation for writing (e.g., struggles with attention, self-regulation, memory).

Students with specific learning disabilities who have difficulty with writing or who are at risk can be explicitly taught transcription skills (i.e., for writing and spelling) and composition skills (i.e., for planning, writing, reviewing, and revising; Berninger & Wolf, 2016; Gillespie & Graham, 2014; Graham et al., 2013).

Graham et al. (2013) completed a meta-analysis of the self-regulated strategy development intervention, which is effective in improving writing quality of students with specific learning disabilities. This intervention includes
- Developing and activating background knowledge,
- Discussing the strategy to be learned,
- Modeling the use of the strategy,
- Memorizing the strategy,
- Providing supports to students as they apply the strategy that are gradually faded, and
- Applying the strategy independently.

Another meta-analysis conducted by Gillespie and Graham (2014) reviewed a broad range of writing interventions and identified 3 additional interventions as effective in improving writing quality of students with learning disabilities: dictation, goal setting, and process writing. For dictation, the student would dictate to a scribe or a tape recorder.

When goal setting, the student would select or receive specific goals related to improving their writing (e.g., using a variety of adjectives). Last, for process writing, the student would participate in the writing process through planning, drafting, revising, editing, and publishing their writing with targeted instruction provided in mini-lessons.

Effective handwriting instruction for students with learning disabilities addresses multiple components, including developing fine motor control and hand strength; explicitly teaching the letter names paired with the motor patterns required for letter formation; practicing writing letters from dictation; supporting transfer by practicing handwriting daily and providing feedback regarding legibility in written assignments; and developing automaticity (Berninger & Wolf, 2016). To teach letter formation, Berninger and Wolf (2016) recommend having students

- Examine a model of the target letter that is presented with numbered arrow cues showing the direction and sequence of strokes,
- Cover the letter and visualize it with eyes closed for a few seconds, and
- Open their eyes, write the letter from memory, then compare their letter with the model.

In addition to developing legible and automatic handwriting, students with specific learning disabilities need to automatically recall letterforms from long-term memory. This can be supported by reinforcing an understanding of alphabetic order through activities such as telling or writing the letter that comes before, after, or between other letters of the alphabet (Berninger & Wolf, 2016).

Occupational therapy practitioners working on handwriting or writing interventions must be aware of the process of writing, not just fine motor or visual–motor skills. (See Chapter 58, "Best Practices in Visual Perception and Visual–Motor Skills to Enhance Participation"; Chapter 49, "Best Practices in Literacy: Handwriting and Written Expression to Enhance Participation"; and Chapter 50, "Best Practices in Literacy: Reading to Enhance Participation.")

SUMMARY

Students with specific learning disabilities experience difficulties with occupational performance in school. School participation may be affected by multiple factors that are within the domain of occupational therapy, including motor, process, and social interaction skills; roles, habits, and routines; and a variety of client factors.

Occupational therapy practitioners use a strengths-based approach when evaluating students with learning disabilities to help teams recognize and draw on individual strengths to support successful participation. They also apply evidence-based interventions to implement individualized and classroom-based interventions, provide curricular and environmental adaptations, and support implementation of universal programs and strategies to optimize successful school experiences for students with learning disabilities.

REFERENCES

American Occupational Therapy Association. (2014a). Guidelines for supervision, roles, and responsibilities during the delivery of occupational therapy services. *American Journal of Occupational Therapy, 68*(Suppl. 3), S16–S22. https://doi.org/10.5014/ajot.2014.686S03

American Occupational Therapy Association. (2014b). Occupational therapy practice framework: Domain and process (3rd ed.). *American Journal of Occupational Therapy, 68*(Suppl. 1), S1–S48. https://doi.org/10.5014/ajot.2014.682006

American Psychiatric Association. (2013). *Diagnostic and statistical manual of mental disorders* (5th ed.). Arlington, VA: American Psychiatric Publishing.

Batorowicz, B., Missiuna, C. A., & Pollock, N. A. (2012). Technology supporting written productivity in children with learning disabilities: A critical review. *Canadian Journal of Occupational Therapy, 79*, 211–224. https://doi.org/10.2182/cjot.2012.79.4.3

Bazyk, S., & Arbesman, M. (2013). *Occupational therapy practice guidelines for mental health promotion, prevention, and intervention for children and youth.* Bethesda, MD: AOTA Press.

Belson, S., Hartmann, D., & Sherman, J. (2013). Digital note taking: The use of electronic pens with students with specific learning disabilities. *Journal of Special Education Technology, 28*(2), 13–24. https://doi.org/10.1177%2F016264341302800202

Berninger, V., Richards, T., & Abbott, R. (2015). Differential diagnosis of dysgraphia, dyslexia, and OWL learning disabilities: Behavioral and neuroimaging evidence. *Reading and Writing: An Interdisciplinary Journal, 28*, 1119–1153. https://doi.org/10.1007/s11145-015-9565-0

Berninger, V., & Wolf, B. J. (2016). *Dyslexia, dysgraphia, OWL learning disabilities, and dyscalculia: Lessons from science and teaching* (2nd ed.). Baltimore: Brookes.

Brooks, B. A., Floyd, F., Robins, D. L., & Chan, W. Y. (2015). Extracurricular activities and the development of social skills in children with intellectual and specific learning disabilities. *Journal of Intellectual Disability Research, 59*, 678–687. https://doi.org/10.1111/jir.12171

Bruhn, A., McDaniel, S., & Kreigh, C. (2015). Self-monitoring interventions for students with behavior problems: A systematic review of current research. *Behavioral Disorders, 40*, 102–121. https://doi.org/10.17988%2FBD-13-45.1

Bryan, T. (2005). Science-based advances in the social domain of learning disabilities. *Learning Disability Quarterly, 28*, 119–121. https://doi/org/10.2307/1593608

Chen, X., Ye, M., Chang, L., Chen, W., & Zhou, R. (2017). Effect of working memory updating training on retrieving symptoms of children with learning disabilities. *Journal of Learning Disabilities, 51*, 507–519. https://doi.org/10.1177%2F0022219417712015

Climie, E., & Henley, L. (2016). A renewed focus on strengths-based assessment in schools. *British Journal of Special Education, 43*, 108–121. https://doi.org/10.1111/1467-8578.12131

Compton, D. L., Fuchs, L. S., Fuchs, D., Lambert, W., & Hamlett, C. (2012). The cognitive and academic profiles of reading and mathematics learning disabilities. *Journal of Learning Disabilities, 45*, 79–95. https://doi.org/10.1177/0022219410393012

Cortiella, C., & Horowitz, S. (2014). *State of learning disabilities: Facts, trends and emerging issues.* New York: National Center for Learning Disabilities.

Council for Exceptional Children. (2017). *High-leverage practices in special education: Foundations for student success.* Arlington, VA: Author.

Dawson, D. R., McEwen, S. E., & Polatajko, H. J. (Eds.). (2017). *Cognitive Orientation to daily Occupational Performance in Occupational Therapy: Using the CO–OP™ approach to enable participation across the lifespan.* Bethesda, MD: AOTA Press.

Education for All Handicapped Children Act of 1975, Pub. L. 94–142, renamed the Individuals with Disabilities Education Improvement Act, codified at 20 U.S.C. §§ 1400–1482.

Ellis, J. (2013). Nonverbal learning disability syndrome. In C. R. Reynolds & E. Fletcher-Janzen (Eds.), *Encyclopedia of special education: A reference for the education of children, adolescents, and adults with disabilities and other exceptional individuals* (Vol. 2, pp. 1850–1851). Hoboken, NJ: Wiley.

Espelage, D., Rose, C., Polanin, J., Houchins, D., & Oakes, W. (2016). Social–emotional learning program to promote pro-social and academic skills among middle school students with disabilities. *Remedial and Special Education, 37,* 323–332. https://doi.org/10.1177%2F0741932515627475

Gillespie, A., & Graham, S. (2014). A meta-analysis of writing interventions for students with learning disabilities. *Exceptional Children, 80,* 454–473. https://doi.org/10.1177%2F0014402914527238

Graham, S., Harris, K., & McKeown, D. (2013). The writing of students with learning disabilities, meta-analysis of self-regulated strategy development writing intervention studies, and future directions. In H. L. Swanson, K. R. Harris, & S. Graham (Eds.), *Handbook of learning disabilities* (pp. 405–438). New York: Guilford Press.

Grajo, L., & Candler, C. (2016). An occupation and participation approach to reading intervention (OPARI) Part II: Pilot clinical application. *Journal of Occupational Therapy, Schools, and Early Intervention, 9,* 86–98. https://doi.org/10.1080/19411243.2016.1141083

Hallahan, D., Pullen, P., & Ward, D. (2013). A brief history of the field of learning disabilities. In H. L. Swanson, K. R. Harris, & S. Graham (Eds.), *Handbook of learning disabilities* (2nd ed., pp. 15–32). New York: Guilford Press.

Handley-More, D. (2008). Developing and using rubrics in occupational therapy. *Journal of Occupational Therapy, Schools, and Early Intervention, 1,* 24–32. https://doi.org/10.1080/19411240802060967

Individuals With Disabilities Education Improvement Act of 2004, Pub. L. 108–446, 20 U.S.C. §§ 1400–1482.

Kaldenberg, E., Ganzeveld, P., Hosp, J., & Rodgers, D. (2016). Common characteristics of writing interventions for students with learning disabilities: A synthesis of the literature. *Psychology in the Schools, 53,* 938–953. https://doi.org/10.1002/pits.21958

Mammarella, I., & Cornoldi, C. (2014). An analysis of the criteria used to diagnose children with nonverbal learning disability (NLD). *Child Neuropsychology, 20,* 255–280. https://doi.org/10.1080/09297049.2013.796920

Milligan, K., Phillips, M., & Morgan, A. (2016). Tailoring social competence interventions for children with learning disabilities. *Journal of Child and Family Studies, 25,* 856–869. https://doi.org/10.1007/s10826-015-0278-4

Morris, M., & Hollenbeck, J. (2016). Evaluating student participation: Focus on strengths in your school-based evaluation. *OT Practice, 21*(1), CE1–CE7.

National Center for Education Statistics. (2017). *Table 204.30: Children 3 to 21 years old served under Individuals With Disabilities Education Act, Part B, by type of disability: Selected years, 1976–77 through 2015–16.* Retrieved from https://nces.ed.gov/programs/digest/d17/tables/dt17_204.30.asp?current=yes

National Center for Learning Disabilities. (2013). *The learning disabilities navigator: Learning disabilities defined.* Retrieved from http://ldnavigator.ncld.org/#/ld-defined

Nelson, J., & Harwood, H. (2011). Learning disabilities and anxiety: A meta-analysis. *Journal of Learning Disabilities, 44,* 3–17. https://doi.org/10.1177%2F0022219409359939

Perelmutter, B., McGregor, K., & Gordon, K. (2017). Assistive technology interventions for adolescents and adults with learning disabilities: An evidence-based systematic review and meta-analysis. *Computers and Education, 114,* 139–163. https://doi.org/10.1016/j.compedu.2017.06.005

Pieters, S., Roeyers, H., Rosseel, Y., Van Waelvelde, H., & Desoete, A. (2015). Identifying subtypes among children with developmental coordination disorder and mathematical learning disabilities, using model-based clustering. *Journal of Learning Disabilities, 48,* 83–95. https://doi.org/10.1177%2F0022219413491288

Polatajko, H., & Mandich, A. (2004). *Enabling occupation in children: The Cognitive Orientation to daily Occupational Performance (CO–OP) approach.* Ottawa: CAOT Publications.

Pullen, P. (2016). Prevalence of LD from parental and professional perspectives: A comparison of the data from the National Survey of Children's Health and the Office of Special Education Programs reports to Congress. *Journal of Learning Disabilities, 50,* 701–711. https://doi.org/10.1177%2F0022219416659447

Pullen, P. C., Lane, H. B., Ashworth, K. E., & Lovelace, S. P. (2017). Specific learning disabilities. In J. M. Kauffman, D. P. Hallahan, & P. C. Pullen (Eds.), *Handbook of special education* (2nd ed., pp. 286–299). Abingdon, England: Taylor & Francis.

Reid, R., Lienemann, T., & Hagaman, J. (2013). *Strategy instruction for students with learning disabilities: What works for special needs learners* (2nd ed.). New York: Guilford Press.

Ruegg, E. (2006). Social skills in children with learning disabilities: Using psychotherapy in the classroom. *Annals of the American Psychotherapy Association, 9*(3), 14–21.

Sahoo, M., Biswas, H., & Padhy, S. (2015). Psychological comorbidity in children with specific learning disorders. *Journal of Family Medicine and Primary Care, 4,* 21–25. https://dx.doi.org/10.4103%2F2249-4863.152243

Swanson, H. (2013). Meta-analysis of research on children with learning disabilities. In H. L. Swanson, K. R. Harris, & S. Graham (Eds.), *Handbook of learning disabilities* (pp. 627–642). New York: Guilford Press.

Tomlinson, C. (2014). *The differentiated classroom: Responding to the needs of all learners* (2nd ed.). Alexandria, VA: Association for Supervision and Curriculum Development.

Wehmeyer, M. L., Shogren, K. A., Toste, J. R., & Mahal, S. (2017). Self-determined learning to motivate struggling learners in reading and writing. *Intervention in School and Clinic, 52,* 295–303. https://doi.org/10.1177%2F1053451216676800

Wendling, B. J., & Mather, N. (2009). *Essentials of evidence-based academic interventions.* Hoboken, NJ: Wiley.

Williams, M. S., & Shellenberger, S. (1996). *How does your engine run? A leader's guide to the Alert Program for self-regulation.* Albuquerque, NM: TherapyWorks.

Zheng, C., Gaumer Erickson, A., Kingston, N., & Noonan, P. (2014). The relationship among self-determination, self-concept, and academic achievement for students with learning disabilities. *Journal of Learning Disabilities, 47,* 462–474. https://doi.org/10.1177/0022219412469688

KEY TERMS AND CONCEPTS

- Closed injury
- Consolidating skills
- Context-sensitive supports
- Direct instruction
- Emerging skills
- Errorless learning
- Established skills
- Open injury
- Postconcussion syndrome
- Posttraumatic amnesia
- Traumatic brain injury

OVERVIEW

The immediate and long-term effects of traumatic brain injury (TBI) hinge on many variables, including the type and severity of injury, age at injury, and psychosocial factors. According to 2009–2010 data (Centers for Disease Control and Prevention [CDC], 2017), adolescents and young adults ages 15–24 years had the second highest incidence of TBI-related emergency room visits. Falls and contact sports were reported as the most frequent mechanisms of injury. Bryan et al. (2016) found that roughly 1–2 million young people age 18 years or younger acquired a postconcussion disorder from a sport- or recreation-related injury. Of this group, fewer than half were seen in a health care setting.

According to the CDC (2017), mild injuries accounted for the majority of pediatric TBI, whereas moderate and severe injuries accounted for approximately 10%. Research has suggested that more than half of those with a severe TBI will require ongoing support to maintain engagement at school (Glang et al., 2018).

The Individuals With Disabilities Education Improvement Act of 2004 (IDEA; Pub. L. 108–446) defines **TBI** as

> an acquired injury to the brain caused by external physical force, resulting in total or partial functional disability or psychosocial impairment, or both, that adversely affects a child's educational performance. The term applies to open or closed head injuries resulting in impairments in one or more areas, such as cognition; language; memory; attention; reasoning; abstract thinking; judgment; problem-solving; sensory, perceptual, and motor abilities; psycho-social behavior; physical functions; information processing; and speech. The term does not apply to brain injuries that are congenital or degenerative, or to brain injuries induced by birth trauma. (300.8[c][12])

Given occupational therapy practitioners'[1] health science knowledge and expertise, they are well positioned to work with students, families, educational teams, and community providers to support students with TBI in the school setting. The primary role of school practitioners is to facilitate the student's independence in areas of academics and performance in the school setting and minimize any adverse effect associated with the TBI.

ESSENTIAL CONSIDERATIONS

Diagnostic conditions and other factors affect a student's long-term outcomes after a TBI.

Classification of Injury

TBIs can be classified as open or closed. An **open injury** (or *penetrating injury*) is one in which the brain is exposed; it typically occurs as a result of a gunshot wound or a severe injury with open skull fracture. It often causes localized brain damage; deficits can be predicted in relation to the specific area of the brain that was injured (Ballantyne et al., 2008). In contrast, a **closed injury** is one in which the skull

---

[1] *Occupational therapy practitioner* refers to both the occupational therapist and the occupational therapy assistant. The American Occupational Therapy Association (2014, p. S18) states, "The occupational therapist is responsible for all aspects of occupational therapy service delivery and is accountable for the safety and effectiveness of the occupational therapy service delivery process" and "must be directly involved in the delivery of services during the initial evaluation and regularly throughout the course of intervention. . . . The occupational therapy assistant delivers safe and effective occupational therapy services under the supervision of and in partnership with the occupational therapist."

Copyright © 2019 by the American Occupational Therapy Association. All rights reserved. To reuse this content, contact www.copyright.com.
https://doi.org/10.7139/2019.978-1-56900-591-0.038

and dura mater remain intact. A closed head injury typically results from a motor vehicle accident, a fall, or being struck by an object. It often causes diffuse damage, with less predictable and more global patterns of deficit compared with an open injury (Jacobs et al., 2007).

In addition to type of injury, TBI is classified according to severity. The Glasgow Coma Scale (Teasdale & Jennett, 1974) is always used at the time of hospital admission to classify a TBI as mild, moderate, or severe. Scores are assigned on the basis of motor, verbal, and eye responses: Scores of 3–8 reflect a severe injury; 9–12, a moderate injury; and 13–15, a mild injury. In addition, the length of time that a child is in posttraumatic amnesia (PTA) is predictive of long-term cognitive and behavioral outcome, with longer periods of PTA indicating more severe injuries (Taylor, 2010). *PTA* refers to the period immediately after injury characterized by disorientation to time, place, and person; lack of continuous memory; and inability to lay down new memories (Taylor, 2010).

The effect of TBI on skill development varies among children. Childhood is a time of rapid growth and development, with cognitive, communication, and motor skills evolving to allow a student to engage in increasingly more complex academic and social activities. Anderson et al. (2011) proposed that children injured early in life who sustain damage to developing neurological systems are most vulnerable to long-term difficulties.

Berman and Graham (2018) described 3 phases of learning: established, consolidating, and emerging:

- *Established skills* are those that a student is able to competently demonstrate across multiple environments and tasks.
- *Consolidating skills* are those that a student is able to demonstrate most of the time; however, the student may need support with these skills in new environments, and skill quality may be inconsistent.
- *Emerging skills* are those that have not yet begun to develop.

Catroppa et al. (2016) found that TBI appears to have the greatest effect on skills that have yet to develop and that those that are well established are most resistant to disruption. Longitudinal studies of children injured early in life demonstrated that children continue to acquire and develop cognitive skills, but these skills develop at a slower rate than those of same-age peers (Anderson et al., 2012; Catroppa et al., 2009).

Participation at School After TBI

In the past 10 years, research has increasingly focused on participation challenges for students with TBI. Bedell (2004) found that children (ages 3–21 years) with a TBI participated less in managing daily schedules and social and play activities than peers without disabilities. Students with more severe brain injuries were also less adaptive in getting along with other children, engaged in fewer social activities, and demonstrated lower performance in the school environment than those with moderate injuries (Bedell, 2004; Galvin et al., 2010; van Tol et al., 2011).

Van Tol et al. (2011) concluded that school-age students with more severe brain injuries demonstrated lower levels of social competence than same-age peers and those with less severe injuries. These lower levels of competence were associated with a decrease in participation in academic and social activities.

Of the most commonly reported environmental issues, the following are directly related to limitations at school:

- Inadequate information about brain injury,
- Inadequate services or programs at school,
- Lack of support with schoolwork, and
- Lack of assistance or equipment at school (Bedell, 2004; Galvin et al., 2010).

Cognitive and Behavioral Impact of TBI

Cognitive and behavioral difficulties are the most common difficulties experienced after TBI. Development of attention skills is a significant problem after TBI; those sustaining severe injuries are most at risk (Anderson et al., 2005). Yeates and Enrile (2005) reported difficulties with selective attention 4 years after injury for children ages 10–16 years; deficits persisted in children with both moderate and severe injuries, but greater deficits were noted in those with more severe injuries. Difficulty with attention to task is a particular challenge to learning and participation in the classroom.

Children with severe injuries typically have great difficulty performing tasks that require cognitive flexibility and following a plan to achieve set goals. Executive function (EF) skills are important in determining goal-directed behaviors and are one of the areas most affected by pediatric TBI (Babikian & Asarnow, 2009; Nadebaum et al., 2007). Children with severe injuries typically perform worse than their same-age peers and children with mild or moderate injuries in tasks requiring executive planning and organization (Anderson et al., 2005).

Problems with attention and EF limit the development of specific academic skills; however, socioeconomic status also influences skill acquisition (Yeates et al., 2002). Catroppa et al. (2009) reported that students with severe TBI demonstrated poorer reading, spelling, and arithmetic skills than their same-age peers. Although evidence showed that skills improve in the first 6 months after injury, deficits were likely to persist, and the gap in skills between students with TBI and their peers widened over time (Anderson et al., 1999; Catroppa & Anderson, 1999; Mangeot et al., 2002).

On the basis of specific cognitive skill deficits that affect classroom performance, Ylvisaker et al. (2001) suggested that students with TBI require support to develop the cognitive skills necessary to participate in the classroom and additional support to learn the academic content being presented to them. (For more information, see Chapter 54, "Best Practices in Cognition and Executive Functioning to Enhance Participation.")

As many as 75% of those with moderate or severe TBI have changes in personality, social cognition, and behavior (Turkstra et al., 2008), and as many as 25% demonstrate aggressive behaviors (Dooley et al., 2008). A recent study of mental health after brain injury suggested that adolescents with brain injury were more likely to attempt suicide than their peers and were nearly twice as likely to be bullied at school or online (Ilie et al., 2014).

Behavioral changes have been reported as the most challenging to adjust to, and rehabilitation teams must work closely with school staff to manage these changes and promote social inclusion in the school setting (Gauvin-Lepage &

Lefebvre, 2010). An effective strategy for students with TBI, context-sensitive supports, has been used to monitor and measure behavior to determine factors that support positive behaviors and those that contribute to maladaptive behaviors (Feeney & Ylvisaker, 2006). ***Context-sensitive supports*** are directly and immediately tied to the context, task, or activity in which the student is engaging (Feeney & Ylvisaker, 2006).

Return to School After a Mild TBI

The terms *mild TBI* and *concussion* are often used interchangeably in the research literature (Prince & Bruhns, 2017). Most children recover from a mild TBI within 2 weeks; for some children, however, ongoing symptoms of dizziness, headache, and cognitive and behavioral changes persist. This is commonly referred to as ***postconcussion syndrome.*** For children who have sustained a mild TBI—particularly those who have ongoing symptoms of postconcussion syndrome and need modifications and accommodations but not specialized instruction for academics—implementation of a 504 plan may be appropriate. Section 504 of the Rehabilitation Act of 1973, as amended (2008; Pub. L. 93–112) has a broader definition of disability than IDEA (2004; see Chapter 27, "Best Practices in Supporting Students With a 504 Plan"). If the student has academic or behavioral needs requiring special instruction, then pursuing a referral to determine special education eligibility is recommended.

Guidelines developed by CanChild (2018) highlight the need to allow the brain time to recover after a concussion. Proactive management of concussion includes identification of the original injury followed by rest, along with modification of academic tasks and a graded return to full classroom and schoolyard participation. In addition, the implementation of supportive interventions, such as psychoeducation regarding the effect of mild TBI, has been shown to assist in reducing the effect of postconcussive symptoms.

Return to School After a Moderate or Severe TBI

The task of returning to school typically begins while the student is in the rehabilitation hospital and involves sharing of information between school and hospital teams. Sharing of information is crucial to ensure that educators understand the effect of TBI (DePompei & Glang, 2018); however, recent studies have highlighted the inconsistency of current practices (Todis et al., 2018).

Initially, the focus is on the student's interaction with others and ability to manage classroom and school routines rather than on academic achievement. For students who have motor difficulties, ensuring they are able to access the school environment is an essential component of planning for school return. The school occupational therapist may provide an evaluation of the environment as it relates to the returning student. For students who are likely to demonstrate cognitive and behavioral challenges, identifying appropriate areas for them to have a rest or time away from the noise and activity of the classroom is an important consideration.

Cognitive fatigue is common after TBI and is frequently expressed as loss of concentration, increased distractibility, slower processing of information, and excessive emotional and behavioral responses (Crichton et al., 2017). Fatigue is also cumulative over time (Ziino & Ponsford, 2006). The initial return to school should be graded to allow for frequent short visits that are closely monitored to reduce the effect of fatigue. Managing fatigue by adjusting workloads and time spent at school is an important component of successful return to school. Ongoing monitoring of fatigue is also important at times of transition, such as beginning a new grade, transferring to a different school, or changing teachers.

Emotional Impact on Other Students

In some schools, with the family's permission, it is standard practice to provide education sessions about brain injury for classmates of the student with TBI in which they learn how to help their classmate when the classmate returns to school. Anecdotal experience suggests this information is most constructive when presented using age-appropriate language and answering all questions in a nonjudgmental way.

BEST PRACTICES

An occupation-based approach that supports the student's optimal performance across changing environments throughout the day is essential. The research to support specific interventions and best practices in the area of pediatric TBI is inconsistent and is frequently based on extrapolation of findings from research on adult TBI and from other areas of practice. Best practices for evaluation and intervention for students with TBI supports responding to current needs but also proactively planning and intervening to develop the skills required in later years of schooling.

Evaluate the Student to Identify Strengths and Needs

An occupational therapy evaluation focuses on identifying the strengths and needs of the student with TBI. The evaluation must address academic and functional requirements of school.

The evaluation begins with a thorough review of information provided by the family and medical facilities as well as a review of the student's academic record preinjury. Current vision and hearing assessments should also be reviewed. Vision loss or double vision may be common and must be addressed to avoid frustration during academic work. Observations of the student in the classroom and other areas of the school are essential to obtain a full occupational profile in the academic environment. In addition to reviewing information on and observing the student, the occupational therapist may evaluate a student's academic performance, occupational performance, and participation. This information could identify a student's strengths and needs for intervention planning.

Academic performance assessments

Students with TBI typically experience difficulty with EF. Difficulties with attention, memory, and speed of processing are common, so standardized assessments of IQ and isolated cognitive functions are less likely to provide an accurate summary of academic performance (Ylvisaker et al., 2002). Ecological assessments of EF measure the student's ability to plan and organize responses and provide information to identify learning challenges and inform development of strategies for the classroom (Chevignard et al., 2012).

Occupation-based assessments

The Perceived Efficacy and Goal Setting System (PEGS; Missiuna et al., 2004) and the Canadian Occupational Performance Measure (COPM; Law et al., 2014) are reliable and valid measures of occupational performance (Carswell et al., 2004). The COPM is for children ages 10 years or older. It uses a numerical scale to rate a child's performance and satisfaction with self-chosen occupations in the areas of self-care, productivity, and leisure. The PEGS is for children ages 10 years or younger; it uses picture cards to allow the child to rate their own performance and identify goals for treatment (Missiuna & Pollock, 2000).

In addition, the Child Occupational Self-Assessment (COSA; Keller et al., 2005), based on the Model of Human Occupation (Kielhofner, 2007), uses either a card-sort or a checklist that includes tasks from home, school, or the community to rate a child's competence across domains. The COSA also provides an opportunity to engage the child in identifying areas of performance that need improvement.

Participation assessments

Two assessments of participation, the Child and Family Follow-Up Survey (CFFS; Bedell, 2004) and the School Function Assessment (SFA; Coster et al., 1998), are frequently used for students with TBI. The CFFS was specifically developed to describe participation difficulties of students with brain injuries at home, school, and in the community. The SFA was designed to measure and describe elementary school students' functional task performance in academic and social domains at school.

Evaluation of performance skills

Research on performance skills for students with TBI has largely focused on cognitive outcomes, with less research available on motor and sensory outcomes. The presence of upper limb motor impairments is typically observed in students with moderate or severe TBI, with changes in tone and quality of movement most frequently observed (Wallen et al., 2001). More recently, deficits have been identified in high-level coordination tasks for students with moderate or severe injuries. High-level coordination deficits may affect the speed and quality of tasks requiring fine motor control (Davis et al., 2010).

Visual and perceptual deficits are common sequelae of TBI that can diminish the ability to learn the motor patterns and shapes required for handwriting. In addition, children with brain injuries often have difficulty with sensory processing (Galvin et al., 2009), which may affect their ability to perceive important information occurring in their environment. Careful observation and assessment of performance

in real-world settings is important because isolated skills often seem within the typical range, but when the cognitive demands and complexity of a task increase, reduced skill performance is observed (Chevignard et al., 2012).

Provide Effective Interventions

Although cognitive and academic outcomes for students with TBI and the factors that contribute to these outcomes have been studied extensively over the past 20 years, little research has been done on interventions that are effective in improving cognitive and academic performance. Despite this, several common themes have emerged from qualitative studies and review articles that can guide interventions to support students with brain injuries in the classroom.

The following section describes the key aspects of occupational therapy intervention for students with TBI and focuses on 4 areas of intervention in the classroom:
1. Performance skills interventions;
2. Occupation-based interventions;
3. School environment, instruction, and curriculum interventions, including collaborative communication; and
4. Task modification.

Performance skills interventions

Component-based approaches target the performance skills that underlie a student's academic challenges. Studies of students with TBI have investigated attempts to remediate specific cognitive skills, with some support shown for improved performance in areas targeted by the intervention. Wilson et al. (2009) implemented a system of computerized reminders via pager with children and adolescents with TBI, and participants showed improved ability to recall information and events in their daily lives. Similar improvements in time management and organization have been noted through the use of a paper notebook (Kerns & Thomson, 1998). With the increasing availability of smartphones and other online technologies, the use of electronic diaries and other reminder systems is becoming a mainstream way of supporting the planning and organization abilities of students with TBI that does not separate them from their peers.

Van t'Hooft et al. (2005) demonstrated improvements in memory and in sustained and selective attention of 38 children with TBI ages 9–16 years after a 30-minute training session each day for 17 weeks. A Cochrane review that aimed to assess the effects of technology-based interventions for children and adolescents with TBI found some evidence that technological aids did improve the EF of adolescents; however, studies contained low numbers of participants and low-quality evidence, meaning that their results should be interpreted with caution (Linden et al., 2016). The use of technology has great potential for students with brain injury, but individual outcomes should be monitored carefully to ensure that technology is meeting the overall goal of improving occupational performance.

Occupation-based interventions

Occupation-based interventions aim to improve student performance on a task or activity rather than address the component deficits that may affect performance. Emerging evidence has suggested that the use of metacognitive strategies such as the Cognitive Orientation to daily Occupational Performance (CO–OP; Dawson et al., 2017; Missiuna et al., 2010) is effective in improving specific goal-directed behaviors. CO–OP teaches children a global problem-solving strategy—the Goal–Plan–Do–Check approach—that supports children in identifying solutions and strategies and evaluating their effectiveness. Missiuna et al. (2010) found that children with TBI were able to use CO–OP's problem-solving strategy effectively to improve their performance on self-selected goals, but they could not generalize the strategy to tasks beyond those specifically addressed in therapy.

Chan and Fong (2011), taking a similar approach, implemented a metacognitive strategy over 6 weeks and demonstrated improvements in task performance in children with TBI. Although children demonstrated improvements in tasks that were identified at baseline, they were not able to generalize the problem-solving strategy to other tasks. The ability to improve performance suggests that metacognitive strategies are useful interventions that can be targeted to assist students to learn strategic behaviors that support their classroom performance.

Direct instruction promotes successful learning for students with learning difficulties similar to those demonstrated by students with TBI. Rather than helping the student develop problem-solving abilities, this approach focuses on teaching specific academic skills and tasks by systematically presenting new information in clear and simple steps. Direct instruction includes the concept of *errorless learning:* A task is divided into small and achievable steps, and support is gradually reduced as the student's independence increases (Glang et al., 2008). An approach that incorporates these key principles is typically suggested for students with TBI, although this recommendation is primarily based on clinical experience rather than research evidence.

Medical clearance is essential before the student returns to sports and outdoor play. Research has shown that students with TBI have the most difficulty engaging in sporting and social activities that are unstructured (Bedell, 2004; Galvin et al., 2010). The occupational therapy practitioner can address this difficulty in sports and physical education classes by focusing on skill-based drills and then integrating these drills into structured, clearly defined games with small groups of students. The practitioner can help structure social interactions by organizing small-group activities and rehearsing conversation starters and promoting the development of appropriate social behaviors.

Circle of Friends (2012) is a program used to link students with disabilities and their general education peers. Although the program has no specific research behind it, it may support social inclusion of students with TBI.

School-based interventions

An essential first step to providing appropriate services and supports is identifying the student with TBI (Mealings et al., 2012). Kahn et al. (2018) and others have noted that teachers are frequently not aware that a student in their class has had a TBI. Communication, particularly at times of transition, is essential to sharing knowledge that will support teachers in providing an optimal learning environment.

School occupational therapists may need to provide educators with professional development to share knowledge and information about TBI and its likely effect on the student's ability to perform in school (Glang et al., 2010). Across studies, the largest barrier to participation identified by students and their parents was school staff's perceived lack of knowledge about TBI and its consequences (Kahn et al., 2018; Turkstra et al., 2008).

To help in sharing information about students with TBI between school years and between different settings, the use of transition videos, which are based on self-advocacy videos (Ylvisaker & Feeney, 2002), has been proposed (Shanahan, 2004). Occupational therapy practitioners work with students to plan what information will be shared with their teachers in the following year. The practitioner provides an outline that prompts students to describe their time in the hospital and what is different now; strategies that help them learn; and ways that teachers and other students can help and what to do when students are feeling sad, angry, or stuck. However, students are free to plan their video with information that they believe is most useful for others. In a single case study, the use of a transition video was found to reduce the practitioner's need to provide school staff with information about and behavioral support for a student with TBI from weekly to quarterly (Shanahan, 2004).

A review by Hux et al. (2010) sought the opinions of students, teachers, and health care professionals about strategies that support success in the school environment. Preparation and accommodation were seen as essential. Bedell et al. (2005) identified strategies that professionals and parents viewed as most effective in supporting students with TBI in the classroom. Three major themes were established:

1. Routine, repetition, and consistency;
2. Supports and models; and
3. Curriculum and environmental modifications.

In qualitative studies of students' experience of return to school, similar themes were found (Mealings et al., 2012). There is little quantitative evidence on which of these strategies are the most effective; however, recommendations described next are supported by an understanding of common cognitive deficits and reports from students.

One of the most effective ways of assisting students with cognitive difficulties is to engage them in routine activities and tasks and be consistent with expectations. Students report that they have more difficulty when expectations change from one class to the next. This change in expectations is why transition between year levels can be so challenging. Having the same teacher and daily schedule allows students to understand the expectations for their performance. In addition, creating checklists for students to check off tasks, or steps of tasks, that have been completed gives them structure and helps them anticipate what will happen next.

The use of daily schedules and planners supports awareness of deadlines and helps the student to prepare for tasks that need to be completed. Electronic diaries and smartphones can provide auditory cues to remind the student when work needs to be completed or equipment needs to be taken to school. Kindergarten and elementary school students may benefit from visually based planners and will require adult assistance to set up and maintain them, whereas middle or high school students can work toward independently managing the planner to organize studies, activities, and schedules.

Students with TBI typically report that to gain knowledge and learn new skills, they need to repeat information and practice tasks more regularly than was required before their injury (Hux et al., 2010; Mealings et al., 2012). Modifications to the curriculum to allow more time for repetition and practice are often necessary. The use of study periods to provide additional opportunities to repeat and rehearse key information from classes is also an important strategy. Elementary school students will likely require an adult to support their learning of new tasks, whereas older students may require less direct assistance but will benefit from having a key person to monitor progress and assist with the organizational aspects of the curriculum.

Task modification

Task modification is an important strategy to support learning for students with TBI, particularly in elementary and middle school because these students may be consolidating their abilities in key academic skills. Using a modification approach, occupational therapy practitioners and teachers identify the key elements of learning for an activity, including motor and cognitive skills, and help students focus on developing these component skills. For example, when a student with TBI is learning to write, they may be able to write letters and words but may find the cognitive and planning demands overwhelming. By identifying that the key element the student is missing is the cognitive task of creating and structuring a story, not the physical task of writing, practitioners and teachers can focus their support on those skills.

Task modification can involve reducing the amount of work that the student is required to complete or allowing additional time to complete assigned tasks. Reducing study loads to minimize cognitive fatigue can support learning in students with TBI. Allowing them additional time to complete written work, particularly exams, is an important compensatory strategy to overcome decreased ability to sustain attention, slowed processing skills, fatigue, and difficulties with executive organization (Mealings et al., 2012).

SUMMARY

Students with TBI benefit from a school program that provides structure and routine and from clear and consistent expectations for academic performance and behavior. TBI includes a range of cognitive and motor deficits that may affect all areas of a student's school performance and participation. These students can learn and achieve academically, but they typically require greater repetition and practice than their classmates. Brain injury affects learning and development in the period immediately after the injury and throughout schooling. Occupational therapy practitioners implement effective strategies to create a supportive learning environment for students with TBI.

REFERENCES

American Occupational Therapy Association. (2014). Guidelines for supervision, roles, and responsibilities during the delivery of occupational therapy services. *American Journal of Occupational Therapy, 68*(Suppl. 3), S16–S22. https://doi.org/10.5014/ajot.2014.686S03

Anderson, V., Catroppa, C., Godfrey, C., & Rosenfeld, J. V. (2012). Intellectual ability 10 years after traumatic brain injury in infancy and childhood: What predicts outcome? *Journal of Neurotrauma, 29*, 143–153. https://doi.org/10.1089/neu.2011.2012

Anderson, V. A., Catroppa, C., Morse, S. A., & Haritou, F. (1999). Functional memory skills following traumatic brain injury in young children. *Pediatric Rehabilitation, 3*, 159–166. https://doi.org/10.1080/136384999289423

Anderson, V., Catroppa, C., Morse, S., Haritou, F., & Rosenfeld, J. (2005). Attentional and processing skills following traumatic brain injury in early childhood. *Brain Injury, 19*, 699–710. https://doi.org/10.1080/02699050400025281

Anderson, V., Spencer-Smith, M., & Wood, A. (2011). Do children really recover better? Neurobehavioural plasticity after early brain insult. *Brain, 134*, 2197–2221. https://doi.org/10.1093/brain/awr103

Babikian, T., & Asarnow, R. (2009). Neurocognitive outcomes and recovery after pediatric traumatic brain injury: Meta-analytic review of the literature. *Neuropsychology, 23*, 283–296. https://doi.org/10.1037/a0015268

Ballantyne, A. O., Spilkin, A. M., Hesselink, J., & Trauner, D. A. (2008). Plasticity in the developing brain: Intellectual, language and academic functions in children with ischemic perinatal stroke. *Brain, 131*, 2975–2985. https://doi.org/10.1093/brain/awn176

Bedell, G. M. (2004). Developing a follow-up survey focused on participation of children and youth with acquired brain injuries after discharge from inpatient rehabilitation. *NeuroRehabilitation, 19*, 191–205.

Bedell, G. M., Cohn, E. S., & Dumas, H. M. (2005). Exploring parents' use of strategies to promote social participation of school-age children with acquired brain injuries. *American Journal of Occupational Therapy, 59*, 273–284. https://doi.org/10.5014/ajot.59.3.273

Berman, J., & Graham, L. (2018). *Learning intervention: Educational casework and responsive teaching for sustainable learning.* Abingdon, England: Routledge.

Bryan, M. A., Rowhani-Rahbar, A., Comstock, R. D., & Rivara, F. (2016). Sports- and recreation-related concussions in US youth. *Pediatrics, 138*, e20154635. https://doi.org/10.1542/peds.2015-4635

CanChild. (2018). *Resources: Concussion/mild traumatic brain injury guideline brochures.* Retrieved from https://www.canchild.ca/en/resources/249-concussion-mild-traumatic-brain-injury-guideline-brochures

Carswell, A., McColl, M. A., Baptiste, S., Law, M., Polatajko, H., & Pollock, N. (2004). The Canadian Occupational Performance Measure: A research and clinical literature review. *Canadian Journal of Occupational Therapy, 71*, 210–222. https://doi.org/10.1177%2F000841740407100406

Catroppa, C., & Anderson, V. (1999). Recovery of educational skills following paediatric traumatic brain injury. *Pediatric Rehabilitation, 3*, 167–175. https://doi.org/10.1080/136384999289432

Catroppa, C., Anderson, V., Beauchamp, M., & Yeates, K. (2016). *New frontiers in pediatric traumatic brain injury.* New York: Routledge.

Catroppa, C., Anderson, V. A., Muscara, F., Morse, S. A., Haritou, F., Rosenfeld, J. V., & Heinrich, L. M. (2009). Educational skills: Long-term outcome and predictors following paediatric traumatic brain injury. *Neuropsychological Rehabilitation, 19,* 716–732. https://doi.org/10.1080/09602010902732868

Centers for Disease Control and Prevention. (2017). *Traumatic brain injury and concussion.* Retrieved from http://www.cdc.gov/traumaticbraininjury/

Chan, D. Y., & Fong, K. N. (2011). The effects of problem-solving skills training based on metacognitive principles for children with acquired brain injury attending mainstream schools: A controlled clinical trial. *Disability and Rehabilitation, 33,* 2023–2032. https://doi.org/10.3109/09638288.2011.556207

Chevignard, M. P., Soo, C., Galvin, J., Catroppa, C., & Eren, S. (2012). Ecological assessment of cognitive functions in children with acquired brain injury: A systematic review. *Brain Injury, 26,* 1033–1057. https://doi.org/10.3109/02699052.2012.666366

Circle of Friends. (2012). *Program description.* Retrieved from http://www.circleofriends.org/

Coster, W., Deeney, T., Haltiwanger, J., & Haley, S. (1998). *School Function Assessment: User's manual.* San Antonio: Therapy Skill Builders.

Crichton, A. J., Babl, F., Oakley, E., Greenham, M., Hearps, S., Delzoppo, C., . . . Anderson, V. A. (2017). Prediction of multidimensional fatigue after childhood brain injury. *Journal of Head Trauma Rehabilitation, 32,* 107–116. https://doi.org/10.1097/HTR.0000000000000248

Davis, E., Galvin, J., & Soo, C. (2010). Reliability of the Assisting Hand Assessment (AHA) for children and youth with acquired brain injury. *Brain Impairment, 11,* 113–124. https://doi.org/10.1375/brim.11.2.113

Dawson, D. R., McEwen, S. E., & Polatajko, H. J. (Eds.). (2017). *Cognitive Orientation to daily Occupational Performance in occupational therapy: Using the CO-OP Approach™ to enable participation across the lifespan.* Bethesda, MD: AOTA Press.

DePompei, R., & Glang, A. (2018). Have we made progress with educational services for students with TBI? *NeuroRehabilitation, 42,* 255–257. https://doi.org/10.3233/NRE-180001

Dooley, J. J., Anderson, V., Hemphill, S. A., & Ohan, J. (2008). Aggression after paediatric traumatic brain injury: A theoretical approach. *Brain Injury, 22,* 836–846. https://doi.org/10.1080/02699050802425444

Feeney, T., & Ylvisaker, M. (2006). Context-sensitive cognitive–behavioural supports for young children with traumatic brain injury: A replication study. *Brain Injury, 20,* 629–645. https://doi.org/10.1080/02699050600744194

Galvin, J., Froude, E. H., & Imms, C. (2009). Sensory processing abilities of children who have sustained traumatic brain injuries. *American Journal of Occupational Therapy, 63,* 701–709. https://doi.org/10.5014/ajot.63.6.701

Galvin, J., Froude, E. H., & McAleer, J. (2010). Children's participation in home, school and community life after acquired brain injury. *Australian Occupational Therapy Journal, 57,* 118–126. https://doi.org/10.1111/j.1440-1630.2009.00822.x

Gauvin-Lepage, J., & Lefebvre, H. (2010). Social inclusion of persons with moderate head injuries: The points of view of adolescents with brain injuries, their parents, and professionals. *Brain Injury, 24,* 1087–1097. https://doi.org/10.3109/02699052.2010.494593

Glang, A., Todis, B., Ettel, D., Wade, S. L., & Yeates, K. O. (2018). Results from a randomized trial evaluating a hospital–school transition support model for students hospitalized with traumatic brain injury. *Brain Injury, 32,* 608–616. https://doi.org/10.1080/02699052.2018.1433329

Glang, A., Todis, B., Sublette, P., Brown, B. E., & Vaccaro, M. (2010). Professional development in traumatic brain injury for educators: The importance of context. *Journal of Head Trauma and Rehabilitation, 25,* 426–432. https://doi.org/10.1097/HTR.0b013e3181fb8f45

Glang, A., Ylvisaker, M., Stein, M., Ehlhardt, L., Todis, B., & Tyler, J. (2008). Validated instructional practices: Application to students with traumatic brain injury. *Journal of Head Trauma and Rehabilitation, 23,* 243–251. https://doi.org/10.1097/01.HTR.0000327256.46504.9f

Hux, K., Bush, E., Zickefoose, S., Holmberg, M., Henderson, A., & Simanek, G. (2010). Exploring the study skills and accommodations used by college student survivors of traumatic brain injury. *Brain Injury, 24,* 13–26. https://doi.org/10.3109/02699050903446823

Ilie, G., Mann, R. E., Boak, A., Adlaf, E. M., Hamilton, H., Asbridge, M., Rehm, J., & Cusimano, M. D. (2014). Suicidality, bullying and other conduct and mental health correlates of traumatic brain injury in adolescents. *PLoS ONE, 9*(4), e94936. https://doi.org/10.1371/journal.pone.0094936

Individuals With Disabilities Education Improvement Act of 2004, Pub. L. 108–446, 20 U.S.C. §§ 1400–1482.

Jacobs, R., Harvey, A. S., & Anderson, V. (2007). Executive function following focal frontal lobe lesions: Impact of timing of lesion on outcome. *Cortex, 43,* 792–805. https://doi.org/10.1016/S0010-9452(08)70507-0

Kahn, L. G., Linden, M. A., McKinlay, A., Gomez, D., & Glang, A. (2018). An international perspective on educators' perceptions of children with traumatic brain injury. *NeuroRehabilitation, 42,* 299–309. https://doi.org/10.3233/NRE-172380

Keller, J., Kafkes, A., & Kielhofner, G. (2005). Psychometric characteristics of the Child Occupational Self Assessment (COSA), Part 1: An initial examination of psychometric properties. *Scandinavian Journal of Occupational Therapy, 12,* 118–127. https://doi.org/10.1080/11038120510031752

Kerns, K. A., & Thomson, J. (1998). Implementation of a compensatory memory system in a school age child with severe memory impairment. *Pediatric Rehabilitation, 2,* 77–87. https://doi.org/10.3109/17518429809068159

Kielhofner, G. (2007). *Model of Human Occupation: Theory and application* (4th ed.). Chicago: Lippincott Williams & Wilkins.

Law, M., Baptiste, S., Carswell, A., McColl, M. A., Polatajko, H., & Pollock, N. (2014). *Canadian Occupational Performance Measure* (5th ed.). Ottawa: CAOT Publications.

Linden, M., Hawley, C., Blackwood, B., Evans, J., Anderson, V., & O'Rourke, C. (2016). Using technology to rehabilitate children and adolescents with acquired brain injury. *Cochrane Database of Systematic Reviews, 2016,* CD011020. https://doi.org/10.1002/14651858.CD011020.pub2

Mangeot, S., Armstrong, K., Colvin, A. N., Yeates, K. O., & Taylor, H. G. (2002). Long-term executive function deficits in children with traumatic brain injuries: Assessment using the Behavior Rating Inventory of Executive Function (BRIEF). *Child Neuropsychology, 8,* 271–284. https://doi.org/10.1076/chin.8.4.271.13503

Mealings, M., Douglas, J., & Olver, J. (2012). Considering the student perspective in returning to school after traumatic brain injury: A literature review. *Brain Injury, 26,* 1165–1176. https://doi.org/10.3109/02699052.2012.672785

Missiuna, C., DeMatteo, C., Hanna, S., Mandich, A., Law, M., Mahoney, W., & Scott, L. (2010). Exploring the use of cognitive intervention for children with acquired brain injury. *Physical and Occupational Therapy in Pediatrics, 30,* 205–219. https://doi.org/10.3109/01942631003761554

Missiuna, C., & Pollock, N. (2000). Perceived efficiency and goal setting in young children. *Canadian Journal of Occupational Therapy, 67,* 101–109. https://doi.org/10.1177%2F000841740006700303

Missiuna, C., Pollock, N., & Law, M. (2004). *PEGS: The Perceived Efficacy and Goal Setting System manual.* San Antonio: Harcourt Assessment.

Nadebaum, C., Anderson, V., & Catroppa, C. (2007). Executive function outcomes following traumatic brain injury in young children: A five-year follow-up. *Developmental Neuropsychology, 32,* 703–728. https://doi.org/10.1080/87565640701376086

Prince, C., & Bruhns, M. E. (2017). Evaluation and treatment of mild traumatic brain injury: The role of neuropsychology. *Brain Sciences, 7*(8). https://doi.org/10.3390/brainsci7080105

Rehabilitation Act of 1973, Pub. L. 93–112, 29 U.S.C. §§ 701–796l.

Section 504 of the Rehabilitation Act of 1973, as amended, 29 U.S.C. § 794 (2008).

Shanahan, L. (2004). Self-advocacy videos at periods of transition: A powerful rehabilitation tool for children with brain injury. *Acquiring Knowledge in Speech, Language and Hearing, 6*(1), 26–29.

Taylor, H. G. (2010). Neurobehavioural outcomes of pediatric traumatic brain injury. In V. Anderson & K. O. Yeates (Eds.), *Pediatric traumatic brain injury: New frontiers in clinical and translational research.* Cambridge, England: Cambridge University Press.

Teasdale, G., & Jennett, B. (1974). Assessment of coma and impaired consciousness: A practical scale. *Lancet, 304,* 81–84. https://doi.org/10.1016/S0140-6736(74)91639-0

Todis, B., McCart, M., & Glang, A. (2018). Hospital to school transition following traumatic brain injury: A qualitative longitudinal study. *NeuroRehabilitation, 42,* 269–276. https://doi.org/10.3233/NRE-172383

Turkstra, L. S., Williams, W. H., Tonks, J., & Frampton, I. (2008). Measuring social cognition in adolescents: Implications for students with traumatic brain injury returning to school. *NeuroRehabilitation, 23,* 501–509.

Van 't Hooft, I., Andersson, K., Bergman, B., Sejersen, T., Von Wendt, L., & Bartfai, A. (2005). Beneficial effect from a cognitive training programme on children with acquired brain injuries demonstrated in a controlled study. *Brain Injury, 19,* 511–518. https://doi.org/10.1080/02699050400025224

van Tol, E., Gorter, J. W., DeMatteo, C., & Meester-Delver, A. (2011). Participation outcomes for children with acquired brain injury: A narrative review. *Brain Injury, 25,* 1279–1287. https://doi.org/10.3109/02699052.2011.613089

Wallen, M. A., Mackay, S., Duff, S. M., McCartney, L. C., & O'Flaherty, S. J. (2001). Upper-limb function in Australian children with traumatic brain injury: A controlled, prospective study. *Archives of Physical Medicine and Rehabilitation, 82,* 642–649. https://doi.org/10.1053/apmr.2001.22620

Wilson, B. A., Emslie, H., Evans, J. J., Quirk, K., Watson, P., & Fish, J. (2009). The NeuroPage system for children and adolescents with neurological deficits. *Developmental Neurorehabilitation, 12,* 421–426. https://doi.org/10.3109/17518420903200573

Yeates, K. O., & Enrile, B. G. (2005). Implicit and explicit memory in children with congenital and acquired brain disorder. *Neuropsychology, 19,* 618–628. https://doi.org/10.1037/0894-4105.19.5.618

Yeates, K. O., Taylor, H. G., Wade, S. L., Drotar, D., Stancin, T., & Minich, N. (2002). A prospective study of short- and long-term neuropsychological outcomes after traumatic brain injury in children. *Neuropsychology, 16,* 514–523. https://doi.org/10.1037/0894-4105.16.4.514

Ylvisaker, M., & Feeney, T. (2002). Executive functions, self-regulation, and learned optimism in paediatric rehabilitation: A review and implications for intervention. *Pediatric Rehabilitation, 5,* 51–70. https://doi.org/10.1080/1363849021000041891

Ylvisaker, M., Hanks, R., & Johnson-Greene, D. (2002). Perspectives on rehabilitation of individuals with cognitive impairment after brain injury: Rationale for reconsideration of theoretical paradigms. *Journal of Head Trauma Rehabilitation, 17,* 191–209.

Ylvisaker, M., Todis, B., Glang, A., Urbanczyk, B., Franklin, C., DePompei, R., . . . Tyler, J. S. (2001). Educating students with traumatic brain injury: Themes and recommendations. *Journal of Head Trauma Rehabilitation, 16,* 76–93.

Ziino, C., & Ponsford, J. (2006). Selective attention deficits and subjective fatigue following traumatic brain injury. *Neuropsychology, 20,* 383–390. https://doi.org/10.1037/0894-4105.20.3.383

Best Practices in Supporting Students With Visual Impairments

Jessica Lampert, OTR, PhD, COMS, CLVT

KEY TERMS AND CONCEPTS

- Certified orientation and mobility specialists
- Expanded core curriculum
- Soft skills
- Teachers of visually impaired children
- Visual impairment

OVERVIEW

Visual impairment (including blindness), as defined by the Individuals With Disabilities Education Improvement Act of 2004 (IDEA; Pub. L. 108–446), is "any impairment in vision that even with correction adversely affects a child's educational performance" (34 C.F.R. 300.8[c][13]). The definition includes conditions caused by any etiology, including ocular pathology as well as brain injury and oculomotor issues (Office of Special Education and Rehabilitation Services, 2017).

According to the American Printing House for the Blind (2017), which maintains a national registry of students eligible to receive materials purchased with Federal Quota money, there were 63,357 students with visual impairment in the United States in 2016. Students are eligible to receive materials when they meet the definition of *legal blindness* (i.e., acuity of 20/200 or less, visual field of 20° or less) or have "visual performance reduced by brain injury or dysfunction when visual function meets the definition of blindness as determined by an eye care specialist or neurologist . . ." (American Printing House for the Blind, n.d., para. 3).

Teachers of visually impaired children (TVIs) and *certified orientation and mobility specialists* (COMSs) are primary members of the student's special education team and are usually the first to address the needs of students with visual impairments in public schools. TVIs address the disability-specific educational needs of students with visual impairments. COMSs address the disability-specific skills and adapted techniques needed for understanding and safely navigating the environment, including school campus, home, and community. Occupational therapy practitioners[1] often become part of this team when a student's

difficulty with motor skills or other occupational performance is identified. In some cases, the occupational therapy practitioner may be the first to suspect a student has a visual impairment and raise the concern with the student's team. Often, these instances occur with students who have multiple disabilities (which may be associated with visual impairment) or oculomotor issues.

ESSENTIAL CONSIDERATIONS

The presence of visual impairment can present distinctive challenges to participation across the life course and across contexts. Occupational therapy practitioners working with students who have visual impairments should become aware of the potential challenges and barriers to participation in school and in transition to postschool life faced by students and their families.

Effects of Visual Impairment on Participation

Occupational performance of students with visual impairments can be influenced by many factors. Students with severe visual impairments may experience delays or challenges in motor, communication, and social skills, all of which may affect participation in daily routines. The effects of visual impairment on development are influenced by age at onset, with congenital visual impairment and blindness potentially associated with greater delays in more areas than acquired visual impairment. The presence of disabilities in addition to visual impairment may influence the

---

[1]*Occupational therapy practitioner* refers to both the occupational therapist and the occupational therapy assistant. The American Occupational Therapy Association (AOTA; 2014a, p. S18) states, "The occupational therapist is responsible for all aspects of occupational

therapy service delivery and is accountable for the safety and effectiveness of the occupational therapy service delivery process" and "must be directly involved in the delivery of services during the initial evaluation and regularly throughout the course of intervention. . . . The occupational therapy assistant delivers safe and effective occupational therapy services under the supervision of and in partnership with the occupational therapist."

Copyright © 2019 by the American Occupational Therapy Association. All rights reserved. To reuse this content, contact www.copyright.com.
https://doi.org/10.7139/2019.978-1-56900-591-0.039

young student's progression through motoric milestone sequences more than the severity of the visual impairment (Ferrell et al., 2014).

Participation of young students

Delays and challenges in motor, communication, and social skills in early childhood can influence later function. School occupational therapy practitioners need to be aware of these challenges to design effective interventions. Positional motor milestones for students with severe visual impairments tend to emerge at the same time as those for sighted peers; dynamic skills that require moving through space or visual direction may be delayed (Bambring, 2006; Celeste, 2006). Young students with visual impairments and motor delays may experience difficulty understanding space beyond their bodies. If a student experiences challenges in moving through space and has vision insufficient for noticing and accurately interpreting physical environmental features, then the student may have difficulty relating objects to each other and to self.

Young students with severe visual impairments may have difficulty with pragmatic language skills (James & Stojanovik, 2007; Tadić et al., 2010). In addition, some young students with visual impairments may demonstrate echolalia for longer periods than their typically sighted peers, have difficulty understanding another person's perspective, and have difficulty initiating and sustaining conversations (Erin, 2006; Fazzi & Klein, 2002).

Students with visual impairments have been found to participate in fewer activities and with less frequency than their typically sighted peers (Engel-Yeger & Hamed-Dahmer, 2013). Because they may not see or accurately interpret social cues such as facial expressions and body language, young students with severe visual impairments may not understand or be aware of typical classroom behaviors (e.g., raising one's hand and waiting to be called on) and social rules (e.g., personal space and distance). A visual impairment can limit a student's ability to access social and environmental information, so they may require explicit teaching to understand social skills and build their knowledge about the physical environment (Erin, 2006).

Participation of adolescents

Adolescents who are visually impaired have been found to have fewer social interactions (i.e., they have smaller social networks), engage in a narrower range of activities, and engage less frequently in these activities than their sighted peers. They also tend to choose more passive activities and spend more time in solitary activity than their sighted peers (Gold et al., 2010; Kroksmark & Nordell, 2001; Pinquart & Pfeiffer, 2013).

Adolescents in a study by Salminen and Karhula (2014) identified challenges to participation, including mobility, embarrassment at using adapted equipment, and difficulty making friends. Lampert (2016) also found that adolescents with visual impairments reported barriers to social participation, including lack of access to information (social cues and difficulty obtaining academic information in accessible formats), reluctance to use accommodations and assistive technology (AT), and mobility. Jessup et al. (2017) reported

that although most of the participants in their study felt accepted and included as members of their schools much of the time, some also described feeling different: They had to work harder and took more time to accomplish tasks than peers who were typically sighted. Students with disabilities in addition to a visual impairment did not feel as included as their peers who had a visual impairment only.

Participation in transition to postschool life

When students with visual impairments experience challenges in their participation during high school, these challenges can continue into postschool life. Even when their academic performance level is equivalent to that of typically sighted peers, success rates for independent living and employment are much lower (Connors et al., 2014; McDonnall, 2011; McDonnall & O'Mally, 2012; Newman et al., 2011; Shaw et al., 2007). This occurs even when students with visual impairments spend more time in general education classrooms and receive more instruction in life skills after graduation than students with other disabilities (Newman et al., 2011).

BEST PRACTICES

The occupational therapy literature has a paucity of evidence for effective occupational therapy interventions and outcomes with students who are visually impaired. A database search for studies published within the past 20 years using the terms *visual impairment, low vision,* and *blindness* with *occupational therapy, children,* and *pediatrics* yielded few results. Most items found dealt with identifying challenges to participation (Engle-Yeager & Hamed-Dahmer, 2013; Ferziger, 2017; Ryan-Bloomer et al., 2016; Salminen & Karhula, 2014). Studies and articles focusing on occupational therapy intervention for students with visual impairments included investigations of visual stimulation methods (Tsai et al., 2013, 2016) and intervention for social skills (Uysal & Düger, 2012).

A guiding concept in education for students with visual impairments is the **expanded core curriculum,** which consists of 9 areas of disability-specific skills necessary for successful school life and transition to adulthood (Allman & Lewis, 2014; Huebner et al., 2004):

1. AT
2. Career education
3. Compensatory skills for accessing information (e.g., Braille, use of optical devices, communication, specialized instruction or adaptations)
4. Independent living skills
5. Orientation and mobility
6. Recreation and leisure
7. Self-determination
8. Sensory efficiency (e.g., vision, hearing, touch, proprioceptive, vestibular)
9. Social interaction skills.

Many of these areas align with occupation categories listed in AOTA's (2014b) *Occupational Therapy Practice Framework: Domain and Process* (3rd ed.). Given that school occupational therapists address client factors, contextual and environmental factors, and engagement in occupation, they can work collaboratively with TVIs and COMSs in assessment of and intervention for expanded core curriculum areas. Occupational therapy practitioners can equally benefit from TVIs and COMSs sharing their knowledge of and expertise in visual impairments and associated disabilities.

Evaluate Students With Visual Impairments

TVIs are charged with assessing the student's use of vision (functional vision assessment) and best media for learning (functional learning or media assessment) as well as all areas of the expanded core curriculum. Occupational therapists can support these assessments by contributing expertise in positioning and movement, fine motor and sensory skills development and function, sequencing skills, and understanding of literacy as occupation. The occupational therapist may also use occupation-based assessments, such as the School Function Assessment (Coster et al., 1998) or Canadian Occupational Performance Measure (Law et al., 2014), to provide additional information to the team.

The student and family are important members of the team and contribute to the evaluation by identifying the student's strengths and family's concerns. Questions regarding how the student uses available vision, how the student's vision loss affects participation in family and community activities, patterns and routines of performance at home, the family's and student's expectations and hopes for the future, the family's and student's perception of how the student's vision impairment affects performance and function at school, and the student's and family's perception of barriers and supports can give useful insight regarding the student's occupational performance.

In gathering data for the student's occupational profile collaboratively with the TVI and COMS as they address the areas of the expanded core curriculum, the occupational therapist can further address supports and barriers to occupational performance. It is important for the occupational therapist to assess performance patterns and consider ways in which they may be influenced by visual impairment. Issues including the student's understanding and use of social rules, classroom behaviors, and gesture or body language; ability to initiate play and other interaction with peers; and self-care, including the ability to carry items such as a loaded cafeteria tray, locate food on a plate, open food and drink packages, or manage clothing for toileting and for changing conditions (e.g., putting on or taking off a jacket) should be addressed. Addressing skills such as identifying topics of interest to peers, initiating and maintaining conversation with peers, and obtaining information about trends and styles in hair, clothing, and makeup are also important in determining supports and barriers to participation.

Physical environmental factors to address include lighting (with attention to ambient light, task lighting, and glare), physical organization of the classroom and school (materials in a consistent location and accessible to the student, including cafeteria line and seating areas), and location of student's desk within the classroom. Social environmental factors to address include supports and barriers to understanding social rules and classroom behaviors (e.g., if the teacher or other students rely greatly on nonverbal communication, the student with visual impairment will not have access to this social information) and adult expectations for the student's responsibility, autonomy, and independent function.

Few standardized assessments exist that specifically address the development of students with visual impairment (Ferrell et al., 2014; Visser et al., 2012). When attempting to determine the functional performance of a student with visual impairment using standardized tests, it is important to be aware of the visually dependent tasks used as milestones and how they may affect the results of testing (Ferreira & Albuquerque, 2017). If the therapist is using standardized assessments to determine functional performance, it is important to collaborate with the TVI or COMS, who can assist in interpreting the effects vision loss may have on the student's performance on specific skill items.

Provide Effective Interventions With Students With Visual Impairments

There is currently little research on the effectiveness of occupational therapy interventions specific to students with visual impairments. Most research has focused on visual skills training in some form.

Tsai et al. (2013, 2016) described improvements in visual acuity after a systematic intensive vision stimulation program. Participants in each study were able to respond to directions and interact (some with assistance) with equipment and examiners. The intervention of vision stimulation provided in a planned and ordered way for cortical or cerebral visual impairment is supported in the educational and ophthalmological literature (Lueck & Dutton, 2015; Roman-Lantzy, 2007). Cohen-Maitre and Haerich (2005) found attentional advantages for movement and color in visual targets used with children who had cortical visual impairment. This result was consistent with Baker-Nobles and Rutherford's (1995) description of color and movement preferences in children with cortical visual impairment.

Roman-Lantzy (2007) advocated intervention on the basis of the characteristic visual behaviors of children with cortical visual impairment and strategies to obtain and sustain visual attention in accordance with these behaviors while integrated into functional daily activities. In collaboration with TVIs and COMSs, occupational therapy practitioners can support students with cortical visual impairment by incorporating these strategies to enhance the students' visual attention, function, and engagement in educational and other activities.

Occupational therapy practitioners in schools aim to optimize students' participation in school occupations. For students with visual impairment, the occupational therapy practitioner may need to adapt tasks or strategically teach students how to compensate for their vision loss. Activities may include locating food on a plate, locating a seat in the cafeteria, identifying clothing, playing on playground equipment, or organizing materials.

Intervention scenarios

The following fictional scenarios describe examples of occupational therapy intervention in the school setting.

Kindergarten intervention. Sara had a diagnosis of optic nerve hypoplasia with light perception only. She started receiving support from a TVI and a COMS when she was 6 months old. She had independent skills in undressing, except for fasteners, and would let adults know when she needed to use the toilet. Sara's team, including her mother, requested an occupational therapy evaluation because she did not use a spoon for eating. Her mother fed her or let her eat with her fingers at home, but she did not want to continue this because it was quite messy. The team agreed that finger feeding alone was not sufficient for school.

The school occupational therapist collaborated with Sara's mother, TVI, COMS, and classroom teacher to establish a priority of self-feeding. During the evaluation, Sara demonstrated the fine motor skills needed for holding a spoon and scooping but had difficulty locating food on her plate. The occupational therapist, working with Sara during school meals, developed a routine for locating food and shared this information with Sara's mother and teacher so they could implement the routine throughout the week.

The routine consisted of Sara's being told the location of each item, with descriptions always starting with food at the top of the plate and progressing in a clockwise manner. At the same time, she was encouraged to explore her plate gently and systematically with her fingers. Although her classroom teacher and mother were familiar with the clock method (e.g., describing items as being at 3:00 or 6:00), they did not use it with Sara because she did not yet have experience with or a concept of a clock face. In addition, Sara was taught to use a cracker in her left hand to stabilize food as she used the spoon to scoop with her right. With consistent implementation of the routine across contexts (i.e., home, school cafeteria, classroom), Sara developed independent spoon skills.

Elementary intervention. Tamika was in 3rd grade and had a diagnosis of retinopathy of prematurity, with a visual acuity of 20/600. She participated in most classroom activities and took her turn in gathering and passing out materials to other students. Her COMS noted that Tamika had difficulty manipulating her handheld monocular telescope during lessons, and the educational team wondered whether underlying fine motor challenges were the barrier. On evaluation, the school occupational therapist noted that Tamika demonstrated difficulty with in-hand manipulation skills that affected her ability to manage her telescope.

The occupational therapist collaborated with the COMS, first to learn how to use the monocular telescope and then, after analyzing Tamika's fine motor skills needed for the task, to support the COMS in helping Tamika develop those skills. The therapist worked with Tamika on her fine motor skills, and Tamika identified activities she wanted to do with the telescope. As Tamika improved her fine motor skills and subsequently skills with managing the telescope, she achieved her goals, including using the telescope on lessons with the COMS.

Middle school intervention. Jill was in 7th grade and totally blind. She was often slow to turn in assignments. Although she could manage her work electronically, she frequently misplaced assignments once they were printed out. She could not identify organizational methods, such as use of folders or sectioned files, and she could not describe how

to organize her locker. In collaboration with the TVI, the school occupational therapy practitioner addressed organizational systems such as use of binder clips, Braille dividers and files, and Braille labels for her locker shelf.

High school (transition) intervention. Sam was 16 and had albinism, with an acuity of 20/200. As he and his team prepared for his transition from high school, Sam had not yet identified a career path, although he knew he wanted to go to college. The school occupational therapist assisted by introducing interest inventories and, in collaboration with the family, COMS, and TVI, helped identify community volunteer opportunities that would allow Sam to explore his interests. The COMS addressed Sam's ability to get to his volunteer site independently, and the TVI addressed his need for AT on the site.

These scenarios are small examples of the ways in which the school occupational therapist and occupational therapy assistant (in collaboration with the therapist) may be involved in addressing issues of engagement in school occupations with students who have visual impairments.

Address social participation

Social participation is an area that affects and is affected by all other areas. Many educators advocate social skills instruction for this population because visual impairment may prevent a student from learning skills that their typically sighted peers learn incidentally through vision (Wolffe, 2006). A student with visual impairment may need instruction in nonverbal communication, how to initiate and maintain friendships, and how to access social information (e.g., determining what styles of dress or hair are fashionable), transportation options (particularly when typically sighted peers are learning to drive), and soft skills that affect obtaining and maintaining employment (Celeste, 2006; Sacks & Wolffe, 2006).

Address nonverbal communication. Students with visual impairment may not notice or accurately interpret others' facial expressions and gestures. In addition, they may not be aware of what their own body language communicates. For example, Linda, a 13-year-old with severe visual impairment, often maintained a downward head tilt during class. She knew that her teacher sounded irritated with her but did not understand why. The teacher mentioned to the occupational therapy practitioner working with Linda that she kept her head down and was not paying attention in class. Linda was surprised to learn why her teacher was upset. The occupational therapy practitioner worked with Linda on monitoring her head position and understanding the implications of turning toward or away from the person speaking. Linda noticed that when she practiced these skills, her teachers and peers responded to her more positively.

In another scenario, Liam, a 17-year-old with congenital blindness, was amused to learn that his peers with typical vision often used hand and arm gestures when speaking and that this helped others maintain interest. Because he wanted to do as well as possible on his debate team, with occupational therapy support he asked his coach to show him how and when to make effective gestures.

Address how to initiate and maintain friendships.
Students with visual impairment may have difficulty understanding social distances, judging the best time to join a group, taking others' perspectives, or determining how to make small talk. Mara, 14 and totally blind, often stood near groups of typically sighted peers as they were seated at lunch. She would smile when jokes were made, yet she would never speak to the group. Her peers did not understand what Mara wanted and were uncomfortable with her standing nearby.

The occupational therapy practitioner, in collaboration with the TVI and COMS, worked with Mara on knowing when the group was approachable (e.g., lulls in conversation), knowing where to stand, and coming up with opening lines to enter the conversation. In addition, the educational team in collaboration with the occupational therapist organized a weekly lunch group with the peers and Mara and facilitated social interactions and exchange of information. The peers began greeting her and inviting her to join them when she entered the cafeteria.

Address accessing social information and obtaining transportation. Students with visual impairments may not be aware of trends in makeup, clothing, or movement (e.g., the way a student smooths clothing when sitting, the way a student "fist dabs"). They may not be aware of "hot" topics, may miss information about social events on fliers, and may have difficulty traveling to events after school. Joe, age 17, who had a progressive eye condition, was told about a party at a peer's home but could not drive. He did not want to ask his parents to take him because it embarrassed him. He was also worried about asking for rides from his friends too often. With his occupational therapy practitioner and COMS, Joe discussed alternatives and decided that he could offer to pay gas money in return for rides, arrange a door-to-door car service with his family's permission, and work more on community travel with his COMS.

Address development of soft skills. **Soft skills** include communication, accountability, problem solving, and team participation, among others. Eddie, age 12 years and with low vision, was embarrassed to use his optical devices (i.e., magnifier and telescope) in class because he felt it made him different. As a result, he did not see an assignment due date on the board, missed the deadline, and received a low grade. His occupational therapist and TVI worked with him on ways to disclose his disability to his teacher and peers, on educating his peers about his optical devices (most wanted to try them out), and on problem-solving ways to ensure he had assignment information when he did not use available adaptations. The TVI arranged for Eddie to meet an adult who used optical devices at his job. The occupational therapist and TVI also worked with the classroom teacher on requiring Eddie to meet deadlines and to allow him to experience natural consequences (she felt guilty giving him a low grade) when he did not use available adaptations or request assistance.

When preparing students for adulthood, school occupational therapy practitioners in partnership with others on the educational team focus on students acquiring skills for "further education, employment and independent living" (IDEA, 2004, §1400[d][1][A]). Wolffe and Kelly (2011)

found that instruction in an expanded core curriculum, particularly career education and instruction in social skills, correlated positively with employment after graduation. Other predictors of successful transition or employment include having multiple jobs, finding one's own job (rather than relying on school personnel), having good orientation and mobility skills, demonstrating academic competence, and using social skills (Botsford, 2013; Cmar, 2015; Connors et al., 2014; McDonnall, 2011; McDonnall & Crudden, 2009; McDonnall & O'Mally, 2012).

SUMMARY

Challenges to participation for students who have visual impairments have been identified through research in other fields as well as occupational therapy. Limited research currently exists on occupational therapy's role and contributions to the success of students with visual impairments in school outcomes. Establishing an evidence base for interventions will help demonstrate the distinct value of occupational therapy for students with visual impairments. Best practices indicate that school occupational therapy practitioners should focus on access, participation, and school performance.

REFERENCES

Allman, C., & Lewis, S. (2014). *ECC essentials—Teaching the expanded core curriculum to students with visual impairments.* New York: AFB Press.

American Occupational Therapy Association. (2014a). Guidelines for supervision, roles, and responsibilities during the delivery of occupational therapy services. *American Journal of Occupational Therapy, 68*(Suppl. 3), S16–S22. https://doi.org/10.5014/ajot.2014.686S03

American Occupational Therapy Association. (2014b). Occupational therapy practice framework: Domain and process (3rd ed.). *American Journal of Occupational Therapy, 68*(Suppl. 1), S1–S48. https://doi.org/10.5014/ajot.2014.682006

American Printing House for the Blind. (n.d.). *What is federal quota?* Retrieved from http://www.aph.org/federal-quota/what-is-federal-quota/

American Printing House for the Blind. (2017). *2017 annual report, fiscal year October 1, 2016–September 30, 2017.* Retrieved from https://www.aph.org/files/annual-reports/APH-Annual-Report-FY17.pdf

Baker-Nobles, L., & Rutherford, A. (1995). Understanding cortical visual impairment in children. *American Journal of Occupational Therapy, 49,* 899–903. https://doi.org/10.5014/ajot.49.9.899

Bambring, M. (2006). Divergent development of gross motor skills in children who are blind or sighted. *Journal of Visual Impairment and Blindness, 100,* 620–634. Retrieved from https://www.afb.org/jvib/newjvibabstract.asp?articleid=jvib001008

Botsford, K. D. (2013). Social skills for youths with visual impairment: A meta-analysis. *Journal of Visual Impairment and Blindness, 107,* 497–508. Retrieved from https://www.afb.org/jvib/Newjvibabstract.asp?articleid=jvib070610

Celeste, M. (2006). Play behaviors and social interactions of a child who is blind: On theory and practice. *Journal of Visual Impairment and Blindness, 100,* 75–90. Retrieved from https://www.afb.org/afbpress/newpubjvib.asp?DocID=jvib960305

Cmar, J. L. (2015). Orientation and mobility skills and outcome expectations as predictors of employment for young adults with visual impairments. *Journal of Visual Impairment and Blindness, 109*, 95–106. Retrieved from https://www.afb.org/afbpress/newpubjvib.asp?DocID=jvib090204

Cohen-Maitre, S. A., & Haerich, P. (2005). Visual attention to movement and color in children with cortical visual impairment. *Journal of Visual Impairment and Blindness, 99*, 478–485. Retrieved from https://www.afb.org/afbpress/newpubjvib.asp?DocID=jvib990702

Connors, E., Curtis, A., Wall Emerson, R., & Dormitorio, B. (2014). Longitudinal analysis of factors associated with successful outcomes for transition-age youths with visual impairment. *Journal of Visual Impairment and Blindness, 108*, 95–106. Retrieved from https://www.afb.org/afbpress/newpubjvib.asp?DocID=jvib080202

Coster, W., Deeny, T. A., Haltiwanger, J. T., & Haley, S. M. (1998). *School Function Assessment: User's manual*. San Antonio: Therapy Skill Builders.

Engel-Yeager, B., & Hamed-Dahmer, S. (2013). Comparing participation in out of school activities between children with visual impairments, children with hearing impairments, and typical peers. *Research in Developmental Disabilities, 34*, 3124–3132. Retrieved from https://doi.org/10.1016/j.ridd.2013.05.049

Erin, J. (2006). Teaching social skills to elementary and middle school students with visual impairments. In S. Z. Sacks & K. E. Wolffe (Eds.), *Teaching social skills to students with visual impairments: From theory to practice* (pp. 364–404). New York: AFB Press.

Fazzi, D. L., & Klein, M. D. (2002). Cognitive focus: Developing cognition, concepts, and language. In R. L. Pogrund & D. L. Fazzi (Eds.), *Early focus: Working with young children who are blind or visually impaired and their families* (2nd ed., pp. 107–153). New York: AFB Press.

Ferreira, V., & Albuquerque, C. P. (2017). Adaptation of a developmental test to accommodate young children with low vision. *Journal of Visual Impairment and Blindness, 111*, 97–111. Retrieved from https://www.afb.org/afbpress/newpubjvib.asp?DocID=jvib110202

Ferrell, K. A., Bruce, S., & Luckner, J. (2014). *Evidence-based practices for students with sensory impairments*. Retrieved from http://ceedar.education.ufl.edu/tools/innovation-configurations

Ferziger, N. (2017). Assessment of gaze responses of children with cerebral palsy and cerebral visual impairment: Implementation of a computerized video coding system. *American Journal of Occupational Therapy, 71*, 7111500021. https://doi.org/10.5014/ajot.2017.71S1-PO1138

Gold, D., Shaw, A., & Wolffe, K. E. (2010). The social lives of Canadian youths with visual impairments. *Journal of Visual Impairment and Blindness, 104*, 431–443. Retrieved from https://www.afb.org/afbpress/newpubjvib.asp?DocID=jvib040706

Huebner, K. M., Merk-Adam, B., Stryker, D., & Wolffe, K. (2004). *The national agenda for the education of children and youths with visual impairment, including those with multiple disabilities*. Retrieved from http://www.afb.org/info/national-agenda-for-education/importance-of-the-goals/25

Individuals With Disabilities Education Improvement Act of 2004, Pub. L. 108–446, 20 U.S.C. §§ 1400–1482.

James, D. M., & Stojanovik, V. (2007). Communication skills in blind children: A preliminary investigation. *Child: Care, Health and Development, 33*, 4–10. https://doi.org/10.1111/j.1365-2214.2006.00621.x

Jessup, G., Bundy, A., Broom, A., & Hancock, N. (2017). The social experiences of high school students with visual impairments. *Journal of Visual Impairment and Blindness, 111*, 5–19. Retrieved from https://www.afb.org/afbpress/newpubjvib.asp?DocID=jvib110102

Kroksmark, U., & Nordell, K. (2001). Adolescence: The age of opportunities and obstacles for students with low vision in Sweden. *Journal of Visual Impairment and Blindness, 95*, 213–225. Retrieved from https://www.afb.org/jvib/newjvibabstract.asp?articleid=JVIB950403

Lampert, J. (2016). *Social participation perspectives: The lived experiences of adolescents who have visual impairments* (Doctoral dissertation). Retrieved from https://twu-ir.tdl.org/twu-ir/handle/11274/8309

Law, M., Baptiste, S., Carswell, A., McColl, M. A., Polatajko, H., & Pollock, N. (2014). *Canadian Occupational Performance Measure* (5th ed.). Ottawa: CAOT Publications.

Lueck, A. H., & Dutton, G. N. (Eds.). (2015). *Vision and the brain: Understanding cerebral visual impairment in children*. New York: AFB Press.

McDonnall, M. C. (2011). Predictors of employment for youths with visual impairments: Findings from the Second National Longitudinal Transition Study. *Journal of Visual Impairment and Blindness, 105*, 453–466. Retrieved from https://www.afb.org/jvib/Newjvibabstract.asp?articleid=jvib050802

McDonnall, M. C., & Crudden, A. (2009). Factors affecting the successful employment of transition-age youths with visual impairments. *Journal of Visual Impairment and Blindness, 103*, 329–341. Retrieved from https://www.afb.org/jvib/newjvibabstract.asp?articleid=jvib030603

McDonnall, M. C., & O'Mally, J. (2012). Characteristics of early work experiences and their association with future employment. *Journal of Visual Impairment and Blindness, 106*, 133–144. Retrieved from https://www.afb.org/afbpress/newpubjvib.asp?DocID=jvib060302

Newman, L., Wagner, M., Knokey, A.-M., Marder, C., Nagle, K., Shaver, D., & Wei, X. (2011). *The post-high school outcomes of young adults with disabilities up to 8 years after high school: A report from the National Longitudinal Transition Study–2* (NCSER 2011-3005). Retrieved from https://ies.ed.gov/ncser/pubs/20113005/pdf/20113005.pdf

Office of Special Education and Rehabilitation Services. (2017). *Memorandum: Eligibility determinations for children suspected of having a visual impairment including blindness under the Individuals With Disabilities Education Act*. Retrieved from https://sites.ed.gov/idea/files/letter-on-visual-impairment-5-22-17.pdf

Pinquart, M., & Pfeiffer, J. P. (2013). Perceived social support in adolescents with and without visual impairment. *Research in Developmental Disabilities, 34*, 4125–4133. https://doi.org/10.1016/j.ridd.2013.08.004

Roman-Lantzy, C. (2007). *Cortical visual impairment: An approach to assessment and intervention*. New York: AFB Press.

Ryan-Bloomer, K., Detten, L., Mahoney, A., McCue, A., McNamara, K., Gerstenkorn, A., & Bundy, A. (2016). Play and playfulness in older children with visual impairment: A mixed-method study. *American Journal of Occupational Therapy, 70*, 7011505100. https://doi.org/10.5014/ajot.2016.70S1-PO1046

Sacks, S. Z., & Wolffe, K. E. (2006). *Teaching social skills to students with visual impairments: From theory to practice*. New York: AFB Press.

Salminen, A. L., & Karhula, M. E. (2014). Young persons with visual impairment: Challenges of participation. *Scandinavian Journal of*

Occupational Therapy, 21, 267–276. https://doi.org/10.3109/110 38128.2014.899622

Shaw, A., Gold, D., & Wolffe, K. E. (2007). Employment-related experiences of youths who are visually impaired: How are these youths faring? *Journal of Visual Impairment and Blindness, 101,* 7–21. Retrieved from https://www.afb.org/jvib/newjvibabstract .asp?articleid=jvib010103

Tadíc, L., Pring, L., & Dale, N. (2010). Are language and social communication intact in children with congenital visual impairment at school age? *Journal of Child Psychology and Psychiatry, 51,* 696–705. https://doi.org/10.1111/j.1469-7610.2009.02200.x

Tsai, L.-T., Hsu, J. L., Wu, C.-T., Chen, C.-C., & Su, Y.-C. (2016). A new vision simulation program for improving visual acuity in children with visual impairment. *Frontiers in Human Neuroscience, 10.* https://doi.org/10.3389/fnhum.2016.00157

Tsai, L.-T., Meng, L. F., Wu, W. C., Jang, Y., & Su, Y.-C. (2013). Effect of visual rehabilitation on a child with severe visual impairment. *American Journal of Occupational Therapy, 67,* 437–447. https:// doi.org/19.5014/ajot.2013.007054

Uysal, S. A., & Düger, T. (2012). Visual perception training on social skills and activity performance in low-vision children. *Scandinavian Journal of Occupational Therapy, 19,* 33–41. https://doi.org/10 .3109/11038128.2011.582512

Visser, L., Ruiter, S. A. J., Van der Meulen, B. F., Ruijssenaars, W. A. J. J. M., & Timmerman, M. E. (2012). A review of standardized developmental assessment instruments for young children and their applicability for children with social needs. *Journal of Cognitive Education and Psychology, 11,* 102–127. https://doi .org/10.1891/1945-8959.11.2.102

Wolffe, K. E. (2006). Teaching social skills to adolescents and young adults with visual impairments. In S. Z. Sacks & K. E. Wolffe (Eds.), *Teaching social skills to students with visual impairments: From theory to practice* (pp. 405–440). New York: AFB Press.

Wolffe, K. E., & Kelly, S. M. (2011). Instructions in areas of the expanded core curriculum linked to transition outcomes for students with visual impairments. *Journal of Visual Impairment and Blindness, 105,* 340–349. https://www.afb.org/afbpress/new pubjvib.asp?DocID=jvib050605

SECTION IV.

Evidence-Guided Practices: Service-Level Considerations to Support Participation

Best Practices in School Occupational Therapy Evaluation and Planning to Support Participation

40

Gloria Frolek Clark, PhD, OTR/L, BCP, SCSS, FAOTA, and Joyce E. Rioux, EdD, OTR/L, SCSS

KEY TERMS AND CONCEPTS

- Analysis of occupational performance
- Assessment
- Child Find
- Evaluation
- Multi-tiered systems of support
- Occupational profile
- Screening
- Strengths-based approach
- Student-centered approach
- Synthesis
- Top-down approach

OVERVIEW

All occupational therapy evaluations should identify the student's strengths and needs regarding access and participation in their educational program. Such an evaluation requires school occupational therapists[1] to apply their professional knowledge and skills with best-practice evaluation processes to gather meaningful information and assist education teams in determining educationally relevant and necessary programming for students.

Evaluations can vary in complexity. Students may be receiving general education instruction in addition to having a 504 plan or an individualized education program (IEP). They may have learning challenges, physical disabilities, behavior disabilities, developmental delays, or health and wellness concerns that affect their engagement in meaningful and important student occupations. Considering these multilayered components, school occupational therapists need to understand their role in evaluating students in educational systems, follow guiding principles for occupational therapy based on laws and standards of practice, and remain occupation centered.

ESSENTIAL CONSIDERATIONS

In the educational setting, an occupational therapy screening or evaluation is often requested to identify the barriers and facilitators that affect a student's access to and participation in relevant and necessary school occupations (e.g., academics, functional life skills, extracurricular activities,

postsecondary preparation). Whether conducting an evaluation or screening, the occupational therapist needs to understand and adhere to state regulatory acts (e.g., licensure), professional standards, and education laws.

Terminology: *Assessment* or *Evaluation*

The term *assessment* is often incorrectly used interchangeably with *evaluation*. **Evaluation** refers to the process used to obtain and interpret data required for intervention (American Occupational Therapy Association [AOTA], 2015b) and is directed toward identifying the student's strengths and needs to participate in school and perform academic and nonacademic activities. **Assessment** refers to a specific tool or measure used during the evaluation process (AOTA, 2015b). Administering an assessment should never be interpreted as conducting an evaluation.

Requests for Occupational Therapy Screening or Evaluation

A screening under early intervening services may be requested for students in general education under multi-tiered systems of support (MTSS). Evaluations may be requested to determine whether the student is eligible for services and accommodations under Section 504 of the Rehabilitation Act of 1973, as amended (2008; Pub. L. 93–112), or whether a student is eligible for special education and related services (e.g., occupational therapy) under the Individuals With Disabilities Education Improvement Act of 2004 (IDEA; Pub. L. 108–446). Under each law, the role and focus of the occupational therapist would be different (see Table 40.1).

Multi-tiered systems of support

When the school district uses **MTSS**—an education initiative prioritized by the Every Student Succeeds Act (2015; Pub. L. 114–95) to target support for struggling students in general education—the focus of screening is to identify

---

[1]The term *occupational therapist* is used throughout this chapter on evaluation because the occupational therapist must be directly involved in services during the initial occupational therapy evaluation process. An occupational therapy assistant may assist under the supervision of and in partnership with the occupational therapist. See Chapter 7, "Best Practices for Occupational Therapy Assistants in Schools."

Copyright © 2019 by the American Occupational Therapy Association. All rights reserved. To reuse this content, contact www.copyright.com.
https://doi.org/10.7139/2019.978-1-56900-591-0.040

TABLE 40.1.   Various Evaluation Roles of the Occupational Therapist

LAW	OCCUPATIONAL THERAPIST'S ROLE AND FOCUS
ESSA	*Specialized instructional support personnel:* Assist in program evaluation to provide insights into strengthening education for all students.
IDEA—early intervening services (MTSS)	*Consultant:* Assist with selection or administration of universal screenings or conduct an individual screening to determine student-specific instructional strategies that others implement in general education.
	Service provider (in states that allow student-specific prereferral activities): Analyze research to practice to determine appropriate interventions, strategies, or both to enhance general education performance.
IDEA—initial evaluations and reevaluations	*Educational team member and service provider:* Provide input in determining whether the student is a student with an educational disability and requires special education and related services, identifying the student's present level of performance in academic and nonacademic areas and developing or revising a student's IEP on the basis of the results of the occupational therapy evaluation.
Section 504	*Building team member and service provider:* Gather information, administer assessments when necessary, and contribute to the determination of whether a student suspected of having a disability has equal opportunity to participate in academic, nonacademic, and extracurricular activities similar to peers who are nondisabled.

Note. May vary depending on state licensure acts or state regulations. ESSA = Every Student Succeeds Act; IDEA = Individuals With Disabilities Education Improvement Act of 2004; IEP = individualized education program; MTSS = multi-tiered systems of support.

students at risk. As described by IDEA (2004), a ***screening*** is used "to determine appropriate instructional strategies for curriculum implementation" (§ 1414[1][E]). Screening may include universal (classroom wide) or individual screenings.

Universal screenings. As part of MTSS, universal screenings help to identify students at risk for learning difficulties (e.g., math, reading, behavior). As the term *universal* implies, all students are screened, although a parent may opt their child out of the screening process in accordance with procedures established under the Protection of Pupil Rights Amendment of 1978 (20 U.S.C. § 1232h; 34 C.F.R. Part 98). In some systems, an occupational therapist's expertise may be sought to assist in selecting or administering a universal screening tool as part of a larger team (e.g., behavioral and mental health screening).

Individual screenings. Individual screenings are student specific. Some states may have established procedures for obtaining parental consent to conduct an individual screening with a student. Either way, best practice is for the person requesting the screening to contact a parent to obtain their consent before the occupational therapist conducts the screening. The purpose of an individual screening is to identify individualized instructional strategies that can be implemented by the teacher or other school staff. At no time would a screening be used to determine eligibility for special education or the need for related services (IDEA, 2004). Occupational therapists working in schools must realize that IDEA uses the term *screen* to describe actions done for the intention of enhancing general education instructional strategies (for more information, see Chapter 26, "Best Practices in Multi-Tiered Systems of Support").

Child Find and full and individual initial evaluations

Child Find is the part of IDEA (2004) that requires states to find and evaluate children to determine if they are a child

with disabilities. Child Find procedures require that when students are suspected of having an educational disability, they must receive a full and individual initial evaluation (34 C.F.R., § 300.111[c][1]). Child Find's focus is to determine a student's eligibility for special education and need for related services.

Once set procedures have been followed to obtain informed written consent from the parent or legal guardian, a full and individual initial evaluation can be conducted. The evaluation must examine "all areas related to the suspected disability including, if appropriate, health, vision, hearing, social and emotional status, general intelligence, academic performance, communicative status, and motor abilities" (IDEA, 2004, 34 C.F.R. § 300.304). In addition, the evaluation must be individualized to the particular student. Results from the evaluations will help the team determine whether the student meets both of these factors required for eligibility for special education: The student

- Has an educational disability that adversely affects their participation and performance in general education and
- Needs special education and possibly related services.

Once a student has met eligibility requirements, teams determine whether related services (e.g., occupational therapy) are needed. There are no additional federal requirements for eligibility for related services.

To assist the team in determining a student's eligibility for special education and need for related services, the occupational therapist is responsible for identifying supports or barriers related to performance and participation in occupations (e.g., educational performance, daily life skills, play, leisure, rest, social interaction) across all settings (e.g., classroom, playground, bathroom, hallway). The occupational therapist should inquire about all areas related to the student's occupational performance, at least during an interview and possibly further, through observation and test administration based on identified concerns.

In addition to identifying the student's performance strengths and difficulties within and across school settings, the evaluation should examine contextual factors (e.g., cultural, personal, temporal, virtual). Observing a student in natural contexts may uncover potential opportunities and barriers to educational access or optimal performance. These factors will be relevant in developing an effective IEP.

Section 504

Sometimes a student has a medical condition or suspected disability that adversely affects their participation and performance in general education, but the student does not require specialized instruction. For example, a student with cerebral palsy may require a computer to complete written work, or a student with attention deficit disorder may need a quiet setting to take a quiz. The occupational therapist may be a member of the building-level team to identify necessary services, modifications, and accommodations so students can participate in the general education program.

Instruction, Curriculum, Environment, and the Student

Applying an occupation-centered approach to evaluation, occupational therapists need to examine the interplay of the instruction and curriculum expectations, the environmental demands, and a learner's skills (referred to as *ICEL*).

> *Instruction* refers to how the content is taught, *curriculum* refers to what content is taught, *environment* refers to the context and conditions for learning, and *learner* refers to the student's unique capacities and traits. The learner is listed last on purpose; if the first three domains are "just right," the learner will learn. (Frolek Clark et al., 2015, p. 12, *italics added*)

Using a top-down, student-centered, strengths-based approach aligns with the core philosophy of IDEA, Section 504, and MTSS and promotes an occupation-centered evaluation. By understanding the expectations and peer performance in a classroom, the occupational therapist is able to identify supports for or barriers to learning and participation. For example, a kindergarten teacher who is frustrated because many students cannot cut a 1-inch picture box may welcome a simple suggestion to enlarge the sheet. With the boxes enlarged, more students may be successful and independently complete the task.

Engaging Parents

IDEA identifies parents (or legal guardians) as part of the IEP team; therefore, facilitating parent involvement early in the evaluation process is important. Parents are the experts on their child and may have information about health issues or concerns that no one may have asked about, yet are critical for decision making. For example, while interviewing the parent, an occupational therapist discovers that the child who becomes aggressive during prereading and fine motor activities fell out of a window at age 2 years and fractured his skull; by calling a parent to inquire about a child's handwriting, which has become progressively worse, the occupational therapy assistant learns that the parent was recently diagnosed with cancer; or the parent shares through an interview that the student with attention

challenges has been talking about killing himself. Therapists should respect the parent's role as a vital member of the student's team.

Handling Team Issues

At times, conflicts arise—including inappropriate evaluation referrals, late referrals, or recommendation for occupational therapy services without an evaluation. The school occupational therapist needs to be well versed in laws, procedures, and best practices to address conflicts as they arise.

Inappropriate referrals

Appropriate referrals to occupational therapy should include both of the following components:
- The identified concern is interfering with the student's ability to participate in their educational program (e.g., academic, functional, extracurricular).
- The identified concern is within the role or domain of the school occupational therapist.

Parents, school staff, the educational team, or others may initiate a referral for an occupational therapy evaluation. If there is no evidence of adverse effect on the student's educational day or if the area appears to be the domain of another professional, this should be discussed with the person making the referral. When the referral is declined for lack of evidence, this determination must be formally documented.

For example, the parents whose child experienced difficulty completing fine motor work contacted the school to request an occupational therapy evaluation. During a meeting with the parents to discuss their concerns, the classroom teacher shared that the student finished his work on Scout days when he needed to leave school early but not on other days. Because the student had the skills to finish his work but lacked the motivation to complete his work on some days, the school psychologist offered to investigate further with the teacher, and the parents agreed. This was documented on the parent notice form (giving them notice that the occupational therapy evaluation would not occur as well as the reason for the decline).

In some instances, the identified concern may already be the target of an IEP goal and is being addressed through specialized instruction. Referrals should never be generated solely on the basis of a medical diagnosis or educational classification. The presence of a negative effect of the medical or educational condition on the student's educational program should always be the primary consideration when referring the student for an occupational therapy evaluation.

IDEA specifically lists exclusionary factors for considering eligibility for special education services. These factors include lack of instruction in an area (reading and math are specifically stated in the law) and limited English proficiency (IDEA, 2004, § 1414[b][5][A]). Evaluating students to determine whether they need special education without first providing them specific instruction in that area is not appropriate. For example, a student whose school does not have handwriting instruction may have illegible handwriting because of a lack of instruction. That is not a special education issue; it is an instruction issue. The occupational therapist must be aware of the student's curriculum, instruction, and attempts to enhance performance before making any recommendations for services.

When a school uses MTSS, the occupational therapist may apply this approach by monitoring the student's performance during short-term interventions (i.e., provided by school staff or the occupational therapist, when applicable). Data obtained on the student's performance should inform whether an occupational therapy evaluation is needed.

Late referrals

IDEA requires the IEP to be completed within 60 calendar days (state timelines may vary) from the date the parent signed consent for evaluation. During this time, team members may determine that the occupational therapist should also evaluate the student. This is not an issue when there is sufficient time; however, when there is not sufficient time or significant people are unavailable, the evaluation may not be adequately completed.

The IEP meeting must be held; the occupational therapist should attend to gather and share information but may have to decline determining service needs until the evaluation is fully completed. This will require gathering the team at a later date; unfortunately, that is the consequence of late referrals. This may be a learning opportunity for the team to contact the occupational therapist earlier in the process.

Teams recommending occupational therapy services without an evaluation by an occupational therapist

An IEP team determines the student's needs, goals, and services. When the team is discussing occupational therapy services, IDEA requires that the therapist attend or notify the family and school before the meeting. The parents and local educational agency (LEA) staff must consent to the excusal of the occupational therapist, and the therapist must submit input in writing for the development of the IEP before the meeting (IDEA, 2004, § 1414[d][1][C]). If a team records occupational therapy as a service on a student's IEP without the knowledge of an occupational therapist, then the team is not following IDEA requirements for team members in attendance (§ 1414[d][1][C]).

In addition, state occupational therapy regulatory acts and professional standards (AOTA, 2015b) require an occupational therapist to conduct an evaluation and determine the need for occupational therapy intervention before providing services. Occupational therapy services outlined in a student's IEP without a prior evaluation of that student should be disregarded because they are out of compliance with state and federal laws. Immediate steps to correct the situation should be discussed with the student's case manager.

BEST PRACTICES

Occupational therapists must use multiple methods of data collection during the evaluation process. These data should focus on the student's access, engagement, and participation in the educational program. This section provides an operational approach for conducting evaluations that applies AOTA's (2014) *Occupational Therapy Practice Framework: Domain and Process* (3rd ed.; *OTPF–3*), state practice act requirements, educational law requirements, and best practices in schools.

Plan the Evaluation

Taking the time to ensure that proper procedures have been followed, understanding the referral request, preplanning the approach to gather information, and scheduling the various components at the onset of referral will put the evaluation on the proper course. Gather information about the student's performance so that suggestions can be made to the team regarding curriculum (what the student needs to learn), instruction (how the student should be taught), and environment (physical and social aspects of the environment to enhance learning).

Receive the referral

Referrals may be made by anyone, so the occupational therapist must identify the source of the referral, the presenting concern(s), and prior attempts to alleviate the problem. In addition, the occupational therapist should identify whether the process followed the expected procedures and that a signed consent to evaluate was obtained from the parent or guardian. When expected procedures are not followed, the administrator should be informed immediately so that action steps can be determined.

Establish clear reasons for referral

An evaluation is more likely to yield valid and useful information when it is directed to answer specific questions about the student's participation and performance. Questions should begin with a broad focus and include multiple settings:
- How is this student participating in the major school activity settings?
- How is this student performing routine school activities (e.g., self-care, play or leisure, interactions with others, academics, extracurricular activities)?
- What aspects of the environment pose challenges for access or performance?

Preplan your approach

Once the questions are established, the occupational therapist will need to determine the best approach to gathering meaningful information.

Top-down. A ***top-down approach*** means that concerns are initially defined at a broad level in relation to the student's engagement in important and meaningful school occupations (Coster, 1998). The critical roles that the student is required to fulfill, the activities and occupations in which the student needs to engage, and the context in which the student needs to participate are identified. In addition, those areas that facilitate or impede the student's participation are gathered before determining whether assessment tools need to be administered to answer the referral questions.

Student-centered. A ***student-centered approach*** values and respects the student's priorities. This approach is a core principle of occupational therapy practice. In schools, although most information is gathered from adults in the student's environment, the student's perspective should also be considered as part of the evaluation process. Students may offer insight into behaviors that have puzzled others or an alternative explanation that could be helpful in suggesting intervention approaches. For example, a student may explain that he gets confused and anxious when the teacher gives "too much information," clarifying why he often starts fiddling in his desk when instructions are given.

Strengths-based. Increasingly, authors in many disciplines have advocated a shift from a problem-focused to a strengths-based approach to evaluation and intervention (Dunn et al., 2013; King, 2009; Morris & Hollenbeck, 2016), a position that is consistent with a collaborative student-centered approach. A *strengths-based approach* requires that the evaluation systematically search out the student's and context's assets and resources so that they can be maximally used to accomplish desired changes. This may include asking the student how they have solved other problems or challenges or asking for an example of something they can do well. It may also include careful observation in the classroom to identify potential resources and supports, such as a peer who positively interacts with the student.

Schedule to collect data

A comprehensive evaluation must include multiple data sources (IDEA, 2004; Section 504, 2008). These data sources should include record review, interview, observation, and, when necessary, assessments. At the planning stage, begin to consider what information will be sought from these data sources, who needs to be interviewed, where and when observations need to take place, how long different components may require, and what assessments may provide meaningful data to answer the referral questions. Schedule time to accomplish each of these tasks with respect to the evaluation timeline.

Conduct the Evaluation

The occupational therapy evaluation process recommended by AOTA (2014) begins with the development of the occupational profile and proceeds to the analysis of occupational performance.

Develop the occupational profile

As applied in the school setting, the *occupational profile* is a summary of the student's school history and experiences, medical history, performance skills and patterns, interests, values, and perceived needs. Information is gathered from the student's perspective when appropriate and from members of the student's educational team, including the student's family. This information gathering can be achieved through record review and formal or informal interviews. Information gathered from the occupational profile may shape and target the next steps of the evaluation process, that is, analysis of occupational performance. AOTA (2017) has published an occupational profile template that can be used and examples that can be referred to during this process (see Appendix B, "AOTA Occupational Profile Template").

Review records. A review of a student's education file often provides information pertaining to the student's school history (e.g., grades, attendance, disciplinary referrals, previous evaluations; Frolek Clark et al., 2015). Additional records to review might include the student's health file, classroom portfolio, report cards, and grade standards. Record reviews can be done before observation to help sharpen the therapist's focus on when and what to observe or afterward to promote an unbiased observation.

Regardless of the timing, a record review provides important information, such as an overall history of the student (e.g., changed schools multiple times, significant medical history, received prior services); an overview of school performance to date, which may show changes in performance across time; and summaries from previous assessments, which may be useful in suggesting areas to reevaluate or compare with current performance.

Interview. An interview, whether with the teacher, classroom assistant, school personnel, family, or, when appropriate, the student, provides information that is otherwise difficult to obtain, particularly in understanding student performance over time. The occupational therapist should inquire and document information about ADLs, play and leisure, and social participation in addition to classroom performance at least during an interview and specifically as part of the full evaluation when concerns are present. This information can direct the evaluation process toward appropriate areas and may provide insight that is highly relevant to interpretation of findings and intervention design. An interview with the student's teacher may reveal critical concerns, identify strategies that have been tried, or discern student behaviors that are consistent or seem to vary. Parents may provide insight into their child that the rest of the educational team may not be able to.

When conducting an interview, a positive approach is preferred, emphasizing that the interviewee is the expert on the student. The purpose of the interview is to gain perspectives into how the student learns, gets along with other children, and solves problems. The use of open-ended questions should result in rich information. Questions or prompts might include "What things help or make it harder for this student to participate in a specific classroom activity?" or "Think of a time when this student faced a challenge, and tell me how they handled it."

Analyze occupational performance

Analysis of occupational performance is the examination of the dynamic interaction among the student's presenting abilities, the learning or activity expectations, and the environmental demands. Authentic data can be obtained through observation and combined with data obtained through record review and interviews to better understand the student's engagement in school occupations. Through observation and, when necessary, administration of assessment tools, the occupational therapist can gather important and meaningful information to answer the referral questions developed at the beginning of the process.

Observe the student. In accordance with IDEA (2004), students must be observed in the area of suspected difficulty to get a sense of the multiple factors that may play a role in the student's challenges as well as strengths that the student may display in other areas. Observing students in settings in which they are also successful may be helpful in capturing a holistic picture. Occupational therapists use formal (i.e., planned) and informal (i.e., incidental) observations to analyze the student's performance in the environment and context to identify supports and constraints for learning and performance (AOTA, 2015a).

Observation of students in their natural context involves recording the person, environment, and task or occupation features that describe the situation and help clarify how the student's behavior is both similar to and different from that of peers. One way to organize this process is around three key questions:

1. What are students supposed to be doing (i.e., occupation focus)?
2. What are other students doing, and what is this student doing (i.e., person focus)?
3. What factors in the environment support or challenge the student's performance (i.e., environment focus)?

Comparing the student with peers may be documented through qualitative data (e.g., "appeared to move around the room while others were working") or quantitative data (e.g., "student worked for 1 minute before leaving chair, peers worked for 10 minutes before putting their work away"). Activity analysis within the observation allows therapists to consider the classroom instruction and curriculum. How were instructions and expectations presented to the class? Were any additional supports for understanding provided (e.g., written instructions, visual cues)? How structured is the work environment? How is expected or unexpected behavior addressed?

Structuring observations to capture quantitative data (i.e., measurements that are counted or timed) can create a clear description of a student's performance in context. In addition, these data can serve as a baseline against which progress can be measured should intervention be provided. For example, an occupational therapist may record the number of seconds a student remains engaged in a fine motor activity. Another example is to calculate the number of times over opportunities a student completed classroom work in a day (for more information, see Chapter 45, "Best Practices in School Occupational Therapy Documentation and Data Collection").

Select assessment tools. As the occupational therapist gathers data, the therapist begins to formulate hypotheses about factors that are likely to be contributing to problems. Ideally, these hypotheses are grounded in theory and knowledge of current evidence. For example, current evidence linking discrete hand skills or particular pencil grips to handwriting quality is not very strong (Schwellnus et al., 2012). An occupational therapist aware of this evidence would consider alternative explanations for observed difficulties and would, in turn, look for assessment tools that could be used to test the alternative hypotheses.

IDEA (2004), the *OTPF–3* (AOTA, 2014), and test publications outline specific components that must be followed when administering assessments:

- The selection and administration of nondiscriminatory assessments must be conducted in the student's primary language to yield accurate and unbiased information.
- The evaluator must have the qualifications, experience, and competence to administer the selected assessment measure.
- Selected tools must be technically sound and administered so results are valid and reliable.
- The results of a single assessment tool or method should be interpreted with caution and not used as the sole determining factor for decision making.

When selecting assessments, the occupational therapist should consider tools to identify supports and barriers to a student's participation in learning and school activities. Assessment tools—particularly those grounded in occupation—allow the examiner to apply professional reasoning and theoretical concepts to understand a student's current occupational strengths and participation challenges. These tools often provide insight into how and why a student engages in activities. Criterion-referenced tools are designed to examine a student's performance in relation to set criteria. Norm-referenced tools are meant to be diagnostic and provide comparison with a normative group. Scores obtained through norm-referenced tools may provide insight into underlying diagnostic concerns yet do not translate or predict school participation or performance. (For a sample of assessment tools commonly used by school occupational therapists, see Appendix F, "Selected Assessment Tools for Analysis of Students' Occupational Performance.")

Using assessment scores as the sole determining factor for educational decision making would be contrary to the IDEA process, as well as the *Standards for Educational and Psychological Testing* (American Educational Research Association et al., 2014). More important, these standards specify that when a particular cut score is used for decision-making purposes, evidence must be presented to substantiate this use. In particular, there should be empirical data showing the relationship of test performance to the identified concern.

Although most standardized tests have high reliability, it does not follow that they are necessarily valid for the evaluation purpose; however, many schools have an unfortunate tendency to view standardized tests as the only credible sources of evaluation data. For example, a test of motor development may yield highly reliable (i.e., replicable) norm-referenced scores, but the scores from the test may or may not be valid indicators of a student's functional motor coordination or ability to complete motor tasks during their educational program. The test may not be sensitive to occupational performance demands related to the cognitive aspects of organization and execution of movement, which might be better identified through careful observation in the natural context (e.g., during classroom instruction).

To select the appropriate test and to justify this choice to others, occupational therapists need a thorough understanding of the strengths and limitations of the various instruments that are available. Building this knowledge may begin with existing reviews (e.g., Asher, 2014; Law et al., 2005) but should also include careful review of the test manual and relevant original literature, particularly studies that have examined the validity of the measure for assessing school-related difficulties and for assessing particular populations (e.g., students with developmental coordination disorder). Some examples of relevant questions to investigate are as follows:

- What is the relation between scores on this test and performance of school-relevant tasks?
- When a relation exists, is it strong enough to specifically interpret as a major contributor to school functioning?
- Does this relationship exist across all school ages?
- Have studies looked at whether factors other than the primary construct affect a student's performance on the test? For example, could difficulty understanding spoken instructions account for poor performance on motor items?

Because validity testing of instruments is an ongoing process, practitioners should routinely review the literature to see whether new evidence has been published related to frequently used instruments.

Synthesize Data and Document the Process

Documentation of evaluation findings should be well organized, clear, concise, and an accurate record of the evaluation process in terms understood by parents and other team members. The primary focus of the report should connect the occupational therapist's professional reasoning to answer the referral questions. That is, the occupational therapist should synthesize and provide insights into how the data inform, explain, or clarify those barriers and supports to the student's performance, student's strengths and needs in context, and potential interventions to improve student outcomes.

Synthesizing is distinctly different from summarizing data. A *summary* captures key points of each data source, whereas a *synthesis* details the professional reasoning of the occupational therapist while combining ideas and drawing meaning from multiple data sources (Mulligan, 2014). The evaluation process described by AOTA (2014) and presented in this chapter lends itself to a top-down approach and a natural progression for synthesizing information and answering the referral questions.

School occupational therapists must adhere to their state's regulatory acts and professional practice standards, such as AOTA's (2015b) *Standards of Practice* and *Guidelines for Documentation in Occupational Therapy* (AOTA, 2018), when writing the evaluation report. Some school teams use a team evaluation report that blends everyone's documents. When using a standard team template, occupational therapists need to ensure that the report provides individualized information and recommendations to the team that are student specific, age appropriate, and relevant.

State regulatory acts may stipulate that the occupational therapy evaluation report delineate the therapist's findings and recommendations. Because the team report would not explicitly comply with such a regulation, the occupational therapist should write an occupational therapy report and could cut and paste information into the team report. Both reports would be considered documents covered by the Family Educational Rights and Privacy Act of 1974 (Pub. L. 93–380) and would become part of the student's educational record, given that they were used to determine eligibility and services as appropriate.

Provide recommendations to the team

As data are shared through the IEP process, decisions about the student's strengths and needs are identified. These needs are then used to develop the student's goals (based on current performance) as well as program and related service needs. Arriving at the meeting with draft goals is a common way to save time; however, this gives the appearance that the school is driving the decisions rather than engaging parents in goal setting for their child. One strategy is to talk with the family beforehand about goals they would like for their child and come prepared with suggestions of specific, meaningful education-related goals that appear achievable on the basis of the evaluation but that are not framed in terms of occupational therapy services. These suggested goals or focus areas would be drafted for the purpose of guiding effective team discussion and decision making.

Disseminate the report before meeting

Providing all team members with a copy of the evaluation report several days before the meeting allows them time to read the report. Districts or states may or may not have established procedures for providing copies ahead of time. The therapist should follow the established practice for their setting. In accordance with IDEA § 300.613(a), districts need to provide copies of the evaluation report when a parent makes a request.

Attend the IEP Meeting to Assist in Team Planning

As a member of the student's IEP team, the occupational therapist should make every effort to attend the IEP meeting (or gain parent and LEA consent to be excused if unable to attend), contribute to discussions (in person or in writing), and assist in the development or revision of the IEP.

Present evaluation findings

The student's team has a responsibility to consider all "relevant functional, developmental and academic information including information provided by the parent" (IDEA, 2004, § 1414[b][2][A]). Ideally, the evaluation report would be reviewed with the family before the IEP meeting. When a parent elects to provide medical reports, recommendations from outside providers, or clinical occupational therapy reports, the team must consider this information along with other gathered information in determining eligibility for special education. If the student is deemed eligible, then an IEP is designed to meet the student's needs and should be contextually based, educationally relevant, educationally necessary, and aligned with the overall profile derived from evaluations.

Develop student goals

The student's IEP team combines information from the evaluation reports and other sources of information to identify the student's overall strengths and needs and prioritizes those needs to address in the student's program, with goals aimed at optimizing student participation in the educational program. Goals are student specific, not discipline specific (i.e., they are not therapy goals). The occupational therapy intervention plan (AOTA, 2015b), required in accordance with professional standards, reflects therapy-specific goals and approaches to be used as directed by the occupational therapist (see Appendix C, "Occupational Therapy Intervention Plan").

IDEA stipulates that the student's measurable annual goals include academic and functional goals designed to enable the student to be involved in and make progress in the general education curriculum (§ 1414[d][A][II]). Goals typically include the timeline, conditions, student's name, performance expected, and criteria, in some order. For example, "By November 25, 20XX, during a 15-minute recess on the playground, Bella will play with peers and the equipment, for at least 10 minutes, without redirection from an adult."

Once student goals are established, the IEP team determines whether related services, accommodations, modifications, and supports are necessary to implement the IEP. In determining related services, the team will need to contemplate whether related services are educationally relevant and educational necessary. The following questions may guide the team's decision making when determining need for related services:

- Does the student have an IEP goal or objective that requires the expertise of the occupational therapy practitioner?
- Can another educational provider adequately meet the needs of the student?
- Will the student experience educational benefit without the provision of occupational therapy?
- Does a member of the student's educational team require training, supports, or routine problem solving to implement the IEP and ensure that the student has access to an appropriate education?

Determine Plan for Ongoing Evaluation

Evaluation is a continuous process, not a one-time event. Therefore, ongoing monitoring of the student's performance is needed for effective intervention. Ongoing evaluation should stay focused on whether the educational goal has been reached, not on whether component abilities are normalized. Occupational therapists should annually summarize these data in a report. When new information is needed, a parent must give consent to a reevaluation.

SUMMARY

Occupational therapists conduct evaluations of a student's academic, behavior, and functional performance using multiple methods: record review, interview, observation, and administration of tools. Analysis and interpretation of these data provides information to the referring team (parents included) about the environment, instruction, curriculum, and student's performance in the context of the student's education.

REFERENCES

American Educational Research Association, American Psychological Association, National Council on Measurement in Education, Joint Committee on Standards for Educational and Psychological Testing. (2014). *Standards for educational and psychological testing.* Washington, DC: American Educational Research Association.

American Occupational Therapy Association. (2014). Occupational therapy practice framework: Domain and process (3rd ed.). *American Journal of Occupational Therapy, 68*(Suppl. 1), S1–S48. https://doi.org/10.5014/ajot.2014.682006

American Occupational Therapy Association. (2015a). Occupational therapy's perspective on the use of environments and contexts to support health, well-being, and participation in occupations. *American Journal of Occupational Therapy, 69*(Suppl. 3), 6913410050. https://doi.org/10.5014/ajot.2015.696S05

American Occupational Therapy Association. (2015b). Standards of practice for occupational therapy. *American Journal of Occupational Therapy, 69*(Suppl. 3), 6913410057. https://doi.org/10.5014/ajot.2015.696S06

American Occupational Therapy Association. (2017). AOTA occupational profile template. *American Journal of Occupational Therapy, 71*(Suppl. 2), 7112420030. https://doi.org/10.5014/ajot.2017.716S12

American Occupational Therapy Association. (2018). Guidelines for documentation in occupational therapy. *American Journal of Occupational Therapy, 72*(Suppl. 2), 7212410010. https://doi.org/10.5014/ajot.2018.72S203

Asher, I. E. (Ed.). (2014). *Occupational therapy assessment tools: An annotated index* (4th ed.). Bethesda, MD: AOTA Press.

Coster, W. J. (1998). Occupation-centered assessment of children. *American Journal of Occupational Therapy, 52,* 337–344. https://doi.org/10.5014/ajot.52.5.337

Dunn, W., Patten Koenig, K., Cox, J., Sabata, D., Pope, E., Foster, L., & Blackwell, A. (2013). Harnessing strengths: Daring to celebrate everyone's unique contributions, Part 1. *Developmental Disabilities Special Interest Section Quarterly, 36*(1), 1–3.

Every Student Succeeds Act, Pub. L. 114–95, 129 Stat. 1802 (2015).

Family Educational Rights and Privacy Act of 1974, Pub. L. 93–380, 20 U.S.C. § 1232g; 34 CFR Part 99.

Frolek Clark, G., Cahill, S. M., & Ivey, C. (2015). School practice documentation: Documenting and organizing quantitative data. *OT Practice, 20*(15), 12–15.

Individuals With Disabilities Education Improvement Act of 2004, Pub. L. 108–446, 20 U.S.C. §§ 1400–1482.

King, G. (2009). A relational goal-oriented model of optimal service delivery to children and families. *Physical and Occupational Therapy in Pediatrics, 29,* 384–408. https://doi.org/10.3109/01942630903222118

Law, M., Baum, C. M., & Dunn, W. (2005). *Measuring occupational performance: Supporting best practice in occupational therapy* (2nd ed.). Thorofare, NJ: Slack.

Morris, M., & Hollenbeck, J. (2016). Evaluating student participation: Focus on strengths in your school-based evaluation. *OT Practice, 21*(1), CE-1–CE-8.

Mulligan, S. E. (2014). *Occupational therapy evaluation for children: A pocket guide* (2nd ed.). Philadelphia: Lippincott Williams & Wilkins.

Protection of Pupil Rights Amendment of 1978, 20 U.S.C. § 1232h; 34 C.F.R. Part 98.

Rehabilitation Act of 1973, Pub. L. 93–112, 29 U.S.C. §§ 701–796l.

Schwellnus, H., Carnahan, H., Kushki, A., Polatajko, H., Missiuna, C., & Chau, T. (2012). Effect of pencil grasp on the speed and legibility of handwriting in children. *American Journal of Occupational Therapy, 66,* 718–726. https://doi.org/10.5014/ajot.2012.004515

Section 504 of the Rehabilitation Act of 1973, as amended, 29 U.S.C. § 794 (2008).

Best Practices in School Occupational Therapy Interventions to Support Participation

41

Gloria Frolek Clark, PhD, OTR/L, BCP, SCSS, FAOTA, and Jan Hollenbeck, OTD, OTR

KEY TERMS AND CONCEPTS

- Accommodations
- Coaching
- Collaboration
- Coteaching
- Embedded services
- Least restrictive environment
- Modifications
- Occupations

OVERVIEW

Under the Individuals With Disabilities Education Improvement Act of 2004 (IDEA; Pub. L. 108–446), school occupational therapy practitioners[1] support access, participation, and progress in the educational program for eligible students with disabilities and at-risk students. They facilitate successful interactions among the student, activities and occupations, and the environment and context to promote participation in functional and educational activities (e.g., academic, social–behavioral, and daily life skills within the school program; American Occupational Therapy Association [AOTA], 2014b).

Federal education laws and regulations guide and influence school practice (e.g., IDEA; Every Student Succeeds Act [2015; Pub. L. 114–95]; Section 504 of the Rehabilitation Act of 1973, as amended [2008; Pub. L. 93–112]) and provide many roles for occupational therapy practitioners (see Table 41.1). In addition, occupational therapy practitioners must follow state professional regulations (e.g., licensure, certification), which take precedence over education laws. Throughout the process, the occupational therapist is responsible for all aspects of provision of services and the safety of the client[2] and may delegate tasks to the occupational therapy assistant, as appropriate (AOTA, 2014a).

---

[1]*Occupational therapy practitioner* refers to both the occupational therapist and the occupational therapy assistant. The American Occupational Therapy Association (AOTA; 2014a, p. S18) states, "The occupational therapist is responsible for all aspects of occupational therapy service delivery and is accountable for the safety and effectiveness of the occupational therapy service delivery process" and "must be directly involved in the delivery of services during the initial evaluation and regularly throughout the course of intervention. . . . The occupational therapy assistant delivers safe and effective occupational therapy services under the supervision of and in partnership with the occupational therapist."

[2]*Client* may include individual (student, teacher, parent), group (classroom), or population (school district).

IDEA (2004) requires services to be individualized and selected on the basis of students' educational needs with consideration of the *least restrictive environment* (LRE) mandate (e.g., that students to receive their education, to the maximum extent appropriate, with nondisabled peers) and focused on participation in natural school contexts. Occupational therapy practitioners provide a continuum of collaborative services based on the individual needs of the student, including services provided on behalf of the student (e.g., training, education, consultation with educational staff) and services provided directly with the student when indicated (e.g., working in natural school contexts and, in some situations, working with the student in a separate setting). School occupational therapy practitioners use the best available evidence to guide their practice in alignment with their profession, state regulatory requirements, and education laws.

This chapter describes a collaborative continuum of occupational therapy interventions to support and promote student participation in functional and academic activities and access to school environments.

ESSENTIAL CONSIDERATIONS

Occupational therapists are responsible for implementing occupational therapy services documented in the student's individualized education program (IEP) and gathering ongoing assessment data to determine effectiveness of interventions provided. The evaluation process is covered in a previous chapter (see Chapter 40, "Best Practices in School Occupational Therapy Evaluation and Planning to Support Participation"). There are no specific federal eligibility criteria for occupational therapy. Students who are eligible for special education may access occupational therapy services *if the IEP team determines these services are required* to assist the student to benefit from their educational program.

The team collaboratively identifies the student's prioritized needs, and these needs become the student's IEP goals. Goals are not specific to an educational team member or

Copyright © 2019 by the American Occupational Therapy Association. All rights reserved. To reuse this content, contact www.copyright.com. https://doi.org/10.7139/2019.978-1-56900-591-0.041

TABLE 41.1. Various Intervention Roles of the Occupational Therapy Practitioner

LAW	PRACTITIONER'S ROLE AND FOCUS
ESSA	*Specialized instructional support personnel:* Provide professional expertise and skilled contributions for all students, use schoolwide system of supports, provide professional development and training for staff, share information.
IDEA—early intervening services (MTSS)	*Consultant and service provider (if state allows):* Collaborative teaming; professional development and training of teachers and other staff directed toward systems, classroom, or students to facilitate successful general education learning environments (AOTA, 2012).
Section 504	*Building team member and service provider:* Collaborative teaming, suggest modifications, strategies, and accommodations; provide student-centered services.
IDEA—special education	*Educational team member and service provider:* Collaborative teaming, services on behalf of the student, suggest modifications, accommodations, and supports to school personnel; provide services directly with the student; provide ongoing monitoring of performance.

Note. May vary depending on state licensure acts or state regulations. AOTA = American Occupational Therapy Association; ESSA = Every Student Succeeds Act; IDEA = Individuals With Disabilities Education Improvement Act of 2004; MTSS = multi-tiered systems of support.

service; there are no occupational therapy goals in the IEP. Rather, the occupational therapy practitioner works with the educational team to ensure that the student meets their goals (i.e., goals are student specific, not therapy specific). Therapy-specific goals, although not included in the IEP, are included in the occupational therapy intervention plan, discussed in the next section.

Focus on Participation in Occupations

"Occupational therapy intervention focuses on creating or facilitating opportunities to engage in occupations that lead to participation in desired life situations" (AOTA, 2014b, p. S4). *Occupations* are meaningful, valued activities that students choose or need to engage in during their school program. The student's strengths and needs, in addition to the contextual supports and barriers relative to the student's ability to participate in desired and needed occupations in school, are gathered during the occupational therapy evaluation process (e.g., interviews, observations) and used to establish the student's goals and to make recommendations for intervention.

To effectively facilitate participation, the practitioner must be knowledgeable about building-level factors (e.g., school culture, building wide initiatives), classroom-level factors (e.g., classroom culture, curriculum, routine, teacher's instructional methods), the environments and contexts of the school (e.g., access to the building, social values, peer interactions), and individual student factors (e.g., current performance, student's learning style, effect of the student's disability on performance).

Students may have underlying challenges (e.g., client factors) that do not affect their access to and participation or progression in school; therefore, they would not need services from the school occupational therapy practitioner. For example, a student may have below-age-level scores on a test of visual–motor skills and yet be able to participate without difficulty in school tasks requiring these skills (e.g., writing, copying); a student may have spastic hemiplegia that results in mild right-sided weakness and coordination challenges, yet use school tools and manipulate objects necessary for effective school participation. When evaluation

data support the team decision that occupational therapy is necessary for a student, the role of the school occupational therapy practitioner is to address student needs that affect school access, participation, and educational progress.

Client-Centered and Individualized Intervention

AOTA's (2014b) *Occupational Therapy Practice Framework: Domain and Process* (3rd ed.; *OTPF–3*) identifies *clients* as persons, groups, and populations. In school settings, possible clients may include students, teachers, parents, other team members, classrooms, or the school district. Individualizing the intervention on the basis of the student's goals, values, and interests is a critical part of occupational therapy and IDEA (2004).

LRE and Continuum of Services

IDEA mandates that services be provided in the LRE with nondisabled peers to the maximum extent appropriate. LRE is a mandate, not a choice, and applies not only to the student's program placement but also to any services the student receives. The IEP team determines the student's educational placement and also considers the LRE when establishing where and how each service on the student's IEP will be provided.

The first choice for direct student intervention should be within the general education setting or other natural environment whenever appropriate (i.e., LRE). Student goals should be focused on school participation. Whenever possible, interventions (and outcome measures) should take place within the natural school contexts in which participation occurs. The *OTPF–3* (AOTA, 2014b) supports occupational therapy interventions in natural contexts as important to achieving participation and meaningful occupational performance. When students are pulled from their environment, they miss critical instruction and peer interactions.

The team may choose to modify or accommodate aspects of the curriculum, instruction, or environment. For educators, the term *modifications* refers to the academic curriculum and is used when reducing the learning expectations

TABLE 41.2. Occupational Therapy in Natural School Contexts: Summary of Benefits

STUDENT BENEFITS	TEACHER BENEFITS	OT AND OTA BENEFITS
▪ Generalize skills in natural routines ▪ Remain in class for instruction, activities, and social interaction ▪ Create more opportunities for authentic practice ▪ Experience fewer unnecessary transitions ▪ Build skills that are essential and applicable to school participation ▪ Learn with classmates and gain a sense of belonging to school community	▪ Foster collaboration between teacher and OT or OTA ▪ Solve problems in real time and actual context to address teacher concerns ▪ See how OT or OTA contributes to student programming ▪ Allow modeling and better carryover	▪ Acquire knowledge about classroom curriculum, instruction, expectations, peers, and environment ▪ Determine whether strategies are feasible and work for the student right away ▪ Solve problems and collaborate with classroom staff in the moment ▪ Address meaningful student participation

Note. OT = occupational therapist; OTA = occupational therapy assistant.

(e.g., an easier reading passage, simplified vocabulary, less complex math problems; Strom, n.d.). ***Accommodations*** do not reduce the learning expectations but refer to physical or environmental changes to provide access to learning for a student with a disability (e.g., extended time, different seating, allowing use of spell-check for completion of non–spelling assignments, a visual checklist; Strom, n.d.). Using these educational terms, occupational therapy practitioners typically provide suggestions for accommodations directed at how the student accesses and participates, whereas modifications to the curriculum and what is being taught are primarily the domain of educators.

Following LRE, occupational therapy practitioners must consider intervention from least to more restrictive on the basis of the individual student's needs: services on behalf of the student, services directly with the student in natural school contexts, and services directly with the student outside of the natural school context. Intervention often includes more than 1 type of service and ebbs and flows based on student participation needs over time. Always providing direct services to students without considering other options is not in compliance with IDEA (see Table 41.2).

Working in schools requires occupational therapy practitioners to understand the school culture and curriculum as well as the values and beliefs of administrators and staff. A clear understanding and ability to apply the requirements of IDEA (2004) and other pertinent federal and state legislation (e.g., state licensure requirements) are necessary. Occupational therapy practitioners must use professional documents and the best available research evidence to advocate for student participation and best practices in intervention.

AOTA Guidelines Documents

Intervention guidance is provided in the following AOTA professional documents:
- *Guidelines for Documentation of Occupational Therapy* (AOTA, 2018);
- *Guidelines for Occupational Therapy Services in Early Intervention and Schools* (AOTA, 2017);
- *Guidelines for Supervision, Roles, and Responsibilities During the Delivery of Occupational Therapy Services* (AOTA, 2014a);
- *Occupational Therapy Code of Ethics (2015)* (AOTA, 2015a);

- *OTPF–3* (AOTA, 2014b); and
- *Standards of Practice for Occupational Therapy* (AOTA, 2015c).

BEST PRACTICES

Occupational therapy practitioners collaborate with parents and educational staff to provide services with students, teams, or systems and to modify and adapt the school context for participation (Frolek Clark, 2016). Occupational therapy practitioners are not directly responsible for the student's academic instruction; delivery of the curriculum is the role of the teacher. Collaborating with the student's teams (e.g., teachers, family), the occupational therapy practitioner supports and enhances the student's access to and participation and progress in their educational program.

Key practices that are supported by evidence include creating a collaborative environment, providing services in natural school contexts, altering the activity, and altering the environment or context to enhance performance. Best practices for interventions in supporting school participation include planning and designing interventions on the basis of the best available evidence, implementing the intervention focused on occupational therapy domains while monitoring ongoing progress, and reevaluating the intervention plan and need for ongoing services (AOTA, 2014b).

Plan and Design Interventions

School occupational therapists use evidence-based research, knowledge, and professional judgment to design and implement effective interventions (see Appendix C, "Occupational Therapy Intervention Plan"). With this in mind, practitioners should establish a pattern of examining current research and evidence to support decision making.

Resources for evidence-based information are included in Table 41.3.

Implement Intervention

The *OTPF–3* (AOTA, 2014b) provides occupational therapy practitioners with several intervention approaches (create or promote, establish or restore, maintain, modify, prevent) that are described in Chapter 2, "The *OTPF–3:* Communicating Occupational Therapy in Schools." These intervention approaches address context and environment, activities, and

TABLE 41.3.   Locating Evidence-Based Resources

RESOURCE	EXAMPLE
AOTA (https://www.aota.org)	Peer-reviewed journals ▪ *American Occupational Therapy Journal* ▪ Access to *British Occupational Therapy Journal* ▪ Access to *Canadian Occupational Therapy Journal* Evidence-based practice and research ▪ Information on children and youth, mental health, toolkits, systematic reviews, and other evidence-based resources (https://bit.ly/2AQcbbQ) Publications through AOTA Press AOTA Continuing Education
AOTF (https://www.aotf.org/Programs/Other-Resources-for-OT-Research/Pathfinders)	AOTF Pathfinders ▪ Guides to information sources on specific topics often researched by occupational therapists, including cerebral palsy, environmental modification and universal design, low vision, obesity, serious mental illness
NBCOT® (https://www.nbcot.org)	Research tools for NBCOT certificants ▪ *Proquest:* Database to locate evidence-based articles ▪ *RefWorks:* Tool to organize evidence articles and references
Google Scholar (https://scholar.google.com/)	Search engine for scholarly articles, theses, books, abstracts, and court opinions from academic publishers, professional societies, online repositories, universities, and other websites
PubMed (https://www.ncbi.nlm.nih.gov/pubmed/)	Repository for biomedical literature from MEDLINE, life science journals, and online books; citations may include links to full-text content from PubMed Central and publisher websites
Library access	Alumni access ▪ Many universities offer campus library access and some offer off-campus access to databases and library resources to alumni. Local university library access ▪ Search and locate evidence and make copies. Local public library network ▪ Most public libraries are part of a larger network and offer online search engines, access to some ejournals and other resources, and interlibrary loan options.

Note. AOTA = American Occupational Therapy Association; AOTF = American Occupational Therapy Foundation; NBCOT = National Board for Certification in Occupational Therapy.

clients (e.g., students, teachers, families, classrooms, school districts). Examples are provided in a hierarchy of least restrictive to more restrictive service provision.

Prevent barriers to participation

Occupational therapy practitioners can provide information to school districts, building teams, and classrooms that may address the needs of general education students who are at risk by using multi-tiered systems of support (see Chapter 26, "Best Practices in Multi-Tiered Systems of Support"). With this in mind, occupational therapy practitioners can provide resources to school districts that support the physical and emotional needs, mental health, and social competence of all students and contribute to schoolwide initiatives (e.g., antibullying, social–emotional learning, positive behavior intervention and supports) to enhance student health and well-being (Handley-More et al., 2013).

Make modifications and accommodations

Occupational therapy practitioners working in schools are in a student's natural environment and should address occu-

pational performance in context. Observing and providing services to students in the natural contexts and routines of the school day increases retention and generalization of skills (Baranek, 2002) and is consistent with the purpose of occupational therapy (AOTA, 2014b, 2015b) and the intent of IDEA (2004).

The *OTPF–3* (AOTA, 2014b) identifies 4 contexts—cultural, personal, temporal, and virtual—and 2 environments—physical and social. An example of intervening at the personal context level might be an occupational therapy practitioner advocating for 2 students who are homeless to have access to the locker-room showers before the start of the school day. Examples of physical environments might include the classroom, bathroom, library, lunchroom, gymnasium, hallway, field trips, and bus. Social environments might include persons or groups with whom the student comes in contact (e.g., friends, classmates, principal, custodian).

Activities are components of occupations necessary for participation. Interventions to change the activity or environment may be necessary to enhance access (e.g., ability to open locker using a touch rather than a rotary lock) or participation (e.g., moving student's chair to a quieter location in the room).

The required actions and performance skills, space demands, sequencing and timing, and other aspects of an activity or occupation may be a barrier to participation. For example, a student with sensitivity to soft materials may scream or gag when expected to use clay in art education. The occupational therapy practitioner can work with the teacher to address this student's needs by suggesting other, more tolerable materials so that the student is able to complete the project with peers.

Occupational therapy practitioners may create enriched contexts, environments, or activities for students. This is done in the natural routine and may include giving the teacher suggestions to create a physical arrangement that promotes social interactions for the students. Another example may be working with the teacher to implement a program that promotes self-regulation for students in the classroom.

Occupational therapy practitioners consider the effect of activities and environmental factors on student performance and can work to change these for enhanced student participation. Research has linked environmental accommodations with improvements in student participation (Dietz et al., 2002; Handley-More et al., 2003; Kinnealey et al., 2012). For example, Kinnealey et al. (2012) found that the use of sound-absorbing walls and halogen lighting benefited students with auditory and visual hypersensitivity by improving their attention and engagement in the classroom. The use of compensatory strategies and changes to the environment is often preferred over direct service focused on remediation of student skill deficits because they are often likely to have a more immediate effect on a student's ability to participate (Egilson & Traustadottir, 2009).

Changes to the context, environment, or activity are achieved through ***collaboration*** with other team members and can work in the moment to enhance student performance, unlike intervention directed at changing the student, which can take time and in some situations may not be possible. For example, a student with hemiplegia due to cerebral palsy may always have challenges with bilateral skills that affect performance of tasks such as managing lunch containers and stabilizing paper while writing. In this situation, the occupational therapy intervention would be compensatory in nature (e.g., providing a type of food storage container that the student can manage 1-handed, providing a clipboard to stabilize the paper while writing).

These compensatory changes to activities or environments require collaboration with other adults (e.g., parent, lunch monitor, teacher) to be effective. The importance of collaboration when making changes to activities or environments cannot be overstated. In addition to collaboration, observing student performance in context is an important aspect of evaluation and intervention necessary to determine accommodations and strategies to enhance participation.

Promote student participation in natural school contexts and routines

Occupational therapy services are provided to enhance access and participation in the student's educational program. A continuum of least to more restrictive services is provided in Figure 41.1. Removal from the LRE should occur only when necessary and must be documented on the student's IEP and collectively reported in each state's annual

---

FIGURE 41.1. Continuum of occupational therapy services in schools, least to more restrictive.

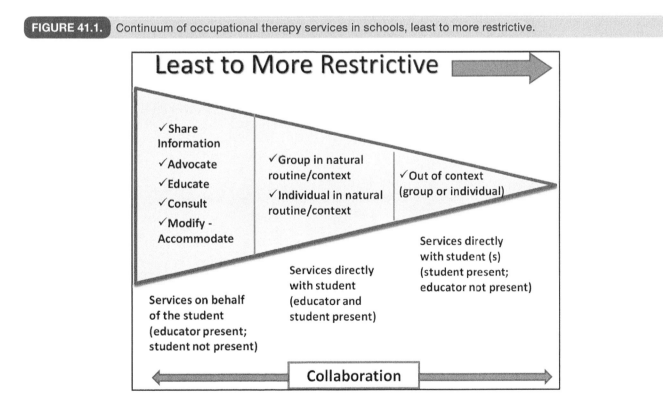

Source. Used with permission from Gloria Frolek Clark and Jan Hollenbeck (2017).

performance report to the U.S. Department of Education's Office of Special Education Programs. When it is necessary to remove a student from the natural contexts and routines of the day (e.g., to teach a skill or strategy), these services should be finite, with a plan to generalize performance to the natural context. When a student is pulled out of the classroom or other natural school context for isolated therapy, the classroom book that was read aloud, the discussion regarding yesterday's assignment, the directions for the next project, and the socialization that occurred on the playground are all missed.

Establish student skills and abilities

IDEA allows services to be provided directly with or on behalf of the student. Occupational therapists should determine the least restrictive method of intervention to meet the student's IEP goals.

Interventions on behalf of the student. Services provided on behalf of the student may include training, educating, or providing resources to the team; consulting collaboratively with teachers on accommodations and strategies to support learning in the classroom; working with equipment vendors; and other tasks to support student participation that do not require the student to be present. Research has indicated that translating knowledge to adults working with students provides them with other strategies and perspectives (Barnes & Turner, 2001; Dunn, 1990; Hanft & Place, 1996; Hanft & Shepherd, 2016; Kemmis & Dunn, 1996; Sayers, 2008; Villeneuve, 2009).

Support to school personnel is imperative to build their capacity to educate and support students with diverse needs. Students should not be "lifers" on the occupational therapy workload; instead, services with students should change in approach, frequency, and duration (e.g., discontinued when appropriate) to match the needs of students in their educational program. For instance, a student may not require the expertise of an occupational therapy practitioner to access instruction, yet the educational staff may need training in specific strategies so that they can effectively educate and support the student. The student's team would list this specific training on the student's IEP.

Direct services embedded in context and routines. Services with students may occur individually or in small or large groups embedded in natural routines *(embedded services).*

Direct services with individual students in natural routines are often occupation based (e.g., moving through the cafeteria to eat lunch, pulling up pants during toileting, writing during journal time). The occupational therapy practitioner supports student participation in the activities, routines, and structure of the classroom or other school setting.

Although the teachers are responsible for the student's instruction, occupational therapy practitioners may use their knowledge and skills to plan and provide whole-class learning activities with the educator (sometimes referred to as *coteaching* or *embedded learning*) to provide and model

strategies or supports to facilitate the participation of students with disabilities.

Coaching is another type of evidence-based approach to build capacity and support for educators. The occupational therapy practitioner coaches the staff member on 1 or more specific skills they would like to learn (e.g., feeding techniques, using a specific handwriting program) to support students with disabilities. These methods involve collaboration and shared responsibility between the occupational therapy practitioner and educator for activities and occupations that occur within the classroom. Research has indicated that a collaborative approach to intervention is effective in improving student performance, enhancing teacher satisfaction and implementation of practitioners' suggestions, and ensuring carryover of student gains in the classroom (Dreiling & Bundy, 2003; Kientz & Dunn, 2012; Sayers, 2008; Villeneuve, 2009).

Bazyk et al. (2009) found that when occupational therapists focused on planning and consultation with teachers for fine motor and emergent literacy skills with kindergarteners in 2 classrooms, children with and without disabilities made statistically significant changes on fine motor and emergent literacy assessments. Occupational therapists may assist the classroom teacher in planning and instructing handwriting and writing programs (e.g., coteaching) in which the teacher is responsible for delivery of curriculum and the occupational therapist is responsible for identifying, providing, and modeling strategies and accommodations to facilitate student handwriting success.

Case-Smith et al. (2012) cotaught handwriting and writing programs in 1st-grade classrooms, including students with disabilities, which resulted in improved legibility, speed, and writing fluency. Case-Smith et al. (2014) embedded a handwriting program into 4 classrooms cotaught by the teacher and occupational therapist. Legibility, speed, and writing fluency were more improved in the group that was cotaught than in the group receiving standard instruction.

Villeneuve (2009) cautioned occupational therapy practitioners to find time to educate teachers about the role of school occupational therapy and collaborate with teachers about school policies, curriculum, and classroom practices. The aim is to develop educationally relevant approaches when providing occupational therapy with students in natural contexts.

Services out of context. Provide direct services out of context or routine only when unable to support students in natural contexts or routines. Services outside of natural school contexts may be necessary to develop methods and strategies, to practice at the activity level without environmental distractions, and when preparatory methods are needed to prepare the student for actual participation in context. Intervention that involves removal of the student from the natural school context should occur only as long as necessary to facilitate participation, and strategies for generalization of skills back into the context should be explicit. More frequency or intensity of service is not necessarily better when it comes to direct services (Giangreco et al., 2001). This is especially true of services that remove a student from the natural school setting (see Exhibit 41.1 for alternatives to removing students).

EXHIBIT 41.1. Alternatives to Pulling Students Out of Natural Routines of Environment

Removing students from their educational routines, resulting in a loss of academic instruction and social engagement, should not be considered as an option when less restrictive but equally or more effective methods may be provided. These methods may include *coteaching* (e.g., teacher and occupational therapist collaborate to develop lesson plans, the teacher provides the curriculum, and the occupational therapy practitioner works with the teacher and class 20 minutes a week to provide strategies and to model for the teacher so that strategies can be implemented throughout the week when the practitioner is not present) or *consultation* (e.g., student has daily practice for 15 minutes in the classroom, and occupational therapy practitioner and teacher consult 15 minutes every 2 weeks). Beginning with services that are the least restrictive and have greater effect on access and participation is essential and is mandated by law.

Ensure Strategies Are Implemented With Fidelity

Occupational therapy practitioners realize that opportunities to enhance participation and skill development exist throughout the day in schools. Translating knowledge to adults working with the student gives them other strategies and perspectives appropriate to their level of skill (Hanft & Place, 1996; Knippenberg & Hanft, 2004). Providing strategies and training to teachers and paraeducators allows the student to have multiple opportunities to practice skills or increase performance throughout the day.

For example, a student working with an occupational therapy practitioner to learn a consistent strategy for organizing a binder would develop independence more quickly if the practitioner provided training for the classroom staff in the strategy being used as well as the types of prompts to provide to the student to facilitate independence. This provides many more opportunities during the school week when the student can practice and develop independence in use of this organizational strategy.

Delivering instruction or strategy implementation in the way it was designed is *fidelity of implementation* (Gresham et al., 2000). To ensure that the strategy (or program) is implemented with fidelity, the practitioner should provide training and written instructions. Frequent monitoring by the practitioner is also important (e.g., observe the person implementing the strategy or carrying out the program to be sure it is completed as designed). In addition, the educational staff should document their instruction or implementation of the strategy (e.g., check boxes for each step, date on data log).

Review Intervention

Reviewing the occupational therapy intervention plan, effectiveness of services, and progress toward the IEP goals is a continuous process (AOTA, 2014b). Team discussion and collaboration are vital to enhancing student participation and performance. For information about data collection procedures, see Chapter 45, "Best Practices in School Occupational Therapy Documentation and Data Collection."

Document the Intervention Process

Documentation is an essential component throughout the intervention process and provides a legal record of therapy provision. "Intervention plans and consistent documentation of occupational therapy interventions, student responses and data collection guide therapy decision-making while progress reports, annual reports, and discharge summaries help to communicate to others the impact of occupational therapy services on student progress" (Frolek Clark & Handley-More, 2017, p. 74).

SUMMARY

School occupational therapy practitioners provide a continuum of collaborative supports and services for students with disabilities to facilitate access, participation, and progress in school. Collaboration among practitioners, students, family, and educational staff is essential for effective interventions. Practitioners are equipped to provide a continuum of services and intervention based on consideration of LRE; providing services and addressing occupational performance in natural contexts; addressing the individual needs of the student within the school program; providing services on behalf of the student, including training and consultation; and providing accommodations and strategies to enhance student participation.

REFERENCES

American Occupational Therapy Association. (2012). *AOTA practice advisory on occupational therapy in response to intervention.* Retrieved from https://www.aota.org/-/media/corporate/files/practice/children/browse/school/rti/aota%20rti%20practice%20adv%20final%20%20101612.pdf

American Occupational Therapy Association. (2014a). Guidelines for supervision, roles, and responsibilities during the delivery of occupational therapy services. *American Journal of Occupational Therapy, 68*(Suppl. 3), S16–S22. https://doi.org/10.5014/ajot.2014.686S03

American Occupational Therapy Association. (2014b). Occupational therapy practice framework: Domain and process (3rd ed.). *American Journal of Occupational Therapy, 68*(Suppl. 1), S1–S48. https://doi.org/10.5014/ajot.2014.682006

American Occupational Therapy Association. (2015a). Occupational therapy code of ethics (2015). *American Journal of Occupational Therapy, 69*(Suppl. 3), 6913410030. https://doi.org/10.5014/ajot.2015.696S03

American Occupational Therapy Association. (2015b). Occupational therapy's perspective on the use of environments and contexts to facilitate health, well-being, and participation in occupations. *American Journal of Occupational Therapy, 69*(Suppl. 3), 6913410050. https://doi.org/10.5014/ajot.2015.696S05

American Occupational Therapy Association. (2015c). Standards of practice for occupational therapy. *American Journal of Occupational Therapy, 69*(Suppl. 3), 6913410057. https://doi.org/10.5014/ajot.2015.696S06

American Occupational Therapy Association. (2017). Guidelines for occupational therapy services in early intervention and schools. *American Journal of Occupational Therapy, 71*(Suppl. 2), 7112410010. https://doi.org/10.5014/ajot.2017.716S01

American Occupational Therapy Association. (2018). Guidelines for documentation of occupational therapy. *American Journal of Occupational Therapy, 72*(Suppl. 2), 7212410010. https://doi.org/10.5014/ajot.2018.72S203

Baranek, G. T. (2002). Efficacy of sensory and motor interventions for children with autism. *Journal of Autism and Developmental Disorders, 33,* 397–422. https://doi.org/10.1023/A:1020541906063

Barnes, K. J., & Turner, K. D. (2001). Team collaborative practices between teachers and occupational therapists. *American Journal of Occupational Therapy, 55,* 83–89. https://doi.org/10.5014/ajot.55.1.83

Bazyk, S., Michaud, P., Goodman, G., Papp, P., Hawkins, E., & Welch, M. A. (2009). Integrating occupational therapy services in a kindergarten curriculum: A look at the outcomes. *American Journal of Occupational Therapy, 63,* 160–171. https://doi.org/10.5014/ajot.63.2.160

Case-Smith, J., Holland, T., Lane, A., & White, S. (2012). Effect of a coteaching handwriting program for first graders: One-group pretest–posttest design. *American Journal of Occupational Therapy, 66,* 396–405. https://doi.org/10.5014/ajot.2012.004333

Case-Smith, J., Weaver, L., & Holland, T. (2014). Effects of a classroom-embedded occupational therapist–teacher handwriting program for first grade students. *American Journal of Occupational Therapy, 68,* 690–698. https://doi.org/10.5014%2Fajot.2014.011585

Dietz, J., Swinth, Y., & White, O. (2002). Powered mobility and preschoolers with complex developmental delays. *American Journal of Occupational Therapy, 56,* 86–96. https://doi.org/10.5014/ajot.56.1.86

Dreiling, D., & Bundy, A. (2003). A comparison of consultative model and direct–indirect intervention with preschoolers. *American Journal of Occupational Therapy, 57,* 566–569. https://doi.org/10.5014/ajot.57.5.566

Dunn, W. (1990). A comparison of service provision models in school-based occupational therapy services: A pilot study. *Occupational Therapy Journal of Research, 10,* 300–320. https://doi.org/10.1177%2F153944929001000505

Egilson, S. T., & Traustadottir, R. (2009). Participation of students with physical disabilities in the school environment. *American Journal of Occupational Therapy, 63,* 264–272. https://doi.org/10.5014/ajot.63.3.264

Every Student Succeeds Act, Pub. L. 114–95, 129 Stat. 1802 (2015).

Frolek Clark, G. (2016). Collaborating within the *Paces:* Structures and routines. In B. Hanft & J. Shepherd (Eds.), *Collaborating for student success: A guide for school-based occupational therapy* (2nd ed., pp. 177–207). Bethesda, MD: AOTA Press.

Frolek Clark, G., & Handley-More, D. (2017). *Best practices for documenting occupational therapy in schools.* Bethesda, MD: AOTA Press.

Giangreco, M. F., Edelman, S. W., Broer, S. M., & Doyle, M. B. (2001). Paraprofessional support of students with disabilities: Literature from the past decade. *Exceptional Children, 68,* 45–63. https://doi.org/10.1177/001440290106800103

Gresham, F., MacMillan, D., Beebe-Frankenberger, M., & Bocian, K. (2000). Treatment integrity in learning disabilities intervention research: Do we really know how treatments are implemented? *Learning Disabilities Research and Practice, 15,* 198–205. https://doi.org/10.1207/SLDRP1504_4

Handley-More, D., Dietz, J., Billingsley, F., & Coggins, T. (2003). Facilitating written work using computer word processing and word prediction. *American Journal of Occupational Therapy, 57,* 139–151. https://doi.org/10.5014/ajot.57.2.139

Handley-More, D., Hollenbeck, J., Orentlicher, M. L., & Wall, E. (2013). Education reform initiatives and school-based practice. *Early Intervention and School Special Interest Section Quarterly, 20*(3), 1–4.

Hanft, B., & Place, P. (1996). *The consulting therapist: A guide for OTs and PTs in schools.* San Antonio: Therapy Skill Builders.

Hanft, B., & Shepherd, J. (2016). *Collaborating for student success: A guide for school-based occupational therapy* (2nd ed.). Bethesda, MD: AOTA Press.

Individuals With Disabilities Education Improvement Act of 2004, Pub. L. 108–446, 20 U.S.C. §§ 1400–1482.

Kemmis, B. L., & Dunn, W. (1996). Collaborative consultation: The efficacy of remedial and compensatory interventions in school contexts. *American Journal of Occupational Therapy, 50,* 709–717. https://doi.org/10.5014/ajot.50.9.709

Kientz, M., & Dunn, W. (2012). Evaluating the effectiveness of contextual intervention for adolescents with autism spectrum disorders. *Journal of Occupational Therapy, Schools, and Early Intervention, 5,* 196–208. https://doi.org/10.1080/19411243.2012.737271

Kinnealey, M., Pfeiffer, B., Miller, J., Roan, C., Shoener, R., & Ellner, M. L. (2012). Effect of a classroom modification on attention and engagement of students with autism or dyspraxia. *American Journal of Occupational Therapy, 66,* 511–519. https://doi.org/10.5014/ajot.2012.004010

Knippenberg, C., & Hanft, B. (2004). The key to educational relevance: Occupation throughout the school day. *School System Special Interest Section Quarterly, 11*(4), 1–3.

Rehabilitation Act of 1973, Pub. L. 93–112, 29 U.S.C. §§ 701–796l.

Sayers, B. (2008). Collaboration in school settings: A critical appraisal of the topic. *Journal of Occupational Therapy, Schools, and Early Intervention, 1,* 170–179. https://doi.org/10.1080/19411240802384318

Section 504 of the Rehabilitation Act of 1973, as amended, 29 U.S.C. § 794 (2008).

Strom, E. (n.d.). *The difference between accommodations and modifications.* Retrieved from https://www.understood.org/en/learning-attention-issues/treatments-approaches/educational-strategies/the-difference-between-accommodations-and-modifications

Villeneuve, M. (2009). A critical examination of school-based occupational therapy collaborative consultation. *Canadian Journal of Occupational Therapy, 76,* 206–218. https://doi.org/10.1177%2F000841740907600s05

Best Practices in Providing Group Interventions to Support Participation

42

Ellenmarie Brady, OTD, OTR/L, RN

KEY TERMS AND CONCEPTS

- Collaborative consultation
- Differentiated instruction
- Group protocol
- Health promotion
- Process oriented
- Station teaching
- Task oriented
- Team teaching

OVERVIEW

Occupational therapy has an extensive history of using groups to provide intervention services. Group intervention includes "use of leadership techniques . . . to facilitate learning and acquisition . . . of skills for participation" (American Occupational Therapy Association [AOTA], 2014b, p. S42).

Occupational therapy preservice education prepares practitioners in group interventions (Accreditation Council for Occupational Therapy Education, 2018, Standard B.5.4, p. 44). Applying the group process in schools requires knowledge of the school environment, the curriculum, instruction, and the student's educational, physical health, and mental health conditions as well as physical, cognitive, social, and communication abilities. Occupational therapy practitioners[1] draw on their experience and skills to facilitate students' learning and engagement in occupations.

Occupational therapy practitioners implement a continuum of service models, including group interventions, when providing therapy in schools under the Individuals With Disabilities Education Improvement Act of 2004 (IDEA; Pub. L. 108–446). Regardless of disabilities, students have the right to placement and service in the least restrictive environment (LRE), accessing their education with peers to the greatest extent possible. Removal from

---

[1]*Occupational therapy practitioner* refers to both the occupational therapist and the occupational therapy assistant. AOTA (2014a, p. S18) states, "The occupational therapist is responsible for all aspects of occupational therapy service delivery and is accountable for the safety and effectiveness of the occupational therapy service delivery process" and "must be directly involved in the delivery of services during the initial evaluation and regularly throughout the course of intervention. . . . The occupational therapy assistant delivers safe and effective occupational therapy services under the supervision of and in partnership with the occupational therapist."

class for individual or group interventions can result in the loss of a sense of continuity for the student because the class may have moved on to a different topic in the student's absence. For some students, this may create anxiety and a loss of social experiences (e.g., missed birthday party, missed shared reading).

Providing services in the student's natural setting allows the occupational therapy practitioner to understand the school culture and expectations as well as the academic, physical, and social environment. If service provision involves removing a student from the class, the practitioner should consider the necessary steps to progress the student from a separate location to a small group outside of the classroom routine, to individual services within the classroom routine, and to full classroom participation.

ESSENTIAL CONSIDERATIONS

Participation as part of a group, whether within or outside of the class, can provide a sense of camaraderie, joint goals, the opportunity for modeling behavior and skills, the opportunity for immediate peer feedback, and a source of motivation.

Group Intervention Supported by Research

In a critical appraisal of studies related to occupational therapy collaboration in the classroom, Sayers (2008) found no significant differences reported in student performance between those seen individually or in small groups. Occupational therapy provided in the classroom resulted in greater implementation of recommendations and a higher level of satisfaction with those services. This finding suggests that students may acquire the targeted skills when seen individually, yet they can achieve the same progress in small groups. Implementation of therapeutic recommendations throughout the day promotes mastery and generalization of skills through consistent practice in the student's natural environment.

Copyright © 2019 by the American Occupational Therapy Association. All rights reserved. To reuse this content, contact www.copyright.com.
https://doi.org/10.7139/2019.978-1-56900-591-0.042

On the basis of the student's educational goals, the occupational therapist determines the type of occupational therapy intervention (AOTA, 2017) for service in collaboration with the educational team. The group intervention model allows for an accessible option for the student in a social context, provides opportunities for collaboration with classroom teachers, and affords improved understanding by educators of the supporting role of the related service provider (i.e., the occupational therapy practitioner) and improved understanding by the occupational therapy practitioner of the educator's roles, instruction, and the academic curriculum. Boshoff and Stewart (2013) noted 4 principles to improve collaboration between educational staff and occupational therapists: "Form a committed team; identify and work on a common problem; communicate your role effectively; and lead the way" (p. 145).

Benefits of Group Interventions

Working collaboratively in the school environment can heighten the focus on promoting function rather than remediation of impairment. *Collaborative consultation* is an interactive problem-solving process to generate solutions to identified concerns (Idol et al., 1994). When occupational therapy practitioners are providing group interventions in the classroom (e.g., assisting with journal writing, coteaching handwriting class), they may provide collaborative consultation on various aspects of the curriculum, instruction, environment, or student. By understanding the environments (e.g., physical, social) and contexts (e.g., cultural, personal, temporal, virtual) in which students' occupations occur and what the students can initiate and complete, practitioners gain insights into underlying influences on students' engagement in their educational program (AOTA, 2014b, 2017).

- Are students able to function (e.g., focus on task, recall multistep directions, initiate actions, complete tasks, organize materials, maintain appropriate self-regulation) as environmental demands and distractions increase?
- Do students demonstrate social awareness when interacting with peers? Can students participate comfortably with group processes?
- Are students able to voice their opinions in a group?
- Are there signs of problems with performance skills?
- Are there biomechanical or positioning issues that interfere with performance?

A review of literature relating to collaborative consultation between teachers and therapists concluded that a shared focus and ongoing communication could yield educationally pertinent results that foster student achievement (Villeneuve, 2009). Successful collaboration requires a mutual understanding of roles, curriculum, and classroom routines to identify desirable approaches and time to communicate. Parent and teacher involvement is important to the generalization of skills (Riethmuller et al., 2009). Wilson (2014, p. 3) listed the following 10 reasons for supporting collaboration:

1. Infuses fresh ideas,
2. Expands resources,
3. Increases effectiveness,
4. Reduces barriers,
5. Keeps things real,
6. Spreads the wealth,
7. Forges good relationships,
8. Boosts self-esteem,
9. Lowers anxiety, and
10. Increases excitement and fun.

Another benefit to group interventions is providing services with educators or other professionals (e.g., school nurses, guidance counselors, social workers). Working together may provide deeper problem solving and analysis of the student's needs and strengths.

Working with groups through multi-tiered systems of support (MTSS) allows occupational therapy practitioners to contribute to students in the classroom, students at risk, and students with disabilities. These interventions may prevent referrals for special education services (see Chapter 26, "Best Practices in Multi-Tiered Systems of Support").

Barriers to Group Interventions

Understanding the barriers allows the occupational therapy practitioner to address these issues upfront. Scheduling, space constraints, financial compensation, resistance to change, and pressure from administrators can adversely affect occupational therapy services with students for group intervention.

Scheduling group interventions

Occupational therapy practitioners, particularly when itinerant, often run into limited timeframes for services. Some groups must occur at a specific time on the basis of the teacher's schedule (e.g., language arts, morning meeting), whereas other groups can be scheduled in collaboration with the teacher on the basis of students' and practitioner's availability.

When groups are cofacilitated with the teacher, scheduling may be an issue when the teacher's plan for the day changes. School and class events often affect daily schedules. Occupational therapy practitioners may not have the flexibility to readily shift their schedule to accommodate changes and must address this with the teacher, principal, and their supervisor.

If students must be separated from the classroom for groups because of needs that require intensive skill building or because the group cannot occur within the routine of the day (e.g., classroom students have silent reading), the occupational therapy practitioner needs to coordinate with the teacher.

Space constraints

Whether one is working with a small group in the natural routine or removing the student from the classroom for a group, space is required. The practitioner should address this with the team to identify where services will occur. For example, when the class is working on a cutting, coloring, and gluing task, the occupational therapy practitioner may sit at a classroom table with the student receiving occupational therapy services and 3 peers. While the whole group is working, the occupational therapy practitioner can provide verbal and physical assistance as needed by the student and peers, allowing the student to observe peers and gain instruction from the occupational therapy practitioner to perform the task. Sometimes the occupational therapy practitioner may use the library as a group location with students from multiple classrooms who need to work on similar goals. The type of activity performed by the group influences the possible location of services.

Financial compensation

School administrations must recognize the expertise, time, and effort of practitioners to implement a group intervention model. When intermediary agencies provide occupational therapy staff, the service agreement or contract needs to reflect the workload, billing structure, documentation time, and service time. A practitioner using group interventions is responsible for multiple students. For example, if the practitioner runs 2 groups every day with 3 different students in each group, that practitioner is providing services to 30 students each week, just within those group timeframes. The occupational therapist (and occupational therapy assistant under the occupational therapist's supervision) is also responsible for planning, implementing, and documenting the intervention as well as attending the individualized education program (IEP) meetings for all students involved. When students receive services in a group, Medicaid billing must be recorded at a group rate to avoid fraud, which also requires documentation in each student's individual record.

The key to resolving many of these issues is education and communication. Occupational therapy practitioners should educate administrators and educational staff about the role of occupational therapy in schools and types of interventions. Once there is a clearer understanding of the potential contributions from occupational therapy practitioners, discussions about the importance of the particular issues confronted in individual school settings may be more productive. Discussions might include the benefits of a workload versus caseload approach to service, which could mediate problems with contracts, scheduling, resistance to change, and job structure (see Chapter 14, "Best Practices in Determining a Workload Approach").

Resistance to change

Sometimes practitioners and educators have established routines and are not open to change. It can be helpful to find one teacher who is open to exploring group intervention options for services. Options may include implementing full classroom coinstruction programs, small group participation in the classroom, or establishing various centers in the classroom to work on skills (e.g., the development and implementation of a cutting or dexterity center by the occupational therapy practitioner).

Group interventions can be particularly effective during lessons in which the class breaks into groups for differentiated instruction. *Differentiated instruction* involves periods in which students with mixed abilities break into groups so the teacher can modify instruction to the skill levels and needs of each group (Dixon et al., 2014). During literacy, social studies, and science blocks, practitioners may provide instruction on the use of graphic organizers, sequencing, highlighting key and unknown terms, numbering passages, techniques such as reading questions before text, and more.

Practitioners can intervene during math lessons to assist with strategies to track and align numbers, perceptually grasp the concepts of direction and more or less using number lines, and adapt classroom tools for use.

Pressure from administrators

Administrators may attempt to impose blanket directives to use group interventions as a means to circumvent therapist shortages and respond to budgetary constraints. This is neither ethical nor legal. Occupational therapists must use their professional expertise to determine the intervention approach and type of intervention (e.g., use of occupations and activities, education and training, group interventions; AOTA, 2014b) as well as the setting that is appropriate for meeting the student's needs. Occupational therapy practitioners must provide services that adhere to their state regulatory laws (e.g., state practice acts; licensure) and professional ethics (AOTA, 2015) rather than a directive to save money.

Types of Groups

On the basis of students' needs, groups may be task oriented, process oriented, or a blend of both. *Task-oriented* groups focus on a specific skill or performance component. An example of such a group is a cotaught handwriting group in the classroom. Students work in a parallel, independent manner to gain mastery of the skill or performance expected. A *process-oriented* group focuses more on the interaction of the group members. An example would be social skills groups. The social interaction among group members may be the objective in itself, or it may be supportive of other skills. For example, a group focused on social skills may involve participation in an enjoyable activity while supporting fundamental elements such as eye contact, reciprocal communication, and sharing of materials.

Groups with adolescents that focus on preparing for transition to postschool employment may use the group to practice skills such as interview techniques or customer service situations. Finally, groups may blend elements of both, such as a handwriting club, which might involve learning and practice of skills followed by an activity in which the group works together to write a letter or story.

BEST PRACTICES

This section covers individualized student evaluation, determining need for occupational therapy, and identifying whether the student is appropriate for a group.

Evaluate Each Student

Before determining whether a student is eligible for special education and needs related services, an evaluation must be conducted (IDEA, 2004). Through this process, the team determines whether the student has an educational disability and needs instructional support; if so, an IEP is developed. When determining group participation for occupational therapy services, it is necessary to evaluate the student in terms of function within the classroom (see Chapter 40, "Best Practices in School Occupational Therapy Evaluation and Planning to Support Participation").

One outcome measure that looks at a student's function within the classroom is the Short Child Occupational Profile (Version 2.2; SCOPE; Bowyer et al., 2008), which is appropriate for ages birth through 21 years. The SCOPE, based on the Model of Human Occupation, is a brief assessment that can be used to examine a student's performance skills (e.g., volition, habituation, communication, process, motor, environment factors). The SCOPE is a systematic evaluation used in schools to identify a student's participation strengths and limitations, along with environmental barriers pertaining to daily activities, response to transitions, physical and social environments, process skills, and student roles.

Occupational therapy practitioners may find that students who have difficulty with classroom routines exhibit challenges with self-regulation and social skills. Outcome measures that assess self-regulation and sensory processing include the Sensory Profile 2™ (Dunn, 2014). This tool helps determine sensory processing styles of students ages 3–14 years, 11 months, in the context of home, school, and community activities.

The School Function Assessment (Costner et al., 2008) assists occupational therapists in collaboration with educational team members to assess a student's ability to meet the functional curriculum. Separate measures of a student's current level of participation in school settings, performance of functional activities, and the supports they need to perform functional tasks are gained. This information can be directly linked to program planning determinations.

Direct observation in the classroom and interviews with the teachers for their perspectives are critical. Questions to consider during professional reasoning include the following:

- What are the barriers to student achievement?
- What strengths and weaknesses are notable?
- Can students focus on required tasks and, if not, why?
- Can students handle interactions with peers in small and large group situations?
- Can students initiate and complete a task independently?
- Can students organize their thoughts and belongings?
- Are there environmental factors that interfere with students' participation?
- Are impulse control and lack of inhibition issues present?
- Are students able to identify and respond to social cues?

Implement Effective Group Interventions

The basis of recommendation for participation in group intervention, type of group, size of group, and location of group is analysis by the occupational therapist of results of assessment tools used, observations, teachers' reports, and the realities of the particular school environment to determine the least restrictive way to address students' needs and support their strengths.

Group interventions for students

Group design varies according to the level of support, ages and developmental status of the students, and individual school environment. As the level of support increases, the same techniques are often appropriate in smaller group settings, with modifications and grading as needed.

Social skills and promotion of mental health. Groups with an emphasis on health promotion can incorporate many themes. **Health promotion** focuses on educating students regarding behaviors and choices that are conducive to general well-being and the ability to learn. Examples include nutrition, exercise, stress management, sleep, and self-care. A systematic review of studies related to occupational therapy and mental health within MTSS (Arbesman et al., 2013) examined the effectiveness of multiple interventions within the 3 themes of social skills, promotion of health, and play or recreational activities. Occupational therapy practitioners should be aware of licensure requirements for education and service provision for groups or individuals without previous evaluation.

Health promotion in general education (Tier 1). Occupational therapy practitioners may provide education to school staff or may coinstruct whole classroom groups with school social workers, education staff, or others with a social–emotional or mental health focus. Strong research supports implementation of programs that address stress management and coping skills, social–emotional learning, and antibullying (with a parent education component) to improve students' social, emotional, and coping skills and reduce students' stress, problematic behaviors, and victimization.

Some schools have begun incorporating mindfulness and yoga into their classrooms, with moderate evidence of support that yoga increases physical fitness and cardiorespiratory health (training is required to implement with fidelity). Ferreira-Vorkapic et al. (2015) examined the effectiveness of yoga in schools, summarizing the results as promising for positive effect size in mood change, tension, anxiety, memory, and self-esteem. Strong evidence exists for the positive effects of an obesity program in reducing body mass in 6- to 12-year-old students. Moderate evidence was found that participation in performing arts activities improved social interaction and skills.

Health promotion in general education and supplemental assistance (Tier 2). Occupational therapy practitioners may coinstruct a group of students at risk for academic failure or advocate for social skills education to improve interaction, acceptance, and social standing. Social skills training has been found to reduce unexpected behaviors and improve social and functional skills for students with learning disabilities. There is strong evidence that social and life skills training for students with intellectual and developmental disabilities improved reciprocal communication, self-management, social initiation, and expected behaviors. Strong evidence has indicated that playgroups for students who experienced neglect, abuse, or both can increase their play skills and self-esteem while decreasing their unexpected behaviors and isolated play. Participation in music and play activities improved attention to peers and social skills in children with intellectual and language delays (Arbesman et al., 2013).

Health promotion in special education (Tier 3). For children diagnosed as being on the autism spectrum, researchers found strong evidence that social skills training that included self-management techniques, differential reinforcement (e.g., giving reinforcement for appropriate behavior), and modification of instructional content helped improve students' expected behavior, social competence, and self-management. There was also strong evidence that the use of musical activities improved communication skills (Arbesman et al., 2013).

Handwriting groups. Hoy et al. (2011) investigated handwriting programs and found that practice was a critical part of the program. Researchers recommended a minimum of 2 sessions per week for at least 20 sessions. They noted that providing instruction in groups was one viable solution to help supply sufficient practice time.

Cotaught, embedded models for handwriting programs have consistently demonstrated success in skill acquisition. Bazyk et al. (2009, p. 163) examined fully embedding occupational therapy services into the "emergent literacy curriculum" of kindergarten classes, which focused on writing as a means of communicating thoughts and ideas, and examining the functional interrelationship of "reading, doing, speaking, listening, and writing" using both direct and indirect services. Students with disabilities and without (although some were considered at risk) demonstrated improvement in fine motor skills and emergent literacy skills, underscoring the effectiveness of integrated services for addressing the mechanics, content, and purpose of writing.

Case-Smith et al. (2012) used 2 types of coteaching (i.e., station teaching, team teaching) in following the Write Start program for 2 first-grade classrooms. In ***station teaching,*** the occupational therapist and teacher created activity stations in which students rotated. In ***team teaching,*** the occupational therapist and teacher planned and alternately instructed students. The Write Start program involved regular meetings between the occupational therapist and teacher to review students' progress, plan activities for the upcoming week, and discuss and determine adaptations (e.g., slant boards, sensory breaks, special paper) for individual students. After the 12-week program, posttest results demonstrated significant gains in students' legibility, writing speed, writing fluency, and written expression.

In a broader study (Case-Smith et al., 2014), 4 first-grade classes received small-group (i.e., 7–8 students) instruction from either a cotaught 12-week Write Start program or a single teacher addressing a standard handwriting program. The small group design allowed instructors to guide students, give feedback, and promote peer modeling and support. Researchers found immediate significant improvement in writing speed and legibility in all groups, with greater improvements in the Write Start groups. At 6 months after completion of the program, the Write Start group demonstrated significantly more improvement in writing fluency than the group that received standard instruction.

Sensory–motor and movement groups. Occupational therapy practitioners understand the interconnection of body structures and functions with executive functions (EFs) that influence academic performance. Practitioners may work with teachers to lead a class in movement activities that provide sensory input to help students focus on academic tasks. This type of class can be particularly helpful for young children at the start of the school day and

during transitions. Programs such as GoNoodle (https://www.gonoodle.com) provide activities that can engage a class and provide movement, sensory awareness, and mindfulness training.

Sensory processing and self-regulation groups. Students may have sensory challenges. In a systematic review of studies of occupational therapy, cognitive or occupation-based interventions used with children promoted self-regulation (i.e., function and participation) in children with sensory processing or integration issues. Researchers found moderate evidence for the effectiveness of the cognitive-based interventions of the Alert Program for Regulation and use of social stories (Pfeiffer et al., 2017).

Other groups. On the basis of student need, group themes are endless. Groups can address various occupations (e.g., self-care, cooking, prevocational, communication) and specific performance skills (e.g., fine motor, visual–perceptual, visual–motor). Technology groups may assist students who need to enhance academic and executive skills.

Group participation does not need to be limited to the academic day. Practitioners may implement after-school clubs that target necessary skills and support students' ability to function in the academic environment. For example, a practitioner can run a group that includes movement and tabletop games. These groups support social and EF skills (e.g., inhibition, turn-taking, active listening, frustration tolerance, reasoning). Kiluk et al. (2009) found that children with attention deficit hyperactivity disorder who participated on 3 or more sports teams through the year displayed fewer symptoms of anxiety. Advocating for organized group physical activities during the school day may result in benefits in the classroom.

Groups may include parents and caregivers at all stages of a student's education to support a collaborative relationship, provide strategies, educate, and model techniques. Examples include after-school crafts groups to demonstrate fine motor activities to promote strength and dexterity; sensory–motor groups to help parents learn activities and techniques to assist with coordination and regulation skills; and transition preparation groups for graduating high school students to demonstrate techniques and technology, including smartphone apps, that foster self-determination and independence.

Complete All Documentation for Group Interventions

The occupational therapist is responsible for ensuring that proper documentation is complete. Schools may require specific documentation for general education intervention with students (when working with general education students, the occupational therapist must be sure to follow their state practice act regarding evaluation and intervention). For students in special education, IDEA requires specific documents (e.g., referral for evaluation, parent consent forms, IEPs). In addition, maintenance of occupational therapy records and data collection sheets for individual students is necessary. These documents are outlined in AOTA's *Standards of Practice for Occupational Therapy* (AOTA, 2015) and *Guidelines for Documentation of Occupational Therapy*

(AOTA, 2018) and are discussed briefly here as they relate to group services.

Screening, evaluation, reevaluation, intervention, and outcome reports

These reports must be written for each student and placed in each student's education record (per agency policy). Although data may be collected on a form with multiple names, that form would not meet confidentiality requirements for documentation of services. The school typically has a timeline for reports; for example, progress reports might need to be submitted to the parents at the same frequency as the district report card. The contents of reports should meet AOTA guidelines (AOTA, 2018).

Intervention plan

Therapists must develop intervention plans for each person receiving occupational therapy services (AOTA, 2015, 2018). The intervention plan identifies

- Each student's information (e.g., name, date of birth, precautions),
- Intervention goals related to the student's ability to engage in activities and occupations,
- Intervention approaches (e.g., prevent, create, establish, maintain, modify) and types of interventions used (e.g., groups, occupation and activities, preparatory methods and tasks, consultation, education),
- Service information (e.g., provider, location, frequency, duration),
- Plan for discontinuation,
- Outcomes measures, and
- Persons overseeing the plan.

Each student should have a completed intervention plan before intervention is implemented (see Appendix C, "Occupational Therapy Intervention Plan").

Contact report

Each time a student receives service, the practitioner must document this information in the student record or therapy file, depending on agency policy. Examples of data recorded include the types of interventions used, the student's response, any education or training of others, and any persons present. The service provider must sign and date this note. Each student's record (or therapy file) must include a copy of this information.

Develop Group Protocol

A *group protocol* organizes the information about the group to communicate the purpose, objectives, and frame of reference foundational to the plan. This protocol identifies targeted goals and guides intervention sessions. A group protocol can educate school administrators and staff about occupational therapy by providing concrete purposes and interventions. Data gathered from student performance provide evidence of implementation and effectiveness.

A written group protocol keeps the practitioner focused on targeted needs, outlines evidence-based interventions and activities, and provides a means to collect data and assess

progress, all of which support fidelity in intervention. If prepared with other staff (e.g., teachers), the protocol may include educationally based language, data, and information.

Cole (2018) gave excellent information on planning groups, guidelines for groups according to various frames of reference, leadership skills for facilitating groups, group dynamics, and other essential elements to consider. Cole (p. 330) suggested 11 headings to address relevant areas when developing a protocol:

1. Group title,
2. Author,
3. Frame of reference or model,
4. Purpose,
5. Group membership and size,
6. Group goals and rationale,
7. Outcome criteria,
8. Methods,
9. Time and place of meeting,
10. Supplies and cost, and
11. References.

In a school setting, goals listed in the protocol should include group goals and individual goals for each member (e.g., use their IEP goals when applicable). Outcome criteria and methods should include the type and frequency of data collection to demonstrate progress toward goals. The time and place of meeting should also include the duration of the group, which may be time limited or may be for the duration of the school year.

SUMMARY

Use of group interventions in natural routines of the school day addresses the LRE mandate of IDEA and provides curriculum-based support for students. Their use reinforces a team approach and promotes communication and students' successful carryover of learned skills and strategies in their school day.

Group interventions in school settings can be challenging. Practitioners need to carefully assess the policies and constraints under which they work and plan accordingly to maximize the potential for successful implementation of groups. This plan might involve starting a dialogue with administrators and staff to discuss the benefits of a collaborative approach in achieving mutual goals.

REFERENCES

Accreditation Council for Occupational Therapy Education. (2018). 2018 Accreditation Council for Occupational Therapy Education (ACOTE®) standards and interpretive guide (effective July 31, 2020). *American Journal of Occupational Therapy, 72*(Suppl. 2), 7212410005. https://doi.org/10.5014/ajot.2018.72S217

American Occupational Therapy Association. (2014a). Guidelines for supervision, roles, and responsibilities during the delivery of occupational therapy services. *American Journal of Occupational Therapy, 68*(Suppl. 3), S16–S22. https://doi.org/10.5014/ajot.2014.686S03

American Occupational Therapy Association. (2014b). Occupational therapy practice framework: Domain and process (3rd ed.). *American Journal of Occupational Therapy, 68*(Suppl. 1), S1–S48. https://doi.org/10.5014/ajot.2014.682006

American Occupational Therapy Association. (2015). Standards of practice for occupational therapy. *American Journal of Occupational Therapy, 69*(Suppl. 3), 6913410057. https://doi.org/10.5014/ajot.2015.696S06

American Occupational Therapy Association. (2017). Guidelines for occupational therapy services in early intervention and schools. *American Journal of Occupational Therapy, 71*(Suppl. 2), 7112410010. https://doi.org/10.5014/ajot.2017.716S01

American Occupational Therapy Association. (2018). Guidelines for documentation of occupational therapy. *American Journal of Occupational Therapy, 72*(2, Suppl.), 7212410010. https://doi.org/10.5014/ajot.2018.72S203

Arbesman, M., Bazyk, S., & Nochajski, S. M. (2013). Systematic review of occupational therapy and mental health promotion, prevention, and intervention for children and youth. *American Journal of Occupational Therapy, 67,* e120–e130. https://doi.org/10.5014/ajot.2013.008359

Bazyk, S., Michaud, P., Goodman, G., Papp, P., Hawkins, E., & Welch, M. A. (2009). Integrating occupational therapy services in a kindergarten curriculum: A look at the outcomes. *American Journal of Occupational Therapy, 63,* 160–171. https://doi.org/10.5014/ajot.63.2.160

Boshoff, K., & Stewart, H. (2013). Key principles for confronting the challenges of collaboration in educational settings. *Australian Occupational Therapy Journal, 60,* 144–147. https://doi.org/10.1111/1440-1630.12003

Bowyer, P. L., Kramer, J., Ploszaj, A., Ross, M., Schwartz, O., Kielhofner, G., & Kramer, K. (2008). *A user's manual for the Short Child Occupational Profile (SCOPE)* (Version 2.2). Chicago: Model of Human Occupation Clearinghouse.

Case-Smith, J., Holland, T., Lane, A., & White, S. (2012). Effect of a co-teaching handwriting program for first graders: One-group pretest–posttest design. *American Journal of Occupational Therapy, 66,* 396–405. https://doi.org/10.5014/ajot.2012.004333

Case-Smith, J., Weaver, L., & Holland, T. (2014). Effects of a classroom-embedded occupational therapist–teacher handwriting program for first-grade students. *American Journal of Occupational Therapy, 68,* 690–698. https://doi.org/10.5014/ajot.2014.011585

Cole, M. B. (2018). *Group dynamics in occupational therapy: The theoretical basis and practice application of group intervention* (5th ed.). Thorofare, NJ: Slack.

Costner, W., Deeney, T., Haltiwanger, J., & Haley, S. (1998). *School Function Assessment (SFA).* San Antonio: Therapy Skills Builder.

Dixon, F. A., Yssel, N., McConnell, J. M., & Hardin, T. (2014). Differentiated instruction, professional development, and teacher efficacy. *Journal for the Education of the Gifted, 37,* 111–127. https://doi.org/10.1177/0162353214529042

Dunn, W. (2014). *Sensory Profile 2™.* San Antonio: Pearson.

Ferreira-Vorkapic, C., Feitoza, J. M., Marchioro, M., Simões, J., Kozasa, E., & Telles, S. (2015). Are there benefits from teaching yoga at schools? A systematic review of randomized control trials of yoga-based interventions. *Evidence-Based Complementary and Alternative Medicine, 2015,* 345835. https://doi.org/10.1155/2015/345835

Hoy, M. P., Egan, M. Y., & Feder, K. P. (2011). A systematic review of interventions to improve handwriting. *Canadian Journal of Occupational Therapy, 78,* 13–25. https://doi.org/10.2182/cjot.2011.78.1.3

Idol, L., Nevin, A., & Paolucci-Whitcomb, P. (1994). *Collaborative consultation* (2nd ed.). Austin, TX: Pro-Ed.

Individuals With Disabilities Education Improvement Act of 2004, Pub. L. 108–446, 20 U.S.C. §§ 1400–1482.

Kiluk, B. D., Weden, S., & Culotta, V. P. (2009). Sport participation and anxiety in children with ADHD. *Journal of Attention Disorders, 12,* 499–506. https://doi.org/10.1177/1087054708320400

Pfeiffer, B., Frolek Clark, G., & Arbesman, M. (2017). Effectiveness of cognitive and occupation-based interventions for children with challenges in sensory processing and integration: A systematic review. *American Journal of Occupational Therapy, 72,* 7201190020. https://doi.org/10.5014/ajot.2018.028233

Riethmuller, A. M., Jones, R., & Okely, A. D. (2009). Efficacy of interventions to improve motor development in young children: A systematic review. *Pediatrics, 124,* e782–e792. https://doi.org/10.1542/peds.2009-0333

Sayers, B. R. (2008). Collaboration in school settings: A critical appraisal of the topic. *Journal of Occupational Therapy, Schools, and Early Intervention, 1,* 170–179. https://doi.org/10.1080/19411240802384318

Villeneuve, M. (2009). A critical examination of school-based occupational therapy collaborative consultation. *Canadian Journal of Occupational Therapy, 76,* 206–218. https://doi.org/10.1177%2F000841740907600s05

Wilson, D. E. (2014). Ten reasons why classroom collaboration is worth the time: A teacher's perspective. *Early Intervention and School Special Interest Section Quarterly, 21*(2), 1–4.

Best Practices in Providing Telehealth to Support Participation

43

Jayna Fischbach, OTD, OTR/L, BCP

KEY TERMS AND CONCEPTS

- Asynchronous
- E-helper
- Synchronous
- Teleconsultation
- Telehealth
- Telemonitoring
- Telerehabilitation

OVERVIEW

Telehealth is increasingly being used as a mode of service delivery by a variety of professions. Shortages of highly trained professionals are common across the country because of difficulties in attracting professionals to a variety of locations throughout the United States.

Telehealth can be used by occupational therapy practitioners[1] to meet the AOTA (2015a) *Occupational Therapy Code of Ethics (2015)* requirement of justice by increasing clients' access to practitioners, especially ones with specific training; preventing delays in care in areas of need; and decreasing costs of time and travel for clients and practitioners (AOTA, 2018b; Cason, 2012a, 2012b). *Justice* is defined in the Code of Ethics as "fairness and objectivity in the provision of occupational therapy services" (p. 4). An additional consideration of justice is helping individuals who need care to receive care, reducing barriers to access to occupational therapy, and advocating for change to systems that limit occupational therapy services (AOTA, 2015a).

Terminology

AOTA (2018b) defines **telehealth** as "the application of evaluative, consultative, preventative, and therapeutic services delivered through information and communication technology" (ICT; p. 1). The term *telehealth* is used to describe all aspects of occupational therapy care and to reflect the ability to provide occupational therapy services to facilitate engagement in health, well-being, and participation. However, **telerehabilitation** is defined as "the application of ICT specifically for the delivery of rehabilitation and habilitation services" (AOTA, 2018b, p. 1). Telerehabilitation does not cover the scope of occupational therapy in schools, which is why the term *telehealth* is preferred in this practice setting and is used throughout this chapter.

The AOTA definition of *telehealth* closely aligns with that of the American Telemedicine Association (ATA; 2017): "the use of electronic information and telecommunications technologies to support clinical healthcare, patient and professional health-related education, public health and health administration" (p. 2). The ATA is a leading expert in information about telemedicine and telehealth and is a great resource for anyone looking to use telehealth to support students' school performance.

Telehealth Service Delivery Model

Telehealth services may be delivered in multiple formats to support performance, including **synchronous,** meaning that intervention is completed in real time with the occupational therapy practitioner and client engaging together online (AOTA, 2018b), and **asynchronous,** meaning that the practitioner may record, store, and forward a video, pictures, or information that the client watches and engages with or the client may record, store, and forward a video, pictures, or information that the practitioner later views (AOTA, 2018b).

As a mode of service delivery, telehealth can be provided on an individual basis or on a consultative basis, just as in-person services may be delivered. Occupational therapy services provided on a consultative basis via technology are referred to as *teleconsultation.* AOTA (2018b) defines **teleconsultation** as "a virtual consultation that includes

---

[1]*Occupational therapy practitioner* refers to both the occupational therapist and the occupational therapy assistant. The American Occupational Therapy Association (AOTA; 2014a, p. S18) states, "The occupational therapist is responsible for all aspects of occupational therapy service delivery and is accountable for the safety and effectiveness of the occupational therapy service delivery process" and "must be directly involved in the delivery of services during the initial evaluation and regularly throughout the course of intervention.... The occupational therapy assistant delivers safe and effective occupational therapy services under the supervision of and in partnership with the occupational therapist."

Copyright © 2019 by the American Occupational Therapy Association. All rights reserved. To reuse this content, contact www.copyright.com.
https://doi.org/10.7139/2019.978-1-56900-591-0.043

the remote provider and client, with caregiver as appropriate; remote provider and local provider . . . with the client and caregiver, as appropriate; or remote provider and local provider without the client present" (p. 3). Another form of service delivery via technology is **telemonitoring,** in which clients and stakeholders use equipment to monitor functioning and goals or self-report activities toward and changes in functioning and goals (AOTA, 2018b).

Telehealth can be used exclusively with students to meet their educational needs or as part of a hybrid approach supplemented with in-person services (World Federation of Occupational Therapists, 2014). Occupational therapy practitioners working in schools should determine appropriate guidelines with the administration, teachers, parents, and other stakeholders for use of synchronous and asynchronous telehealth, teleconsultation, and telemonitoring to support school performance.

ESSENTIAL CONSIDERATIONS

All practitioners must adhere to the AOTA (2018a) guidelines to ensure that provision of occupational therapy services by telehealth is in the best interest of clients. In addition, these 5 aspects should be considered:
1. Knowledge, skill, and competence of the occupational therapy practitioner
2. Requirements of the practice setting
3. Client's context and environment
4. Complexity of client's condition
5. Nature and complexity of the intervention (AOTA, 2018b).

The determination of a student's fit for telehealth should be continuously monitored as an occupational therapy practitioner works with the student and their school to ensure it remains an acceptable way to meet federal education requirements of related service.

Knowledge, Skill, and Competence of Occupational Therapy Practitioners

When providing occupational therapy in school via telehealth, the practitioner should have a level of knowledge, skill, and competence similar to that of practitioners working on-site.

Practitioner

Occupational therapy practitioners using telehealth as a method of service provision should be competent in the practice area, be culturally competent with regard to the setting and client population, and follow all state and federal regulations. They should also be able to communicate in clear and concise statements.

The practitioner may be employed by an educational agency or contracted by an outside agency to provide services under the Individuals With Disabilities Education Improvement Act of 2004 (IDEA; Pub. L. 108–446). In both cases, the practitioner must understand all of the laws that affect services (see Chapter 3, "Laws That Affect Occupational Therapy in Schools") and adhere to professional standards and ethics (AOTA, 2015a, 2015b) regarding evaluation and intervention (AOTA, 2014b), documentation of services (AOTA, 2018a), confidentiality of interactions, privacy, security of records, and supervision (AOTA, 2014a).

Occupational therapy practitioners using telehealth must remain up to date on evidence to support or refute the use of telehealth with a variety of client factors and performance skills. In this way, an occupational therapy practitioner maintains the Principle of Veracity, that is, "occupational therapy personnel shall provide comprehensive, accurate, and objective information when representing the profession" (AOTA, 2015a, p. 6). The current state of the literature is limited, although more and more research is being produced. This should be communicated to stakeholders, balanced with statements about why and how telehealth will benefit the student (AOTA, 2018b).

Competency using software programs and web-based systems. Occupational therapy practitioners must be familiar with navigating technical challenges. There should be written guidelines for contacting additional support to troubleshoot any technical difficulties with software or web-based systems that are interrupting occupational therapy services. This is vital to ensure that students receive services when a practitioner has scheduled times with students and educational staff.

The occupational therapy practitioner should have training and mentorship in providing services via telehealth before working with students. Training includes attending continuing education events, reading research articles and practice guidelines, obtaining training from an established company that provides telehealth services, and practicing with mock clients to gain experience in virtual interaction with students. The level of training required depends on the practitioner's comfort with technology and understanding of telehealth practices.

The Accreditation Council for Occupational Therapy Education (2018) requires telehealth to be taught as part of entry-level occupational therapy education to prepare all levels of students to have the skills needed to provide services using telehealth.

Skillful in working with others. The use of someone to assist with occupational therapy sessions is best practice to support student performance in school and can be essential, depending on the student's age and condition. When determining fit for services, work with the school to identify an individual to serve as the e-helper. The **e-helper's** role will be to assist during treatment sessions and also to assist in ensuring that suggestions are carried over into multiple school settings. Examples of appropriate e-helpers may include paraeducators, special education teachers, general education teachers, librarians, and classroom support personnel.

The goal is to select an e-helper who will engage with the student in settings beyond the occupational therapy sessions and help carry over accommodations, supports, and skills into multiple settings with fidelity. Use of an e-helper in the general education classroom is essential to ensure a student is receiving services in the least restrictive environment (LRE).

State regulations

Occupational therapy practitioners are required to be licensed in the state in which they are providing services, whether they are physically located in that state or not. Some state practice regulations may also require that the practitioner reside in the state in which they provide telehealth services. It is best practice for practitioners to be licensed in their state of residence and follow the regulations regarding telehealth (AOTA, 2018b). When state guidelines differ, the occupational therapy practitioner should adhere to the stricter guidelines to maintain ethical commitments of the occupational therapy practitioner's license (AOTA, 2018b). AOTA has resources for state regulations that are updated regularly, but the best place to obtain accurate information is the state licensing board. When a state board does not have specific guidelines for telehealth services, AOTA (2018b) recommends contacting the state board directly; do not use the absence of regulations as permission to provide services using telehealth.

In addition, some state Department of Education rules require related service providers, such as occupational therapists, to be registered with the educational licensure board (e.g., fingerprinted, background check) in addition to state occupational therapy licensure board requirements. Practitioners are responsible for being aware of and complying with these requirements. An understanding of the state occupational therapy licensing guidelines and educational billing systems is important for all telehealth practitioners.

Supervision of an occupational therapy assistant

AOTA's guidelines for supervision of occupational therapy assistants support telehealth as an effective means to implement clients' plans of care carried out by occupational therapy assistants (AOTA, 2014a). Some states require the occupational therapist to directly supervise occupational therapy assistants, completing a session together after a specific period of time. This direct supervision may be completed via telehealth by having the occupational therapist join a session from their physical location to view the session, as long as the state regulations do not require the occupational therapy assistant and occupational therapist to be in the same physical location. Supervision of an occupational therapy assistant who is using telehealth should be performed by an occupational therapist who has experience with telehealth so that they can engage in a respectful and beneficial relationship that promotes optimal outcomes for students.

Payer sources

Local educational agencies (LEAs) may seek cost recovery for health services (i.e., in person or telehealth) through Medicaid, private insurance, or both. The use of these must be voluntary, and services cannot be denied if parents refuse to authorize the use of Medicaid or private insurance. Parents cannot incur any financial cost (e.g., risk of loss of eligibility for waiver program, increase in premiums or discontinuation of insurance coverage, copayment, deductible, reduction of an annual or lifetime cap on coverage; Special Ed Connection, 2018). IDEA (2004) requires that LEAs notify parents and obtain their one-time consent to access their billing information; after that, LEAs must provide parents with annual written notice that they are accessing that information (some LEAs may require a higher frequency). The school must also inform the parent about any potential consequences to billing their insurance

and notify the parent that their refusal to consent does not deny their child services.

Providing occupational therapy services via telehealth is considered the same as occupational therapy provided in person; therefore, it is billed in the same way as in-person services are billed (AOTA, 2018b). When consultative services are being provided via teleconsultation, they are also billed the same as in-person consultation. Any practitioner invoicing Medicaid or an insurance company must be aware of current coding and billing requirements, insurance rules, and regulations because they change frequently. All sessions should be documented to provide a written record of what was provided, the student's response, and progress. Documentation must comply with professional guidelines (AOTA, 2018a). Documentation for telehealth services can happen in a variety of formats, much like in-person services.

Standards and Requirements for Practice

Although the Family Educational Rights and Privacy Act of 1974 (FERPA; Pub. L. 93–380) applies to all education services, the Health Insurance Portability and Accountability Act of 1996 (HIPAA; Pub. L. 104–191) establishes guidelines that require high levels of security for technology being used to store health care information and to engage in services by health care providers, whether those services are provided in person or via technology.

All documentation of services provided—evaluations, contact reports, progress reports, individualized education programs (IEPs), and others—must be stored on a secured system, just as for in-person services. Any documents that contain protected health information must be sent via a secured method (HIPAA, 1996). For example, when an occupational therapy practitioner's email contains confidential student health information, the information must be sent via a secure email server with safeguards in place (usually requiring encrypted passwords). It is important to work with legal counsel, a privacy and security officer, and technology experts to determine appropriate platforms for this type of information. Other considerations are included in Table 43.1.

Student's Context and Environment

Technological considerations can help practitioners provide services in the LRE to support engagement in school (IDEA, 2004). This can be done through asynchronous or synchronous modes. An example of using an asynchronous occupational therapy intervention would be providing the student with videos of how to form letters correctly while writing sentences during class to increase success and allow the student to demonstrate their highest cognitive abilities. An example of a synchronous intervention would be having the student trial a variety of writing tools and writing surfaces in the classroom during a writing activity while the e-helper sets up the student's environment on the basis of feedback from the occupational therapy practitioner.

Space and materials must be established before the session. The occupational therapy practitioner should work with a contact at the school (e.g., e-helper, teacher) to determine the location of the occupational therapy session. It is important

TABLE 43.1.   Considerations of Technology When Providing Telehealth Services

CONSIDERATIONS	RECOMMENDATIONS
HIPAA and FERPA compliant	Video interactions and storage must adhere to these laws and consider all students in the classroom. Some states may require students or their families to give consent for photos or video recording to occur. Recording and saving a session require compliance with more regulations than completion of a session without recording the students.
Internet capabilities	Must be strong enough so synchronous sessions can occur with minimal to no lag; consider effects of inclement weather on speeds or high computer use times in building.
Device with student	Must allow access to video conferencing platforms, secure communication technologies, and other technology platforms vital to service provision. Screen size for viewing practitioner should be based on each individual student's needs. There must be a way to provide a stable video feed and easy manipulation of the camera to change the field of view (e.g., wider lens, a tablet or laptop that can be moved or mounted on a tripod, system to control camera movement).
Device of practitioner	Device must allow for stable video feed that can be manipulated to allow student and e-helper to view practitioner performing desired activities.
Viewing in natural environment	Must consider the student's context, environment, and occupations. Space needs to be "safe."

Note. FERPA = Family Educational Rights and Privacy Act of 1974; HIPAA = Health Insurance Portability and Accountability Act of 1996.

that this space be safe for the e-helper and student, just as it would be important for an in-person session.

Materials needed for the session should be discussed ahead of time so the e-helper has time to locate them. For example, when students need modifications to their chair to provide them adequate support, a list of potential items needed should be drafted by the occupational therapy practitioner and discussed with the e-helper before the session to determine what is available at the school and what potentially needs to be purchased. Another example is collaboration between the practitioner and e-helper to obtain small materials or games to use with a student receiving services to enhance cutting, coloring, and dexterity skills.

Complexity of Student's Condition

Every student should be assessed for the ability to engage appropriately in telehealth services to meet their educational needs. AOTA (2015a) defines *Beneficence* as "a concern for the well-being and safety of the recipients of services" (p. 2); this Principle should be considered when evaluating the student's needs and whether telehealth is able to meet these needs.

It is also important when determining the appropriate e-helper for the student. The e-helper should be trained in emergency response procedures in case an emergency medical situation arises during a session. These procedures should already be established with the school. The occupational therapy practitioner should also be aware of any procedures or contacts they need to make to assist the student, as appropriate, similar to what would occur if a student had a medical emergency during an in-person occupational therapy service.

Autonomy is defined as "the right of the individual to self-determination, privacy, confidentiality, and consent" (AOTA, 2015a, p. 4). This Principle is especially important when using telehealth to provide services. The student, their parents, and all other stakeholders should be informed about how occupational therapy services via telehealth will look and meet the student's needs. All stakeholders need to

agree to receive occupational therapy services via telehealth to meet the standard of autonomy for that student. An occupational therapy practitioner using telehealth should discuss the risks and benefits of any intervention method to be used and respect the wishes of the student and e-helper about engagement in any of the services, just as in-person occupational therapy practitioners would do to maintain client autonomy.

Telehealth may observe the Principle of Justice by matching a student with an occupational therapy practitioner with an understanding of a student's cultural background or primary language to be able to communicate better with family. Occupational therapy practitioners must also maintain the Principle of Fidelity, that is, "treat clients, colleagues, and other professionals with respect, fairness, discretion, and integrity" (AOTA, 2015b, p. 7). An occupational therapy practitioner needs to respect the decisions of all stakeholders involved in a student's school life and address concerns as they arise.

Nature and Complexity of Intervention

In schools, occupational therapy (e.g., in person or telehealth) focuses on students increasing their access to and participation in learning and school activities. For telehealth, e-helpers should be considered vital persons for the therapy team because they will help to increase carryover of adaptive techniques and students' practice of emerging skills to enhance participation. Safety should be the main focus of determining ability to engage in an intervention. The student, e-helper, school setting, environment, and requirements of services provided in a school should help inform an occupational therapy practitioner's decision to use telehealth with a student.

Another consideration of the Principle of Beneficence is ensuring that the occupational therapy practitioner is up to date on current evidence for working with students and using different types of intervention (AOTA, 2015a, 2015b). Telehealth may be a viable solution to secure a practitioner with specialized knowledge and skills to work with a student with a unique condition and intervention need. A student can be matched with a specialist via telehealth to achieve the best outcomes.

In rural areas, many school occupational therapy practitioners work alone in their school districts. Telehealth may allow practitioners to network with each other to develop new knowledge and skills to improve outcomes for students.

BEST PRACTICES

Best practices for occupational therapy practitioners working in schools using telehealth should mirror best practices for in-person services. This section discusses the actual process of evaluation and intervention using telehealth service delivery.

Best practices in telehealth are rapidly evolving, as minimal research currently exists. Practitioners engaging in telehealth should remain up to date with the latest evidence to support or refute the use of telehealth. Practitioners should also review the literature on coaching because this model of intervention can be implemented via telehealth.

Communicate With Schools and E-Helpers

Collaboration with stakeholders is critical for student success, whether therapy is being delivered via telehealth or in person. This collaboration and communication take on a new significance when the occupational therapy practitioner is not physically entering the building to provide services. Developing communication plans that meet the needs of each student and their school is critical to success. Occupational therapy practitioners may plan to virtually attend school district meetings to discuss therapy services. An occupational therapy practitioner could provide a teacher in-service via telehealth to assist in a schoolwide antibullying program or a schoolwide fine motor skill development program for young students.

Quarterly progress notes are an important way to communicate with schools, parents, and other important stakeholders on how the student is progressing toward meeting their IEP goals. Communication happens regularly with the e-helper during a therapy session. Although this individual may help to communicate therapy focus and progress, they should not be solely responsible for this communication. The occupational therapy practitioner may send an email to the teacher regarding strategies that were helpful, using pictures or a short video from the therapy session to remind the teacher to set up adaptive techniques on a daily basis. Keeping the parents informed about therapy services and the student's performance is important.

Appropriate communication with school staff initiating telehealth services may need to be at a higher level than with those who have experience using this type of service delivery. Occupational therapy practitioners should carry out this high level of communication to help the school become comfortable with the services their students are receiving. When done well, communication allows individuals to have an important role in providing multiple opportunities for students to practice learned strategies and assist them in meeting their goals.

Conduct Screening and Evaluation of Student Participation From a Distance

Under early intervening services (IDEA, 2004), occupational therapists may conduct screenings with general education students to recommend instructional strategies for general education staff. (*Note:* This is not allowed in all states, based on state occupational therapy licensure). This screening can easily be completed via telehealth by having someone set up a device for the occupational therapist to view the student in comparison with classroom peers and provide informed recommendations. (*Note:* Because other students in the environment would also be videotaped or viewed, some districts require parent notification, consent, or both.)

For the evaluation process, occupational therapists should follow AOTA official documents, including the position paper on telehealth (AOTA, 2018b), *Occupational Therapy Code of Ethics (2015)* (AOTA, 2015a), and the *Occupational Therapy Practice Framework: Domain and Process* (3rd ed.; AOTA, 2014b). Record review could be completed using a FERPA- and HIPAA-compliant online system, which is commonly used for in-person services. Interviewing students, parents, and other educational team members can take place via video conferencing and can increase access to parents, who do not have to go to the school to participate.

The occupational therapist needs to ensure the evaluation and assessment methods are appropriate to address the student's access, participation, and performance in school. Therefore, the therapist should determine the assessment to be used with the student on the basis of the occupations of concern (e.g., using classroom materials, preparing for transition, caring for self).

Using a standardized assessment that requires a set of standardized manipulatives to administer the assessment is a challenge via telehealth. A few studies have examined interrater reliability by comparing a telehealth model with face-to-face administration of an assessment (Baker & Jacobs, 2013; Dreyer et al., 2001; Durfee et al., 2007; Palsbo et al., 2007). The research is limited, and additional evidence on assessment administration is needed. The American Speech–Language–Hearing Association's (2017) statement on assessment procedures says, "Assessment and therapy procedures and materials may need to be modified or adapted to accommodate the lack of physical contact with the client. These modifications should be reflected in the interpretation and documentation of the service" ("Practice Areas," para. 5).

The e-helper may be vital to adhering as closely as possible to standardized administration of an assessment. One way to achieve minimal modifications is to mail the assessment manipulatives to the school along with an administration manual. Before the student joins the session, the occupational therapist should teach the e-helper how to set up the different aspects of the assessment. The occupational therapist should also explain the importance of the e-helper's setting up the assessment correctly and what level of communication is appropriate, based on the assessment's administration manual.

During administration of the assessment, the occupational therapist will provide instructions to the student while the e-helper sets up the assessment. All modifications (e.g., administration via telehealth) to a standardized

EXHIBIT 43.1. Resources for Online Assessments

General information: Pearson and WPS have systems that allow parents, teachers, and other school personnel to complete measures online. Each tool has a different level of interpretation of results and abilities to assist with intervention planning, based on the student's results. Pearson and companies may pay for these services at the level needed to support evaluation of student performance using telehealth.

- Pearson has a telepractice website that provides helpful information from a variety of sources about use of their products via telehealth ("Telepractice," n.d.).
- Pearson also has Q-global® (2013), a site that allows occupational therapy practitioners to access a variety of tools for online administration.
- WPS (2017) has the WPS Online Evaluation System, which allows online administration of assessments such as the Sensory Processing Measure.
- Developers of assessment tools, such as the Peabody Developmental Motor Scales (Folio & Fewell, 2000), are creating computer-assisted assessments to improve adherence to administration protocols and allow assessment administration via telehealth (Janes et al., 2016).

assessment must be included in documentation of the assessment results. The reliability and validity of an assessment may not be applicable to telehealth administration. For this reason, occupational therapists need to be informed about current research and the assessment being used. Assessment producers are continuing to develop assessments and guidelines for telehealth administration. See Exhibit 43.1 for assessment resources.

Occupational therapists administering assessments must select tools that meet the needs of the student, whether providing services via telehealth or in person. Selecting an assessment that does not provide all needed information as a result of telehealth use restrictions may mean a student is not appropriate for telehealth at the time. Occupational therapists must stay current with the latest literature on assessment to know whether evidence has been produced to support administration via telehealth. An assessment can be carried out by an occupational therapy assistant under the supervision of an occupational therapist via telehealth, just as completed in person (see Chapter 7, "Best Practices for Occupational Therapy Assistants in Schools").

Plan Interventions

Nonmaleficence, defined as "refrain[ing] from actions that cause harm" (AOTA, 2015a, p. 3), should be considered throughout the occupational therapy process. The focus of Nonmaleficence is that an occupational therapy practitioner not cause harm, pain with intervention, or negative emotional feelings, even if the potential of long-term benefits seems to outweigh the acute negative experience (AOTA, 2015b). Safety should be discussed with the e-helper to make sure they understand harm is not acceptable for the student engaging in therapy at any point. It is important to consider nonmaleficence when determining fit of the student to telehealth.

Self-care is within occupational therapy's scope of practice and should be addressed in school to support independence and engagement in educational activities (AOTA, 2014b, 2014c). An occupational therapy practitioner addressing self-care may work on self-toileting strategies with a student to improve their skills and abilities to be independent.

Placing a student on camera in a compromised position would be inappropriate. More reasoned options would be to simulate the self-care activity with the student seated on the toilet fully dressed, to assess the student's height and access, or to have the e-helper assist the student in completing the self-care activity and provide input to the occupational therapy practitioner. The e-helper would be in the bathroom with the student to report difficulties, with the camera positioned outside the bathroom. In this way, collaboration and coaching can be used to meet the student's needs without putting the student on camera.

Be Present in the LRE

Occupational therapy practitioners need to select intervention methods that support students in the LRE and their ability to participate in their school day more actively. Telehealth can support and hinder this goal in a variety of ways. When students have an e-helper who is a paraeducator, it may be easy to add a tablet device to the student's desk to work on a skill with minimal distraction to the rest of the room and without putting an additional person in a small space.

At times, difficulties may arise when the e-helper does not understand what the occupational therapy practitioner intends. To overcome this difficulty, the practitioner may have items on their end to model what they want the e-helper and student to carry out. Occupational therapy practitioners may even need to change their position on camera to ensure that the e-helper and student can understand what performance skills are desired from the student when working on a variety of occupations and activities. Portions of a session may be captured by video and provided to the e-helper, paraeducator, teacher, parent, or other stakeholder to promote carryover and target desired outcomes.

Occupational therapy practitioners using telehealth should be sure to communicate ahead of time with the student's e-helper about plans for the session, using input from all parties. The plan provided to the e-helper should include an outline of skills to be worked on and activities planned as well as any needed equipment and plans for the space in which the session will be conducted (e.g., general education classroom, student desk). Because various schooling options exist, occupational therapy practitioners may need to provide intervention with students in online academies or home schools. The student's e-helper may be the parent, who would assist with acquisition and carryover of skills in meaningful activities. There is some evidence to support the use of telehealth to improve handwriting for students completing online education (Criss, 2013).

In schools using multi-tiered systems of support, occupational therapy practitioners engaging in Tier 1 or Tier 2 services should consider the nature of the intervention and how telehealth may support or hinder this level of service. Providing Tier 1 and Tier 2 services also requires collaboration and preplanning with the school and identifying the e-helper role. The occupational therapy practitioner should determine what the appropriate support would be (this may not be different from in-person services).

For example, a Tier 1 program to promote healthy living choices in elementary students may require the occupational therapist to collaborate with the head of food services and communicate with all teachers to determine implementation and plans for the program. In another example, the occupational therapist may collaborate with the home economics teacher to design and implement a Tier 2 group program that would support teens with disabilities looking to transition to supported or independent living after graduation.

Assist With Transition Planning

Occupational therapy practitioners working in schools consider transition planning for all students. In accordance with IDEA (2004), an individualized transition plan must be developed and implemented when a student turns age 16 years (some states may regulate a younger age). The occupational therapy practitioner should work with the student, their family, and the school to determine the plan for the student after completing their education.

An advantage of using telehealth would be the occupational therapy practitioner's ability to "travel" to a student's potential secondary education site, employment, or living location even when it is far away. The occupational therapy practitioner could help the student and family solve identified barriers and supports to being as independent as possible in the new settings. Asynchronous technologies can be applied to develop video or media supports to help the student to complete ADLs, organization of responsibilities, or aspects of their job tasks and used as needed at these locations.

Propose Discontinuation and Provide Supports

Proposing discontinuation of telehealth services should mirror in-person services, with communication among student, the family, teachers, and other stakeholders vital to student success before the IEP meeting. Asynchronous supports that were initially developed to support the student during therapy may continue to be used by the student to support their ongoing independence. Plans to follow up with the student, teachers, parents, and other stakeholders are important to ensure that the student remains successful after discontinuation. This follow-up is even more important when using telehealth because the occupational therapy practitioner is not visiting the school and may not communicate with those people again without a plan in place.

SUMMARY

Occupational therapy services in schools provided via telehealth should mirror the services delivered in person as much as possible. The occupational therapy practitioner should partner with an e-helper to reduce the barriers established by the use of telehealth and support students in their educational goals. Students, their goals, and their school should be individually considered and continually assessed for their fit to receive school supports via telehealth. If in-person therapy becomes necessary, steps should be taken to ensure this is possible.

Occupational therapy practitioners engaging in telehealth must adhere to AOTA's guidelines provided in current and future documents on telehealth and continue to review new research on telehealth to inform their practice. Occupational therapy practitioners using telehealth should also consider ways to contribute to the body of knowledge about telehealth to support development of the profession and this service delivery mode.

REFERENCES

Accreditation Council for Occupational Therapy Education. (2018). 2018 Accreditation Council for Occupational Therapy Education (ACOTE®) standards and interpretive guide. *American Journal of Occupational Therapy, 72*(Suppl. 2), 7212410005. https://doi.org/10.5014/ajot.2018.72S217

American Occupational Therapy Association. (2014a). Guidelines for supervision, roles, and responsibilities during the delivery of occupational therapy services. *American Journal of Occupational Therapy, 68*(Suppl. 3), S16–S22. https://doi.org/10.5014/ajot.2014.686S03

American Occupational Therapy Association. (2014b). Occupational therapy practice framework: Domain and process (3rd ed.). *American Journal of Occupational Therapy, 68*(Suppl. 1), S1–S48. https://doi.org/10.5014/ajot.2014.682006

American Occupational Therapy Association. (2014c). Scope of practice. *American Journal of Occupational Therapy, 68*(Suppl. 3), S34–S40. https://doi.org/10.5014/ajot.2014.686S04

American Occupational Therapy Association. (2015a). Occupational therapy code of ethics (2015). *American Journal of Occupational Therapy, 69*(Suppl. 3), 6913410030. https://doi.org/10.5014/ajot.2015.696S03

American Occupational Therapy Association. (2015b). Standards of practice for occupational therapy. *American Journal of Occupational Therapy, 64*(Suppl. 3), S106–S111. https://doi.org/10.5014/ajot.2010.64S106

American Occupational Therapy Association. (2018a). Guidelines for documentation of occupational therapy. *American Journal of Occupational Therapy, 72*(Suppl. 2), 7212410010. https://doi.org/10.5014/ajot.2018.72S203

American Occupational Therapy Association. (2018b). Telehealth in occupational therapy. *American Journal of Occupational Therapy, 72*(Suppl. 2), 7212410059. https://doi.org/10.5014/ajot.2018.72S219

American Speech–Language–Hearing Association. (2017). *Telepractice.* Retrieved from https://www.asha.org/prpprinttemplate.aspx?folderid=8589934956

American Telemedicine Association. (2017). *Principles for delivering telerehabilitation services.* Retrieved from https://www.americantelemed.org/main/membership/ata-members/ata-sigs/telerehabilitation-sig

Baker, N., & Jacobs, K. (2013). The feasibility and accuracy of using a remote method to assess computer workstations. *Human Factors, 56,* 784–788. https://doi.org/10.1177/0018720813503985

Cason, J. (2012a). An introduction to telehealth as a service delivery model within occupational therapy. *OT Practice, 17*(7), CE-1–CE-8.

Cason, J. (2012b). Telehealth opportunities in occupational therapy through the Affordable Care Act. *American Journal of Occupational Therapy, 66,* 131–136. https://doi.org/10.5014/ajot.2012.662001

Criss, M. J. (2013). School-based telerehabilitation in occupational therapy: Using telerehabilitation technologies to promote improvements in student performance. *International Journal of*

Telerehabilitation, 5(1), 39–46. https://doi.org/10.5195/ijt.2013 .6115

Dreyer, N. C., Dreyer, K. A., Shaw, D. K., & Wittman, P. (2001). Efficacy of telemedicine in occupational therapy: A pilot study. *Journal of Allied Health, 30,* 39–42.

Durfee, W. K., Savard, L., & Weinstein, S. (2007). Technical feasibility of teleassessments for rehabilitation. *IEEE Transactions of Neural Systems and Rehabilitation Engineering, 15,* 23–29. https://doi.org/10.1109/TNSRE.2007.891400

Family Educational Rights and Privacy Act of 1974, Pub. L. 93–380, 20 U.S.C. § 1232g; 34 C.F.R. Part 99.

Folio, M. R., & Fewell, R. R. (2000). *Peabody Developmental Motor Scales* (2nd ed.). Austin, TX: Pro-Ed.

Health Insurance Portability and Accountability Act of 1996 (HIPAA), Pub. L. 104–191, 42 U.S.C. § 300gg, 29 U.S.C. §§ 1181–1183, and 42 U.S.C. §§ 1320d–1320d9.

Individuals With Disabilities Education Improvement Act of 2004, Pub. L. 108–446, 20 U.S.C. §§ 1400–1482.

Janes, W. E., Persch, A., Schwartz, J., & Cason, J. (2016). Current trends in assessment and technology. *SIS Quarterly Practice Connections, 1*(3), 12–14.

Palsbo, S. E., Dawson, S. J., Savard, L., Goldstein, M., & Heuser, A. (2007). Televideo assessment using Functional Reach Test and European Stroke Scale. *Journal of Rehabilitation Research and Development, 44,* 659–664. https://dx.doi.org/10.1682/JRRD .2006.11.0144

Q-global® web-based administration, scoring, and reporting. (2013). Retrieved from https://images.pearsonclinical.com/images /qglobal/

Special Ed Connection. (2018). *Smartstart: Financial responsibility— Use of public insurance.* Retrieved from https://www.specialed connection.com/LrpSecStoryTool/index.jsp?contentId=10005 &chunkid=335185&query=((PUBLIC+INSURANCE))&listnum =0&offset=0&topic=Main&chunknum=1

Telepractice. (n.d.). Retrieved from http://www.pearsonclinical .com/psychology/RelatedInfo/telepractice.html

World Federation of Occupational Therapists. (2014). World Federation of Occupational Therapists' position statement on telehealth. *International Journal of Telerehabilitation, 6*(1), 37–39. https://doi.org/10.5195/ijt.2014.6153

WPS. (2017). *Online evaluation system.* Retrieved from https:// platform.wpspublish.com/account/login

Best Practices in Providing Services in Nonpublic Schools and Homeschooling

44

Alyssa M. Fagan, OTD, OTR/L, LMT

KEY TERMS AND CONCEPTS

- Free appropriate public education
- Homeschooling
- Parentally placed private school students with disabilities
- Private school
- Public school
- Publicly placed private school students with disabilities
- Unilateral placement

OVERVIEW

The role of the occupational therapy practitioner[1] specific to service provision in nonpublic schools and homeschooling may vary considerably from that of practitioners working in public education. Moreover, occupational therapy services may be different in the realms of nonpublic schools and homeschooling. The primary factors influencing the role and practice of occupational therapy practitioners in these settings may include the source of funding that the school or institution receives, the federal and state legislative requirements, and the decision-making process at the local level. Performance patterns, contextual issues, and environmental factors may also affect services in these settings, such as the type of school, the school mission statement, the culture of the school or home, and the physical and social environments of the nonpublic school and home (AOTA, 2014b).

Occupational therapy services in nonpublic schools are more customary than they have been in the recent past (AOTA, 2016), and the prevalence of families choosing an education through homeschooling is increasing (Redford et al., 2017). Occupational therapy practitioners working with students should familiarize themselves with the various legislative, funding, and contextual factors that may affect service provision in nonpublic schools and homeschooling to promote the application of and advocacy for best practices in each of these settings.

ESSENTIAL CONSIDERATIONS

For occupational therapy practitioners working with students in nonpublic schools and homeschooling, understanding the factors that have the potential to influence service in these settings is essential in promoting best practices.

What Are Nonpublic Schools and Homeschooling?

In the areas of nonpublic schools and homeschooling, there are many types of schools and related terminology. Some terminology may be regional, so it is vital to familiarize oneself with the lexicon that is used most frequently in one's practice locale. For this chapter, we use the term *private school* to represent a nonpublic school.

Private schools

Families seeking an alternative to public education for their child may pursue a private school education. The term ***private school*** broadly encompasses many types of institutions, such as traditional, independent, religious, boarding, private special education, language immersion, and those that focus on a specific pedagogy (e.g., Montessori, Reggio Emilia, Waldorf; Barrington, 2017).

The National Center for Education Statistics (NCES; n.d.) forecast that 9% of students (more than 5,000,000) would enroll in private schools during the 2017–2018 school year, which indicates a decline. In the 1995–1996 school year, 12% of all students enrolled in private schools, whereas only 10% enrolled in these institutions during the 2013–2014 school year (NCES, 2017). Despite these statistics, AOTA (2016) included this area in its emerging niche

---

[1]*Occupational therapy practitioner* refers to both the occupational therapist and the occupational therapy assistant. The American Occupational Therapy Association (AOTA; 2014a, p. S18) states, "The occupational therapist is responsible for all aspects of occupational therapy service delivery and is accountable for the safety and effectiveness of the occupational therapy service delivery process" and "must be directly involved in the delivery of services during the initial evaluation and regularly throughout the course of intervention. . . . The occupational therapy assistant delivers safe and effective occupational therapy services under the supervision of and in partnership with the occupational therapist."

Copyright © 2019 by the American Occupational Therapy Association. All rights reserved. To reuse this content, contact www.copyright.com.
https://doi.org/10.7139/2019.978-1-56900-591-0.044

series in 2011, asserting that working in a private school was one developing field for school occupational therapy practitioners. Although statistics are not currently available, AOTA (2016) now considers this practice area to be more commonplace.

Private schools differ from public schools in many ways. **Public schools** are financed by federal, state, and local funds and taxes (NCES, 2017) and therefore must follow legislation at those respective levels. Conversely, individuals or corporations may own and operate private schools as either for-profit or nonprofit institutions (Kennedy, 2017). Private schools are generally not eligible for public aid for their operations (although states may vary in their provision of transportation, textbooks, testing services, and technology; U.S. Department of Education [U.S. DOE], 2009). Of importance to this chapter, **publicly placed private school students with disabilities** (i.e., students placed in private schools per mutual agreement between parent and school district) would occur at public expense as a means of providing a *free appropriate public education* (FAPE) in accordance with the Individuals With Disabilities Education Improvement Act of 2004 (IDEA; Pub. L. 108–446; U.S. DOE, 2009). FAPE ensures that students with disabilities receive educational services and supports individualized to their identified needs through public funding. These IDEA funds would require the private school to follow proceedings in the same manner as those in the public sector.

The enrollment process highlights another discrepancy between public and private schools. Public school enrollment typically depends on the location of the student's residence, whereas private school student enrollment may depend on the type of education a family chooses or a public agency determines (e.g., local educational agency [LEA] in collaboration with the individualized education program [IEP] team and family) and the admissions process (Chen, 2017). The admissions process of a private school often requires families to fill out an application, participate in an interview, and provide additional paperwork (e.g., report cards, progress reports, clinical evaluations). Occasionally, observations of the student in their current school or the potential private school occur to ensure the appropriate placement.

In public schools, the education that students receive is free for families, and special education and related services are also available at no cost to students who are eligible (U.S. DOE, 2016a). Private schools are often tuition based, with the responsibility for payment typically falling on the student's guardian or LEA (U.S. DOE, 2011). LEA's responsibilities vary depending on whether the student was publicly placed or parentally placed. When a student is publicly placed, the LEA funds special education and related services. When parentally placed, the LEA is obligated to spend a proportionate amount of IDEA funds to provide equitable services. In some cases, LEAs may expend more than their proportionate share. Some private schools may offer scholarships or financial aid. The tuition for a private school education can vary depending on the location and type of private school (e.g., religious, elementary, high school; U.S. DOE, 2016b).

Most private schools do not have the same extent of supports and services for students with special needs as do public schools. Of 34,576 identified private schools in the United States during the 2015–2016 school year, only 5% specialized in students with special education needs (Broughman et al., 2017). Tuition is typically much higher for schools that educate specific populations, such as students with autism, learning disabilities, or emotional disabilities.

Homeschooling

Homeschooling refers to families who choose to educate their children at home. Terminology and regulations regarding homeschooling may vary from state to state (U.S. DOE, 2009).

The percentage of students who receive education through homeschooling is on the rise. In 2012, the National Household Education Surveys Program conducted a survey to gather information about students receiving an education through homeschooling (Redford et al., 2017). Of 17,563 identified students, 2.2% families chose homeschooling in 2003 compared with 3.4% in 2012. For families who pursued homeschooling in 2012, 91% cited environmental concerns as the most important rationale for doing so. Redford et al. (2017) further discovered that 16% of families cited special needs as the rationale for homeschooling. Mental or physical health concerns were the reason for 15% of the same group of families.

Federal Legislation

The No Child Left Behind Act of 2001 (Pub. L. 107–110), a reauthorization of the Elementary and Secondary Education Act of 1965 (Pub. L. No. 89–313), provided specific options for families who sought alternatives to traditional public school settings, such as charter schools, magnet schools, private schools, and homeschooling (U.S. DOE, 2013). The more recent reauthorization of the Elementary and Secondary Education Act, the Every Student Succeeds Act (ESSA; 2015; Pub. L. 114–95), no longer explicitly defines school choice for families, thereby placing the responsibility for determining these options at the state and local levels (Burke & Corona, 2016).

ESSA (2015) promoted fair and reasonable access to high-quality education and proportional funding as well as adequate follow-through from a team supporting the student on a local level (Council for American Private Education, 2016). More specific to occupational therapy, ESSA urged practitioners working in the public arena to influence schools at the system or population level (AOTA, 2017a). This legislation does not affect occupational therapy service in a private school that does not receive government funding. However, system-level supports and influence in a private school are still aspects of best practice.

IDEA and Section 504 of the Rehabilitation Act of 1973, as amended (2008; Pub. L. 93–112), ensure that school-age students receive FAPE. Families have the choice to select a private school or homeschooling over a public school education. When families independently choose either of these options (i.e., there is no concern about FAPE), they are opting out of the certainty of federal funding that would support their child and their child's individual and specific needs in a public school environment (Coalition for Responsible Home Education, n.d.). Despite losing certain supports, families who independently forgo a public education for their child continue to have certain rights under IDEA (U.S. DOE, 2015). In general, when FAPE is not a concern, the process for determining and implementing service is considerably different than that in the public domain.

Parentally placed private school students with disabilities

The U.S. DOE (2011) uses the term **parentally placed private school students with disabilities** for families who independently choose a private school for their child when FAPE is not a concern. Under IDEA, LEAs are required to locate, identify, and evaluate students who are thought to have disabilities (i.e., Child Find activities; U.S. DOE, 2011). The location of the private school, not the residence of the student's guardian, determines which LEA would conduct Child Find activities, conclude whether the child is eligible for special education and related services, and provide a service plan (similar to an IEP; U.S. DOE, 2011).

State educational agencies oversee LEAs' spending of funds from IDEA "to ensure equitable participation . . . in programs assisted by or carried out under the equitable participation requirements" (U.S. DOE, 2011, p. 1). However, students who are parentally placed in private schools may not have an individual right to all or even some of the individualized services that they would have access to in a public school or when publicly placed in a private school, if found eligible.

Consultation is a crucial aspect of the process of providing equal involvement for a parentally placed private school student with disabilities. The consultation process occurs between the LEA where the school is located and delegates from both the private school and the student's family (U.S. DOE, 2011). The goal of the deliberation between these individuals aims to resolve several issues. These issues include finding and assessing eligible students; determining the amount and allocation of funds that will assist the parentally placed student with disabilities in a private school placement; establishing the logistics of any interventions or supports that they may deem necessary (e.g., type, frequency, location of service); and reporting on the timing and documentation of the involved processes (U.S. DOE, 2011).

When families choose a private education, the consultation between the LEA and the delegates of the parentally placed student with disabilities also aids in creating service plans for students who are eligible for special education and related services (U.S. DOE, 2011). Service plans are akin to IEPs but are not as in-depth. These plans may include the type and location of special education and related services offered (Morin, n.d.), present level of performance, goals, signatures of the individuals involved in creating the service plan, and transition information (State of New Jersey

Department of Education, n.d.). Implementation of service plans requires parental consent.

In some cases, families may pursue a **unilateral placement**—that is, they may pursue a private school placement when they consider a public school placement inadequate for meeting FAPE (Coleman Tucker, n.d.). Families may engage in due process to resolve disputes and seek tuition reimbursement by the LEA. The burden of proof is variable among states, falling on either the LEA or the family (Shipman & Goodwin, 2005).

Some schools that primarily educate students through unilateral placement may have an alternative and internal plan in place that is like an IEP, whereas others have no internal guiding document (U.S. DOE, 2011). Some of these schools may choose to reference the IEP to aid recommendations for a student or to assist in general decision making about supports and service needs. As a result, private schools may vary greatly in the internal procedures and practices that influence occupational therapy service provision.

Publicly placed private school students with disabilities

In some instances, an LEA, in collaboration with the family and IEP team, may determine that a private school placement is the appropriate setting for a student in consideration of FAPE. The LEA in which the student's guardian resides would be responsible for funding the student's private education. Publicly placed private school students with disabilities are eligible for the same type and extent of services and supports as a student attending public school. The public school would be required to follow the student's IEP. Decisions agreed on at IEP meetings determine and direct the implementation of services in these settings just as in the public arena.

State Legislation

State education laws and regulations regarding private school and homeschooling are incredibly variable. *State Regulation of Private Schools* (U.S. DOE, 2009) is an excellent resource for exploring each state's specific requirements and statutes for private schools and homeschooling.

Private schools

According to the U.S. DOE (2009), regulations for the provision of special education and related services in private schools differ significantly among states. Some states do not have special education policies about private schools. Other states have statutes that may specify student assessment and placement, fund distributions, transportation, eligibility for special education services, and when and how public schools have arrangements with private schools or nonprofit corporations. Several states specify the ability of public schools to contract services with nonprofit corporations (U.S. DOE, 2009).

Staying informed about changes in laws is extremely important. For example, in New York, the education law changed in 2011 (Education Law Amendments of 2011). The law required corporations that operate private schools and educate students with special needs to obtain a waiver for licensed related service providers to practice in their institutions (New York State Education Department, 2018). Corporations without this waiver are now out of compliance with the law, and licensed service providers should no longer be working in these settings. Anyone who continues to do so would potentially put their professional license at risk as well as compromise the Vercity and Fidelity of their professional ethics (AOTA, 2015a).

Homeschooling

States vary greatly in how they define *homeschooling*. Some states provide specific supports, whereas others may have statutes that require specific procedures or documentation for students educated through homeschooling (U.S. DOE, 2009). Several states do not have any laws regarding homeschooling (U.S. DOE, 2009); others consider homeschooling as a private school education (U.S. DOE, 2013). In the latter case, students may be eligible for services on the basis of statutes that apply to private schools (U.S. DOE, 2015). Some states allow parents to dual-enroll their children in public school and homeschool. Parents may choose dual enrollment so their child may participate in sports, music, and special education.

Accreditation

Accreditation of private schools from an external or state institution ensures that schools meet specific qualifications and standards. Accreditation is not a federal requirement (U.S. DOE, 2015). According to the U.S. DOE (2009), it is often optional and not required at the state level. For example, accreditation is voluntary in California, Colorado, Illinois, Pennsylvania, Utah, and Minnesota. The requirement for accreditation is absent altogether in Delaware, Georgia, Maine, Massachusetts, New Jersey, and New York. In certain states, such as Iowa, accreditation may be an additional requirement in granting students with disabilities the same rights as those in public school (Iowa Department of Education, 2014).

Employment and Salary in Private Schools and Homeschooling

Occupational therapy practitioners may work with a student in private school or homeschooling settings in numerous ways. LEAs may contract with practitioners who work for a public school, a cooperative education service, or an outpatient clinic or in private practice to work with students in private schools or homeschooling. Some private schools may employ occupational therapy practitioners directly for that setting.

Occupational therapy practitioners working with students in a private school setting or homeschooling may find variations in payment, salary, and benefits depending on where and how they provide services. Practitioners working for a business entity (e.g., clinic, private practice) and contracted with the school may have different billing structures, such as per diem rates, insurance billing, and direct pay from schools. For school occupational therapists and occupational therapy assistants who are employed directly

by a public or private school, there are more specific reports of salary averages (see U.S. Department of Labor, 2018a, 2018b, 2018c, 2018d, 2018e).

Occupational therapy practitioners working in private schools earn wages approximately 3% higher than those of their colleagues in public schools (U.S. Department of Labor, 2018a, 2018b, 2018d). Despite the higher average salary in private schools, occupational therapists and occupational therapy assistants working in public schools may have additional benefits that may be unavailable in the private sector. These benefits may include accessing comprehensive employer-paid benefits, acquiring a pension after a period of employment, receiving debt relief for school loans, and gaining certain protections and supports through a teachers' union.

Cultural Considerations

School occupational therapy practitioners working in the private sector may find contextual factors and performance patterns that are different from those in the public arena (AOTA, 2014b).

Private schools

The type of private school and its values may also influence specific practices. For example, a private school educating students with special needs may have more system supports in place for students (e.g., therapeutic programming, assistive technology [AT], specialized curricula, environmental modifications) than do schools that do not have this type of mission. Consequently, practitioners in this setting may find greater opportunities to address the needs of the student population using multi-tiered systems of support.

Schools with a religious affiliation or those that focus on a specific pedagogy may have different practices, routines, and curricula that place demands on a student's occupational performance during the school day that are not apparent in public schools. For example, students in a religious school may need to sit for a relatively extended period for religious services. Schools that have a specific pedagogy with specific core values may have certain practices related to the curriculum that they follow. For instance, Montessori schools promote autonomy and self-monitoring by requiring students to work continuously and at their own pace during various activities (American Montessori Society, n.d.).

In both instances, an occupational therapy practitioner may find these demands to be unique to private schools and problematic for students with special needs. Practitioners may address these types of factors when working with students to improve or enhance occupational performance in these settings (AOTA, 2014b).

Private schools may also have additional duties and responsibilities that influence an occupational therapy practitioner's experience in this setting. Some private schools may require practitioners to attend regular meetings for professional development, interprofessional collaboration and consultation, or general school updates and planning. In some instances, these sessions may occur before or after typical school hours. Practitioners also may need to participate in events during the school year to promote parent–practitioner interaction and collaboration, such as Back-to-School Night meetings and parent–teacher conferences. Some private schools seeking to maintain accreditation may involve practitioners in the review process through written departmental progress reports and interviews with the accrediting body.

Private schools may also require or strongly encourage occupational therapy practitioners to provide additional support on the basis of demands during the school day or year. For example, some practitioners may have to perform lunch and recess duty on a regular or semiregular basis; schools may require the practitioner's assistance during the arrival or dismissal process, or practitioners may be required to act as proctor for examinations. Other opportunities to support the school may occur on a volunteer basis and infrequently include a stipend. These types of opportunities may include being a part of a crisis intervention team; being an active member of a committee (e.g., service, leadership, wellness, school event planning); running a student club; assisting in fundraising efforts; acting as chaperone for a school dance; coaching students (e.g., sports, play practice, talent show); and leading after-school enrichment groups.

Homeschooling

Cultural factors in homeschooling are unique to each state, local school district, and family. Variations in requirements and recommendations at state and local levels influence the location of occupational therapy services. As mentioned previously, services may occur in the student's home, an outpatient clinic, or a public school. When working in a student's home, cultural factors will be unique to each family's situation—values and beliefs of the family, the socioeconomic status (SES) of the family, the presence and involvement of other family members in the home, the physical home environment, and the neighborhood or community in which the family resides.

Advocating for Occupational Therapy in Private Schools

To promote best practices in private schools, occupational therapy practitioners often need to take on the role of advocate. A lack of awareness of the role of occupational therapy in schools may hinder and reduce the success of specific practices, such as the collaboration between practitioners and school faculty (Benson, 2013; Kennedy & Stewart, 2012; Villeneuve, 2009). The lack of understanding and awareness of the potential role of an occupational therapy practitioner may also limit the potential scope of practice in a school setting (Sonday et al., 2012). In addition, those who supervise occupational therapy practitioners in schools are often unfamiliar with factors that influence occupational therapy practice (AOTA, 2017a).

Occupational therapy practitioners working in private education may need to educate supervisors, administrators, and policymakers regarding best practices and the potential scope and role of occupational therapy practitioners in these types of settings. Because non–government-funded private schools often have more freedom regarding service delivery, the need for advocacy is paramount. Prospects for supporting students and educating stakeholders from the individual to the population level in private schools and homeschooling support the sentiment of the profession's *Vision 2025* (AOTA, 2017b).

BEST PRACTICES

Best practices in private schools and homeschooling should not differ immensely from best practices in public schools. However, because of discrepancies in legislation, funding, and other contextual factors in each of these domains, occupational therapy practitioners may find variability in practice patterns in these settings. At the very least, best practices in private schools and homeschooling should be determined by numerous professional guidelines.

AOTA provides multiple documents and publications that serve to direct practitioners and their practices, such as the

- *Guidelines for Supervision, Roles, and Responsibilities During the Delivery of Occupational Therapy Services* (AOTA, 2014a);
- *Occupational Therapy Practice Framework: Domain and Process* (3rd ed.; AOTA, 2014b);
- *Guidelines for Documentation of Occupational Therapy* (AOTA, 2018);
- *Occupational Therapy Code of Ethics (2015)* (AOTA, 2015a);
- *Standards for Continuing Competence* (AOTA, 2015b);
- *Guidelines for Occupational Therapy Services in Early Intervention and Schools* (AOTA, 2017a); and
- *Standards of Practice for Occupational Therapy* (AOTA, 2015c).

Best practices in evaluation, intervention, and outcomes should align with all professional documents.

Beyond the professional guiding documents, state licensure statutes provide practitioners with regulations regarding scope of practice and service that must be followed. Moreover, evidence-based practices help practitioners make the soundest decisions regarding evaluation, intervention, and outcomes processes.

Conduct Evaluation to Gather a Variety of Data

Best practices in the evaluation of students in the private school and homeschooling domains should consist of a process that gathers information in a range of ways so that an occupational therapist may develop an occupational profile, assess occupational performance, and contribute to the student's service plan (AOTA, 2015c). More specifically, this process includes the review of any available records (e.g., previous evaluations, report cards); observation of a student in various school-related contexts; administration of standardized and nonstandardized assessments when appropriate; and interviewing school faculty (e.g., teachers, paraeducators, administrators, previous practitioners), families, and any practitioners who are currently working with the student outside of school.

Evaluations may take place in the home, in a private or public school, or in an outpatient clinic. Observations of and administration of assessments to the student may occur in the educational environment that they are most familiar with (e.g., private school, home) or one that may be novel for the student (e.g., public school, outpatient clinic). Gathering information from individuals in various settings via interview or by proxy may be necessary to create a more comprehensive intervention plan. Occupational therapists working directly for a private school may find more opportunities to obtain observations of a student in various contexts throughout the school day, in comparison with those evaluating a student in other settings.

Evaluation procedures and requirements may differ when the local school district hires an occupational therapist compared with one working directly for a private school. More specifically, the location, timing, and documentation of the evaluation may be unique to the policies, procedures, and decision-making process of either the LEA or the private school. Some private schools may not have formal policies and procedures in place regarding the evaluation process; in that case, the individual therapist or therapy department bears the onus of implementing best evaluation practices.

Implement Evidence-Based Interventions

Best practices in intervention for private schools and homeschooling domains should consist of executing and modifying an intervention plan on the basis of the results of the evaluation and sound clinical reasoning as well as engaging in proper documentation during the intervention period (AOTA, 2015c). In general, a good amount of research supports occupation-based, in-context, and collaborative interventions for all school occupational therapy practitioners (Bazyk et al., 2009; Benson, 2013; Campbell et al., 2012; Case-Smith et al., 2014; Sonday et al., 2012; Zylstra & Pfeiffer, 2016).

Occupational therapy practitioners employed by private schools may find themselves providing services in innovative ways. For example, practitioners may co-instruct a class with another school professional (e.g., speech–language pathologist, occupational therapist, physical therapist, counselor, physical education teacher, art teacher). In other cases, occupational therapists may take on more of a leadership role in curriculum or program development, such as creating a life skills curriculum; establishing an AT process; or performing a needs assessment for a new or existing program at an elementary, middle, or high school.

Processes that determine occupational therapy services in homeschooling are unique because of the consultation between LEAs and delegates from the private school and families (U.S. DOE, 2011). Depending on the service plan, intervention may occur in the home, at a clinic, or in a public school. In comparison with working in a school or clinic setting, practitioners working in homeschooling may find unique affordances and barriers when providing intervention with a student in the home environment (e.g., presence of family members or caretakers, SES, equipment options, space, travel requirements, professional boundaries). Each situation will be distinctive on the basis of the student, the family situation, and the decision-making process at the local level.

Establish Outcomes

The various types of outcomes in occupational therapy in the realm of private schools and homeschooling are not different from those undertaken in the public arena. An occupational therapy practitioner has the potential to pursue outcomes from the individual level to the population level in a school setting, especially when the practitioner works directly for the private school. As with other aspects of service provision, the unique processes of local school districts or private schools may influence the documentation and discontinuation proceedings. At the very least, practitioners should abide by professional guidelines to promote best practices in these settings regarding outcomes (AOTA, 2015c).

Practitioners working in private schools that do not follow IEPs may not need to report evaluation results, progress on goals and objectives, or present level of student performance in the same manner or with the same frequency as those working in a public school, a government-funded private school, or a private school that is chosen by an LEA to provide FAPE for a student. Without the need to follow IEP regulations, practitioners may also find greater allowances and ease in changing the frequency and type of service. In private schools, paperwork requirements may align with semester or trimester reporting in contrast to reporting based on IEP requirements in public schools.

In general, there may be considerable irregularity across states or lack of formal procedures for evaluation, intervention, goal and objective setting, outcomes, discontinuation of service, and paperwork requirements in private schools. Documentation in homeschooling aligns with the distinct requirements based on the decisions at the local level. As mentioned previously, occupational therapy practitioners must rely on their state's practice guidelines and the core professional documents that align with professional and ethical practice.

SUMMARY

The increased trend in homeschooling and the inclination for occupational therapy practitioners to work in private schools emphasize the importance of becoming familiar with the factors that influence occupational therapy practice in nonpublic schools and homeschooling. Occupational therapy practitioners working in these settings may encounter different practice patterns compared with service in public schools. Complexities in the nonpublic and homeschooling domains may also be quite apparent because of the variability in funding sources and legislation influencing service provision, the determination of services at the local level, and contextual factors within each of the domains.

Occupational therapy practitioners who choose to work in these areas must maintain awareness of updates in professional practice and keep informed of changes in legislation at all levels. Opportunities for education and advocacy regarding the role, scope, and practice requirements of occupational therapy are essential aspects of promoting best practices in private schools and homeschooling.

REFERENCES

American Montessori Society. (n.d.). *Core components of Montessori education.* Retrieved from https://amshq.org/Montessori -Education/Introduction-to-Montessori/Core-Components -of-Montessori-Education

American Occupational Therapy Association. (2014a). Guidelines for supervision, roles, and responsibilities during the delivery of occupational therapy services. *American Journal of Occupational Therapy, 68*(Suppl. 3), S16–S22. https://doi.org/10.5014/ajot.63.6.797

American Occupational Therapy Association. (2014b). Occupational therapy practice framework: Domain and process (3rd ed.). *American Journal of Occupational Therapy, 68*(Suppl. 1), S1–S48. https://doi.org/10.5014/ajot.2014.682006

American Occupational Therapy Association. (2015a). Occupational therapy code of ethics (2015). *American Journal of Occupational Therapy, 69*(Suppl. 3), 6913410030. https://doi.org/10.5014/ajot.2015.696S03

American Occupational Therapy Association. (2015b). Standards for continuing competence. *American Journal of Occupational Therapy, 69*(Suppl. 3), 6913410055. https://doi.org/10.5014/ajot.2015.696S16

American Occupational Therapy Association. (2015c). Standards of practice for occupational therapy. *American Journal of Occupational Therapy, 69*(Suppl. 3), S106–S111. https://doi.org/10.5014/ajot.2010.64S106

American Occupational Therapy Association. (2016). *Broader scope in schools.* Retrieved from http://www.aota.org/practice/children-youth/emerging-niche/broader-scope-in-schools.aspx

American Occupational Therapy Association. (2017a). Guidelines for occupational therapy services in early intervention and schools. *American Journal of Occupational Therapy, 71*(Suppl. 2), 7112410010. https://doi.org/10.5014/ajot.2017.716S01

American Occupational Therapy Association. (2017b). Vision 2025. *American Journal of Occupational Therapy, 71,* 7103420010. https://doi.org/10.5014/ajot.2017.713002

American Occupational Therapy Association. (2018). Guidelines for documentation of occupational therapy. *American Journal of Occupational Therapy, 72*(Suppl. 2), 7212410010. https://doi.org/10.5014/ajot.2018.72S203

Barrington, K. (2017). *A quick guide to U.S. public and private school options.* Retrieved from https://www.publicschoolreview.com/blog/a-quick-guide-to-us-public-and-private-school-options

Bazyk, S., Michaud, P., Goodman, G., Papp, P., Hawkins, E., & Welch, M. A. (2009). Integrating occupational therapy services in a kindergarten curriculum: A look at the outcomes. *American Journal of Occupational Therapy, 63,* 160–171. https://doi.org/10.5014/ajot.63.2.160

Benson, J. (2013). School-based occupational therapy practice: Perceptions and realities of current practice and the role of occupation. *Journal of Occupational Therapy, Schools, and Early Intervention, 6,* 165–178. https://doi.org/10.1080/19411243.2013.811348

Broughman, S. P., Rettig, A., & Peterson, J. (2017). *Characteristics of private schools in the United States: Results from the 2015–16 private school universe survey.* Retrieved from https://nces.ed.gov/pubs2017/2017073.pdf

Burke, L., & Corona, B. (2016, February 16). ESSA and what it means for school choice [Blog post]. Retrieved from https://www.edchoice.org/blog/essa-and-what-it-means-for-school-choice/

Campbell, W. N., Missiuna, C. A., Rivard, L. M., & Pollock, N. A. (2012). "Support for everyone": Experiences of occupational therapists delivering a new model of school-based service. *Canadian Journal of Occupational Therapy, 79,* 51–59. https://doi.org/10.2182/cjot.2012.79.1.7

Case-Smith, J., Holland, T., & White, S. (2014). Effectiveness of a co-taught handwriting program for first grade students. *Physical and Occupational Therapy in Pediatrics, 34,* 30–43. https://doi.org/10.3109/01942638.2013.783898

Chen, G. (2017, July 12). Public school vs. private school [Blog post]. Retrieved from https://www.publicschoolreview.com/blog/public-school-vs-private-school

Coalition for Responsible Home Education. (n.d.). *Disabilities.* Retrieved from https://www.responsiblehomeschooling.org/policy-issues/current-policy/special-needs/

Coleman Tucker, G. (n.d.). *Unilateral placement: Moving from public to private school.* Retrieved from https://www.understood.org/en/school-learning/choosing-starting-school/finding-right-school/unilateral-placement-moving-from-public-to-private-school

Council for American Private Education. (2016). *Private schools and the Every Student Succeeds Act.* Retrieved from http://www.capenet.org/pdf/ESSACAPE.pdf

Education Law Amendments of 2011, N.Y. Comp. Codes R. & Regs. 8 § 581-6503-b (West 2018).

Elementary and Secondary Education Act of 1965, Pub. L. No. 89–313, 20 U.S.C. §§ 2701–3386.

Every Student Succeeds Act, Pub. L. 114–95, 129 Stat. 1802 (2015).

Individuals With Disabilities Education Improvement Act of 2004, Pub. L. 108–446, 20 U.S.C. §§ 1400–1482.

Iowa Department of Education. (2014, March 3). *Private schools.* Retrieved from https://www.educateiowa.gov/sites/files/ed/documents/10.%20PRIVATE%20SCHOOLS.pdf

Kennedy, R. (2017, March 23). For profit vs. not for profit schools [Blog post]. Retrieved from https://www.privateschoolreview.com/blog/for-profit-vs-not-for-profit-schools

Kennedy, S., & Stewart, H. (2012). Collaboration with teachers: A survey of South Australian occupational therapists' perceptions and experiences. *Australian Occupational Therapy Journal, 59,* 147–155. https://doi.org/10.1111/j.1440-1630.2012.00999.x

Morin, A. (n.d.). *The difference between IEPs and service plans.* Retrieved from https://www.understood.org/en/school-learning/special-services/special-education-basics/the-difference-between-ieps-and-service-plans

National Center for Education Statistics. (2017). *Private school enrollment.* Retrieved from https://nces.ed.gov/programs/coe/pdf/Indicator_CGC/coe_cgc_2017_05.pdf

National Center for Education Statistics. (n.d.). *Fast facts: Back to school statistics.* Retrieved from https://nces.ed.gov/fastfacts/display.asp?id=372

New York State Education Department. (2018). *Waivers from corporate practice restrictions for special education schools and early intervention agencies.* Retrieved from http://www.op.nysed.gov/waiver-ei-info.htm

No Child Left Behind Act of 2001, Pub. L. 107–110, 20 U.S.C. §§ 6301–8962.

Redford, J., Battle, D., & Bielick, S. (2017). *Homeschooling in the United States: 2012.* Retrieved from https://nces.ed.gov/pubs2016/2016096rev.pdf

Rehabilitation Act of 1973, Pub. L. 93–112, 29 U.S.C. §§ 701–796l.

Section 504 of the Rehabilitation Act of 1973, as amended, 29 U.S.C. § 794 (2008).

Shipman & Goodwin. (2005). *Recent Supreme Court decisions—Schaffer v. Weast.* Retrieved from http://www.shipmangoodwin.com/recent-supreme-court-decision-schaffer-v-weast

Sonday, A., Anderson, K., Flack, C., Fisher, C., Greenhough, J., Kendal, R., & Shadwell, C. (2012). School-based occupational clinicians: An exploration into their role in a Cape Metropole full service school. *South African Journal of Occupational Therapy, 42*(1), 2–6. http://www.sajot.co.za/index.php/sajot/article/view/120

State of New Jersey Department of Education. (n.d.). *Service plan components.* Retrieved from http://www.nj.gov/education/specialed/form/np/

U.S. Department of Education. (2009). *State regulation of private schools.* Retrieved from https://www2.ed.gov/admins/comm/choice/regprivschl/regprivschl.pdf

U.S. Department of Education. (2011). *The Individuals With Disabilities Education Act: Provisions related to children with disabilities enrolled by their parents in private schools.* Retrieved from https://www2.ed.gov/admins/lead/speced/privateschools/idea.pdf

U.S. Department of Education. (2013). *Choices for parents.* Retrieved from https://www2.ed.gov/nclb/choice/index.html

U.S. Department of Education. (2015). *ONPE general issues frequently asked questions related to nonpublic schools.* Retrieved from https://www2.ed.gov/about/offices/list/oii/nonpublic/faqgeneral.html?src=preview#3

U.S. Department of Education. (2016a). *Free appropriate public education (FAPE).* Retrieved from https://www2.ed.gov/about/offices/list/ocr/frontpage/pro-students/issues/dis-issue03.html

U.S. Department of Education. (2016b, December 2). *Statistics about nonpublic education in the United States.* Retrieved from https://www2.ed.gov/about/offices/list/oii/nonpublic/statistics.html

U.S. Department of Labor. (2018a). *May 2017 national occupational employment and wage estimates by ownership: NAICS 611100–elementary and secondary schools, local government-owned.* Retrieved from https://www.bls.gov/oes/current/611100_3.htm

U.S. Department of Labor. (2018b). *May 2017 national occupational employment and wage estimates by ownership: NAICS 611100–elementary and secondary schools, privately owned.* Retrieved from https://www.bls.gov/oes/current/611100_5.htm

U.S. Department of Labor. (2018c). *May 2017 national occupational employment and wage estimates by ownership: NAICS 611100–elementary and secondary schools, state government-owned.* Retrieved from https://www.bls.gov/oes/current/611100_2.htm

U.S. Department of Labor. (2018d). *Occupational employment and wages, May 2017: 29-1122 occupational therapists.* Retrieved from https://www.bls.gov/oes/current/oes291122.htm

U.S. Department of Labor. (2018e). *Occupational employment and wages: May 2017, 31-2011 occupational therapy assistants.* Retrieved from https://www.bls.gov/oes/current/oes312011.htm

Villeneuve, M. (2009). A critical examination of school-based occupational therapy collaborative consultation. *Canadian Journal of Occupational Therapy, 76,* 206–218. https://doi.org/10.1177%2F000841740907600s05

Zylstra, S. E., & Pfeiffer, B. (2016). Effectiveness of a handwriting intervention with at-risk kindergarteners. *American Journal of Occupational Therapy, 70,* 7003220020. https://doi.org/10.5014/ajot.2016.018820

Best Practices in School Occupational Therapy Documentation and Data Collection

45

Gloria Frolek Clark, PhD, OTR/L, BCP, SCSS, FAOTA

KEY TERMS AND CONCEPTS

- Contact report
- Documentation
- Evaluation
- Goal attainment scaling
- Intervention
- Intervention plan
- Outcomes
- Progress monitoring
- Reevaluation
- Referral
- Rubrics

OVERVIEW

In addition to the requirements of state regulatory boards (SRBs; licensure), occupational therapy practitioners[1] must follow documentation guidelines and standards for the profession established by AOTA (2015, 2018). Documentation by occupational therapy practitioners is required whenever professional services are provided to students and their family, school staff, teams, and others (AOTA, 2018). In addition, federal and state laws have forms and documentation that are required to be completed before and during service provision. Supervisors of occupational therapy practitioners are often not occupational therapists, so practitioners must provide them with copies of SRB rules and standards as well as official documents from AOTA to enhance their understanding of occupational therapy.

Documentation communicates client information from the perspective of occupational therapy; articulates the rationale for services (e.g., reflects the practitioner's clinical reasoning and professional judgment); and provides a chronological, legal record of the client's status, services provided, and the client's response (AOTA, 2018). "Documentation represents the quality of one's professional work; recording one's information, decision making, and outcomes demonstrates the professional's willingness to be accountable for the work" (Hopkins & Smith, 1993, as cited in Linder & Frolek Clark, 2000, p. 135). Occupational therapy practitioners working with students collect data from multiple sources for the purpose of decision making, establishing goals, monitoring progress, and promoting effective outcomes (Frolek Clark et al., 2015). Data-based decision making uses quantitative data collected in a systematic manner to enhance problem-solving collaboration and demonstrate the effectiveness of occupational therapy interventions (Frolek Clark & Handley-More, 2017; Frolek Clark & Miller, 1996).

This chapter reviews AOTA guidelines and documents and requirements under the Individuals With Disabilities Education Improvement Act of 2004 (IDEA; Pub. L. 108–446) for documentation at various points in the occupational therapy process in school practice. This information can help school occupational therapy practitioners adhere to legal and ethical requirements.

ESSENTIAL CONSIDERATIONS

Practitioners are expected to know and follow occupational therapy professional rules and standards in addition to those related to their work setting.

Professional Guidelines for Documentation

Professional documentation requires compliance with various laws and regulations and following basic fundamentals. Occupational therapy practitioners must be knowledgeable of any conflicts between their state professional requirements and work requirements and work to resolve these issues with state professional organizations and public agency administrators.

For example, some state occupational therapy regulatory rules and regulations do not allow occupational therapy practitioners to work with clients unless they have been evaluated; other SRBs view general education multi-tiered systems of support as screening because the students have not been

---

[1]*Occupational therapy practitioner* refers to both the occupational therapist and the occupational therapy assistant. The American Occupational Therapy Association (AOTA; 2014a, p. S18) states, "The occupational therapist is responsible for all aspects of occupational therapy service delivery and is accountable for the safety and effectiveness of the occupational therapy service delivery process" and "must be directly involved in the delivery of services during the initial evaluation and regularly throughout the course of intervention. . . . The occupational therapy assistant delivers safe and effective occupational therapy services under the supervision of and in partnership with the occupational therapist."

Copyright © 2019 by the American Occupational Therapy Association. All rights reserved. To reuse this content, contact www.copyright.com.
https://doi.org/10.7139/2019.978-1-56900-591-0.045

identified as needing an evaluation. Practitioners working in the latter group of states may see students for short-term interventions while identifying strategies for the general education teacher to use; however, those in the former set of states may provide information to the teachers but not specifically for the student. Some SRBs have changed their regulations to allow services for health and wellness or ongoing screenings because under education law, the term *evaluation* is restricted to determining eligibility for special education (SE) and related services (e.g., occupational therapy).

Fundamental Information About Documentation

The student's occupational therapy record is a permanent file that should be maintained in a legal and professional manner (AOTA, 2018). Documentation should be well organized, provide an accurate and complete account of the services or communication that occurred, and follow fundamental elements of documentation (see Exhibit 45.1). Documentation should be

- *Objective:* State information in brief, nonderogatory language, and use complete sentences. Any contact or service should be documented (e.g., email, phone calls, trainings, home recommendations).
- *Legible and grammatically correct:* Documentation should be written in a professional manner using clear language for others (e.g., medical and profession-specific jargon kept to a minimum).
- *Timely:* Complete all documentation in accordance with agency or payer requirements (e.g., Medicaid). Record date and time of service.
- *Signed and dated:* Use your first initial (or name), full last name, and credentials, as well as the date the document was signed.
- *Completed in ink or electronically:* Do not use pencil. Do not leave blank lines or extra blank spaces on the document (draw a line through the area, when necessary). If using electronic records, then indicate below your signature that this is the end of the record.
- *Corrected appropriately:* Information is not erased. Changes to documents should be done in ink by drawing a straight line through the error and writing the correction next to the line or above the line. Write your initials

above or next to the error. When electronic records are used, the system must have the ability to track changes with the original entry still viewable. The current date and time and the name of the person making the change should be entered. Correction fluid is not to be used on permanent or official records.

Electronic records

Many educational agencies have switched to electronic documentation. Occupational therapy practitioners working in agencies that use electronic records should ensure that these formats comply with state professional licensure documentation requirements and are securely stored. Although electronic records have several advantages, such as improved legibility, secured storage in one location, and easy access for team members or administrators, they have disadvantages as well. Electronic records must be signed (requires electronic signature), allow the ability to make corrections or changes without deleting previous information (see earlier information regarding corrections), and require additional time and access for people providing services in multiple settings or areas with weak or no Wi-Fi capabilities.

Destruction of records

Occupational therapy practitioners often question how long student occupational therapy records must be kept. Some state licensure laws provide guidance for student's records, such as storing them for a minimum of 3 years after the client reaches the age of majority under state law or 5 years after the date on which therapy is discontinued, whichever is longer. Medicaid may require longer timelines for retention. Check your local state licensure and payer requirements.

IDEA (2004) states that the parents must be informed when "personally identifiable information collected, maintained, or used under this part is no longer needed to provide educational services to the child" (34 CFR § 300.624). Under the Family Educational Rights and Privacy Act of 1974 (FERPA; Pub. L. 93–380), the rights of parents regarding educational records are transferred to the student at age 18 years unless legal guardianship has been obtained

---

| **EXHIBIT 45.1.** | Fundamentals of Occupational Therapy Documentation |

- Documentation practices and storage and disposal of documentation must meet all state and federal regulations and guidelines, payer and facility requirements, practice guidelines, and confidentiality requirements.
- Client's full name, date of birth, gender, and case number, if applicable, are included on each page of the documentation.
- Identification of type of documentation and the date on which service is provided and documentation is completed are included in the documentation.
- Acceptable terminology, acronyms, and abbreviations are defined and used within the boundaries of the setting.
- Clear rationale for the purpose, value, and necessity of skilled occupational therapy services is provided. The client's diagnosis or prognosis is not the sole rationale for occupational therapy services.
- Professional signature (first name or initial, last name) and credential; cosignature and credential when required for documentation of supervision; and, when necessary, signature of the recorder are included with each documentation entry.
- All errors are noted and initialed or signed.

Note. From "Guidelines for Documentation of Occupational Therapy," by the American Occupational Therapy Association, 2018, *American Journal of Occupational Therapy, 72*(Suppl. 2), 7212410010, p. 2. https://doi.org/10.5014/ajot.2018.72S203. Copyright © 2018 by the American Occupational Therapy Association. Reprinted with permission.

or appointed to another adult through probate court. A request for these records may occur before or after the person graduates, so education agencies that provided services must produce evidence of these records. Because the destruction of records must occur in ways that protect confidentiality, shredding of records is common.

Confidentiality

Occupational therapy practitioners must adhere to federal, state, and local confidentiality requirements. Any document with personally identifiable data, information, or records must be protected. Education records are protected under FERPA; if the agency or school bills Medicaid or insurance, the Health Insurance Portability and Accountability Act of 1996 (Pub. L. 104–191) must also be followed. To disclose any personal information to other agencies (e.g., health care providers, day care providers), signed consent from the family must be obtained and updated on a regular basis (form should state date when authorization begins and ends). Parents have the right to inspect and review their child's education records. The occupational therapy practitioner's records of a student are generally part of this education record.

Depending on state rules, personal documentation kept in the sole possession of the practitioner and not accessible to others except for a substitute may not be open for inspection unless kept in the office or shared with others. Emails and texts may be considered part of the student's education record and be requested by parents during hearings. The U.S. District Court for the Eastern District of California (in *S. A. v. Tulare County Office of Education*, 2009) held that emails are only considered an education record under FERPA when the student is personally identifiable and the email is placed in the student's permanent file (IDEA, 2004, 34 CFR § 300.613[b]). (*Note:* District court rulings may be binding only in those districts.) Practitioners should follow state licensure and public agency procedures regarding confidentiality and management of records under FERPA.

Billing Medicaid and Private Insurance

Practitioners must know and follow the rules of their state for billing services in schools. Ethical issues can arise with medical billing unless practitioners understand the rules (see Exhibit 45.2). Practitioners are responsible for services and billing that they complete. They are advised to obtain a copy of billing procedures and identify a contact person

at the state level (e.g., Department of Education personnel, Medicaid official) to answer questions about Medicaid services and billing. Some states have made clear distinctions that Medicaid is not billed when occupational therapy services are solely educationally necessary and not medically necessary or if the student is not in the room.

Occupational therapy practitioners must document only facts that they can substantiate and store the documents in the student's record. Practitioners should *only* sign their name for services that they provided, even when pressured by their agency to sign records for another practitioner's services. The government considers billing for services that are not provided as fraud. If pressured by a public educational agency to put students on an individualized education program (IEP) so it can bill Medicaid or private insurance, the occupational therapist must present unbiased data to the team for a decision about the student's need for occupational therapy. Although a public agency may be fined for fraud, practitioners may be fined, jailed, or lose their license. An occupational therapist is responsible for all aspects of occupational therapy services and should be aware of services and billing conducted by occupational therapy assistants under their supervision (AOTA, 2014a). For more information, see Chapter 16, "Best Practices in Medicaid Cost Recovery." Exhibit 45.2 provides information about billing insurance and Medicaid.

IDEA Requirements for Documentation

SRBs set rules and regulations for occupational therapy within that state. Most state practice acts use medical-based language, which does not align with IDEA. For example, an occupational therapy evaluation would not occur under IDEA unless eligibility for special education was being considered. Under IDEA, occupational therapy is a related service and is provided to students with disabilities in special education programs (note that some state Department of Education rules identify occupational therapy as specially designed services so they can be the sole service on a student's IEP). IDEA and AOTA use different terms, which can be confusing. Table 45.1 compares the different processes, many of which require documentation. Practitioners must adhere to their professional guidelines and requirements as well as those under IDEA.

IDEA has several documentation requirements, many of which are intended to provide safeguards for families and students. Each state educational agency or school district may develop forms to meet these requirements. Occupational

---

EXHIBIT 45.2. Using Insurance and Medicaid to Bill for Part B Services

- LEAs may use the parent's insurance or the child's Medicaid to pay for related services required under IDEA Part B; however, this must be voluntary, and services may not be denied if parents decline the request.
- Parents may not be required to enroll in SE and related service programs so that LEAs can be billed for Part B services.
- Parents may not incur a financial cost (increased premiums, copay, deductible; decreased lifetime coverage; discontinuation of insurance or Medicaid because of billing; or risk loss of eligibility of waivers).
- Parents must be notified when billing occurs.
- LEAs must inform parents about any potential consequences to billing their insurance and that their refusal to consent does not deny their child services.

Note. IDEA = Individuals With Disabilities Education Improvement Act of 2004; LEA = local educational agency; SE = special education.

TABLE 45.1.   Comparing AOTA and IDEA Occupational Therapy Processes Requiring Documentation

PROCESS	AOTA	IDEA
Screening	Screening is obtaining and reviewing data relevant to a person to determine the need for further evaluation and intervention (AOTA, 2015).	Child Find identifies and evaluates students who may be eligible for SE services (§ 300.111). Some states may include a universal screening as part of their initial Child Find activities. EIS allow screening for instructional purposes and are not to be considered an evaluation for special education or related services (§ 300.302).
Evaluation and reevaluation	*Evaluation* is the "process of obtaining and interpreting data necessary for intervention" (AOTA, 2015, p. 2). *Reevaluation* is the reappraisal of the client's performance and goals to determine the type and amount of change that has taken place (AOTA, 2014b, p. S45).	*Full and individual initial evaluation* is completed as a team to determine whether a child is "a child with a disability" under IDEA and eligible for SE and related services (§ 1414[a], § 1414[b]). This evaluation may include an *occupational therapy evaluation* to determine effect of functional, behavioral, and academic performance on health and participation and to identify need for occupational therapy services. *Reevaluation* (at least every 3 years) reviews ongoing need for SE and related services (§ 1414[c]); occupational therapy reevaluation may result in continuation or discontinuation of services.
Determining need for services	Need for services is based on data gathered during the occupational profile and analysis of occupational performance; the occupational therapist uses professional judgment regarding appropriateness of occupational therapy or a need to refer to other services (AOTA, 2015, 2018).	Determination of eligibility for SE is made by the team; if eligible, student may receive related services, as needed (§ 1414[c]).
Outcomes and educational goals	*Outcomes* are the end result of the occupational therapy process: what clients can achieve through occupational therapy intervention (AOTA, 2014b, p. S44).	The team develops the IEP to identify student's functional, academic, and behavioral performance; prioritize needs; and establish student goals and services. Transition plans are included, when appropriate (§ 1414[d]). The team conducts an IEP review to review the student's goals and identify additions or deletions in services, based on current needs and goals (§ 1414[d][4]).
Intervention	*Intervention* is the "process and skilled actions taken by occupational therapy practitioners in collaboration with the client to facilitate engagement in occupation related to health and participation" (AOTA, 2015, p. 2).	*Implementation of the IEP* includes a description of how the student's progress toward the goal will be measured; periodic reports on student's progress are given to the family (§ 1414[d][1][A]).
Transition and discharge plan	Transition is "actions coordinated to prepare for or facilitate a change, such as from one functional level to another, from one life [change] to another, from one program to another, or from one environment to another" (AOTA, 2015, p. 2). The occupational therapist is responsible for preparing and implementing a transition or discontinuation report.	*Transition services* are a coordinated set of activities focused on improving the academic and functional achievement of the student to move from school to postschool activities (e.g., postsecondary education, vocational education, integrated employment, continuing and adult education, adult services, independent living, or community participation; § 1401[34]). *Discontinuation of related services:* Whether the IEP team or the parents decide to discontinue services, a public agency cannot discontinue services until prior written notice has been provided to the parents (§ 300.503). Parents must be given a reasonable time to receive the information, fully consider the change, and determine whether they have any questions or concerns. Parents are not required to give reasons for revoking consent.

Note. AOTA = American Occupational Therapy Association; EIS = early intervening services; IDEA = Individuals With Disabilities Education Improvement Act of 2004; IEP = individualized education program; SE = special education.

TABLE 45.2.   Common Documents Required Under IDEA

EIS	NEEDED TO DETERMINE ELIGIBILITY	AFTER ELIGIBILITY DETERMINED
▪ Report on number of children receiving EIS and number who subsequently receive SE and related services during the preceding 2-year period (§ 1413[f][3])	▪ Written parental consent for initial evaluation to determine eligibility for SE (§ 1414[a][1][D]) ▪ Parent notice of any evaluation procedure proposed by agency (§ 1414[b]) ▪ Parent notice of meeting ▪ Evaluation report and documentation of determination of eligibility provided to parent (§ 1414[b][4][b]) ▪ Due process procedural safeguards available for parents (§ 300.500) ▪ Written notice to parent within a reasonable time before public agency proposes (or refuses) to initiate or change the identification, evaluation, or educational placement of the child (§ 300.503)	▪ Excusal form signed by parent and LEA to excuse member of the IEP team from attending part or all of the meeting that involves a modification or discussion of that related service (§ 1414[d][C]) ▪ IEP (§ 1414[d]) ▪ Written parental consent for services before providing SE and related services to child (§ 1414[a][1][E]) ▪ IEP transition plan (§ 1414[d][1][A][VIII]) ▪ Review and revision of the IEP (§ 1414[d][2][F][4]) ▪ Written parental consent for reevaluation (§ 1414[c][3])

Note. EIS = early intervening services; IDEA = Individuals With Disabilities Education Improvement Act of 2004; IEP = individualized education program; LEA = local educational agency; SE = special education.

therapy practitioners must be aware of the process and forms to document the actions. Some common examples are listed in Table 45.2.

Document Student Goals on the IEP

To develop student goals (never called "OT goals"), the team should consider the student performance desired and establish the criteria to achieve it. The occupational therapist may collaboratively develop and monitor goals for the student with other team members. A systematic method of writing student IEP goals should be followed (Frolek Clark, 2005; see Table 45.3).

Collect Data to Document Effectiveness of Services

IDEA requires annual goals to be measurable and the student's progress to be reported through the use of quarterly or other periodic reports (concurrent with the school's report cards). Ongoing data collection to monitor the

student's progress toward the goals is essential to determine the effectiveness of services (Frolek Clark et al., 2015; Frolek Clark & Handley-More, 2017). Occupational therapy practitioners working in schools commonly use *progress monitoring,* a scientifically based practice that systematically assesses student performance and can be used for decision making (Frolek Clark & Miller, 1996); *goal attainment scaling* (GAS), a systematic method of measuring progress based on current and progressive performance; and *rubrics,* a scoring tool that sets criteria for performance and has gradations of quality for each of the criteria listed. They are explained in more detail in the next section.

BEST PRACTICES

The occupational therapist is responsible for all aspects of occupational therapy service provision, including documentation, and may receive assistance from the occupational therapy assistant (AOTA, 2014a). Practitioners are always responsible for knowing and complying with their professional requirements (e.g., licensure law, ethics, standards

TABLE 45.3.   Systematic Method of Writing Student IEP Goals

STEP	EXAMPLE
1. Gather information through the occupational profile.	The 1st-grade teacher would like Stacy to perform cutting, coloring, and writing tasks (fine motor) independently in the classroom. Stacy has difficulty with motor planning and fine motor dexterity. She becomes frustrated and cuts through the paper or tears it up. Currently she completes 28% of the activities. $$\text{Formula}: \frac{\textit{Number of activities completed}}{\textit{Number of opportunities provided}}$$
2. Define the desired performance.	[What] Stacy will complete all cutting, coloring, and writing activities.
3. Identify the conditions.	[When] By 3-9-20, [where] in the classroom [other conditions] during class cutting, coloring, or writing activities.
4. Establish the criterion.	[How will we know it is met] Complete each activity independently 75% of the opportunities.

Completed goal: By 3-9-20, in the classroom during class work time, Stacy will complete cutting, coloring, and writing activities independently 75% of the opportunities.

Note. IEP = individualized education program.

of practice). In addition, documentation requirements of IDEA and other educational laws must be followed; therefore, practitioners must find efficient ways to manage all documentation. Documentation may include services with clients (e.g., students, teachers, classrooms, school teams, district). To assist in problem solving and to determine the effectiveness of services, practitioners must be proficient in methods of ongoing data collection.

Complete Documentation

The *Guidelines for Documentation of Occupational Therapy* (AOTA, 2018) list 8 types of reports typically used by occupational therapy practitioners:
1. Screening report,
2. Evaluation report,
3. Reevaluation report,
4. Intervention plan,
5. Contact report,
6. Progress report,
7. Transition plan, and
8. Discontinuation report.

Depending on the setting, these reports may be named differently or combined and reorganized, but occupational therapy practitioners should always record services including screening, evaluation, intervention, and discontinuation of services. Information typically included in these reports is outlined in a format that can be used as a personal guide or program audit (see Appendix E, "Full or Partial Audit of Occupational Therapy Documentation") to ensure content is included (AOTA, 2018).

The process begins with a **referral,** which has a different meaning in clinical and school settings. Under IDEA, a referral or request for evaluation may occur when initiated by the parent to determine whether the student is eligible for SE, when the team suspects a student may have a disability and needs SE, or to identify the need for related services (e.g., occupational therapy). Whenever an occupational therapist is asked to see a student (whether as a request for general education EIS, if allowed by state occupational therapy licensure, or as a referral for occupational therapy evaluation), the following items should be documented:
- Who initiated the referral or request, including their phone number and agency or district;
- Date of the referral or request; and
- Why they are seeking services from occupational therapy (i.e., expectation, outcome).

Occupational therapy screening or evaluation report

A report to document the screening and results should be written whenever the occupational therapist provides student-specific information to enhance general education instruction. The report may be simple (e.g., check boxes), but it will need to capture the screening process and results. Before conducting screenings, the therapist should check their state licensure law and LEA procedures.

The occupational therapy evaluation report may be separate or included in a team report. When the team report is blended (e.g., information is provided under topics without identifying names and specific information from the evaluator), a separate occupational therapy report may be needed to meet state licensure requirements for an occupational therapy evaluation. Occupational therapists should check their licensure law to determine whether a separate report is necessary.

After summarizing and analyzing results, the occupational therapist can answer the following questions to determine the need for occupational therapy expertise or services from others on the educational team:
- What does the student need to learn (e.g., to transition independently from preschool, to chew foods, to complete work at a prevocational site)?
- What type of instruction works best (e.g., provide models, provide multiple opportunities)?
- What context and conditions support learning (e.g., physical assistance to set up computer, special equipment for sitting in group, quiet area in back of room for independent work)?
- What other supports does this student need for learning (e.g., access to a switch to activate computer, support in classroom to prompt them to finish a task)?
- Do these data support the need for the expertise of an occupational therapist to assist this student with participation in their educational program?

Occupational therapy reevaluation report

The reevaluation report should describe new information on the same areas or new areas of occupations. An occupational therapy reevaluation should be conducted when the student's performance has changed greatly and may warrant an increase, decrease, or discontinuation of services.

Occupational therapy intervention plan

The occupational therapist is responsible for developing, documenting, and implementing the intervention plan on the basis of the evaluation, client goals, best available evidence, and professional and clinical reasoning (AOTA, 2015). The **intervention plan** is a professional document, separate from the IEP, that includes information about occupational therapy service provision. This intervention plan is developed in collaboration with the student (family, educational staff) on the basis of their needs and priorities and is modified throughout the intervention process (AOTA, 2015). The occupational therapy assistant may assist in the development of the intervention plan as well. See Appendix C, "Occupational Therapy Intervention Plan."

Service contact report

The **contact report** provides a chronological record of student–practitioner interactions and is often used in legal situations. If interactions are not documented, then there is no record that contact occurred. Contacts between occupational therapy practitioners and the student (family, educational staff), including interventions, phone calls, and formal or informal meetings, must be documented. Many practitioners find that using the student's IEP review as a time to begin a new contact report keeps documentation more organized (i.e., contact report matches frequency and goals of the new IEP) and saves time at the start or end of the academic year by not having to add new contact reports for all students on the occupational therapy practitioner's workload.

Some occupational therapy practitioners complete a short summary of the intervention and suggested strategies that is shared with educators and families through a shared notebook or form. This communication builds partnerships and provides simple activities that can be performed to enhance progress toward the student's IEP goal. The practitioner should keep the original communication (e.g., therapy note form) and send home a copy. When a shared notebook is used, a copy of correspondence should be maintained as well.

Progress reports

There are 2 types of progress reports: (1) progress on IEP goals and (2) occupational therapy progress report. IDEA requires that a student's progress toward IEP goals be shared with the family using the same period as report cards (e.g., quarterly, trimester). Occupational therapists may collaborate with educators on completing these periodic progress reports for families.

Occupational therapists, with the assistance of the occupational therapy assistant, summarize the occupational therapy services and document student progress at least annually. This is a professional standard and best practice. Rather than completing progress summaries at the end of each year on the entire caseload, occupational therapists may write the occupational therapy progress report before each student's annual IEP meeting to provide current information for the meeting. Completing the report at this time, rather the end of the year, aligns with the IEP timelines.

Occupational therapy transition plan

The occupational therapy transition plan is written to coordinate change (e.g., student moving to another school district, changing schools). When a student is moving to another school district or graduating, a transition plan and discontinuation report may be combined. The intent of the report is to summarize the student's current performance in occupations, what approaches to intervention and types of intervention have been used, and their efficiency.

Occupational therapy discontinuation report

When students will continue to attend school in the same district or program but occupational therapy services are being discontinued, a discontinuation report summarizes the onset and ending of services. Discontinuation might occur when

- Services are no longer educationally relevant;
- Goal has been met, and no additional goals that require occupational therapy intervention are appropriate;
- Skill and expertise of occupational therapy are no longer required to meet student's educational needs;
- Therapy is contraindicated; or
- Parents (or student at age of consent) decline ongoing goals or service in that area.

Be Proficient in Ongoing Data Collection to Measure Effectiveness of Interventions

"Attention to accountability has been increasing in all settings and programs where occupational therapists practice"

FIGURE 45.1. Stacy's progress monitoring chart.

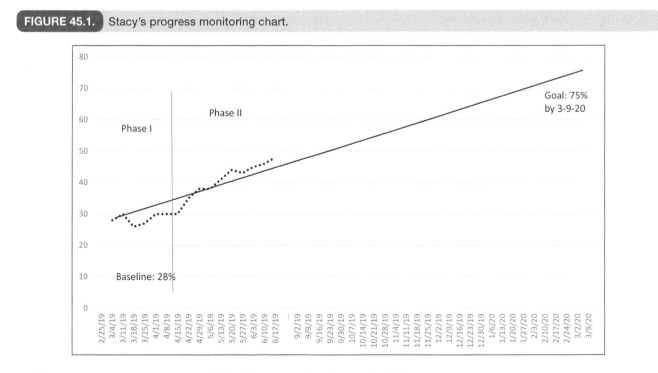

Note. Dotted line indicates child performance; solid line indicates expected performance (goal line).

EXHIBIT 45.3.	Ty's Sample Goal Attainment Scale	

BASELINE: –2 EXPECTED OUTCOME: 0

SCORE	DESCRIPTION	OBJECTIVE
+2	Much more than expected	Cuts 100% of the shape on the border line
+1	Somewhat more than expected	Cuts at least 90% of the shape on the border line
0	Expected level of outcome	Cuts at least 90% of the shape within 1/8 of an inch of the border line
–1	Progress	Cuts at least 50% of shape within 1/4 inch from the border line
–2	Baseline (present level of performance)	Cuts shape on regular paper without any regard to border line (e.g., cuts circle in half)
–3	Regression from baseline	Refuses to cut

(Frolek Clark, 2010, p. 743). IDEA requires a statement of the student's present levels of academic and functional performance (baseline), measurable annual goals, and how the student's progress will be measured and reported to families (§ 1414[d][1][A][I–III]). Several methods commonly used by school occupational therapy practitioners are discussed next, including progress monitoring, GAS, and rubrics. Occupational therapy practitioners can learn more about these methods of data collection from Frolek Clark and Handley-More (2017).

Progress monitoring

Progress monitoring is a scientifically based practice that uses student performance data to evaluate the effectiveness of instruction and interventions. If the team identifies a baseline and establishes a measurable goal, then the student's performance can be monitored by counting or timing the student's performance. Progress monitoring can be used to measure any performance or skill that can be counted or measured.

Figure 45.1 is a sample of a progress monitoring chart for the goal "Stacy will complete at least 75% of classroom cutting, coloring, and writing activities independently." After the student's baseline was graphed (28%), an expected goal (75%) was placed on the chart; then a solid line was added to connect those points. This goal line indicates the rate of progress that Stacy must achieve to meet the goal within the

timeline set. Student performance data were systematically collected each week and plotted on the graph (Phase I). The 4 data point rule was applied for decision making by reviewing 4 consecutive data points (Stacy's performance line).

Stacy's performance was improving but not enough to meet her goal by the timeline established by the team (her data are the dotted line). In other words, the current intervention did not appear to be effective in meeting the goal in the time allotted. The intervention was changed, and Phase II was begun. During that phase, Stacy's performance data were above and below the goal line, indicating she was beginning to increase her rate of progress. When the data were reviewed after 4 additional consecutive data points, no changes were made to the intervention. She finished by meeting her goal on time.

Goal attainment scaling

GAS, a systematic method of describing clients' current and progressive performance, has been used by occupational therapists in goal setting, measuring progress toward intervention outcomes, and effectively measuring research (Mailloux et al., 2007). Advantages to GAS include individualized goals that are measurable and realistic.

Exhibit 45.3 provides an example of using GAS for a student who has difficulty with cutting. The goal is to increase Ty's ability to cut shapes on the line (border)—specifically that he can cut within 1/8 of an inch from the border for at

EXHIBIT 45.4.	Rubric for Grading Rudd's Social Skills			

TASK COMPONENT	1: UNACCEPTABLE	2: WITH ASSISTANCE	3: ACCEPTABLE (EXPECTED)	4: EXCEEDS EXPECTATIONS
Turn taking	Refuses to share equipment or allow another student to have a turn	Shares or allows other student to take a turn after adult verbal prompting	Spontaneously shares equipment or allows other student to take a turn	Encourages a student to go first or to use equipment first
Manage stress	Screams or hits others if he does not get his way	Within 2 seconds of adult verbal cue, will stop screaming or hitting others	Will understand that he must wait or share without adult intervention	Will state his feelings in a way that conveys coping ("I want to go first, but it is his turn")

TABLE 45.4. OSEP Part B Indicators for Students From Kindergarten Through Graduation

NO. AND INDICATOR	DESCRIPTION
1. Graduation rates	Percentage of youth with IEPs graduating from high school with a regular diploma
2. Dropout rates	Percentage of youth with IEPs dropping out of high school
3. Participation and performance on statewide assessments	Participation and performance of children with IEPs on statewide assessments: A. Percentage of the districts with a disability subgroup that meet the state's minimum *n* size AYP targets for the disability subgroup B. Participation rate for children with IEPs C. Proficiency rate for children with IEPs against grade level and modified and alternate academic achievement standards
4. Suspensions and expulsions	Rates of suspension and expulsion: A. Percentage of districts that have a significant discrepancy in the rate of suspensions and expulsions of more than 10 days in a school year for children with IEPs and B. Percentage of districts that have (1) A significant discrepancy, by race or ethnicity, in the rate of suspensions and expulsions of more than 10 days in a school year for children with IEPs and (2) Policies, procedures, or practices that contribute to the significant discrepancy and do not comply with requirements relating to the development and implementation of IEPs, the use of positive behavioral interventions and supports, and procedural safeguards.
5. Participation or time in general education settings (LRE)	Percentage of children with IEPs ages 6–21 years served: A. Inside the regular class 80% or more of the day, B. Inside the regular class less than 40% of the day, and C. In separate schools, residential facilities, or homebound or hospital placements.
8. Parental involvement	Percentage of parents with a child receiving SE services who report that schools facilitated parent involvement as a means of improving services and results for children with disabilities
9. Disproportionate representation in SE (inappropriate identification)	Percentage of districts with disproportionate representation of racial and ethnic groups in SE and related services that is the result of inappropriate identification
10. Disproportionate representation in SE (specific disability categories)	Percentage of districts with disproportionate representation of racial and ethnic groups in specific disability categories that is the result of inappropriate identification
11. Evaluation timeframe	Percentage of children who were evaluated within 60 days of receiving parental consent for initial evaluation or, if the state establishes a timeframe within which the evaluation must be conducted, within that timeframe
12. Part C to B transition	Percentage of children referred by Part C before age 3 years, who are found eligible for Part B, and who have an IEP developed and implemented by their 3rd birthday
13. Postschool transition goals in IEP	Percentage of youth with IEPs ages 16 years or older with an IEP that includes appropriate measurable postsecondary goals that are annually updated and based on an age-appropriate transition assessment; transition services, including courses of study, that will reasonably enable the student to meet those postsecondary goals; and annual IEP goals related to the student's transition services needs; there also must be evidence that the student was invited to the IEP team meeting at which transition services were discussed and evidence that, if appropriate, a representative of any participating agency was invited to the IEP team meeting with the prior consent of the parent or student who had reached the age of majority
14. Participation in postsecondary settings	Percentage of youth who are no longer in secondary school, had IEPs in effect at the time they left school, and were A. Enrolled in higher education within 1 year of leaving high school B. Enrolled in higher education or competitively employed within 1 year of leaving high school C. Enrolled in higher education or in some other postsecondary education or training program or competitively employed or in some other employment within 1 year of leaving high school.

Note. Indicators 6 and 7 are omitted from the tables because they apply to preschool; 15–20 because they are systems focused. AYP = adequate yearly progress; IEP = individualized education program; LRE = least restrictive environment; OSEP = Office of Special Education Programs; SE = special education.

least 90% of the shape (0 on GAS). Currently, he picks up the paper and cuts straight across the shape, without any regard for the square or circle outline (–2 on GAS). Although this skill is worked on daily, the teacher and occupational therapist use the GAS to measure Ty's performance quarterly to inform parents of his progress.

Rubrics

Rubrics are tools that assess student performance on the basis of gradations of criteria for each task. "Well-written rubrics help students learn classroom expectations, recognize what they need to do to improve their performance, and evaluate the quality of their work" (Handley-More, 2008, p. 32). Rubrics specifically state the expectations for the task and are based on accepted standards; however, occupational therapy practitioners should confirm the standard (expected performance) with the teacher for each of the components.

Exhibit 45.4 is an example of a junior high student with autism spectrum disorder who has difficulty with coping and social skills during noon recess when students meet outside or in the gym to play ball. Although Rudd is good at playing ball, he does not understand turn taking or sharing and becomes very upset when he has to wait. The occupational therapist suggested to the teacher that they use a simple rubric to measure Rudd's performance over recess. A score of 6 (i.e., 3 + 3) is expected of Rudd (goal) and other students; Rudd's baseline is 2 (i.e., 1 + 1).

Document Outcomes, Part B Indicators, and State-Identified Measurable Results

Accountability is critical. Several ways that data are used to identify the results of programming include using the *Occupational Therapy Framework: Domain and Process* (3rd ed.; *OTPF–3*; AOTA, 2014b) outcomes, Office of Special Education (OSEP) Part B indicators, and State-Identified Measurable Results (SIMR). Each of these is discussed as they pertain to school occupational therapy services.

OTPF–3 outcomes

The *OTPF–3* (AOTA, 2014b, p. S34) describes outcomes as "what the clients achieve through occupational therapy interventions" (p. S16). These outcomes are described in Chapter 2, "The *OTPF–3*: Communicating Occupational Therapy in Schools," and Table 2.3 lists the various *OTPF–3* outcomes with examples.

Outcomes should be documented in the occupational therapy intervention plan as well as the occupational therapy discontinuation report. An occupational therapist may document that the student is now able to engage in fine motor activities in the classroom (participation outcome) or to socially interact and contribute to a group project with peers (role competence).

Part B Indicators

SEAs must measure and report statewide performance on 20 Part B indicators. The indicators that pertain to students from kindergarten to graduation are listed in Table 45.4.

Omitted from the table are Indicators 6 and 7 because they pertain to preschool and Indicators 15–20 because they are system indicators (e.g., resolution of written complaints, due process timelines, the timelines and accuracy of state data). These indicators are part of the State Performance Report and Annual Performance Report that are submitted to OSEP so that OSEP can monitor and supervise state implementation in specific areas.

States are assigned a rating on the basis of meeting compliance and performance data set by OSEP. Ratings include the following:
- Meets the requirements and purposes of IDEA,
- Needs assistance in implementing the requirements of IDEA,
- Needs intervention in implementing the requirements of IDEA, or
- Needs substantial intervention in implementing the requirements of IDEA (U.S. Department of Education, 2018).

SIMR

In response to OSEP's initiative regarding results-driven accountability, many states submitted drafts in their state systematic improvement plan focused on specific outcomes, known as SIMR. The majority of the outcomes for Part B focus on assessment data (aligned to Indicator 3), whereas others are targeting graduation rates.

SUMMARY

Reports and other documentation by school occupational therapy practitioners are legal documents. Lawyers may subpoena these documents to use at hearings. With increasing workloads, practitioners must find ways to provide quality documentation in less time. Using templates that allow check marks or evaluation templates that can be cut and pasted may allow practitioners to stay informed about their documentation requirements. Documentation is an important—and required—part of providing school occupational therapy services.

REFERENCES

American Occupational Therapy Association. (2014a). Guidelines for supervision, roles, and responsibilities during the delivery of occupational therapy services. *American Journal of Occupational Therapy, 68*(Suppl. 3), S16–S22. https://doi.org/10.5014/ajot.63.6.797

American Occupational Therapy Association. (2014b). Occupational therapy practice framework: Domain and process (3rd ed.). *American Journal of Occupational Therapy, 68*(Suppl. 1), S1–S48. https://doi.org/10.5014/ajot.2014.682006

American Occupational Therapy Association. (2015). Standards of practice for occupational therapy. *American Journal of Occupational Therapy, 69*(Suppl. 3), 6913410057. https://doi.org/10.5014/ajot.2015.696S06

American Occupational Therapy Association. (2018). Guidelines for documentation of occupational therapy. *American Journal of Occupational Therapy, 72*(Suppl. 2), 7212410010. https://doi.org/10.5014/ajot.2018.72S203.

Family Educational Rights and Privacy Act of 1974, Pub. L. 93–380, 20 U.S.C. § 1232g; 34 C.F.R. Part 99.

Frolek Clark, G. (2005). Developing appropriate student IEP goals. *OT Practice, 10*(14), 12–15.

Frolek Clark, G. (2010). Using data to guide your decisions. In H. M. Kuhaneck & R. Watling (Eds.), *Autism: A comprehensive occupational therapy approach* (3rd ed., pp. 743–776). Bethesda, MD: AOTA Press.

Frolek Clark, G., Cahill, S., & Ivy, C. (2015). School practice documentation: Documenting and organizing quantitative data. *OT Practice, 20*(15), 12–15.

Frolek Clark, G., & Handley-More, D. (2017). *Best practices for documenting occupational therapy services in schools.* Bethesda, MD: AOTA Press.

Frolek Clark, G., & Miller, L. (1996). Providing effective occupational therapy services: Data-based decision making in school-based practices. *American Journal of Occupational Therapy, 50,* 701–708. https://doi.org/10.5014/ajot.50.9.701

Handley-More, D. (2008). Developing and using rubrics in occupational therapy. *Journal of Occupational Therapy, Schools, and Early Intervention, 1,* 24–32. https://doi.org/10.1080/19411240802060967

Health Insurance Portability and Accountability Act of 1996, Pub. L. 104–191, 42 U.S.C. § 300gg, 29 U.S.C. §§ 1181–1183, and 42 U.S.C. §§ 1320d–1320d9.

Hopkins, H., & Smith, H. (Eds.). (1993). *Willard and Spackman's occupational therapy* (8th ed., pp. 387–390). Philadelphia: Lippincott.

Individuals With Disabilities Education Improvement Act of 2004, Pub. L. 108–446, 20 U.S.C. §§ 1400–1482.

Linder, J., & Frolek Clark, G. (2000). Best practices in documentation. In W. Dunn (Ed.), *Best practice occupational therapy: In community service with children and families* (pp. 135–145). Thorofare, NJ: Slack.

Mailloux, Z., May-Benson, T., Summers, C. S., Miller, L. J., Brett-Green, B., Burke, J. P., . . . Schoen, S. A. (2007). Goal attainment scaling as a measure of meaningful outcomes for children with sensory integration disorders. *American Journal of Occupational Therapy, 61,* 254–259. https://doi.org/10.5014/ajot.61.2.254

S. A. v. Tulare County Office of Education, 2009 WL 3126322 (E.D. Cal. 2009).

U.S. Department of Education. (2018). *2018 Determination letters on state implementation of IDEA.* Retrieved from http://dataserver.lrp.com/DATA/servlet/DataServlet?fname=2018+Determination+Letters+on+State+Implementation+of+IDEA.pdf

SECTION V.

Evidence-Guided Practices: Supporting Occupations to Enhance Student Participation

Best Practices in ADLs to Enhance Participation

46

Jayne Shepherd, MS, OTR/L, FAOTA

KEY TERMS AND CONCEPTS

- Activity or task analysis
- Backward chaining
- Coaching
- Cognitive Orientation to daily Occupational Performance
- Collaborative goals
- Context-focused therapy
- Ecological assessment process
- Forward chaining
- Functional performance
- Instructional cues or prompts
- Occupational profile
- Partial participation
- Routines
- Social Stories™
- Video modeling of others
- Video self-modeling

OVERVIEW

ADLs occur throughout the student's life, including dressing, personal hygiene and grooming, toilet hygiene (including bowel and bladder management), personal device care, bathing and showering, functional and personal mobility, and expressing sexual needs (American Occupational Therapy Association [AOTA], 2014b). Feeding and eating are also ADLs and are addressed separately in Chapter 47, "Best Practices in School Mealtimes to Enhance Participation."

As defined in the *Federal Register* ("Assistance to States for the Education of Children With Disabilities and Preschool Grants for Children With Disabilities," 2006), *functional performance* "refer[s] to skills or activities that are not considered academic or related to a child's academic achievement. Instead, 'functional' is often used in the context of routine activities of everyday living" (p. 46661). Functional performance includes ADLs and is documented, when appropriate, in the individualized education program (IEP) and as a summary of performance. Working with students in school settings, teams assess students' ADL performance and determine whether goals are for independence or partial participation. *Partial participation* occurs when a student completes or directs part of the ADL sequence and the adult or peer completes the other part of the ADL task (e.g., student puts on their coat while adult or peer completes the fasteners; Shepherd & Ivey, in press; Snell et al., 2015).

Students unable to perform daily self-care have limited peer acceptance; social participation; or engagement in academics, after-school or community activities, or part-time work. They may also struggle with developing healthy habits and relationships; understanding procreation; and knowing how to prevent pregnancy, disease, and exploitation (Krantz et al., 2016; Shepherd & Ivey, in press). Inadequate ADL performance and habits may diminish a student's self-efficacy, health, self-esteem, and self-determination (Dunn et al., 2012).

ESSENTIAL CONSIDERATIONS

School occupational therapy practitioners[1] are vital in promoting each student's functional performance as mandated by the Individuals With Disabilities Education Improvement Act of 2004 (IDEA; Pub. L. 108–446; Hanft & Shepherd, 2016).

Collaborative Goal Setting With Student, Family, and Educational Personnel

School occupational therapy practitioners set *collaborative goals* with students, educational staff, and families by understanding their perspectives to determine which ADL tasks are most important to learn (Hanft & Shepherd, 2016). Parents' and teachers' opinions about needed intervention for a particular ADL task may differ from each other and from the student's (Vroland-Nordstrand et al., 2015). Parents of students with motor challenges often have greater concerns

---

[1]*Occupational therapy practitioner* refers to both the occupational therapist and the occupational therapy assistant. AOTA (2014a, p. S18) states, "The occupational therapist is responsible for all aspects of occupational therapy service delivery and is accountable for the safety and effectiveness of the occupational therapy service delivery process" and "must be directly involved in the delivery of services during the initial evaluation and regularly throughout the course of intervention. . . . The occupational therapy assistant delivers safe and effective occupational therapy services under the supervision of and in partnership with the occupational therapist."

Copyright © 2019 by the American Occupational Therapy Association. All rights reserved. To reuse this content, contact www.copyright.com.
https://doi.org/10.7139/2019.978-1-56900-591-0.046

about ADLs or school tasks than the students themselves (O'Brien et al., 2009; Vroland-Nordstrand et al., 2015).

Goals are achievable and motivating when they are student centered and task oriented with daily opportunities for practice (Novak et al., 2013; Vroland-Nordstrand et al., 2015). The team determines when and where ADL tasks are done, the rules of safety in self-care, the expectations of others, and when self-care tasks are done independently or with assistance. The amount of assistance teachers and paraeducators give a student is discussed with the team to evaluate whether it is beneficial or necessary.

Routines for ADLs in the Classroom and Throughout the Day

Routines or patterns of observable behaviors provide a predictable structure to complete ADLs and develop future healthy habits (automatic behaviors) for students (AOTA, 2014b; Persch et al., 2015). By evaluating typical routines at school or at home and collaborating with team members, the occupational therapist ensures that routines match student, family, and teacher values and the time available to practice or complete ADLs in the natural environment (Shepherd & Ivey, in press). Together, the team chooses how and when to embed ADLs during the school day so routines are practical, effective, and consistent (Frolek Clark, 2016). Some routines are imposed by others or the environment, and others develop through trial and error while trying new strategies for efficiency (Pfeiffer et al., 2017).

Contextually relevant routines (e.g., hanging up coats when first entering the classroom; washing hands before having a snack, lunch, or toileting), and cues (e.g., Social Stories, visual schedules, electronic reminders for toileting breaks or wheelchair pushups) are helpful for students. When students need to meet different demands in new environments, accommodations within routines may be necessary as well as more time to practice and refine new routines. Habits, such as handwashing, may help maintain health, but a habit can sometimes become an interference when a student perseverates on a particular task (e.g., washing hands 20 times a day; AOTA, 2014b; Shepherd & Ivey, in press).

Effect of Various Health Conditions

A student's health, disability status, and performance skills may affect ADLs. For example, the amount of time it takes for a student to complete an ADL task, the severity of fatigue or pain, and the level of effort needed as well as the team's satisfaction with a student's performance influence the choice of ADL goals. Goals may not be warranted when ADL performance is so time consuming or tiring that a student cannot concentrate on academics or participate in after-school activities or when a student has a progressive disability that makes performance unlikely to improve. Physical ability often predicts a student's capacity to complete ADLs (Phipps & Roberts, 2012), especially hand function when completing everyday activities in the natural environment (Kee et al., 2014).

Occupational therapists need to ask, "Is a particular self-care or mobility goal achievable for a student, or should a student use partial participation or modifications to the task method, materials, or environment to take part in self-care or mobility?" As a student ages, ADL goals on the IEP may need modifying (e.g., either removed if the task has not been learned or added when a student enters puberty, such as menstrual hygiene, shaving, dressing for physical education class, or expressing sexuality).

Students with developmental coordination disorder are often disorganized in sequencing ADLs and may take an excessive amount of time to learn and complete them (Thornton et al., 2016). Students with sensory sensitivity may avoid or perform ADLs according to their sensory preferences (e.g., type and amount of clothes worn; tolerating touching of the face; approaches to diapering, handwashing, hair brushing, or tooth brushing; Bagby et al., 2012; Schaaf et al., 2014). Learning new tasks may take more time for students with intellectual disabilities because they may lack the receptive or expressive language to understand directions or make their preferences known, or they may have difficulty with problem solving and generalizing learning (Barnes & Beck, 2011). Students with emotional regulation issues may lack frustration tolerance, which limits persistence to complete a task, ability to express needs, or having a sense of control. Many students who have had painful injuries or medical procedures in the past may have high anxiety that interferes with ADL routines or performance (Shepherd & Ivey, in press).

Students who do not understand the social routines or norms of ADLs may leave the restroom half-dressed, comb their hair in the lunchroom, or discuss toileting or a recent sexual education lesson at inappropriate times. In addition, students may fear failure or excessively ask for help. As their behavior unfolds, negative interactions with peers often occur. All students with disabilities are at risk for abuse (Stalker & McArthur, 2012). If a student has been previously sexually abused while performing dressing, toileting, or showering tasks, then they may have negative feelings, reactions, or fear when acquiring or practicing these ADLs with others.

BEST PRACTICES

Evaluation and intervention ADL strategies for students with disabilities are critical responsibilities for school occupational therapists and require multifaceted approaches. As students with disabilities perform ADL occupations in school, home, and community contexts, they are viewed more positively by themselves and others.

Evaluate Student

Occupational therapists begin the evaluation by gathering the *occupational profile* (what are the concerns, what occupations are supported or hindered, does the environment or context support or impede performance). Evaluating ADL skills requires a multilevel approach using interviews, observations within natural environments, checklists, or other formal ADL assessment tools. If they are available and appropriate, reviewing reports from a student's physician is helpful.

Assess environment and context

ADL tasks occur in a variety of environments and contexts throughout the school day. Practitioners use an *ecological assessment process* by observing ADL tasks where they naturally occur in the school environment, not in separate therapy spaces, unless privacy is an issue. Typical tasks to observe include getting off and on the bus; moving from class to class; toileting routines; putting on and taking off coats or personal devices, such as splints, hearing aids, or glasses; dressing and grooming for a physical education class or a band performance; and observing relationships with peers during and outside of class.

Certain physical attributes of schools may impede ADLs, such as cluttered classrooms and hallways, heavy doors, long distances between activities, steep ramps, large thresholds or no curb cuts, rough or uneven sidewalks, carpeting, or lack of stable seating. In addition, consider the space available, terrain, accessibility, type of assistive technology (AT) used, and signage to and in the classroom. Other physical attributes not directly related to the school environment (e.g., inclement weather requiring quick transitions between activities) may limit students with motor disabilities (e.g., getting on and off the bus, recess, field trips, changing classes within a campus; Egilson & Traustadottir, 2009). The sensory environment is evaluated (e.g., visual, auditory, tactile, vestibular, kinesthetic, proprioceptive, olfactory qualities) using observations or evaluations such as the Classroom Sensory Environment Assessment (Miller-Kuhaneck & Kelleher, 2015) or the Participation and Sensory Environment Questionnaire: Teacher Version (Piller et al., 2017).

When evaluating the school's social environment, the occupational therapist considers the following questions:

- What are the classroom routines for self-care?
- Is the social environment conducive to independence in ADLs?
- Is the student fitting in or accepted by the class (not ridiculed)?
- Are appropriate role models and supports available?

After identifying supports and barriers and considering cultural preferences, the activity demands in the physical and social environments are assessed. Do the student's actions, sequencing, and timing meet the expectations in the school environment? The Participation and Environment Measure for Children and Youth (Coster et al., 2010) is a teacher-report assessment that may provide more information about the student's participation in school and in home and community environments.

Context-focused therapy concentrates on modifications to the ADL task or environment rather than remediating the performance skills of the child. It is supported by research for children with autism spectrum disorder (ASD; Darrah et al., 2011; Dunn et al., 2012) and children with cerebral palsy (CP; Novak et al., 2013). Occupational therapists assess the supports and barriers of the environment or context that influence student participation and concentrate on modifications (Anaby et al., 2014; Coster et al., 2013). Therapists evaluate ADL task demands (i.e., objects and properties, space, sequencing and timing, required actions, body functions and structures) that are interwoven with a student's interactions with the environment and context (e.g., physical, social, cultural, personal, temporal, virtual conditions; AOTA, 2014b). Working in the context reinforces skills and routines to promote, establish, and maintain ADLs.

Evaluate specific student's strengths and needs

Perspectives on a student's ADL performance are gathered through interviews with a student, teacher, paraeducator or other team members, and a parent or caregiver to set meaningful, contextually relevant goals (Dunn et al., 2012; Law et al., 2011). Students, teachers, and parents often know what works. This valuable input helps embed ADL opportunities into the routines at school and home (Pfeiffer et al., 2017). This top-down approach to evaluation focuses on self-care tasks needed to participate in school and community environments, not a student's performance skills (e.g., motor, process, or social interaction) or body functions or structures (e.g., strength, sensory, praxis).

Use Effective ADL Interventions

Many strategies for ADL interventions are based on education and psychological research, but not all have evidence-based research to support their use. A multifaceted approach to and research on outcomes in ADLs and the effectiveness of intervention strategies for students are needed.

Alter task, materials, method, or environment

An *activity or task analysis* breaks an ADL task into even or equal numbers of steps that are observable and logical to a student and school staff (Snell & Brown, 2011). The clarity of the ADL and desired outcome is improved when team members have input into the activity analysis, including the number of steps; wording of instructional cues; and the amount, type, and timing of cues. Steps from activity analyses often are placed on a data collection sheet to monitor student progress and are graphed to demonstrate progress (Frolek Clark, 2016). Practitioners systematically use their knowledge of activity analysis and grading techniques to alter task demands, materials, methods, instruction, or the environment to facilitate a student's independence and participation in ADLs at school (Barnes & Beck, 2011; Darrah et al., 2011).

Planning is done in collaboration with the student and team so that changes are acceptable, valued, and more likely to be used by all. By embedding ADL skills in everyday environments and routines, practice of skills may occur more often while being reinforced in natural contexts (Chien et al., 2014). Note that students may reject strategies that call attention to their disability or that do not fit in the physical or social environment. Trialing proposed approaches and collecting data to determine whether the student is more efficient with adaptations and whether the student and educational personnel will use them are recommended (Hemmingsson et al., 2009).

Alter task or materials

Grading techniques include changing the sequence or number of steps in the ADL task; increasing or decreasing the level of difficulty of the task or the amount of time to do the task; modifying or fading the amount of prompting or physical assistance given; and modifying the tools, materials, or equipment used. If AT is chosen, it must fit the needs of a student in the context of school and home; data are collected to determine the AT's effectiveness and efficiency, as well as team satisfaction with the method.

Practitioners generally begin with low technology, such as color cues (e.g., back of shirt or pants), checklists, or visual schedules to promote on-task behaviors before moving to high-technology electronic devices. *Low-technology devices* that augment performance of ADLs include buttonhooks, elastic shoelaces, built-up tools, mobility devices, transfer boards, tongs, and reachers. Portable memory aids (e.g., checklists, voice-activated recorders), medication alarm pill boxes, watches with specialized features (e.g., talking, alarms, schedules), alarm organizers, pagers, and simple switches that program up to 3 steps are also task materials that may enhance ADL independence.

In *video modeling of others,* a student watches a video of an adult or peer performing the ADL task (e.g., wiping mouth, tying shoes, brushing teeth) on a TV, tablet, or handheld device and then attempts the task. In *video self-modeling,* a student performs the task during numerous taping sessions; then a 2- to 3-minute video is spliced together of the student performing the task correctly, which is used to prompt ADL performance (Bereznak et al., 2012).

Video modeling of others and video self-modeling are evidence-based practices for students with ASD and developmental disabilities to learn social (Domire & Wolfe, 2014; Meister & Salls, 2015) and functional ADLs, such as tooth brushing (Cihak et al., 2016; Popple et al., 2016) and handwashing (Lee & Lee, 2014; Rosenberg et al., 2010). These methods support what therapists and parents have known for years: Seeing a friend or peer eat or dress a certain way or do different ADLs as a role model is helpful and motivates students to try or complete these activities themselves. When video modeling is used with students with ASD, the strongest effects were with elementary (ages 5–9 years) and adolescent to adult students (age 16 years to young adult; Hong et al., 2016). Video modeling of others completing an ADL task is an easy, fast, and practical instructional strategy to acquire new behaviors or improve already acquired skills with technology that all students can use and does not require reading.

Modify task method or strategies used

The team decides on the appropriate method or strategy to use, the amount of participation expected, and what practice opportunities are available. Graduated guidance requires task analysis aimed to shape a desired behavior by either doing the steps of a task from beginning to end (*forward chaining*) or ending with the task and working backward (*backward chaining*) while giving cues, either through positive reinforcement or error correction. Several toileting programs for students with ASD and intellectual disabilities have successfully used a combination of these techniques (Kroeger & Sorensen-Burnworth, 2009).

Instructional cues or prompts are used purposefully and judiciously and are antecedents designed to increase the likelihood that a student will complete an ADL task (Snell & Brown, 2011; Snell et al., 2015). Prompts are given before or during a task, beginning with the least invasive prompt

possible and progressing to the most invasive prompt. A system of least prompts to most prompts is as follows:

- Opportunity cues (indirect nonverbal cues such as a raised eyebrow)
- Natural cues or consequences (e.g., leave the brush near the sink as a reminder to brush)
- Indirect verbal ("What comes next?")
- Gestural guidance (pointing, pretending to brush teeth)
- Visuals (e.g., words, checklists, pictures, computer-aided checklists with pictures, video modeling)
- Direct verbal instructions ("Pick up the brush")
- Modeling
- Physical assistance (e.g., shadowing, 2-finger prompting, hand under hand, manual physical guidance)
- Partial participation by child in the task
- Full physical assistance of others (Snell & Brown, 2011).

Educational personnel continually evaluate the effectiveness and practicality of cues by collecting data and feedback from the student and team members and graphing progress when possible (Ault & Griffen, 2013). Once a student has acquired the task, cues are decreased in saliency, amount, or proximity to a student; combined (e.g., gestural prompt with verbal prompt); or faded (e.g., delaying the time before a cue is given or eliminate the cue; Snell & Brown, 2011). Note that cues do not work when they are incorrectly used, when they are overused, or when attitudes do not support their use (e.g., by a professional who dislikes suggested cues or thinks that the reinforcement system is too hard to do).

Alter environment

Occupational therapy practitioners collaborate with team members to alter the environment where ADLs occur while considering the culture of the classroom and the people involved. Student success in ADLs may improve by altering sensory characteristics, work surfaces, positioning and accessibility options, and time schedules and expectations and involving peers when appropriate (Shepherd & Ivey, in press).

In the virtual context, electronic devices such as computers, tablets, MP3 players, personal digital assistants, and phones are used effectively as cognitive prosthetic devices for visual schedules, prompting hierarchies, Social Stories, and video modeling (den Brok & Sterkenburg, 2015). These devices may augment instructions from others or be self-controlled while giving the visual, auditory, and tactile prompts needed to initiate, sequence, sustain, and complete ADLs at school and home (Bimbrahw et al., 2012; den Brok & Sterkenburg, 2015; Kagohara et al., 2013).

Educate Students, Parents, and Educational Personnel

Attempting ADLs in new environments is often stressful and anxiety producing for students, families, and educational personnel. Education to prevent or avoid ADL issues has merit.

Use Social Stories to prepare students for ADLs

Social Stories may decrease students' frustration, fear, or anxiety while using the school or public bathrooms, showering after physical education, riding the bus to school, getting to class independently, or changing routines. *Social Stories*™ consist of a short story with or without pictures that is written for a student for a particular situation, according to Gray's (2015) story criteria.

Students with ASD, behavior issues, or intellectual disabilities benefit from Social Stories, and they are easy to make and to implement and use in a variety of situations. Social Story sentences have the recommended following ratio: For every directive sentence given, at least 2–5 sentences should be affirmative, descriptive, or perspective-giving (Gray, 2015). These stories may be on paper (low technology) or on a tablet, computer, or handheld device so students can review them before performing a task. Data collection to assess the effectiveness, social validity, and procedural reliability of Social Stories is needed (Test et al., 2010).

Plan ahead and use cognitive strategies

By anticipating problems, parents or teachers plan for the unexpected. Parents often use this approach with their school-age students with brain injury and ASD to avoid meltdowns during ADLs (Kirby et al., 2016; Pfeiffer et al., 2017). Strategies may include using modeling, prompts, video modeling, or Social Stories bringing a change of clothes or using simple fasteners on physical education days. When able to do so, students also generate possible solutions for the unexpected ahead of time.

The ***Cognitive Orientation to daily Occupational Performance*** (CO–OP; Dawson et al., 2017) is a cognitive-based problem-solving model collectively known as Goal–Plan–Do–Check (Polatajko et al., 2001). Application of this 4-step model demonstrated improvement in task performance (some ADLs) for students with developmental coordination disorder (Thornton et al., 2016), brain injury (Missiuna et al., 2010), ASD (Rodger et al., 2009), and CP (Cameron et al., 2017). After using this technique, children changed strategies and reduced the time they took to do a task (Rodger & Brandenburg, 2009). CO–OP group intervention was effective for parents of children with CP who successfully applied these strategies at home (Jackman et al., 2017) and for group intervention for children with motor coordination difficulties (Anderson et al., 2017). CO–OP embeds learning in the natural environment and is used mostly with students who have adequate receptive and expressive communication and cognition to participate.

Coach students, parents, and educational personnel within the school context

Coaching is an interaction style that promotes collaborative partnerships and allows self-discovery by all parties (Rush & Shelden, 2011). Instead of giving directives, therapists encourage self-reflection through open-ended questions while sharing ideas. This education approach is evidence based and appears effective when occupational therapy practitioners work with students and educational personnel in their natural environments (Darrah et al., 2011; Skiffington et al., 2011; Wilson et al., 2012) or with families and their children with ASD, attention deficit hyperactivity

disorder, or CP (Dunn et al., 2012; Graham et al., 2013; Law et al., 2011; Zwi et al., 2011).

Team members learn from each other while supporting students, families, and personnel through communicating, problem solving together, and providing hands-on support. Coaching is effective when a structured process is used to set goals with team members who describe the preobservation (what do you anticipate will happen), observe what happened (with video when possible), and then reflect about what is or is not working (Skiffington et al., 2011). Better designed outcome measures to support the coaching model are needed (Miller-Kuhaneck & Watling, 2018).

Outcomes

Intervention aims to improve ADL performance for student participation in school, after-school, and work activities. Outcome measures for ADLs in schools are chosen according to team preferences and must be valid for the student evaluated (Gleason & Coster, 2012). These measures objectively establish the student's baseline performance and identify change after intervention.

James et al. (2013) reviewed 26 measures of ADL performance and determined that for young children, the Pediatric Evaluation of Disability Inventory (PEDI; Haley et al., 1992) was the best predictive measure of ADL capabilities for children with CP ages 6 months–7.5 years. The Pediatric Evaluation of Disability Inventory Computer Adaptive Test (PEDI–CAT; Haley et al., 2012) is used in multiple environments to assess ADL outcomes through parent report and is based on the *International Classification of Functioning, Disability and Health* model (Kao et al., 2012). The Assessment of Motor and Process Skills (AMPS; ages 3 or older; Fisher & Bray Jones, 2012, 2013) is the best measure of ADL performance for children with CP because it links motor and process skills to ADL outcomes (James et al., 2013). A training and calibration process is required for evaluators to use the AMPS.

The School Function Assessment (Coster et al., 1998) is an outcome measure used by a team to rate a student's participation in 6 different environments: transportation, transitions, classroom, cafeteria, bathroom, and playground. ADL assessment is a portion of the entire evaluation for children ages 5–12 years. The Kohlman Evaluation of Living Skills (Kohlman Thomson & Robnett, 2016) for adolescents and the Adaptive Behavior Assessment System (Harrison & Oakland, 2015) are other valid and standardized assessments that evaluate ADL outcomes. Goal attainment scaling is a practical way to measure small changes in ADL outcomes and is being used in therapy research in conjunction with other client-centered measurements, such as the Canadian Occupational Performance Measure (Dunn et al., 2012; Law et al., 2005; Schaaf et al., 2014).

Positive outcomes for learning ADLs through the previously described intervention methods are numerous. They may increase student competency and self-esteem, increase teacher and family competency and efficacy, improve student relationships at home and school, provide more time for all parties to participate in other activities, and improve a student's quality of life (Bendixen et al., 2011; Dunn et al., 2012; Graham et al., 2013).

SUMMARY

Occupational therapy practitioners have a strong role in promoting each student's functional performance. The occupational therapist's evaluation of ADL skills would guide the team's decision-making process for identifying a student's functional needs in the educational setting.

  Occupational therapy practitioners may provide intervention throughout the student's participation in school, especially when they enter new phases of expectations. Using appropriate outcome measures and a top-down approach to evaluation, therapists observe students in natural environments while considering the influence of student, teacher, and caregiver preferences as well as goals, classroom routines, and specific characteristics of the student and environment. Altering the task, materials, methods, and environment and using an education approach are recommended. Evidence supports embedding ADL instruction in the school context and routines, using a variety of instructional techniques while collaboratively coaching students, teachers, paraeducators, and caregivers.

REFERENCES

American Occupational Therapy Association. (2014a). Guidelines for supervision, roles, and responsibilities during the delivery of occupational therapy services. *American Journal of Occupational Therapy, 68*(Suppl. 3), S16–S22. https://doi.org/10.5014/ajot.2014.686S03

American Occupational Therapy Association. (2014b). Occupational therapy practice framework: Domain and process (3rd ed.). *American Journal of Occupational Therapy, 68*(Suppl. 1), S1–S48. https://doi.org/10.5014/ajot.682006

Anaby, D., Law, M., Coster, W., Bedell, G., Khetani, M., Avery, L., & Teplicky, R. (2014). The mediating role of the environment in explaining participation of children and youth with and without disabilities across home, school and community. *Archives of Physical Medicine and Rehabilitation, 95,* 908–917. https://doi.org/10.1016/j.apmr.2014.01.005

Anderson, L., Wilson, J., & Williams, G. (2017). Cognitive Orientation to daily Occupational Performance (CO–OP) as group therapy for children living with motor coordination difficulties: An integrated literature review. *Australian Occupational Therapy Journal, 64,* 170–184. https://doi.org/10.1111/1440-1630.12333

Assistance to States for the Education of Children With Disabilities and Preschool Grants for Children With Disabilities, 71 Fed. Reg. 46539 (August 14, 2006) (to be codified at 34 C.F.R. 300, 301).

Ault, M., & Griffen, A. (2013). Teaching with the system of least prompts: An easy method for monitoring progress. *TEACHING Exceptional Children, 45*(3), 46–53.

Bagby, M. S., Dickie, V. A., & Baranek, G. (2012). How sensory experiences of children with and without autism affect family occupations. *American Journal of Occupational Therapy, 66,* 78–86. https://doi.org/10.5014/ajot.2012.000604

Barnes, K. J., & Beck, A. J. (2011). Enabling performance and participation for children with developmental disabilities. In C. H. Christiansen & K. M. Matuska (Eds.), *Ways of living: Intervention strategies to enable participation* (4th ed., pp. 131–170). Bethesda, MD: AOTA Press.

Bendixen, R. M., Elder, J. H., Donaldson, S., Kairalla, J. A., Valcante, G., & Ferdig, R. E. (2011). Effects of a father-based in-home intervention on perceived stress and family dynamics in parents of children with autism. *American Journal of Occupational Therapy, 65,* 679–687. https://doi.org/10.5014/ajot.2011.001271

Bereznak, S., Ayres, K. M., Alexander, J. L., & Mechling, L. C. (2012). Video self-prompting and mobile technology to increase daily living and vocational independence for students with autism spectrum disorders. *Journal of Developmental and Physical Disabilities, 24,* 269–285. https://doi.org/10.1007/s10882-012-9270-8

Bimbrahw, J., Boger, J., & Mihailidis, A. (2012). Investigating the efficacy of a computerized prompting device to assist children with autism spectrum disorder with activities of daily living. *Assistive Technology, 24,* 286–298. https://doi.org/10.1080/10400435.2012.680661

Cameron, D., Craig, T., Edwards, B., Missiuna, C., Schwellnus, H., & Polatajko, H. (2017). Cognitive Orientation to daily Occupational Performance (CO–OP): A new approach for children with cerebral palsy. *Physical and Occupational Therapy in Pediatrics, 37,* 183–198. https://doi.org/10.1080/01942638.2016.1185500

Chien, C.-W., Brown, T., McDonald, R., & Yu, M.-L. (2014). The contributing role of real-life hand skill performance in self-care function of children with and without disabilities. *Child: Care, Health and Development, 40,* 134–144. https://doi.org/10.1111/j.1365-2214.2012.01429.x

Cihak, D. F., Moore, E. J., Wright, R. E., McMahon, D. D., Gibbons, M. M., & Smith, C. (2016). Evaluating augmented reality to complete a chain task for elementary students with autism. *Journal of Special Education Technology, 31,* 99–108. https://doi.org/10.1177/0162643416651724

Coster, W. J., Deeney, T., Haltiwanger, J., & Haley, S. (1998). *School Function Assessment.* San Antonio: Psychological Corporation.

Coster, W., Law, M., & Bedell, G. (2010). *Participation and Environment Measure for Children and Youth (PEM–CY).* Boston: Boston University.

Coster, W., Law, M., Bedell, G., Liljenquist, K., Kao, Y.-C., Khetani, M., & Teplicky, R. (2013). School participation, supports, and barriers of students with and without disabilities. *Child: Care, Health and Development, 39,* 535–543. https://doi.org/10.1111/cch.12046

Darrah, J., Law, M., Pollock, N., Wilson, B., Russell, D., Walter, S., . . . Galuppi, B. (2011). Context therapy: A new intervention approach for children with cerebral palsy. *Developmental Medicine and Child Neurology, 53,* 615–620. https://doi.org/10.1111/j.1469-8749.2011.03959.x

Dawson, D. R., McEwen, S. E., & Polatajko, H. J. (Eds.). (2017). *Cognitive Orientation to daily Occupational Performance in occupational therapy: Using the CO–OP Approach™ to enable participation across the lifespan.* Bethesda, MD: AOTA Press.

den Brok, W., & Sterkenburg, P. (2015). Self-controlled technologies to support skill attainment in persons with an autism spectrum disorder and/or an intellectual disability: A systematic literature review. *Disability and Rehabilitation, 10,* 1–10. https://doi.org/10.3109/17483107.2014.921248

Domire, S., & Wolfe, P. (2014). Effects of video prompting techniques on teaching daily living skills to children with autism spectrum disorders: A review. *Research and Practice for Persons With Severe Disabilities, 39,* 211–226. https://doi.org/10.1177%2F1540796914555578

Dunn, W., Cox, J., Foster, L., Mische-Lawson, L., & Tanquary, J. (2012). Impact of a contextual intervention on child participation and parent competence among children with autism spectrum disorders: A pretest–posttest repeated measures design. *American Journal of Occupational Therapy, 66,* 520–528. https://doi.org/10.5014/ajot.2012.004119

Egilson, S. T., & Traustadottir, R. (2009). Participation of students with physical disabilities in the school environment. *American Journal of Occupational Therapy, 63,* 264–272. https://doi.org/10.5014/ajot.63.3.264

Fisher, A. G., & Bray Jones, K. (2012). *Assessment of Motor and Process Skills: Vol. 1. Development, standardization, and administration manual* (7th rev. ed.). Fort Collins, CO: Three Star Press.

Fisher, A. G., & Bray Jones, K. (2014). *Assessment of Motor and Process Skills: Vol. 2. User manual* (8th ed.). Fort Collins, CO: Three Star Press.

Frolek Clark, G. (2016). Collaborating within the *Paces*: Structures and routines. In B. Hanft & J. Shepherd (Eds.), *Collaborating for student success: A guide for school-based occupational therapy* (2nd ed., pp. 177–208). Bethesda, MD: AOTA Press.

Gleason, K., & Coster, W. (2012). An ICF–CY-based content analysis of the Vineland Adaptive Behavior Scales–II. *Journal of Intellectual and Developmental Disability, 37,* 285–293. https://doi.org/10.3109/13668250.2012.720675

Graham, F., Rodger, S., & Ziviani, J. (2013). Effectiveness of occupational performance coaching in improving children's and mothers' performance and mothers' self-competence. *American Journal of Occupational Therapy, 67,* 10–18. https://doi.org/10.5014/ajot.2013.004648

Gray, C. (2015). *The new social story book: Illustrated edition.* Arlington, TX: Future Horizons.

Haley, S. M., Coster, W. J., Dumas, H. M., Fragile-Pinkham, M. A., & Moed, R. (2012). *PEDI–CAT: Development, standardization, and administration manual.* Boston: Boston University.

Haley, S. M., Coster, W. J., Ludlow, L. H., Haltiwanger, J. T., & Andrellos, P. J. (1992). *Pediatric Evaluation of Disability Inventory (PEDI).* San Antonio: Psychological Corporation.

Hanft, B., & Shepherd, J. (Eds.). (2016). *Collaborating for student success: A guide for school-based occupational therapy* (2nd ed.). Bethesda, MD: AOTA Press.

Harrison, P., & Oakland, T. (2015). *Adaptive Behavior Assessment System* (3rd ed.). Los Angeles: Western Psychological Services.

Hemmingsson, H., Lidstrom, H., & Nygard, L. (2009). Use of assistive technology devices in mainstream schools: Students' perspective. *American Journal of Occupational Therapy, 63,* 463–472. https://doi.org/10.5014/ajot.63.4.463

Hong, E. R., Ganz, J. B., Mason, R., Morin, K., Davis, J. L., Ninci, J., . . . Gilliland, W. D. (2016). The effects of video modeling in teaching functional living skills to persons with ASD: A meta-analysis of single-case studies. *Research in Developmental Disabilities, 57,* 158–169. https://doi.org/10.1016/j.ridd.2016.07.001

Individuals With Disabilities Education Improvement Act of 2004, Pub. L. 108–446, 20 U.S.C. §§ 1400–1482.

Jackman, M., Novak, I., Lannin, N., & Froude, E. (2017). Parents' experience of undertaking an intensive Cognitive Orientation to daily Occupational Performance (CO–OP) group for children with cerebral palsy. *Disability Rehabilitation, 39,* 1018–1024. https://doi.org/10.1080/09638288.2016.1179350

James, S., Ziviani, J., & Boyd, R. (2013). A systematic review of activities of daily living measures for children and adolescents with cerebral palsy. *Developmental Medicine and Child Neurology, 56,* 233–244. https://doi.org/10.1111/dmcn.12226

Kagohara, D. M., van der Meer, L., Ramdoss, S., O'Reilly, M. F., Lancioni, G. E., Davis, T. N., . . . Sigafoos, J. (2013). Using iPods and iPads in teaching programs for individuals with developmental disabilities: A systematic review. *Research in Developmental Disabilities, 34,* 147–156. https://doi.org/10.1016/j.ridd.2012.07.027

Kao, Y.-C., Kramer, J. M., Liljenquist, K. S., & Coster, W. J. (2015). Association between impairment, function, and daily life task management in children and youth with autism. *Developmental Medicine and Child Neurology, 57,* 68–74. https://doi.org/10.1111/dmcn.12562

Kee, E. G., Chien, C.-W., Rodger, S., & Copley, J. (2014). Examining the association between children's hand skill performance and participation in everyday life. *Journal of Occupational Therapy, Schools, and Early Intervention, 7,* 246–259. https://doi.org/10.1080/19411243.2014.979598

Kirby, A. V., Little, L. M., Schultz, B., Watson, L. R., Zhang, W., & Baranek, G. T. (2016). Brief Report—Development and pilot of the Caregiver Strategies Inventory. *American Journal of Occupational Therapy, 70,* 7004360010. https://doi.org/10.5014/ajot.2016.019901

Kohlman Thomson, L., & Robnett, R. (2016). *Kohlman Evaluation of Living Skills* (4th ed.). Bethesda, MD: AOTA Press.

Krantz, G., Tolan, V., Pontarelli, K., & Cahill, S. (2016). What do adolescents with developmental disabilities learn about sexuality and dating? A potential role for occupational therapy. *Open Journal of Occupational Therapy, 4*(2), Article 5. https://doi.org/10.15453/2168-6408.1208

Kroeger, K. A., & Sorensen-Burnworth, R. (2009). Toilet training individuals with autism and other developmental disabilities: A critical review. *Research in Autism Spectrum Disorders, 3,* 607–618. https://doi.org/10.1016/j.rasd.2009.01.005

Law, M., Baptiste, S., Carswell, A., McColl, M. A., Polatajko, H., & Pollock, N. (2005). *Canadian Occupational Performance Measure* (4th ed.). Ottawa: CAOT Publications.

Law, M., Darrah, J., Pollock, N., Wilson, B., Russell, D. J., Walter, S. D., . . . Galuppi, B. (2011). Focus on function: A cluster, randomized controlled trial comparing child- versus context-focused intervention for young children with cerebral palsy. *Developmental Medicine and Child Neurology, 53,* 621–629. https://doi.org/10.1111/j.1469-8749.2011.03962.x

Lee, R., & Lee, P. (2014). To evaluate the effects of a simplified hand washing improvement program in school children with mild intellectual disability: A pilot study. *Research in Developmental Disabilities, 35,* 3014–3025. https://doi.org/10.1016/j.ridd.2014.07.016

Meister, C., & Salls, J. (2015). Video modeling for teaching daily living skills to children with autism spectrum disorder: A pilot study. *Journal of Occupational Therapy, Schools, and Early Intervention, 8,* 307–318. https://doi.org/10.1080/19411243.2015.1107005

Miller-Kuhaneck, H. M., & Kelleher, J. P. (2015). Development of the Classroom Sensory Environment Assessment. *American Journal of Occupational Therapy, 69,* 6906180040. https://doi.org/10.5014/ajot.2015.019430

Miller-Kuhaneck, H., & Watling, R. (2018). Parental or teacher education and coaching to support function and participation of children and youth with sensory processing and sensory integration challenges: A systematic review. *American Journal of Occupational Therapy, 72,* 7201190030. https://doi.org/10.5014/ajot.2018.029017

Missiuna, C., DeMatteo, C., Hanna, S., Mandich, A., Law, M., Mahoney, W., & Scott, L. (2010). Exploring the use of cognitive intervention for children with acquired brain injury. *Physical and Occupational Therapy in Pediatrics, 30,* 205–219. https://doi.org/10.3109/01942631003761554

Novak, I., McIntyre, S., Morgan, C., Campbell, L., Dark, L., Morton, N., . . . Goldsmith, S. (2013). A systematic review of interventions for children with cerebral palsy: State of the evidence. *Developmental Medicine and Child Neurology, 55,* 885–910. https://doi.org/10.1111/dmcn.12246

O'Brien, J., Bergeron, A., Duprey, H., Oliver, C., & St. Onge, H. (2009). Children with disabilities and their parents' views of occupational participation needs. *Occupational Therapy in Mental Health, 25,* 164–180. https://doi.org/10.1080/01642120902859196

Persch, A., Lamb, A., Metzler, C., & Fristad, M. (2015). Healthy habits for children: Leveraging existing evidence to demonstrate value. *American Journal of Occupational Therapy, 69,* 6904090010. https://doi.org/10.5014/ajot.2015.694001

Pfeiffer, B., Coster, W., Snethen, G., Derstine, M., Piller, A., & Tucker, C. (2017). Caregivers' perspectives on the sensory environment and participation in daily activities of children with autism spectrum disorder. *American Journal of Occupational Therapy, 71,* 7104220020. https://doi.org/10.5014/ajot.2017.021360

Phipps, S., & Roberts, P. (2012). Predicting the effects of cerebral palsy severity on self-care, mobility, and social function. *American Journal of Occupational Therapy, 66,* 422–429. https://doi.org/10.5014/ajot.2012.003921

Piller, A., Fletcher, T., Pfeiffer, B., Dunlap, K., & Pickens, N. (2017). Reliability of the Participation and Sensory Environment Questionnaire: Teacher version. *Journal of Autism and Developmental Disorders, 47,* 3541–3549. https://doi.org/10.1007/s10803-017-3273-3

Polatajko, H. J., Mandich, A. D., Miller, L. T., & Macnab, J. J. (2001). Cognitive Orientation to daily Occupational Performance (CO–OP): Part II—The evidence. *Physical and Occupational Therapy in Pediatrics, 20,* 83–106. https://doi.org/10.1080/J006v20n02_06

Popple, B., Wall, C., Flink, L., Powell, K., Discepolo, K., Keck, D., . . . Shic, F. (2016). Brief Report: Remotely delivered video modeling for improving oral hygiene in children with ASD: A pilot study. *Journal of Autism and Developmental Disorders, 46,* 2791–2796. https://doi.org/10.1007/s10803-016-2795-4

Rodger, S., & Brandenburg, J. (2009). Cognitive Orientation to (daily) Occupational Performance (CO–OP) with children with Asperger's syndrome who have motor-based occupational performance goals. *Australian Occupational Therapy Journal, 56,* 41–50. https://doi.org/10.1111/j.1440-1630.2008.00739.x

Rodger, S., Pham, C., & Mitchell, S. (2009). Cognitive strategy use by children with Asperger's syndrome during intervention for motor-based goals. *Australian Occupational Therapy Journal, 56,* 103–111.

Rosenberg, N. E., Schwartz, I. S., & Davis, C. A. (2010). Evaluating the utility of commercial videotapes for teaching hand washing to children with autism. *Education and Treatment of Children, 33,* 443–455. https://doi.org/10.1353/etc.0.0098

Rush, D., & Shelden, M. (2011). *Coaching families and colleagues in early childhood.* Baltimore: Brookes.

Schaaf, R. C., Benevides, T., Mailloux, Z., Faller, P., Hunt, J., van Hooydonk, E., . . . Kelly, D. (2014). An intervention for sensory difficulties in children with autism: A randomized trial. *Journal of Autism and Developmental Disorders, 44,* 1493–1506. https://doi.org/10.1007/s10803-013-1983-8

Shepherd, J., & Ivey, C. (in press). Activities of daily living, sexuality, and sleep and rest. In J. O'Brien & H. Miller-Kuhaneck (Eds.), *Case-Smith's occupational therapy for children and adolescents* (8th ed.). St. Louis: Elsevier.

Skiffington, S., Washburn, S., & Elliott, K. (2011). Instructional coaching: Helping preschool teachers reach their full potential. *Young Children, 66*(3), 12–20.

Snell, M. E., & Brown, F. (2011). Selecting teaching strategies and arranging educational environments. In M. E. Snell & F. Brown (Eds.), *Instruction of students with severe disabilities* (7th ed., pp. 122–185). Upper Saddle River, NJ: Prentice-Hall.

Snell, M., Delano, M., & Walker, V. (2015). Teaching self-care skills. In F. Brown, M. E. Snell, & J. McDonnell (Eds.), *Instruction of students with severe disabilities* (8th ed.). Upper Saddle River, NJ: Prentice Hall.

Stalker, K., & McArthur, K. (2012). Child abuse, child protection and disabled children: A review of recent research. *Child Abuse Review, 21*(1), 24–40. https://doi.org/10.1002/car.1154

Test, D. W., Richter, S., Knight, V., & Spooner, F. (2010). A comprehensive review and meta-analysis of the Social Stories literature. *Focus on Autism and Other Developmental Disabilities, 26,* 49–62. https://doi.org/10.1177%2F1088357609351573

Thornton, A., Licari, M., Reid, S., Armstrong, J., Fallows, R., & Elliott, C. (2016). Cognitive Orientation to (daily) Occupational Performance intervention leads to improvements in impairments, activity and participation in children with developmental coordination disorder. *Disability and Rehabilitation, 38,* 979–986. https://doi.org/10.3109/09638288.2015.1070298

Vroland-Nordstrand, K., Eliasson, A.-C., Jacobsson, H., Johansson, U., & Krumlinde-Sundholm, L. (2015). Can children identify and achieve goals for intervention? A randomized trial comparing two goal-setting approaches. *Developmental Medicine and Child Neurology, 58,* 58–96. https://doi.org/10.1111/dmcn.12925

Wilson, K. P., Dykstra, J. R., Watson, L. R., Boyd, B. A., & Crais, E. R. (2012). Coaching in early education classrooms serving children with autism: A pilot study. *Journal of Early Childhood Education, 40,* 97–105. https://doi.org/10.1007/s10643-011-0493-6

Zwi, M., Jones, H., Thorgaard, C., York, A., & Dennis, J. (2011). Parent training interventions for attention deficit hyperactivity disorder (ADHD) in children aged 5 to 18 years. *Cochrane Database of Systematic Reviews, 2011,* CD003018. https://doi.org/10.1002/14651858.CD00301

Best Practices in School Mealtimes to Enhance Participation

Winifred Schultz-Krohn, PhD, OTR/L, BCP, SWC, FAOTA, and Gloria Frolek Clark, PhD, OTR/L, BCP, SCSS, FAOTA

47

KEY TERMS AND CONCEPTS

- Dysphagia
- Eating
- Feeding
- Feeding plan
- Fiberoptic endoscopic evaluation of swallowing
- Food selectivity
- Fussy eaters
- Picky eaters
- Swallowing
- Tube feeding
- Videofluoroscopy swallow study

OVERVIEW

School districts are responsible for students' safety and nutrition and hydration needs so that students can participate in school. School mealtimes may include breakfast, snack, and lunch. School breakfast and lunch programs (Healthy, Hunger-Free Kids Act of 2010; Pub. L. 111–296) are regulated by the U.S. Department of Agriculture (USDA), which has developed guidelines to require schools to substitute or modify school meals for students with disabilities (USDA, 2017). Federal laws that address mealtime supports in schools include

- Supreme Court rulings requiring school districts to provide supportive services for a student to attend school and benefit from education (*Cedar Rapids Community School District vs. Garret F.*, 1999; *Irving Independent School District v. Tatro*, 1984);
- The Individuals With Disabilities Education Improvement Act of 2004's (IDEA; Pub. L. 108–446) reference to students' functional performance (e.g., skills used during routine ADLs); and
- Section 504 of the Rehabilitation Act of 1973, as amended (2008; Pub. L. 93–112), which does not allow students to be excluded from participation in school activities (including mealtimes) solely on the basis of a disabling condition (Power-deFur & Alley, 2008).

Occupational therapy practitioners,[1] as related service providers under IDEA, work with school districts to modify foods and adapt environments for students with special needs as well as provide services directly with students. Eighty percent of students with disabilities and 25%–45% of typically developing children have feeding and swallowing disorders, making a team approach essential (Arvedson, 2008).

Common Terms and Definitions

Broad definitions applied in this chapter are primarily from the AOTA (2017) document *The Practice of Occupational Therapy in Feeding, Eating, and Swallowing*. **Feeding** is "the process of bringing food to the mouth, sometimes called self-feeding" when completed by the individual; **eating** is "keeping and manipulating food or liquid in the mouth and swallowing it"; and **swallowing** is "moving the food from the mouth to the stomach" (AOTA, 2017, p. 2). **Dysphagia,** as defined by Lefton-Greif and Arvedson (2008), is a disorder of swallowing.

Three terms used for children who refuse food are *picky eaters, fussy eaters,* and *children with food selectivity*. **Picky eaters** are defined as those who consume "small amounts of food and . . . a limited variety of food" (Kim et al., 2011, p. 1364). Picky eaters often exhibit tantrums regarding food selection, slow eating, and food refusal of both familiar and novel foods (Lafraire et al., 2016). **Fussy eaters** describes children who reject foods and food textures and exhibit tantrums regarding food selection, slow eating, and food refusals of both familiar and novel foods (Lafraire et al., 2016).

---

[1]*Occupational therapy practitioner* refers to both the occupational therapist and the occupational therapy assistant. The American Occupational Therapy Association (AOTA; 2014, p. S18) states, "The occupational therapist is responsible for all aspects of occupational therapy service delivery and is accountable for the safety and effectiveness of the occupational therapy service delivery process" and "must be directly involved in the delivery of services during the initial evaluation and regularly throughout the course of intervention. . . . The occupational therapy assistant delivers safe and effective occupational therapy services under the supervision of and in partnership with the occupational therapist."

Copyright © 2019 by the American Occupational Therapy Association. All rights reserved. To reuse this content, contact www.copyright.com.
https://doi.org/10.7139/2019.978-1-56900-591-0.047

Children with *food selectivity* are those with more serious eating and feeding problems than picky eaters; they typically display the following characteristics: refusing food, limiting food choices, and having a high frequency of "single food intake" (Bandini et al., 2010, p. 260). The majority of children who are seen as picky or fussy eaters no longer exhibit these behaviors after age 6 years (Cano et al., 2015).

Tube feeding is the feeding of a liquid formula administered through a tube passed through the nose (nasogastric) or inserted into the stomach (gastric; Arvedson & Brodsky, 2002). *Fiberoptic endoscopic evaluation of swallowing* (FEES) is an instrumental assessment of the swallow (Arvedson & Lefton-Greif, 2017); a flexible tube is inserted in the nasal canal and threaded through the oropharynx to observe the swallowing process as the child eats or drinks. *Videofluoroscopy swallow study* (VFSS) is an instrumental assessment of the pharyngeal and esophageal phases using barium (Arvedson & Brodsky, 2002). This instrumental assessment can identify dysphagia, aspiration, and gastroesophageal reflux disease (GERD).

ESSENTIAL CONSIDERATIONS

Difficulties in participation during mealtimes may be caused by a variety of factors, such as environmental (e.g., too noisy, smell of foods, poor seating), activity or occupation (e.g., texture of food not safe, refuses a food on their plate), or student (e.g., poor oral–motor skills, dysphagia). Limited participation may result in poor nutrition, which lowers students' energy and alertness level; unsafe conditions; students' inability to join in social settings, such as eating lunch in the cafeteria; and behavioral issues, which can negatively affect the interaction among students and peers.

Safety and Nutrition During Mealtimes Are Critical

All students must safely receive adequate nutrition and hydration during school meals. Complex medical conditions, such as traumatic brain injury or cerebral palsy (CP), increase the risk for dysphagia in neurological conditions. Difficulties with swallowing foods, particularly novel foods, may result in increased coughing, choking, or restricted food or fluid intake (Lefton-Greif et al., 2006).

Inadequate nutrition is detrimental to a student's physical and mental health and results in poor school performance (Fiese et al., 2011; Jackson et al., 2017), such as significantly lower math and reading scores than peers in food-secure households (Jyoti et al., 2005). Inadequate nutrition is also a problem for students with poor eating behaviors, such as food selectivity and fear of trying new foods, and students with poor oral–motor skills who are unable to safely consume table foods and liquids. However, modifications and accommodations to school foods, per recommendations from a physician or dietitian, can help these students to receive proper nutrition (USDA, 2017).

Diagnostic Conditions That Affect Mealtime Performance

Students may have a diagnosis that carries secondary conditions that affect mealtime participation.

Autism spectrum disorder

Feeding and eating challenges are a recognizable part of mealtime for children with autism spectrum disorder (ASD; Emond et al., 2010; Provost et al., 2010), possibly for as many as 90% (Kodak & Piazza, 2008). Students with ASD have substantial food refusal, food restriction problems, and oral–sensory sensitivities compared with peers without ASD (Chistol et al., 2018; Provost et al., 2010), including acceptance of only a few food textures and varieties. Rituals (e.g., specific food preparation or packaging, food types) often interfere with eating both familiar and unfamiliar foods. Children with ASD who have feeding problems tend to have a greater frequency of food selectivity, such as refusing particular meats or vegetables, than children with feeding and eating disorders who do not have ASD (Cermak et al., 2010; Chistol et al., 2018; Emond et al., 2010; Field et al., 2003). Students with ASD may also exhibit oral–motor delay and dysphagia.

Food acceptance was significantly limited in all children with ASD, regardless of the severity of ASD, when compared with peers (Martins et al., 2008). Although 25%–35% of typically developing children have feeding and eating problems similar to those seen in children with ASD, these problems tend to be less severe in typically developing children and of shorter duration (Rogers et al., 2012). Children with ASD display food selectivity that persists into the teenage years, and the limited number of foods consumed does not substantially change as the child ages (Bandini et al., 2017). Children with ASD have fewer self-feeding skills, greater food avoidance, and more fear of trying new foods compared with peers (Martins et al., 2008). Children with ASD had lower body mass index and poorer nutritional intake compared with typically developing peers (Mari-Bauset et al., 2015).

CP

Calis et al. (2008) found only 1% of children (*N* = 166) ages 2–19 years (mean age = 9 years) diagnosed with CP and intellectual disability did not have dysphagia. On the basis of results with the Dysphagia Disorders Survey, Baladin et al. (as cited in Calis et al., 2008) found that 76% of the children had moderate to severe dysphagia, whereas 15% had profound dysphagia (e.g., no food by mouth); however, parents did not report dysphagia in their children. When dysphagia is suspected, the student should be referred for a medical evaluation, such as a VFSS or FEES. Symptoms such as persistent coughing, choking, or aspiration secondary to exhaustion with a long feeding session (e.g., more than 30 minutes) may indicate difficulty with oral–motor and swallowing skills.

A student with severe CP and substantial eating and swallowing problems will often experience nutritional deficits that decrease school performance (e.g., inability to pay attention, remain alert, stay healthy). A review of the nutritional status of children with CP (mean age = 6–7 years) found a high frequency of feeding problems and a high proportion of undernourished children, with oral–motor dysfunction as a contributing factor (Dahlseng et al., 2011). Children who have CP may require additional time to coordinate oral structures when eating, and the caloric value of food may need to be increased to compensate for the potential decreased quantity of food consumed.

To identify a relationship between the severity of CP and the severity of oral–motor dysfunction, Erkin et al. (2010) studied children with CP (average age = 6 years) and found a positive correlation: The more severe the CP symptoms, the more severe the eating dysfunction. Although the use of feeding tubes is often necessary for children with CP because they have reduced oral–motor skills, Erkin et al. reported that tube feedings increased the prevalence of overweight children with CP. In addition, the feeding, eating, and drinking problems appeared to remain fairly consistent over time in children with CP (Clancy & Hustad, 2011).

Gastrointestinal issues

Gastrointestinal (GI) problems include constipation, diarrhea, and GERD. GERD is most often associated with food refusal (Field et al., 2003). In addition, 85% of children with ASD had reported GI problems that were not related to restricted diet yet contributed to a poor appetite (Gorrindo et al., 2012). Nonverbal students may express discomfort through aggression or screaming. Research proving or disproving inadequate digestion of gluten and casein does not exist.

Genetic and medical conditions

Genetic and medical conditions may result in oral–motor delays or lack of fine motor skills needed for self-feeding (Lewis & Kritzinger, 2004). Children who have Down syndrome often have a reduced oral cavity size with a small jaw and low muscle tone, which contributes to problems with tongue protrusion, poor tongue control, and drooling. These issues diminish a student's ability to control the food bolus in the mouth and control fluid during drinking, which can lead to choking and potential aspiration. Although self-feeding skills are typically present by school age, food selectivity, food refusal, or restricting specific textures may interfere with eating (Field et al., 2003). Children with Down syndrome have a comorbidity (50%) of congenital heart disease, which can contribute to poor endurance for feeding, eating, and drinking.

Other disorders associated with feeding and eating problems include Pierre Robin sequence, Williams syndrome, Prader–Willi syndrome, Rett syndrome (Brown et al., 2008), and Noonan syndrome (Fonteles et al., 2013). Challenges may include difficulty chewing and swallowing foods, which may compromise the endurance and participation in the educational setting of these students. Students with esophageal atresia (e.g., the esophagus and stomach are not connected) have persistent swallowing difficulties that compromise weight gain and growth (Menzies et al., 2017). Students with myelomeningocele and an Arnold–Chiari II malformation frequently have eating and feeding dysfunction because the malformation compresses the cranial nerves in the brain stem involved with swallow coordination. Students with these disorders may have persistent difficulties with safely coordinating chewing and swallowing foods and liquids.

Mealtime Environment and Social Interactions

School lunch is often a time of social interaction, yet the school environment may be overwhelming with noise, smell, and movement. Students who are stressed during mealtimes in school may refuse to eat or not eat enough, resulting in inadequate nutrition to fully participate in the educational program (Lefton-Greif & Arvedson, 2008). Students with ASD often have eating and feeding challenges related to difficulties processing sensory information and may benefit from sitting with a few classmates in a quieter area of the cafeteria (Tomchek & Dunn, 2007). Adults who sit near or feed students with significant physical or cognitive limitations should encourage social interactions between the student and peers as much as possible. The use of a communication device during mealtime allows the student to converse with peers.

BEST PRACTICES

School occupational therapy practitioners support students in the educational setting to promote success in achieving educationally related and functional goals. These goals may include functional independence in daily living skills such as the mealtime skills of eating, feeding, and drinking, which are necessary for proper nutrition to perform in school programs.

Partner With Community, Family, and School Team

School and community-based teams must collaborate with the parents to coordinate information and develop a comprehensive mealtime plan for the student (Schultz-Krohn, 2006). The occupational therapist may help the student's individualized education program (IEP) team understand the evaluation results and implement recommendations in the student's school program. Even students who are primarily tube fed have been successfully transitioned to oral feeding in the school setting with collaboration among the family, school, and medical personnel (McKirdy et al., 2008).

Communicating with the student's health care provider for medical guidance for the student's safety (e.g., family requests oral feedings for a student with a feeding tube, student appears to be aspirating foods or liquids, student has severe reflux, student fails to gain weight) is an ethical and professional responsibility. Although occupational therapists can evaluate the physiological factors of feeding, eating, and swallowing as well as the psychosocial, cultural, and environmental factors involved in mealtime, when aspiration is suspected, a referral should be made for evaluation by appropriate medical personnel to identify aspiration using procedures such as VFSS or FEES.

Evaluate Student's Strengths and Needs During Mealtimes

Occupational therapists typically interview the parent and teacher regarding the student's strengths and needs; review educational and health records and reports; observe the student during snack, lunch, or both; and use informal or formal methods of documenting functional eating skills during participation in mealtimes. A more in-depth evaluation may be needed to determine oral–motor skills, oral–sensory skills, behavioral issues related to eating and self-feeding skills, environmental supports, and equipment needs (Aldridge et al., 2010; Ramsay et al., 2011).

This evaluation begins with gathering data for the occupational profile. During this process, the therapist identifies environmental (e.g., physical, social) supports and challenges and any specialized positioning or feeding equipment needed. Evaluation questions include

- What are the concerns or problems, and when do the problems occur?
- What factors support or limit participation in mealtimes and performance of feeding, eating, and swallowing skills in the school setting?

Record review

The occupational therapist should review the student's educational records to determine whether the child is frequently absent (e.g., chronic illness) and assess overall performance in school. The school nurse typically has health information about the student that can be accessed by the occupational therapist. With written consent from the family, best practice is to contact the student's physician, dietitian, or gastroenterologist to gain understanding about the student's ability to safely swallow foods and fluids. Instrumental assessments such as VFSS or FEES can provide discrete information about the mechanics of the student's swallow. When a family declines to authorize this communication, the IEP team (including the school nurse) must identify appropriate steps for the safety of the student's eating, feeding, and swallowing at school. For students who receive nutrition nonorally, teams should not attempt oral feedings without medical authorization.

Interview

Interviewing family and educational staff provides information about the client factors, environment (e.g., cultural, physical, social), and activity (e.g., what materials are used, what is expected). Arvedson (2008, p. 120) designed the following questions to identify eating and feeding problems and prioritize interventions:

- How long does it take for the child to eat a meal or be fed?
- Is the child dependent on others for eating and drinking? If yes, what can the child do independently or with modifications?
- Does the child refuse foods? If yes, are they proteins? Carbohydrates? Fruits? Vegetables?
- Are mealtimes stressful? If yes, what causes the stress?
- Has the child slowed or stopped weight gain during the previous 2–3 months?
- Does the child have respiratory distress?
- Does the child regularly vomit, gag, or cough during or after meals?
- Does the child become irritable or lethargic during mealtimes?

Answers to these questions, combined with a student's history of eating and feeding problems as well as evaluation data, provide a good foundation.

Observation

Observations should occur during a meal and identify the supports and barriers in the context and environment (e.g., routine lunch vs. special luncheon, size of room, seating, noises, smells, lighting, nearness of peers), the activity (e.g., food and liquid being served, utensils used), and the student (e.g., body functions and structure, performance skills, performance habits). Observation of the student's oral structure (e.g., asymmetries of the lips, jaw, tongue, or teeth that could negatively affect the ability to eat), oral–motor control (e.g., lips, tongue, jaw, cheek movements), muscle tone, endurance needed to eat an entire meal, respiration (e.g., monitor breathing while swallowing foods or liquids), and oral–sensory skills (e.g., preferred and nonpreferred textures, acceptance and refusal of temperatures or flavors) should be made to determine what supports or interferes with student participation in mealtimes.

Assessment tools

Several formal assessment tools may be used to systematically evaluate oral–motor and behavioral issues related to eating and feeding. Originally designed for persons with severe or profound intellectual disabilities, the Screening Tool of Feeding Problems (STEP; Matson et al., 2008; Matson & Kuhn, 2001) identifies feeding problems in 5 areas:
1. Risk of aspiration,
2. Food selectivity,
3. Feeding skills,
4. Food refusal, and
5. Nutritional behaviors that affect eating and feeding.

A recent study using the STEP found that 97% of children with severe or profound intellectual disabilities living at home had a much greater chance of aspiration and problems with feeding and eating skills than children with moderate or mild intellectual disabilities (Gal et al., 2011).

A modified version of the STEP that can be used for children ages 2–18 years with a wide range of diagnostic conditions is the Screening Tool of Feeding Problems for Children (STEP–CHILD; Seiverling et al., 2011). This parent report instrument has good reliability and validity, assessing 6 areas related to eating and feeding behaviors:
1. Chewing problems,
2. Rapid eating,
3. Food refusal,
4. Food selectivity,
5. Vomiting, and
6. Stealing food.

Seiverling et al. (2011) posited that children who have problems chewing typical table foods and are not given successive opportunities to chew table foods might have difficulties developing these skills.

The Brief Autism Mealtime Behavior Inventory (BAMBI; Lukens & Linscheid, 2008) was specifically developed to identify mealtime behaviors that compromise feeding skills for children with autism, ages 3–11 years. Parents use this inventory to rate mealtime behaviors on 18 items using a 5-point Likert-type scale. The items are clustered into 3 areas: limited variety, food refusal, and features of ASD. Lukens and Linscheid (2008) demonstrated the validity and reliability of this instrument as a sensitive tool to assess mealtime behaviors in children with ASD.

The Brief Assessment of Mealtime Behavior in Children (BAMBIC) was developed to serve a wider range of children with mealtime issues (Hendy et al., 2013; Seiverling et al., 2016). This instrument includes 3 subscales—Limited Variety, Food Refusal, and Disruptive Behavior—and is a parent questionnaire modified from the BAMBI for wider clinical use.

The Eating Profile (Nadon et al., 2011) is a parent report instrument developed for children with ASD. It consists of 60 items addressing a child's dietary history, health and mealtime behaviors, food preferences, and eating skills, as well as the effect of feeding in daily life. When the Eating Profile was combined with the first edition of the Short Sensory Profile (SSP; Dunn, 1999), the researchers found that 87% of the children had sensory processing problems; 65% of that subgroup had a score in the "definite difference" category and had statistically more eating problems than children with a typical performance on the SSP.

The Picky Eating Behavior Questionnaire is a parental report that provides a systematic approach to collecting data about eating behaviors for children ages 1–5 years (Kwon et al., 2017). The definition of *picky eating* used for this questionnaire is focused on 2 main elements: eating small quantities of food and eating a limited variety of foods. This questionnaire was developed to meet the need to assess the unique characteristics of children who exhibit picky eating through parental report.

Design Student's Mealtime Plan as a Team

After data have been collected from multiple sources, the occupational therapist analyzes them to determine the student's strengths and needs. Recommendations are made to the student's IEP team. Collaboration between the occupational therapy practitioner and other members of the IEP team, including the family, school personnel, and community providers, is key to successfully addressing eating and feeding problems in students with disabilities. The team develops the student's goal and identifies the need for related services.

In addition to services provided to the student, services on behalf of students may be provided by giving input on food texture and temperature, rate of presentation and amount of food, and positioning of a student to ensure the student's safety during a meal or snack (AOTA, 2017). When a student has difficulty swallowing, the practitioner educates and trains the family and school personnel to optimize these factors to facilitate safe swallowing. For some students, a *feeding plan,* which identifies the necessary equipment, positioning, and range of foods, is essential (Frolek Clark, 2003).

Implement Safe and Effective Mealtime Interventions

On the basis of professional development to establish and maintain competence in this area, occupational therapy practitioners use many effective and evidence-based interventions to enhance mealtime skills. Improving mealtime skills may require interventions that address the student (e.g., oral–motor, oral–sensory, behavioral needs), the occupation (modifications to the foods), and the environment (e.g., positioning, noise).

Biomechanical strategies for proper positioning

Many investigations have supported the use of correct sitting alignment as an initial intervention for students who have oral–motor dysfunction that limits eating and feeding skills (Ekberg, 1986; Gisel et al., 2000; West & Redstone, 2004). When a student is sitting in an upright position with the hips and trunk aligned and with the head and neck in slight flexion, the student may have more efficient oral movement and improved oral–motor control (Gisel et al., 2000). Correct alignment reduces the potential for aspiration and improves oral–motor coordination. Evidence has shown that slight neck flexion reduces the risk of aspiration for children with diminished oral–motor control (Ekberg, 1986). Moreover, environmental modifications such as adjusting table and chair height can support a student's ability to eat and self-feed.

Modifications to food

School occupational therapists often work with the family, cafeteria workers, and a student's physician to modify school meals by substituting menu items (e.g., allergy, substituting foods that do not puree well); modifying recipes (e.g., low sugar, high fiber); and changing food texture (e.g., thick liquids, pureed foods, ground foods, chopped foods), temperature, and portion size (Frolek Clark & Jost, 1999). Certification from a physician or other health care provider may be requested for food modifications (USDA, 2017). When a student receives nutrition via tube feedings, the team should determine whether blended foods or formula is necessary.

Adaptive equipment to enhance participation

Occupational therapy practitioners are knowledgeable about the skills of eating, feeding, and swallowing in the school environment and understand how equipment supports or interferes with function; therefore, their input to the educational team is crucial in addressing the needs of students (Lane, 2012). They should determine whether adaptive equipment, such as modified utensils, plates, cups, and straws, is needed to support a student's participation in meals and snacks in the educational setting (AOTA, 2017). In addition, practitioners are responsible for training school personnel in the use of equipment.

Social Stories

Occupational therapy practitioners understand the importance of a student's ability to socialize during lunch. Social Stories are an opportunity for the occupational therapy practitioner and student to write a brief scenario about the lunchroom setting and what to expect (Twachtman-Reilly et al., 2008). The practitioner and student can write a Social Story (Gray, 2000; Gray & Garand, 1993) about the cafeteria, the interaction with friends, and how to respond to the smells by asking to use the bathroom when the sensory experience becomes overwhelming. A series of systematic supports can be used to allow the student to develop the habits and skills needed to eat in the school cafeteria on a consistent basis by using a series of Social Stories to cover a variety of situations during mealtime.

Hands on with student and education of adults

Occupational therapy practitioners use clinical reasoning to apply these strategies and to educate and train others in their use.

Oral–motor strategies. Oral–motor strategies include changing food texture; allowing more time for eating, biting, and chewing opportunities; and strategies for lip, tongue, jaw, and cheek movements. Gisel and Alphonce (1995) found that children with severe oral–motor problems required longer eating times for both solid and pureed foods, children with moderate oral–motor impairments had some difficulties with solids but primarily with pureed foods, and children with mild oral–motor deficits ate soft solids at a slower rate. School occupational therapy practitioners should recommend particular types of food and time needed for eating for students with oral–motor difficulties.

Students with CP, particularly with those with severe motor impairments, benefited from oral–motor intervention to foster improved lip closure and chewing (Baghbadorani et al., 2014; Gisel, 2008). These improvements translated into more efficient intake of food during meals. Specific oral sensorimotor exercises practiced 3 times per week across 24 sessions resulted in improved lip closure on the spoon during eating, control of food during swallowing, and chewing (Baghbadorani et al., 2014). Oral–motor therapy has also been effective in improving strength of lingual musculature, control of the bolus, and improved lip closure during oral transit (Fonteles et al., 2013).

Strategies for food refusal. The interventions described to improve eating and feeding skills specific to food refusal are the results of systematic programs implemented in home or clinical settings. Judicious use of these strategies in the school setting may be beneficial:

- Improve attention and in-seat behavior so student can participate in the meal. May need short break (e.g., get a straw and return); use visual schedule.
- Establish food routines. Toomey (2002) recommended each meal consist of 1 protein, 1 starch, and 1 fruit or vegetable; Janzen (2003, p. 419) recommended eating sequences such as "take a bite, chew, swallow; take a bite."
- Choose small portions; combine new foods with familiar foods; select new foods that are close in flavor, appearance, or texture to preferred foods. Use peer modeling (Ernsperger & Stegen-Hanson, 2004).
- Expand range of acceptable foods through oral exploration (e.g., taste, temperature, texture). Add condiments to increase vegetable consumption (Ahearn, 2003).
- Provide motivators for eating appropriately (e.g., social praise, attention, stickers) and follow eating with preferred activities (Janzen, 2003).
- Provide specific strategies to manage sensory sensitivities (see next section).

Specific sensory sensitivity strategies. Sensory sensitivity strategies can be used when students exaggerate sensory responses related to the environment (e.g., too much sensory stimulation) or to food (e.g., certain smells, visual images, textures, temperatures) that affect their feeding and eating behavior or are barriers to eating (Ernsperger & Stegen-Hanson, 2004). Occupational therapy practitioners can use systematic sensory strategies to expand the student's range of acceptable foods (Schultz-Krohn, 1997), such as placing 2 similar foods, 1 preferred and 1 less preferred, on the same plate. The student selects the preferred food while being exposed to a less preferred food.

This process of approximation has been used successfully to introduce oral feeding to children who have had prolonged tube feedings (Harding et al., 2010). This approach can be effective in reducing the fear and anxiety often seen in students with sensory sensitivities related to foods and eating.

SUMMARY

School occupational therapy practitioners have a critical role in mealtime skills for students with special needs. Occupational therapists evaluate physiological, psychosocial, cultural, and environmental factors that support or limit mealtime performance, specifically feeding, eating, or swallowing. Interventions provide strategies as well as food and equipment modifications, adaptive equipment, environmental adaptations for safe eating and drinking habits, and education or training for families and others (AOTA, 2017). These services focus on improving the student's ability to participate in snacks and meals served in the school and foster independence in self-feeding skills as needed.

REFERENCES

Ahearn, W. A. (2003). Using simultaneous presentation to increase vegetable consumption in a mildly selective child with autism. *Journal of Applied Behavioral Analysis, 36,* 361–365. https://doi.org/10.1901/jaba.2003.36-361

Aldridge, V. K., Dovey, T. M., Martin, C. I., & Meyer, C. (2010). Identifying clinically relevant feeding problems and disorders. *Journal of Child Health Care, 14,* 261–270. https://doi.org/10.1177%2F1367493510370456

American Occupational Therapy Association. (2014). Guidelines for supervision, roles, and responsibilities during the delivery of occupational therapy services. *American Journal of Occupational Therapy, 68*(Suppl. 3), S16–S22. https://doi.org/10.5014/ajot.2014.686S03

American Occupational Therapy Association. (2017). The practice of occupational therapy in feeding, eating, and swallowing. *American Journal of Occupational Therapy, 71*(Suppl. 2), 7112410015. https://doi.org/10.5014/ajot.2017.716S04

Arvedson, J. C. (2008). Assessment of pediatric dysphagia and feeding disorders: Clinical and instrumental approaches. *Developmental Disabilities Research Reviews, 14,* 118–127. https://doi.org/10.1002/ddrr.17

Arvedson, J. C., & Brodsky, L. (2002). *Pediatric swallowing and feeding: Assessment and management* (2nd ed.). New York: Singular.

Arvedson, J. C., & Lefton-Greif, M. A. (2017). Instrumental assessment of pediatric dysphagia. *Seminars in Speech and Language, 38,* 135–146. https://doi.org/10.1055/s-0037-1599111

Baghbadorani, M. K., Soleymani, Z., Dadgar, H., & Salehi, M. (2014). The effect of oral sensorimotor stimulations on feeding performance in children with spastic cerebral palsy. *Acta Medica Iranica, 52,* 899–904.

Bandini, L. G., Anderson, S. E., Curtin, C., Cermak, S., Evans, E. W., Scampini, R., . . . Must, A. (2010). Food selectivity in children with autism spectrum disorders and typically developing children. *Journal of Pediatrics, 157,* 259–264. https://doi.org/10.1016/j.jpeds.2010.02.013

Bandini, L. G., Curtin, C., Phillips, S., Anderson, S. E., Maslin, M., & Must, A. (2017). Changes in food selectivity in children with autism spectrum disorder. *Journal of Autism and Developmental Disorders, 47,* 439–446. https://doi.org/10.1007/s10803-016-2963-6

Brown, L. C., Copeland, S., Dailey, S., Downey, D., Petersen, M. C., Stimson, C., & Van Dyke, D. C. (2008). Feeding and swallowing dysfunction in genetic syndromes. *Developmental Disabilities Research Reviews, 14,* 147–157. https://doi.org/10.1002/ddrr.19

Calis, E. A. C., Veugelers, R., Sheppard, J. J., Tibboel, D., Evenhuis, H. M., & Penning, C. (2008). Dysphagia in children with severe generalized cerebral palsy and intellectual disability. *Developmental Medicine and Child Neurology, 50,* 625–630. https://doi.org/10.1111/j.1469-8749.2008.03047.x

Cano, S. C., Tiemeier, H., van Hoeken, D., Tharner, A., Jaddoe, V. W., Hofman, A., . . . Hoek, H. W. (2015). Trajectories of picky eating during childhood: A general population study. *International Journal of Eating Disorders, 48,* 570–579. https://doi.org/10.1002/eat.22384

Cedar Rapids Community School District v. Garret F., 526 U.S. 66 (1999).

Cermak, S. A., Curtin, C., & Bandini, L. G. (2010). Food selectivity and sensory sensitivity in children with autism spectrum disorders. *Journal of the American Dietetic Association, 110,* 238–246. https://doi.org/10.1016%2Fj.jada.2009.10.032

Chistol, L. T., Bandini, L. G., Must, A., Phillips, S., Cermak, S. A., & Curtin, C. (2018). Sensory sensitivity and food selectivity in children with autism spectrum disorder. *Journal of Developmental Disorders, 48,* 583–591. https://doi.org/10.1007/s10803-017-3340-9

Clancy, K. J., & Hustad, K. C. (2011). Longitudinal changes in feeding among children with cerebral palsy between the ages of 4 and 7 years. *Developmental Neurorehabilitation, 14,* 191–198. https://doi.org/10.3109/17518423.2011.568467

Dahlseng, M. O., Finbraten, A., Juliusson, P. B., Skranes, J., Andersen, G., & Vik, T. (2011). Feeding problems, growth and nutritional status in children with cerebral palsy. *Acta Pediatrica, 101,* 92–98. https://doi.org/10.1111/j.1651-2227.2011.02412.x

Dunn, W. (1999). *The Sensory Profile manual.* San Antonio: Psychological Corporation.

Ekberg, O. (1986). Posture of the head and pharyngeal swallowing. *Acta Radiologica Diagnosis, 27,* 691–696. https://doi.org/10.1177%2F028418518602700612

Emond, A., Emmett, P., Steer, C., & Golding, J. (2010). Feeding symptoms, dietary patterns, and growth in young children with autism spectrum disorders. *Pediatrics, 126,* 337–342. https://doi.org/10.1542/peds.2009-2391

Erkin, G., Cuhla, C., Ozel, S., & Kirbiyik, E. G. (2010). Feeding and gastrointestinal problems in children with cerebral palsy. *International Journal of Rehabilitation Research, 33,* 218–224. https://doi.org/10.1097/MRR.0b013e3283375e10

Ernsperger, L., & Stegen-Hanson, T. (2004). *Just take a bite: Easy, effective answers to food aversions and eating challenges.* Arlington, TX: Future Horizons.

Field, D., Garland, M., & Williams, K. (2003). Correlates of specific childhood feeding problems. *Journal of Paediatric Child Health, 39,* 299–304. https://doi.org/10.1046/j.1440-1754.2003.00151.x

Fiese, B. H., Gundersen, C., Koester, B., & Washington, L. (2011). Household food insecurity: Serious concerns for child development. *Social Policy Report, 25*(3), 1–19.

Fonteles, C. S. R., Mota, A. C. M., Lima, R. A., Borges, P. C., & Silveira, A. (2013). Conservative management of severe open bite and feeding difficulties in patient with Noonan syndrome. *Cleft-Palate-Craniofacial Journal, 50,* 242–248. https://doi.org/10.1597/11-214

Frolek Clark, G. (2003). What's for lunch? *OT Practice, 8*(22), 17–20.

Frolek Clark, G., & Jost, M. (1999). Addressing student's feeding and eating needs. *OT Practice, 4*(6), 33–36.

Gal, E., Hardal-Nasser, R., & Engel-Yeger, B. (2011). The relationship between the severity of eating problems and intellectual developmental deficit level. *Research in Developmental Disabilities, 32,* 1464–1469. https://doi.org/10.1016/j.ridd.2010.12.003

Gisel, E. (2008). Interventions and outcomes for children with dysphagia. *Developmental Disabilities Research Reviews, 14,* 165–173. https://doi.org/10.1002/ddrr.21

Gisel, E. G., & Alphonce, E. (1995). Classification of eating impairments based on eating efficiency in children with cerebral palsy. *Dysphagia, 10,* 268–274. https://doi.org/10.1007/BF00431421

Gisel, E. G., Alphonce, E., & Ramsay, M. (2000). Assessment of ingestive and oral praxis skills: Children with cerebral palsy vs. controls. *Dysphagia, 15,* 236–244. https://doi.org/10.1007/s004550000033

Gorrindo, P., Williams, K. C., Lee, E. B., Walker, L. S., McGrew, S. G., & Levitt, P. (2012). Gastrointestinal dysfunction in autism: A parental report, clinical evaluation and associated factors. *Autism Research, 5,* 101–108. https://doi.org/10.1002/aur.237

Gray, C. (2000). *Writing Social Stories with Carol Gray: Accompanying workbook to video.* Arlington, TX: Future Horizons.

Gray, C. A., & Garand, J. D. (1993). Social Stories: Improving responses of students with autism with accurate social information. *Focus on Autistic Behavior, 8*(1), 1–10. https://doi.org/10.1177%2F108835769300800101

Harding, C., Faiman, A., & Wright, J. (2010). Evaluation of an intensive desensitization, oral tolerance therapy, and hunger provocation program for children who have had prolonged periods of tube feeds. *International Journal of Evidence-Based Healthcare, 8,* 268–276. https://doi.org/10.1111/j.1744-1609.2010.00184.x

Healthy, Hunger-Free Kids Act of 2010, Pub. L. 111–296, 124 Stat. 3183.

Hendy, H. M., Seiverling, L., Lukens, C. T., & Williams, K. E. (2013). Brief Assessment of Mealtime Behavior in Children: Psychometrics and association with child characteristics and parent responses. *Children's Health Care, 42,* 1–14. https://doi.org/10.1080/02739615.2013.753799

Individuals With Disabilities Education Improvement Act of 2004, Pub. L. 108–446, 20 U.S.C. §§ 1400–1482.

Irving Independent School District v. Tatro, 468 U.S. 883 (1984).

Jackson, J. A., Smit, E., Branscum, A., Gunter, K., Harvey, M., Manore, M. M., & John, D. (2017). The family home environment, food insecurity, and body mass index in rural children. *Health Education and Behavior, 44,* 648–657. https://doi.org/10.1177/1090198116684757

Janzen, J. (2003). *Understanding the nature of autism* (2nd ed.). San Antonio: Therapy Skill Builders.

Jyoti, D. F., Frongillo, E. A., & Jones, S. J. (2005). Food insecurity affects school children's academic performance, weight gain, and social skills. *Journal of Nutrition, 135,* 2831–2839. https://doi.org/10.1093/jn/135.12.2831

Kim, J. E., Kim, J., & Mathai, R. A. (2011). Associations of infant feeding practices and picky eating behaviors of pre-school children. *Journal of the American Dietetic Association, 111,* 1363–1368. https://doi.org/10.1016/j.jada.2011.06.410

Kodak, T., & Piazza, C. C. (2008). Assessment and behavioral treatment of feeding and sleeping disorders in children with autism spectrum disorders. *Child and Adolescent Psychiatric Clinics of North America, 17,* 887–905. https://doi.org/10.1016/j.chc.2008.06.005

Kwon, K. M., Shim, J. E., Kang, M., & Paik, H.-Y. (2017). Association between picky eating behaviors and nutritional status in early childhood: Performance of a picky eating behavior questionnaire. *Nutrients, 9,* 463. https://doi.org/10.3390/nu9050463

Lafraire, J., Rioux, C., Giboreau, A., & Picard, D. (2016). Food rejections in children: Cognitive and social/environmental factors involved in food neophobia and picky/fussy eating behavior. *Appetite, 96,* 347–357. https://doi.org/10.1016/j.appet.2015.09.008

Lane, S. J. (2012). Disorders of eating and feeding and disorders following prenatal substance abuse. In S. J. Lane & A. Bundy (Eds.), *Kids can be kids: A childhood occupations approach* (pp. 417–436). Philadelphia: F. A. Davis.

Lefton-Greif, M. A., & Arvedson, J. C. (2008). Schoolchildren with dysphagia associated with medically complex conditions. *Language, Speech, and Hearing Services in Schools, 39,* 237–248. https://doi.org/10.1044/0161-1461(2008/023)

Lefton-Greif, M. A., Carroll, J. L., & Loughlin, G. M. (2006). Long-term follow-up of oropharyngeal dysphagia in children without apparent risk factors. *Pediatric Pulmonology, 41,* 1040–1048. https://doi.org/10.1002/ppul.20488

Lewis, E., & Kritzinger, A. (2004). Parental experiences of feeding problems in their infants with Down syndrome. *Down Syndrome Research and Practice, 9*(2), 45–52. https://doi.org/10.3104/reports.291

Lukens, C. T., & Linscheid, T. R. (2008). Development and validation of an inventory to assess mealtime behavior in children with autism. *Journal of Autism and Developmental Disorders, 38,* 342–352. https://doi.org/10.1007/s10803-007-0401-5

Mari-Bauset, S., Gonzales, A. L., Garcia, I. Z., Mari-Sanchis, A., & Varela, M. M. S. (2015). Nutritional status of children with autism spectrum disorders (ASDs): A case-controlled study. *Journal of Autism and Developmental Disorders, 45,* 203–212. https://doi.org/10.1007/s10803-014-2205-8

Martins, Y., Young, R. L., & Robson, D. C. (2008). Feeding and eating behaviors in children with autism and typically developing children. *Journal of Autism and Developmental Disorders, 38,* 1878–1887. https://doi.org/10.1007/s10803-008-0583-5

Matson, J. L., Fodstad, J. C., & Boisjoli, J. A. (2008). Cutoff scores, norms and patterns of feeding problems for the Screening Tool of Feeding Problems (STEP) for adults with intellectual disabilities. *Research in Developmental Disabilities, 29,* 363–372. https://doi.org/10.1016/j.ridd.2007.06.001

Matson, J. L., & Kuhn, E. D. (2001). Identifying feeding problems in mentally retarded persons: Development and reliability of the Screening Tool of Feeding Problems (STEP). *Research in Developmental Disabilities, 21,* 165–172. https://doi.org/10.1016/S0891-4222(01)00065-8

McKirdy, L. S., Sheppard, J. J., Osbourne, M. L., & Payne, P. (2008). Transition from tube to oral feeding in the school setting. *Language, Speech, and Hearing Services in Schools, 39,* 249–260. https://doi.org/10.1044/0161-1461(2008/024)

Menzies, J., Hughes, J., Leach, S., Belessis, Y., & Krishnan, U. (2017). Prevalence of malnutrition and feeding difficulties in children with esophageal atresia. *Journal of Pediatric Gastroenterology and Nutrition, 64,* e100–e105. https://doi.org/10.1097/MPG.0000000000001436

Nadon, G., Feldman, D. E., Dunn, W., & Gisel, E. (2011). Association of sensory processing and eating problems in children with autism spectrum disorders. *Autism Research and Treatment, 2011,* 541926. https://doi.org/10.1155/2011/541926

Power-deFur, L., & Alley, N. S. N. (2008). Legal and financial issues associated with providing services in schools to children with swallowing and feeding disorders. *Language, Speech, and Hearing Services in Schools, 39,* 160–166. https://doi.org/10.1044/0161-1461(2008/016)

Provost, B., Crowe, T. K., Osbourn, P. L., McClain, C., & Skipper, B. J., (2010). Mealtime behaviors of preschool children: Comparison of children with autism spectrum disorder and children with typical development. *Physical and Occupational Therapy in Pediatrics, 30,* 220–233. https://doi.org/10.3109/01942631003757669

Ramsay, M., Martel, C., Porporino, M., & Zygmuntowicz, C. (2011). The Montreal Children's Hospital Feeding Scale: A brief bilingual screening tool for identifying feeding problems. *Paediatrics and Child Health, 16,* 147–151.

Rehabilitation Act of 1973, Pub. L. 93–112, 29 U.S.C. §§ 701–7961.

Rogers, L. G., Magill-Evans, J., & Rempel, G. R. (2012). Mothers' challenges in feeding their children with autism spectrum disorder—Managing more than just picky eating. *Journal of Developmental and Physical Disabilities, 24,* 19–33. https://doi.org/10.1007/s10882-011-9252-2

Schultz-Krohn, W. (1997). Early intervention: Meeting the unique needs of parent–child interaction. *Infants and Young Children, 10,* 47–60.

Schultz-Krohn, W. (2006). Feeding and eating for infants and toddlers. *OT Practice, 11*(9), 16–20.

Seiverling, L., Hendy, H. M., & Williams, K. (2011). The Screening Tool of Feeding Problems applied to children (STEP–CHILD): Psychometric characteristics and associations with child and parent variables. *Research in Developmental Disabilities, 32,* 1122–1129. https://doi.org/10.1016/j.ridd.2011.01.012

Seiverling, L. J., Williams, K. E., Hendy, H. M., Adams, K., Fernandez, A., . . . Hart, S. (2016). Validation of the Brief Assessment of Mealtime Behavior in Children (BAMBIC) for children in a non-clinical sample. *Children's Health Care, 45,* 165–176. https://doi.org/10.1080/02739615.2014.979925

Tomchek, S. D., & Dunn, W. (2007). Sensory processing in children with and without autism: A comparative study using the Short Sensory Profile. *American Journal of Occupational Therapy, 61,* 190–200. https://doi.org/10.5014/ajot.61.2.190

Toomey, K. A. (2002). *When children won't eat: The SOS approach to eating.* Denver: Author.

Twachtman-Reilly, J., Amaral, S. C., & Zebrowski, P. P. (2008). Addressing feeding disorders in children on the autism spectrum in school-based settings: Physiological and behavioral issues. *Language, Speech, and Hearing Services in Schools, 39,* 261–272. https://doi.org/10.1044/0161-1461(2008/025)

U.S. Department of Agriculture. (2017). *Accommodating children with disabilities in the school meal programs: Guidance for school* *food service professionals.* Washington, DC: Author. Retrieved from https://fns-prod.azureedge.net/sites/default/files/cn/SP40 -2017a1.pdf

West, J. F., & Redstone, F. (2004). Alignment during feeding and swallowing: Does it matter? A review. *Perceptual and Motor Skills, 98,* 349–358. https://doi.org/10.2466/pms.98.1 .349-358

48

Best Practices in IADLs to Enhance Participation

Shannon Corkrean, MOT/L, and Deborah B. Schwind, DHSc, MEd, OTR/L

KEY TERMS AND CONCEPTS

- Community-based instruction
- Community mobility
- Constant time delay
- Functional skills
- Health management and maintenance
- Independent living skills
- Life skills
- Most-to-least prompt schedule
- Self-determination

OVERVIEW

IADLs are "activities to support daily life within the home and community that often require more complex interactions than those used in ADLs" (American Occupational Therapy Association [AOTA], 2014b, p. S19). IADLs include care of others, care of pets, child rearing, use of communication devices, community mobility and navigation, financial management, health management and maintenance, home establishment and management, meal preparation and cleanup, religious observance, safety and emergency maintenance, and shopping (AOTA, 2014b).

In school settings, IADLs are typically referred to as ***independent living skills*** or ***life skills.*** The Individuals With Disabilities Education Improvement Act of 2004 (IDEA; Pub. L. 108–446) uses the term ***functional skills*** to describe "the context of routine activities of everyday living" ("Assistance to States for the Education of Children With Disabilities and Preschool Grants for Children With Disabilities," 2006, p. 46661). Many IADL skills are addressed through the student's transition individualized education program (IEP) under the area of "living" and should be inclusive of home, school, and community participation. Facilitating independence in IADLs is a central tenet of the occupational therapy profession. For occupational therapy practitioners[1] working

in schools, promoting students' autonomy in IADLs is an important area of practice.

ESSENTIAL CONSIDERATIONS

Occupational therapy practitioners use ADLs to help students develop the self-care, home management, work, school, leisure, and social skills necessary to live and work in their community (Brollier et al., 1994). Safety and competence in home and community life skills are critical to the success of independent living.

Promoting Access, Participation, and Independence

When students can manage some or all IADLs, they may have more success in social situations, regard safety as a priority, experience some fiscal independence, and manage home and health situations adequately. The ability to perform certain IADLs can correlate to vocational skills. For example, making sandwiches can correlate to a job in a cafeteria, fixing hot chocolate to a job in a coffee shop, or caring for a pet to a job in a pet store or veterinarian's office.

Wehman (2013) showed that social skills, workplace behaviors, self-determination, inclusive practices in the school community, and parental involvement are associated with better postsecondary outcomes. These skills can be addressed through school IADL interventions. A research study by Dymond et al. (2017) determined that even for students with disabilities who go to college, IADLs (e.g., time management, medication management, study skills, social skills, social interaction, self-advocacy) affect success in college.

Walker et al. (2010) suggested that development of IADL skills should begin as early as elementary school to allow for repetition. The extra time to acquire skills with scaffolding of the tasks and modifications to the environment builds success. Research conducted by Wertalik and Kubina

---

[1]*Occupational therapy practitioner* refers to both the occupational therapist and the occupational therapy assistant. AOTA (2014a, p. S18) states, "The occupational therapist is responsible for all aspects of occupational therapy service delivery and is accountable for the safety and effectiveness of the occupational therapy service delivery process" and "must be directly involved in the delivery of services during the initial evaluation and regularly throughout the course of intervention. . . . The occupational therapy assistant delivers safe and effective occupational therapy services under the supervision of and in partnership with the occupational therapist."

Copyright © 2019 by the American Occupational Therapy Association. All rights reserved. To reuse this content, contact www.copyright.com.
https://doi.org/10.7139/2019.978-1-56900-591-0.048

(2017) indicated that IADLs are critical skills to learn in high school for postschool success. Behaviors such as finishing an IADL task, keeping hands to oneself, and displaying appropriate behaviors while performing an IADL are soft skills that can generalize to a job for postschool success.

Self-determination in students and their families can be addressed at any age. Wehmeyer and Schalock (2001) defined *self-determination* as making choices and decisions free from outside influences and accepting responsibility for the outcome. Introducing characteristics of self-determination into family dynamics early on will help build a culture of independence and can be done by incorporating chores into the home routine. Doing IADLs in the familiar and predictable home environment develops independence with routine tasks and interests in specific activities. Students can advocate to do chores they like as a way to build self-determination and self-advocacy skills.

Functional living skills are among the 8 predictors of postschool success identified by Ohio Employment First (n.d.-b):

1. A collaborative transition team with family participation;
2. An individualized career plan based on interests and strengths;
3. Community experiences;
4. Social skills, including work behaviors;
5. Academic, vocational, and occupational preparation, including functional living skills;
6. Parental involvement with expectations;
7. Self-determination skills, including instruction in independent living skills; and
8. Personal management as well as engagement and participation in inclusive practices and programs.

By addressing IADLs and functional living skills, occupational therapy practitioners can affect students' postschool success and create career interests.

IADLS and Postschool Success

Students with disabilities may need more intense instruction with IADLs, and this specialized instruction should be reflected in their transition IEP under the area of "living." Research conducted by Walker et al. (2010) indicated that functional life skills training may not be emphasized in school because of a focus on the general education curriculum. However, functional living skills lead to success beyond school and should be explicitly and systematically taught in natural environments. A research study by Wertalik and Kubina (2017) found that students with autism spectrum disorder, specifically, have very low rates of independent living and should be taught IADLs in school for postschool success and improved quality of life.

Even students on the autism spectrum who are considered high functioning and go to college have significant deficits with functional living skills (Dymond et al., 2017); higher IQ scores do not protect them from demands placed on them (Kraper et al., 2017). In addition, Kraper et al. (2017) showed that the gaps between IQ and functional living skills can affect mental health, causing anxiety and depression and leading to poor engagement in IADLs.

Occupational therapy practitioners' expertise in modifying materials or providing adaptive equipment for curricular access and participation is vital to independence. Performing task analysis, arranging workspaces, adapting utensils, creating adapted tools, modifying tasks, using technology, and teaching energy conservation and work simplification are ways in which practitioners can promote independence in IADLs.

These life skills should be included in IEPs as early as possible (Bal et al., 2015) because some students need a significant amount of time to develop their skills (Chiang et al., 2017). Evidence-based interventions identified by Ohio Employment First (n.d.-a) include

- Chaining the task,
- Community-based instruction for generalization of knowledge in an authentic environment,
- Use of technology,
- Mnemonics,
- Self-monitoring and self-management of behaviors,
- Video modeling,
- Prompting,
- Self-determination and self-advocacy,
- Use of visual supports, and
- Simulation of tasks.

Occupational therapy practitioners can use these strategies in school practice. Performing a task with repetition prevents stress and anxiety, especially in new environments with new tasks, novel people, and novel demands (Orentlicher & Olson, 2010). Repetition requires less executive functioning (EF) skill and builds automaticity.

School occupational therapy services may be provided on behalf of (e.g., consulting and training others, modifying the environment) or directly with the student. The level of occupational therapy service is based on many factors, such as the student's diagnosis, age, strengths, educational needs, level of discrepancy from age or intellectual expectations, and rate of progress.

Functional Life Skills Curriculum

A functional curriculum is one that will best meet the needs of students striving to increase independence in IADLs. *Functional curriculum* is a relative term, and the implementation of such a model is frequently done sporadically, in moment-to-moment interactions (Bouck, 2008). Many special education programs do not adhere to a functional life skills curriculum per se but instead adopt a curriculum that combines academic and independent living skills in a manner that meets the particular needs of the student. The Functional Curriculum for Teaching Students With Disabilities (Valletutti et al., 2008) can be used to assess and instruct students in a significant number of skills associated with IADL mastery in the school setting.

IEP teams may also capitalize on impromptu teaching opportunities that happen across a variety of settings, such as community outings, work-based learning opportunities, and social interactions with peers and adults. Students should be included in general education classes such as family and consumer science courses that teach IADL skills. Darrah et al. (2010) noted that the current model of social inclusion and a focus on academic testing may not prepare students in special education with the functional skills needed for transition on graduation. Occupational therapy practitioners can provide input to the team to identify functional skills on the basis of student's strengths, interests, and preferences.

Community-Based Instruction

Community-based instruction (CBI) is an evidence-based practice that allows students of all ages to generalize information from the classroom to authentic, real-world applications (Kluth, 2000). The community becomes the classroom for practical IADL instruction in which academics (e.g., literacy, money, time, numeracy skills) can be embedded functionally. Communities can include the school and larger environments in which the student lives. When implementing CBI in the school environment, a collaborative approach that includes all staff in the building (e.g., media specialist, maintenance worker, cafeteria helper, librarian) is best to provide real-life experiences for students. School IADLs may include being a library helper and collecting books for return to the library or assisting with raising and lowering the flag outside the school building each day.

Expectations for Elementary School Students

For elementary-age students, IADLs can be explored through pretend play (e.g., playing house, pretending to be a veterinarian, using play money to buy things) or social play (e.g., being a leader, being a member of a group, negotiating play). Occupational therapy practitioners need to understand and communicate the importance of IADLs for students in the school setting (Chapparo & Hooper, 2005).

Students with disabilities often associate self-care tasks with tedious and laborious work. This is in contrast to persons without disabilities who render these tasks quickly and simply. Gaining information from the student, family, and teacher about barriers to performing occupations can guide intervention planning. Without this information, the student and teacher may overlook skills necessary to complete these tasks, which affect participation and independence. The more complex nature of IADLs necessitates open and frequent communication among home, community supports, and school.

Expectations for Secondary School Students

In the secondary setting, there needs to be an increased expectation for independence, which can best occur when there has been previous exposure. Students in special education require more time to learn these skills and may need more scaffolding of the task or the environment. An IADL curriculum using a CBI approach may allow for perspective taking on career interests. For example, taking a high school student to the grocery store to shop and pay may allow the student to understand that they could work at the grocery store. Social skills, self-determination skills, and work behaviors can be embedded in IADL instruction for purposeful, functional application. Research conducted by Pillay and Brownlow (2017) indicated that performing IADLs independently can predict employment outcomes.

CBI programming can be expanded in high school with greater expectations. Internships or volunteer positions that incorporate IADL skills can occur in the school community and might include working in the school store, being a helper in the library or in the office, volunteering

in the preschool classroom at a local elementary school, or serving food as a school cafeteria helper. These positions provide inclusive opportunities that are meaningful and purposeful for socialization and relationship building, and they can further reinforce social skills, soft skills, and self-determination skills that lead to better outcomes (Wehman, 2013).

In preparation for college, students should learn how to schedule their day, set an alarm clock, have a grooming routine, prepare light meals, learn medication schedules, and self-advocate; these are important nonacademic skills to learn in high school (Dymond et al., 2017).

Networking and Team Collaboration

The school occupational therapy practitioner's partnership with educational team members and school organizations can create IADL opportunities for students. For example, the parent–teacher association may have a request to count money after a dance, a club may need brochures distributed in mailboxes, or items may need to be stocked in the school store. Practicing functional living skills in the community should be the goal for generalization. Community integration that models the real world helps with meaningful inclusion beyond school in the larger community.

More than 68% of individuals ages 18 years or older with a mobility aid (e.g., cane, crutches, walker, wheelchair) have 1 or more IADL limitations, compared with only 5.5% of individuals who do not use a mobility aid (Kaye et al., 2000). Although there are no comparable data for school-age students, occupational therapy practitioners should consider screening IADLs for students with mobility aids. Whether a remediation or an adaptive intervention approach is used, close collaboration with a physical therapist and other team members is essential to facilitate independence in mobility and, consequently, independence in IADLs.

BEST PRACTICES

Occupational therapy practitioners provide a variety of evaluation and intervention services to address the strengths and needs of the student. Occupational therapy practitioners can help students develop self-determination and self-advocacy skills, teach self-management or functional living skills using modifications or technology, and help develop accommodations for community living (Jirikowic et al., 2013). In accordance with best practice, training should occur in natural contexts and community settings to promote generalization of IADL skills (Case-Smith & Weaver, 2015).

Plan and Conduct Student Evaluation

During the evaluation process, the occupational therapist should interview parents, teachers, support staff, the school nurse, and the student when appropriate. Discerning what IADLs are important to the student and team, as well as the student's strengths, needs, and short- and long-term expectations will all be necessary in the decision-making process.

Observing the student when performing IADLs in the natural environment is a key factor to help determine strengths and needs. When possible, observations should be conducted within the normal routine and include familiar settings and materials. For example, observe the student when grocery shopping in a familiar store or accessing online shopping using familiar technology.

Occasions may arise when additional formative assessment data are needed to identify underlying performance skill deficits (e.g., motor and praxis skills, sensory–perceptual skills)—for example, administering a visual–perceptual assessment to confirm or rule out potential deficits that might interfere with the student's ability to move around the community. When necessary and when consent is given, the occupational therapist can use formal assessments to evaluate the student's IADL skills. Examples of assessments that evaluate IADLs include the Adaptive Behavior Assessment System (Harrison & Oakland, 2003), Do–Eat (Goffer et al., 2009), Functional Independence Measure for Children (Hamilton & Granger, 1991), Roll Evaluation of Activities of Life (Roll & Roll, 2013), Scales of Independent Behavior–Revised (Bruininks et al., 1996), School Function Assessment (Coster et al., 1998), and Vineland Adaptive Behavior Scales–II (Sparrow et al., 2005). For additional assessments, see Appendix F, "Selected Assessment Tools for Analysis of Students' Occupational Performance."

Provide Effective Interventions and Strategies for School-Age IADLs

Occupational therapy practitioners in the school setting have an important role to play in the area of IADL instruction as it affects future functioning. Instruction may be provided in a group or individually in the classroom or larger community for practical application using evidence-based strategies such as video modeling, visuals, visual schedules, interactive books or stories, simulation, systematic instruction, grading or scaffolding tasks, and chunking tasks and providing sensory supports or behavioral supports to ensure success with IADLs. The specific IADL areas discussed in this section can be used to help create functional life skills curricular opportunities in the school setting.

Care of others (including selecting and supervising caregivers)

Multiple ways exist to actively assist others in the school. Caring for others could come in a role as student ambassador or manager of a sports team. School administrations typically hire and train paraeducators for students; however, input from an adolescent with a disability regarding desired characteristics in a paraeducator and helping to develop a training module that captures the tasks involved in caring for the student gives an older student a sense of empowerment. Older elementary, middle, or high school students engaging in work-based learning may have a role working in the preschool classroom performing tasks, such as wiping down tables after a snack, helping with a snack by opening containers, helping students unpack backpacks, or helping with dismissal routines.

Care of community

Research by Wehman (2013) indicated that being part of a community should be encouraged. Participation and engagement in the school community can have effects on health and well-being (Erikkson et al., 2007). Being part of a community gives students roles and responsibilities and can promote awareness and acceptance. The community could be the classroom, with jobs such as line leader, table wiper, chair stacker, snack helper, or sweeper. These roles build competence, increase independence, show a student's abilities, and affect self-esteem. Jobs can give a sense of purpose and a feeling of responsibility.

CBI can be slowly expanded to include the school and then the off-campus community. Inclusive community practices promote acceptance of those with all abilities, and these classroom IADLs can generalize to the home and larger community. Having students as young as elementary school age organize the school's Lost and Found would benefit the entire school community, afford an opportunity for students to develop functional living skills, and provide social participation. Learning to hang up clothes can translate into independence at home but can also generalize to employment in a clothing store, in a dry cleaning business, or at venues that have coat checks.

Another opportunity for older students to give back to their community is to get involved in their school's community service or service cord program. Unfortunately, students with disabilities rarely participate in these volunteer programs. There are many benefits to involvement in community volunteer efforts. By extending care and compassion to others in their community, the student experiences empathy for others who may be less fortunate. In addition, the student gains an opportunity to be an agent of change and have a positive effect on their community. Finally, integrated volunteer work with others in the community helps build positive work relationships and work skills. The school occupational therapy practitioner, in collaboration with the student, family, and school staff, can encourage the student to identify, schedule, and complete accessible and manageable community volunteer experiences.

Care of pets or plants

Many elementary classrooms and homes have a pet that allows students the opportunity to understand how to care for animals. Initial exposure to IADLs may occur during feeding, cleaning, and caring for a pet. At the high school level, students interested in animals can volunteer or participate in a work-based learning opportunity where these interests and strengths can be further developed. High school vocational programs may include horticulture programs in which students plant, water, harvest, and sell plants. Programs such as these have also been seen in middle and elementary schools. Students can develop a sense of confidence when they are being relied on to perform a task and know that this is their role. These roles can also help students to develop their identity, develop interests, and create a sense of purpose.

Child rearing

Preparation for adult roles should not ignore the possibility of becoming a parent or caring for a child. Students with disabilities should learn caregiving strategies that align with their strengths and needs. For example, a student with hemiplegia may need assistance to learn how to safely pick up an infant. The occupational therapy practitioner may consider working with parents and school health programs to address sexuality at the appropriate cognitive level of the student with a disability.

Communication management to enhance IADLs

When a student requires an augmentative communication device, the speech–language pathologist (SLP) and occupational therapy practitioner may collaborate to identify the student's motor, sensory, and cognitive abilities to access and use the device. Families and students may choose a communication device for social and emergency needs.

During the teen years, increased autonomy may lead to an increased desire to connect with friends and, perhaps more important, a means of communicating during an emergency. Augmentative communication systems, apps, and low-tech visual schedules or interactive books can be used to help teach IADLs. Communication about the steps of the tasks and specific vocabulary programmed for socialization can be incorporated with the SLP. It is important for students to use communication to perform an IADL, but it is equally as important to use the communication system to express likes, the need for help, frustration when they cannot perform an IADL, and their personal goals and desires.

Community mobility, navigation, and personal safety

The relatively new "gig economy" has had a profound effect on transportation for persons with disabilities. Location-based ride-sharing apps have leveled the playing field for people with disabilities and offer cost-effective ways to access community mobility. Some of the ride-sharing apps feature vehicles with wheelchair lifts and ramps for transport of a person in a wheelchair. The most natural way to embed *community mobility* (e.g., using public transportation, calling a taxi) into the school setting is during planned field trips, scheduled community outings to teach community mobility (e.g., restaurant, grocery stores), or travel to community work settings. Students should be exposed to various places in the community, such as the neighborhood library, gym, or grocery store, to build familiarity. Safety would include following street signs and road signs and navigating sidewalks as well as obstacles.

Community mobility includes transportation, and high school students can begin to set that up. Students can be responsible for locating the phone number to the school bus garage, calling the bus garage, and communicating the date and time the ride is needed. Students can gather this information and rehearse the conversation before the call is made. Phone numbers can be preprogrammed into cell phones, and students can be taught how to access information. Internet safety in the virtual community should also be taught. Smart wheelchairs equipped with GPS may contribute to independence with community mobility.

In the community setting, the occupational therapy practitioner may identify areas of support and barriers to participation and collaboratively consult with the teacher (or team) about strategies to enhance participation. For example,

students with physical disabilities may go to a grocery store to purchase food for a classroom meal. The practitioner may be asked to accompany the class on this trip and solve ways to navigate through the store, obtain necessary items, put them in a basket, and pay for them.

Community mobility should include the school building. Orientation to the school and classroom should be provided, especially at the beginning of the school year and when there is a transition to a new building. Inclusive opportunities in the school for those with powered mobility or assisted mobility such as walkers can be created to build socialization skills with typical peers. A student in a power wheelchair can pull a wagon full of recess supplies to the playground or take books to the library. Some schools provide food for the weekend in backpacks or bags, and students can deliver these items to specific classrooms. These meaningful contributions would showcase students' abilities and create opportunities for awareness, acceptance, compassion, empathy, and understanding that all people have abilities.

Financial management

Many life skills programs embed money manipulation and money cards into the curriculum. Physically handling an automated lunch card or student identification card can be comparable to handling a debit or credit card. The occupational therapy practitioner can modify this task on the basis of the student's needs. For example, if the lunch card is attached to a retractable lanyard that tucks away, the student can manage independently, without fear of dropping it.

A functional living skill for primary grades may be counting money in the school store and assuming the role of banker. This graded task can be expanded on in secondary grades to money or ticket exchange at school events such as sports or musical productions. The secondary school goal could also be independently buying items at a store or restaurant or collecting and depositing a paycheck.

Health management and maintenance

As a member of the student's team, the occupational therapy practitioner facilitates independence with *health management and maintenance* (e.g., scheduling doctor's appointments, taking medication, eating a balanced diet). During medication disbursement, the student should be taught what medication is being taken, its purpose, possible side effects, and what to do if a dose is skipped. Time in the nurse's office may be used to care for teeth, cleaning eyeglasses, and skin care. Students should be expected to perform these tasks as independently as possible. Occupational therapy practitioners are often asked to assist with problem solving for students with physical, intellectual, or behavioral disabilities who may need equipment or alternative methods because of poor motor control or judgment.

Using a body chart may help students indicate where they hurt. Exploring the nurse's medical tools may eliminate the fear they have in an unfamiliar doctor's office. Students can visit the doctor's office when they are not sick to build familiarity and comfort in that environment. Sensory supports can be discussed with the doctor's office, such as having beanbags in the exam room and soft lights or dimmable lights. Stories or videos about the doctor's office using pictures from the office can be created so students understand what will happen and be familiar with what it will look like. Medication management can be taught through apps, through the use of medicine containers that have auditory feedback, or through low-tech visuals.

Home establishment and management

Classrooms with a functional living curriculum may have appliances (e.g., washer, dryer, dishwasher, microwave, oven). Students may learn how to use these appliances or learn how to self-advocate when they are not accessible. Generalizing these skills into the student's home is necessary for success in natural environments. Talking with families about chores that the student can do at home is important and should begin in elementary school with classroom jobs or simple home chores as a way to scaffold the tasks and responsibilities. These skills are important to learn for independent living.

Similar to other IADLs, chores can begin early with simple tasks and can increase in complexity with systematic instruction and modifications or accommodations to ensure success. Occupational therapy practitioners can guide the student and family as to which chores are appropriate. Students with special needs often take longer to accomplish tasks, so embedding some chores on the weekends or during school breaks when more time is available may be the most reasonable way to initiate and successfully learn those tasks.

Chores not only build routines and responsibilities but also allow participation in the family community, and they can be done from an early age. Families can be provided with a list of chores that can be done as part of a regular routine over the summer. Chores can be simple, such as

- Getting the mail,
- Sorting silverware,
- Carrying bags in from the grocery store,
- Putting away canned items in the pantry,
- Washing fruit,
- Watering plants, or
- Feeding the family pet.

More complex chores would involve more steps, such as making a sandwich, washing a car, vacuuming, washing dishes, and folding clothes.

Meal preparation and cleanup

Meal preparation and cleanup encompasses a wide variety of skill levels. The occupational therapy practitioner can assist the special education teacher and paraeducator in grading the steps for meal preparation. A student with physical or intellectual disabilities who is preparing a fruit salad may start with cutting soft fruit before moving on to tougher fruits. Adapting and modifying utensils to ensure increased independence is another way in which occupational therapy practitioners can use their expertise.

Many schools have implemented a school café or school coffee shop managed and operated by students. Not only does this serve to address many IADLs, it has an important vocational component to it as well. These environments provide opportunities for social integration, meaningful inclusion, work experience, and generalization of classroom IADL skills to the community.

When teaching students with intellectual disabilities a simple cooking task (e.g., heating premade soup from a can), research has shown that using a ***constant time delay*** (amount of time between general task direction and needed follow-up prompts) and a ***most-to-least prompt schedule*** (phasing out prompts on the basis of success in previous tasks) are equally effective in teaching and retaining daily living skills (Aykut, 2012). In addition, the time delay procedure is an evidence-based, response-prompting procedure that is effective in teaching chained tasks and discrete skills across settings (Collins, 2007; Schuster et al., 1998; Wolery et al., 1992).

Religious observance

Occupational therapy practitioners can help build students' skills for participation in religious rituals and routines that are part of the family routine or part of the parochial school. Finding meaningful roles and responsibilities for students during a religious service is important. For example, if a student with hemiplegia is a greeter and needs to be able to distribute bulletins to worshippers as they enter the place of worship, the occupational therapy practitioner can provide strategies so the student is as self-sufficient as possible.

Safety and emergency maintenance

Perhaps the biggest source of worry for school staff and families is that a student could experience a situation that is life threatening. Taking a proactive approach to safety is critical. Teach students at an early age to understand when they should not talk to strangers, how to safely cross the street with the help of the school crossing guard, and what to share when they are lost (e.g., name, address, emergency card).

Technology can serve as a resource in safety situations. When used appropriately, cell phones, texting, phone calls, and video conferencing can be links between the student and responsible adults when home alone or in the community. Parents should ensure that emergency contacts are programmed into their children's phones. Also, most phones have a medical identification app that can be accessed on a locked phone. In the event of an emergency, a first responder can access the owner's name, medical condition, emergency contacts, and organ donor status through the medical identification screen. Occupational therapy practitioners, in conjunction with the student and family, can help facilitate programming of this information onto the phone and instruct them in how to access and edit the information as needed.

GPS can be another technology resource for students with the propensity to elope. Activating the GPS on a student's smartphone will allow caregivers and family members to locate them in the event they elope or wander away.

Even with the medical identification app on most phones, having a medical alert bracelet is a sound idea. As older students transition out of the school setting and into the community, fewer people will be aware of their medical conditions. For students who experience seizures or diabetes, for example, having a bracelet that alerts a first responder to the condition and a caregiver's contact information is prudent. The occupational therapy practitioner, in conjunction with the student and family, can be a resource in initiating this type of medical alert.

Shopping

Online grocery shopping and delivery is a relatively new service that has had a positive impact for people of all abilities but especially for people with disabilities. Having the opportunity to order groceries, toiletries, and over-the-counter medication online and have them delivered to one's home has made this IADL much more accessible. For persons with EF difficulties, ordering necessary items online from the comfort of their own home helps to alleviate distractions, stay focused, and possibly avoid impulse buys. Not only can online shoppers stay on budget, they can be less likely to forget an item.

A school occupational therapist can work with the special education teacher and older student to introduce the concept of online grocery shopping, help set up an account, and navigate the website. Proactively introducing this service to older students will help create an increased sense of self-reliance.

During traditional grocery shopping outings, occupational therapy practitioners who accompany a student on a shopping trip will likely witness several IADLs concurrently. Planning a shopping trip also requires skills that can be addressed by the occupational therapy practitioner, including problem solving what students need and generating a list (e.g., written, electronic, pictorial). They may look up prices before they go to ensure they have the correct amount of money or find sales on the items they are looking for.

The actual shopping experience may require the student to navigate the community, apply financial management, observe safety awareness, complete the shopping task, and engage in social interactions. Assistive technology or augmentative and alternative communication devices may also be used. Shopping at various community sites (e.g., grocery store, bakery, post office, department store) provides different experiences and should be considered. Sensory supports or behavior charts may also need to be considered in the larger community setting when appropriate.

SUMMARY

School occupational therapy practitioners have a vital role in supporting students and the IEP team so that the student can be as independent as possible with IADLs. Students should develop functional living skills and possibly vocational interests for positive employment outcomes and greater independence as an adult.

REFERENCES

American Occupational Therapy Association. (2014a). Guidelines for supervision, roles, and responsibilities during the delivery of occupational therapy services. *American Journal of Occupational Therapy, 68*(Suppl. 3), S16–S22. https://doi.org/10.5014/ajot.2014.686S03

American Occupational Therapy Association. (2014b). Occupational therapy practice framework: Domain and process (3rd ed.). *American Journal of Occupational Therapy, 68*(Suppl. 1), S1–S48. https://doi.org/10.5014/ajot.2014.682006

Assistance to States for the Education of Children With Disabilities and Preschool Grants for Children With Disabilities, 71 Fed. Reg. 46539 (August 14, 2006) (to be codified at 34 C.F.R. 300, 301).

Aykut, Ç. (2012). Effectiveness and efficiency of constant-time delay and most-to-least prompt procedures in teaching daily living skills with intellectual disabilities. *Educational Sciences: Theory and Practice, 12,* 366–373.

Bal, V. H., Kim, S.-H., Cheong, D., & Lord, C. (2015). Daily living skills in individuals with autism spectrum disorder from 2 to 21 years of age. *Autism, 19,* 774–784. https://doi.org/10.1177/1362361315575840

Bouck, E. C. (2008). Exploring the enactment of functional curriculum in self-contained cross-categorical programs: A case study. *Qualitative Report, 133,* 495–530.

Brollier, C., Shepherd, J., & Flick Markley, K. (1994). Transition from school to community living. *American Journal of Occupational Therapy, 48,* 346–353. https://doi.org/10.5014/ajot.48.4.346

Bruininks, R. H., Woodcock, R. W., Weatherman, R. F., & Hill, B. K. (1996). *Scales of Independent Behavior–Revised.* Itasca, IL: Riverside.

Case-Smith, J., & Weaver, L. (2015). *Critically appraised topic: Evidence-based interventions targeting ADL, IADL and sleep for persons with autism spectrum disorder.* Bethesda, MD: American Occupational Therapy Association. Retrieved from https://www.aota.org/Practice/Children-Youth/Evidence-based/CAT-IADL-ADL-sleep-ASD.aspx

Chapparo, C., & Hooper, E. (2005). Self-care at school: Perceptions of 6-year-old children. *American Journal of Occupational Therapy, 59,* 67–77. https://doi.org/10.5014/ajot.59.1.67

Chiang, H.-M., Ni, X., & Lee, Y.-S. (2017). Life skills training for middle school and high school students with autism. *Journal of Autism and Developmental Disorders, 47,* 1113–1121. https://doi.org/10.1007/s10803-017-3028-1

Collins, B. C. (2007). *Moderate to severe disabilities: A foundational approach.* Upper Saddle River, NJ: Merrill/Prentice Hall.

Coster, W., Deeney, T. A., Haltiwanger, J. T., & Haley, S. M. (1998). *School Function Assessment user's manual.* San Antonio: Therapy Skill Builders.

Darrah, J., Magill-Evans, J., & Galambos, N. L. (2010). Community services for young adults with motor disabilities: A paradox. *Disability and Rehabilitation, 32,* 223–229. https://doi.org/10.3109/09638280903071834

Dymond, S. L., Meadan, H., & Pickens, J. L. (2017). Postsecondary education and students with autism spectrum disorders: Experiences of parents and university personnel. *Journal of Developmental and Physical Disabilities, 29,* 809–825. https://doi.org/10.1007/s10882-017-9558-9

Erikkson, L., Welander, J., & Granlund, M. (2007). Participation in everyday school activities for children with and without disabilities. *Journal of Developmental and Physical Disabilities, 19,* 485–502. https://doi.org/1007/s10882-007-9065-5

Goffer, A., Josman, N., & Rosenblum, S. (2009). *Do–Eat: Performance-based assessment tool for children.* Haifa, Israel: University of Haifa.

Hamilton, B. B., & Granger, C. U. (1991). *Functional Independence Measure for Children (WeeFIM).* Buffalo: Research Foundation of the State University of New York.

Harrison, P., & Oakland, T. (2003). *Adaptive Behavior Assessment System–School: Manual* (2nd ed.). San Antonio: Psychological Corporation.

Individuals With Disabilities Education Improvement Act of 2004, Pub. L. 108–446, 20 U.S.C. §§ 1400–1482.

Jirikowic, T., Campbell, J., DiAmico, M., Frauwith, S., & Mahoney, W. (2013). *Students with disabilities in postsecondary education settings: How occupational therapy can help.* Retrieved from https://www.aota.org/About-Occupational-Therapy/Professionals/CY/Postsecondary-Education.aspx

Kaye, H. S., Kang, T., & LaPlante, M. P. (2000). *Mobility device use in the United States* (Disability Statistics Report No. 14). Washington, DC: U.S. Department of Education, National Institute on Disability and Rehabilitation Research.

Kluth, P. (2000). Community-referenced learning and the inclusive classroom. *Remedial and Special Education, 21,* 19–26. https://doi.org/10.1177%2F074193250002100103

Kraper, C. K., Kenworthy, L., Popal, H., Martin, A., & Wallace, G. L. (2017). The gap between adaptive behavior and intelligence in autism persists into young adulthood and is linked to psychiatric co-morbidities. *Journal of Autism and Developmental Disorders, 47,* 3007–3017. https://doi.org/10.1007/s10803-017-3213-2

Ohio Employment First. (n.d.-a). *Evidence based practices for transition youth.* Retrieved from http://www.ohioemploymentfirst.org/up_doc/Evidence_Based_Practices_for_Transition_youth_2017-09-07.pdf

Ohio Employment First. (n.d.-b). *Evidence based predictors for post-school success.* Retrieved from http://www.ohioemploymentfirst.org/up_doc/Evidence_Based_Predictors_for_Post_school_Success3_25_15.pdf

Orentlicher, M. L., & Olson, L. J. (2010). Transition from school to adult life for students with an autism spectrum disorder. In H. M. Kuhaneck & R. Watling (Eds.), *Autism: A comprehensive occupational therapy approach* (pp. 665–700). Bethesda, MD: AOTA Press.

Pillay, Y., & Brownlow, C. (2017). Predictors for successful employment outcomes for adolescents with autism spectrum disorders: A systematic literature review. *Review Journal of Autism and Developmental Disorders, 4*(1), 1–11. https://doi.org/10.1007/s40489-016-0092-y

Roll, K., & Roll, W. (2013). *The REAL: The Roll Evaluation of Activities of Life.* New York: Pearson.

Schuster, J. W., Morse, T. E., Ault, M. J., Doyle, P. M., Crawford, M. R., & Wolery, M. (1998). Constant time delay and chained tasks: A review of literature. *Education and Treatment of Children, 21,* 74–106.

Sparrow, S., Balla, D., & Cicchetti, D. (2005*). Vineland Adaptive Behavior Scales–II* (2nd ed.). Circle Pines, MN: American Guidance Service.

Valletutti, P. J., Bender, M., Hoffnung, A. S., & Baglin, C. A. (2008). *Functional curriculum for teaching students with disabilities* (4th ed.). Austin, TX: Pro-Ed.

Walker, A. R., Richter, S., Uphold, N. M., & Test, D. W. (2010). Review of the literature on community-based instruction across grade levels. *Education and Training in Autism and Developmental Disabilities, 45,* 242–267.

Wehman, P. (2013). Transition from school to work: Where are we and where do we need to go? *Career Development and Transition for Exceptional Individuals, 36,* 58–66. https://doi.org/10.1177/2165143413482137

Wehmeyer, M., & Schalock, R. (2001). Self-determination and quality of life: Implications for special education services and supports. *Focus on Exceptional Children, 33*(8), 1–16. https://doi.org/10.17161/foec.v33i8.6782

Wertalik, J. L., & Kubina, R. M., Jr. (2017). Interventions to improve personal care skills for individuals with autism: A review of literature. *Review Journal of Autism and Developmental Disorders 4,* 50–60. https://doi.org/10.1007/s40489-016-0097-6

Wolery, M., Ault, M. J., & Doyle, P. M. (1992). *Teaching students with moderate to severe disabilities.* New York: Longman.

Best Practices in Literacy: Handwriting and Written Expression to Enhance Participation

49

Naomi Weintraub, PhD, OTR

KEY TERMS AND CONCEPTS

- Dysgraphia
- Keyboarding
- Language by ear
- Language by eye
- Language by hand
- Language by mouth
- Legibility
- Simple view of writing

OVERVIEW

Writing enables people to communicate and express their knowledge, thoughts, feelings, and experiences. It is used for various purposes such as corresponding, engaging in social media, and writing lists or reports. In academic settings, students perform different writing activities, including taking notes and writing essays, stories, or tests, that enable them to develop and express their ideas and knowledge (Graham et al., 2016). The different tasks are facilitated through the use of handwriting and keyboarding.

Writing is considered 1 of 4 language systems (Berninger, 2000). First, children develop an aural language for processing the language they hear (*language by ear*). Next, they develop an oral language for producing the language they speak (*language by mouth*). Then they learn to read (*language by eye*). Finally, children learn to handwrite (*language by hand*). The 4 languages develop in parallel, but they also overlap, and thus they are interrelated.

Therefore, handwriting is a linguistic and cognitive or metacognitive activity (Graham et al., 2016) as well as a perceptual–motor activity. It requires the mastery of basic lower level skills, including spelling, handwriting or keyboarding (i.e., transcription), and the conventions of writing, along with the knowledge of grammar and sentence construction, that form the foundations for expressing oneself in writing (Graham & Harris, 2013).

Handwriting is acquired in the early years of school through direct instruction and many hours of practice (Santangelo & Graham, 2016) and is used throughout the school years. As the use of digital media increases, *keyboarding* is gradually becoming an important medium for writing (e.g., on tablets or word processors). Similar to handwriting, efficient keyboarding requires systematic instruction (e.g., touch-typing) and practice. Otherwise, students' keyboarding may be slower and less accurate than that of those who learned to touch-type (Logan et al., 2016).

Difficulties in handwriting and written expression may have negative ramifications on students' participation in different life situations. In addition, the presentation of written text, including spelling errors, poor legibility, and disorganization, may influence teachers' or other readers' judgments of the quality of the written text (Greifeneder et al., 2011), thus affecting the students' academic achievement and consequently their self-esteem and motivation (Engel-Yeger et al., 2009; Graham & Harris, 2013). Handwriting difficulties are one of the most common reasons for referrals to occupational therapy practitioners[1] working in schools.

ESSENTIAL CONSIDERATIONS

The role of occupational therapy practitioners working in the school system is to enhance students' participation in school activities. Writing is an essential activity that enables students to engage in different academic activities. Therefore, it is important that occupational therapy practitioners understand writing and handwriting processes.

Process of Written Expression

The first and most influential model explaining the writing process was described by Hayes and Flowers (1980). Berninger and colleagues (Berninger, 2000; Berninger et al., 1995) expanded this model, known as the *simple view of writing.* According to this model, the writing process

---

[1] *Occupational therapy practitioner* refers to both the occupational therapist and the occupational therapy assistant. The American Occupational Therapy Association (AOTA; 2014a, p. S18) states, "The occupational therapist is responsible for all aspects of occupational therapy service delivery and is accountable for the safety and effectiveness of the occupational therapy service delivery process" and "must be directly involved in the delivery of services during the initial evaluation and regularly throughout the course of intervention. . . . The occupational therapy assistant delivers safe and effective occupational therapy services under the supervision of and in partnership with the occupational therapist."

Copyright © 2019 by the American Occupational Therapy Association. All rights reserved. To reuse this content, contact www.copyright.com.
https://doi.org/10.7139/2019.978-1-56900-591-0.049

consists of 3 components that need to be carefully orchestrated. The first is *transcription* (e.g., spelling, handwriting, keyboarding), in which internal language representations are transformed into visible, external language (e.g., words, phrases, sentences). The second is *text generation* or *composing,* in which ideas are transformed (translated) into language and maintained in working memory. The third component requires higher level cognitive skills (executive functions [EF]), including planning (setting writing goals and generating and organizing ideas), monitoring, and reviewing or revising.

The acquisition of the writing process requires direct strategy instruction relating to each stage of the writing process (Graham & Harris, 2013). The complexity of the writing process may explain why students may experience writing as difficult and frustrating. This frustration, in turn, may affect their motivation and self-efficacy (Graham & Harris, 2009). In addition, the writing model demonstrates the reciprocal relationship between written expression and transcription, including spelling and handwriting.

Process of Handwriting

Handwriting is not a simple activity to acquire and perform. Van Galen (1991) developed one of the first models describing the handwriting process of adults, which was later revised by Graham et al. (2006). In this model, handwriting is described as a hierarchical process that includes several stages that occur both sequentially and in parallel. The first 3 stages are psycholinguistic processes (generating ideas, translating them into words, and constructing sentences). Next, phoneme-to-grapheme translation (spelling) occurs. The graphemes are then translated into allographs (i.e., the specific forms of letters: upper- or lowercase, manuscript or cursive), and the motor programs corresponding to each allograph are activated. Next, the writer decides where to position the letters on the line in relation to other letters (spacing). The writer then sets the parameters for executing the motor programs (letter size) and carries out the program.

Measuring Handwriting Performance

When evaluating handwriting performance, occupational therapists need to consider both the process and the written product.

Process (speed, fluency, and automaticity)

The main measures of the handwriting process are speed and automaticity. Speed is commonly measured as the number of letters or words written per minute (Rosenblum et al., 2003). Handwriting is considered automatic when it is produced with minimal conscious attention and effort, which is usually achieved by 3rd–5th grade. It reflects students' ability to activate the correct sensory–motor maps of each letter efficiently while relying on sensory rather than on visual feedback (Kandel & Perret, 2015). Handwriting automaticity (often measured as the speed of writing the alphabet letters from memory) is one of the best predictors of handwriting speed as well as of the quality and quantity of written compositions (Feng et al., 2017).

Handwritten product (legibility)

The main focus of the handwritten product is **legibility.** Legible handwriting enables students to communicate their knowledge and thoughts. Illegible handwritten outputs are prone to *legibility bias*, in which students' grades may be negatively affected by their poor legibility, even when the content of the text is of high quality (Greifeneder et al., 2011).

One method for rating overall legibility is based on the evaluator's perception. However, this method may be biased against boys (Greifeneder et al., 2011). The second method is a functional approach, often operationalized as the percentage of readable words in a text (Brossard-Racine et al., 2012). This approach is more ecologically valid (D'Amato et al., 2005) because it taps the purpose of legible handwriting. Yet neither method provides information about the reason why handwriting is less legible (i.e., the intactness of its components).

The readability of handwriting is influenced by various factors, including letter formation (i.e., whether the letter is identifiable and written in the correct direction and allograph), spatial organization (e.g., letter size, spaces, slant), neatness, erasures, and spelling errors (Graham et al., 2006). Each component is usually judged separately using predetermined criteria (Amundson, 1995; Rosenblum et al., 2003). Analysis provides important information about students' strengths and weaknesses in each of these elements and often serves as the basis for developing intervention goals.

Handwriting Tasks

Students engage in a variety of activities that require different functions (Rosenblum et al., 2003). Copying (both near- and far-point) entails visual attention and tracking as well as orthographic (visual) encoding of the text and translating it to a written output (Feng et al., 2017). Writing to dictation requires auditory attention, phonological encoding, phonemes-to-grapheme conversion, and orthographic–motor integration (DeCoste, 2014). Composition has elements similar to dictation but involves higher order cognitive functions and may reflect students' handwriting performance in a more demanding writing context.

Performing these tasks requires the acquisition of prewriting skills, including knowledge of the alphabet (both upper- and lowercase), the ability to write one's name, and the ability to copy letters and write them from memory (Frolek Clark, 2016). Therefore, it is important to determine that students have acquired these basic skills. Moreover, measuring handwriting performance should include the different writing tasks described here to increase the ecological validity of the measurement.

Body Functions Related to Handwriting Performance

The biopsychosocial model delineated in the *International Classification of Functioning, Disability and Health* (World Health Organization [WHO], 2001) asserted that handwriting performance may be affected by students' body structure and functions. Therefore, occupational therapy practitioners should be aware of these factors and their possible effect on students' handwriting performance.

Cognitive and psychosocial functions

Initially, students need to acquire basic literacy skills (Frolek Clark, 2016), such as the rules of written languages, alphabet knowledge, and phonological awareness (see Chapter 17, "Best Practices in Literacy and STEM Skills to Enhance Participation at the District and Building Levels"). The handwriting process also requires various cognitive skills, including attention and EF such as planning, organizing, and working memory (Feng et al., 2017; Peverly et al., 2013). Psychosocial functions such as emotional disposition while writing, self-efficacy, and motivation (Engel-Yeger et al., 2009; Lahav et al., 2014) are additional important aspects that may affect students' attitudes toward handwriting and the effort they exert while writing. These aspects may affect their performance and participation in classroom activities that involve handwriting.

Sensory–perceptual functions

Sensory perception guides people's movement and motor execution. It plays an important role in learning to write and in providing feedback to proficient handwriters (Yu et al., 2012). Although most studies have not found a significant relationship between visual perception (of forms) and handwriting performance (Prunty et al., 2016), a medium correlation between visual–motor integration and handwriting legibility has been noted among students in their earlier stages of handwriting acquisition (Brown & Link, 2016; Prunty et al., 2016). With practice, handwriting becomes automatic, and writers rely primarily on kinesthetic, tactile, and haptic perception for feedback. These sensory functions were found to be predictors of handwriting speed and legibility for 1st- and 2nd-grade students (Yu et al., 2012).

Motor functions and pencil grip

Handwriting execution occurs through the motor system, including gross and fine motor functions. Postural control is important for stabilizing the body while enabling controlled and precise movement of the hand, and it has been shown to differentiate between students with poor and good handwriting (Parush et al., 1998). Moreover, fine motor skills, including in-hand manipulation and motor control, were found to be related to handwriting speed and legibility (Brown & Link, 2016). Occupational therapy practitioners assist in developing these skills, which are important in many daily activities, specifically while gripping and manipulating the pencil or pen while writing.

Most studies reported that pencil grip pattern does not affect students' legibility or speed (Rosenblum et al., 2006; Schwellnus et al., 2012). However, pencil grip may affect the amount of pressure students exert while writing, causing fatigue and pain (Baur et al., 2009). Therefore, even though at the early stages of handwriting students' performance may not be affected by pencil grip, in later years, as writing demands increase, their grip may affect their writing durability.

Contextual Factors Related to Handwriting

Students' writing occurs in various personal (e.g., age, gender) and environmental contexts (WHO, 2001), which may serve as barriers to or facilitators of students' handwriting performance. Therefore, it is important that occupational therapy practitioners be aware of them and their effect on students' handwriting.

Personal factors

Age and gender may affect students' handwriting performance. Handwriting improves with age, but the course of development is not linear. It appears that the greatest improvement occurs during elementary school, followed by a gradual but slower improvement during middle school (Graham et al., 1998). In addition, most studies have reported gender differences in handwriting performance; girls have usually been found to write more legibly and fluently (Greifeneder et al., 2011; Weintraub & Graham, 2000).

In contrast, the evidence of the effect of hand preference is equivocal, and most studies have not found differences between right- and left-handed students in handwriting performance (Graham & Weintraub, 1996). Nevertheless, Hawkyard et al. (2014) investigated the handwriting experience of left-handed elementary school students, who raised the need for specialized equipment (e.g., pencils, pencil grips). Awareness of the specific needs of left-handed students may enhance their participation in classroom activities.

Environmental factors

The physical and sociocultural (linguistic) environments may also affect students' performance and participation in handwriting activities. The physical environment related to writing (ergonomic factors) may include the writing tools, surfaces, and furniture (desk and chair height or proportion) as well as the students' sitting placement (e.g., distance to the blackboard; Feder & Majnemer, 2007). To support students' postural control, students should have proper seating that enables them to sit with feet flat on the floor, hips and low back supported against the chair back, knees flexed to approximately 90°, and elbows slightly flexed with forearms resting comfortably on the desk surface.

The evidence of the effect of writing tools is limited. On the basis of a literature review, Graham and Weintraub (1996) concluded that the different writing utensils (e.g., primary pencils, regular pencil with and without triangular grip) had their advantages and disadvantages and did not affect handwriting performance. Therefore, students should be allowed to use a variety of instruments when learning to write and select the one that is most comfortable for them. Similarly, students should experience various types of paper (e.g., with and without lines, different widths of lines).

The linguistic context is also important while writing. Worldwide, there are students who are bilingual (either through the home or through the educational setting). Studies have shown that bilingualism is often beneficial for students and may enhance their linguistic and cognitive skills

(Genesee, 2015). Yet learning a second language, and specifically handwriting in itself, may place additional demands on students because they need to learn a new set of phoneme-grapheme correspondence. Moreover, if the second language is not based on the same written language forms (e.g., Latin based), then students need to acquire a new (additional) set of letterforms and corresponding motor programs. Therefore, it is essential that occupational therapy practitioners be aware of students' linguistic background and proficiency in other languages.

Handwriting Difficulties

Studies have reported that 5%–44% of students may encounter handwriting difficulties (Feng et al., 2017), often referred to as *dysgraphia* (Berninger et al., 2017). The manifestations of handwriting difficulties vary and may include slow writing, poor legibility, pain, and fatigue (Graham et al., 2016). Writing and handwriting difficulties are often experienced by students with different neurodevelopmental disabilities, including dyslexia (Berninger et al., 2015), attention deficit hyperactivity disorder (Berninger et al., 2017; Graham et al., 2016), developmental coordination disorder (Prunty et al., 2016), and autism spectrum disorder (Dirlikov et al., 2017). They may be the result of deficits in linguistic, cognitive, perceptual, sensory, and motor functions (Donica et al., 2013) as well as contextual constraints. All of these factors need to be considered when treating students with writing and handwriting problems.

BEST PRACTICES

Occupational therapy practitioners provide services with students who are referred because of possible writing difficulties. This process is best applied when practitioners follow a client-centered approach and collaborate with students, parents, and teachers with the purpose of enhancing students' performance and participation in school activities (AOTA, 2014b).

Evaluate Writing

Congruent with the biopsychosocial model (WHO, 2001), best practice in occupational therapy suggests using an occupation-based assessment approach to evaluate students' performance and participation in a relevant context (van Hartingsveldt et al., 2011). Therefore, it is first important to establish whether students have writing difficulties and, if so, how they affect their performance and participation in classroom activities. Second, occupational therapists need to understand the nature of the impairments in body structure and function that may be contributing to the limitation in students' performance and participation. Finally, it is necessary to examine the possible effects of the contextual factors (supports and barriers; AOTA, 2014b).

Informal data collection

Initially, it is important to gather information on the student's occupational profile from the perspectives of the student, parents, teachers, and significant others. This information gathering may be achieved through interviews and informal questionnaires relating to the student's occupational history and experiences in general and specifically relating to writing; their use of handwriting in educational and daily activities; and their attitude toward writing, as well as their reasons for seeking services (AOTA, 2014b). It is also important to establish the student's perception and awareness of their handwriting performance. A useful tool for this purpose may be Here's How I Write, a pictorial self-report suitable for 2nd- to 5th-grade students. It is also helpful in jointly developing intervention goals (Cermak & Bissell, 2014; Goldstand et al., 2013).

In addition, occupational therapy practitioners are encouraged to observe students in their classroom during instruction and writing activities. Observation should include their ability to engage in and perform the activities independently (e.g., initiate, complete), such as copying from the blackboard or writing a story. It is also important to note the students' sitting position while writing, their use of the nondominant hand to stabilize the page, and the instruction strategies presented.

Furthermore, occupational therapists should note the contextual factors and their contribution in enabling or limiting the student's writing performance, including ergonomic factors such as their sitting placement in the classroom, desk and chair height, writing tools, level of light, and classroom curriculum and activities (Rosenblum et al., 2006; van Hartingsveldt et al., 2011). Informal data collection should also include reviewing the students' records, such as their folders, writing samples, and individualized education program, so as to understand their academic and psychosocial performance over the years (Frolek Clark & Giroux, 2013).

Formal assessments

Standardized assessments enable the occupational therapist to systematically identify students' handwriting difficulties in a reliable and valid manner and to compare their performance across tasks and writing modes and with that of their peers. They may also serve as intervention outcome measures and are the basis for establishing eligibility for services or accommodations required (DeCoste, 2014).

Van Hartingsveldt et al. (2011) described 12 standardized handwriting readiness tools. All but 1, the Writing Essential Skill Screener–Preschool version (WESS–P; Erford, 1997), focused on body functions related to handwriting. The WESS–P consists of 4 activities: (1) copying simple geometric shapes, (2) copying letters, (3) copying numbers, and (4) name writing. For older students, occupational therapists may use screening tools as part of the evaluation, such as the Handwriting Without Tears Screener of Handwriting Proficiency (Olsen & Knapton, 2008) or the Handwriting Proficiency Screening Questionnaire (Rosenblum, 2008).

Several formal handwriting assessments have also been found to have sound psychometric properties. For the earlier levels (Grades 1–3), commonly used measures include the Children's Handwriting Scale (Phelps et al., 1985), Minnesota Handwriting Test (Reisman, 1993), and the Evaluation Tool of Children's Handwriting–Manuscript (Amundson, 1995). For older students, the Evaluation Tool of Children's Handwriting–Cursive (Amundson, 1995; Duff & Goyen, 2010) may be used.

An additional valuable tool that may assist occupational therapists in their decision-making process is the DeCoste

Writing Protocol (DeCoste, 2014). This is a comprehensive assessment that is meant to identify factors that affect students' ability to produce writing. It enables a comparison of the student's performance across handwriting and keyboarding tasks and examines spelling performance and writing skills. On the basis of this information, occupational therapists can make informed decisions about instructional strategies and the appropriate accommodations required.

When selecting a handwriting assessment, several factors should be considered, including the assessment's psychometric properties (validity and reliability), its sensitivity to developmental changes in the main handwriting measures (speed and legibility), and the appropriateness of the texts and tasks (e.g., alphabet writing, numeral writing, near- and far-point copying, dictation, and free writing [composition]; Salameh-Matar et al., 2016).

Computerized handwriting assessments

The use of (digitizer-based) computers for assessing handwriting performance is steadily increasing. Until recently, such methods were limited both because of the equipment and software they required and because of their limited psychometric properties and ecological validity. However, in a recent study, Dirlikov et al. (2017) compared the use of the Minnesota Handwriting Test (Reisman, 1993) in a computerized versus a conventional form in discriminating between students with and without dysgraphia. Their results indicated that both assessment forms differentiated between the 2 groups of students and provided an understanding of their handwriting difficulties. However, the computerized evaluation provided more precise and additional data relating to pen pressure and letter form (size, fluidity, and angles). Therefore, computerized handwriting may assist occupational therapy practitioners in better understanding students' handwriting process.

Assessing body functions related to handwriting

If the information gathered so far indicates that the student is encountering handwriting difficulties, congruent with the biopsychosocial model (WHO, 2001) and using a clinical reasoning process, occupational therapists can postulate the underlying causes of these difficulties, including deficits in specific body functions (e.g., linguistic, cognitive, sensory–motor) and contextual barriers. These hypotheses should then be verified through additional formal assessments of body functions.

Various tools measure body functions that have been found to be related to handwriting performance. For linguistic functions, the Alphabet Writing Test measures handwriting automaticity and orthographic–motor integration (Berninger et al., 1992; Christensen, 2004). Visual–motor integration may be measured using the Developmental Test of Visual–Motor Integration (Beery & Beery, 2010) and the Developmental Test of Visual Perception (3rd ed.; the Copying subscale; Hammill et al., 2014). Fine motor skills may be measured using the Test of In-Hand Manipulation–Revised (Pont et al., 2008) and the Motor

Coordination subtest of the Developmental Test of Visual–Motor Integration.

After integrating the information gathered through the different measures, the occupational therapist can draw conclusions as to the profile of the student's handwriting performance as well as the factors supporting and limiting their participation in classroom activities. This information may assist in developing intervention goals and a plan.

Provide Effective Writing Intervention

The purpose of occupational therapy intervention is to enhance students' performance and participation in school activities. With the move toward the Common Core Standards Initiative and multi-tiered systems of support, there is a greater awareness of the need for individualized and evidence-based instruction and intervention, in general, and specifically relating to handwriting (Asher & Estes, 2016; Graham & Harris, 2013). Intervention programs may be delivered through different approaches, such as creation, prevention, restoration, or modification (AOTA, 2014b). Occupational therapy practitioners should select the intervention approach on the basis of the students' needs and the context within which the program is implemented.

Creation and prevention

In the school system, the purposes of the creation and prevention approaches are to enhance all students' handwriting acquisition and performance as well as to prevent or diminish handwriting difficulties. Occupational therapy practitioners may be an important resource for implementing such programs by providing workshops, consulting team members, and co-teaching or collaborating with general or special education staff. In each intervention model, occupational therapists should apply effective, evidence-based handwriting readiness programs (e.g., phonological awareness, fine motor development, proper body structure, letter and number recognition; Donica et al., 2013) and handwriting programs (Asher & Estes, 2016).

On the basis of a recent meta-analysis of 25 studies related to handwriting instruction, Santangelo and Graham (2016) concluded that providing instruction (regardless of the specific program) versus not providing instruction resulted in enhanced handwriting performance. Moreover, handwriting instruction was found to have positive effects on composition length and quality. However, there was no sufficient evidence supporting a specific program over another (e.g., D'Nealian Handwriting Program, Handwriting Without Tears, Loops and Other Groups, Zaner–Bloser Handwriting Program) in developing handwriting skills (Asher & Estes, 2016; Santangelo & Graham, 2016).

Nevertheless, a few general methods were found to be effective, including direct, systematic, and individualized handwriting instruction; having students self-evaluate their handwriting performance; and use of technology such as digitized tablets (Santangelo & Graham, 2016). In addition, writing letters from memory and the use of haptic and visual perception were also found to enhance students' learning of letter forms (Bara & Gentaz, 2011; Berninger et al., 1997).

Providing direct intervention (restoration)

In cases in which students experience handwriting difficulties despite receiving evidence-based instructional programs, restoration or modification intervention methods may be helpful. On the basis of a systematic review of handwriting intervention programs, Hoy et al. (2011) concluded that handwriting intervention programs that did not include handwriting practice were ineffective. Moreover, effective programs required practice at least twice a week for a total of at least 20 sessions.

Most effective handwriting intervention programs either were based on cognitive approaches or implemented cognitive strategies combined with a task-oriented approach in which students practiced writing letters and texts in ecologically valid activities (e.g., journals, birthday invitations).

Thornton et al. (2016), for example, found that a 10-week intervention program based on the Cognitive Orientation to daily Occupational Performance Approach™ improved handwriting performance of elementary school students with developmental coordination disorder. Other studies found that using visual cues (e.g., arrows) with or without the support of mnemonics was effective in students' acquisition of letter formation and handwriting automaticity (Berninger et al., 1997; Weintraub et al., 2009). A few intervention programs used self-evaluation strategies (e.g., students monitored their work or selected their best-performed work) to increase their awareness of their writing performance (Denton et al., 2006; Weintraub et al., 2009).

Modifications and accommodations

Whereas many students with handwriting difficulties may benefit from direct intervention programs, some students will also require modifications or accommodations to fully participate in school activities. Modifications may include writing fewer or shorter answers. Accommodations, such as extended time or dictating their responses while taking tests, have also been found to assist students in expressing their knowledge. In addition, students may also benefit from the use of assistive technology (DeCoste, 2014).

The use of technology to enhance students' school participation is described in Chapter 21, "Best Practices in the Use of Assistive Technology to Enhance Participation." Occupational therapy practitioners should be aware of the advantages of word processing for writing. For example, Christensen (2004) noted that after keyboarding instruction, the quantity and quality of students' written output were enhanced when compared with writing using paper and pencil. However, effective use of word processors requires automatic keyboarding and proficiency in word processing. It is essential that students systematically learn touch-typing; just providing them with a computer is not enough.

Occupational therapists should be aware of different touch-typing instructional programs, such as the comprehensive program Keyboarding Without Tears®, designed for kindergarten to 5th-grade students (Learning Without Tears, 2017). When necessary, they should incorporate such programs in their intervention plans. They should also take into account that keyboarding may not be beneficial for all students. Therefore, occupational therapy practitioners

should know about different modifications and accommodations, the methods for establishing what technology or other accommodations may assist the students, and how they may benefit from them (DeCoste, 2014).

SUMMARY

Writing is an essential school activity that students use throughout their academic years. As with any learned motor activity, acquisition of handwriting requires educators to provide systematic instruction and practice. When problems arise in writing, a request for an occupational therapy evaluation is made to gather information using formal and informal methods with respect to the student's performance and contextual supports and barriers.

Using a professional reasoning process, the occupational therapist develops an intervention program. This program needs to be client centered and match the student's abilities and needs and the family's preferences. In addition, consideration needs to be given to the school's curriculum, instructional methods, and environment. Evidence indicates that occupation-based intervention that includes handwriting practice is most effective. Finally, collaborating with school staff is important for long-term effective outcomes.

REFERENCES

American Occupational Therapy Association. (2014a). Guidelines for supervision, roles, and responsibilities during the delivery of occupational therapy services. *American Journal of Occupational Therapy, 68*(Suppl. 3), S16–S22. https://doi.org/10.5014/ajot.2014.686S03

American Occupational Therapy Association. (2014b). Occupational therapy practice framework: Domain and process (3rd ed.). *American Journal of Occupational Therapy, 68*(Suppl. 1), S1–S48. https://doi.org/10.5014/ajot.2014.682006

Amundson, S. J. (1995). *Evaluation Tool of Children's Handwriting: ETCH examiner's manual.* Homer, AK: O.T. Kids.

Asher, A., & Estes, J. (2016). Handwriting instruction in elementary schools: Revisited! *Journal of Occupational Therapy, Schools, and Early Intervention, 9,* 353–365. https://doi.org/10.1080/19411243.2016.1239560

Bara, F., & Gentaz, E. (2011). Haptics in teaching handwriting: The role of perceptual and visuo-motor skills. *Human Movement Science, 30,* 745–759. https://doi.org/10.1016/j.humov.2010.05.015

Baur, B., Fürholzer, W., Jasper, I., Marquardt, C., & Hermsdörfer, J. (2009). Effects of modified pen grip and handwriting training on writer's cramp. *Archives of Physical Medicine and Rehabilitation, 90,* 867–875. https://doi.org/10.1016/j.ampr.2008.10.015

Beery, K. E., & Beery, N. A. (2010). *The Beery–Buktenica Developmental Test of Visual–Motor Integration* (6th ed.). Parsippany, NJ: Modern Curriculum Press.

Berninger, V. W. (2000). Development of language by hand and its connections with language by ear, mouth and eye. *Topics in Language Disorders, 20,* 65–84.

Berninger, V., Abbott, R., Cook, C. R., & Nagy, W. (2017). Relationships of attention and executive functions to oral language, reading, and writing skills and systems in middle childhood and early adolescence. *Journal of Learning Disabilities, 50,* 434–449. https://doi.org/10.1177/0022219415617176

Berninger, V. W., Abbott, R. D., Whitaker, D., Sylvester, L., & Nolen, S. B. (1995). Integrating low- and high-level skills in instructional protocols for writing disabilities. *Learning Disabilities Quarterly, 18,* 293–309. https://doi.org/10.2307%2F1511235

Berninger, V. W., Richards, T. L., & Abbott, R. D. (2015). Differential diagnosis of dysgraphia, dyslexia, and OWL LD: Behavioral and neuroimaging evidence. *Reading and Writing, 28,* 1119–1153. https://doi.org/10.1007/s11145-015-9565-0

Berninger, V. W., Vaughan, K. B., Abbott, R. D., Abbott, S. P., Rogan, L. W., Brooks, A., . . . Graham, S. (1997). Treatment of handwriting problems in beginning writers: Transfer from handwriting to composition. *Journal of Educational Psychology, 89,* 652–666. https://doi.org/10.1037/0022-0663.89.4.652

Berninger, V., Yates, C., Cartwright, A., Rutberg, J., Remy, E., & Abbott, R. (1992). Lower-level developmental skills in beginning writing. *Reading and Writing, 4,* 257–280. https://doi.org/10.1007/BF01027151

Brossard-Racine, M., Mazer, B., Julien, M., & Majnemer, A. (2012). Validating the use of the Evaluation Tool of Children's Handwriting–Manuscript to identify handwriting difficulties and detect change in school-age children. *American Journal of Occupational Therapy, 66,* 414–421. https://doi.org/10.5014/ajot.2012.003558

Brown, T., & Link, J. (2016). The association between measures of visual perception, visual–motor integration, and in-hand manipulation skills of school–age children and their manuscript handwriting speed. *British Journal of Occupational Therapy, 79,* 163–171. https://doi.org/10.1177/0308022615600179

Cermak, S. A., & Bissell, J. (2014). Content and construct validity of Here's How I Write (HHIW): A child's self-assessment and goal setting tool. *American Journal of Occupational Therapy, 68,* 296–306. https://doi.org/10.5014/ajot.2014.010637

Christensen, C. A. (2004). Relationship between orthographic–motor integration and computer use for the production of creative and well-instructured written text. *British Journal of Educational Psychology, 74,* 551–564. https://doi.org/10.1348/0007099042376373

D'Amato, R. C., Crepeau-Hobson, F., Huang, L. V., & Geil, M. (2005). Ecological neuropsychology: An alternative to the deficit model for conceptualizing and serving students with learning disabilities. *Neuropsychology Review, 15,* 97–103. https://doi.org/10.1007/s11065-005-7092-5

DeCoste, D. C. (2014). *DeCoste Writing Protocol.* Volo, IL: Don Johnston.

Denton, P. L., Cope, S., & Moser, C. (2006). The effects of sensorimotor-based intervention versus therapeutic practice on improving handwriting performance in 6- to 11-year-old children. *American Journal of Occupational Therapy, 60,* 16–27. https://doi.org/10.5014/ajot.60.1.16

Dirlikov, B., Younes, L., Nebel, M. B., Martinelli, M. K., Tiedemann, A. N., Koch, C. A., . . . Mostofsky, S. H. (2017). Novel automated morphometric and kinematic handwriting assessment: A validity study in children with ASD and ADHD. *Journal of Occupational Therapy, Schools, and Early Intervention, 10,* 185–201. https://doi.org/10.1080/19411243.2017.1304841

Donica, D. K., Goins, A., & Wagner, L. (2013). Effectiveness of handwriting readiness programs on postural control, hand control, and letter and number formation in Head Start classrooms. *Journal of Occupational Therapy, Schools, and Early Intervention, 6,* 81–93. https://doi.org/10.1080/19411243.2013.810938

Duff, S., & Goyen, T. (2010). Reliability and validity of the Evaluation Tool of Children's Handwriting–Cursive (ETCH) using general scoring criteria. *American Journal of Occupational Therapy, 64,* 37–46. https://doi.org/10.5014/ajot.64.1.376

Engel-Yeger, B., Nagauker-Yanuv, L., & Rosenblum, S. (2009). Handwriting performance, self-reports, and perceived self-efficacy among children with dysgraphia. *American Journal of Occupational Therapy, 63,* 182–192. https://doi.org/10.5014/ajot.63.2.182

Erford, B. T. (1997). Reliability and validity of the Writing Essential Skill Screener–Preschool version (WESS–P). *Assessment for Effective Intervention, 23,* 213–223. https://doi.org/10.1177%2F153450849702300104

Feder, K. P., & Majnemer, A. (2007). Handwriting development, competency, and intervention. *Developmental Medicine and Child Neurology, 49,* 312–317. https://doi.org/10.1111/j.1469-8749.2007.00312.x

Feng, L., Lindner, A., Ji, X. R., & Joshi, R. M. (2017). The roles of handwriting and keyboarding in writing: A meta-analytic review. *Reading and Writing,* 1–31. https://doi.org/10.1007/s11145-017-9749-x

Frolek Clark, G. (2016). The occupations of literacy: Occupational therapy's role. *Journal of Occupational Therapy, Schools, and Early Intervention, 9,* 27–37. https://doi.org/10.1080/19411243.2016.1152835

Frolek Clark, G., & Giroux, P. (2013). Best practices in handwriting and writing skills to enhance participation. In G. Frolek Clark & B. Chandler (Eds.), *Best practices for occupational therapy in schools* (pp. 483–497). Bethesda, MD: AOTA Press.

Genesee, F. (2015). Myths about early childhood bilingualism. *Canadian Psychology, 56,* 6–15. https://doi.org/10.1037/a0038599

Goldstand, S., Gevir, D., Cermak, S., & Bissell, J. (2013). *Here's How I Write: A child's self-assessment of handwriting and goal setting tool.* Framingham, MA: Therapro.

Graham, S., Berninger, V., Weintraub, N., & Schafer, W. (1998). Development of handwriting speed and legibility in Grades 1–9. *Journal of Educational Research, 92,* 42–52. https://doi.org/10.1080/00220679809597574

Graham, S., Fishman, E. J., Reid, R., & Hebert, M. (2016). Writing characteristics of students with attention deficit hyperactive disorder: A meta-analysis. *Learning Disabilities Research and Practice, 31,* 75–89. https://doi.org/10.1111/ldrp.12099

Graham, S., & Harris, K. R. (2009). Almost 30 years of writing research: Making sense of it all with *The Wrath of Khan. Learning Disabilities Research and Practice, 24,* 58–68. https://doi.org/10.1111/j.1540-5826.2009.01277.x

Graham, S., & Harris, K. R. (2013). Common core state standards, writing, and students with LD: Recommendations. *Learning Disabilities Research and Practice, 28,* 28–37. https://doi.org/10.1111/ldrp.12004

Graham, S., Struck, M., Santoro, J., & Berninger, V. W. (2006). Dimensions of good and poor handwriting legibility in first and second graders: Motor programs, visual–spatial arrangement, and letter formation parameter setting. *Developmental Neuropsychology, 29,* 43–60. https://doi.org/10.1207/s15326942dn2901_4

Graham, S., & Weintraub, N. (1996). A review of handwriting research: Progress and prospects from 1980 to 1994. *Educational Psychology Review, 8,* 7–87. https://doi.org/10.1007/BF01761831

Greifeneder, R., Zelt, S., Seele, T., Bottenberg, K., & Alt, A. (2011). Towards a better understanding of the legibility bias in performance assessments: The case of gender-based inferences. *British Journal of Educational Psychology, 82,* 361–374. https://doi.org/10.1111/j.2044-8279.2011.02029.x

Hammill, D. D., Pearson, N. A., & Voress, J. K. (2014). *Developmental Test of Visual Perception* (3rd ed.). Austin, TX: Pro-Ed.

Hawkyard, R., Dempsey, I., & Arthur-Kelly, M. (2014). The handwriting experiences of left-handed primary school students in a digital age: Australian data and critique. *Australian Journal of Education, 58,* 123–138. https://doi.org/10.1177/0004944114530062

Hayes, J., & Flowers, L. (1980). Identifying the organization of writing. In L. W. Gregg & E. R. Steinberg (Eds.), *Cognitive processes in writing* (pp. 3–30). Hillsdale, NJ: Erlbaum.

Hoy, M. M. P., Egan, M. Y., & Feder, K. P. (2011). A systematic review of interventions to improve handwriting. *Canadian Journal of Occupational Therapy, 78,* 13–25. https://doi.org/10.2182/cjot.2011.78.1.3

Kandel, S., & Perret, C. (2015). How do movements to produce letters become automatic during writing acquisition? Investigating the development of motor anticipation. *International Journal of Behavioral Development, 39,* 113–120. https://doi.org/10.1177/0165025414557532

Lahav, O., Maeir, A., & Weintraub, N. (2014). Gender differences in students' self-awareness of their handwriting performance. *British Journal of Occupational Therapy, 77,* 614–618. https://doi.org/10.4276/030802214X14176260335309

Learning Without Tears. (2017). *Keyboarding Without Tears.* Retrieved from http://www.lwtears.com/kwt

Logan, G. D., Ulrich, J. E., & Lindsey, D. R. (2016). Different (key) strokes for different folks: How standard and nonstandard typists balance Fitts' law and Hick's law. *Journal of Experimental Psychology: Human Perception and Performance, 42,* 2084–2102. https://doi.org/10.1037/xhp0000272

Olsen, J. Z., & Knapton, E. F. (2008). *Handwriting Without Tears pre-K teachers guide.* Cabin John, MD: Handwriting Without Tears.

Parush, S., Levanon-Erez, N., & Weintraub, N. (1998). Ergonomic factors influencing handwriting performance. *Work, 11,* 295–305. https://doi.org/10.3233/WOR-1998-11306

Peverly, S. T., Vekaria, P. C., Reddington, L. A., Sumowski, J. F., Johnson, K. R., & Ramsay, C. M. (2013). The relationship of handwriting speed, working memory, language comprehension and outlines to lecture note-taking and test-taking among college students. *Applied Cognitive Psychology, 27,* 115–126. https://doi.org/10.1002/acp.2881

Phelps, J., Stempel, L., & Speck, G. (1985). The Children's Handwriting Scale: A new diagnostic tool. *Journal of Educational Research, 79,* 46–50. https://doi.org/10.1080/00220671.1985.10885646

Pont, K., Wallen, M., Bundy, A., & Case-Smith, J. (2008). Reliability and validity of the Test of In-Hand Manipulation in children ages 5 to 6 years. *American Journal of Occupational Therapy, 62,* 384–392. https://doi.org/10.5014/ajot.62.4.384

Prunty, M., Barnett, A. L., Wilmut, K., & Plumb, M. (2016). Visual perceptual and handwriting skills in children with developmental coordination disorder. *Human Movement Science, 49,* 54–65. https://doi.org/10.1016/j.humov.2016.06.003

Reisman, J. E. (1993). Development and reliability of the research version of the Minnesota Handwriting Test. *Physical and Occupational Therapy in Pediatrics, 13,* 41–55. https://doi.org/10.1080/J006v13n02_03

Rosenblum, S. (2008). Development, reliability, and validity of the Handwriting Proficiency Screening Questionnaire (HPSQ). *American Journal of Occupational Therapy, 62,* 298–307. https://doi.org/10.5014/ajot.62.3.298

Rosenblum, S., Goldstand, S., & Parush, S. (2006). Relationships among biomechanical ergonomic factors, handwriting product quality, handwriting efficiency, and computerized handwriting process measures in children with and without handwriting difficulties. *American Journal of Occupational Therapy, 60,* 28–39. https://doi.org/10.5014/ajot.60.1.28

Rosenblum, S., Weiss, L., & Parush, P. (2003). Product and process evaluation of handwriting difficulties. *Educational Psychology Review, 15,* 41–81. https://doi.org/10.1023/A:1021371425220

Salameh-Matar, A., Basal, N., Nashef-Tali, B., & Weintraub, N. (2016). Development and validity of the Arabic Handwriting Assessment for elementary school students. *British Journal of Occupational Therapy, 79,* 212–219. https://doi.org/10.1177/0308022615616819

Santangelo, T., & Graham, S. (2016). A comprehensive meta-analysis of handwriting instruction. *Educational Psychology Review, 28,* 225–265. https://doi.org/10.1007/s10648-015-9335-1

Schwellnus, H., Carnahan, H., Kushki, A., Polatajko, H., Missiuna, C., & Chau, T. (2012). Effect of pencil grasp on the speed and legibility of handwriting in children. *American Journal of Occupational Therapy, 66,* 718–726. https://doi.org/10.5014/ajot.2012.004515

Thornton, A., Licari, M., Reid, S., Armstrong, J., Fallows, R., & Elliott, C. (2016). Cognitive Orientation to (daily) Occupational Performance intervention leads to improvements in impairments, activity and participation in children with developmental coordination disorder. *Disability and Rehabilitation, 38,* 979–986. https://doi.org/10.3109/09638288.2015.1070298

van Galen, G. P. (1991). Handwriting: Issues for a psychomotor theory. *Human Movement Science, 10,* 165–191. https://doi.org/10.1016/0167-9457(91)90003-G

van Hartingsveldt, M. J., De Groot, I. J., Aarts, P., & Nijhuis-van Der Sanden, M. W. (2011). Standardized tests of handwriting readiness: A systematic review of the literature. *Developmental Medicine and Child Neurology, 53,* 506–515. https://doi.org/10.1111/j.1469-8749.2010.03895.x

Weintraub, N., & Graham, S. (2000). The contribution of gender, orthographic, finger function, and visual–motor processes to the prediction of handwriting status. *OTJR: Occupation, Participation and Health, 20,* 121–140. https://doi.org/10.1177%2F153944920002000203

Weintraub, N., Yinon, M., Hirsch, I. B. E., & Parush, S. (2009). Effectiveness of sensorimotor and task-oriented handwriting intervention in elementary school-aged students with handwriting difficulties. *OTJR: Occupation, Participation and Health, 29,* 125–134. https://doi.org/10.3928/15394492-200909611-05

World Health Organization. (2001). *International classification of functioning, disability and health.* Geneva: Author.

Yu, T. Y., Hinojosa, J., Howe, T. H., & Voelbel, G. T. (2012). Contribution of tactile and kinesthetic perceptions to handwriting in Taiwanese children in first and second grade. *OTJR: Occupation, Participation and Health, 32,* 87–94. https://doi.org/10.3928/15394492-20111209-02

Best Practices in Literacy: Reading to Enhance Participation

50

Lenin C. Grajo, PhD, EdM, OTR/L

KEY TERMS AND CONCEPTS

- Cognitive Orientation to daily Occupational Performance
- Cooperative Learning Strategy
- Double-deficit hypothesis of dyslexia
- Dyslexia
- Functional cognition
- Functional literacy
- Functional reading
- Inhibition
- Learning Together Approach
- Magnocellular theory of dyslexia
- Occupation and Participation Approach to Reading Intervention
- Peer-Assisted Learning Strategies
- Phonological processing deficit of dyslexia
- Rapid automatic switching
- Set shifting

OVERVIEW

The latest statistics from the National Center for Learning Disabilities (Horowitz et al., 2017) on 4th-grade students report that 27% of students without disabilities, 69% of students with disabilities, and 85% of students with specific learning disabilities fall below basic levels of literacy. Literacy problems, particularly reading disorders (including *dyslexia*), are defined and understood from a variety of theoretical and neuroscientific perspectives. The most widely recognized theory is the *phonological processing deficit of dyslexia,* which is the core of reading failure (Snowling, 2005). This deficit makes it difficult for children to form and dissect letter blends to pronounce words.

Significant neuroscientific research has been conducted on intervention programs in reading, with phonology-based skills remediation as its primary emphasis (e.g., Krafnick et al., 2011; Odegard et al., 2008). These reading programs are delivered primarily by traditional classroom and special education teachers, reading specialists, and speech–language pathologists (SLPs).

An emergence of neuroscientific dyslexia studies happened in the late 1990s. These studies suggested that phonology deficits alone do not explain the plethora of other problems children with specific reading difficulties experience (Stein & Walsh, 1997). These studies support existing educational and behavioral psychology theories and hypotheses that might explain causes of reading challenges beyond phonological processing.

The *double-deficit hypothesis of dyslexia* states that children may experience markedly slower rates of naming a sequence of serially presented visual stimuli, such as letters, numbers, and objects (O'Brien et al., 2012). The double-deficit hypothesis focuses on explaining why children who have difficulties in reading show labored, slow, and dysfluent performance in various reading tasks.

Another theory is the *magnocellular theory of dyslexia,* which hypothesizes that auditory, visual, and motor deficits compound existing phonological deficits that cause reading problems (Stein, 2001). Aberrant magnocellular systems in the brain lead to slower visual discrimination and letter and letter–pattern discrimination, which affect automatic decoding of words.

Newer neuroscience studies are also emerging that propose the critical role of visual–perceptual skills in reading abilities. Other studies have also explored the relationship language and literacy development have with the socioemotional and intentionality centers of the brain. Hruby et al. (2011) explained the presence of cortical connections in brain areas for affect regulation and socioemotional response that develop early in childhood. Binney et al. (2010) also found connections in the brain areas that regulate emotional control and semantic memory and the reading and language centers.

The newly emerging hypotheses about the complexity of reading disorders support findings that for 30% of children with dyslexia and as many as 50% of children with disabilities, phonological deficits are not the sole cause of reading challenges. Moreover, these children may not respond to phonology-based remediation alone (Laycock & Crewther, 2008). Landmark studies, such as the meta-analysis conducted by the National Reading Panel (2000), have comprehensively examined more than 100,000 publications on reading and reading intervention. The meta-analysis recommended a more holistic approach to reading intervention beyond language processing. Occupational therapy

Copyright © 2019 by the American Occupational Therapy Association. All rights reserved. To reuse this content, contact www.copyright.com.
https://doi.org/10.7139/2019.978-1-56900-591-0.050

practitioners[1] can provide this multidimensional perspective in reading intervention from the viewpoint of occupational participation.

ESSENTIAL CONSIDERATIONS

This section presents a definition of functional reading and an overview of non–language-based performance skills needed for effective reading participation. Occupational therapy practitioners have vital roles in the development of cognitive, executive functions (EFs), and sensory processing skills as prerequisite skills to support reading.

Defining Functional Reading: A Proposed Definition From Functional Cognition

Literacy components such as reading, writing, and social participation are critical to a person's performance in home, community, school, and work settings (Frolek Clark, 2016). Grajo and Gutman (2019) have proposed to name and frame literacy within occupational participation as *functional literacy.*

Functional literacy is defined as the ability to interpret and process common written materials that one needs to effectively carry out basic daily life skills, participate in meaningful occupations and social roles, and live independently in communities. The term was adapted and expanded from Kirsch and Guthrie's (1977–1978) definition of *functional reading* as the ability to read and understand materials that are directly related to everyday living. However, since its first inception, the term *functional reading* has been rarely used in contemporary educational literature.

The concept of functional literacy has its roots in *functional cognition,* defined by AOTA (2015) as the thinking and processing skills needed to accomplish complex everyday activities, such as

- Home, financial, and medication management;
- Work, school, and volunteer activities; and
- Driving and community navigation.

By applying this concept in schools, occupational therapy practitioners can address functional literacy as a means to ensure that all students

- Are able to access and optimally participate in occupations in schools;
- Are able to live in and be part of a community;
- Maintain physical and mental health and well-being; and
- Feel socially connected with peers, school personnel, families, and other meaningful others.

---

[1]*Occupational therapy practitioner* refers to both the occupational therapist and the occupational therapy assistant. The American Occupational Therapy Association (AOTA; 2014, p. S18) states, "The occupational therapist is responsible for all aspects of occupational therapy service delivery and is accountable for the safety and effectiveness of the occupational therapy service delivery process" and "must be directly involved in the delivery of services during the initial evaluation and regularly throughout the course of intervention. . . . The occupational therapy assistant delivers safe and effective occupational therapy services under the supervision of and in partnership with the occupational therapist."

How functional literacy can be specifically applied in the domains of occupational therapy practice is discussed in the "Best Practices" section of this chapter.

Cognition and reading performance

Siegel and Mazabel (2013) have synthesized literature describing several cognitive processes that affect reading performance. Table 50.1 summarizes some of these cognitive processes. Children with reading difficulties have been shown to have

- Difficulties with sentence correction and sentence completion tasks, demonstrating difficulties with syntactic awareness;
- Difficulties with recalling words presented in serial sentences, demonstrating working memory (WM) challenges (Siegel & Ryan, 1988);
- Poor morphological awareness, which may contribute to reading and spelling difficulties (Arnbak & Elbro, 2000); and
- Difficulties understanding word structures, which also contribute to spelling difficulties (Olson et al., 1985).

Several studies, however, have found that children and adults with orthographic processing difficulties have learned to rely on and use their visual skills to compensate for deficient language skills needed for effective reading (Shafrir & Siegel, 1991).

Executive functioning

Dawson and Guare (2010) identified EFs as the high-level cognitive processes that people need to plan and direct activities. Planning involves determining what factors are most relevant to a need. To effectively formulate a goal and a path to that goal, people require EFs involving organization, time management, WM, and metacognition—or the ability to reflect on one's own progress.

Helland and Asbjørnsen (2000) used an attention model to analyze the ability of children with dyslexia to execute responses, sustain focus, and shift attention when performing reading-related tasks. They found that children with dyslexia had a greater frequency of impaired EFs in these areas. These impairments were consistent with more severe accompanying language deficits than is typical for children with literacy problems who do not have dyslexia.

Altemeier et al. (2008) used the terms *inhibition, set shifting,* and *rapid automatic switching* to refer to EFs related to reading. Their study defined **inhibition** as the ability to inhibit automatic responses to engage in strategic processes in favor of a long-term goal (e.g., being able to read in a library with a lot of people). They defined **set shifting** as the ability to flexibly shift attention as task demands change. **Rapid automatic switching** is the ability to shift varying linguistic information, such as scanning across lines, sequencing within lines, and integrating visual and verbal codes.

Altemeier et al. (2008) found that

- Inhibition and rapid automatic switching contributed to reading and writing achievement among typically developing readers and writers;

TABLE 50.1. Cognitive Processes in Reading Disabilities

COGNITIVE PROCESS	DEFINITION
Morphological awareness	Morphemes are the smallest units of meaning within words; they help make word pronunciation predictable and preserve the semantic relationship between words (Shaywitz, 2003). Morphological awareness is the conscious awareness of the morphemic structure of words and the ability to reflect on and manipulate this structure.
Orthographic processing	The awareness of the structure of the words in a language.
Syntactic awareness	The ability to understand the basic grammatical structure of language used.
Working memory	The ability to retain information in short-term memory while processing new information.

- EFs predicted literacy outcomes in the elementary grades for children with and without dyslexia when the authors used measures without a timed component; and
- For both populations, EF skills affected performance in timed reading tasks.

Vision and reading performance

People need effective vision and visual processing skills for optimal participation in tasks that require decoding of letters and words. There is, however, much debate in neuroscience about the impact of vision intervention among children with reading difficulties. The American Academy of Pediatrics (AAP) Section on Ophthalmology et al. (2009) released a joint statement synthesizing scientific studies on the relationship of vision, visual skills, and reading difficulties.

Despite the assertion of the AAP et al. (2009), there is currently a lack of consensus among health practitioners on the role of vision in effective reading. Table 50.2 presents a synthesis of study findings and relevant citations from the AAP et al.'s statement.

Sensory processing

Researchers have suggested the importance of integrating sensory information and being able to process this information at an appropriate speed as important prerequisites to effective reading (Conlon et al., 2011). Of a sample of

70 children with dyslexia, Wright and Conlon (2009) identified sensory processing deficits among 20%–30%, which may constitute a separate or additional risk factor for reading failure. Children with dyslexia may have difficulties accessing and copying a well-defined sensory representation of reading stimuli to a domain-specific (auditory or visual) WM buffer, thus making reading difficult.

Sensory deficits affect the way stimuli presented at various speeds and durations and stimuli with multielement sequences are processed in the brain (Conlon et al., 2011). Thus, sensory deficits may explain the struggles of a child with dyslexia when pressured to read aloud unfamiliar words in the classroom or during group reading activities.

Contextual Factors That Influence Effective Reading Participation

Reading can be a challenging task, and various demands brought about by social contexts of the home and school can impose additional stress on struggling readers that may significantly affect literacy, particularly reading development. The demand for students to complete assignments, perform well on standardized tests, read independently, read with peers, and read aloud at school can lead to increasingly frequent feelings of frustration, agitation, withdrawal, and social isolation (Fleming et al., 2004). Such feelings and behaviors commonly place students at risk for depression and social anxiety, substance use, and school dropout (Quiroga et al., 2013).

TABLE 50.2. Synthesis of Findings on Visual Skills and Reading Difficulties

VISUAL SKILL	RELATIONSHIP TO LEARNING DISABILITY, DYSLEXIA, AND READING DIFFICULTIES	RELEVANT CRITICAL AND SEMINAL STUDIES
Saccadic eye movements (short-duration, high-velocity jumping movements of the eyes)	Atypical saccadic patterns seen among children with dyslexia are a result of but not the cause of reading disability.	American Academy of Ophthalmology (2001), Olitsky & Nelson (2003)
Visual tracking	Children with dyslexia often lose their place while reading because of difficulties with word decoding and comprehension but not because of deficient visual tracking skills.	Hutzler et al. (2006)
Convergence, divergence, visual perception, visual sequencing, visual memory	Word reversals and skipping words, which are seen in readers with dyslexia, have been shown to result from linguistic deficiencies rather than visual–perceptual disorders.	Vellutino et al. (2004)

Note. Findings are from the American Academy of Pediatrics Section on Ophthalmology et al. (2009).

Several studies have shown that the language environment in the home and the quality of language and social interaction and learning experiences with the parent are directly and significantly associated with children's cognitive and language development and emergent literacy competence (Dickinson & Tabors, 2001; Foster et al., 2005). Parent–child shared reading activities, frequency of access to books and other print material in the home, and the social learning opportunities in and away from the home contribute to children's language and literacy competence and set the stage for subsequent school success (Payne et al., 1994).

Downer et al. (2007) have also synthesized the literature to understand classroom and school context factors that influence learning and literacy achievement. Some of these factors include

- The quality of social and behavioral engagement in learning,
- Instructional and global learning conditions in the classroom,
- The amount of work done in big groups vs. small groups vs. individual tasks,
- Direct teaching or analytical and inferential type of instruction,
- The quality of interaction with peers, and
- The ability to meet the needs of students at risk for problems.

Reading Intervention From a Participation Perspective: Occupation and Participation Approach to Reading Intervention

Grajo and Candler (2016a) developed the *Occupation and Participation Approach to Reading Intervention* (OPARI; Grajo & Candler, 2016a) to identify a role for occupational therapy practitioners to support children with reading difficulties within the scope of practice of occupational therapy. Occupational therapists are not reading specialists. What the OPARI suggests is a holistic approach in addressing and supporting children with reading challenges beyond prerequisite literacy skills (e.g., visual–perceptual skills, EF skills, sensory processing abilities).

The OPARI advocates for addressing increased participation in reading as an occupation. Practitioners using the OPARI focus on creating therapeutic contexts that facilitate children's development of meaningful reading goals and strategies that will facilitate reading with mastery and competence. Practitioners also collaborate with families and school personnel to increase the child's sense of enjoyment and self-initiation of meaningful reading occupations (Grajo & Candler, 2016a).

BEST PRACTICES

Best practices gleaned from the literature support 6 essential elements:

1. Need to measure reading participation,
2. Focus on participation and engagement,
3. Use of self-generated strategies,
4. Collaboration with families and the interprofessional team,
5. Use of natural contexts, and
6. Emphasis on mastery and competence.

Measure Reading Participation

Resources defining and measuring reading as a meaningful activity that children participate in have been scarce. However, expansive amounts of literature exist that explore and document the reasons why children read, how they read, and what motivates them to read. Wigfield et al. (2004) found that when children were given opportunities to choose what they read, to decide which questions to pursue about what they read, and to interact with other students in the process of reading, their level of curiosity, acceptance of challenge, reading frequency, and self-efficacy improved significantly.

De Naeghel et al. (2012) found that children's autonomous reading motivation (e.g., "I read in my free time because I really like it" and "I read in my free time because it's fun to read") was directly and positively associated with reading frequency, engagement, and comprehension compared with children's controlled motivation (e.g., "I read in my free time because I have to prove myself that I can get good reading grades" and "I read in my free time because I can be proud of myself if I get good reading grades").

How reading is performed as an occupation may be different for children with reported reading difficulties. Kent et al. (2012) found that students at risk for reading difficulties spent only about half of the scheduled reading instructional block in schools participating in literacy activities. Increased anxiety levels have also been documented among children with dyslexia (Carroll & Iles, 2006), and this anxiety may affect active engagement in structured reading tasks.

Children who have reading disabilities often believe that their reading ability is controlled by external factors and that reading is difficult and something they cannot master (Kirby et al., 2011). Meltzer et al. (2004) found that students who perceived themselves as struggling in the academic domains of reading, writing, and spelling reported less effort and less consistent use of strategies with their schoolwork, which therefore affected participation.

Occupational therapists, from a prerequisite skill perspective, can use standardized and nonstandardized tools to assess vision-related, sensory processing, cognitive, motor, and coping and adaptive performance skills students need for effective reading. Grajo et al. (2016) suggested the use of nonstandardized tools, functional observation, and interview methods to determine patterns of reading participation of children with reading difficulties.

Using data gathered from determining the psychometric properties of an occupation-based questionnaire on reading participation, Grajo et al. (2016) found value in

- Identifying the different kinds of reading materials children access at home, at school, and in communities;
- Determining perceptions about the level of difficulty of reading materials;
- Determining perceptions about the child's level of mastery when engaging with different reading materials;
- Identifying motivating factors for reading; and
- Determining the frequency of reading participation, the social supports available for reading, and the resources

available to freely participate in reading occupations to provide a holistic perspective to the child's reading participation.

Focus on Participation and Engagement

Occupational therapy practitioners supporting students with reading challenges must aim to increase students' participation and engagement in self-chosen and structured reading occupations (Grajo & Candler, 2016a). When addressing reading participation, practitioners can use the following approaches:

- Create opportunities for students to choose reading materials they want to work on at home and in classrooms.
- Promote students' control of the reading environment to make it more engaging, more interactive, and less stressful.
- Incorporate a variety of play-based and social classroom activities, such as writing and reading letters to friends, parents, and siblings; playing board games; ordering food from a menu; making fun class announcements; doing arts and crafts; and participating in sports activities.
- Collaborate with classroom teachers to determine ways to combine structured and less structured activities that support reading and comprehension goals.

Facilitating children's reading participation requires the skillful use of facilitative techniques rather than direct instruction (Grajo & Candler, 2016b). Occupational therapy practitioners can use principles from the *Cognitive Orientation to daily Occupational Performance* (CO–OP; Dawson et al., 2017; Polatajko & Mandich, 2004) to support children in self-generating strategies to use when they encounter challenging reading tasks. The CO–OP Approach™, originally developed for children with developmental coordination disorder, is an individualized, client-centered approach focused on strategy-based skills acquisition.

CO–OP emphasizes skills acquisition, cognitive strategy development, and generalization and transfer of skills and strategies. CO–OP has been pilot tested for children with reading difficulties (Grajo & Candler, 2016b). Table 50.3 provides examples of specific approaches practitioners can take when using cognitive strategy development to enhance reading participation.

Collaborate With Families and School Personnel

Because literacy is an emerging area of occupational therapy practice in schools, it is not uncommon for members of the reading intervention team (e.g., teachers, reading specialists, school psychologists, SLPs) to be unfamiliar with how occupational therapy practitioners can support children with reading difficulties in schools. It has been well documented (Truong & Hodgetts, 2017) that teachers are often confused about the scope of occupational therapy practice, express desire for more open and reciprocal communication, and want to have a better understanding of needs and constraints in the classroom setting.

Using a case study, Asher and Nichols (2016) outlined some best practices in collaborating and working with interprofessional teams in schools to address the literacy needs of students:

- Identify shared philosophy.
- Define discipline-specific roles, understand the scope of practice of interprofessional team members, and be willing to compromise with responsibilities.

TABLE 50.3. Techniques to Facilitate Development of Cognitive Strategies to Support Reading Participation

FACILITATIVE TECHNIQUE	SPECIFIC APPROACH
Explore, through guided questioning, strategies that can be used during reading participation.	Provide opportunities for students to explore and identify task-specific strategies during reading activities. Instead of a direct teaching approach, therapists must use guided series of questions and facilitative prompts to allow discovery of strategies that might work for the student. Examples of task-specific strategies may include use of tools to allow proper scanning and reading of lines of text, strategies to calm and organize the body in preparation for challenging reading, and techniques to detect and recognize errors in reading.
Allow students to name and label their own strategies.	Allowing students to name and label strategies facilitates better recall and use of the strategy. Encourage students to name strategies using words that are simple, engaging, unique, and easy to remember.
Allow for trial and error. Strategy development is an iterative process.	Strategy development is an iterative process that is best developed by starting with small, achievable goals. When setting reading-related goals, start with smaller goals that will allow the student to experience success (e.g., read 2 sentences from a page of a student-chosen book using specific strategies). Strive to gain mastery of the simpler goal and go through an iterative process of trying out different strategies before progressing to a goal with a higher level of complexity or degree of difficulty.
Allow for exploration of strategies that may seem ineffective.	During the iterative process of goal achievement and strategy use, students may explore the use of strategies that therapists might immediately perceive as ineffective (e.g., "When I encounter a difficult reading word, I will just skip the sentence"). Instead of immediately dismissing the strategy or directly telling the student that the strategy will be ineffective, provide the opportunity to explore and try the strategy. Use facilitative questions to guide the student to modify, simplify, expand, or completely revise strategies that did not achieve goal completion (e.g., "When you skip sentences, I notice that you misunderstand the story. What can you do to change your skipping strategy? Instead of full sentences, what can you skip to allow you to still read more words or sentences?").

- Determine shared responsibilities and foster situational leadership.
- Establish equal and mutual respect and clear methods of communication.

When providing interventions in the student's natural contexts (e.g., the classroom) to enhance participation in reading, occupational therapy practitioners have 2 important considerations: working collaboratively with the classroom teacher and optimizing the student's social environment. Bazyk et al. (2009) reported that occupational therapy services provided in natural contexts can concurrently address the occupational performance needs of students with disabilities and of those at risk of delay.

Several intervention programs based on cooperative learning have been found to be effective and can be used by occupational therapists in collaboration with the classroom teacher:

- The ***Learning Together Approach*** (Johnson & Johnson 1994) is an activity-based reading intervention that includes whole-group discussions, hands-on activities, games, and individual worksheets. The approach works by rewarding groups on the basis of each member's performance, guiding students to encourage and facilitate each other's achievement, holding individuals accountable for learning skills, using interpersonal skills, and reflecting on how well the group functions.
- The ***Cooperative Learning Strategy*** (Klingner & Vaughn, 1996) is a classroom approach whereby students are taught to use reciprocal teaching comprehension strategies (e.g., prediction, summarization, question generation, clarification) while reading text. The facilitator models the strategies by "thinking aloud" when reading a passage, then leads students in text-related discussions.
- ***Peer-Assisted Learning Strategies*** (Fuchs et al., 1997) is a cooperative learning program in which students work in pairs, taking turns reading aloud to one another and engaging in summarization and prediction activities.

Emphasize Mastery and Competence

When addressing reading from the perspective of occupational participation, the occupational therapist provides opportunities for the child with reading difficulties to feel a sense of mastery and competence. The therapist can do this by

- Carefully grading and adapting activities so the student experiences the just-right challenge;
- Gradually introducing chunks of structured reading tasks to increase the student's adaptive capacity and feeling of competence with reading tasks;
- Guiding the student to set realistic reading goals (e.g., reading 1 page of a storybook in 5 minutes); and
- Working with the interprofessional team and discussing with the student a mechanism for monitoring emotions during reading participation, such as a chart or sticker book.

Strategies for self-monitoring might enable the student to develop insights about reading participation and adapt better when feeling overwhelmed or frustrated.

SUMMARY

Occupational therapy practitioners support students with reading difficulties using a holistic and participation approach. Although it is essential for practitioners to address the prerequisite skills students need for effective reading, these skills must be related to the goal of increasing meaningful participation in reading activities at school, at home, and in the community. Occupational therapy practitioners work toward students acquiring functional literacy skills to effectively fulfill daily life needs and participate in meaningful occupations and social roles.

REFERENCES

Altemeier, L. E., Abbott, R. D., & Berninger, V. W. (2008). Executive functions for reading and writing in typical literacy development and dyslexia. *Journal of Clinical and Experimental Neuropsychology, 30,* 588–606. https://doi.org/10.1080/1380 3390701562818

American Academy of Ophthalmology. (2001). *Complementary therapy assessment: Vision therapy for learning disabilities.* Retrieved from https://aapos.org/client_data/files/2011/331_aao complementarytxassessmentvtforld.pdf

American Academy of Pediatrics Section on Ophthalmology, Council on Children With Disabilities, American Academy of Ophthalmology, American Association for Pediatric Ophthalmology, and Strabismus, & American Association of Certified Orthoptists. (2009). Learning disabilities, dyslexia, and vision. *Pediatrics, 124,* 837–844. https://doi.org/10.1542/peds .2009-1445

American Occupational Therapy Association. (2014). Guidelines for supervision, roles, and responsibilities during the delivery of occupational therapy services. *American Journal of Occupational Therapy, 68*(Suppl. 3), S16–S22. https://doi.org/10.5014 /ajot.2014.686S03

American Occupational Therapy Association. (2015). *Role of occupational therapy in assessing functional cognition.* Retrieved from https://www.aota.org/Advocacy-Policy/Federal-Reg-Affairs /Medicare/Guidance/role-OT-assessing-functional-cognition.aspx

Arnbak, E., & Elbro, C. (2000). The effects of morphological awareness training on the reading and spelling skills of young dyslexics. *Scandinavian Journal of Educational Research, 44,* 229–251. https://doi.org/10.1080/00313830050154485

Asher, A., & Nichols, J. D. (2016). Collaboration around facilitating emergent literacy: Role of occupational therapy. *Journal of Occupational Therapy, Schools, and Early Intervention, 9,* 51–73. https://doi.org/10.1080/19411243.2016.1156415

Bazyk, S., Michaud, P., Goodman, G., Papp, P., Hawkins, E., & Welch, M. A. (2009). Integrating occupational therapy services in a kindergarten curriculum: A look at the outcomes. *American Journal of Occupational Therapy, 63,* 160–171. https://doi .org/10.5014/ajot.63.2.160

Binney, R. J., Embleton, K. V., Jefferies, E., Parker, G. J. M., & Ralph, M. A. L. (2010). The ventral and inferolateral aspects of the anterior temporal lobe are crucial in semantic memory: Evidence from a novel direct comparison of distortion-corrected fMRI, rTMS, and semantic dementia. *Cerebral Cortex, 20,* 2728–2738. https://doi.org/10.1093/cercor /bhq019

Carroll, J. M., & Iles, J. E. (2006). An assessment of anxiety levels in dyslexic students in higher education. *British Journal of Educational Psychology, 76,* 651–662. https://doi.org/10.1348/000709905X66233

Conlon, E. G., Wright, C. M., Norris, K., & Chekaluk, E. (2011). Does a sensory processing deficit explain counting accuracy on rapid visual sequencing tasks in adults with and without dyslexia? *Brain and Cognition, 76,* 197–205. https://doi.org/10.1016/j.bandc.2010.10.014

Dawson, D. R., McEwen, S. E., & Polatajko, H. J. (Eds.). (2017). *Cognitive Orientation to daily Occupational Performance in occupational therapy: Using the CO–OP approach to enable participation across the lifespan.* Bethesda, MD: AOTA Press.

Dawson, P., & Guare, R. (2010). *Executive skills in children and adolescents: A practical guide to assessment and intervention* (2nd ed.). London: Guilford Press.

De Naeghel, J., Van Keer, H., Vansteenkiste, M., & Rosseel, Y. (2012). The relation between elementary students' recreational and academic reading motivation, reading frequency, engagement, and comprehension: A self-determination theory perspective. *Journal of Educational Psychology,* 104, 1006–1021. https://doi.org/10.1037/a0027800

Dickinson, D. K., & Tabors, P. O. (2001). *Beginning literacy with language.* Baltimore: Brookes.

Downer, J. T., Rimm-Kaufman, S. E., & Pianta, R. C. (2007). How do classroom conditions and children's risk for school problems contribute to children's behavioral engagement in learning? *School Psychology Review, 36,* 413–432.

Fleming, C. B., Harachi, T. W., Cortes, R. C., Abbott, R. D., & Catalano, R. F. (2004). Level and change in reading scores and attention problems during elementary school as predictors of problem behavior in middle school. *Journal of Emotional and Behavioral Disorders, 12,* 130–144. https://doi.org/10.1177/10634266040120030101

Foster, M. A., Lambert, R., Abbott-Shim, M., McCarty, F., & Franze, S. (2005). A model of home learning environment and social risk factors in relation to children's emergent literacy and social outcomes. *Early Childhood Research Quarterly, 20,* 13–36. https://doi.org/10.1016/j.ecresq.2005.01.006

Frolek Clark, G. (2016). The occupations of literacy: Occupational therapy's role. *Journal of Occupational Therapy, Schools, and Early Intervention, 9,* 27–37. https://doi.org/10.1080/19411243.2016.1152835

Fuchs, D., Fuchs, L. S., Mathes, P. G., & Simmons, D. (1997). Peer-assisted learning strategies: Making classrooms more responsive to diversity. *American Educational Research Journal, 34,* 174–206. https://doi.org/10.2307/1163346

Grajo, L., & Candler, C. (2016a). An Occupation and Participation Approach to Reading Intervention (OPARI) Part I: Defining reading as an occupation. *Journal of Occupational Therapy, Schools, and Early Intervention, 9,* 74–85. https://doi.org/10.1080/19411243.2016.1141082

Grajo, L., & Candler, C. (2016b). An Occupation and Participation Approach to Reading Intervention (OPARI) Part II: Pilot clinical application. *Journal of Occupational Therapy, Schools, and Early Intervention, 9,* 86–98. https://doi.org/10.1080/19411243.2016.1141083

Grajo, L. C., Candler, C., Bowyer, P., Schultz, S., Thomson, J., & Fong, K. (2016). Determining the internal validity of the Inventory of Reading Occupations: An assessment tool of children's reading participation. *American Journal of Occupational Therapy, 70,* 7003220010. https://doi.org/10.5014/ajot.2016.017582

Grajo, L., & Gutman, S. (2019). The role of occupational therapy in functional literacy. *Open Journal of Occupational Therapy, 7*(1), Article 13.

Helland, T., & Asbjørnsen, A. (2000). Executive functions in dyslexia. *Child Neuropsychology, 6*(1), 37–48. https://doi.org/10.1076/0929-7049(200003)6:1;1-B;FT037

Horowitz, S. H., Rawe, J., & Whittaker, M. C. (2017). *The state of learning disabilities: Understanding the 1 in 5.* New York: National Center for Learning Disabilities.

Hruby, G., Goswami, U., Frederiksen, C., & Perfetti, C. (2011). Neuroscience and reading: A review for reading education researchers. *Reading Research Quarterly, 46,* 156–172. https://doi.org/10.1598/RRQ.46.2.4

Hutzler, F., Kronbichler, M., Jacobs, A. M., & Wimmer, H. (2006). Perhaps correlational but not causal: No effect of dyslexic readers' magnocellular system on their eye movements during reading. *Neuropsychologia, 44,* 637–648. https://doi.org/10.1016/j.neuropsychologia.2005.06.006

Johnson, R. T., & Johnson, R. T. (1994). *Learning together and alone.* Boston: Allyn & Bacon.

Kent, S. C., Wanzek, J., & Al Otaiba, S. (2012). Print reading in general education kindergarten classrooms: What does it look like for students at-risk for reading difficulties? *Learning Disabilities Research and Practice, 27*(2), 56–65. https://doi.org/10.1111/j.1540-5826.2012.00351.x

Kirby, J. R., Ball, A., Geier, B. K., Parrila, R., & Wade-Woolley, L. (2011). The development of reading interest and its relation to reading ability. *Journal of Research in Reading, 34,* 263–280. https://doi.org/10.1111/j.1467-9817.2010.01439.x

Kirsch, I., & Guthrie, J. T. (1977–1978). The concept and measurement of functional literacy. *Reading Research Quarterly, 13,* 485–507. https://doi.org/10.2307/747509

Klingner, J. K., & Vaughn, S. (1996). Reciprocal teaching of reading comprehension strategies for students with learning disabilities who use English as a second language. *Elementary School Journal, 96,* 275–293. https://doi.org/10.1086/461828

Krafnick, A. J., Flowers, D. L., Napoliello, E. M., & Eden, G. F. (2011). Gray matter volume changes following reading intervention in dyslexic children. *NeuroImage, 57,* 733–741. https://doi.org/10.1016/j.neuroimage.2010.10.062

Laycock, R., & Crewther, S. G. (2008). Towards an understanding of the role of the "magnocellular advantage" in fluent reading. *Neuroscience and Biobehavioral Reviews, 32,* 1494–1506. https://doi.org/10.1016/j.neubiorev.2008.06.002

Meltzer, L., Katzir, T., Miller, L., Reddy, R., & Roditi, B. (2004). Academic self-perceptions, effort, and strategy use in students with learning disabilities: Changes over time. *Learning Disabilities Research and Practice, 19,* 99–108. https://doi.org/10.1111/j.1540-5826.2004.00093.x

National Reading Panel. (2000). *Report of the National Reading Panel: Teaching children to read: An evidence-based assessment of the scientific research literature on reading and its implications for reading instruction.* Washington, DC: National Institute of Child Health and Human Development, National Institutes of Health. Retrieved from https://www.nichd.nih.gov/publications/pubs/nrp/smallbook

O'Brien, B. A., Wolf, M., & Lovett, M. W. (2012). A taxometric investigation of developmental dyslexia subtypes. *Dyslexia, 18*(1), 16–39. https://doi.org/10.1002/dys.1431

Odegard, T., Ring, J., Smith, S., Biggan, J., & Black, J. (2008). Differentiating the neural response to intervention in children with developmental dyslexia. *Annals of Dyslexia, 58*(1), 1–14. https://doi.org/10.1007/s11881-008-0014-5

Olitsky, S. E., & Nelson, L. B. (2003). Reading disorders in children. *Pediatric Clinics of North America, 50*(1), 213–224.

Olson, R. K., Kliegl, R., Davidson, B. J., & Foltz, G. (1985). Individual and developmental differences in reading disability. In G. E. MacKinnon & T. G. Waller (Eds.), *Reading research: Advances in theory and practice* (Vol. 4, pp. 1–64). New York: Academic Press.

Payne, A. C., Whitehurst, G. J., & Angell, A. L. (1994). The role of home literacy environment in the development of language ability in preschool children from low-income families. *Early Childhood Research Quarterly, 9,* 427–440. https://doi.org/10.1016/0885-2006(94)90018-3

Polatajko, H. J., & Mandich, A. (2004). *Enabling occupation in children: The Cognitive Orientation to daily Occupational Performance (CO–OP) Approach.* Ottawa: CAOT Publications ACE.

Quiroga, C. V., Janosz, M., Bisset, S., & Morin, A. J. (2013). Early adolescent depression symptoms and school dropout: Mediating processes involving self-reported academic competence and achievement. *Journal of Educational Psychology, 105,* 552–560. https://doi.org/10.1037/a0031524

Shafrir, U., & Siegel, L. (1991). Preference for visual scanning versus phonological rehearsal in university students with reading disabilities. *Journal of Learning Disabilities, 27,* 583–588. https://doi.org/10.1177/002221949402700907

Shaywitz, S. (2003). *Overcoming dyslexia: A new and complete science-based program for reading problems at any level.* New York: Vintage.

Siegel, L. S., & Mazabel, S. (2013). Basic cognitive processes and reading disabilities. In H. L. Swanson, K. R. Harris, & S. Graham (Eds.), *Handbook of learning disabilities* (2nd ed., pp. 186–213). New York: Guilford Press.

Siegel, L. S., & Ryan, E. B. (1988). Development of grammatical-sensitivity, phonological, and short-term memory in normally achieving and learning disabled children. *Developmental Psychology, 24,* 28–37. https://doi.org/10.1037/0012-1649.24.1.28

Snowling, M. J. (2005). Phonological processing and developmental dyslexia. *Journal of Research in Reading, 18,* 132–138. https://doi.org/10.1111/j.1467-9817.1995.tb00079.x

Stein, J. (2001). The magnocellular theory of developmental dyslexia. *Dyslexia, 7*(1), 12–36. https://doi.org/10.1002/dys.186

Stein, J., & Walsh, V. (1997). To see but not to read: The magnocellular theory of dyslexia. *Trends in Neurosciences, 20,* 147–152. https://doi.org/10.1016/S0166-2236(96)01005-3

Truong, V., & Hodgetts, S. (2017). An exploration of teacher perceptions toward occupational therapy and occupational therapy practices. *Journal of Occupational Therapy, Schools, and Early Intervention, 10,* 121–136. https://doi.org/10.1080/19411243.2017.1304840

Vellutino, F., Fletcher, J., Snowling, M., & Scanlon, D. (2004). Specific reading disability (dyslexia): What have we learned in the past four decades? *Journal of Child Psychology and Psychiatry, 45,* 2–40. https://doi.org/10.1046/j.0021-9630.2003.00305.x

Wigfield, A., Guthrie, J. T., Tonks, S., & Perencevich, K. C. (2004). Children's motivation for reading: Domain specificity and instructional influences. *Journal of Educational Research, 97,* 299–309. https://doi.org/10.3200/JOER.97.6.299-310

Wright, C. M., & Conlon, E. G. (2009). Auditory and visual processing in children with dyslexia. *Developmental Neuropsychology, 34,* 330–355. https://doi.org/10.1080/87565640902801882

Best Practices in Play, Leisure, and Extracurricular Skills to Enhance Participation

51

Elizabeth Richardson, MS, OTR/L

KEY TERMS AND CONCEPTS

- Extracurricular activities
- Integrated playgroup
- Leisure
- Peer-mediated intervention
- Pivotal response training
- Play
- Recess
- Structured activities
- Unstructured activities

Leisure is often playful and play is often leisurely.
—Sellar and Stanley (2010, p. 358)

OVERVIEW

The United Nations (1989) has identified participation in occupations of play and leisure as a universal right of children. Moreover, it is considered to be essential in contributing to a child's acquisition of skills across all developmental areas, ability to learn, and overall well-being (Dahan-Oliel et al., 2012; Holder et al., 2009; Neumayer & Wilding, 2004; Rigby & Rodger, 2006).

Play and leisure are recognized as being within the domain of occupational therapy practice (American Occupational Therapy Association [AOTA], 2014b); therefore, they should be considered by practitioners[1] throughout the course of occupational therapy service provision. Parham and Fazio (1997, as cited in AOTA, 2014b) defined *play* as "any spontaneous or organized activity that provides enjoyment, entertainment, amusement, or diversion" (p. S21) and *leisure* as "nonobligatory activity that is intrinsically motivated and engaged in during discretionary time, that is, time not committed to obligatory occupations such as work, self-care, or sleep" (p. S21). Recreation and leisure are classified as informal or organized arts and culture, crafts, hobbies, play, sports, and socializing (World Health Organization [WHO], 2007).

People with a disability are provided fewer or limited access to opportunities for engagement in all areas of participation, including the occupations of play and leisure, despite their recognized importance (Imms et al., 2008, 2009; King et al., 2009; Majnemer et al., 2008). Several barriers to participation in these areas have been identified, including

- Exclusion from school and social contexts where play and leisure take place;
- Cultural attitudes or stereotypes that are hostile toward people with disabilities;
- Communication challenges; and
- Lack of or inadequate access to physical spaces, transportation, or needed technology (UN Committee on the Rights of the Child, 2013).

Students with a physical, sensory, or cognitive impairment are at risk of experiencing restrictions or limited opportunities to engage in play in part because a greater emphasis is placed on attending to other needs (McDonald & Brown, 2009). Students with a disability are often limited in the types of activities they participate in and where those activities take place, and they participate less often and with decreased intensity than typically developing peers (Imms, 2008).

Students with a disability are also more likely to engage in leisure activities by themselves or with their parents because of dependence for support (Shikako-Thomas et al., 2008). Often, these students experience reduced participation in leisure activities as they get older or have greater motor and mobility limitations (Welsh et al., 2006). A report by the U.S. Government Accountability Office (2010) found that students with a disability participated in athletics at lower rates than students without a disability because of limited resources and information made available to schools.

---

[1] *Occupational therapy practitioner* refers to both the occupational therapist and the occupational therapy assistant. The American Occupational Therapy Association (AOTA; 2014a, p. S18) states, "The occupational therapist is responsible for all aspects of occupational therapy service delivery and is accountable for the safety and effectiveness of the occupational therapy service delivery process" and "must be directly involved in the delivery of services during the initial evaluation and regularly throughout the course of intervention. . . . The occupational therapy assistant delivers safe and effective occupational therapy services under the supervision of and in partnership with the occupational therapist."

Copyright © 2019 by the American Occupational Therapy Association. All rights reserved. To reuse this content, contact www.copyright.com.
https://doi.org/10.7139/2019.978-1-56900-591-0.051

ESSENTIAL CONSIDERATIONS

The American Academy of Pediatrics (2015) has recommended that children and adolescents (ages 6 years or older) engage in 60 minutes or more of physical activity a day; this can include unstructured play and leisure activities. Quality of life (QoL) improves with both spontaneous and structured leisure activities (Dahan-Oliel et al., 2012).

Play, Leisure, and Extracurricular Activities

The profession of occupational therapy has a long history of addressing the occupations of play and leisure (Primeau, 2014). Understanding the value and added benefits of students' access to and participation in play, leisure, and extracurricular activities is critical.

Play

Play is holistic and promotes all dimensions of health: physical, social, emotional, mental, environmental, and spiritual (Bruce et al., 2010). Play enhances children's well-being, resilience, and ability to cope by allowing children to gain an understanding of different emotions through practice and experience (Children's Society, 2014). These attributes support the child in successfully navigating stressful situations (Yogman et al., 2018).

Pretend play is important to the development of literacy, language development, and social competence (Stagnitti, 2009). Through play, a child can develop "creativity, imagination, self-confidence, self-efficacy and physical, social, cognitive and emotional strength and skills" (International Play Association, 2013, p. 2). However, play experiences are often centered on physical health, including promoting physical and outdoor activity and creating safe play environments (UN Committee on the Rights of the Child, 2013).

Leisure

Participation in leisure activities includes participation in sports, arts, entertainment, social, self-improvement, and religious activities (Dahan-Oliel et al., 2012). Leisure activities can be further distinguished as those that are structured and unstructured. **Structured activities** are organized by adults around specific goals, whereas **unstructured activities** emerge more spontaneously on the basis of what is going on in a child's life (Fletcher et al., 2003).

Engagement in leisure activities provides time away from the various responsibilities and demands of everyday life, which has been found to result in numerous health benefits (Neumayer & Wilding, 2004). Structured leisure activities, such as sports or hobbies, enhance children's well-being through self-actualization, self-enrichment, self-expression, and self-renewal.

Extracurricular activities

In the school setting, **extracurricular activities,** such as athletics or special interest groups or clubs, offer students an opportunity to explore various leisure activities. Participation in extracurricular activities promotes the development of
- Teamwork values;
- Individual and group responsibility;
- Physical health and fitness; and
- A sense of culture and community, which increases engagement and attachment to school and decreases the likelihood of failure and dropout (U.S. Government Accountability Office, 2010).

Through extracurricular activities, concepts from the classroom can be reinforced through application in real-time contexts. Participation in sports and clubs is associated with higher academic grades and higher ratings of social competence and psychosocial maturity (Fletcher et al., 2003).

Laws Ensuring Equal Access to Play, Leisure, and Extracurricular Activities

Certain laws provide protections for students with disabilities to participate in play, leisure, and extracurricular activities (U.S. Department of Education, Office of Civil Rights, 2016). Section 504 of the Rehabilitation Act of 1973, as amended (2008; Pub. L. 92–112) requires that all students receive and all school districts provide nonacademic services and activities in a manner that provides students with disabilities an equal opportunity for participation in extracurricular athletics, special interest groups, or clubs (34 C.F.R. § 104.37[a][c]; 34 C.F.R. § 104.4[b][1]).

Under the Individuals With Disabilities Education Improvement Act of 2004 (Pub. L. 108–446), schools are required to take steps to provide students with disabilities an opportunity to participate in nonacademic and extracurricular services and activities in a manner equal to that of other students. This requirement includes the provision of supplementary aids and services determined appropriate and necessary (34 C.F.R. § 300.117).

Physical Activity and Health Initiatives

WHO's (2004) *Global Strategy on Diet, Physical Activity and Health* states, "School policies and programmes should support the adoption of healthy diets and physical activity" (para. 49). The Healthy People 2020 initiative (Office of Disease Prevention and Health Promotion, 2008) includes nutrition, physical activity, and obesity as leading health indicators. It also includes physical activity and health-related QoL and well-being as topics with specific objectives that can be measured in each area. The objectives are broad and include 3 domains:
1. Self-rated physical and mental health,
2. Overall well-being, and
3. Participation in society.

Physical activity objectives that target young children include addressing the importance of recess and physical education in schools.

The Convention on the Rights of Persons With Disabilities (UN General Assembly, 2006) identified the right to full and effective participation and inclusion in recreation, leisure, and sport. Article 30 requires that actions be taken to

encourage and promote the participation, to the fullest extent possible, of persons with disabilities in mainstream sporting activities at all levels [and] . . . ensure that persons with disabilities have an opportunity to organize, develop and participate in disability specific sporting and recreational activities and, to this end, encourage the provision, on an equal basis with others, of appropriate instruction, training and resources. (para. 5)

Despite the significant evidence that highlights the value of play and leisure, the child's rights to participation in these activities is frequently misunderstood and disregarded (Family & Community Services, 2015). The time available for participation in play and leisure activities is often limited as a result of increased pressures to spend more time in structured academic work or because of the practice of withholding recess as a consequence for undesired behavior (Ramstetter et al., 2010). In addition, limited access to outdoor space, increased parental involvement, increased use of technology and virtual spaces, and changes in play and leisure environments because of risk and safety concerns further contribute to a reduction in play and leisure participation (Rigby & Rodger, 2006; Sturgess, 2003). To target these concerns, the UN Committee on the Rights of the Child (2013) issued a comment to challenge states to provide necessary policy frameworks and resources.

Physical Education and Physical Activity

Physical education can provide students with an opportunity to explore and engage in structured play and leisure activities designed to promote physical activity. Physical education programs teach students lifelong skills to keep them healthy. A systematic review completed for the American College of Sports Medicine by Donnelly et al. (2016) found evidence that supports the associations among physical activity, fitness, cognition, executive function, and academic achievement.

Recess: Definitions and Guidelines

Definitions of and guidelines for recess vary depending on the source. However, one important tenet is present across all sources: *Recess* should be unstructured time dedicated to physical activity and play (Centers for Disease Control and Prevention, 2017). Other important aspects that are highlighted include

- The significance of recess as an educational support that promotes social, emotional, physical, and cognitive development;
- Overall health;
- Academic achievement; and
- School connectedness.

Although recess is often considered to be available only in elementary schools, designated time to break from academic work during the school day and participate in physical activity should be integrated into middle and high school schedules.

Physical, Social, and Cultural Environments

The environment is a critical factor affecting engagement in play and leisure activities. Occupational therapy practitioners must consider the fit among the individual, the environment, and the play or leisure activity to ensure successful engagement. The physical environment should reflect a universal design that supports accessibility for students of all abilities and ensures safety. Elements of a supportive physical environment include

- Sufficient space,
- Absence of physical barriers,
- Adjustable or adapted equipment, and
- Accessible modes of transport from 1 place to another.

Spending time in natural physical environments can produce a restorative effect that may lead to increased relaxation and decreased stress associated with daily life (Gill, 2014). Other benefits may include improved

- Physical activity, fitness, and competence;
- Self-confidence;
- Creativity;
- Emotional regulation;
- Learning; and
- Academic achievement.

Creating a social environment that promotes interactions with peers supports a student's development (Rigby & Rodger, 2006). In addition, students with delayed play skills may benefit by learning new skills while interacting with typically developing peers (Tanta et al., 2005).

The cultural environment encompasses shared perceptions and common values, attitudes, beliefs, and actions among a group of individuals that are learned through instruction and imitation (Fitzgerald, 2010). For children, the development of cultural competence often occurs through play. When aspects of a student's culture are incorporated into play experiences, the student may be more motivated to participate (Hinman, 2003). The student's parents are a valuable resource for understanding family routines, rituals, and cultural values that can be connected through play. In addition, occupational therapy practitioners must be aware of their own cultural beliefs as well as those of students, teachers, and parents, because they may influence access to and engagement in play and leisure activities.

Movement and Learning

Movement increases blood and oxygen flow, which enhances cognitive development and mental and physical health. There are many linkages between learning and movement during play or leisure activities. Providing breaks to help with attention has been researched. Pelligrini and Holmes (2006) found students paid more attention to academics after a recess (an unstructured break). In China and Japan, students are given short breaks every 50 minutes (Stevenson & Lee, 1990) and have become high achievers.

There are other benefits that affect learning. Studies found that children who engaged in frequent pretend play had stronger self-regulation skills (Lillard et al., 2013). Wolfgang et al. (2001) tracked block play by 4-year-old children and their high school academic performance. They found that the complexity of block play predicted high school mathematic achievements, even when the child's IQ was controlled. Hanline et al. (2010) conducted a longitudinal study and found a predictive relationship for higher reading abilities and faster rate of growth in reading abilities among early elementary students, but they found no relationship with math skills. Preschoolers who play with blocks in more sophisticated ways seem to build higher complex thinking.

BEST PRACTICES

Do not keep children to their studies by compulsion but by play.—Plato, *The Republic*

Participation in play and leisure activities is essential to the development of important life skills and promotes healthy relationships between students and their caregivers or peers (Rigby & Rodger, 2006). Students of all abilities should be provided with opportunities to have access to and engage in play and leisure activities to enhance overall QoL.

Evaluate Play and Leisure in the Student's School Day

Evaluation of play and leisure should include gathering information about the student, the specific occupations of play and leisure that are relevant to the student, and the environments in which they do or should occur. Through observation, student and caregiver interviews, file review, and administration of select assessment tools, the occupational therapist can identify goals and priorities. Therapists can use the Canadian Occupational Performance Measure (Law et al., 2014) to establish a foundation on which to direct the student-centered evaluation. Goal attainment scaling is a useful tool in the ongoing assessment of intervention outcomes (Ottenbacker & Cusick, 1990).

Specific assessment tools should be selected on the basis of what aspect of play or leisure needs to be further explored. This process may include looking at individual skills, preferred activities, how the activities are approached, or the environment in which the activity takes place.

Consider assessment tools aimed to measure aspects of play

Most assessment tools for play are designed for use with preschoolers and elementary students. Massey et al. (2018) developed the Great Recess Framework–Observational Tool to examine the recess environment and provide a guide for intervention to enhance recess by gathering information about safety, resources, student engagement, adult engagement, behavior, and student empowerment. The Child Initiated Pretend Play Assessment (Stagnitti, 2007) assesses the quality of a child's (age 3–7 years) ability to self-initiate pretend play.

Consider assessment tools aimed to identify the student's interests

Several tools assess interests and activities for older students. The Pediatric Interest Profiles (Henry, 2008) gather information about a student's play and interests through self-report. They are available for 3 age groups: Kid Play Profile (6–9 years), Preteen Play Profile (9–12 years), and Adolescent Leisure Interest Profile (12–21 years).

The Paediatric Activity Card Sort (Madich et al., 2004) uses pictures and responses to gather information about engagement in different activities, including play. It can be used with students who are developmentally between the ages of 4 and 14 years. The Children's Assessment of Participation and Enjoyment (King et al., 2004) is a child-report measure for children and youth ages 6–21 years old and evaluates their participation, preferences, and enjoyment in structured and unstructured activities.

Consider assessment tools aimed to measure approaches to play and leisure

The Test of Playfulness (Skard & Bundy, 2008), for children and youth ages 6 months–18 years, is an observational tool that evaluates different aspects of playfulness, including intrinsic motivation, internal control, freedom from constraints, and the ability to give and read cues.

Consider assessment tools aimed to measure environmental supports

The Test of Environmental Supportiveness (Skard & Bundy, 2008), for children and youth ages 18 months–15 years, helps to guide the occupational therapy practitioner during observations to gather information about the student's approach to play and how it is supported. The Assistance to Participate Scale (Bourke-Taylor et al., 2009) is completed by the caregiver of children ages 5–18 years and helps the practitioner to identify what support a child might need to enable participation in leisure activities. The Participation Environment Measure for Children and Youth (Coster et al., 2013) includes a web-based survey that is completed by the caregiver of children 5–18 years old. It gathers information about the level of assistance a student needs to participate in play and leisure activities.

Address Engagement Through Intervention

When establishing intervention plans to address engagement in play and leisure activities, the occupational therapy practitioner must consider the fit among the student, environment, and play or leisure activity that the student wants or needs to engage in. Because a student with a disability may have limited opportunities for engagement in play and leisure, the occupational therapy practitioner may need to educate them on choices of play and leisure activities before specific interventions can begin. Different play and leisure approaches have been identified as having high levels of evidence or emerging evidence to support their effectiveness in intervention.

Adapt the occupation

By adapting an activity, the occupational therapy practitioner is able to support a student with a disability to participate in a way that uses their existing skills while considering their challenges. Practitioners can adapt activities by changing or simplifying rules, using different equipment, using assistive technology, or creating a sport or activity with specific capacities in mind (Mackenzie & O'Toole, 2011; McDonald & Brown, 2009).

Acquire play skills

When teaching play skills, maintaining the essential characteristics of play, including keeping a balance between structure and individual choice, is important (Luckett et al., 2007). Practitioners can teach these skills through modeling, encouraging student-directed interactions, and providing opportunities for practice that is fun and motivating (McDonald & Brown, 2009; Stagnitti et al., 2012).

In a systematic review conducted by Jung and Sainato (2013), the authors found that students with autism spectrum disorder (ASD) might improve their play skills, social interactions, and behavioral responses when play activities focused on the student's strengths and interests and when students were engaged with peers. Video modeling used in combination with other approaches, such as pivotal response training, was also found to be effective. *Pivotal response training* is a naturalistic intervention that is based on identifying motivators, providing multiple cues, and encouraging self-management and social initiation (Pierce & Schreibman, 1997).

Despite the stark contrast between the principles of behavioral approaches and the characteristics of play, Luckett et al. (2007) found some evidence that behavioral approaches were effective in changing students' disposition toward play. However, the procedures used varied from the traditional behavioral approach in that

- The practitioners scaffolded the activities by building on students' existing skills,
- Reinforcement was generated by the activity itself rather than external rewards, and
- Students learned to self-monitor.

Engagement in play-based intervention with peers has been found to promote play and social skills among students with and without disabilities. Arbesman et al. (2013) provided evidence that children who experienced abuse or neglect demonstrated improvements in play skills, social–emotional development, and behavioral responses, along with decreases in solitary play, after participation in a playgroup. For children diagnosed with ASD, *integrated playgroups,* in which novice players were paired with expert players, were found to significantly improve children's symbolic and social play (Wolfberg et al., 2015). The goal of this intervention was to engage students in mutually meaningful play experiences that enhanced capacity for socialization, communication, imagination, and play. The activities were guided by a qualified adult who adjusted the amount of support provided on the basis of students' abilities to successfully mediate their own experiences (Wolfberg et al., 2015).

Similarly, *peer-mediated interventions,* which occur in the context of mixed playgroups that include children with and without a disability, resulted in improved responsiveness to peers and behavior for both groups (Frolek Clark & Kingsley, 2013). Improved play skills and social outcomes for children with disabilities were also found. In these groups, students without a disability received training on how to support learning, behavior, and social interactions for students with a disability (Garrison-Harrell et al., 1997; Laushey & Heflin, 2000). Last, play-based interventions that involved pairing a child with attention deficit hyperactivity disorder with a familiar, typically developing child and facilitating play interactions between them resulted in improved play and social skills, which were sustained over time (Wilkes et al., 2011, 2014a, 2014b).

Play-based programs, such as the Learn to Play program, support the development of self-initiated pretend play skills, social interaction, and language (Stagnitti et al., 2012). The program includes video modeling, themed play areas, adult modeling and facilitation, talk about play, imitation, and repetition.

Promote participation

Arbesman et al. (2013) found strong evidence to support the use of social skills programs and engagement in play, leisure, and recreational activities to improve social participation and social skills for children with developmental delays, intellectual disabilities, and learning disabilities. Carter and Hughes (2005) found that students with disabilities who participated in recreation, leisure, and physical education with peers improved in the area of social interaction. Shikako-Thomas et al. (2012) discovered that when students with cerebral palsy (CP) participated in physically active leisure activities, their physical and psychosocial well-being improved. Engaging in meaningful and adapted leisure activities that consider the student's skills and preferences may enhance their QoL.

Create opportunities

When music is incorporated into play, students with intellectual and language impairments can improve social skills and attention to peers (Arbesman et al., 2013). For students with ASD, researchers found that using a structured approach that included social rules, assignment of roles, opportunities to share, and team problem solving to build different LEGO® structures resulted in improvements in social interaction and a decrease in social challenges (LeGoff & Sherman, 2006; Owens et al., 2008).

For children with CP, the use of virtual reality as an intervention approach was found to be effective in promoting playfulness, pleasure, and motivation (Laufer & Weiss, 2011). This approach encouraged engagement in play that resulted in motivation to explore and to practice repetitive activities that supported skill acquisition. For typically developing children ages 5–7 years, playground activities that included opportunities to play with nontraditional items (e.g., recycled materials) were found to have a significant effect on playfulness (Bundy et al., 2008).

Engagement in nature-based activities increases students' physical activity and self-esteem (Bird, 2004; Wells et al., 2007). Natural areas stimulate more diverse and creative play than standard playground play. In addition, nature-based activities are more inclusive and offer students with disabilities greater opportunities to engage in play and leisure (Bird, 2004).

Advocate, Educate, and Collaborate

Occupational therapy practitioners can advocate for and provide education regarding the importance of students' participation in play, leisure, and extracurricular activities. They can do this by sharing evidence on the benefits of recess, play, and physical activities for learning. Educating teachers and administrators on the role of occupational therapy in this area is critical. Collaboration with other school personnel, including physical education teachers, physical therapists, and playground staff, supports students who are experiencing challenges in these areas.

SUMMARY

Occupational therapy practitioners assume many roles in supporting students' participation in play, leisure, and extra-curricular activities in schools. These areas of occupation are often undervalued and overlooked, yet substantial evidence indicates that engagement in these activities results in enhanced performance in all developmental areas as well as learning. Critical to the evaluation and intervention process is consideration of the characteristics of and goodness of fit among the student, their environment, and their preferred play or leisure occupations. Advocacy, education, and collaboration can help to reframe school personnel and caregiver perceptions, attitudes, knowledge, and skills to help them understand the critical link among movement, physical and mental health, and learning.

REFERENCES

American Academy of Pediatrics. (2015). *AAP updates recommendations on obesity prevention: It's never too early to begin living a healthy lifestyle.* Retrieved from https://www.aap.org/en-us /about-the-aap/aap-press-room/pages/AAP-Updates-Recom mendations-on-Obesity-Prevention-It%27s-Never-Too-Early -to-Begin-Living-a-Healthy-Lifestyle.aspx

American Occupational Therapy Association. (2014a). Guidelines for supervision, roles, and responsibilities during the delivery of occupational therapy services. *American Journal of Occupational Therapy, 68*(Suppl. 3), S16–S22. https://doi.org/10.5014 /ajot.2014.686S03

American Occupational Therapy Association. (2014b). Occupational therapy practice framework: Domain and process (3rd ed.). *American Journal of Occupational Therapy, 68*(Suppl. 1), S1–S48. https://doi.org/10.5014/ajot.2014.682006

Arbesman, M., Bazyk, S., & Nochajski, S. M. (2013). Systematic review of occupational therapy and mental health promotion, prevention, and intervention for children and youth. *American Journal Occupational Therapy, 67*, e120–e130. https://doi .org/10.5014/ajot.2013.008359

Bird, W. (2004). *Natural fit: Can green space and biodiversity increase levels of physical activity?* Sandy, England: Royal Society for the Protection of Birds.

Bourke-Taylor, H. M., Law, M., Howie, L., & Pallant, J. F. (2009). Development of the Assistance to Participate Scale (APS) for children's play and leisure activities. *Child: Care, Health and Development, 35*, 738–745. https://doi.org/10.1111/j.1365-2214.2009.00995.x

Bruce, T., Meggitt, C., & Greenier, J. (2010). *Child care and education* (5th ed.). London: Hodder Education.

Bundy, A. C., Luckett, T., Naughton, G. A., Tranter, P. J., Wyver, S. R., Ragen, J., & Spies, G. (2008). Playful interaction: Occupational therapy for all children on the school playground. *American Journal of Occupational Therapy, 62*, 522–527. https://doi .org/10.5014/ajot.62.5.522

Carter, E. W., & Hughes, C. (2005). Increasing social interaction among adolescents with intellectual disabilities and their general education peers: Effective interventions. *Research and Practice for Persons With Severe Disabilities, 30*, 179–193. https://doi.org /10.2511/rpsd.30.4.179

Centers for Disease Control and Prevention. (2017). *Strategies for recess in schools.* Retrieved from https://www.cdc.gov/healthy schools/physicalactivity/pdf/2016_12_16_SchoolRecessStrategies _508.pdf

Children's Society. (2014). *The good childhood report 2014.* London: Author.

Coster, W., Law, M., Bedell, G., Khetani, M., Anaby, D., Teplicky, R., & Lin, C.-Y. (2013). *The Participation Environment Measure for Children and Youth: An innovative measure for home, school and community.* Hamilton, Ontario: CanChild. Retrieved from https://www.canchild.ca/en/resources/228-the-participation -and-environment-measure-for-children-and-youth-pem-cy -an-innovative-measure-for-home-school-and-community

Dahan-Oliel, N., Shikako-Thomas, K., & Majnemer, A. (2012). Quality of life and leisure participation in children with neurodevelopmental disabilities: A thematic analysis of the literature. *Quality of Life Research, 21*, 427–439. https://doi.org/10.1007 /s11136-011-0063-9

Donnelly, J. E., Hillman, C. H., Castelli, C., Etnier, J. L., Lee, S., Tomporowski, P., . . . Szabo-Reed, A. N. (2016). Physical activity, fitness, cognitive function, and academic achievement in children: A systematic review. *Medicine and Science in Sports and Exercise, 48*, 1197–1222. https://doi.org/10.1249/MSS.0000000000000901

Family and Community Services. (2015). *Play and leisure: Practice guide for occupational therapists who support people with disability.* Retrieved from https://www.adhc.nsw.gov.au/sp/delivering _disability_services/core_standards

Fitzgerald, M. H. (2010). Cultural competence. In S. J. Lane & A. C. Bundy (Eds.), *Kids can be kids: A childhood occupations approach* (pp. 194–202). Philadelphia: F. A. Davis.

Fletcher, A. C., Nickerson, P. F., & Wright, K. L. (2003). Structured leisure activities in middle childhood: Links to well-being. *Journal of Community Psychology, 31*, 641–659. https://doi.org /10.1002/jcop.10075

Frolek Clark, G., & Kingsley, K. (2013). *Occupational therapy practice guidelines for early childhood: Birth through 5 years.* Bethesda, MD: AOTA Press.

Garrison-Harrell, L., Kamps, D. M., & Kravits, T. (1997). The effects of peer networks on social-communicative behaviors for students with autism. *Focus on Autism and Other Developmental Disorders, 12*, 241–254. https://doi.org/10.1177/108835769701200406

Gill, T. (2014). The benefits of children's engagement in nature: A systematic literature review. *Children, Youth, and Environments, 24*(2), 10–34.

Hanline, M. F., Milton, S., & Phelps, P. (2010). The relationship between preschool block play and reading and maths abilities in early elementary school: A longitudinal study of children with and without disabilities. *Early Child Development and Care, 180*, 1005–1017. https://doi.org/10.1080 /03004430802671171

Henry, A. D. (2008). Assessment of play and leisure in children and adolescents. In L. D. Parham & L. S. Fazio (Eds.), *Play in occupational therapy for children* (pp. 95–125). St. Louis: Mosby Elsevier.

Hinman, C. (2003). Multicultural considerations in the delivery of play therapy services. *International Journal of Play Therapy, 12*(2), 107–122. https://doi.org/10.1037/h0088881

Holder, M. D., Coleman, B., & Sehn, Z. L. (2009). The contribution of active and passive leisure to children's well-being. *Journal of Health Psychology, 14*, 378–386. https://doi.org/10.1177 /1359105308101676

Imms, C. (2008). Children with cerebral palsy participate: A review of the literature. *Disability and Rehabilitation, 30,* 1867–1884. https://doi.org/10.1080/09638280701673542

Imms, C., Reilly, S., Carlin, J., & Dodd, K. (2008). Diversity of participation in children with cerebral palsy. *Developmental Medicine and Child Neurology, 50,* 363–369. https://doi.org/10.1111/j.1469-8749.2008.02051.x

Imms, C., Reilly, S., Carlin, J., & Dodd, K. J. (2009). Characteristics influencing participation of Australian children with cerebral palsy. *Disability and Rehabilitation, 31,* 2204–2215. https://doi.org/10.3109/09638280902971406

Individuals With Disabilities Education Improvement Act of 2004, Pub. L. 108–446, 20 U.S.C. §§ 1400–1482.

International Play Association. (2013). *Summary United Nations General Comment No. 17 on the right of the child to rest, leisure, play, recreational activities, cultural life and the arts (Article 31).* Sydney, New South Wales, Australia: Author.

Jung, S., & Sainato, D. M. (2013). Teaching play skills to young children with autism. *Journal of Intellectual Developmental Disabilities, 38*(1), 74–90. https://doi.org/10.3109/13668250.2012.732220

King, G., Law, M., King, S., Hurley, P., Hanna, S., Kertoy, M., . . . Young, N. (2004). *Children's Assessment of Participation and Enjoyment (CAPE) and Preferences for Activities of Children (PAC).* San Antonio: Harcourt Assessment.

King, G., Petrenchik, T., Law, M., & Hurley, P. (2009). The enjoyment of formal and informal recreation and leisure activities: A comparison of school-aged children with and without physical disabilities. *International Journal of Disability, Development and Education, 56,* 109–130. https://doi.org/10.1080/10349120902868558

Laufer, Y., & Weiss, P. L. (2011). Virtual reality in the assessment and treatment of children with motor impairment: A systematic review. *Journal of Physical Therapy Education, 25*(1), 59–71. https://doi.org/10.1097/00001416-201110000-00011

Laushey, K. M., & Heflin, L. J. (2000). Enhancing social skills of kindergarten children with autism through the training of multiple peers as tutors. *Journal of Autism and Developmental Disorders, 30,* 183–193. https://doi.org/10.1023/A:1005558101038

Law, M., Baptiste, S., Carswell, A., McColl, M. A., Polatajko, H., & Pollock, N. (2014). *Canadian Occupational Performance Measure* (5th ed.). Ottawa: CAOT Publications.

LeGoff, D. B., & Sherman, M. (2006). Long-term outcome of social skills intervention based on interactive LEGO© play. *Autism, 10,* 317–329. https://doi.org/10.1177/1362361306064403

Lillard, A., Lerner, M., Hopkins, E., Dore, R., Smith, E., & Palmquist, C. (2013). The impact of pretend play on children's development: A review of the evidence. *Psychological Bulletin, 19,* 1–34. https://doi.org/10.1037/a0029321

Luckett, T., Bundy, A., & Roberts, J. (2007). Do behavioural approaches teach children with autism to play or are they pretending? *Autism, 11,* 365–388. https://doi.org/10.1177/1362361307078135

Mackenzie, L., & O'Toole, G. (2011). *Occupation analysis in practice.* Hoboken, NJ: Wiley-Blackwell.

Madich, A., Polatajko, H. J., Miller, L., & Baum, C. (2004). *The Paediatric Activity Card Sort (PACS).* Ottawa: Canadian Association of Occupational Therapists.

Majnemer, A., Shevell, M., Law, M., Birnbaum, R., Chilingaryan, G., Rosenbaum, P., & Poulin, C. (2008). Participation and enjoyment of leisure activities in school-aged children with cerebral palsy. *Developmental Medicine and Child Neurology, 50,* 751–758. https://doi.org/10.1111/j.1469-8749.2008.03068.x

Massey, W. V., Stellino, M. B., Mullen, S. P., Claassen, J., & Wilkison, M. (2018). Development of the Great Recess Framework–Observational Tool to measure contextual and behavioral components of elementary school recess. *BMC Public Health, 18,* 394. https://doi.org/10.1186/s12889-018-5295-y

McDonald, R., & Brown, T. (2009). Challenging bodies: Enabling physically disabled children to participate in play. In K. Stagnitti & R. Cooper (Eds.), *Play as therapy: Assessment and therapeutic interventions* (pp. 205–217). London: Jessica Kingsley.

Neumayer, B., & Wilding, C. (2004). Leisure as commodity. In G. Whiteford & V. Wright-St. Clair (Eds.), *Occupation and practice in context* (pp. 317–331). Amsterdam: Elsevier.

Office of Disease Prevention and Health Promotion. (2008). *Physical activity guidelines for Americans.* Retrieved from https://www.healthypeople.gov/2020/topics-objectives/topic/physical-activity

Ottenbacker, K. J., & Cusick, A. (1990). Goal attainment scaling as a method of clinical service education. *American Journal of Occupational Therapy, 44,* 519–525. https://doi.org/10.5014/ajot.44.6.519

Owens, G., Granader, Y. G., Humphrey, A., & Baron-Cohen, S. (2008). LEGO therapy and the social use of language programme: An evaluation of two social skills interventions for children with high functioning autism and Asperger syndrome. *Journal of Autism and Developmental Disorders, 38,* 1944–1957. https://doi.org/10.1007/s10803-008-0590-6

Pelligrini, A. D., & Holmes, R. M. (2006). The role of recess in primary school. In D. Singer, R. Golinkoff, & K. Hirsh-Pasek (Eds.), *Play = learning: How play motivates and enhances children's cognitive and social–emotional growth* (pp. 36–53). New York: Oxford University Press.

Pierce, K., & Schreibman, L. (1997). Multiple peer use of pivotal response training to increase social behaviors of classmates with autism: Results from trained and untrained peers. *Journal of Applied Behavior Analysis, 30,* 157–160. https://doi.org/10.1901/jaba.1997.30-157

Primeau, L. A. (2014). Play and leisure. In H. S. Willard & B. A. Boyt Schell (Eds.), *Willard and Spackman's occupational therapy* (12th ed., pp. 697–713). Philadelphia: Wolters Kluwer Health/Lippincott Williams & Wilkins.

Ramstetter, C. L., Murray, R., & Garner, A. S. (2010). The crucial role of recess in schools. *Journal of School Health, 80,* 517–526. https://doi.org/10.1111/j.1746-1561.2010.00537.x

Rehabilitation Act of 1973, Pub. L. 93–112, 20 U.S.C. §§ 701–7961.

Rigby, P., & Rodger, S. (2006). Developing as a player. In S. Rodger & J. Ziviani (Eds.), *Occupational therapy with children: Understanding children's occupations and enabling participation* (pp. 177–199). Oxford, England: Blackwell.

Section 504 of the Rehabilitation Act of 1973, as amended, 29 U.S.C. § 794 (2008).

Sellar, B., & Stanley, M. (2010). Leisure. In M. Curtin, M. Mollineaux, & J. Supyk-Mellson (Eds.), *Occupational therapy for physical dysfunction: Enabling occupation* (pp. 357–370). Edinburgh, Scotland: Churchill Livingstone Elsevier.

Shikako-Thomas, S., Dahan-Oliel, N., Shevell, M., Law, M., Brinbaum, P., Powlin, C., & Majneur, A. (2012). Play and be happy? Leisure participation and quality of life in school-aged children with cerebral palsy. *International Journal of Pediatrics, 2012,* 387280. https://doi.org/10.1155/2012/387280

Shikako-Thomas, K., Majnemer, A., Law, M., & Lach, L. (2008). Determinants of participation in leisure activities in children and youth with cerebral palsy: Systematic review. *Physical and*

Occupational Therapy in Pediatrics, 28, 155–169. https://doi.org/10.1080/01942630802031834

Skard, G., & Bundy, A. C. (2008). Test of Playfulness. In L. D. Parham & L. S. Fazio (Eds.), *Play in occupational therapy in children* (pp. 71–93). St. Louis: Mosby Elsevier.

Stagnitti, K. (2007). *The Child Initiated Pretend Play Assessment (ChIPPA)* [Kit]. West Brunswick, Western Australia, Australia: Co-ordinates.

Stagnitti, K. (2009). Children and pretend play. In K. Stagnitti & R. Cooper (Eds.), *Play as therapy: Assessment and therapeutic interventions* (pp. 59–69). London: Jessica Kingsley.

Stagnitti, K., O'Connor, C., & Sheppa, L. (2012). Impact of the Learn to Play program on play, social competence and language for children aged 5–8 years who attend a specialist school. *Australian Occupational Therapy Journal, 59,* 302–311. https://doi.org/10.1111/j.1440-1630.2012.01018.x

Stevenson, H. W., & Lee, S. Y. (1990). Contexts of achievement: A study of American, Chinese, and Japanese children. *Monographs of the Society for Research in Child Development, 55*(1–2), 1–123.

Sturgess, J. (2003). A model describing play as a child-chosen activity—Is this still valid in contemporary Australia? *Australian Occupational Therapy Journal, 50,* 104–108. https://doi.org/10.1046/j.1440-1630.2003.00362.x

Tanta, K. J., Deitz, J. C., White, O., & Billingsley, F. (2005). The effects of peer-play level on initiations and responses of preschool children with delayed play skills. *American Journal of Occupational Therapy, 59,* 437–445. https://doi.org/10.5014/ajot.59.4.437

United Nations. (1989). *Convention on the rights of the child.* Retrieved from www.ohchr.org/EN/ProfessionalInterest/Pages/CRC.aspx.

UN Committee on the Rights of the Child. (2013). *Convention on the rights of the child: General Comment No. 17 (2013) on the right of the child to rest, leisure, play, recreational activities, cultural life and the arts (art. 31).* Retrieved from http://docstore.ohchr.org/SelfServices/FilesHandler.ashx?enc=6QkG1d%2fPPRiCAqhKb7yhsqIkirKQZLK2M58RF%2f5F0vFw58qKy0NsTuVUIOzAukKtwGqGgFkAgArTuTdZZUuSZObAaHCoPsdppxu9L6un29TyD4Jyrk0F22kRyLCMeCVm

UN General Assembly. (2006). *Convention on the rights of persons with disabilities.* Retrieved from http://www.un.org/esa/socdev/enable/rights/convtexte.htm

U.S. Department of Education, Office of Civil Rights. (2016). *Parent and educator resource guide to Section 504 in public elementary and secondary schools.* Retrieved from https://www2.ed.gov/about/offices/list/ocr/docs/504-resource-guide-201612.pdf

U.S. Government Accountability Office. (2010). *Students with disabilities: More information and guidance could improve opportunities in physical education and athletics* (No. GA-10-519). Washington, DC: Author. Retrieved from https://www.gao.gov/assets/310/305770.pdf

Wells, N. M., Ashdown, S. P., Davies, E. H. S., Cowett, F. D., & Yang, Y. (2007). Environment, design, and obesity: Opportunities for interdisciplinary collaborative research. *Environment and Behavior, 39*(1), 6–33. https://doi.org/10.1177/0013916506295570

Welsh, B., Jarvis, S., Hammal, D., & Colver, A. (2006). How might districts identify local barriers to participation for children with cerebral palsy? *Public Health, 120,* 167–175. https://doi.org/10.1016/j.puhe.2005.04.006

Wilkes, S., Cordier, R., Bundy, A., Docking, K., & Munro, N. (2011). A play-based intervention for children with ADHD: A pilot study. *Australian Occupational Therapy Journal, 58,* 231–240. https://doi.org/10.1111/j.1440-1630.2011.00928.x

Wilkes-Gillan, S., Bundy, A., Cordier, R., & Lincoln, M. (2014a). Eighteen-month follow-up of a play-based intervention to improve the social play skills of children with attention deficit hyperactivity disorder. *Australian Occupational Therapy Journal, 61,* 299–307. https://doi.org/10.1111/1440-1630.12124

Wilkes-Gillan, S., Bundy, A., Cordier, R., & Lincoln, M. (2014b). Evaluation of a pilot parent-delivered play-based intervention for children with attention deficit hyperactivity disorder. *American Journal of Occupational Therapy, 68,* 700–709. https://doi.org/10.5014/ajot.2014.012450

Wolfberg, P., DeWitt, M., Young, G. S., & Nguyen, T. (2015). Integrated play groups: Promoting symbolic play and social engagement with typical peers in children with ASD across settings. *Journal of Autism Developmental Disorders, 45,* 830–845. https://doi.org/10.1007/s10803-014-2245-0

Wolfgang, C. H., Stannard, L. L., & Jones, I. (2001). Block play performance among preschoolers as a later school achievement in mathematics. *Journal of Research in Childhood Education, 15,* 173–189. https://doi.org/10.1080/02568540109594958

World Health Organization. (2004). *Global strategy on diet, physical activity and health.* Geneva: Author.

World Health Organization. (2007). *International classification of functioning, disability and health–Children and youth version.* Geneva: Author.

Yogman, M., Garner, A., Hutchinson, J., Hirsh-Pasek, K., & Michnick Golinkoff, R. (2018). The power of play: A pediatric role in enhancing development in young children. *Pediatrics, 142,* 1–16. https://doi.org/10.1542/peds.2018-2058

Best Practices in Driver's Education to Enhance Participation

52

Miriam Monahan, OTD, OTR/L, CDRS, CDI, and Sherrilene Classen, PhD, MPH, OTR/L, FAOTA, FGSA

KEY TERMS AND CONCEPTS

- Advanced driver-assistance system
- Certified driver rehabilitation specialist
- Comprehensive driving evaluation
- Driver rehabilitation specialist
- Hand controls
- In-vehicle information system
- Michon's model of driver behavior
- Operational level
- Pedal guard
- Steering knob
- Strategic level
- Tactical level

OVERVIEW

Teens and young adults typically view getting a driver's license as a right. At an age when assimilating with peers is paramount, teens and young adults with disabilities may perceive earning a driver's license as an important affirmation that they are part of the larger peer group. However, driving remains a privilege that brings independence in mobility as well as risks of adverse events that may range in severity.

To be fit to drive, teens and young adults need to acquire and become proficient in a unique set of visual, cognitive, and motor skills as well as have a foundation of predriving life skills, which include independence in community skills critical for driving (e.g., safely crossing a busy street as a pedestrian; Classen et al., 2013). Without this skill set, adverse events, such as motor vehicle crashes, are the unfortunate and often fatal outcome, as reflected in national statistics of crashes involving teenagers and young adults.

Teen drivers (ages 16–19 years) are 3 times more likely to be involved in a crash than all other age groups (Insurance Institute for Highway Safety, 2016). In 2015, 2,333 teens died (6 deaths per day) and 221,000 were treated and released from emergency rooms as a result of motor vehicle crashes. The crash rates among teen drivers are attributed to various factors, such as novice skills, risk-taking behaviors, peer pressure, and inexperience with recognizing and managing hazards (Centers for Disease Control and Prevention, 2017).

ESSENTIAL CONSIDERATIONS

Several important considerations affect driving as an occupation of teens and young adults with medical conditions or disabilities, such as attention deficit hyperactivity disorder (ADHD), autism spectrum disorder (ASD), spina bifida and hydrocephalus (SBH), and cerebral palsy (CP).

Teens and Young Adults With ADHD and ASD

ADHD is characterized by impaired
- Motor inhibition;
- Attention to task; and
- Executive function (EF), in particular decreased selective attention, impulse control, and judgment (National Institute of Mental Health, 2016).

ASD is characterized by impaired
- Motor coordination (Reed, 2014);
- Interpretation of nonverbal cues; and
- EF, in particular attention shifting (i.e., shifting attention from one stimulus to another), sequencing, and planning (Hill, 2004).

Driving can be challenging for people with ADHD and ASD, because the task requires a level of proficiency with the above-mentioned client factors and performance skills.

ADHD

Teens with ADHD have a 36% higher crash risk and are more likely to engage in risk-taking behaviors, such as driving under the influence of alcohol or drugs, speeding, and driving without a driver's license, than neurotypical peers (Curry, Metzger, et al., 2017; Fischer et al., 2007). The main determinant of risk-taking behaviors among these teens is impaired EFs (Barkley, 2004). Given that their neurotypical peers have the highest population-based crash rate of all groups, the crash propensity of teens with ADHD becomes especially noteworthy, because ADHD presents characteristics that may further impair fitness-to-drive capabilities.

ASD

Approximately 1 in 3 teens with high-functioning ASD (no cognitive impairment) will become licensed drivers by age 21, a rate lower than their peers (83.5%; Curry, Yerys,

Copyright © 2019 by the American Occupational Therapy Association. All rights reserved. To reuse this content, contact www.copyright.com.
https://doi.org/10.7139/2019.978-1-56900-591-0.052

et al., 2017). The process of learning to drive can be more challenging for teens and young adults with ASD, and they may require an extended training period to earn their drivers' license. Once licensed to drive, drivers with ASD self-report more traffic violations than their peers (Daly et al., 2014). The violations may be due in part to difficulty locating and recognizing hazards (Sheppard et al., 2016). The literature is too sparse to make conclusive statements, and much needs to be researched in terms of teens with ASD and driving (Classen & Monahan, 2013).

Dual diagnosis of ASD and ADHD

Teens with co-occurring symptoms of ASD and ADHD may also be at greater risk than their neurotypical peers. Huang et al. (2012) surveyed parents of teens with high-functioning ASD ($N = 297$) about their child's driving status. Approximately half of the parents reported that their child had a dual diagnosis of ASD–ADHD; within that group, more than half reported that their child was a licensed driver.

No primary studies have been published in the English-language literature over the past 10 years to make known the driving risk of teens with this dual diagnosis. However, Classen et al. (2013) found that teens with a dual diagnosis of ASD and ADHD made a greater number of driving errors than neurotypical peers when tested on a driving simulator.

Teens and Young Adults With SBH and CP

SBH is characterized by impaired
- Neurological functioning, which may include complete or incomplete lower extremity (LE) paralysis;
- Memory;
- Attention;
- Visual perception; and
- EF, in particular impaired sequencing, planning, and judgment (Reed, 2014).

CP is characterized by impaired
- Neurological functioning, which may include deficits in motor coordination;
- Memory;
- Attention;
- Visual information processing; and
- EF, in particular impaired attention shifting and planning (Reed, 2014).

Driving can be challenging for people with SBH and CP because the task requires a level of proficiency with the above-mentioned client factors and performance skills.

Teens and young adults with SBH or CP may be at greater risk for a crash in the first years of driving than healthy control participants, despite driving fewer miles (Simms, 1991). Lafrance et al. (2017) surveyed 74 occupational therapists and certified driver rehabilitation specialists (CDRSs) about training people with SBH and CP to drive. The authors identified a longer learning-to-drive duration because of information processing and EF skill deficits, as opposed to learning adaptive driving controls (e.g., hand controls). In addition, 50% of the respondents identified a need for occupational therapists to address predriving or life skills before people with SBH and CP begin learning to drive (Lafrance et al., 2017).

Although the literature on teens with ADHD, ASD, SBH, and CP is limited, these studies suggest that within the

population of drivers, teen drivers are at the highest risk for motor vehicle crashes and fatalities, and teens with medical conditions may experience an even greater risk. It is crucial that occupational therapists are involved in the screening, assessment, and intervention planning of teens' fitness-to-drive abilities. Such actions will help to facilitate driver fitness, mitigate risks, and reverse the death and injury statistics of this population.

Vehicle Technology Advances

With the advent of the autonomous vehicle, society is standing on the brink of a transportation revolution. The last time society faced a similar transformation was between 1903 and 1904, when the Model T Ford automobile started replacing the horse and carriage (Kennedy, 2018). Just as the horseless carriage brought disquiet to society, a similar disruption is expected from autonomous vehicles. Teens and young adults—the segment of the population who are natural assimilators of technology—may very well be the early adopters of the autonomous vehicle. Although autonomous vehicles are becoming a reality, self-driving cars may not be fully integrated until 2030 (Bhuiyan, 2016; Society of Automotive Engineers, 2014).

Two features already included in standard vehicles—advanced driver-assistance systems (ADAS) and in-vehicle information systems (IVIS)—may hold benefits for teen driving. Teens typically have challenges with hazard anticipation, hazard detection, and hazard mitigation (Deery & Fildes, 1999), which may be offset by ADAS and IVIS.

ADAS is an integrated system that can directly help the driver with the control of the vehicle, especially in high-risk situations. These systems may include features, such as an automatic braking system, to help with hazard detection and hazard mitigation (Wilschut, 2009). Likewise, ***IVIS***—technologies aimed at providing information to the driver on traffic congestion or navigation—may help with hazard anticipation. Although these technologies are meant to enhance a driver's control of the vehicle, they are not a replacement for a knowledgeable and attentive driver. Therefore, the increasing availability of ADAS and IVIS may dramatically reduce teen road crashes; however, empirical studies are necessary to support this assumption.

BEST PRACTICES

Occupational therapy practitioners[1] in school systems can play a vital role in identifying teens and young adults who are at risk for pursuing driving, making the appropriate

---

[1]*Occupational therapy practitioner* refers to both the occupational therapist and the occupational therapy assistant. The American Occupational Therapy Association (AOTA; 2014a, p. S18) states, "The occupational therapist is responsible for all aspects of occupational therapy service delivery and is accountable for the safety and effectiveness of the occupational therapy service delivery process" and "must be directly involved in the delivery of services during the initial evaluation and regularly throughout the course of intervention. . . . The occupational therapy assistant delivers safe and effective occupational therapy services under the supervision of and in partnership with the occupational therapist."

referral to driver education, and preparing students for driving through targeted and tailored interventions.

Identify Teens' and Young Adults' Fitness to Drive

To help practitioners understand the complexities of fitness to drive among teens and young adults, we propose the following 4-step framework:
1. Apply a conceptual model to underscore the theoretical postulates of fitness to drive.
2. Understand the client factors and performance skills necessary for fitness to drive.
3. Identify evidence-based assessments to predict fitness to drive.
4. Understand which life skills are prerequisites for teens and young adults who want to learn to drive.

Apply a conceptual model

Driving can be operationalized with Michon's (1989) model of driver behavior. *Michon's model of driver behavior* is a human factors model that defines driving as a hierarchical task occurring on 3 levels:
1. Operational,
2. Tactical, and
3. Strategic.

The *operational level* is basic vehicle control inherent in all routine driving tasks, such as staying in the lane and controlling the vehicle through a turn, down a hill, or during a lane change (Michon, 1989). Skills acquired in driver's education are primarily at the operational level. The *tactical level* requires the driver to make decisions and carry out vehicle maneuvers while driving, such as avoiding obstacles, deciding when to pass during a lane change, and adjusting speed in the context of the driving environment (Michon, 1989). The *strategic level* involves decisions made before driving and requires skills for trip planning (e.g., trip goals, route selection, time of day to drive, risks involved, with whom to drive; Michon, 1989).

When skills at the operational level (lowest level of the hierarchy) are impaired, they can impair the higher level tactical and strategic skills. However, deficits at the tactical and strategic levels may not impair operational skills. The level effect is an important consideration, especially because deficits in the tactical and strategic skills might not be observed during driver's education or driver's licensing examinations. However, such deficits may impair fitness to drive.

Understand client factors and performance skills

For a teen or young adult to be competent with tasks associated with each of Michon's (1989) hierarchical levels, they need to master client factors (e.g., attention, planning, binocular vision abilities, movement functions) and performance skills (e.g., navigational and social relations). Tables 52.1 and 52.2 list client factors and performance skills associated with teens' and young adults' fitness to drive, with examples of potential driving errors that may occur when mastery is not achieved. Knowledge of these client factors (Table 52.1) and performance skills (Table 52.2) will help

occupational therapy practitioners to identify fitness-to-drive challenges among teens and young adults and enable practitioners to articulate such concerns to parents and school administrators.

Identify evidence-based assessment tools

Driving performance tests predictive of fitness to drive for the teen population, and specifically for teens with medical conditions, are extremely limited (Classen & Monahan, 2013). Because of this lack of predictive measurement tools, many occupational therapists practicing in driver rehabilitation have been administering assessments designed for adult and older adult drivers when evaluating the teen population. Two examples are the Clock Test (Freund et al., 2004) and the Trail Making Test Part B (Reitan, 1958), which are not age normed for teens and thus are not generalizable to this population.

School occupational therapists commonly administer tools that can be used to assess fitness to drive among the teen population (Table 52.3). Although the list of assessments is limited for teens with special needs, further research is ongoing to develop tests that may be sensitive and specific to the driving fitness of teens with special needs.

Understand predriving life skills

Many of the motor and process skills that are prerequisites for driving are also inherent in ADLs and IADLs. One could argue that before learning to drive, a teen or young adult should be able to independently navigate familiar surroundings, cross busy streets, and interact with strangers. The teen or young adult should be able to prioritize, sequence, organize, and attend to complex tasks, such as preparing a meal or building a construction project. Likewise, the teen or young adult should be able to evaluate an emergency situation at home or in the community and determine which resources, strategies, and steps are needed to manage the emergency (Monahan, 2012). Occupational therapists may use life skills assessments, such as the Vineland–3 (Sparrow et al., 2016), to identify whether the teen or young adult has achieved the necessary predriving life skills.

Make the Appropriate Referral for Driver Education

School occupational therapists may refer a teen or young adult to a *driver rehabilitation specialist* (DRS) for a comprehensive driving evaluation (CDE), which includes a battery of clinical and behind-the-wheel assessments. Alternatively, they might refer students to a driving school instructor for driver's education. Understanding the roles and credentials of these professionals will further elucidate the path for appropriate referrals.

DRS

A *DRS* provides driver rehabilitation services for people with disabilities who may have impaired visual, cognitive, or physical abilities. These professionals may include occupational therapy practitioners, driving school instructors,

TABLE 52.1.   Client Factors and Potential Driving Challenges

CLIENT FACTORS	EXAMPLES OF DRIVING ERRORS
Mental Functions	
Attention	Teens and young adults who have difficulty with sustained attention, divided attention, or selective attention may have absent or delayed reactions to driving environments. They may be unable to sustain attention on quiet roadways; have difficulty shifting attention from one stimulus to the next; or be challenged by distractors in the environment, such as pedestrians on the sidewalk or passengers in the car.
Judgment	Judgment impairments can be associated with distracted, drunk, or drugged driving. In addition, impulsivity may lead to driving at higher speeds or entering into intersections before assessing the traffic and its complexities.
Problem solving	Teens and young adults with limitations in problem solving may not be able to manage a vehicle breakdown, negotiate unsafe road conditions, or take actions to overcome getting lost.
Mental functions of sequencing complex movement	To avoid debris in the road, a driver may need to check the adjacent lane, adjust their speed, and carry out the steps of a lane change. Teens and young adults with difficulty sequencing complex movements may make a lane change in this situation before looking to see whether the adjacent lane is clear.
Processing speed	Teens and young adults with delayed processing speed may have slowed reactions to traffic lights, regulatory signs, slowing or stopped vehicles, and vehicles entering intersections.
Visual Functions	
Acuity	Teens and young adults with visual acuity impairments may have difficulty reading signs and seeing brake lights or traffic lights.
Visual field	An impaired visual field can limit drivers' ability to see critical roadway information. Size and location of the visual field defect may result in varying degrees of impairment.
Binocular vision	Teens and young adults with impaired binocular vision, such as those with monocular vision, impaired depth perception, or misaligned eyes, may have difficulty maintaining the vehicle in the lane, judging safe gaps in traffic at intersections and during lane changes, or executing parking and backing maneuvers.
Saccadic eye movements	Teens and young adults with impaired targeting accuracy, latency, or nystagmus (i.e., involuntary rapid eye movement) during saccadic eye movements (i.e., glancing at targets) may have difficulty with maintaining their lane position during a lane change because of the demands on saccadic eye movements.
Additional Sensory Functions	
Proprioceptive functions	Teens and young adults with impaired proprioception in the right ankle or knee may have difficulty locating the pedals without visual compensation. Impaired proprioception in the upper extremities may cause difficulty locating the wiper and turn signals or other controls without glancing at the controls.
Touch functions	Teens and young adults with impaired tactile sensation in the right LE may have difficulty applying appropriate pressure on the pedals and locating the pedals without visual compensation.
Neuromusculoskeletal and Movement-Related Functions	
Joint mobility	Teens and young adults with limited range of motion in their spine or UEs or LEs may have difficulty operating standard vehicle equipment. For example, a teen with limited spine rotation may be unable to use side mirrors or turn to check the blind spot during a lane change. A teen with limited shoulder flexion may have difficulty reaching the steering wheel. A teen with limited ankle inversion and eversion may have difficulty effectively moving between the pedals for adequate brake reaction.
Muscle Functions	
Muscle power	For teens and young adults with strength impairments, the resistance of standard vehicle operating equipment (e.g., power steering, electronic pedals) may prove to be too great. Thus, the person may not have the strength to apply the brake fully or rotate the steering wheel adequately.
Movement Functions	
Motor reflexes	A bump in the road or a siren may cause teens with a startle reflex, such as in cerebral palsy, to lose control of the vehicle (Hegberg, 2012). An asymmetric tonic neck reflex may cause a teen to inadvertently change lanes when performing an over-the-shoulder check.

Note. Client factors were selected from the *Occupational Therapy Practice Framework: Domain and Process* (3rd ed.; American Occupational Therapy Association, 2014b). LE = lower extremity; UE = upper extremity.

TABLE 52.2.   Performance Skills and Potential Driving Challenges

PERFORMANCE SKILLS	EXAMPLES OF DRIVING ERRORS
Process Skills	
Navigates	Teens and young adults with navigational impairments may be unable to negotiate their way out of a parking lot or find routine destinations in their community.
Adjusts	Teens and young adults with challenges adjusting to changes in the driving environment may have difficulty negotiating a road closure.
Motor Skills	
Calibrates	Teens and young adults may have difficulty with negotiating hills, curves, and right and left turns. For example, the teen may be unable to regulate the speed or turn the steering wheel to the appropriate rotation (i.e., motor response) to match the degree of a turn on the road (i.e., visual input; Classen et al., 2013).
Paces	Teens and young adults may have difficulty with pacing and timing a motor response, which might cause them to enter intersections with inappropriate speed for the pace of traffic or have ineffective timing.
Communication or Social Interaction Skills	
Notices and responds	Teens and young adults with limitations in nonverbal communication may exhibit 2 problems. First, they may not effectively interpret other road users' actions, particularly when other road users do not follow rules, such as failing to use their turn signal. Second, they may not anticipate how the other drivers or pedestrians may perceive their actions.
Takes turns	Teens and young adults with limitations in social relations may have difficulty coordinating actions with other road users, such as those required for merging lanes or clearing a path in a congested parking lot.

Note. Performance skills were selected from the *Occupational Therapy Practice Framework: Domain and Process* (3rd ed.; American Occupational Therapy Association, 2014b).

driving educators, rehabilitation engineers, and others (Dickerson & Schold Davis, 2012). There are no required training courses to become a DRS. However, some DRSs may elect to enroll in workshops, attend conferences, be mentored on the job, or enroll in a university-based certificate program (e.g., University of Florida; see https://drt.ot.phhp.ufl.edu/).

Some DRSs pursue credentialing to become a ***CDRS*** through the Association for Driver Rehabilitation Specialists (ADED). To become a CDRS, the candidate needs to qualify, with designated years of experience in driver rehabilitation, before taking and passing the certification examination. The expertise of a CDRS can vary. Some CDRSs have evaluation and intervention skills to address the needs of medically at-risk licensed drivers, whereas others may also have expertise with novice drivers (Dickerson & Schold Davis, 2012).

In addition, the expertise of a CDRS or DRS may include
- Knowledge of vehicle equipment assessment,
- Driver training for operating the equipment, and
- Vehicle prescription.

For example, the CDRS may evaluate a teen with spastic diplegia CP with clinical assessments, in addition to an on-road assessment with a specially equipped vehicle.

After the clinical and on-road assessments, the CDRS may recommend that the teen drive with the following equipment:
- ***Hand controls*** (operate the accelerator and brake with the right or left UE)
- ***Steering knob*** (enables single-handed steering)
- ***Pedal guards*** (prevent inadvertent acceleration or braking in the event of an LE spasm in which the foot that is not supposed to be in use comes in contact with the gas or brake pedal; Hegberg, 2012).

The CDRS or DRS may provide the teen with training in operation of the equipment and write a prescription for a vehicle modifier to install equipment in the teen's or family's personal vehicle (ADED, 2016). Some vehicle

TABLE 52.3.   Off-Road Driving Assessments for Teens

ASSESSMENT	RELATED EVIDENCE
Beery–Buktenica Developmental Test of Visual–Motor Integration (Beery et al., 2010)	For teens with ADHD or ASD, poor scores are associated with more driving errors and difficulty with basic vehicle maneuvers (Classen et al., 2013).
Bruininks–Oseretsky Test of Motor Proficiency–Short Form (Bruininks & Bruininks, 2005)	For teens with ADHD or ASD, poor scores are associated with visual scanning errors, such as failing to appropriately scan an intersection before proceeding (Classen et al., 2013).

Note. ADHD = attention deficit hyperactivity disorder; ASD = autism spectrum disorder.

modifiers require a CDRS designation to fill a vehicle prescription.

A CDE is the industry gold standard for driving evaluation and is conducted by a CDRS. The **CDE** entails the use of evidence-based clinical tests and an on-road, in-traffic assessment to evaluate a person's fitness-to-drive capabilities (Di Stefano & Macdonald, 2005). The CDE has 3 possible outcomes:

1. The person passes the on-road assessment, which suggests that they are fit to drive.
2. The person fails the on-road assessment, which suggests that they are unfit to drive.
3. The person requires remediation, which suggests that rehabilitation is necessary before they can be deemed fit to drive (Classen & Monahan, 2013).

Driving school instructors

Driving school instructors provide driver education and training courses. The curriculum includes traffic laws and regulations, skills for hazard avoidance, and an understanding of responsibilities inherent in driving a vehicle. Courses encompass classroom and in-car training (U.S. Department of Transportation, 2017). Some DRSs and CDRSs are also credentialed as driving school instructors. The DRS or CDRS who is credentialed as a driving school instructor is well

positioned to provide the driver education component to teens and young adults with special needs (Monahan, 2012).

When deciding the best course for driver education, occupational therapy practitioners can be aided through the use of a decision tree (see Figure 52.1). When using the decision tree, one needs to recognize that skill deficits can be impairments related to client factors, performance skills, or predriving life skills. These deficits are identified through formal assessment tools and observations. For example, when an occupational therapy practitioner in a school identifies a teen with

- Client factor limitations (e.g., shows limitations in attention, judgment, or problem solving),
- Performance skill limitations (e.g., paces, adjusts, notices, responds), or
- Predriving life skill limitations (e.g., bumps into others when walking in a hallway with a backpack; requires assistance to plan, organize, and sequence school tasks),

they may determine that the teen is not fit to drive.

The next step is to determine whether driving is an appropriate goal in the future. A "yes" answer is appropriate when the teen is likely to benefit from interventions and compensatory strategies to improve and manage the noted deficits and achieve the necessary predriving life skills. A "no" answer is appropriate when the teen is unlikely to benefit from interventions and strategies to facilitate fitness to drive.

For the teen who is a future candidate for driving, the next step for the occupational therapist is to determine what

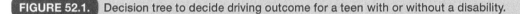

FIGURE 52.1.   Decision tree to decide driving outcome for a teen with or without a disability.

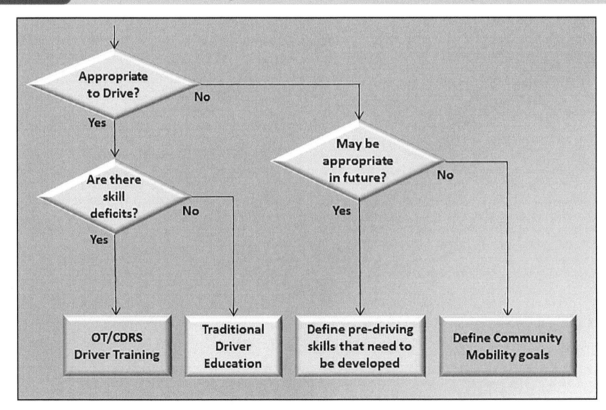

Note. CDRS = certified driver rehabilitation specialist; OT = occupational therapist.

Source. From *Administration and Interpretation of Tests Predicting Driving Errors in Teens With ADHD/ASD Compared to Healthy Controls* [Online continuing education], by M. Monahan and S. Classen, 2012. Gainesville: University of Florida, Department of Occupational Therapy. Used with permission.

predriving life skills need to be developed and to create an intervention plan accordingly. For the teen who is not a candidate for driving in the future, the next step is to determine the appropriate community mobility goals and interventions. Some states provide driver's education in the public school curriculum. In these states, occupational therapy practitioners can advocate for specialized training in the student's individualized education program or Section 504 plan.

Prepare Students for Driving

Activities that increase the potential for driving by addressing client factors, performance skills, and predriving life skills can be incorporated into school settings (see Tables 52.4 and 52.5). School occupational therapy practitioners can use these activities to improve students' driver fitness. These activities can be introduced as early as elementary school

TABLE 52.4. Activities to Improve Driver Fitness in the School Setting

| ACTIVITY | GRADED FOR COMPLEXITY | | RELEVANCE TO DRIVING |
	SIMPLE	COMPLEX	
Navigating school parking lot	While walking through the parking lot, the student identifies when vehicles are backing or braking by the vehicle's motion and lights (e.g., reverse, brake). The practitioner asks the student to identify when the drivers are aware of the student's presence (e.g., driver's eye gaze, vehicle motions).	While walking through the parking lot, the student identifies what the hazards are in the parking lot, classifies them as low or high hazards, and selects the response to the hazard (e.g., stop, continue to walk, move away).	Drivers need to recognize hazards on the roadway and respond appropriately to the level of urgency. Drivers need to anticipate and recognize the actions and intentions of other drivers.
Managing time	The student receives support to manage a daily planner for class schedules and assignments. With support, the student records the time it takes to complete assignments.	The student manages their daily planner and estimates the time it will take to complete assignments. The student records the actual time it takes to complete. Using knowledge of how long the assignment actually took, the student estimates the time to complete other assignments. The practitioner can introduce the concept of adjusting for time on the basis of complexity of the assignments.	In route planning, drivers need to anticipate the time it will take to reach a destination on the basis of traffic and weather conditions to arrive on time for work and appointments.
Planning and executing emergency procedures	The practitioner has the student make a personalized emergency phone list. The student identifies adults (e.g., neighbors, relatives), community emergency services (e.g., police, fire department), and professionals (e.g., doctors) who should be on the list. The practitioner describes different emergency scenarios and asks the student whom they would contact.	The practitioner reviews public safety materials. The student role-plays emergency scenarios.	Drivers need to anticipate and manage emergencies, such as the vehicle's breaking down, being involved in a crash, or getting lost.
Cooperation in sports and games	Students toss a ball to one another on the basis of whose name is called by the occupational therapy practitioner. Students are directed to toss to others only when the receiver of the ball seems ready.	The students run down a field or in the gym, kicking a soccer ball back and forth to each other. The students' goal is to see how many passes they can make to one another before they reach the end of the field or gym.	Drivers need to interact with other drivers by recognizing actions of other drivers, timing responses, or sequentially initiating motor responses at an adequate pace.
Project-based classes: woodshop or culinary arts classes	The student selects an item to make. The student prepares a list of supplies that they will need and takes inventory of items available. Using a provided list of the steps, the student adds details related to their setting.	The student selects an item to make, considering whether they have the time and supplies to complete the task. Students are involved in problem solving when items are not available to complete their project, deciding how to acquire those items or identifying reasonable substitutes.	Drivers need to plan the route to reach a destination in an appropriate order and identify the time they will need to complete the trip. The driver needs to use clear communication with other drivers.

TABLE 52.5. Electronic Activities to Improve Driver Fitness in the School Setting

ACTIVITY	DESCRIPTION
Drive Focus® (Drive Focus, Williston, VT)	Interactive video training that targets identification and prioritization of critical roadway information in addition to reaction speed
Tracking and Perceptual Skills for Occupational Therapists (Vision Education Seminars, Bala Cynwyd, PA)	Interactive software that targets saccadic eye movement and visual–spatial and visual–motor integration skills for children and adults
Wii Fit Plus™, Nintendo Wii (Nintendo, Redmond, WA)	Interactive software that targets bilateral UE and LE coordination, timing of motor response, speed, and steering skills for children and adults.

Note. All electronic activities can be graded from simple to complex. Inclusion in this list is not an endorsement of the product. LE = lower extremity; UE = upper extremity.

and graded to increase in complexity through high school or as the student's skills improve. Note that the activity examples are based on best practices, not empirical findings.

Obtain Professional Development in This Practice Area

Driving is a critical area of practice. School occupational therapy practitioners interested in teen and young adult driving may choose to obtain professional development related to this practice area. AOTA has several resources for transition to community mobility across the life span. The University of Florida offers online continuing education courses and a certificate in driver-rehabilitation therapy (see https://drt.ot.phhp.ufl.edu). For occupational therapy practitioners specializing in driving and community mobility, AOTA has a specialty certification that provides formal recognition of their ongoing professional development, specialized knowledge and skills, and contributions to improved client outcomes (see https://bit.ly/2AQcbbQ).

SUMMARY

Students with special needs may be at greater risk than their peers when taking on the responsibilities of being a licensed driver. School occupational therapy practitioners are uniquely positioned to identify students at risk before they pursue driving, recommend an appropriate course for drivers' education, and develop the fitness-to-drive potential of teens with special needs.

In light of limited driver fitness prediction measures for teens with special needs, occupational therapy practitioners must understand client factors, performance skills, and pre-driving skills underlying the complex task of driving. With such understanding and by using best clinical practices, best clinical reasoning, and best existing evidence, the therapist can make fitness-to-drive recommendations for this population, and the occupational therapy practitioner can implement intervention plans to help develop predriving skills.

REFERENCES

American Occupational Therapy Association. (2014a). Guidelines for supervision, roles, and responsibilities during the delivery of occupational therapy services. *American Journal of Occupational Therapy, 68*(Suppl. 3), S16–S22. https://doi.org/10.5014/ajot.2014.686S03

American Occupational Therapy Association. (2014b). Occupational therapy practice framework: Domain and process (3rd ed.). *American Journal of Occupational Therapy, 68*(Suppl. 1), S1–S48. https://doi.org/10.5014/ajot.2014.682006

Association for Driver Rehabilitation Specialists. (2016). *Best practice guidelines for the delivery of driver rehabilitation services.* Retrieved from https://cdn.ymaws.com/www.aded.net/resource/resmgr/docs/aded_bestpracticeguidelines_.pdf

Barkley, R. A. (2004). Driving impairments in teens and adults with attention-deficit/hyperactivity disorder. *Psychiatric Clinics of North America, 27,* 233–260. https://doi.org/10.1016/S0193-953X(03)00091-1

Beery, K. E., Buktenica, N., & Beery, N. (2010). *Beery–Buktenica Developmental Test of Visual–Motor Integration.* San Antonio: Psychological Corporation.

Bhuiyan, J. (2016). *The complete timeline to self-driving cars: Self-driving cars are coming. The question is when and how.* Retrieved from https://www.recode.net/2016/5/16/11635628/self-driving-autonomous-cars-timeline

Bruininks, R. H., & Bruininks, B. D. (2005). *Bruininks–Oseretsky Test of Motor Proficiency–Short Form* (2nd ed.). San Antonio: Psychological Corporation.

Centers for Disease Control and Prevention. (2017). *Teen drivers: Get the facts.* Retrieved from https://www.cdc.gov/motorvehiclesafety/teen_drivers/teendrivers_factsheet.html

Classen, S., & Monahan, M. (2013). Evidence-based review on interventions and determinants of driving performance in teens with attention deficit hyperactivity disorder or autism spectrum disorder. *Traffic Injury Prevention, 14,* 188–193. https://doi.org/10.1080/15389588.2012.700747

Classen, S., Monahan, M., & Wang, Y. (2013). Driving characteristics of teens with attention deficit hyperactivity and autism spectrum disorder. *American Journal of Occupational Therapy, 67,* 664–673. https://doi.org/10.5014/ajot.2013.008821

Curry, A. E., Metzger, K. B., Pfeiffer, M. R., Elliot, M. R., Winston, F. K., & Power, T. J. (2017). Motor vehicle crash risk among adolescents and young adults with attention-deficit/hyperactivity disorder. *JAMA Pediatrics, 171,* 756–763. https://doi.org/10.1001/jamapediatrics.2017.0910

Curry, A. E., Yerys, B. E., Huang, P., & Metzger, K. B. (2017). Longitudinal study of driver licensing rates among adolescents and young adults with autism spectrum disorder. *Autism, 22,* 479–488. https://doi.org/10.1177/1362361317699586

Daly, B. P., Nicholls, E. G., Patrick, K. E., Brinckman, D. D., & Schultheis, M. T. (2014). Driving behaviors in adults with autism spectrum disorders. *Journal of Autism and Developmental Disorders, 44,* 3119–3128. https://doi.org/10.1007/s10803-014-2166-y

Deery, H. A., & Fildes, B. N. (1999). Young novice driver subtypes: Relationship to high-risk behavior, traffic accident record, and simulator driving performance. *Human Factors, 41,* 628–643. https://doi.org/10.1518/001872099779656671

Dickerson, A. E., & Schold Davis, E. (2012). Welcome to the team! Who are the stakeholders? In M. J. McGuire & E. Schold Davis (Eds.), *Driving and community mobility: Occupational therapy strategies across the lifespan* (pp. 49–77). Bethesda, MD: AOTA Press.

Di Stefano, M., & Macdonald, W. (2005). On-the-road evaluation of driving performance. In J. M. Pellerito (Ed.), *Driver rehabilitation and community principles and practice* (pp. 255–274). St. Louis: Elsevier/Mosby.

Fischer, M., Barkley, R. A., Smallish, L., & Fletcher, K. (2007). Hyperactive children as young adults: Driving abilities, safe driving behavior, and adverse driving outcomes. *Accident Analysis and Prevention, 39,* 94–105. https://doi.org/10.1016/j.aap.2006.06.008

Freund, B., Gravenstein, S., Ferris, R., & Shaheen, E. (2004). Clock drawing test tracks progression of driving performance in cognitively impaired older adults: Case comparisons. *Clinical Geriatrics, 12*(7), 33–36.

Hegberg, A. (2012). Use of adaptive equipment to compensate for impairments in motor performance skills and client factors. In M. J. McGuire & E. Schold Davis (Eds.), *Driving and community mobility: Occupational therapy strategies across the lifespan* (pp. 279–319). Bethesda, MD: AOTA Press.

Hill, E. L. (2004). Evaluating the theory of executive dysfunction in autism. *Developmental Review, 24,* 189–233. https://doi.org/10.1016/j.dr.2004.01.001

Huang, P., Kao, T., Curry, A., & Durbin, D. R. (2012). Factors associated with driving in teens with autism spectrum disorders. *Journal of Developmental Behavior in Pediatrics, 33*(1), 70–74. https://doi.org/10.1097/DBP.0b013e31823a43b7

Insurance Institute for Highway Safety. (2016). *Teenagers: Driving carries extra risk for them.* Retrieved from http://www.iihs.org/iihs/topics/t/teenagers/fatalityfacts/teenagers

Kennedy, R. C. (2018, January 31). *The invader.* Retrieved from http://www.harpweek.com/09Cartoon/BrowseByDateCartoon.asp?Month=November&Date=9

Lafrance, M. E., Benoit, D., Dahan-Oiel, N., & Gelinas, I. (2017). Development of a driving readiness program for adolescents and young adults with cerebral palsy and spina bifida. *British Journal of Occupational Therapy, 80,* 173–182. https://doi.org/10.1177/0308022616672480

Michon, J. A. (1989). Explanatory pitfalls and rule-based driver models. *Accident Analysis and Prevention, 21,* 341–353.

Monahan, M. (2012). Evaluating and treating adolescents with special needs. In M. J. McGuire & E. Schold Davis (Eds.), *Driving and community mobility: Occupational therapy strategies across the lifespan* (pp. 383–410). Bethesda, MD: AOTA Press.

Monahan, M., & Classen, S. (Producers). (2012). *Administration and interpretation of tests predicting driving errors in teens with ADHD/ASD compared to healthy controls* [Online continuing education]. Gainesville: University of Florida, Department of Occupational Therapy.

National Institute of Mental Health. (2016). *Attention deficit hyperactivity disorder (ADHD): The basics.* Retrieved from http://www.nimh.nih.gov/health/publications/attention-deficit-hyperactivity-disorder/complete-index.shtml

Reed, K. L. (2014). *Quick reference to occupational therapy* (3rd ed.). Austin, TX: Pro-Ed.

Reitan, R. M. (1958). Validity of the Trail Making Test as an indicator of organic brain damage. *Perceptual and Motor Skills, 8,* 271–276. https://doi.org/10.2466/pms.1958.8.3.271

Sheppard, E., van Loon, E., Underwood, G., & Ropar, D. (2016). Attentional differences in a driving hazard perception task in adults with autism spectrum disorders. *Journal of Autism and Developmental Disorders, 47,* 405–414. https://doi.org/10.1007/s10803-016-2965-4

Simms, B. (1991). The car use of young drivers with spina bifida and hydrocephalus. *European Journal of Pediatric Surgery, 1*(Suppl. 1), 31–34. https://doi.org/10.1055/s-2008-1042536

Society of Automotive Engineers. (2014). *Taxonomy and definitions for terms related to on-road motor vehicle automated driving systems (J3016_201401).* Warrendale, PA: Author.

Sparrow, S. S., Cicchetti, D. V., & Saulnier, C. A. (2016). *Vineland Adaptive Behavior Scales* (3rd ed.). San Antonio: Pearson.

U.S. Department of Transportation. (2017). *Novice teen driver education and training administrative standards (NTDETAS) 2017 revision.* Washington, DC: National Highway Traffic Safety Administration.

Wilschut, E. S. (2009). *The impact of in-vehicle information systems on simulated driving performance: Effects of age, timing and display characteristics* (Unpublished doctoral dissertation). University of Groningen, the Netherlands.

Best Practices in Enhancing Social Participation

Lisa Crabtree, PhD, OTR/L, FAOTA, and Lorienne Watson, MOT, DrOT, OTR/L

53

KEY TERMS AND CONCEPTS

- Environment-focused intervention
- Peer-mediated intervention
- Social participation
- Supportive context

Just because a child may not be able to speak doesn't mean that he has nothing to say. Just because a person may be overwhelmed in social situations doesn't mean that she doesn't long for friendship. Just because someone has difficulty initiating movement doesn't mean that he doesn't want to participate.—Hussman (2018, p. 1)

OVERVIEW

Social participation is the "interweaving of occupations to support desired engagement in community and family activities as well as those involving peers and friends" (Gillen & Boyt Schell, 2014, cited in American Occupational Therapy Association [AOTA], 2014b, p. S21). Social skills are complex and central to participation, and they develop over a life span of experiences (Orsmond et al., 2013; Tonkin et al., 2014). Interpersonal, communication, decision-making, and problem-solving skills are all critical for participation in school occupations (Kauffman & Kinnealey, 2015).

Occupational therapy practitioners[1] identify social participation as an occupation that supports engagement in activities with one's family, friends, peers, and the community (AOTA, 2014b). To engage in social participation activities with teachers, peers, and other members of the school community, students need to have adequate social skills. They need knowledge of the social and cultural context to participate in a given activity, such as understanding the rules of a game or the expectations of other participants.

Basic social interaction skill components include
- Approaches to start conversations;
- An understanding of nonverbal gestures or looks;
- Fluency in speaking, asking, and responding to questions;
- An ability to take turns in conversations;
- Self-regulation; and
- An understanding of emotional expressions.

Positive social participation experiences in school can contribute to students' social well-being and influence their self-confidence in social interactions in the community (Koegel et al., 2012; Kramer et al., 2012; Tonkin et al., 2014).

Children develop social engagement through early interactions with caregivers by participating in joint attention activities. Typically developing children learn strategies to initiate social interactions with peers, respond appropriately to others, and resolve conflicts while engaging in social play (Case-Smith, 2013). By middle and high school, typically developing students become adept at interpreting and understanding nonverbal cues and gestures, interacting with peers through social media networks, navigating romantic relationships, collaborating with peers on group projects, and communicating effectively with adults (Huyder et al., 2017).

Children and youth with language, motor, and social challenges often do not engage in these typical developmental activities and have fewer opportunities to experience foundational interactions that support social participation (McMaugh, 2011; Milen & Nicholas, 2017). Without frequent, effective social interactions between child and caregiver, the children who may need the most help have fewer opportunities to practice skills to support social engagement.

When children and youth struggle to speak, move, or interact with others, caregivers often respond by meeting the child's needs preemptively, thereby limiting the opportunities for the child to learn to respond in ways that will support development of these critical skills. This process often perpetuates dependency on others for interpreting

---

[1] *Occupational therapy practitioner* refers to both the occupational therapist and the occupational therapy assistant. AOTA (2014a, p. S18) states, "The occupational therapist is responsible for all aspects of occupational therapy service delivery and is accountable for the safety and effectiveness of the occupational therapy service delivery process" and "must be directly involved in the delivery of services during the initial evaluation and regularly throughout the course of intervention. . . . The occupational therapy assistant delivers safe and effective occupational therapy services under the supervision of and in partnership with the occupational therapist."

Copyright © 2019 by the American Occupational Therapy Association. All rights reserved. To reuse this content, contact www.copyright.com.
https://doi.org/10.7139/2019.978-1-56900-591-0.053

communicative intent. Conversely, children and youth who are provided with systematic, scaffolded opportunities to learn alternative communication and social interaction strategies through embedded experiences can have better outcomes (Sutton et al., 2018).

ESSENTIAL CONSIDERATIONS

The distinct value of occupational therapy includes a focus on facilitating participation in everyday living (AOTA, 2018). Participation in all school activities requires use of fundamental social skills as well as supportive contexts that facilitate engagement with others. *Supportive contexts* include culturally appropriate activities that can be embedded in the school environment to support social engagement of children and youth. It is important for occupational therapy practitioners to understand their role in facilitating participation by supporting skill development and inclusive, culturally responsive contexts.

Characteristics That Influence Development of Social Skills

Researchers have identified characteristics that influence the development of social skills for people with mental health and behavioral challenges (e.g., autism spectrum disorder [ASD], anxiety, depression), physical disabilities (e.g., neuromotor disorders, brain injuries), and learning differences (e.g., learning disabilities, attention deficit hyperactivity disorder [ADHD], intellectual and developmental disabilities [IDD]).

In a study conducted by Little et al. (2014), school-age children with ASD participated less frequently than typically developing children in unstructured activities, social activities, and hobbies. In addition, adolescents with ASD participated less frequently in recreational and community activities (e.g., after-school clubs, scouting, 4H) than typically developing peers. The activity demands and social context seemed to be the greatest influencing factors. Activities combined with physical and social demands (e.g., swimming, visiting friends) were highly challenging for these children because of insufficient prerequisite social skills (Kramer et al., 2012).

In a study by Wilkes-Gillan et al. (2016), children with attention difficulties, such as those with ADHD, experienced greater social difficulties than typically developing children in peer-to-peer play interactions and had difficulties in several areas, including

- Sharing,
- Responding to social cues,
- Participating in cooperative play,
- Solving problems,
- Taking others' perspective,
- Exercising empathy, and
- Spontaneously performing skills.

Selanikyo et al. (2017) reported that students with IDD experienced limited participation in school activities because of difficulties in communication, choice making, and initiation. In addition, they depended significantly on others to fully participate in the school environment.

Youth with an acquired brain injury (ABI) also demonstrated challenges with social skills, such as

- Comprehension of social rules and boundaries;
- Understanding of emotions conveyed by facial expressions; and
- Pragmatic communication skills, including staying on topic, asking relevant questions, taking turns, and organizing and expressing thoughts and ideas (Agnihotri et al., 2014).

Finally, children and youth with severe physical disabilities affecting their mobility were dependent on others to move around and explore their environment, which decreased their opportunities for free play, exploration, and social interactions with peers (Guerette et al., 2013). Physical mobility challenges increased the risk of delays in communication, interaction, and socialization. Thus, occupational therapists must consider many factors when evaluating and planning social skills interventions for increased participation of students with disabilities.

Focus on Skills Acquisition

Supporting positive social participation of students with disabilities promotes academic success (Sepanski & Fisher, 2011). When students have challenges in communicating ideas or requests to others, they may express frustration, display negative behaviors, or disrupt their classroom participation to get their needs met (Koegel et al., 2012). Use of motivating activities, integration of low-tech and high-tech assistive technology (AT) solutions, various communication strategies (e.g., Picture Exchange Communication System [Bondy & Frost, 1998], visual boards, sign language), and strategies embedded into classroom programming can support social participation in a school environment (Guerette et al., 2013; Ichikawa et al., 2013; Laugeson et al., 2014; Sutton et al., 2018).

Creating Inclusive Contexts

In addition to supporting students' skills acquisition, providing supportive and inclusive social experiences can influence their social participation (Anaby et al., 2016). Occupational therapy practitioners can use group interventions to provide valuable opportunities to facilitate interactions and practice skills (Tomchek & Koenig, 2016). Also, educating typically developing peers about what it feels like to move or interact differently because of a disability provides them with an understanding of the importance of inclusion in social activities (Leigers & Myers, 2015).

Facilitating co-occupations for students in context changes the culture of the classroom by supporting inclusion of students with disabilities and creating a positive climate for learning (Leigers et al., 2016). Peer interactions provide a connection for practicing social skills and support generalization through social participation in context. Students with disabilities who experience positive peer relationships are less likely to demonstrate behavioral challenges in the classroom (Murray & Greenberg, 2006).

In addition, participation in inclusive school contexts contributes to positive outcomes for adults with disabilities (Woodman et al., 2016). Inclusive contexts require team collaboration to support success. When planning and implementing services that support social participation, occupational therapy practitioners work collaboratively with teachers, administrators, and speech–language therapists. Family collaboration also promotes generalization of skills and contributes to effective, culturally responsive intervention approaches tailored to the individual needs of children and youth.

BEST PRACTICES

Occupational therapists apply evidence-based knowledge to evaluate and provide optimal interventions to support students' social engagement. In collaboration with other team members and the family, occupational therapists determine priorities for intervention through an evaluation process that integrates interviews, observation, records review, and assessment tools, as needed. Intervention strategies are often embedded in inclusive classroom environments through naturalistic strategies that include social peer partners.

Plan and Conduct Evaluations

Evaluation of a student's social participation begins with development of an occupational profile (AOTA, 2014b, 2017) that includes a description of the student's current engagement in social situations and the communication strategies and level of social interaction skills used by the student (e.g., relaying intentions and needs, coordinating social exchanges). Depending on the student's age and context, priorities can include
- Learning basic requests,
- Sharing materials,
- Interacting in small groups, and
- Developing community-based skills (Raghavendra et al., 2012; Selanikyo et al., 2017).

Skilled observation of a student's social engagement with others in the context of the classroom, playground, cafeteria, and transition spaces (e.g., hallways, bus) provides valuable information related to barriers and affordances that occupational therapy practitioners can address (Kreider et al., 2016). In addition to skilled observation, occupational therapists can use a variety of occupation-centered assessment tools to identify specific strengths and needs. They can then integrate results of standardized testing with skilled observations to develop priorities for intervention. Table 53.1 includes a sample of assessment tools that occupational therapists can use to measure these skills to support a comprehensive evaluation process.

Provide Interventions Based on Current Research and Best Practice

Occupational therapy practitioners use evidence-based interventions to support students' social participation, including interventions that are peer mediated, activity based, social, skill focused, and environment focused. This section considers the dynamic interactions among the student's skills, the context (including physical, social, and cultural aspects), and activities in school contexts (e.g., learning, playing, taking care of needs).

Incorporate peer-mediated interventions

Peer-mediated interventions are social play opportunities between typical peers and students with disabilities that occur in the classroom, school, or community environments (Case-Smith, 2013). Occupational therapy practitioners guide activities with peers to encourage effective social participation.

TABLE 53.1. Assessment Tools to Measure Social Participation and Engagement

TOOL	DESCRIPTION
Child Occupational Self-Assessment (Keller et al., 2005)	*Age:* 6–17 years *Purpose:* A self-assessment of how competent children or youth feel engaging in and completing activities and how much they value engagement in activities.
Children's Assessment of Participation and Enjoyment; Preferences for Activities of Children (King et al., 2004)	*Age:* 6–21 years *Purpose:* A self-assessment of participation and preferences for participation for children and youth. Includes a measure of participation in social activities as well as identification of with whom the child or youth participates.
Participation and Environment Measure for Children and Youth (Coster et al., 2014)	*Age:* 5–17 years *Purpose:* An evaluation of participation and environmental factors in the home, at school, and in the community, including measures of socialization.
School Function Assessment (Coster et al., 1998)	*Age:* 5–12 years *Purpose:* A criterion-referenced tool to measure school-related academic and social skills, including participation, task supports, and activity participation.
Social Responsiveness Scale (2nd ed.; Constantino & Gruber, 2012)	*Age:* 2.5 years–adult *Purpose:* A norm-referenced measure of everyday social skills and interactions, including social awareness, social cognition, social communication, social motivation, restricted interests, and repetitive behavior. Practitioners can compare scores over time to measure intervention effectiveness
Social Skills Improvement Systems: Rating Scales (Gresham & Elliott, 2008)	*Age:* 3–18 years *Purpose:* A norm-referenced measure focused on social behavior of students that uses self-assessment, parent, and teacher forms. Has 7 subscales: Communication, Cooperation, Assertion, Responsibility, Empathy, Engagement, and Self-Control

In a systematic review, Case-Smith (2013) identified several evidenced-based peer-mediated interventions, including

- Turn-taking computer-based games to encourage social interactions,
- The use of picture activity schedules to select joint social play activities under the guidance of occupational therapy practitioners, and
- Partnerships between children with disabilities and children at a higher developmental and social competence level during classroom activities.

Tanner et al. (2015) examined the effectiveness of interventions focused on social participation, play, and leisure skills for people with ASD. In their review of peer-mediated interventions, 6 Level I studies reported gains in social skills. The overall strength of evidence for peer-mediated interventions is mixed, given that the outcomes achieved in some studies did not generalize to other contexts. Reichow and Volkmar (2010) reviewed 66 studies of interventions to increase social behavior among people with ASD to identify evidence-based practice strategies. Their review found that evidence supported the use of peer training combined with behavioral skills training strategies focused on social skills.

Engage students in occupations and activities

Interventions that incorporate engagement in the occupation of play to address students' social interactions can improve outcomes. Tanner et al. (2015) found moderate evidence to support participation of individuals with ASD in group activity–based interventions compared with solitary programs focused on development of social skills.

Wilkes-Gillan et al. (2016) conducted a randomized controlled trial of a play-based intervention designed to improve the social participation of children with ADHD. The intervention included play sessions with a typical peer, weekly home modules, and a 1-month home follow-up visit. The authors used the Test of Playfulness to measure the children's peer-to-peer play interactions. The intervention group demonstrated a significant change in their overall play skills in comparison with the control group. Also, the social Test of Playfulness item scores improved significantly from the preintervention to the postintervention period and from the preintervention to the 1-month follow-up period, which demonstrated generalization of skills.

Integrate social interventions in context

Social interventions, including video modeling, social skills groups, social scripts, and Social Stories™, promote social participation when used in preparation for or during embedded activities with others. Raghavendra et al. (2013) examined the effectiveness of AT training to access the Internet with 18 children and adolescents with cerebral palsy, physical disability, and ABI. The children and adolescents learned strategies to socialize online (e.g., games, Facebook, Skype, email, videos) in their home.

Researchers identified clinically significant increases in performance and satisfaction ratings on the Canadian Occupational Performance Measure (COPM; Law et al., 2014).

Using goal attainment scaling, participants achieved 70% of their goals (Raghavendra et al., 2013). Supported online training increased participants' social connections online with existing friends and family, created new online connections, and increased participants' self-esteem and confidence with social communication.

Test et al. (2011) examined Social Stories literature through a comprehensive review of 28 studies and a meta-analysis of 18 studies. Findings suggest that Social Stories may improve social skills, but additional research is needed to verify generalization and continued use of the intervention. However, 12 out of 18 studies in the meta-analysis suggested that using Social Stories alone was an ineffective intervention. Therefore, professional judgment is critical when occupational therapy practitioners are considering the most appropriate contexts for using Social Stories to promote social participation.

Reichow and Volkmar (2010) found limited evidence to support the use of social skills groups as a single intervention; most studies used social skills groups as one component of an intervention program. The authors found that combining visual strategies, such as Social Stories, scripts, and activity schedules, could be effective in enhancing social understanding and structuring communication and social interactions for children with ASD. Finally, video modeling seemed to be an effective method of teaching social skills to people with ASD. However, the evidence was limited, and these strategies need further investigation because they are used with different populations.

Develop performance skills

Interventions focused on performance skills include self-management strategies, problem-solving strategies, and social skills groups to develop targeted skills, such as emotional regulation, social skills, and executive functioning (EF). Wells et al. (2012) examined a neurocognitive habilitation program for children with fetal alcohol syndrome and alcohol-related neurodevelopmental disorder who were adopted or lived in foster care. The curriculum used an adapted Alert Program® with the children and their caregivers over a 12-week period to address EF and emotional regulation skills in the home and school environments.

The curriculum used the ALERT Program's engine speed analogy in all of the sessions and used occupational tasks to target concepts such as emotional awareness, problem solving, social skills, and self-esteem. The caregiver sessions provided education and strategies to generalize the learned skills into the home environment. The children in the intervention group demonstrated significant improvements in executive and emotional functioning in comparison with the control group (Wells et al., 2012).

Missiuna et al. (2012) developed the Partnering for Change model to address the needs of students with developmental coordination disorder in the classroom and school settings. Following this model, occupational therapy practitioners collaborate with and coach teachers in their classrooms to assist them in identifying, accommodating, and supporting children with developmental coordination disorder. The Partnering for Change model uses the concepts of universal design for learning, differentiated instruction, and response to intervention to monitor and accommodate students' needs and to enable teachers and parents to facilitate students' development.

Tanner et al. (2015) reported that group-based social skills training programs for children with ASD were effective in improving social skills and joint engagement on the playground while decreasing solitary play. Group-based social skills training programs for children with ASD conducted in clinic-based and naturalistic settings resulted in increased self-esteem, increased social participation, improved social competency, and improved friendships. There is strong evidence to support the use of group-based programs to improve social interaction skills for children and youth with ASD.

Gutman et al. (2012) used a motor-based role-play intervention to increase social skills for adolescents with ASD. The intervention focused on social skills training in different areas of the school and provided students with opportunities to practice role-playing scenarios that targeted verbal and nonverbal social behaviors with peers. Students improved their verbal and nonverbal behaviors through the role-playing intervention, and anecdotal evidence from teachers, administrators, and parents reported students' generalization of social performance in everyday situations.

Laugeson et al. (2014) examined the social functioning of adolescents with ASD after their participation in the Program for the Education and Enrichment of Relational Skills at school. Teachers implemented the social skills curriculum over a 14-week semester. The researchers found the program to be effective in improving the adolescents' social functioning. Also, in comparison with an active treatment control group, the students demonstrated overall improvement in social responsiveness (e.g., social motivation, social awareness, social communication) on the Social Responsiveness Scale, as reported by their teachers.

Implement environment-focused interventions

In *environment-focused interventions,* the occupational therapy practitioner works collaboratively with the student and the family or school staff to identify environmental barriers and supports to participation in desired activities. The practitioner proposes strategies to remove barriers and builds on the student's strengths and supports to improve participation in these activities (Anaby et al., 2016).

Selanikyo et al. (2017) developed a combined in-service and collaborative consultation intervention program to enhance the social participation of students with moderate IDD in the classroom setting. An occupational therapist provided an in-service to a team of teachers and collaborated individually with each teacher to create activities to increase the social participation of students with IDD in the classroom. The activities consisted of 3 components—communicating, choosing, and initiating—over a 20-week intervention period. Significant improvement was demonstrated in the students' classroom social participation in each of the 3 targeted components in comparison with students in a control group (i.e., students whose teachers received only the in-service training). The authors concluded that the use of a combined intervention model may be an effective method for increasing social participation among students with IDD.

In a study by Anaby et al. (2016), 6 adolescents with a variety of disabilities and their families participated in a 12-week program to address leisure and participation goals through an environment-based and coaching intervention model. The results indicated a clinically significant improvement in performance scores on the COPM for the adolescents.

In addition, a small improvement in participation frequency was noted on the community setting scores of the Participation and Environment Measure for Children and Youth (Anaby et al., 2016). Also on this measure, on average, the mean number of activities in which the adolescents participated increased, the mean number of activities in which the parents desired change decreased, and improvements in the scores in the quality of life domains of autonomy and physical well-being were observed.

Measure Outcomes to Provide Evidence and Plan Modifications to Interventions

Occupational therapy intervention to improve social participation in inclusive school environments can enhance quality of life for students with disabilities, such as greater opportunities for social networking (Koegel et al., 2012; Leigers et al., 2016). The ability to interact with others can be particularly important when students transition out of secondary school and learn to generalize skills to community and work environments (Gutman et al., 2012; Milen & Nicholas, 2017; Orsmond et al., 2013). When occupational therapy interventions are modified with a focus on students' long-term outcomes, they can have a greater impact on facilitating meaningful student outcomes.

SUMMARY

School occupational therapy practitioners have a major role in supporting social participation through the development of communication and social skills for students with disabilities. In collaboration with team members, occupational therapists can identify students' strengths and challenges using a thorough assessment process to prioritize needs and target key roles for occupational therapy intervention. Despite the heterogeneity of abilities of students with disabilities, there is evidence for use of intervention strategies to facilitate increased participation by providing support in inclusive environments and scaffolding skill-building experiences.

Currently, research evidence provides support for peer-mediated, skill-focused, activity-based social and environment-focused interventions. Providing these interventions in an inclusive, collaborative model through partnerships with interprofessional team members institutes best practice intervention focused on social participation.

REFERENCES

Agnihotri, S., Gray, J., Colantonio, A., Polatajko, H., Cameron, D., Wiseman-Hakes, C., . . . Keightley, M. (2014). Arts-based social skills interventions for adolescents with acquired brain injuries: Five case reports. *Developmental Neurorehabilitation, 17,* 44–63. https://doi.org/10.3109/17518423.2013.844739

American Occupational Therapy Association. (2014a). Guidelines for supervision, roles, and responsibilities during the delivery of occupational therapy services. *American Journal of Occupational Therapy, 68*(Suppl. 3), S16–S22. https://doi.org/10.5014/ajot.2014.686S03

American Occupational Therapy Association. (2014b). Occupational therapy practice framework: Domain and process (3rd ed.). *American Journal of Occupational Therapy, 68*(Suppl. 1), S1–S48. https://doi.org/10.5014/ajot.2014.682006

American Occupational Therapy Association. (2017). Guidelines for occupational therapy services in early intervention and schools. *American Journal of Occupational Therapy, 71*(Suppl. 2), 7112410010. https://doi.org/10.5014/ajot.2017.716S01

American Occupational Therapy Association. (2018). Vision 2025. *American Journal of Occupational Therapy, 71*, 7103420010. https://doi.org/10.5014/ajot.2017.713002.

Anaby, D. R., Law, M. C., Majnemer, A., & Feldman, D. (2016). Opening doors to participation of youth with physical disabilities: An intervention study. *Canadian Journal of Occupational Therapy, 83*, 83–90. https://doi.org/10.1177/0008417415608653

Bondy, A., & Frost, L. (1998). The Picture Exchange Communication System. *Seminars in Speech and Language, 19*, 373–389. https://doi.org/10.1055/s-2008-1064055

Case-Smith, J. (2013). Systematic review of interventions to promote social–emotional development in young children with or at risk for disability. *American Journal of Occupational Therapy, 67*, 395–404. https://doi.org/10.5014/ajot.2013.004713

Constantino, J. N., & Gruber, C. P. (2012). *Social Responsiveness Scale–Second Edition (SRS-2)*. Torrance, CA: Western Psychological Services.

Coster, W. J., Deeney, T., Haltiwanger, J., & Haley, S. (1998). *School Function Assessment*. San Antonio: Psychological Corporation.

Coster, W. J., Law, M., Bedell, G., Anaby, D., Khetani, M. A., & Teplicky, R. (2014). *Participation and Environment Measure for Children and Youth (PEM-CY) user's guide*. Hamilton, Ontario: CanChild Centre for Childhood Disability Research.

Gresham, F. M., & Elliott, S. N. (2008). *Social skills improvement system: Rating scales manual*. Bloomington, MN: NCS Pearson.

Guerette, P., Furumasu, J., & Tefft, D. (2013). The positive effects of early powered mobility on children's psychosocial and play skills. *Assistive Technology, 25*, 39–50. https://doi.org/10.1080/10400435.2012.685824

Gutman, S. A., Raphael-Greenfield, E. I., & Rao, A. K. (2012). Effect of a motor-based role-play intervention on the social behaviors of adolescents with high-functioning autism: Multiple-baseline single-subject design. *American Journal of Occupational Therapy, 66*, 529–537. https://doi.org/10.5014/ajot.2012.003756

Hussman, J. (2018). *Presume competence: A guide to successful, evidence-based principles for supporting and engaging individuals with autism*. Retrieved from http://www.hussmanautism.org/wp-content/uploads/pdf/PresumeCompetence_Hussman Institute.pdf

Huyder, V., Nilsen, E. S., & Bacso, S. A. (2017). The relationship between children's executive functioning, theory of mind, and verbal skills with their own and others' behaviour in a cooperative context: Changes in relations from early to middle school-age. *Infant and Child Development, 26*, e2027. https://doi.org/10.1002/icd.2027

Ichikawa, K., Takahashi, Y., Ando, M., Anme, T., Ishizaki, T., Yamaguchi, H., & Nakayama, T. (2013). TEACCH-based group social skills training for children with high-functioning autism: A pilot randomized controlled trial. *BioPsychoSocial Medicine, 7*, Article 14. https://doi.org/10.1186/1751-0759-7-14

Kauffman, N. A., & Kinnealey, M. (2015). Comprehensive social skills taxonomy: Development and application. *American Journal of Occupational Therapy, 69*, 6902220030. https://doi.org/10.5014/ajot.2015.013151

Keller, J., Kafkes, A., Basu, S., Feerico, J., & Kielhofner, G. (2005). *Child Occupational Self-Assessment*. Chicago: University of Illinois at Chicago.

King, G., Law, M., King, S., Hurley, P., Hanna, S., Kertoy, M., . . . Young, N. (2004). *Children's Assessment of Participation and Enjoyment and Preferences for Activities of Children*. San Antonio: Harcourt Assessment.

Koegel, L. K., Vernon, T. W., Koegel, R. L., Koegel, B. L., & Paullin, A. W. (2012). Improving social engagement and initiations between children with autism spectrum disorder and their peers in inclusive settings. *Journal of Positive Behavior Interventions, 14*, 220–227. https://doi.org/10.1177/1098300712437042

Kramer, J. M., Olsen, S., Mermelstein, M., Balcells, A., & Liljenquist, K. (2012). Youth with disabilities' perspectives of the environment and participation: A qualitative meta-synthesis. *Child: Care, Health and Development, 38*, 763–777. https://doi.org/10.1111/j.1365-2214.2012.01365.x

Kreider, C. M., Bendixen, R. M., Young, M. E., Prudencio, S. M., McCarty, C., & Mann, W. C. (2016). Social networks and participation with others for youth with learning, attention, and autism spectrum disorders. *Canadian Journal of Occupational Therapy, 83*, 14–26. https://doi.org/10.1177/0008417415583107

Laugeson, E. A., Ellingsen, R., Sanderson, J., Tucci, L., & Bates, S. (2014). The ABC's of teaching social skills to adolescents with autism spectrum disorder in the classroom: The UCLA PEERS® program. *Journal of Autism and Developmental Disorders, 44*, 2244–2256. https://doi.org/10.1007/s10803-014-2108-8

Law, M., Baptiste, S., Carswell, A., McColl, M. A., Polatajko, H., & Pollock, N. (2014). *Canadian Occupational Performance Measure* (5th ed.). Ottawa: CAOT Publications.

Leigers, K., & Myers, C. (2015). Effect of duration of peer awareness education on attitudes toward students with disabilities: A systematic review. *Journal of Occupational Therapy, Schools, and Early Intervention, 8*, 79–96. https://doi.org/10.1080/19411243.2015.1021067

Leigers, K., Myers, C., & Schneck, C. (2016). Social participation in schools: A survey of occupational therapy practitioners. *American Journal of Occupational Therapy, 70*, 7005280010. https://doi.org/10.5014/ajot.2016.020768

Little, L. M., Sideris, J., Ausderau, K., & Baranek, G. T. (2014). Activity participation among children with autism spectrum disorder. *American Journal of Occupational Therapy, 68*, 177–185. https://doi.org/10.5014/ajot.2014.009894

McMaugh, A. (2011). En/countering disablement in school life in Australia: Children talk about peer relations and living with illness and disability. *Disability and Society, 26*, 853–866. https://doi.org/10.1080/09687599.2011.618740

Milen, M. T., & Nicholas, D. B. (2017). Examining transitions from youth to adult services for young persons with autism. *Social Work in Health Care, 56*, 636–648. https://doi.org/10.1080/00981389.2017.1318800

Missiuna, C. A., Pollock, N. A., Levac, D. E., Campbell, W. N., Sahagian Whalen, S. D., Bennett, S. M., . . . Russell, D. J. (2012). Partnering for Change: An innovative school-based occupational therapy service delivery model for children with developmental coordination disorder. *Canadian Journal of Occupational Therapy, 79*, 41–50. https://doi.org/10.2182/cjot.2012.79.1.6

Murray, C., & Greenberg, M. T. (2006). Examining the importance of social relationships and social contexts in the lives of children with high-incidence disabilities. *Journal of Special Education, 39,* 220–233. https://doi.org/10.1177/00224669060390040301

Orsmond, G. I., Shattuck, P. T., Cooper, B. P., Sterzing, P. R., & Anderson, K. A. (2013). Social participation among young adults with an autism spectrum disorder. *Journal of Autism and Developmental Disorders, 43,* 2710–2719. https://doi.org/10.1007/s10803-013-1833-8

Raghavendra, P., Newman, L., Grace, E., & Wood, D. (2013). "I could never do that before": Effectiveness of a tailored Internet support intervention to increase the social participation of youth with disabilities. *Child: Care, Health and Development, 39,* 552–561. https://doi.org/10.1111/cch.12048

Raghavendra, P., Olsson, C., Sampson, J., McInerney, R., & Connell, T. (2012). School participation and social networks of children with complex communication needs, physical disabilities, and typically developing peers. *Augmentative and Alternative Communication, 28,* 33–43. https://doi.org/10.3109/07434618.2011.653604

Reichow, B., & Volkmar, F. R. (2010). Social skills interventions for individuals with autism: Evaluation for evidenced-based practices within a best evidence synthesis framework. *Journal of Autism and Developmental Disorders, 40,* 149–166. https://doi.org/10.1007/s10803-009-0842-0

Selanikyo, E., Yalon-Chamovitz, S., & Weintraub, N. (2017). Enhancing classroom participation of students with intellectual and developmental disabilities. *Canadian Journal of Occupational Therapy, 84,* 76–86. https://doi.org/10.1177/0008417416661346

Sepanski, B., & Fisher, T. (2011). Psychosocial occupational therapy and school-based practice. *Early Intervention and School Special Interest Section Quarterly, 18*(1), 1–4.

Sutton, B., Webster, A., & Westerveld, M. (2018). A systematic review of school-based interventions targeting social communication behaviors for students with autism. *Autism.* Advance online publication. https://doi.org/10.1177/1362361317753564

Tanner, K., Hand, B. N., O'Toole, G., & Lane, A. E. (2015). Effectiveness of interventions to improve social participation, play, leisure, and restricted and repetitive behaviors in people with autism spectrum disorder: A systematic review. *American Journal of Occupational Therapy, 69,* 6905180010. https://doi.org/10.5014/ajot.2015.017806

Test, D. W., Richter, S., Knight, V., & Spooner, F. (2011). A comprehensive review and meta-analysis of the Social Stories literature. *Focus on Autism and Other Developmental Disabilities, 26*(1), 49–62. https://doi.org/10.1177/1088357609351573

Tomchek, S. D., & Koenig, K. P. (2016). *Occupational therapy practice guidelines for individuals with autism spectrum disorder.* Bethesda, MD: AOTA Press.

Tonkin, B. L., Ogilvie, B. D., Greenwood, S. A., Law, M. C., & Anaby, D. R. (2014). The participation of children and youth with disabilities in activities outside of school: A scoping review. *Canadian Journal of Occupational Therapy, 81,* 226–236. https://doi.org/10.1177/0008417414550998

Wells, A. M., Chasnoff, I. J., Schmidt, C. A., Telford, E., & Schwartz, L. D. (2012). Neurocognitive habilitation therapy for children with fetal alcohol spectrum disorders: An adaptation of the Alert Program®. *American Journal of Occupational Therapy, 66,* 24–34. https://doi.org/10.5014/ajot.2012.002691

Wilkes-Gillan, S., Bundy, A., Cordier, R., Lincoln, M., & Chen, Y.-W. (2016). A randomized controlled trial of a play-based intervention to improve the social play skills of children with attention deficit hyperactivity disorder (ADHD). *PLoS ONE, 11*(8), e0160558. https://doi.org/10.1371/journal.pone.0160558

Woodman, A. C., Smith, L. E., Greenberg, J. S., & Mailick, M. R. (2016). Contextual factors predict patterns of change in functioning over 10 years among adolescents and adults with autism spectrum disorders. *Journal of Autism and Developmental Disorders, 46,* 176–189. https://doi.org/10.1007/s10803-015-2561-z

SECTION VI.

Evidence-Guided Practices: Addressing Performance Skills to Enhance Student Participation

KEY TERMS AND CONCEPTS

- Attention
- Cognition
- Cognitive flexibility
- Cool EF skills
- Executive function
- Hot EF skills
- Memory
- Metacognition
- Theory of mind
- Working memory

OVERVIEW

The ability to gain and retain information is one feature of cognition. Increasingly, literature addressing children's cognitive abilities has focused on another component, called *executive function* (EF; Carlson, 2011; Diamond, 2013). **EF** refers to a variety of higher order processes, including the ability to plan and execute action, modify action in response to environmental demands, and assess the results of action (Payne et al., 2012). Deficits in EF can be seen in difficulties in abstract reasoning and poor

- Problem solving,
- Planning,
- Organizational skills,
- Impulse control, and
- Engagement in flexible thinking (Diamond, 2013).

Students with a history of cognitive deficits may demonstrate myriad problems, including limited EF, difficulty with social skills, poor health, and lack of participation in school and community (Levan et al., 2016; Rosenberg et al., 2017). In addition, students with EF deficits frequently have deficits in visual–perceptual, visual–motor, and motor performance skills (Rosenberg et al., 2017; Ziviani et al., 2008).

The high frequency with which children have both EF and motor coordination problems creates a clear need for occupational therapy practitioners[1] to be included in the evaluation

process. These deficits can negatively affect a child's ability to participate in the educational setting (McDermott et al., 2012).

EF is often conceptualized as inhibitory cognitive functions, with several core elements identified (Diamond, 2013). EF is complex and critical in the completion of ADLs. People need self-control and regulation to avoid impulsive reactions to situations.

Working memory (WM) is the ability to mentally hold information while working with the information in context of another task, as people do during problem-solving tasks. *Cognitive flexibility* refers to the ability to adjust to differing task demands and shift between tasks. EF continues to develop as the child matures from infancy to adulthood, but it can be disrupted or delayed by various exogenous and endogenous factors.

ESSENTIAL CONSIDERATIONS

EF is part of overall cognitive abilities related to future goal-oriented skills (Kouklari et al., 2018). By understanding the terminology and impact on performance, occupational therapy practitioners can support educational participation and enhance cognitive and EF skills through a variety of strategies.

Common Terminology

The following terms are typically used in the literature addressing EF. Brief definitions are provided to assist readers.
- *Attention:* Attention is sustained focus on a task, including concentration and the ability to shift focus between 2 tasks as needed in a setting.
- *Cognition:* This term broadly refers to the mental ability to acquire knowledge and often includes attention, memory, awareness, and reasoning. EF is considered to be a component of cognition.

---

[1]*Occupational therapy practitioner* refers to both the occupational therapist and the occupational therapy assistant. The American Occupational Therapy Association (AOTA; 2014a, p. S18) states, "The occupational therapist is responsible for all aspects of occupational therapy service delivery and is accountable for the safety and effectiveness of the occupational therapy service delivery process" and "must be directly involved in the delivery of services during the initial evaluation and regularly throughout the course of intervention. . . . The occupational therapy assistant delivers safe and effective occupational therapy services under the supervision of and in partnership with the occupational therapist."

Copyright © 2019 by the American Occupational Therapy Association. All rights reserved. To reuse this content, contact www.copyright.com.
https://doi.org/10.7139/2019.978-1-56900-591-0.054

- *Metacognition:* This term is used to explain how a person is able to examine knowledge (e.g., thinking about thinking).
- *Memory:* Memory is the ability to retain information for use at a later time (Payne et al., 2012). Several memory types are discussed in the literature (e.g., episodic, long term, short term, procedural, working), but there is no universally accepted single classification system.
- *Theory of mind:* Theory of mind is the ability to "infer mental/emotional states in order to predict and explain behavior" (Kouklari et al., 2018, p. 1).

Cognition and EF

In schools, there is an expectation that a student can retain and manipulate information effectively in addition to shifting between various demands in the classroom environment. Paying attention to details and using acquired skills are difficult for students with inadequate EF skills. Incidental learning, which often occurs in schools, is also a challenge for students who lack adequate EF skills.

The *Occupational Therapy Practice Framework: Domain and Practice* (3rd ed.; *OTPF–3*; AOTA, 2014b) lists client factors, such as mental functions, that include cognitive skills. Client factors reside within the person and influence occupational engagement. Under the performance skills in the *OTPF–3*, defined as observable elements of action with a specific functional purpose, is a category called *process skills* (e.g., attends, chooses, inquires, initiates), which cover cognitive abilities.

Although the *OTPF–3* clearly indicates that cognitive functioning, particularly as it relates to occupational performance, is within the domain of occupational therapy, this information is often not clearly conveyed to recipients of service (e.g., parents, teachers, team members, administrators). Informing those in the educational setting that EF skills are addressed in the domain of occupational therapy services is important. Occupational therapy practitioners should examine how deficits in EF compromise occupational participation in schools (Connor & Maeir, 2011; Cramm et al., 2013).

Development of Cognitive Function and EF

The prefrontal cortex, which is not fully developed until adolescence, is clearly linked with social behavior and decision making in social settings (Nickel & Gu, 2018). The hippocampal formation, which is part of the limbic system, is closely linked to the prefrontal cortex and contributes to memory formation and consolidation. The increasing process of myelination of the brain contributes to decision making that is based on a wide variety of factors and not merely in response to a situation (Nickel & Gu, 2018).

A study by Insel et al. (2017) found that 13- to 20-year-olds made more differentiated decisions on the basis of outcomes and environmental demands when the stakes (i.e., importance of the outcome) increased as compared with younger teens, who tended to expend comparable effort on the decision-making process, regardless of the outcomes. Insel et al. (2017) postulated that the development of corticostriatal connections supports goal-directed behavior. These connections typically occur later in adolescence.

Students who have deficits in EF frequently display difficulties with foundational educational skills, such as planning and organizing a task, engaging in the task under novel or unfamiliar circumstances, or evaluating the effectiveness of task completion (Carlson, 2011). Educators expect students to acquire skills and then effectively use those skills in novel situations or combine several skills to produce a favorable outcome to a goal-directed task. This requires WM and the ability to inhibit action sufficiently to meet novel task demands (Danielsson et al., 2012), which is problematic for students who have EF deficits.

"Cool" and "Hot" EF Skills

Cool EF skills focus on WM and inhibition of action (analytical properties) and are often used when decisions do not include a personal reward or emotional component, such as remembering a series of digits or words. *Hot EF skills* are influenced by "social/affective aspects and greater attention to the broader social milieu in which EF develops and the consequences for academic achievement" (Carlson, 2011, p. 411). Hot EF skills are more commonly seen during daily decision making in the context of family, friends, and social situations in which emotions, motivation, and environmental context frequently play an important role.

These skills develop at different rates, with the relatively cool EF skills developing earlier, initially seen in early childhood but progressing over time. Hot skills develop over a longer period of time and are seen later in childhood or adolescence (Prencipe et al., 2011; Zelazo et al., 2004). Although both cool and hot EF elements foster goal-directed behavior, they seem to reflect different aspects of EF skills.

EF Deficits and Other Conditions

EF deficits are known to be associated with several childhood conditions as well as limited sleep and poor sleep patterns. These conditions and difficulties are listed in Table 54.1.

BEST PRACTICES

Cognition is a key factor in occupational performance (Law et al., 1997). The intersection of EF and environmental demands is the focus of occupational therapy services in the educational setting.

Identify EF Through Evaluation

The occupational therapist participates in the evaluation of cognitive functioning and EF to identify students with EF problems. Using interviews and observations, the occupational therapist completes the occupational profile (AOTA, 2017) and notes the cognitive aspects of occupational performance. This evaluation requires that the therapist clearly understand the demands of the educational environment and identify how the student's EF affects performance.

Observations and interviews

Interviewing students, family, and others in the student's environment provides information about occupational history, occupations, activities enjoyed, and areas of concern. It is beneficial to screen the student's cognitive status while

TABLE 54.1. Examples of Childhood Conditions and Executive Function Difficulties

CONDITION	RESEARCH FINDINGS
Attention deficit hyperactivity disorder (ADHD)	■ Approximately 50% of students with ADHD have additional EF deficits beyond diminished attention (Lambek et al., 2010) and need additional external supports and structure to use skills in novel situations. ■ One study found that children with ADHD and sleep problems had poorer EF skills and greater difficulties with theory of mind skills to support peer social interactions (Tesfaye & Gruber, 2017).
Autism spectrum disorder (ASD)	■ Children with ASD have greater limitations in cognitive flexibility than typically developing peers and children with nonverbal learning disabilities (Semrud-Clikeman et al., 2014). ■ They tend to have difficulty with planning and organization required for manual dexterity (Schurink et al., 2012). ■ Children with ASD perform significantly below peers on visual–motor and selective attention tasks (e.g., pay attention to specific stimuli and filter extraneous stimuli; Brandes-Aitken et al., 2018).
Developmental coordination disorder (DCD)	■ Children with DCD and EF problems experience difficulties participating in daily activities (Rosenberg et al., 2017). ■ Children with DCD have greater difficulties than peers with tasks of WM, inhibition, planning, and organization skills (Leonard et al., 2015). ■ They also have difficulties with self-regulation of social cues compared with peers (Rahimi-Golkhandan et al., 2016). ■ Children with DCD have widespread deficits in EF skills that persistently and negatively affect academic performance (Bernardi et al., 2018).
Intellectual disabilities (ID)	■ Children with ID have deficits in EF that are unique and not necessarily consistent with their mental age equivalent (Danielsson et al., 2012). ■ They have greater difficulties with inhibition of action given environmental demands, poorer planning, and problems with nonverbal WM (Danielsson et al., 2012). ■ Children with ID, in particular, Down syndrome, are also at risk for poor sleep patterns, which further compromise their EF skills (Esbensen & Hoffman, 2018). ■ Students who have ID frequently exhibit impaired visual processing of information (Boot et al., 2012).
Learning disabilities	■ One study found that students with learning disabilities had significantly more difficulties with visual sequential processing compared with children with ASD and typical peers but had fewer problems with cognitive flexibility compared with children with ASD (Semrud-Clikeman et al., 2014). ■ Difficulties in WM needed for sequential visual–motor tasks compromise many school-related tasks, whether copying assignments, transferring information, or taking notes (Rosen et al., 2014). ■ Children with learning disabilities have difficulties with ability to shift attention during writing from memory or keyboard use (Berninger et al., 2017).
Sleep patterns	■ Sleep problems have been linked to children's poor academic performance (Cho et al., 2015; Gruber et al., 2010), in particular, verbal WM. ■ Children ages 5–17 years old who experienced sleep-disordered breathing had EF problems in WM, inhibition, and shifting (alternating between tasks; Mietchen et al., 2016). ■ Poor sleep quality, with a pattern of falling asleep and then awakening, disrupts EF among adolescents (Kuula et al., 2015). ■ Girls with disordered sleep patterns (more fragmented sleep) had greater difficulties with tasks that required changing responses on the basis of feedback. Boys with disordered sleep had more difficulties with tasks requiring attention to a specific stimulus for an extended time (Kuula et al., 2015). Because many of the girls had reached puberty, as compared with few of the boys, this might have influenced results.
Trauma or abuse history	■ Children with a history of neglect or abuse often display EF deficits (McDermott et al., 2012), with children from orphanages exhibiting poorer inhibition compared with children in foster care or living with their family. ■ One study found that positive parenting skills were significantly correlated to the child's planning skills and that maternal emotion regulation was significantly correlated to the child's ability to use feedback and shift responses (Samuelson et al., 2012). ■ Children prenatally exposed to alcohol (fetal alcohol syndrome) demonstrated EF deficits along with emotional regulation challenges (Wells et al., 2012).

Note. EF = executive function; WM = working memory.

observing the student completing familiar and unfamiliar tasks. Questions that can guide observations regarding aspects of cognition may include the following:

- Does the student attend and maintain attention during the task, inhibiting other stimuli?
- Can the student form a plan and follow through?
- Does the student have difficulty initiating and completing activities?
- Is memory (e.g., short term, long term, working) affected?
- Is the student able to effectively problem solve for their age?
- Does the student self-monitor and correct effectively during tasks?
- Does the student struggle in all academic subjects or perform within average range in some of them?

Observing the student's performance provides the therapist with data about cognitive functioning during routine or school tasks. Classroom peers can sometimes be used for comparison during observations (e.g., 20 of 23 students could initiate the task within 10 seconds of the teacher's request; this student initiated after 30 seconds and 3 verbal cues).

Formal tools to assess EF

The occupational therapist gathers data to develop the occupational profile of the student being evaluated. If the student has EF deficits, the occupational therapist is expected to assess these skills, either informally through observations, interviews, and checklists or formally through assessment tools. Some assessments are often administered by a psychologist or neuropsychologist, but an occupational therapist with sufficient training could also use these tools (see Table 54.2).

Implement Evidence-Based Interventions

Occupational therapy practitioners may use various types of interventions (e.g., environmental adaptations, accommodations, use of occupations and activities, consultation, education and training) and draw on a variety of approaches (e.g., create, establish, modify) to meet the identified outcomes (AOTA, 2014b). There is no one prescribed or preferred service model to support students with EF deficits, but models of choice should serve to improve problem-solving skills and self-regulation.

Cognitive Orientation to daily Occupational Performance (CO–OP)

The CO–OP Approach™ (Dawson et al., 2017; Polatajko & Mandich, 2004) specifically teaches students to use problem-solving and self-regulatory strategies when engaging in self-selected goals (Hyland & Polatajko, 2012; Polatajko & Mandich, 2004). CO–OP was designed to foster the use of cognitive strategies, particularly problem-solving skills (Miller et al., 2001; Polatajko & Mandich, 2004; Polatajko et al., 2001).

This intervention has been effectively used to help with goal setting, planning, execution of the plan, and self-evaluation of the outcome of the action, which are foundational EF skills (Rodger et al., 2007; Taylor et al., 2007). Jokic et al. (2013) used the CO–OP Approach with children diagnosed with developmental coordination disorder (DCD) and saw substantial gains in motor and self-regulatory skills after 10 sessions provided twice a week.

The problem-solving strategies used with the student during the program are Goal, Plan, Do, and Check (Polatajko & Mandich, 2004). These strategies allow the student to systematically engage in organizing (*Goal*) and planning the task (*Plan*), enacting the plan (*Do*), and then self-monitoring performance and assessing the effectiveness of the plan in meeting the desired goal (*Check*). During each step, the occupational therapy practitioner uses probative questions to help the student through the process. The program was initially designed to be offered once to twice a week for a 10-week period, but this approach has been effectively adapted to shorter time frames (Scammell et al., 2016).

TABLE 54.2.   Assessment Tools for Executive Functioning

TEST	DESCRIPTION
Behavior Rating Inventory of Executive Function (Gioia et al., 2000)	Assesses EF in everyday tasks (Qian et al., 2010). Uses parent report of the functional ability of the child. A form of the measure is also available for teachers (Toplak et al., 2009).
Movement Assessment Battery for Children–2 (Henderson et al., 2007)	Used to assess children for motor planning and organizational skills during a comprehensive evaluation of potential EF problems and development coordination disorders (Bernardi et al., 2018; Leonard et al., 2015).
Stroop Color and Word Test (Golden, 1978)	Requires a person to inhibit the interference portion and respond only to the request to identify the color, not the word (e.g., the word *red* might be printed in blue ink).
Tower of London (Shallice, 1982)	The person is given a pegboard with a specific arrangement of colored beads (Anderson et al., 1996) and asked to replicate the pattern. The total number of moves plus the time required to complete the task provide a performance-based score of planning and problem solving.
Trail Making Test (Reitan, 1944)	Requires a person to draw a line to connect numbers in the order in which they are displayed randomly on a single test page.
Wisconsin Card Sorting Test (Nyhus & Barcelo, 2009)	The person sorts a deck of cards with geometric shapes on the basis of feedback from an examiner, who indicates whether the response is correct or a mistake. The person uses problem solving to detect the variable required to sort the stack of cards.

Note. EF = executive function.

Although CO–OP was originally developed for children with DCD, this strategy has been effectively used with children with autism spectrum disorder to address motor planning and social and organizational skills (Rodger & Brandenburg, 2009; Rodger et al., 2008, 2009; Rodger & Vishram, 2010; Skowronski & Engsberg, 2017). An investigation using CO–OP with children diagnosed with cerebral palsy found that this systematic approach fostered improved arm function and positive parental reports (Jackman et al., 2017). This approach can readily be used in the educational setting to help a student develop the EF skills needed to meet classroom demands (Banks et al., 2008).

Alert Program

The Alert Program® is a cognitive intervention based on self-regulatory skills to promote EF. A 12-week adaptation of the Alert Program (Williams & Shellenberger, 1996) was effectively used to improve EF skills among children diagnosed with fetal alcohol syndrome (Wells et al., 2012).

Cognitive skill training

Tamm et al. (2014) used direct training of cognitive skills for young children (preschool to 2nd grade) with attention deficit hyperactivity disorder (ADHD) and EF deficits. Participants demonstrated improved EF skills for attention, WM, and cognitive flexibility. Although this investigation lacked a control group, changes in EF skills were attributed to the short-term intervention of 8 consecutive weeks.

Cognitive–Functional (Cog–Fun)

Students with ADHD often have EF deficits that compromise completion of tasks at school and home (Hahn-Markowitz et al., 2011). Hahn-Markowitz et al. (2011) used a pilot program called Cog–Fun to develop EF skills among children ages 7–8 years with ADHD. The specific focus was on having children and parents develop goal-directed functional skills in the school and home environment. In the program, an occupational therapy practitioner provided specific environmental suggestions to foster improved EF skills, such as arrangement of items in the room and provision of positive feedback. On completion of the 10-week program, the authors noted significant gains in EF skills.

The authors then used the Cog–Fun approach with children ages 5–7 years diagnosed with ADHD (Hahn-Markowitz et al., 2011). After 12 weeks of intervention, significant gains were noted in the group that received the Cog–Fun services compared with the control group. Additional data collected 12 weeks after the intervention indicated that these gains were retained. The Cog–Fun program was also used with children ages 7–10 years who were diagnosed with ADHD (Hahn-Markowitz et al., 2011). Results indicated significant improvements in self-regulation skills and participation in ADLs.

SUMMARY

Students with EF deficits struggle in the educational environment with mastering a skill and, once they have mastered it, have difficulties effectively using that skill in novel settings.

Often, students who have EF deficits also have other diagnoses. After EF needs have been identified, intervention may include adapting the environment and fostering improved EF skills. EF needs must be included when occupational therapists plan interventions with students who have academic, functional, or behavioral needs.

There is an increasing body of evidence supporting occupational therapy intervention approaches to improve the specific EF skills of self-regulation and problem solving as applied to functional daily living tasks. To enhance meaningful learning, development, and performance, occupational therapy practitioners must actively promote the use of these interventions to support students in academic settings.

REFERENCES

American Occupational Therapy Association. (2014a). Guidelines for supervision, roles, and responsibilities during the delivery of occupational therapy services. *American Journal of Occupational Therapy, 68*(Suppl. 3), S16–S22. https://doi.org/10.5014/ajot.2014.686S03

American Occupational Therapy Association. (2014b). Occupational therapy practice framework: Domain and process (3rd ed.). *American Journal of Occupational Therapy, 68*(Suppl. 1), S1–S48. https://doi.org/10.5014/ajot.2014.682006

American Occupational Therapy Association. (2017). AOTA occupational profile template. *American Journal of Occupational Therapy, 71*(Suppl. 2), 7112420030. https://doi.org/10.5014/ajot.2017.716S12

Anderson, P., Anderson, V., & Lajoie, G. (1996). The Tower of London Test: Validation and standardization for pediatric populations. *Clinical Neuropsychologist, 10,* 54–65. https://doi.org/10.1080/13854049608406663

Banks, R., Rodger, S., & Polatajko, H. (2008). Mastering handwriting: How children with developmental coordination disorder succeed with CO–OP. *Occupational Therapy Journal of Research, 28,* 100–109. https://doi.org/10.3928/15394492-20080601-01

Bernardi, M., Leonard, H. C., Hill, E. L., Botting, N., & Henry, L. A. (2018). Executive functions in children with developmental coordination disorder: A 2-year follow-up study. *Developmental Medicine and Child Neurology, 60,* 306–313. https://doi.org/10.1111/dmcn.13640

Berninger, V., Abbott, R., Cook, C. R., & Nagy, W. (2017). Relationships of attention and executive functions to oral language, reading, and writing skills and systems in middle childhood and early adolescence. *Journal of Learning Disabilities, 50,* 434–449. https://doi.org/10.1177/0022219415617167

Boot, F. H., Pel, J. J. M., Evenhuis, H. M., & van der Steen, J. (2012). Factors related to impaired visual orienting behavior in children with intellectual disabilities. *Research in Developmental Disabilities, 33,* 1670–1676. https://doi.org/10.1016/j.ridd.2012.04.007

Brandes-Aitken, A., Anguera, J. A., Rolle, C. E., Desai, S. S., Demopoulos, C., Skinner, S. N., . . . Marco, E. J. (2018). Characterizing cognitive and visuomotor control in children with sensory processing dysfunction and autism spectrum disorders. *Neuropsychology, 32,* 148–160. https://doi.org/10.1037/neu0000404

Carlson, S. M. (2011). Introduction to the Special Issue: Executive function. *Journal of Experimental Child Psychology, 108,* 411–413. https://doi.org/10.1016/j.jecp.2011.01.004

Cho, M., Quach, J., Anderson, P., Mensah, F., Wake, M., & Roberts, G. (2015). Poor sleep and lower working memory in Grade 1 children: Cross-sectional, population-based study. *Academic Pediatrics, 15,* 111–116. https://doi.org/10.1016/j.acap.2014.06.021

Connor, L. T., & Maeir, A. (2011). Putting executive performance in a theoretical context. *OTJR: Occupation, Participation and Health, 31*(Suppl.), S3–S7. https://doi.org/10.3928/15394492-20101108-02

Cramm, H., Krupa, T., Missiuna, C., Lysaght, R. M., & Parker, K. C. H. (2013). Broadening the occupational therapy toolkit: An executive functioning lens for occupational therapy with children and youth. *American Journal of Occupational Therapy, 67,* e139–e147. https://doi.org/10.5014/ajot.2013.008607

Danielsson, H., Henry, L., Messer, D., & Ronnberg, J. (2012). Strengths and weaknesses in executive functioning in children with intellectual disability. *Research in Developmental Disabilities, 33,* 600–607. https://doi.org/10.1016/j.ridd.2011.11.004

Dawson, D. R., McEwen, S. E., & Polatajko, H. J. (Eds.). (2017). *Cognitive Orientation to daily Occupational Performance in occupational therapy: Using the CO–OP Approach™ to enable participation across the lifespan.* Bethesda, MD: AOTA Press.

Diamond, A. (2013). Executive functions. *Annual Review of Psychology, 64,* 135–168. https://doi.org/10.1146/annurev-psych-113011-143750

Esbensen, A. J., & Hoffman, E. K. (2018). Impact of sleep on executive functioning in school-age children with Down syndrome. *Journal of Intellectual Disability Research, 62,* 569–580. https://doi.org/10.1111/jir.12496

Gioia, G. A., Isquith, P. K., Guy, S., & Kenworthy, L. (2000). *BRIEF: Behavior Rating Inventory of Executive Function professional manual.* Lutz, FL: Psychological Assessment Resources.

Golden, C. J. (1978). *Stroop Color and Word Test: A manual for clinical and experimental uses.* Wood Dale, IL: Stoelting.

Gruber, R., Laviolette, R., Deluca, P., Monson, E., Cornish, K., & Carrier, J. (2010). Short sleep duration is associated with poor performance on IQ measures in healthy school-age children. *Sleep Medicine, 11,* 289–294. https://doi.org/10.1016/j.sleep.2009.09.007

Hahn-Markowitz, J., Manor, I., & Maeir, A. (2011). Effectiveness of cognitive–functional (Cog–Fun) intervention with children with attention deficit hyperactivity disorder: A pilot study. *American Journal of Occupational Therapy, 65,* 384–392. https://doi.org/10.5014/ajot.2011.000901

Henderson, S., Sugden, D., & Barnett, A. (2007). *Movement Assessment Battery for Children* (2nd ed.). San Antonio, TX: Psychological Corporation.

Hyland, M., & Polatajko, H. J. (2012). Enabling children with coordination disorder to self-regulate through the use of dynamic performance analysis: Evidence from the CO–OP Approach. *Human Movement Science, 31,* 987–998. https://doi.org/10.1016/j.humov.2011.09.003

Insel, C., Kastman, E. K., Glenn, C. R., & Somerville, L. H. (2017). Development of corticostriatal connectivity constrains goal-directed behavior during adolescence. *Nature Communications, 8,* 1605. https://doi.org/10.1038/s41467-017-01369-8

Jackman, M., Novak, I., Lannin, N., & Froude, E. (2017). Parents' experience of undertaking an intensive Cognitive Orientation to daily Occupational Performance (CO–OP) group for children with cerebral palsy. *Journal of Disability and Rehabilitation, 39,* 1018–1024. https://doi.org/10.1080/09638288.2016.1179350

Jokic, C. S., Polatjko, H., & Whitebread, D. (2013). Self-regulation as a mediator in motor learning: The effect of the Cognitive Orientation to Occupational Performance approach on children

with DCD. *Adapted Physical Activity Quarterly, 29,* 103–126. https://doi.org/10.1123/apaq.30.2.103

Kouklari, E., Tsermentseli, S., & Monks, C. P. (2018). Developmental trends of hot and cool executive function in school-aged children with and without autism spectrum disorder: Links with theory of mind. *Development and Pathopsychology.* Advance online publication. https://doi.org/10.1017/S0954579418000081

Kuula, L., Pesonen, A., Martikaninen, S., Kajantie, E, Lahti, J., Tuovinen, S., . . . Raikkonen, K. (2015). Poor sleep and neurocognitive function in early adolescence. *Sleep Medicine, 16,* 1207–1212. https://doi.org/10.1016/j.sleep.2015.06.017

Lambek, R., Tannock, R., Dalsgaard, S., Trillingsgaard, A., Damm, D., & Thomsen, P. H. (2010). Validating neuropsychological subtypes of ADHD: How do children with and without an executive function deficit differ? *Journal of Child Psychology and Psychiatry, 51,* 895–904. https://doi.org/10.1111/j.1469-7610.2010.02248.x

Law, M., Polatajko, H., Baptiste, S., & Townsend, E. (1997). Core concepts of occupational therapy. In E. Townsend, S. Stanton, M. Law, H. Polatajko, S. Baptiste, T. Thompson-Franson, . . . L. Campanile (Eds.), *Enabling occupation: An occupational therapy perspective* (pp. 29–56). Ottawa: CAOT Publications.

Leonard, H. C., Bernardi, M., Hill, E. L., & Henry, L. A. (2015). Executive functioning, motor difficulties, and developmental coordination disorder. *Developmental Neuropsychology, 40,* 201–215. https://doi.org/10.1080/87565641.2014.997933

Levan, A., Black, G., Mietchen, J., Baxter, L., Kirwan C. B., & Gale, S. D. (2016). Right frontal pole cortical thickness and executive functioning in children with traumatic brain injury: The impact on social problems. *Brain Imaging and Behavior, 10,* 1090–1095. https://doi.org/10.1007/s11682-015-9472-7

McDermott, J. M., Westerlund, A., Zeanah, C. H., Nelson, C. A., & Fox, N. A. (2012). Early adversity and neural correlates of executive function: Implications for academic adjustment. *Developmental Cognitive Neuroscience, 2*(Suppl. 1), S59–S66. https://doi.org/10.1016/j.dcn.2011.09.008

Mietchen, J. J., Bennett, D. P., Huff, T., Hedges, D. W., & Gale, S. D. (2016). Executive function in pediatric sleep-disordered breathing: A meta-analysis. *Journal of the International Neuropsychological Society, 22,* 839–850. https://doi.org/10.1017/S1355617716000643

Miller, L. T., Polatajko, H. J., Missiuna, C., Mandich, A. D., & Macnab, J. J. (2001). A pilot trial of a cognitive treatment for children with developmental coordination disorder. *Human Movement Science, 20,* 183–210. https://doi.org/10.1016/S0167-9457(01)00034-3

Nickel, M., & Gu, C. (2018). Regulation of central nervous system myelination in higher brain functions. *Neural Plasticity, 2018,* 6436453. https://doi.org/10.1155/2018/6436453

Nyhus, E., & Barcelo, F. (2009). The Wisconsin Card Sorting Test and the cognitive assessment of prefrontal executive functions: A critical update. *Brain and Cognition, 71,* 437–451. https://doi.org/10.1016/j.bandc.2009.03.005

Payne, J. M., Arnold, S. S., Pride, N. A., & North, K. N. (2012). Does attention-deficit–hyperactivity disorder exacerbate executive dysfunction in children with neurofibromatosis Type 1? *Developmental Medicine and Child Neurology, 54,* 898–904. https://doi.org/10.1111/j.1469-8749.2012.04357.x

Polatajko, H., & Mandich A. (2004). *Enabling occupation in children: The Cognitive Orientation to daily Occupational Performance (CO–OP) approach.* Ottawa: CAOT Publications.

Polatajko, H. J., Mandich, A. D., Miller, L. T., & Macnab, J. J. (2001). Cognitive Orientation to daily Occupational Performance (CO–OP): Part II—The evidence. *Physical and Occupational Therapy in Pediatrics, 20*(2/3), 83–106. https://doi.org /10.1080/J006v20n02_06

Prencipe, A., Kesek, A., Cohen, J., Lamm, C., Lewis, M. D., & Zelazo, P. D. (2011). Development of hot and cool executive function during the transition to adolescence. *Journal of Experimental Child Psychology, 108,* 621–637. https://doi.org /10.1016/j.jecp.2010.09.008

Qian, Y., Shuai, L., Cao, Q., Chan, R. C. K., & Wang, Y. (2010). Do executive function deficits differentiate between children with attention deficit hyperactivity disorder (ADHD) and ADHD comorbid with oppositional defiant disorder? A cross-cultural study using performance-based tests and the Behavior Rating Inventory of Executive Function. *Clinical Neuropsychologist, 24,* 793–810. https://doi.org/10.1080/13854041003749342

Rahimi-Golkhandan, S., Steenbergen, B., Piek, J., Caeyenberghs, K., & Wilson, P. (2016). Revealing hot executive function in children with motor coordination problems: What's the go? *Brain and Cognition, 106,* 55–64. https://doi.org/10.1016/j.bandc .2016.04.010

Reitan, R. M. (1944). *Trail Making Test.* Washington, DC: U.S. Army, Adjutant General's Office, War Department.

Rodger, S., & Brandenburg, J. (2009). Cognitive Orientation to (daily) Occupational Performance (CO–OP) with children with Asperger syndrome who have motor-based occupational performance goals. *Australian Occupational Therapy Journal, 56,* 41–50. https://doi.org/10.1111/j.1440-1630.2008.00739.x

Rodger, S., Ireland, S., & Vun, M. (2008). Can Cognitive Orientation to daily Occupational Performance (CO–OP) help children with Asperger syndrome master social and organizational goals? *British Journal of Occupational Therapy, 71*(10), 23–32. https://doi.org/10.1177/030802260807100105

Rodger, S., Pham, C., & Mitchell, S. (2009). Cognitive strategy use by children with Asperger's syndrome during intervention for motor-based goals. *Australian Occupational Therapy Journal, 56,* 103–111. https://doi.org/10.1111/j.1440-1630.2007.00719.x

Rodger, S., Springfield, E., & Polatajko, H. J. (2007). Cognitive Orientation for daily Occupational Performance approach for children with Asperger's syndrome: A case report. *Physical and Occupational Therapy in Pediatrics, 27,* 7–22. https://doi .org/10.1080/J006v27n04_02

Rodger, S., & Vishram, A. (2010). Mastering social and organization goals: Strategy use by two children with Asperger's syndrome during Cognitive Orientation to daily Occupational Performance. *Physical and Occupational Therapy in Pediatrics, 30,* 264–276. https://doi.org/10.3109/01942638.2010.500893

Rosen, S. M., Boyle, J. R., Cariss, K., & Forchelli, G. A. (2014). Changing how we think, changing how we learn: Scaffolding executive function processes for students with learning disabilities. *Learning Disabilities, 20,* 165–176.

Rosenberg, L., Jacobi, S., & Bart, O. (2017). Executive functions and motor ability contribute to children's participation in daily activities. *Journal of Occupational Therapy, Schools, and Early Intervention, 10,* 315–326. https://doi.org/10.1080/19411243 .2017.1312660

Samuelson, K. W., Krueger, C. E., & Wilson, C. (2012). Relationships between maternal emotion regulation, parenting, and children's executive functioning in families exposed to intimate partner violence. *Journal of Interpersonal Violence, 27,* 3532–3550. https://doi.org/10.1177/0886260512445385

Scammell, E. M., Bates, S. V., Houldin, A., & Polatajko, H. J. (2016). The Cognitive Orientation to daily Occupational Performance (CO–OP): A scoping review. *Canadian Journal of Occupational Therapy, 83,* 216–225. https://doi.org/10.1177 /0008417416651277

Schurink, J., Hartman, E., Scherder, E. J. A., Houwen, S., & Visscher, C. (2012). Relationship between motor and executive functioning in school-age children with pervasive developmental disorder not otherwise specified. *Research in Autism Spectrum Disorders, 6,* 726–732. https://doi.org/10.1016/j.rasd .2011.10.013

Semrud-Clikeman, M., Fine, J. G., & Bledsoe, J. (2014). Comparison among children with autism spectrum disorder, nonverbal learning disorder and typically developing children on measures of executive functioning. *Journal of Autism and Developmental Disorders, 44,* 331–342. https://doi.org/10.1007 /s10803-013-1871-2

Shallice, T. (1982). Specific impairments of planning. *Philosophical Transactions of the Royal Society B: Biological Sciences, 298,* 199–209. https://doi.org/10.1098/rstb.1982.0082

Skowronski, J. M., & Engsberg, J. R. (2017). Blended Approach to Occupational Performance (BAOP): Guidelines enabling children with autism. *Open Journal of Occupational Therapy, 5,* Article 7. https://doi.org/10.15453/2168-6408.1282

Tamm, L., Nakonezny, P. A., & Hughes, C. W. (2014). An open trial of a metacognitive executive function training for young children with ADHD. *Journal of Attention Disorders, 18,* 551–559. https://doi.org/10.1177/1087054712445782

Taylor, S., Fayed, N., & Mandich, A. (2007). CO–OP intervention for young children with developmental coordination disorder. *Occupational Therapy Journal of Research, 27,* 124–130. https:// doi.org/10.1177/153944920702700402

Tesfaye, R., & Gruber, R. (2017). The association between sleep and theory of mind in school aged children with ADHD. *Medical Sciences, 5*(3), 18. https://doi.org/10.3390/medsci5030018

Toplak, M. E., Bucciarelli, S. M., Jain, U., & Tannock, R. (2009). Executive functions: Performance-based measures and the Behavior Rating Inventory of Executive Function (BRIEF) in adolescents with attention deficit/hyperactivity disorder (ADHD). *Child Neuropsychology, 15,* 53–72. https://doi.org/10.1080/09297 040802070929

Wells, A. M., Chasnoff, I. J., Schmidt, C. A., Telford, E., & Schwartz, L. D. (2012). Neurocognitive habilitation therapy for children with fetal alcohol spectrum disorders: An adaptation of the Alert Program®. *American Journal of Occupational Therapy, 66,* 24–34. https://doi.org/10.5014/ajot.2012.002691

Williams, M. S., & Shellenberger, S. (1996). *"How does your engine run?" A leader's guide to the Alert Program for self-regulation.* Albuquerque, NM: Therapy Works.

Zelazo, P. D., Craik, F. I. M., & Booth, L. (2004). Executive function across the life span. *Acta Psychologica, 115,* 167–183. https://doi.org/10.1016/j.actpsy.2003.12.005

Ziviani, J., Copley, J., Ownsworth, T. L., Campbell, N. E., & Cummins, K. L. (2008). Visual perception abilities and executive functions in children with school-related occupational performance difficulties. *Journal of Occupational Therapy, Schools and Early Intervention, 1,* 246–262. https://doi.org/10 .1080/19411240802589247

Best Practices in Fine Motor Skills to Enhance Participation

55

Charlotte E. Exner, PhD, OT/L, FAOTA, and Amanda C. Jozkowski, PhD, OTR/L

KEY TERMS AND CONCEPTS

- Asymmetrical bilateral activities
- Constraint-induced movement therapy
- Hand–arm bimanual intensive therapy
- In-hand manipulation
- Manual ability
- Simultaneous manipulation
- Strengths-based approach
- Symmetrical bilateral activities

OVERVIEW

Fine motor skills are integral to completion of many school activities that are vital to academic success. Fine motor skills allow for engagement in learning activities both in and outside of the classroom. In the typical classroom, demonstration of learned concepts requires the use of one's hands to perform required actions inherent to an activity (e.g., actions to a song, counting, gesturing) and to interact with and move materials, such as paper, writing tools, computers, notebooks, and class-specific objects.

The importance of fine motor skills for activity engagement and learning experiences is readily apparent in young students' programs at the early elementary school level, when handling materials is a key component of learning activities for approximately half of the school day (Marr et al., 2003). Fine motor skills are also prerequisite to or associated with learning activities throughout elementary school (Cameron et al., 2012; Dinehart & Manfra, 2013), middle school (Fernandes et al., 2016), and high school and are the foundation for participation in post–high school education and in most work settings. Some classes have substantial demands for fine motor skills, with learning materials such as calculators, math and science equipment, art materials, and musical instruments.

Students with fine motor difficulties may encounter other challenges (Dinehart & Manfra, 2013). They may miss key school experiences because they need additional time to complete tasks involving fine motor skills. Proprioceptive and tactile learning that accompanies classroom tasks and supports an in-depth understanding of object properties can be compromised when more complex fine motor skills are difficult. In addition, fine motor skills have been linked with perceived competence and self-efficacy for children (Gaul & Issartel, 2016). Outside the classroom, fine motor difficulties can interfere with navigation (e.g., opening a door, pushing a button on an elevator, signaling someone to wait).

Overall, fine motor skills influence participation in the school environment across a wide range of activities that become more complex over time and require more refined fine motor skills (see Table 55.1). Addressing fine motor difficulties can support the student's school performance and affect future opportunities, including successful transition from school into post–high school roles.

ESSENTIAL CONSIDERATIONS

Many key areas have been found to have a relationship with fine motor performance (Case-Smith et al., 2013). Using this evidence, occupational therapists have a basis for identifying areas for evaluation and potentially for explaining factors associated with certain fine motor challenges (see Table 55.2). Intervention may be designed to concurrently address some of these areas along with fine motor skills.

Research related to relationships among factors associated with fine motor skills is prevalent. However, links between fine motor skills and participation among students and youth seem to be understudied. Although studies that consider relationships between or among variables can be helpful in understanding some of the co-occurring factors, these findings cannot be used directly to plan interventions, unless the occupational therapist has other data to support an intervention.

In addition, few studies have assessed the long-term impact of intervention. Very little research is available relative to high school students, who may be confronting additional challenges in classes with greater demands for higher level fine motor skills and preparing to move into a post–high school education setting or into the work environment.

Another key gap in research evidence is related to measuring outcomes associated with therapeutic interventions that are implemented by others (e.g., teachers, support staff, family members) but designed by therapists. School

Copyright © 2019 by the American Occupational Therapy Association. All rights reserved. To reuse this content, contact www.copyright.com. https://doi.org/10.7139/2019.978-1-56900-591-0.055

TABLE 55.1.   Examples of Typical School Activities Requiring Fine Motor Skills

AREA	ELEMENTARY SCHOOL	MIDDLE AND HIGH SCHOOL
Fine motor control and coordination	Drawing, printing letters, building with interlocking blocks, brushing teeth, manipulating currency, completing arts-and-crafts projects	Opening various containers, handling delicate science tools and objects, using finger isolation for smart technology, using a swipe card
Bimanual skills	Stabilizing paper for writing and erasing, navigating the cafeteria, tying shoes, managing clothing, packing a backpack, filing papers, playing an instrument	Managing more complex personal hygiene and clothing, handling and storing papers and materials, completing class project activities, using science equipment
Visual–motor skills	Coloring, writing, copying from a board, typing and using a computer	Organizing project materials, engaging in employment interests

occupational therapists can evaluate, intervene with both indirect and direct strategies, advocate for accommodations and the student's development of skills in planning for alternative strategies, and model and support students' self-advocacy efforts in schools. Each of these efforts warrants increased attention in the literature to further inform practice in schools.

BEST PRACTICES

Because of the complexity of fine motor skills, a student's quality and efficiency in using these skills can be affected by a wide variety of factors, which must be carefully gathered through the evaluation process. Interventions should address students' ability to participate in their school program.

Evaluate Fine Motor Performance

The occupational therapist uses a strategic combination of formal and informal assessment, observation, and professional reasoning to evaluate a student's fine motor performance skills.

When assessing these skills, the occupational therapist's priority is to determine the impact of the student's competency to effectively accomplish a range of tasks and activities in the school setting. Starting with a top-down approach, the therapist should first consider how fine motor challenges affect the student's school success, participation, and occupational satisfaction. If limitations in occupational performance are identified, therapists can begin to drill down to tease out the multiple factors that may influence fine motor performance.

It is critical not only to assess traditional areas, such as coordination, fine motor dexterity, and visual–motor integration, but also to include assessment of other related areas in the full evaluation report. These areas may include

- Sensory integration and processing,
- Reflex development,
- Core stability, and
- Psychosocial factors.

In addition, fine motor performance should be assessed during different activities (e.g., academic, eating, dressing) and in varied positions (e.g., sitting, standing, walking).

When selecting assessment tools for fine motor evaluation, the school occupational therapist should consider tools that provide reliable, functional information and are sensitive to change for tracking outcomes and progress toward individualized education program (IEP) goals. Therapists

should also endeavor to use a ***strengths-based approach*** for evaluation and reporting. The strengths-based approach focuses on the skills and abilities of the student and their impact on educational performance rather than on the student's diagnosis and deficits.

The IEP team develops the student's goals on the basis of the student's identified strengths and needs. Sources of information used to develop goals include

- Data from observations of the student during school routines,
- Student interviews regarding their goals,
- Teacher and parent interviews, and
- Data from assessments tools.

When students are unable to meet expectations, accommodations may be needed. Such accommodations may include changes to the activity or materials (e.g., using modified scissors), alterations to physical demands (e.g., changing body position), or changes to the environment (e.g., different desk, quieter area).

Determine Intervention Approach to Enhance Fine Motor Performance

Occupational therapists consider the approach to intervention that seems most appropriate for the student and the skills needed. Evidence for fine motor interventions to target specific outcomes, particularly for students across diagnostic categories, is limited. Occupational therapy practitioners[1] may provide intervention in the classroom routine that affects the student's ability to participate, such as drawing or cutting or by focusing on the factors that they have identified as contributing to the difficulties, such as attention, strength, motor planning, or sensory issues (McGlashan et al., 2017). Both approaches may be used together. Thus, the strategies that follow are grouped by area of challenge with

---

[1]*Occupational therapy practitioner* refers to both the occupational therapist and the occupational therapy assistant. The American Occupational Therapy Association (AOTA; 2014, p. S18) states, "The occupational therapist is responsible for all aspects of occupational therapy service delivery and is accountable for the safety and effectiveness of the occupational therapy service delivery process" and "must be directly involved in the delivery of services during the initial evaluation and regularly throughout the course of intervention. . . . The occupational therapy assistant delivers safe and effective occupational therapy services under the supervision of and in partnership with the occupational therapist."

TABLE 55.2.   Relationships Between Fine Motor Performance and Cognitive or Motor Areas

AREA	RESEARCH
Cognitive	
Attention	Motor coordination was negatively affected among students ages 7–14 years with ADHD; errors were more linked to inattention than to hyperactivity (Fenollar-Cortés et al., 2017).
Initiation	Students with DCD may have difficulty planning and starting a motor task (Smits-Engelsman et al., 2013).
Motor learning	Completing a short fine motor training program (2D and 3D tracing for approximately 6 weeks) improved perceptual–motor learning, especially among 7- to 8-year-olds (Snapp-Childs et al., 2015).
Cognitive control and planning	Students with ID and DD were likely to have difficulties with fine manual dexterity and cognitive planning or verbal working memory (Chen et al., 2014).
Energy and motivation	Children with CP receiving a play-focused occupational therapy intervention demonstrated greater improvements in fine motor skills than those who received therapy focused on self-care skills (Senapati, 2017). Focus on a particular goal during therapy was beneficial (Harbourne & Kamm, 2015).
Motor skill and praxis	
Postural stability and mobility	A positive relationship was found between students' postural control and hand skills (Flatters et al., 2014).
Arm and hand stability and mobility	Postural stability and hand skills had a significant but not strong relationship in a study of typically developing students between ages 3 and 11 years (Flatters et al., 2014). Individual finger isolation relies on stability of some fingers while the person differentiates 1 or more fingers for selected movements. Upper limb kinematics do not develop until the later elementary school age range, so younger students are somewhat inconsistent in their reach, grasp, object manipulation, and force control patterns.
In-hand manipulation skills	Case-Smith and Exner (2005) described various types of in-hand manipulation skills that rely on stability in the hand in conjunction with graded control and finger movement differentiation. ***In-hand manipulation*** skills allow the person to position objects in the hand to effectively prepare for a functional activity, such as rotating a paper clip for fastening papers or adjusting a pencil for the fingers to be near the writing end. Greater difficulty of in-hand manipulation skills occurs during manipulation of an object while another object is stabilized in the same hand (Visser et al., 2014). In 1 study, young students who used tablets frequently or who had limited opportunities to use complex fine motor skills had less developed fine motor skills (Lin et al., 2017).
Bilateral coordination and integration	Bimanual coordination includes interaction between the hands. ***Symmetrical bilateral activities*** involve the hands acting together in a similar manner in an activity (e.g., pulling a chair up to a table, catching a ball, carrying a lunch tray). ***Asymmetrical bilateral activities*** involve stabilizing an object with 1 hand while manipulating an object with the other hand. ***Simultaneous manipulation*** may occur with the same or different pattern of movements, such as in shoe tying.
Hand preference and handedness	This is commonly noted as an area of challenge for students with fine motor difficulties. Hand preference is variable among young students, with greater inconsistency among students with a left-hand preference (Scharoun & Bryden, 2014).
Sensory and perceptual skills	Challenges in fine motor skills were associated with increased sensitivity to touch and decreased proprioception among girls with autism (Riquelme et al., 2016). Proprioception difficulties were found among students with DCD (Tseng et al., 2019). Bilateral manipulation was identified as particularly challenging for a student with binocular vision difficulties (Niechwiej-Szwedo et al., 2017). Visual–spatial integration was a key element (in combination with visual–motor coordination and IQ) for writing outcomes (Carlson et al., 2013).

Note. ADHD = attention deficit hyperactivity disorder; CP = cerebral palsy; DCD = developmental coordination disorder; DD = developmental disabilities; ID = intellectual disabilities.

notations specific to degree of difficulties, with the environment first, to facilitate performance.

Address positioning in the environment

General considerations for various fine motor skills often identified for intervention in occupational therapy practice in the schools are outlined next. Occupational therapy practitioners will find more detailed descriptions of intervention strategies in the work of Case-Smith and O'Brien (2015) and Henderson and Pehoski (2005).

School furniture can support postural control or create challenges for students, particularly for students with motor skill challenges. Castellucci et al. (2016) conducted a systematic review of classroom furniture and its impact on students' physical status and performance. They found that furniture fitted to students' body size was essential.

Smith-Zuzovsky and Exner (2004) found that 6- and 7-year-old students seated in appropriately fitted furniture had more effective in-hand manipulation skills. Typical classroom chairs do not allow students to sit with their knees at a 90° bend with feet flat on the floor and the table at elbow height. The authors found that using furniture that fitted students well seemed to result in students using more complex in-hand manipulation skills effectively in comparison with their skill use when seated in typical furniture.

Wingrat and Exner (2005) found that 4th-grade students' attention to classroom tasks, as well as their sitting position, was better when they used chairs and tables that fitted well instead of sitting in the standard classroom furniture. Thus, careful review of the chair and table fit for students across settings is important. If needed, modifications should be made to support function and comfort. Also, although the seated position is used most often in schools, other positions may be more successful during some types of intervention and in supporting the student to generalize skill use.

Applying a critical analysis of the literature, Harbourne and Kamm (2015) concluded that posture and upper extremity function (i.e., reaching to explore and manipulate materials) are linked. Interventions that address reaching skills must include

- Variability and an opportunity to problem solve,
- Challenging activities that incorporate posture and reaching,
- Whole-body movement combined with reaching,
- Consideration of developmental demands, and
- Allowance for error learning.

These principles promote generalization of skills.

General strategies for fine motor skill intervention

Arnould et al. (2014) found that the strongest contributors to the **manual ability** (i.e., hand skills essential for functional tasks) in students with cerebral palsy (6–16 years) were skill in grasp and release of small- to medium-sized objects (and the ability to recognize objects by touch (stereognosis), particularly in the child's preferred hand. Grip strength also seemed to play a role in students' skill in functional activities. Based on their research and review of other studies, Arnould et al. (2014) recommended that practitioners consider addressing hand strengthening (including weakness associated with spasticity), dexterity training, and interventions that emphasize a focus on activities (e.g., constraint-induced movement therapy, hand–arm bimanual intensive therapy).

Specific strategies to consider in fine motor intervention

Using natural, goal-oriented activities with students while addressing fine motor skills supports inclusion and generalization (Chien et al., 2014). Changing the location and orientation of objects can support students' skill development in handling materials for various meaningful activities.

For example, having students place books on a shelf in a vertical orientation encourages external rotation of the arm and sustained forearm supination. This process can also include a bilateral skill component if students use the other hand to separate books and place the books in the correct place on the shelf. Modifying this task for horizontal placement of a book on top of other books can make the task feasible for students who need to use 2 hands to carry or place a book. Another general strategy for classroom use is making various writing tools an acceptable and available option for all students. This approach allows for students' involvement in decision making about which tool will be most comfortable and supports their analysis of best options.

Creating group experiences to practice various fine motor skills also may be an effective strategy for inclusion of students who have difficulties as well as others who could benefit from skill enhancement. Such activities may be helpful for students with mild challenges who can participate in these activities with minimal or no additional support.

General education students who are at risk for fine motor problems. Students in general education programs with fine motor or dexterity issues have benefited from occupational therapy interventions. Examples of interventions for kindergarten students reported as having positive fine motor or dexterity outcomes include the following:

- Fine motor activities with various small tools to grasp and move objects (Stewart et al., 2007)
- Traditional folk games (e.g., playing cat's cradle, using a paper fortune teller, cutting paper lanterns) 3 times a week for 40- to 50-minute sessions for 3 months (Wei, 2016)
- A 10-week general education intervention that included a weekly co-led classroom group (teacher and occupational therapist), a new fine motor center in the classroom each week, and weekly collaborative consultation between the teacher and the occupational therapist (Ohl et al., 2013).

Elementary and middle school students have been shown to benefit from fine motor interventions, such as

- A computerized typing intervention to improve general manual dexterity for 8- to 10-year-olds without delays (McGlashan et al., 2017),
- A motor skill development program for 9- to 12-year-olds to improve bilateral coordination (Africa & Van Deventer, 2015), and
- A visual–motor training study that included students ages 2–12 years old (Snapp-Childs et al., 2015).

Strategies to enhance hand reaching and manipulation. Direct intervention strategies include changes to objects used in therapy—for example, selecting objects on the basis of size, shape, and texture—that result in optimal performance for the student and gradually increasing task complexity. Exploring positions in which the forearm is supported by a surface when combining reach and grasp may allow more effective use of finger and thumb mobility. Students with moderate or greater difficulties may benefit from intervention for index finger or another individual finger control to support access to technology devices. Assistive technology, such as switches, environmental controls, and wearables, may be needed for students with limited hand skills to foster engagement and learning activities (Perelmutter et al., 2017).

Supporting development of reaching skills is dependent on an analysis of the degree of stability that the student has in the trunk and throughout the arm. Reaching can be facilitated through use of different body positions, with consideration of the need for postural control. Reaching coupled with touching an object is less complex than reaching and grasping, and reaching with grasp is less challenging if the object is closer to the student's body and if forearm pronation can be used. Reach and grasp of small objects or unstable objects are a more advanced skill.

The student's body stability can affect the quality of in-hand manipulation skills (Smith-Zuzovsky & Exner, 2004), so students should be seated on a well-fitted chair at a table with an appropriate height for hand use, especially when skills are emerging. The general developmental sequence of in-hand manipulation skills coupled with small-sized objects is recommended as a starting point for intervention planning. In-hand manipulation skills that do not involve concurrent stabilization of another object in the hand are easier to use.

In selecting objects for in-hand manipulation practice, practitioners should note that larger objects require more control of the palmar arches; very small objects require precision with fingertip control and greater regulation of pressure on the object during manipulation. Manipulating unstable objects (e.g., shoelaces) is more challenging than manipulating more stable objects. Visual or verbal cueing may promote use of more complex in-hand manipulation skills (Exner, 1990).

Visual–motor skills. Practitioners should address visual–motor skills in both 2D and 3D activities. Interventions should consider any visual–perceptual, motor, and motor planning challenges. One study found that students (7–8 years old) demonstrated enhanced 3D performance and improved 2D drawing with tracing (Snapp-Childs et al., 2015). For more information, see Chapter 58, "Best Practices in Visual Perception and Visual–Motor Skills to Enhance Participation."

Visual attention and fine motor skills. Attention and fine motor performance may be linked, given findings that students with attention difficulties are likely to show fine motor problems (Fenollar-Cortés et al., 2017). Addressing fine motor performance, especially with activities that are engaging and require focus on detail and precision, may also support attention skills. During intervention, use of an age-appropriate, highly engaging, goal-directed fine motor activity is recommended.

Clinical interventions. Occupational therapy practitioners in schools should be aware of interventions common to clinical settings. Having a general awareness will allow school practitioners to
- Better collaborate with clinical providers,
- Educate team members when parents choose clinical services for their child, and
- Delineate why various interventions should be provided in a clinical setting instead of being offered in an educational setting.

Constraint-induced movement therapy (CIMT) and *hand–arm bimanual intensive therapy* (HABIT) are 2 interventions that might be offered in a clinical setting. Some students with significant hand skill problems may receive CIMT through their clinical services. CIMT intervention is rigorous; it focuses on restricting the use of the child's less involved hand and facilitating the use of their more involved hand in bilateral activities as well as unilateral activities (Case-Smith, 2015; Cohen-Holzer, Katz-Leurer, et al., 2017; Cohen-Holzer, Sorek, et al., 2017; Hung et al., 2011). Durand et al. (2018) conducted a systematic review of use of CIMT with children, provided at home or in a group setting, and found positive outcomes in use of the arm involved and functional activities.

Hung et al. (2011) compared CIMT with HABIT to determine which program was more effective in improving 4- to 10-year-olds' use of the more involved hand. HABIT requires intensive bimanual training (e.g., 90 hours), typically in a group format, with an emphasis on bimanual activities. In Hung et al.'s (2011) study, the HABIT group had significantly more gains in using both hands together and improved timing of hand movements.

Collaborate on Fine Motor Skills

In addition to collaborating with the student with fine motor challenges, school occupational therapy practitioners should keep in mind the value and importance of communicating with teachers, family members, and others regarding the evaluation and intervention of fine motor skills in schools (Koelbl et al., 2016). Finally, occupational therapy practitioners should strive to be mindful of the ultimate goal of skill generalization, which has been supported by research as critical to occupational well-being across contexts. Fine motor opportunities must be translated, rehearsed, and supported in other settings both inside and outside the school, so that generalization of skills can occur. This allows the student to participate in daily occupations across contexts.

SUMMARY

Occupational therapy practitioners provide interventions for students who present with fine motor performance challenges that affect their participation in school. A group approach can be favorable for young students to build their fine motor skills through play and functional activities. Currently, research on fine motor interventions is limited; therefore, occupational therapists need to use their professional judgment and best available evidence to design intervention plans and monitor student progress. As data are collected, interventions can be adjusted to optimize student performance. School occupational therapy practitioners are encouraged to contribute to scholarly works and share interventions that produce meaningful outcomes for students.

ONLINE RESOURCES FOR FINE MOTOR IDEAS, ACTIVITIES, AND CONTINUING EDUCATION

- **AOTA's Resources for School-Based OT Practitioners** (https://bit.ly/2H7AojK): List of AOTA-approved documents related to occupational therapy practice in the schools, including policy issues and statements on inclusion

- **The Inspired Treehouse's Resources for Therapists** (https://bit.ly/2QISCat): Activity ideas, products, and helpful articles on issues such as seating, "push-in" vs. "pull-out" models in schools, and classroom strategies
- **Mama OT** (http://www.mamaot.com) **and Kids Play Smarter** (https://kidsplaysmarter.com) weblogs: Two weblogs published by occupational therapists that provide helpful tips on activities to do with students at home; categorized by area of intervention, information about sensory processing, toy and gift guides, developmental milestones, and links to other books and resources
- **NewGradOccupationalTherapy's "60 Effective School-Based Apps for Occupational Therapy"** (https://bit.ly /2Fn65nt): List of mobile apps for therapy in schools; includes links to and descriptions of apps to address a range of functional areas, including fine motor, handwriting, and life skills
- **OccupationalTherapy.com's Finger and Hand Fun for School Based Therapists** (https://bit.ly/2sq9pp8): Continuing education course with emphasis on writing and other fine motor demands related to current Common Core educational standards
- **OT Mom Learning Activities** (https://www.ot-mom -learning-activities.com/): A weblog published by an occupational therapist who homeschools her children; includes excellent step-by-step and visual instructions for developing a range of fine and visual–motor skills relevant to students, as well as printables and recommended products
- **Pediatric Occupational Therapists Facebook group** (https://www.facebook.com/groups/80351866792/): International group of occupational therapy practitioners and occupational therapy students formed to share resources, problem solve challenging cases, and discuss issues related to pediatric practice
- **Tools to Grow: Resources for Pediatric Therapists** (https://www.toolstogrowot.com/): Thousands of free and subscription-based resources for fine motor intervention ideas

REFERENCES

Africa, E. K., & Van Deventer, K. L. (2015). Balance and bilateral skills of selected previously disadvantaged children aged 9 to 12 years. *South African Journal for Research in Sport, Physical Education and Recreation, 37*(3), 1–13.

American Occupational Therapy Association. (2014). Guidelines for supervision, roles, and responsibilities during the delivery of occupational therapy services. *American Journal of Occupational Therapy, 68*(Suppl. 3), S16–S22. https://doi.org/10.5014 /ajot.2014.686S03

Arnould, C., Bleyenheuft, Y., & Thonnard, J. L. (2014). Hand functioning in children with cerebral palsy. *Frontiers in Neurology, 5,* Article 48. https://doi.org/10.3389/fneur.2014.00048

Cameron, C. E., Brock, L. L., Murrah, W. M., Bell, L. H., Worzalla, S. L., Grissmer, D., & Morrison, F. J. (2012). Fine motor skills and executive function both contribute to kindergarten achievement. *Child Development, 83,* 1229–1244. https://doi .org/10.1111/j.1467-8624.2012.01768.x

Carlson, A. G., Rowe, E., & Curby, T. W. (2013). Disentangling fine motor skills' relations to academic achievement: The relative contributions of visual–spatial integration and visual–motor coordination. *Journal of Genetic Psychology, 174,* 514–533. https://doi.org/10.1080/00221325.2012.717122

Case-Smith, J. (2015). Best practices in fine motor and visual–motor skills to enhance participation. In G. F. Clark & B. E. Chandler (Eds.), *Best practices for occupational therapy in schools* (pp. 443–457). Bethesda, MD: AOTA Press.

Case-Smith, J., & Exner, C. E. (2015). Hand function evaluation and intervention. In J. Case-Smith & J. C. O'Brien (Eds.), *Occupational therapy for children and adolescents* (7th ed., pp. 225–227). St. Louis, MO: Elsevier.

Case-Smith, J., Frolek Clark, G. J., & Schlabach, T. L. (2013). Systematic review of interventions used in occupational therapy to promote motor performance for children ages birth–5 years. *American Journal of Occupational Therapy, 67,* 413–424. https:// doi.org/10.5014/ajot.2013.005959

Case-Smith, J., & O'Brien, J. C. (2015). *Occupational therapy for children and adolescents* (7th ed.). St. Louis: Mosby.

Castellucci, I., Arezes, P. M., Molenbroek, J. F. M., & Viviani, C. (2016). The influence of school furniture on students' performance and physical responses: Results of a systematic review. *Ergonomics, 60,* 93–110. https://doi.org/10.1080/00140139.2016 .1170889

Chen, C.-C., Ringenbach, S. D. R., Albert, A., & Semken, K. (2014). Fine motor control is related to cognitive control in adolescents with Down syndrome. *International Journal of Disability, Development and Education, 61*(1), 6–15. https://doi.org /10.1080/1034912X.2014.878532

Chien, C.-W., Brown, T., McDonald, R., & Yu, M.-L. (2014). The contributing role of real-life hand skill performance in self-care function of children with and without disabilities. *Child: Care, Health and Development, 40,* 134–144. https://doi.org /10.1111/j.1365-2214.2012.01429.x

Cohen-Holzer, M., Katz-Leurer, M., Meyer, S., Green, D., & Parush, S. (2017). The effect of bimanual training with or without constraint on hand functions in children with unilateral cerebral palsy: A non-randomized clinical trial. *Physical and Occupational Therapy in Pediatrics, 37,* 516–527. https://doi.org /10.1080/01942638.2017.1280871

Cohen-Holzer, M., Sorek, G., Kerem, J., & Katz-Leurer, M. (2017). The impact of combined constraint-induced and bimanual arm training program on the perceived hand-use experience of children with unilateral cerebral palsy. *Developmental Neurorehabilitation, 20,* 355–360. https://doi.org/10.1080/17518423.2016 .1238017

Dinehart, L., & Manfra, L. (2013). Associations between low-income children's fine motor skills in preschool and academic performance in second grade. *Early Education and Development, 24,* 138–161. https://doi.org/10.1080/10409289.2011 .636729

Durand, E., Plante, P., Pelletier, A.-A., Rondeiau, J., Simard, F., & Voisin, J. (2018). At-home and in-group delivery of constraint-induced movement therapy in children with hemiparesis: A systematic review. *Annals of Physical and Rehabilitation Medicine, 61,* 245–261. https://doi.org/10.1016/j.rehab .2017.10.004

Exner, C. E. (1990). The zone of proximal development in in-hand manipulation skills of nondysfunctional 3- and 4-year old children. *American Journal of Occupational Therapy, 44,* 884–891. https://doi.org/10.5014/ajot.44.10.884

Fenollar-Cortés, J., Gallego-Martínez, A., & Fuentes, L. J. (2017). The role of inattention and hyperactivity/impulsivity in the fine motor coordination in children with ADHD. *Research in Developmental Disabilities, 69,* 77–84. https://doi.org/10.1016/j.ridd.2017.08.003

Fernandes, V. R., Scipiao Riberio, M. L., Melo, T., Maciel-Pinheiro, P. T., Guimaraes, T. T., Araujo, . . . Deslandes, A. C. (2016). Motor coordination correlates with academic achievement and cognitive function in children. *Frontiers in Psychology, 7,* 318. https://doi.org/10.3389/fpsyg.2016.00318

Flatters, I., Mushtaq, F., Hill, L. J. B., Holt, R. J., Wilkie, R. M., & Mon-Williams, M. (2014). The relationship between a child's postural stability and manual dexterity. *Experimental Brain Research, 239,* 2907–2917. https://doi.org/10.1007/s00221-014-3947-4

Gaul, D., & Issartel, J. (2016). Fine motor skill proficiency in typically developing children: On or off the maturation track? *Human Movement Science, 46,* 78–85. https://doi.org/10.1016/j.humov.2015.12.011

Harbourne, R., & Kamm, K. (2015). Upper extremity function: What's posture got to do with it? *Journal of Hand Therapy, 28,* 106–113. https://doi.org/10.1016/j.jht.2015.01.008

Henderson, A., & Pehoski, C. (2005). *Hand function in the child: Foundations for remediation* (2nd ed.). St. Louis: Mosby.

Hung, Y. C., Casertano, L., Hillman, A., & Gordon, A. M. R. (2011). The effect of intensive bimanual training on coordination of hands in children with congenital hemiplegia. *Research in Developmental Disabilities, 32,* 2724–2731. https://doi.org/10.1016/j.ridd.2011.05.038

Koelbl, H., Myman, Y., Wuestefeld, A. C., Elenko, B., & Ohl, A. (2016). Occupational therapist's perceptions of STEPS–K: A response to intervention (RtI) program. *Journal of Occupational Therapy, Schools, and Early Intervention, 9,* 269–280. https://doi.org/10.1080/19411243.2016.1207213

Lin, L.-Y., Cherng, R.-J., & Chen, Y.-J. (2017). Effect of touch screen tablet use on fine motor development of young children. *Physical and Occupational Therapy in Pediatrics, 37,* 457–467. https://doi.org/10.1080/01942638.2016.1255290

Marr, D., Cermak, S., Cohn, E. S., & Henderson, A. (2003). Fine motor activities in Head Start and kindergarten classrooms. *American Journal of Occupational Therapy, 57,* 550–557. https://doi.org/10.5014/ajot.57.5.550

McGlashan, H. L., Blanchard, C. C., Sycamore, N. J., Lee, R., French, B., & Holmes, N. P. (2017). Improvement in children's fine motor skills following a computerized typing intervention. *Human Movement Science, 56*(Part B), 29–36. https://doi.org/10.1016/j.humov.2017.10.013

Niechwiej-Szwedo, E., Alramis, F., & Christian, L. W. (2017). Association between fine motor skills and binocular visual function in children with reading difficulties. *Human Movement Science 56*(Part B), 1–10. https://doi.org/10.1016/j.humov.2017.10.014

Ohl, A. M., Graze, H., Weber, K., Kenny, S., Salvatore, C., & Wagreich, S. (2013). Effectiveness of a 10-week Tier-1 response to intervention program in improving fine motor and visual–motor skills in general education kindergarten students. *American Journal of Occupational Therapy, 67,* 507–514. https://doi.org/10.5014/ajot.2013.008110

Perelmutter, B., McGregor, K. K., & Gordon, K. R. (2017). Assistive technology interventions for adolescents and adults with learning disabilities: An evidence-based systematic review and meta-analysis. *Computers and Education, 114,* 139–163. https://doi.org/10.1016/j.compedu.2017.06.005

Riquelme, I., Hatem, S. M., & Montoya, P. (2016). Abnormal pressure pain, touch sensitivity, proprioception, and manual dexterity in children with autism spectrum disorders. *Neural Plasticity, 2016,* 1723401. https://doi.org/10.1155/2016/1723401

Scharoun, S. M., & Bryden, P. J. (2014). Hand preference, performance abilities, and hand selection in children. *Frontiers in Psychology, 5,* 82. https://doi.org/10.3389/fpsyg.2014.00082

Senapati, B. (2017). The effectiveness of play activities and functional activities on fine motor skills in children with spastic diplegic cerebral palsy. *Indian Journal of Physiotherapy and Occupational Therapy, 11*(1), 85–89. https://doi.org/10.5958/0973-5674.2017.00017.X

Smith-Zuzovsky, N., & Exner, C. E. (2004). The effect of seated positioning quality on typical 6- and 7-year-old children's object manipulation skills. *American Journal of Occupational Therapy, 58,* 380–388. https://doi.org/10.5014/ajot.58.4.380

Smits-Engelsman, B. C. M., Blank, R., Van Der Kaay, A.-C., Mosterd-Van Der Meijs, R., Vlugt-Van Den Brand, E., Polatajko, H. J., & Wilson, P. H. (2013). Efficacy of interventions to improve motor performance in children with developmental coordination disorder: A combined systematic review and meta-analysis. *Developmental Medicine and Child Neurology, 55,* 229–223. https://doi.org/10.1111/dmcn.12008

Snapp-Childs, W., Fath, A. J., Watson, C. A., Flatters, I., Mon-Williams, M., & Bingham, G. P. (2015). Training to improve manual control in 7–8 and 10–12 year old children: Training eliminates performance differences between ages. *Human Movement Science, 43,* 90–99. https://doi.org/10.1016/j.humov.2015.07.006

Stewart, R., Rule, A., & Giordano, D. (2007). The effect of fine motor skill activities on kindergarten student attention. *Early Childhood Education Journal, 35,* 103–109.

Tseng, Y.-T., Tsai, C.-L., Chen, F.-C., & Konczak, J. (2019). Position sense dysfunction affects proximal and distal arm joints in children with developmental coordination disorder. *Journal of Motor Behavior, 51,* 49–58. https://doi.org/10.1080/00222895.2017.1415200

Visser, M., Nel, M., deVries, J., Klopper, E., Olen, K., & van Coller, J. (2014). In-hand manipulation of children aged four and five-years old: Translation, rotation and shift movements. *South African Journal of Occupational Therapy, 44*(2), 22–28.

Wei, W. (2016). Research on the boost of development on young children's fine motor by folk games. *International Education Studies, 9*(9), 111–119. https://doi.org/10.5539/ies.v9n9p111

Wingrat, J. K., & Exner, C. E. (2005). The impact of school furniture on fourth grade children's on-task and sitting behavior in the classroom: A pilot study. *Work, 25,* 263–272.

Best Practices in Motor Skills to Enhance Participation

56

Jan Hollenbeck, OTD, OTR/L; Virginia Spielmann, MSOT; and Lucy Jane Miller, PhD, OTR

KEY TERMS AND CONCEPTS

- Activity-level evaluation
- Least restrictive environment
- Motor performance skills
- Motor skills
- Performance skills

OVERVIEW

Quality motor performance is necessary whenever a student interacts with objects, people, or the environment. Limitations in motor skills can affect a student's ability to participate in their educational program in a multitude of ways. Occupational therapy practitioners[1] consider motor abilities in the broader context of social skills, client factors, contextual and environmental features, and expectations when determining how best to facilitate student participation and occupational performance for school success.

Motor skills are embedded in occupational performance and support a student's ability to participate in all occupations across school activities and contexts. For example, to prepare for math class, Jason must position himself in close proximity to his locker, bend and reach to grip and lift his math textbook, then transport the book as he walks through the hallway to math class. Jason must also have the underlying client factors necessary to support this myriad motor skills (e.g., postural control, balance to stand and bend, gait patterns to walk, fine motor control and strength to grip the textbook). Jason must also adjust his motor performance on the basis of the context of the busy hallway between classes, including

- The physical environment (e.g., negotiating around other students),
- The social conventions (e.g., using the right amount of force to high-five a friend), and

- The institutional expectations (e.g., walking on the right). The interaction of the individual, the task, and the environment contributes to the organization of functional movement (Shumway-Cook & Wollacott, 2017) and influences occupational performance.

ESSENTIAL CONSIDERATIONS

Motor skill deficits occur in many conditions, including
- Attention deficit hyperactivity disorder (ADHD),
- Autism spectrum disorder (ASD),
- Developmental coordination disorder (DCD),
- Developmental delay, and
- Other conditions more commonly categorized as physical disabilities (see Chapter 36, "Best Practices in Supporting Students With Physical Disabilities").

Recent research on motor performance among children with common conditions is summarized in this section, and implications for participation and practice are discussed. The occupational therapy practitioner must consider the influence of motor skills on all aspects of school participation and intervene to enhance participation for students with motor skill deficits.

Definitions

Motor skills are one aspect of performance skills in the *Occupational Therapy Practice Framework: Domain and Process* (3rd ed., or *OTPF–3*; AOTA, 2014b). Social interaction skills and process skills also fall under the performance domain and should therefore be included in any attempt to determine the impact of motor skills on occupational performance.

Performance skills are observable, goal-directed actions used to engage in meaningful occupations. They are learned over time and situated in specific environments and contexts. The *OTPF-3* (AOTA, 2014b) defines *motor performance skills* as observable elements of action, such as stabilizing, reaching, gripping, manipulating, and walking, that are embedded in purposeful activity and occupational performance. Additional motor capacities, such as

---

[1]*Occupational therapy practitioner* refers to both the occupational therapist and the occupational therapy assistant. The American Occupational Therapy Association (AOTA; 2014a, p. S18) states, "The occupational therapist is responsible for all aspects of occupational therapy service delivery and is accountable for the safety and effectiveness of the occupational therapy service delivery process" and "must be directly involved in the delivery of services during the initial evaluation and regularly throughout the course of intervention. . . . The occupational therapy assistant delivers safe and effective occupational therapy services under the supervision of and in partnership with the occupational therapist."

Copyright © 2019 by the American Occupational Therapy Association. All rights reserved. To reuse this content, contact www.copyright.com.
https://doi.org/10.7139/2019.978-1-56900-591-0.056

those related to body functions and structures (e.g., postural reactions, muscle strength, eye–hand coordination, gross motor control, praxis), are identified as client factors and can affect motor performance skills and occupational performance.

Impact of Motor Skills on School Participation Through the Grades

The occupational therapy practitioner must consider the influence of motor skills on a student's school participation and occupational performance in the curriculum and across all activities and contexts in the school day. The practitioner uses this information to understand how these participatory demands and expectations change as the student moves through the educational system.

In elementary school, students participate in activities such as riding a school bus, negotiating hallways, moving through the lunch line, sitting at a table and socializing with peers while eating lunch, climbing on play structures at recess, and participating in ball games in physical education. Motor skill demands change as students move into middle school, where the curriculum becomes more complex, and students must manage multiple contexts (e.g., use a locker, maintain a schedule, transition between classes, carry books, change into athletic clothes). Students have to negotiate a variety of new environments (e.g., bleachers for school events, science labs, after-school clubs and activities).

High school affords another increase in complexity, with even more varied classes, teachers, rules, and expectations. Students may need to use public transportation and deal with a more complex and less predictable schedule. Transition to adulthood activities and expectations is part of the curriculum, including preparation for work and community access.

The list of contextual school tasks that may be affected by impaired motor skills becomes longer and more varied as students progress through school. Students with motor performance deficits who once could compensate to achieve success at school often find that they require novel or additional strategies and methods to sustain school success as demands change with each increasing grade. The occupational therapy practitioner must adapt to a changing role to support students as they progress through the grades.

Common Conditions, Motor Abilities, and Implications for School Participation

Much has been learned in the past few years about motor performance (and contributing client factors) in common conditions (Kaiser et al., 2015), and it is possible to provide only a brief overview of some critical findings, for a select few diagnoses, within the scope of this chapter. Notable throughout recent research into the neurobiology of conditions is an increased understanding that the causation and presentation of disorders vary immensely from person to person. Often, a confluence of factors—including but not limited to genetics, neurodevelopment, and environment—contribute to a diagnostic profile, creating a range of vulnerabilities (Curatolo et al., 2010).

Therefore, the occupational therapy practitioner is encouraged to look beyond diagnostic categorization toward thinking about motor abilities in the context of client factors, performance skills, context, and environment (AOTA, 2014b). Indeed, the occupational therapy practitioner is uniquely prepared to help the school team understand this complex interplay of factors as they relate to academic achievement and the student's ability to participate in the life of the school. The recent research on motor performance among children with ADHD, ASD, and DCD is summarized below. However, the list is not exhaustive, and other conditions warrant their own literature reviews.

ADHD (all subtypes)

More than 50% of children with ADHD have difficulties with gross motor and fine motor skills (Kaiser et al., 2015). Children with ADHD (inattentive subtype) may present with more impairment of fine motor skills, slow reaction time, and feedback and feedforward motor plan adaptation during complex tasks (Kaiser et al., 2015). Children with ADHD have differences from typically developing children in prevalence of neurological soft signs:

- Increased overflow movements,
- Dysrhythmia, and
- Slowness in execution of timed movements (Pitzianti et al., 2017).

Those with ADHD (hyperactive subtype) have impaired response inhibition, which contributes to decreased accuracy in motor tasks (Fenollar-Cortés et al., 2017; Kaiser et al., 2015).

In a study, children with ADHD and motor skills deficits experienced greater psychological distress (i.e., symptoms of depression and anxiety) than typically developing peers (Missiuna et al., 2014). Children with ADHD also have been found to exhibit a high prevalence of dysgraphia (Mayes et al., 2017). Students' awareness of differences between their ability and that of peers may lead them to feel excluded from shared activities with high motor demands.

Motor skill deficits are often missed among children with ADHD, and therefore intervention is not offered (Fliers et al., 2010). Prescribed medication can improve motor problems for some children but does not resolve the issues and may not improve difficulties with participation (Kaiser et al., 2015). Even when medication is effective, students still need to learn how to best use improved attentional capacities (Lange et al., 2007). Individuals with ADHD should be routinely screened for comorbid DCD (Lange, 2017). Support for social skills development is also indicated (Missiuna et al., 2014), with opportunities for peer interactions in which motor skill prowess is deemphasized and the student is set up for success (Lange, 2017).

ASD

Children with ASD have marked difficulties in

- Imitation praxis,
- Vestibular bilateral integration,
- Somatosensory perception, and
- Sensory reactivity,

with relative strengths in visual praxis (Smith-Roley et al., 2015). Motor planning is typically impaired as well (Becchio

& Castiello, 2012; Izawa et al., 2012). Ocular–motor challenges are common (Johnson et al., 2016).

A central, profound difficulty with motor skills may impede the ability of a student with ASD to make meaning of motor gestures, motor experiences, and facial expressions and thereby reduce their understanding of others' experiences (Trevarthen & Delafield-Butt, 2013). In the school context, motor performance deficits may directly disrupt a student's ability to infer meaning from their teacher's facial expressions or tone of voice and from peers' complex social interactions.

Individuals with ASD should be assessed for comorbid DCD (Caçola et al., 2017). The central role of motor performance in ASD suggests that a crucial aspect of intervention is support and education of the school team about these motor challenges and how to accommodate and adapt activities and environments for enhanced student participation.

DCD

Children with DCD often exhibit poor postural control, associated with

- Poor visual–vestibular–somatosensory integration,
- Abnormal recruitment of postural muscles,
- Slow muscle contraction, and
- Atypical lower limb muscle strength and patterns of recruitment (Fong et al., 2018).

Researchers have also observed deficits in proprioception, motor programming, and the timing or sequencing of movements, as well as deficits imitating meaningful and novel gestures (Reynolds et al., 2015). Children with DCD have difficulty adapting motor plans (Wade & Kazeck, 2016) and have atypical walking patterns, with decreased anticipatory mechanisms and control (Wilmut & Barnett, 2017). Researchers have often noted ideation and anticipatory motor planning deficits as well as weaknesses in perceptual and sensory integration and processing (Gomez & Sirigu, 2015).

The psychosocial impacts of dyspraxia (i.e., anxiety, depression) as secondary to motor performance skill deficits are considered the most disabling aspects of DCD (Zwicker et al., 2013). In the school setting, this may mean that students referred for social challenges also have underlying motor performance deficits. Conversely, it may also indicate that students referred for problems with participation related to motor performance skills may also struggle in the social interaction domain.

A recent systematic review demonstrated that both activity-oriented and body-function–oriented interventions can have a positive effect on motor function and skills and on participation (Smits-Engelsman et al., 2018). Handwriting challenges may be due to motor issues rather than visual–perceptual challenges (Prunty et al., 2016). Camden et al. (2015), in a scoping review, found that children with DCD can learn and retain new motor skills. The authors recommended that classroom adaptations and therapeutic intervention allow more time for

- Processing of movement and practice of new motor skills,
- Consideration of different techniques for learning motor skills, and
- Support to address maladaptive motor planning.

The occupational therapist must understand the disabling conditions and the associated client factors relative to motor function to conduct meaningful evaluations and provide effective intervention plans. Occupational therapy practitioners must stay current with related intervention-effectiveness research, including complications of specific conditions that might influence practice.

Importance of Regulation

Motor skills are transactional; thus, social interactions and process skills are critical to successful motor achievements. In addition, research suggests that motor abilities have a key role in developing self-regulation, social–emotional abilities, and executive functioning (Sigurdsson et al., 2002). Occupational therapy practitioners should consider that social–emotional factors may impede client motor factors, including balance (Hainaut et al., 2011), ocular–motor control (Staab, 2014), and praxis along with overall motor performance (Ekornås et al., 2010). Practitioners should consider the impact of potential social–emotional and regulation factors when evaluating and intervening with students who have motor skills challenges.

BEST PRACTICES

Best practices for school occupational therapy practitioners focus on the student's school participation in natural school contexts (Handley-More et al., 2013).

Identify Students' Participation Strengths, Challenges, and Motor Issues

Motor skills are embedded in occupational performance, and therefore the school occupational therapist should evaluate students' motor skills during purposeful actions in natural school contexts (AOTA, 2014b; Kovic & Schultz-Krohn, 2013). They should consider academic, behavioral, and functional aspects of the school program across all school contexts. The therapist should begin the evaluation process by identifying participation concerns through referral information and interviews with the parent or guardian, the educational staff, and the student.

The occupational therapist seeks to identify not only concerns focusing on areas where participation is problematic but also the student's strengths and desired outcomes. The desired outcomes inform the therapist about what is meaningful to the student and other clients (e.g., teacher, parents or guardians), which is important for goal development and intervention. By identifying and understanding the student's strengths and the resources available, the therapist can enhance the student's school participation and help them achieve desired outcomes (Morris & Hollenbeck, 2016).

The occupational therapist then conducts observations of the student in natural school contexts, paying particular attention to those contexts in which the student struggles but also observing contexts in which the student performs well. The therapist observes and evaluates the student's motor performance skills, which are embedded in occupational performance. Through these contextual observations, the therapist can see firsthand the participation-based challenges the student is experiencing and can gather information that informs their hypothesis about the cause of the participation challenges (see Exhibit 56.1).

Participation-level assessment tools may identify challenges related to the student's school participation (Coster, 1998). Examples of participation-level tools include

- The School Function Assessment (Coster et al., 1998),
- The Canadian Occupational Performance Measure (Law et al., 2005),
- The Children's Assessment of Participation and Enjoyment and Preferences for Activities of Children (King et al., 2004), and
- The Miller Function and Participation Scale's Classroom Observation Checklist (Miller, 2006).

For more information, see Chapter 40, "Best Practices in School Occupational Therapy Evaluation and Planning to Support Participation."

After interviewing stakeholders (e.g., parents, teacher, student), observing the student participating in daily school activities and routines, and administering any suitable participation-based evaluation tools, the occupational therapist develops a hypothesis as to what factors might contribute to the student's reported and observed challenges with school participation. The hypothesis then drives the selection of additional assessment tools and evaluation methods. If the therapist hypothesizes that motor skills are affecting a student's participation (occupational performance), they will administer tools and methods to further examine motor skills and client factors.

Activity-level evaluations (outside of the natural context) can provide useful information about the student's motor abilities; however, practitioners should use caution in generalizing these results to make assumptions about a student's school participation. A student may be able to use scissors to cut out a shape, put on a jacket, or carry a loaded tray in the isolated testing situation but may struggle in contexts in which they routinely perform these activities (e.g., art room, hallway, cafeteria) because of contextual factors.

For example, classroom cutting activities may use different materials and tools (e.g., a different type of scissors, thicker paper, a desk that is too high or low for optimal student performance) or a different time of day (e.g., the

student is tired when art occurs at the end of the day). Conversely, when a student is challenged to perform an activity in an isolated setting, it does not necessarily mean that they are experiencing a problem in context with the same activity. There may be contextual supports that allow greater success in the natural environment that are not present in the testing environment (see Exhibit 56.2).

The Goal-Oriented Assessment of Lifeskills (Miller et al., 2013) and the Miller Function and Participation Scales (Miller, 2006) are norm-referenced tools that assess at the activity level, can be used to support evaluation of participation, and are appropriate for school use. Underlying client factors, such as range of motion, strength, tone, and coordination, may be evaluated with standardized tools, such as

- The Peabody Developmental Motor Scales (2nd ed.; Folio & Fewell, 2000),
- Clinical Observations of Motor and Postural Disorders (2nd ed.; Wilson et al., 2001), or
- The Bruininks–Oseretsky Test of Motor Proficiency (2nd ed.; Bruininks & Bruininks, 2005; Dietz et al., 2007).

These tools assess body structures and functions (client factors). Although these tools are not used to make inferences about school participation, it can be helpful for the occupational therapist to have an understanding of the underlying factors contributing to the already identified participation-based problems. With this information, the therapist can select appropriate interventions and strategies to facilitate the student's participation in the most efficient manner (see Exhibit 56.3).

Outcomes measurement should include goals related to the student's participation in the educational program, and progress and outcome data should be taken in natural school contexts and routines. Throughout the evaluation process, the occupational therapist considers what strategies, supports, and services will be effective to facilitate the student's participation in and performance of school-related tasks successfully and efficiently.

Intervene When Deficits in Motor Skills Interfere With School Participation

Intervention in natural school contexts is considered best practice; however, the school occupational therapy practitioner has available to them a full range of collaborative

---

EXHIBIT 56.1. Evaluation Method: Classroom Observation of Devin

The **occupational therapist** observes **Devin,** a 1st-grade student with hemiplegia, getting ready for recess alongside his classmates. Devin struggles to align and stabilize himself to reach for, grasp, and lift his coat from the hook. He holds onto the wall for stability and loses his balance when removing his coat from the hook. A peer helps him regain his balance and hands him his coat. Devin slowly coordinates his arm movements to successfully insert each arm into the sleeves, taking about 2 minutes to put on his coat, compared with his 18 classmates, who took between 10 and 30 seconds to put on their coats. Devin joins his classmates in line but is unable to hook the zipper of his coat, which his teacher does for him. Two other students require teacher assistance to hook their zipper. The therapist gleans substantial information about supports and barriers to Devin's occupational performance and motor skills through observing in natural contexts.

EXHIBIT 56.2. Evaluation Method: Assessment Tool

The **evaluator** administers the Goal-Oriented Assessment of Lifeskills (Miller et al., 2013) to **Sara,** a middle school student. Sara presents with significant trouble carrying items on a tray during administration of the measure. To gain contextual data, the evaluator determines that an observation of Sara while she is getting her lunch in the cafeteria is warranted. In the cafeteria, the observation reveals that Sara is able to carry her tray because the trays have handles, and she is able to slide the tray along the runners while selecting food items. Although Sara may have underlying motor coordination deficits, she is able to perform the school-relevant activity of managing her tray to get through the lunch line with her lunch and tray intact. It would be inappropriate to base intervention solely on activity-level assessment without identifying challenges in participation.

EXHIBIT 56.3.	Considerations in the Use of Standardized Tools

Occupational therapy practitioners should exercise caution when using standardized tools designed to test underlying client factors. These tools should only be used when participation-based challenges have been identified (through interview, contextual observation, and participation-level tools) and have led to the hypothesis that underlying body structures and functions may be contributing to the student's challenges with occupational performance. In addition, practitioners should be aware that standardized tools that measure underlying motor-related client factors are not designed to measure progress or outcomes in the school setting. For some students, standardized assessments are not useful to identify changes in performance. In addition, some stakeholders might inappropriately interpret low scores as an indication that the student needs therapy services to fix the deficit area; this, in turn, might misalign the focus of school services. In many instances, altering the environment and activities to remove barriers and support the student's performance in the classroom optimizes their participation and learning.

intervention options. The Individuals With Disabilities Education Improvement Act of 2004 (IDEA; Pub. L. 108–446), through its least restrictive environment (LRE) mandate, and the *OTPF–3* (AOTA, 2014b) both support interventions that occur in natural school contexts to support student participation in the school day.

Occupational therapy intervention may involve working directly with the student, working with the teachers and other adults who are in more consistent daily contact with the student, or both. Services on behalf of the student include

- Information sharing,
- Training,
- Consulting,
- Coaching, and
- Providing strategies to adapt activities and environments for student success.

A collaborative relationship with the teacher and other involved adults is critical to working effectively as a team to address school participation challenges. Although direct service remediation of motor skills is acceptable when the educational team believes that this approach is necessary to achieve school participation, compensatory strategies and environmental adaptations are often preferred because they are likely to have a more immediate impact on participation (Bonnard & Anaby, 2015; Egilson & Traustadottir, 2009).

The occupational therapy practitioner should use a top-down, participation-based approach in the school setting to support student participation in context (Coster, 1998), based on the premise that movement is influenced by the interaction of the individual, the task, and the environment (Shumway-Cook & Wollacott, 2017). Contemporary theories of motor control and motor learning (Shumway-Cook & Wollacott, 2017), including Dynamic Systems Theory (Thelen & Smith, 1996), support a top-down approach. By intervening and measuring progress in natural school contexts, the occupational therapy practitioner can address meaningful student participation and ensure educational relevance and necessity.

Change activity, environment, and context to support participation

Students use motor skills throughout their daily life and across school activities, environments, and contexts. Playing at recess, moving through the hallways and classrooms, working at a desk while maintaining an upright body position, and using tools are just a few of the many motor-based activities the student might engage in daily in school. Aspects or features of these activities and the environments and contexts in which they occur can influence a student's ability to participate (e.g., time of day, number of peers in the immediate area, noise level, lighting level, style of teacher, organization of materials, type of seating, length of time students are expected to be seated).

Occupational therapy practitioners focus intervention on modifying or manipulating these factors to remove barriers and to facilitate student participation (AOTA, 2015; Bonnard & Anaby, 2015). The breadth of intervention strategies varies tremendously, based on the individual features of the student and the context in which difficulties are observed. Therefore, practitioners must understand each context in which the student is struggling so that they can develop and implement effective intervention strategies.

Occupational therapy practitioners should develop interventions collaboratively with educational personnel and the student. For example, for a student with motor challenges, the practitioner can consult with recess monitors to provide strategies to enhance participation in desired recess activities, provide movement experiences, and facilitate interaction with peers. For a student with postural issues, a practitioner might collaborate with the classroom teacher to

- Reduce or break up seated work time required in each class segment,
- Encourage and design options for alternative positions in the classroom (e.g., standing, kneeling on chair, sitting on a therapy ball during "seated" work),
- Adjust the size of the desk and chair to fit the student,
- Teach self-regulation strategies to alleviate postural fatigue, and
- Identify activities outside school that will promote postural abilities.

When designing an intervention plan, the occupational therapist should consider what will allow the student to access and participate in the educational program in the most efficient and least restrictive and disruptive manner.

Develop motor skills in context

As described throughout this chapter, deficits in school participation and occupational performance related to motor skills should be addressed in the naturally occurring and meaningful school context. Through collaborative consultation with the educational staff, the occupational therapy practitioner can guide and contribute to the selection of strategies, accommodations, and other supports to implement in the classroom and other school contexts.

The occupational therapy practitioner can also design routines and programs that will promote the student's skill development and independence, and they can provide training to the educational staff so that these programs may be implemented on a consistent daily basis whether or not the practitioner is present. These routines and programs define the type and degree of assistance or prompting that the student requires and include data collection systems for classroom staff. The consulting practitioner may also intervene in the natural contexts to periodically monitor and modify these programs or to directly support the student in the natural activities in the moment (see Exhibit 56.4).

Provide a continuum of services

IDEA mandates intervention based on a continuum of service delivery in the **LRE** in existing school routines whenever possible. Strategies should be based on what the team determines to be the LRE for each individual student and are listed in the following hierarchical order from least to most restrictive:

- Provide services on behalf of the student through information sharing, accommodations, and consultation to help classroom staff and others working directly with the student to understand and decrease the impact of motor skill problems on school performance.
- Conduct intervention with the student in the naturally occurring contexts of the school day where the student is experiencing performance problems (e.g., classroom, physical education, recess on the playground, cafeteria, transitions through the hallways, in the bathroom). Providing services in naturally occurring contexts is advantageous, because it eliminates the need for generalization of skills back into the context where they are used; reduces the number of transitions the student must negotiate during the school day; provides opportunities for modeling and training classroom staff in the moment when the student is experiencing performance problems; and, if done well, decreases stigmatization of the student. It also allows the student to participate in all class activities because they are not removed from the classroom to attend an occupational therapy session in isolation.
- Intervention with the student removed from the context of their school program may be considered necessary in some instances but is never the first choice (e.g., to teach a motor skill, to maintain privacy, to ensure safety, to avoid embarrassing the student). For example, the team might recommend that the occupational therapy practitioner work with a student on negotiating the bleachers in the gym for pep rallies and other student gatherings. Intervention might first occur when the gym and bleachers

are empty (natural setting, but out of context) to develop strategies (e.g., identifying the most easily accessible location, creating strategies for climbing the bleachers to reduce potential trips and falls) and then transfer those strategies to the actual context when an event is occurring in the gym. Students are removed from their peers and educational context only when other, less restrictive options are determined to be ineffective.

SUMMARY

Motor skills support a student's ability to participate in occupations across school activities and contexts. The occupational therapist, and occupational therapy assistant when applicable, evaluates and intervenes in natural school contexts to observe and address motor skills as they are embedded in occupational performance. Occupational therapy intervention for students with motor skill challenges addresses the impact of these challenges on participation in the educational program, including academic, social, and functional aspects of the educational program and school experience.

REFERENCES

American Occupational Therapy Association. (2014a). Guidelines for supervision, roles, and responsibilities during the delivery of occupational therapy services. *American Journal of Occupational Therapy, 68*(Suppl. 3), S16–S22. https://doi.org/10.5014/ajot.2014.686S03

American Occupational Therapy Association. (2014b). Occupational therapy practice framework: Domain and process (3rd ed.). *American Journal of Occupational Therapy, 68*(Suppl. 1), S1–S48. https://doi.org/10.5014/ajot.2014.682006

American Occupational Therapy Association. (2015). Occupational therapy's perspective on the use of environments and contexts to facilitate health, well-being, and participation in occupations. *American Journal of Occupational Therapy, 69*(Suppl. 3), 6913410050. https://doi.org/10.5014/ajot.2015.696S05

Becchio, C., & Castiello, U. (2012). Visuomotor resonance in autism spectrum disorders. *Frontiers in Integrative Neuroscience, 6,* 110. https://doi.org/10.3389/fnint.2012.00110

Bonnard, M., & Anaby, D. (2015). Enabling participation of students through school occupational therapy services: Towards a broader scope of practice. *British Journal of Occupational Therapy, 79,* 188–192. https://doi.org/10.1177/0308022615612807

Bruininks, R., & Bruininks, B. (2005). *Bruininks–Oseretsky Test of Motor Proficiency* (2nd ed.). Minneapolis: NCS Pearson.

Caçola, P., Miller, H. L., & Williamson, P. O. (2017). Behavioral comparisons in autism spectrum disorder and developmental coordination disorder: A systematic literature review. *Research in Autism Spectrum Disorders, 38,* 6–18. https://doi.org/10.1016/j.rasd.2017.03.004

Camden, C., Wilson, B., Kirby, A., Sugden, D., & Missiuna, C. (2015). Best practice principles for management of children with developmental coordination disorder (DCD): Results of a scoping review. *Child: Care, Health and Development, 41*(1), 147–159. https://doi.org/10.1111/cch.12128

Coster, W. (1998). Occupation-centered assessment of children. *American Journal of Occupational Therapy, 52,* 337–344. https://doi.org/10.5014/ajot.52.5.337

EXHIBIT 56.4. Intervention Implementation: Training and Monitoring for Devin

The **occupational therapy practitioner** develops a program for **Devin** to put on a coat (i.e., steps, sequence, prompt and assistance levels, data collection). The practitioner trains **classroom staff** to implement the program each day with fidelity and to record data on student performance. The practitioner follows up with consultation and periodic observation of staff implementing the program, answers questions, and adapts the program on the basis of student progress.

Coster, W., Deeney, T., Haltiwanger, J., & Haley, S. (1998). *School Function Assessment.* San Antonio: Psychological Corporation.

Curatolo, P., D'Agati, E., & Moavero, R. (2010). The neurobiological basis of ADHD. *Italian Journal of Pediatrics, 36*(1), 79. http://doi.org/10.1186/1824-7288-36-79

Dietz, J., Kartin, D., & Kopp, K. (2007). Review of the Bruininks–Oseretsky Test of Motor Proficiency, Second Edition (BOT–2). *Physical and Occupational Therapy in Pediatrics, 27*(4), 87–102. https://doi.org/10.1080/J006v27n04_06ß

Egilson, S. T., & Traustadottir, R. (2009). Participation of students with physical disabilities in the school environment. *American Journal of Occupational Therapy, 63,* 264–272. https://doi.org/10.5014/ajot.63.3.264

Ekornås, B., Lundervold, A. J., Tjus, T., & Heimann, M. (2010). Anxiety disorders in 8–11-year-old children: Motor skill performance and self-perception of competence. *Scandinavian Journal of Psychology, 51,* 271–277. https://doi.org/10.1111/j.1467-9450.2009.00763.x

Fenollar-Cortés, J., Gallego-Martínez, A., & Fuentes, L. J. (2017). The role of inattention and hyperactivity/impulsivity in the fine motor coordination in children with ADHD. *Research in Developmental Disabilities, 69,* 77–84. https://doi.org/10.1016/j.ridd.2017.08.003

Fliers, E. A., Franke, B., Lambregts-Rommelse, N. N., Altink, M. E., Buschgens, C. J., Nijhuis van der Sanden, M. W., . . . Buitelaar, J. K. (2010). Undertreatment of motor problems in children with ADHD. *Child and Adolescent Mental Health, 15*(2), 85–90. https://doi.org/10.1111/j.1475-3588.2009.00538.x

Folio, M. R., & Fewell, R. R. (2000). *Peabody Developmental Motor Scales* (2nd ed.). Austin, TX: Pro-Ed.

Fong, S. S. M., Chung, L. M. Y., Bae, Y., Vackova, D., Ma, A. W. W., & Liu, K. P. Y. (2018). Neuromuscular processes in the control of posture in children with developmental coordination disorder: Current evidence and future research directions. *Current Developmental Disorders Reports, 5*(1), 43–48. https://doi.org/10.1007/s40474-018-0130-9

Gomez, A., & Sirigu, A. (2015). Developmental coordination disorder: Core sensori-motor deficits, neurobiology and etiology. *Neuropsychologia, 79*(Part B), 272–287. https://doi.org/10.1016/j.neuropsychologia.2015.09.032

Hainaut, J. P., Caillet, G., Lestienne, F. G., & Bolmont, B. (2011). The role of trait anxiety on static balance performance in control and anxiogenic situations. *Gait and Posture, 33,* 604–608. https://doi.org/10.1016/j.gaitpost.2011.01.017

Handley-More, D., Wall, E., Orentlicher, M. L., & Hollenbeck, J. (2013). Working in early intervention and school settings: Current views of best practice. *Early Intervention and School Special Interest Section Quarterly, 20*(2), 1–4.

Individuals With Disabilities Education Improvement Act of 2004, Pub. L. 108–446, 20 U.S.C. §§ 1400–1482.

Izawa, J., Pekny, S. E., Marko, M. K., Haswell, C. C., Shadmehr, R., & Mostofsky, S. H. (2012). Motor learning relies on integrated sensory inputs in ADHD, but over-selectively on proprioception in autism spectrum conditions. *Autism Research, 5,* 124–136. https://doi.org/10.1002/aur.1222

Johnson, B. P., Lum, J. A. G., Rinehart, N. J., & Fielding, J. (2016). Ocular motor disturbances in autism spectrum disorders: Systematic review and comprehensive meta-analysis. *Neuroscience and Biobehavioral Reviews, 69,* 260–279. https://doi.org/10.1016/j.neubiorev.2016.08.007

Kaiser, M., Schoemaker, M. M., Albaret, J., & Geuze, R. H. (2015). What is the evidence of impaired motor skills and motor control among children with attention deficit hyperactivity disorder (ADHD)? Systematic review of the literature. *Research in Developmental Disabilities, 36,* 338–357. https://doi.org/10.1016/j.ridd.2014.09.023

King, G., Law, M., King, S., Hurley, P., Hanna, S., Kertoy, M., . . . Young, N. (2004). *Children's Assessment of Participation and Enjoyment (CAPE) and Preferences for Activities of Children (PAC).* San Antonio: Harcourt Assessment.

Kovic, M., & Schultz-Krohn, W. (2013). Performance skills: Definitions and evaluation in the context of the occupational therapy framework. In H. Pendleton & W. Schultz-Krohn (Eds.), *Pedretti's occupational therapy: Practice skills for physical dysfunction* (7th ed., pp. 450–460). St. Louis: Elsevier.

Lange, K. W., Tucha, L., Walitza, S., Gerlach, M., Linder, M., & Tucha, O. (2007). Interaction of attention and graphomotor functions in children with attention deficit hyperactivity disorder. In M. Gerlach, J. Deckert, K. Double, & E. Koutsilier (Eds.), *Neuropsychiatric disorders: An integrative approach* (pp. 249–259). Vienna: Springer.

Lange, S. M. (2017). ADHD and comorbid developmental coordination disorder: Implications and recommendations for school psychologists. *Contemporary School Psychology, 22*(1), 30–39. https://doi.org/10.1007/s40688-017-0122-5

Law, M., Baptiste, S., Carswell, A., McColl, M. A., Polatajko, H., & Pollock, N. (2005). *Canadian Occupational Performance Measure* (4th ed.). Ottawa: CAOT Publications.

Mayes, S. D., Breaux, R. P., Calhoun, S. L., & Frye, S. S. (2017). High prevalence of dysgraphia in elementary through high school students with ADHD and autism. *Journal of Attention Disorders.* Advance online publication. https://doi.org/10.1177/1087054717720721

Miller, L. J. (2006). *Miller Function and Participation Scales.* San Antonio: Harcourt Assessment.

Miller, L. J., Oakland, T., & Hertzberg, D. (2013). *Goal-Oriented Assessment of Lifeskills (GOAL).* Los Angeles: Western Psychological Corporation.

Missiuna, C. A., Cairney, J., Pollock, N., Campbell, W., Russell, D. J., Macdonald, K., . . . Cousins, M. (2014). Psychological distress in children with developmental coordination disorder and attention-deficit hyperactivity disorder. *Research in Developmental Disabilities, 35,* 1198–1207. https://doi.org/10.1016/j.ridd.2014.01.007

Morris, M., & Hollenbeck, J. (2016). Evaluating student participation: Focus on strengths in your school-based evaluation. *OT Practice, 21*(1), CE-1–CE-8.

Pitzianti, M., Grelloni, C., Casarelli, L., D'Agati, E., Spiridigliozzi, S., Curatolo, P., & Pasini, A. (2017). Neurological soft signs, but not theory of mind and emotion recognition deficit distinguished children with ADHD from healthy control. *Psychiatry Research, 256,* 96–101. https://doi.org/10.1016/j.psychres.2017.06.029

Prunty, M., Barnett, A. L., Wilmut, K., & Plumb, M. (2016). Visual–perceptual and handwriting skills in children with developmental coordination disorder. *Human Movement Science, 49,* 54–65. https://doi.org/10.1016/j.humov.2016.06.003

Reynolds, J. E., Thornton, A. L., Elliott, C., Williams, J., Lay, B. S., & Licari, M. K. (2015). A systematic review of mirror neuron system function in developmental coordination disorder: Imitation, motor imagery, and neuroimaging evidence. *Research in Developmental Disabilities, 47,* 234–283. https://doi.org/10.1016/j.ridd.2015.09.015

Shumway-Cook, A., & Wollacott, M. H. (2017). *Motor control: Translating research into clinical practice* (5th ed.). Philadelphia: Wolters Kluwer.

Sigurdsson, E., Van Os, J., & Fombonne, E. (2002). Are impaired childhood motor skills a risk factor for adolescent anxiety? Results from the 1958 U.K. birth cohort and the National Child Development Study. *American Journal of Psychiatry, 159,* 1044–1046. https://doi.org/10.1176/appi.ajp.159.6.1044

Smith-Roley, S., Mailloux, Z., Parham, L. D., Schaaf, R. C., Lane, C. J., & Cermak, S. (2015). Sensory integration and praxis patterns in children with autism. *American Journal of Occupational Therapy, 69,* 6901220010. https://doi.org/10.5014/ajot.2015.012476

Smits-Engelsman, B., Vinçon, S., Blank, R., Quadrado, V. H., Polatajko, H., & Wilson, P. H. (2018). Evaluating the evidence for motor-based interventions in developmental coordination disorder: A systematic review and meta-analysis. *Research in Developmental Disabilities, 74,* 72–102. https://doi.org/10.1016/j.ridd.2018.01.002

Staab, J. P. (2014). The influence of anxiety on ocular motor control and gaze. *Current Opinion in Neurology, 27,* 118–124. https://doi.org/10.1097/WCO.0000000000000055

Thelen, E., & Smith, L. B. (1996). *A dynamic systems approach to the development of cognition and action.* Cambridge: Massachusetts Institute of Technology.

Trevarthen, C., & Delafield-Butt, J. T. (2013). Autism as a developmental disorder in intentional movement and affective engagement. *Frontiers in Integrative Neuroscience, 7,* 49. https://doi.org/10.3389/fnint.2013.00049

Wade, M. G., & Kazeck, M. (2016). Developmental coordination disorder and its cause: The road less travelled. *Human Movement Science, 57,* 489–500. https://doi.org/10.1016/j.humov.2016.08.004

Wilmut, K., & Barnett, A. L. (2017). When an object appears unexpectedly: Anticipatory movement and object circumvention in individuals with and without developmental coordination disorder. *Experimental Brain Research, 235,* 1531–1540. https://doi.org/10.1007/s00221-017-4901-z

Wilson, B., Kaplan, B., Pollock, N., & Law, M. (2001). *Clinical observations of motor and postural disorders* (2nd ed.). Framingham, MA: Therapro.

Zwicker, J. G., Harris, S. R., & Klassen, A. F. (2013). Quality of life domains affected in children with developmental coordination disorder: A systematic review. *Child: Care, Health and Development, 39,* 562–580. https://doi.org/10.1111/j.1365-2214.2012.01379.x

KEY TERMS AND CONCEPTS

- Coaching
- Dunn's model
- Dunn's Sensory Processing Framework
- Goal attainment scaling
- Self-regulation continuum
- Sensory processing
- Threshold

OVERVIEW

Sensory processing is the ability to make meaning out of sensory input; it may support or interfere with a student's ability to participate. Other team members have come to understand that sensory processing is an area of expertise for occupational therapy practitioners.[1] Practitioners consider many factors that may support or interfere with school participation; sensory processing is an area people count on occupational therapy practitioners to address (Dunn, 2011a).

Sensory processing knowledge is an important contribution to the school team's planning because evidence indicates that students who are vulnerable (e.g., students with autism spectrum disorder [ASD] or developmental conditions) are more likely to have differences in sensory experiences in everyday life (e.g., Abele-Webster et al., 2012; Backhouse et al., 2012; Ben-Sasson, Hen, et al., 2009; Brockevelt et al., 2013; Cheung & Siu, 2009; Dunn, 2011; Engel-Yeger et al., 2011; Hildenbrand & Smith, 2012; Kern, Garver, et al., 2007; Kern, Trivedi, et al., 2007; Patten et al., 2013; Provost et al., 2009; Tomchek & Dunn, 2007; van der Linde et al., 2013). These differences, in turn, affect coping, behavior, and performance throughout the school day (Ashburner et al., 2008; Gere et al., 2009; Jirikowic et al., 2008; Reynolds et al., 2011; Rodger et al., 2010; Tomchek et al., 2014). This chapter

---

[1]*Occupational therapy practitioner* refers to both the occupational therapist and the occupational therapy assistant. The American Occupational Therapy Association (AOTA; 2014, p. S18) states, "The occupational therapist is responsible for all aspects of occupational therapy service delivery and is accountable for the safety and effectiveness of the occupational therapy service delivery process" and "must be directly involved in the delivery of services during the initial evaluation and regularly throughout the course of intervention. . . . The occupational therapy assistant delivers safe and effective occupational therapy services under the supervision of and in partnership with the occupational therapist."

presents the contributions of sensory processing knowledge by occupational therapy practitioners to the team problem-solving process to support students' success at school.

ESSENTIAL CONSIDERATIONS

Participation at school depends on one's sensory processing patterns. ***Dunn's Sensory Processing Framework*** (also referred to as ***Dunn's model***; Dunn, 2014) provides a structure to relate school behavior to sensory processing.

Sensory Processing Concepts

Data across the life span indicate that all people exhibit sensory patterns that reflect their experiences with everyday life. Researchers have reported distinct physiological markers related to particular sensory patterns (e.g., Davies et al., 2009).

First, the nervous system operates on the basis of ***thresholds,*** which are the points at which the nervous system has enough information to react. With low thresholds, it takes very little excitation to activate the nervous system; with high thresholds, it takes a lot of excitation to activate the nervous system. Second, a person also operates along a ***self-regulation continuum*** to meet individual needs. At one end of this continuum, a person is more passive (i.e., letting things happen and then reacting); at the other end of this continuum, a person behaves in an active way to meet needs throughout the day.

In Dunn's model, these 2 continua yield 4 basic patterns of sensory processing:
1. Seekers,
2. Avoiders,
3. Sensors, and
4. Bystanders (Dunn, 2014).
Studies suggest that these differences can influence effectiveness and satisfaction in everyday experiences (Ashburner et al., 2008; Ben-Sasson, Carter, & Briggs-Gowan, 2009; Dunn, 2011; Jirikowic et al., 2008; Lane et al., 2010; Minshew

---

Copyright © 2019 by the American Occupational Therapy Association. All rights reserved. To reuse this content, contact www.copyright.com.
https://doi.org/10.7139/2019.978-1-56900-591-0.057

& Hobson, 2008). An important feature of Dunn's model is that it describes everyone's sensory processing patterns. Dunn's model is a strengths-based model that invites discussion about every person's inherent characteristics and how to make all settings and activities accessible to all students and teachers so the classroom milieu is useful for everyone.

In Dunn's model, a difference score is synonymous with the 2 ends of the bell curve. A difference score does not mean something is automatically dysfunctional or disordered with those persons or their performance. In a representative sample of elementary-school students (N = 925), Ben-Sasson, Carter, and Briggs-Gowan (2009, 2010) reported that 16% of students were sensitive to at least 4 touch or sound sensations. Their findings reflect the bell curve, just like the standardization sample (Dunn, 2014).

Dunn's model invites professionals to consider how a person's sensory patterns interact with settings and activities to support participation. Even among children with expected development, those with "difference" scores in sensory processing preferred more active physical activities (Engel-Yeger, 2008). Some settings and activities provide intense sensory input; these circumstances are more useful for someone who needs sensory input and more challenging for someone who is easily overwhelmed by that same sensory input.

Jasmin et al. (2009) reported that even when they controlled for cognitive levels, there was a significant relationship among environmental reactivity, sensory avoiding, and participants' ability to perform daily living skills. For example, bus rides to school are typically noisy, students bump into each other, and movements are continuous and unpredictable. Students who love or need sound, touch, or movement (seekers and bystanders, respectively) will thrive during the ride to school, whereas students who are easily overwhelmed by these sensations will find the ride challenging. A sensory processing approach is a specific application of the Person–Environment–Occupation models in occupational therapy (Baum et al., 2015; Law et al., 1996).

Impact of Sensory Processing Concepts at School

Minshew and Hobson (2008) found a relationship between sensory sensitivities and perceptual errors among children with ASD. In a study by Jirkowic et al. (2008), children with fetal alcohol spectrum disorder had more challenges with adaptability, problem behaviors, and academic performance paired with differences in sensory processing patterns. Watson et al. (2011) found positive relationships between challenging social–communication skills and both hyporesponsiveness and pattern seeking among children with ASD. Others have reported that children with hyperresponsiveness were less competent in adaptive skills, social activities, and school performance (Ashburner et al., 2008; Ben-Sasson, Carter, & Briggs-Gowan, 2009).

Researchers also have found significant relationships between sensitivity to sensory input and maladaptive behaviors (Dean et al., 2017; Lane et al., 2010). Dean et al. (2016) found that children who displayed externalizing behaviors were significantly more likely to have low-threshold sensory patterns (avoiding and sensitivity). Zimmer and Desch (2012) found that children with ASD had a higher sensitivity to pitch, which may contribute to reduced social interactions

and repetitive behaviors to manage the effects of the sounds. They suggested providing earplugs or headphones for noisy environments, such as the gym or the lunchroom at school. However, this should not be a long-standing solution because overprotection of the ears can lead to lifelong difficulties (Stiegler & Davis, 2010). Gere et al. (2009) found similar sensitivity among children who were gifted; they linked sensitivity to superior problem-solving ability and challenges with social relationships. Taken together, these findings suggest a relationship between sensory responsiveness and school participation.

Teachers do not usually pay attention to sensory aspects of children's behavior (Dunn, 2008b), so occupational therapy practitioners must take the lead. For example, skilled observation during school lunchtime can be the best tool to recognize how sensory patterns affect how much a student eats, how the student manages the lunchroom routines, and how peer interactions are affected. Evidence suggests that there is a relationship among food preferences, eating challenges, and sensory processing.

Smith et al. (2005) found that children who were "picky eaters" had poor appetites, had a limited food repertoire, gagged and bit their lips more often, and had difference scores on the Sensory Profile. In another study, children with ASD had significantly narrower food choices when compared with siblings (Nadon et al., 2011).

Sensory processing knowledge can inform patterns of behavior among students, which illustrates the importance of the occupational therapy practitioner as a related service professional on the school team. Occupational therapists can support learning at school by structuring environments and activities to promote adaptive and reduce challenging behaviors.

BEST PRACTICES

Occupational therapy practitioners have the responsibility to apply evidence-based knowledge in their practices. This section discusses strategies for applying sensory processing knowledge during the occupational therapy process.

Identify Sensory Processing Patterns at School

School occupational therapy practitioners must make their work relevant to the educational setting. Sensory processing knowledge contributes to the information the interdisciplinary team needs to plan effective interventions. Using standardized assessment measures to identify a student's and teacher's sensory patterns provides information about what approaches are likely to support them in the teaching and learning process. Information from interviews and skilled observations allows therapists to create a planning culture that considers sensory aspects of all parts of the day. In concert, these methods ensure that professionals verify hypotheses about how sensory processing might affect participation.

Standardized assessment

In education, evaluations serve to
- Establish eligibility,
- Identify information for planning, and
- Check progress.

Standardized assessments such as the Sensory Profile 2 (Dunn, 2014) cannot establish eligibility alone, because a difference score does not mean something is wrong. These scores only reflect the student's patterns in relation to peers; how patterns affect performance is another matter.

Professionals do not use standardized sensory processing testing to check progress. Occupational therapists, as members of educational teams, are concerned with the student's participation, so the only progress that matters is the student's increased effectiveness at school. Therapists use knowledge about sensory patterns to examine participation in settings and activities across the school day to determine what supports or interferes with the student's effectiveness. Making sure a student's sensory patterns support participation is essential, so progress monitoring must focus on changes in participation rather than changes in sensory processing.

Interviews

Interviews provide a way to learn everyone's narrative about how the day goes; what is easy or hard; and what matters to the teacher, the student, parents, or even peers. From a sensory point of view, occupational therapists listen for sensory features of activities and settings as each person explains their point of view.

For example, when a teacher talks about a student having a meltdown, it is important to find out what behaviors constitute melting down to that teacher. For one teacher, a student huffing off could qualify, whereas another teacher might reserve this term for a student who screams, throws things, or falls down. It is also important to find out in what settings and activities the student has this reaction because something in the setting might trigger the behavior. For a student with sensitivities to sound, another student tapping a pencil on their desk can be too much of a distraction.

Conversely, a teacher might think a student who has bystander sensory patterns is uninterested in learning. In this case, interviews can reveal what sensory intensity might be necessary to get that student's attention.

Even difficult behavior may be adaptive in the sense that the student is attempting to manage what they perceive as an overwhelming situation. Insightful interviewing reveals what might create the sense of being overwhelmed. A teacher's classroom decorations might be distracting, contributing to a student's agitation across the day. Air fresheners or hand lotion might have an aroma that overloads the student's olfactory threshold, leading to difficult interactions with peers.

When teachers understand relationships such as these, they feel more competent to manage classroom behaviors. By pointing out these possibilities, occupational therapy practitioners contribute to mindfulness about how environmental stimuli affect behavior. This mindfulness reduces the belief that students are being defiant and increases the chance that the teacher will handle disruptions in a more acceptable way.

Skilled observation

In addition to informative interviews, occupational therapists conduct skilled observations to obtain more detailed and contextually relevant information about how sensory experiences affect behavior. Because occupational therapists are primed to notice sensory aspects, skilled observations can reveal relationships between sensory events and students' behavior. Occupational therapists also have the advantage that during observations, classroom management is not their responsibility, so their attention is devoted to students in their contexts.

Therapists should keep 2 components in mind when conducting a skilled observation related to sensory processing. First, document what sensory events occur in the setting and activity (e.g., background noises, people bumping into each other, frequent movement). Second, detect whether these sensory events affect the target student. A student who is a bystander may not notice movement around the room, even though there is a lot of activity; at the extreme, this student may not notice that others are lining up and leaving the classroom for another activity. A student who is a sensor may notice all the movements, such that seatwork goes incomplete. Do not assume that if you notice and feel bothered by something, this is automatically a bothersome stimulus for the student or the teacher.

By finding opportunities to link sensory observations with teachers' and students' behaviors, occupational therapists infuse sensory knowledge into the teachers' considerations. Skilled observations provide data to support a teacher's strengths as well as identify what a particular student's needs might be.

When a teacher makes adjustments or demonstrates attentiveness to a student's needs (e.g., moving the student to another work space because others are distracting), the occupational therapist uses sensory perspectives to point out why that was a great strategy. For example, a therapist might say, "I noticed that you moved Tommy to the table that faces away from the class project area. That was a great strategy because it reduced Tommy's access to the other students' movements and consequent bumping, both of which are distracting inputs for Tommy."

Occupational therapists should observe all of the school's environments. Walk around the school. Stop in various settings and notice what sensory experiences are inherent in these settings and activities. What behaviors do students and teachers engage in to indicate that a particular sensory feature makes no difference (i.e., they don't regard the feature), is helpful (i.e., energizes them to engage), or interferes (i.e., stops participation)? The team must sort out when sensory features contribute to the behaviors exhibited (see Case Example 57.1).

Craft Evidence-Based Interventions

After interpreting information from multiple sources, occupational therapists design interventions that are within the student's and teacher's routines.

Prepare for interdisciplinary dialogue

Before exploring specific intervention methods, practitioners prepare for the team's conversations. Occupational therapy practitioners focus on interventions that are embedded into the student's routines and focused on

CASE EXAMPLE 57.1. KASUKA: 3RD GRADER WHO NEEDS TO COMPLETE WORK EFFICIENTLY

Kasuka is a 3rd grader who has done well in school until now. With the increasing demands of independent work productivity, the teacher is concerned that Kasuka is falling behind his capability. During skilled observation, the occupational therapist notices that Kasuka gets up a lot, although he still seems to know what is going on in class. Interviews with the teacher and testing confirm that Kasuka needs a lot of movement and joint input throughout the day. Taking a strengths perspective, the therapist points out that Kasuka is doing a great job trying to regulate his own state of arousal, even though his behavior choices interfere with learning.

The teacher, mom, and therapist meet to consider ways to make adjustments throughout Kasuka's daily routines. Using coaching approaches, which require the therapist to reflect, ask questions, and wonder about options (Dunn et al., 2012, 2018) rather than tell the others what to do, they explore options that will fit into the home and school routines. Exhibit 57.1 provides an excerpt from the plan they developed, illustrating ways they captured Kasuka's need for movement (i.e., to maintain arousal) in needed routines to improve participation. By looking at the routines and settings aimed toward opportunities to move, the team came up with creative ways to meet Kasuka's sensory needs while supporting his participation.

EXHIBIT 57.1.   Portion of Kasuka's Activity Analysis to Determine Sensory Processing Options

Activity: What Kasuka currently does to get movement and joint input
Options: Options for meeting sensory needs within these activities

7:30 a.m.: Gets up and gets ready for school
Activity: Gets up quickly when called; runs throughout the house, fleeing his bedroom, where his clothes are
Options: Set up clothing in different parts of the house so Kasuka moves to gather his underwear, socks, and so forth to move his muscles and joints within the "getting dressed" routine (e.g., higher so he has to stretch, clothing in hall closet)

8:30 a.m.: Rides to school on the bus
Activity: Looks out windows, slides back and forth on his seat, sometimes falls into the aisle
Options: Give him a list of things to look out for on the way; place his book bag on the aisle side so he can lean against it in the seat

9:00 a.m.: Participates in the arrival routine
Activity: Very fidgety in his chair, disrupts lessons, sometimes gets up while the teacher is starting the day
Options: Assign Kasuka to point to items as the teacher talks; have Kasuka hold books (to provide weight as the teacher talks)

9:30 a.m.: Completes seatwork and participates in small-group instruction
Activity: Gets up while the teacher is with other groups, fidgets during small-group instruction
Options: Break his seatwork into multiple parts (e.g., each row of work is cut apart, so he gets up to submit each row and get the next; provide a movable cushion so he can fidget without getting up, provide a "standing" place for Kasuka to complete his work)

Noon: Eats lunch
Activity: Eats quickly and enjoys a healthy diet, leaves the lunch area frequently
Options: Choose foods that take longer to prepare (e.g., opening containers) and eat (e.g., more chewing) to provide resistance to Kasuka's hands and mouth; have him replace younger students' trays when they are done eating so he can move and carry throughout the lunch period

---

participation (Rodger et al., 2010). Koenig and Rudney (2010) recommended that practitioners take more active roles in social and community participation aspects of learning, on the basis of their finding of a moderate relationship between sensory processing and these aspects of daily life. This sentiment is also reflected in the AOTA Practice Guidelines about serving people who have ASD (Tomchek et al., 2016).

Rodger et al. (2010) suggested that occupational therapy practitioners must emphasize their occupation-centered focus, reminding us that sensory processing is not our core identity. For example, if someone says, "I read that sensory approaches were not effective," practitioners can say, "There is a lot of controversy about specific sensory interventions. Here at school, we are looking for times and places that the student's sensory patterns are helping or interfering so we can make adjustments to support learning for that student. Evidence suggests that applying our ideas to the student's routines is an effective way to support participation" (Dunn, 2014; Pilkington, 2002; Spagnola & Fiese, 2007).

AOTA has developed several systematic reviews in this area (e.g., Bodison & Parham, 2017; May-Benson & Koomar, 2010; Pfeiffer et al., 2017; Weitlauf et al., 2017). The reviewed studies have found variable results, including some interventions that addressed intermediate features (e.g., self-regulation), but there is little application to school practice.

Apply sensory processing knowledge within school routines and settings

In the school context, occupational therapy practitioners support teachers' priorities about learning, motivation,

CASE EXAMPLE 57.2. FATIMA: 3RD GRADER WHO NEEDS TO COMPLETE HER WORK

Fatima is a 3rd grader who loves school. **Her teacher, Mr. Polk,** has become more concerned about Fatima's ability to get her work completed. If the **occupational therapist** as coach can explore with Mr. Polk what he sees as the barriers, then Mr. Polk will be more likely to implement the therapeutic intervention options on Fatima's (and his) behalf.

The therapist knows how adjustments in Fatima's routines make it easier for her to complete her work, as well as that Fatima is a bystander (Dunn, 2014). She also understands coaching evidence; the therapist listens for opportunities to provide reflective guidance to build insight and discover a workable solution. Table 57.1 presents a coaching dialogue between Mr. Polk and the therapist. In this coaching intervention, one can see that the therapist guides Mr. Polk toward a solution that fits with the current routines of his classroom.

The therapist could have given Mr. Polk 2–3 strategies to keep Fatima focused on her work, but in doing so, she might have made incorrect assumptions about the situation. She could have presumed that Mr. Polk thought of Fatima as lazy or incapable. Alternatively, she might have assumed she knew why Fatima was not completing her work and made suggestions that did not fit Mr. Polk's classroom routines. For example, if Fatima does not complete her work because of daydreaming, the therapist might make different suggestions than if Fatima does not complete her work because she frequently leaves her seat.

By taking the time to find out Mr. Polk's perspective, the therapist identifies the precise way a therapeutic intervention could be embedded into the class routine that suits Mr. Polk's teaching methods and is consistent with why Fatima is not completing her work.

TABLE 57.1. Analysis of Coaching Conversation

COACHING CONVERSATION	ANALYSIS
Mr. Polk: "Fatima has started to have incomplete work." **Occupational therapist:** "What is happening during work time right now?"	Promotes *awareness* of the task
Mr. Polk: "At this time of year, we start to give students more independence with parts of their work. Fatima did okay when I provided step-by-step instructions; as the students have taken on some responsibility, Fatima seems lost." **Occupational therapist:** "So, with other children, taking on more responsibility for the work is effective, and with Fatima, this change has not been so helpful. Do you have ideas about what might make it work better?"	Points out that Mr. Polk is *analyzing*—making comparisons—and asks him to consider options and *alternatives*
Mr. Polk: "Well, I tried repeating the directions to Fatima directly, but as soon as I am not right there, she doesn't complete the work." **Occupational therapist:** "That was a good idea to try. . . . I wonder whether you can think of a time when Fatima was able to complete some work independently."	Invites Mr. Polk to make comparisons (*analysis*)
Mr. Polk: "Hmmm . . . you know what? When I let her stand at the counter to work a while back, she did complete the project on her own!" **Occupational therapist:** "This is a great insight. You know the testing we did indicated that Fatima misses a lot more cues than other students; she gets more input to her body when standing to work. That counter by the window is visually bright and interesting, so perhaps we need to think about other times she can stand to work at that counter. Are there specific times that you could give Fatima a place to work at the counter so she could get experience working independently?"	Works on a plan (*action*); tries to expand thinking about classroom possibilities
Mr. Polk: "Well, I don't want to single her out or make it obvious that she gets to do something that others don't get to do." **Occupational therapist:** "Good point. I appreciate that you are astute about the class dynamics. Are there ways we could use this idea of standing to work that won't single her out?"	*Affirms* Mr. Polk; tries to generate *alternatives* so they can move to an *action* plan
Mr. Polk: "You know what? I think there are a couple of other students who might do better standing up, and I have 2 counters in my room. I could ask who wants to try standing to work so it becomes just part of our class routine, and no one will think anything of it." **Occupational therapist:** "Are you willing to try this and take note of how it works for you, Fatima, the other students, and the class? It seems to be a good match, but we can think some more if it doesn't work like you need it to. Let's check in about this by phone in a couple of days."	Gets a commitment to an *action* plan; provides an opening for considering *alternatives* next time
Mr. Polk: "Thanks so much. This has been helpful. I have so much to do all day, I cannot spend all my time providing individual instruction to 1 student. I do want Fatima to be more independent before she gets to 4th grade."	

classroom management, and social interactions. Sensory processing knowledge applied within a teacher's routines offers a powerful tool to increase the teacher's effectiveness in all areas. When a teacher understands that voice volume, moving around or standing still, and even one's hand lotion can affect students, that teacher can make changes accordingly.

The challenges that matter to teachers are those that interfere with learning and getting along in the classroom routines. Teachers have sensory patterns to contend with, just like their students. When observing in a classroom, occupational therapy practitioners can detect the teacher's patterns:

- How is the room organized?
- What are the class rules?
- What does the teacher point out as concerning behaviors?

The teacher sets the context for students, so noticing these factors for planning will create both useful and effective interventions.

Teachers can also create an acceptance of diversity while using sensory processing knowledge. When the occupational therapy practitioner gives teachers and students ways to explain their own reactions to situations, the class develops both knowledge of and approval for individual differences. A teacher can say, "I get overwhelmed by everyone talking at once. Does that bother anyone else?" This can lead to a productive discussion of individual differences. Eventually, students can say, "That bothers me," as modeled by the teacher.

Apply evidence-based methods using sensory processing knowledge

Evidence suggests that coaching practices are an effective way to provide services (Graham et al., 2010; Knight, 2009; Little et al., 2018; Miller-Kuhaneck & Watling, 2017; Rush & Shelden, 2008). *Coaching* is a very compatible method when practitioners are using sensory processing knowledge to solve problems at school. It is critical that the person being coached is an active participant in problem solving.

As a coach, the occupational therapy practitioner

- Listens to the teacher's descriptions of successful and challenging situations,
- Asks questions,
- Reflects back to the teacher,
- Wonders what might be possible, and
- Inquires when the child is effective during the school day.

Case Example 57.2 illustrates effective coaching.

Create evidence in your practice

Even with all the evidence presented in this chapter, each practitioner has the responsibility to collect data about students at school. The data support decision making about that student and make it clear that even substantial evidence in the literature does not substitute for finding out whether that evidence is applicable to a particular situation. Participation is the only outcome that matters for students in schools (see Law et al., 2017). With data about that particular student, the occupational therapy practitioner can design specific methods to measure the precise participation that matters to the student, family, and teacher (see Dunn, 2008a, 2011).

Use goal attainment scaling

Goal attainment scaling (GAS) is a fruitful way to document changes in participation (Dunn et al., 2012; Graham et al., 2010; Mailloux et al., 2007). When using GAS, the occupational therapy practitioner and teacher describe current and desired behaviors with questions such as, "What will it look like when Kaitlin is participating in her small groups?" GAS provides a way to be very specific about what behavior changes matter to the teacher and the situation and is another way to create insight relevant to the students served in school practice. For more information, see Chapter 45, "Best Practices in School Occupational Therapy Documentation and Data Collection."

SUMMARY

Sensory processing is a powerful body of knowledge that contributes to insights about a student's and teacher's behaviors. With these insights, occupational therapy practitioners can support the teacher and student to make adjustments that are respectful of sensory patterns and of the classroom routines. Research has flourished to show how sensory processing affects children's lives; some studies have shown us the effectiveness of interventions that incorporate sensory knowledge into plans. More intervention research in authentic contexts, such as schools, will guide occupational therapy practices to support students and their teachers.

REFERENCES

Abele-Webster, L. A., Magill-Evans, J. E., & Pei, J. R. (2012). Sensory processing and ADHD in children with fetal alcohol spectrum disorder. *Canadian Journal of Occupational Therapy, 79,* 60–63. https://doi.org/10.2182/cjot.2012.79.1.8

American Occupational Therapy Association. (2014). Guidelines for supervision, roles, and responsibilities during the delivery of occupational therapy services. *American Journal of Occupational Therapy, 68*(Suppl. 3), S16–S22. https://doi.org/10.5014/ajot.2014.686S03

Ashburner, J., Ziviani, J., & Rodger, S. (2008). Sensory processing and classroom emotional, behavioral, and educational outcomes in children with autism spectrum disorder. *American Journal of Occupational Therapy, 62,* 564–573. https://doi.org/10.5014/ajot.62.5.564

Backhouse, M., Harding, L., Rodger, S., & Hindman, N. (2012). Investigating sensory processing patterns in boys with Duchenne muscular dystrophy using the Sensory Profile. *British Journal of Occupational Therapy, 75,* 271–280. https://doi.org/10.4276/030802212X13383757345148

Baum, C. M., Christiansen, C. H., & Bass, J. D. (2015). The Person–Environment–Occupation–Performance (PEOP) model. In C. H. Christiansen, C. M. Baum, & J. D. Bass (Eds.), *Occupational therapy: Performance, participation, and well-being* (4th ed., pp. 49–56). Thorofare, NJ: Slack.

Ben-Sasson, A., Carter, A. S., & Briggs-Gowan, M. J. (2009). Sensory over-responsivity in elementary school: Prevalence and social-emotional correlates. *Journal of Abnormal Child Psychology, 37,* 705–716. https://doi.org/10.1007/s10802-008-9295-8

Ben-Sasson, A., Carter, A. S., & Briggs-Gowan, M. J. (2010). The development of sensory over-responsivity from infancy to elementary school. *Journal of Abnormal Child Psychology, 38,* 1193–1202. https://doi.org/10.1007/s10802-010-9435-9

Ben-Sasson, A., Hen, L., Fluss, R., Cermak, S. A., Engel-Yeger, B., & Gal, E. (2009). A meta-analysis of sensory modulation symptoms in individuals with autism spectrum disorders. *Journal of Autism and Developmental Disorders, 39,* 1–11. https://doi.org/10.1007/s10803-008-0593-3

Bodison, S., & Parham, D. (2017). Specific sensory techniques and sensory environmental modifications for children and youth with sensory integration difficulties: A systematic review. *American Journal of Occupational Therapy, 72,* 7201190040. https://doi.org/10.5014/ajot.2018.029413

Brockevelt, B. L., Nissen, R., Schweinle, W. E., Kurtz, E., & Larson, K. J. (2013). A comparison of the Sensory Profile scores of children with autism and an age- and gender-matched sample. *South Dakota Medicine, 66,* 463–465.

Cheung, P., & Siu, A. (2009). A comparison of patterns of sensory processing in children with and without developmental disabilities. *Research in Developmental Disabilities, 30,* 1468–1480. https://doi.org/10.1016/j.ridd.2009.07.009

Davies, P., Chang, W., & Gavin, W. (2009). Maturation of sensory gating performance in children with and without sensory processing disorders. *International Journal of Psychophysiology, 72,* 187–197. https://doi.org/10.1016/j.ijpsycho.2008.12.007

Dean, E., Little, L., Tomchek, S., & Dunn, W. (2017). Sensory processing in the general population: Adaptability, resiliency, and challenging behavior. *American Journal of Occupational Therapy, 72,* 7201195060. https://doi.org/10.5014/ajot.2018.019919

Dean, E., Tomchek, S., Dunn, W., & Little, L. (2016). Sensory processing and challenging behavior in the general population. *American Journal of Occupational Therapy, 70*(Suppl. 4), 7011500003. https://doi.org/10.5014/ajot.2016.70S1-RP202C

Dunn, W. (2008a). *Bringing evidence into everyday practice: Practical strategies for healthcare professionals.* Thorofare, NJ: Slack.

Dunn, W. (2008b). Harnessing teacher's wisdom for evidence-based practice: Standardization data from the Sensory Profile School Companion. *Journal of Occupational Therapy, Schools, and Early Intervention, 1,* 206–214. https://doi.org/10.1080/19411240802589106

Dunn, W. (2011). *Best practice occupational therapy for children and families in community settings* (2nd. ed.). Thorofare, NJ: Slack.

Dunn, W. (2014). *Sensory Profile 2: Strengths based approach to assessment and planning.* San Antonio: Pearson.

Dunn, W., Cox, J., Foster, L., Mische-Lawson, L., & Tanquary, J. (2012). Impact of a contextual intervention on child participation and parental competence among children with autism spectrum disorders (ASD): A pretest–posttest repeated-measures design. *American Journal of Occupational Therapy, 66,* 520–528. https://doi.org/10.5014/ajot.2012.004119

Dunn, W., Little, L., Pope, E., & Wallisch, A. (2018). Establishing fidelity of occupational performance coaching. *OTJR: Occupation, Participation and Health, 38,* 96–104. https://doi.org/10.1177/1539449217724755

Engel-Yeger, B. (2008). Sensory processing patterns and daily activity preferences of Israeli children. *Canadian Journal of Occupational Therapy, 75,* 220–229. https://doi.org/10.1177/000841741007700207

Engel-Yeger, B., Hardal-Nasser, R., & Gal, E. (2011). Sensory processing dysfunctions as expressed among children with different severities of intellectual developmental disabilities. *Research in Developmental Disabilities, 32,* 1770–1775. https://doi.org/10.1016/j.ridd.2011.03.005

Gere, D., Capps, S., Mitchell, W., & Grubbs, E. (2009). Sensory sensitivities of gifted children. *American Journal of Occupational Therapy, 63,* 288–295. https://doi.org/10.5014/ajot.63.3.288

Graham, F., Rodger, S., & Ziviani, J. (2010). Enabling occupational performance of children through coaching parents: Three case reports. *Physical and Occupational Therapy in Pediatrics, 30,* 4–15. https://doi.org/10.3109/01942630903337536

Hildenbrand, H. L., & Smith, A. C. M. (2012). Analysis of the Sensory Profile in children with Smith-Magenis Syndrome. *Physical and Occupational Therapy in Pediatrics, 32,* 48–65. https://doi.org/10.3109/01942638.2011.572152

Jasmin, E., Couture, M., McKinley, P., Reid, G., Fombonne, E., & Gisel, E. (2009). Sensori-motor and daily living skills of preschool children with autism spectrum disorders. *Journal of Autism and Developmental Disorders, 39,* 231–241. https://doi.org/10.1007/s10803-008-0617-z

Jirikowic, T., Olson, C., & Kartin, D. (2008). Sensory processing, school performance and adaptive behavior of young school-age children with fetal alcohol spectrum disorders. *Physical and Occupational Therapy in Pediatrics, 28*(2), 117–136. https://doi.org/10.1080/01942630802031800

Kern, J. K., Garver, C. R., Carmody, T., Andrews, A. A., Trivedi, M. H., & Mehta, J. A. (2007). Examining sensory quadrants in autism. *Research in Autism Spectrum Disorders, 1,* 185–193. https://doi.org/10.1016/j.rasd.2006.09.002

Kern, J. K., Trivedi, M. H., Grannemann, B. D., Garver, C. R., Johnson, D., Andrews, A. A., . . . Schroeder, J. (2007). Sensory correlations in autism. *Autism, 11,* 123–134. https://doi.org/10.1177/1362361307075702

Knight, J. (2009). Coaching: The key to translating research into practices lies in continuous, job-embedded learning with ongoing support. *Journal of Staff Development, 30*(1), 18–22.

Koenig, K. P., & Rudney, S. G. (2010). Performance challenges for children and adolescents with difficulty processing and integrating sensory information: A systematic review. *American Journal of Occupational Therapy, 64,* 430–442. https://doi.org/10.5014/ajot.2010.09073

Lane, A., Young, R., Baker, A., & Angley, M. (2010). Sensory processing subtypes in autism: Association with adaptive behavior. *Journal of Autism and Developmental Disorders, 40,* 112–122. https://doi.org/10.1007/s10803-009-0840-2

Law, M., Baum, C., & Dunn, W. (2017). *Measuring occupational performance: Supporting best practice in occupational therapy* (3rd ed.). Thorofare, NJ: Slack.

Law, M., Cooper, B., Strong, S., Stewart, D., Rigby, P., & Letts, L. (1996). The Person–Environment–Occupation Model: A transactive approach to occupational performance. *Canadian Journal of Occupational Therapy, 63,* 9–23. https://doi.org/10.1177/000841749606300103

Little, L., Pope, E., Wallisch, A., & Dunn, W. (2018). Occupation-based coaching by means of telehealth for families of young children with autism spectrum disorder. *American Journal of Occupational Therapy, 72,* 7202205020. https://doi.org/10.5014/ajot.2018.024786

Mailloux, Z., May-Benson, T., Summers, C. A., Miller, L., Brett-Green, B., Burke, J. P., . . . Schoen, S. A. (2007). Goal attainment scaling as a measure of meaningful outcomes for children with sensory integration disorders. *American Journal of Occupational Therapy, 61*, 254–259. https://doi.org/10.5014/ajot.61.2.254

May-Benson, T. A., & Koomar, J. A. (2010). Systematic review of the research evidence examining the effectiveness of interventions using a sensory integrative approach for children. *American Journal of Occupational Therapy, 64*, 403–414. https://doi.org/10.1177/1362361313517762

Miller-Kuhaneck, H., & Watling, R. (2017). Parental or teacher education and coaching to support function and participation of children and youth with sensory processing and sensory integration challenges: A systematic review. *American Journal of Occupational Therapy, 72*, 7201190030. https://doi.org/10.5014/ajot.2018.029017

Minshew, N., & Hobson, J. (2008). Sensory sensitivities and performance on sensory perceptual tasks in high functioning individuals with autism. *Journal of Autism and Developmental Disorders, 38*, 1485–1498. https://doi.org/10.1007/s10803-007-0528-4

Nadon, G., Feldman, D., Dunn, W., & Gisel, E. (2011). Association of sensory processing and eating problems in children with autism spectrum disorders. *Autism Research and Treatment, 2011*, 541926. https://doi.org/10.1155/2011/541926

Patten, E., Ausderau, K. K., Watson, L. R., & Baranek, G. T. (2013). Sensory response patterns in nonverbal children with ASD. *Autism Research and Treatment, 2013*, 436286. https://doi.org/10.1155/2013/436286

Pfeiffer, B., Frolek Clark, G., & Arbesman, M. (2017). Effectiveness of cognitive and occupation-based interventions for children with challenges in sensory processing and integration: A systematic review. *American Journal of Occupational Therapy, 72*, 7201190020. https://doi.org/10.5014/ajot.2018.028233

Pilkington, K. M. (2002). The natural environment II: Uncovering deeper responsibilities within relationship-based services. *Infants and Young Children, 15*(2), 78–84.

Provost, B., Crowe, T. K., Acree, K., Osbourn, P. L., & McClain, C. (2009). Sensory behaviors of preschool children with and without autism spectrum disorders. *New Zealand Journal of Occupational Therapy, 56*(2), 9–17.

Reynolds, S., Bendixen, R., Lawrence, T., & Lane, S. (2011). A pilot study examining activity participation, sensory responsiveness, and competence in children with high functioning autism spectrum disorder. *Journal of Autism and Developmental Disorders, 41*, 1496–1506. https://doi.org/10.1007/s10803-010-1173-x

Rodger, S., Ashburner, J., Cartmill, L., & Bourke-Taylor, H. (2010). Helping children with autism spectrum disorders and their families: Are we losing our occupation-centered focus? *Australian Occupational Therapy Journal, 57*, 276–280. https://doi.org/10.1111/j.1440-1630.2010.00877.x

Rush, D., & Shelden, M. (2008). Script for explaining an evidence-based early intervention model. *Family, Infant and Preschool Program, 1*(3), 1–5.

Smith, A., Roux, S., Naidoo, T., & Venter, D. (2005). Food choice of tactile defensive children. *Nutrition, 21*(1), 14–19.

Spagnola, M., & Fiese, B. (2007). Family routines and rituals: A context for development in the lives of young children. *Infants and Young Children, 20*, 284–299. https://doi.org/10.1097/01.IYC.0000290352.32170.5a

Stiegler, L. N., & Davis, R. (2010). Understanding sound sensitivity in individuals with autism spectrum disorders. *Focus on Autism and Other Developmental Disabilities, 25*(2), 67–75. https://doi.org/10.1177/1088357610364530

Tomchek, S. D., & Dunn, W. (2007). Sensory processing in children with and without autism: A comparative study using the Short Sensory Profile. *American Journal of Occupational Therapy, 61*, 190–200. https://doi.org/10.5014/ajot.61.2.190

Tomchek, S., Huebner, R., & Dunn, W. (2014). Patterns of sensory processing in children with an autism spectrum disorder. *Research in Autism Spectrum Disorders, 8*, 1214–1224. https://doi.org/10.1016/j.rasd.2014.06.006

Tomchek, S., Koenig, K. P., Arbesman, M., & Lieberman, D. (2016). Occupational therapy interventions for adolescents with autism spectrum disorder. *American Journal of Occupational Therapy, 71*, 7101395010. https://doi.org/10.5014/ajot.2017.711003

van der Linde, J., Franzsen, D., & Barnard-Ashton, P. (2013). The Sensory Profile: Comparative analysis of children with specific language impairment, ADHD and autism. *South African Journal of Occupational Therapy, 43*(3), 34–40

Watson, L. R., Patten, E., Baranek, G. T., Poe, M., Boyd, B. A., Freuler, A., & Lorenzi, J. (2011). Differential associations between sensory response patterns and language, social, and communication measures in children with autism or other developmental disabilities. *Journal of Speech, Language, and Hearing Research, 54*, 1562–1576. https://doi.org/10.1044/1092-4388(2011/10-0029)

Weitlauf, A. S., Sathe, N., McPheeters, M. L., & Warren, Z. E. (2017). Interventions targeting sensory challenges in autism spectrum disorder: A systematic review. *Pediatrics, 139*, e20170347. https://doi.org/10.1542/peds.2017-0347

Zimmer, M., & Desch, L. (2012). Sensory integration therapies for children with developmental and behavioral disorders. *Pediatrics, 129*, 1186–1189. https://doi.org/10.1542/peds.2012-0876

Best Practices in Visual Perception and Visual–Motor Skills to Enhance Participation

58

Colleen Schneck, SCD, OTR/L, FAOTA

KEY TERMS AND CONCEPTS

- Depth perception
- Figure ground perception
- Form constancy
- Object perception
- Orthographics
- Sight vocabulary
- Spatial perception
- Topographic orientation
- Visual attention
- Visual closure
- Visual cognitive component
- Visual efficiency
- Visual integrity
- Visual memory
- Visual perception
- Visual receptive component
- Visual–motor integration
- Visual–spatial orientation

OVERVIEW

Visual deficits were found in 68% of typical 7th-grade participants in a study by Goldstand et al. (2005). Nonproficient readers had significantly poorer academic performance, vision screening scores, and visual perception scores than proficient readers, which emphasizes the importance of providing support services and intervention for students who are experiencing academic difficulties.

Visual perception is a complex process responsible for reception and cognition of visual stimuli. The sensory function, or *visual receptive component,* is the process of extracting and organizing information from the environment. The specific mental functions, which constitute the *visual cognitive component,* provide the capacity to organize, structure, and interpret visual stimuli, giving meaning to what one sees. Together, these two components enable students to understand what they see, and both are necessary for functional vision.

In addition, the student's current abilities and the context influence visual perception. When people interpret a visual image, their culture, education, and prior experience all interact with sensory receptors and brain activity to interpret the image (Coté, 2015).

Visual–perceptual skills, which include the recognition and identification of shapes, objects, colors, and other qualities, allow a person to make accurate judgments about the size, configuration, and spatial relationships of objects. As described in the *Occupational Therapy Practice Framework: Domain and Process* (3rd ed.; American Occupational Therapy Association [AOTA], 2014b), visual receptive components fall under client factors of sensory functions, and visual cognitive components are described under specific mental functions.

A review of the literature reveals support for perceptual and perceptual–motor skills as important aspects of academic performance, such as reading, writing, and other desktop tasks (National Early Literacy Panel, 2008). For example, print awareness has a moderate relationship to reading comprehension, and concepts about print have a moderate to strong relationship with decoding and reading comprehension.

Occupational therapy practitioners[1] focus on individuals' engagement in ADLs, IADLS, education, work, play, leisure, and social participation. The focus on the client factor of visual perception and its effects on performance skills, including literacy, can be critical. Literacy is embedded in all areas of occupational performance, from functional life skills (e.g., reading recipes) to education (e.g., taking notes in class) and social participation (e.g., reading bus schedules).

The Every Student Succeeds Act (2015; Pub. L. 114–195) outlines a direct and sustained approach to improving literacy achievement by supporting states in developing high-quality literacy instruction. It also details a continuum of interventions and support for students at risk for reading and writing failure in subject areas and across grade levels. With a student of any age, occupational therapy practitioners can support literacy in many ways,

---

[1]*Occupational therapy practitioner* refers to both the occupational therapist and the occupational therapy assistant. The American Occupational Therapy Association (AOTA; 2014a, p. S18) states, "The occupational therapist is responsible for all aspects of occupational therapy service delivery and is accountable for the safety and effectiveness of the occupational therapy service delivery process" and "must be directly involved in the delivery of services during the initial evaluation and regularly throughout the course of intervention. . . . The occupational therapy assistant delivers safe and effective occupational therapy services under the supervision of and in partnership with the occupational therapist."

Copyright © 2019 by the American Occupational Therapy Association. All rights reserved. To reuse this content, contact www.copyright.com.
https://doi.org/10.7139/2019.978-1-56900-591-0.058

including providing services to enhance visual perception and visual–motor skills.

ESSENTIAL CONSIDERATIONS

This section outlines terminology associated with visual perception and reviews the impact of visual–perceptual and visual–motor deficits on students' occupations and participation in school.

Definitions

The following operational definitions are applied in this chapter.

Visual receptive skills

In a hierarchical model, visual receptive skills form the foundation of all visual cognitive functions. **Visual integrity** includes visual acuity, refractive abilities, and eye health. *Visual acuity* is the ability to discriminate the fine details of objects in the visual field. A vision measurement of 20/20 means that a person is considered to have normal ability to see small details at a tested distance of 20 feet. Refractive and eye health disorders can decrease visual integrity, thus possibly compromising visual–perceptual and visual–motor skills.

Visual efficiency includes accommodation (the ability of each eye to compensate for a blurred image), binocular vision (the ability to mentally combine the images from the 2 eyes into a single percept), and ocular motility (efficient eye movements).

Visual cognitive skills

Visual attention, visual memory, and visual information processing or visual perception, when combined, contribute to the visual cognitive process (Matthews & Martin, 2009). **Visual attention** is the ability to attend to visual stimuli. Attention directs the eyes to gather specific details or to choose an interpretation of those details that is relevant to the task (Gilbert & Li, 2013). It involves alertness, selective attention, vigilance, and divided attention. People need visual attention to attend to correct information, encode it into new knowledge, and then act on it or store it in memory (Gilbert & Li, 2013).

As a student reads, they must be able to visually attend to text for a finite period of time while both filtering out and monitoring other visual stimuli in their environment. Research on visual attention and reading has pinpointed visual deficits in several areas that may contribute to reading difficulties, including

- Insufficiencies in visual pathways that are important to spatial–temporal attributes of visual attention (Matthews & Martin, 2009), and
- Reduced ability in the rapid visual processing needed for fluent reading (Solan et al., 2007).

Visual memory is the integration of visual information with previous experiences. It includes 2 subcomponents:
1. Visual working memory (WM; limited information for a very limited time)
2. Long-term visual memory (infinite amounts of information that is permanent).

Several recent studies have identified the unique contribution that visual memory makes to the reading process (Magi et al., 2018; Menghini et al., 2011; Ram-Tsur et al., 2008).

Visual perception is the skill used to distinguish the features of visual stimuli (Schneck, 2010; Woodrome & Johnson, 2007). Visual perception, as it relates to reading, includes the ability to recognize the particular features of letters, match letter shapes to the same or similar letter shapes, and categorize similarities and differences among letters and words. It incorporates visual constructs of the form of objects and how they relate spatially. Studies have underscored the important role that visual perception plays in the facilitation of acquiring letter knowledge (Woodrome & Johnson, 2007), which has been shown to have a correlation with success in learning to read (National Early Literacy Panel, 2008).

Types of Visual Perception

Object and spatial visual perception are different. **Object perception** is the visual identification of objects by color, texture, shape, and size (what things are). **Spatial perception** is the visual location of objects in space (where things are); it responds to motor input and seems to be integral to egocentric localization during visual–motor tasks.

As visual information is processed by the occipital lobe, it follows two main pathways: ventral (the "what pathway") or dorsal (the "how pathway"; Lauwereyns, 2012). The ventral pathway travels to the temporal lobe and is identified with object identification and recognition (foveal vision). The dorsal pathway terminates in the parietal lobe and is involved in processing an object's spatial location (parafoveal vision). This pathway is also important in reading fluency, because the perceptual span (amount of text vision a student can sense at one point) increases with experience (Schotter et al., 2012).

Visual information about object characteristics permits the formation of long-term perceptual representations that support object identification and visual learning. Spatial perception provides information about the location of object qualities that people need to guide their action, such as adjusting the hand during reach to the size and orientation of an object. These two types of perceptions are discussed in more detail.

Form (object) perception

There are 3 types of form perception: (1) form constancy, (2) visual closure, and (3) figure ground. **Form constancy** is the recognition of forms and objects as the same in various environments, positions, and sizes. For example, a student can identify the letter *A* whether it is typed, written in manuscript, written in cursive, written in uppercase or lowercase letters, or italicized.

Visual closure is the identification of forms or objects from incomplete presentations. For example, a high school student working at their desk can distinguish a pencil from a pen, even when both are partly hidden under some papers. **Figure ground perception** is the differentiation between foreground or background forms and objects. For example, a middle school student can visually find a textbook needed for class in their locker, their socks in a cluttered drawer, or the sleeve of a monochromatic shirt.

Spatial (vision) perception

Object-focused spatial abilities focus on the spatial relations of objects regardless of the individual who is viewing them. *Depth perception* is the determination of the relative distance between objects, figures, or landmarks and the observer as well as changes in planes of surfaces. *Topographic orientation* is the determination of the location of objects and settings and the route to the location. For example, the student can leave the classroom for a drink of water from the water fountain down the hall and then return to their desk.

Position in space, or *visual–spatial orientation,* is the determination of the spatial relationship of figures and objects to oneself or other forms and objects. This skill is important to understanding directional language concepts, such as *in, out, up, down, in front of, behind, between, left,* and *right,* as well as providing the ability to differentiate among letters and sequences of letters in a word or in a sentence. Knowing how to place letters equal spaces apart and touching the line and how to recognize letters that extend below the line, such as *p* or *q,* is an example of this skill.

Visual–Motor Integration

Visual–motor integration combines visual–perceptual and motor skills in performance of various occupational activities, including handwriting, keyboard skills, and throwing or catching a ball. In a study by Carlson et al. (2013), visual–motor integration, which the authors measured using a copy figure task, explained significant variance in children's math and written expression achievement throughout childhood and adolescence. Visual–motor integration also showed significant relations with the quality of handwriting in another study (Kaiser et al., 2009).

Impact on Learning and Participation

Visual perception and visual–motor deficits can influence students' occupational performance, such as
- Play;
- Self-care;
- Education through reading, spelling, handwriting, and math; and
- Other visual–motor activities across grade levels.

Play and leisure activities

The student may demonstrate difficulty with
- Playing games and sports,
- Drawing and coloring,
- Cutting with scissors,
- Pasting,
- Constructing manipulatives, and
- Doing puzzles.

The student may experience teasing by other students if they are unable to catch the ball during playground games, for example. In turn, the student may stop participating in difficult activities, therefore not getting the further practice to develop the needed visual–perceptual and visual–motor skills inherent in natural contexts.

Self-care

Students with visual–perceptual problems may demonstrate difficulty with self-care and daily living skills (e.g., finding items in their desk, using a brush and mirror to style their hair, applying toothpaste to the toothbrush, putting on and removing clothing, tying shoes). Skilled use of handwriting, phones, computers, and communication devices may all present difficulty for the student with visual–perceptual problems. IADLs, such as home management, may present problems (e.g., difficulty sorting and folding clothes). Community mobility may be difficult because the student is unable to locate objects and navigate their environment.

Education

Students with visual–perceptual challenges may have difficulty with educational activities, such as reading and literacy activities, spelling, handwriting, and math. Classroom activities (e.g., cutting, drawing, writing, keyboarding) may be affected, as well as social interactions with peers and others, because the student may not be able to move through space efficiently.

Reading and literacy. Understanding the contribution of visual perception to the reading process is important. Kavale and Forness (2000) investigated the involvement of a variety of visual–perceptual skills in reading achievement. The skills of
- Visual discrimination,
- Visual memory,
- Visual closure,
- Visual–spatial relationships,
- Visual–motor integration,
- Visual association,
- Figure ground perception, and
- Visual–auditory integration

were all found to make a significant contribution. Together, they accounted for 6%–20% of reading abilities (depending on the reading variable).

Learning the concepts of directionality of print (i.e., left page before right page, first and last, top and bottom) is reliant on visual–spatial perceptual ability. Letter knowledge contributes significantly to reading and should be measured in preschool, kindergarten, and 1st grade (National Early Literacy Panel, 2008).

The characteristics of printed (written) information make reading possible. These include a word's
- Visual configuration,
- Orthography (order of letters),
- Phonology (sounds represented), and
- Semantics (meaning).

The student benefits from these multiple simultaneous cues in reading. If the student has difficulty with one characteristic, they can rely on their perception of the other characteristics to extract the meaning.

In early reading, students first encounter the visual configuration (graphics) and orthographics of a printed word. *Orthographics* is the standardized system for using script to write a particular language. It includes rules of spelling and other elements of written language, such as capitalization, word breaks, and punctuation.

The student then must break the written word into its component phonemes (*phonology*), hold them in active WM, and synthesize and blend the phonemes to form recognizable words (*semantics*). Visual word recognition seems to involve a subphonemic level of processing, the ability to hear the difference between 2 sounds that differ acoustically and phonetically.

After practice, this step is skipped, and the word is added to the student's growing sight vocabulary. It can then be dealt with as a gestalt (i.e., in its entirety) rather than letter by letter. **Sight vocabulary** consists of words that are instantly recognized as gestalts. As a student's reliance on sight vocabulary increases, decoding takes less time, and the student develops automaticity, which allows them to begin to concentrate on comprehension and retention.

Understanding sentences requires adding 2 more variables—*context* (i.e., word order) and *syntax* (i.e., grammatical construction)—to the skills previously discussed. For reading paragraphs, chapters, and texts, it is assumed that decoding is automatic. A hierarchy can be assumed such that any developmental dysfunctions that impair decoding or sentence comprehension impede text reading.

The segmenting of written words in early reading calls for a variety of skills. First, students must be able to recognize individual letter symbols. This requires visual attention, memory, and discrimination. Two aspects of word reading are important for comprehension: (1) accuracy and (2) speed. The more attentional resources are consumed by lower level processes (e.g., word identification), the fewer resources are available for comprehension.

Students with visual perception challenges may not be able to recognize symbols and therefore may be slow to master the alphabet and numbers. Their relatively weak grasp of constancy of forms may make visual discrimination an inefficient process. Some students cannot readily discern the differences between visually similar symbols. Confusion among the letters *p, q,* and *g* and between *a* and *o* may result, as well as letter reversals, such as the differentiation between *b* and *d*. Form perception and spatial perception are somewhat less important at advanced stages of reading acquisition than they are during the initial stages.

Confusion over directionality and other spatial characteristics of a word may result in weak registration in visual memory, which, again, may cause significant delays in the consolidation of sight vocabulary. Even frequently encountered words need to be analyzed anew each time they appear. A student with visual–spatial deficits has difficulty with map reading and interpretation of instructional graphics, such as charts and diagrams.

Graphic representations require the student to

- Integrate,
- Extract the most salient elements from,
- Condense, and
- Organize

large numbers of stimuli presented at once. The student may not have difficulty with the perceptual content, but the amount of information to be assimilated simultaneously may be more than the student can integrate and remember.

Memory deficits affect reading in several ways. Students with visual memory problems may be unable to remember the visual shape of letters and words. Such students may also demonstrate an inability to associate these shapes with letters, sounds, and words. Students with weaknesses of visual–verbal associative memory have difficulty establishing easily retrievable or recognizable sound–symbol associations. They are unable to associate the sound, visual configuration, or meaning of the word with what they see or hear.

Students who have difficulty with active WM also may have difficulty holding one aspect of the reading process in suspension while pursuing another component. This ability is closely related to perceptual span, or the ability to recall the beginning of the sentence while reading the end of it. The student must take a second look at the beginning of a sentence after reading the end of it.

With severe dysfunction, recognition of words may be impaired, which interferes with the acquisition of sight vocabulary. The occupational therapy practitioner might suspect problems with visual perception if a student seems to be better at understanding what they read than at actually decoding the words. This student has good language abilities but some trouble processing written words. Reading should also be conceptualized not just as the product of decoding symbols and text, scanning and tracking letters, processing information, and comprehending the meaning but also as a process that involves active participation and motivation (Grajo & Candler, 2016; see Chapter 50, "Best Practices in Literacy: Reading to Enhance Participation").

Spelling skills. Spelling may depend more on visual recognition or visual imagery ability than visual memory. Students with impaired processing of simultaneous visual stimuli may have difficulty with spelling. Their inability to visualize words may result from indistinct or distorted initial visual registration. Such students who have strong sound–symbol association may spell the word phonetically (e.g., *lite* for *light*) yet incorrectly.

Handwriting. Handwriting requires the ability to integrate the visual image of letters or shapes with the appropriate motor response, called **visual–motor integration.** (For more information, see Chapter 49, "Best Practices in Literacy: Handwriting and Written Expression to Enhance Participation.") Visual cognitive abilities may affect writing in a variety of situations, including difficulty with correct letter formation; spelling; and the mechanics of grammar, punctuation, and capitalization.

Students may have difficulty formulating the sequential flow of ideas necessary for written communication or recalling the shape and formation of letters and numbers, or they might need a model to write. For students to spontaneously write, they must be able to visualize letters and words without visual cues. Other problems seen among students with poor visual memory include mixing lowercase and capital letters in a sentence, writing the same letter many different ways on the same page, and being unable to print the alphabet from memory.

Clark (2010) found that kindergartners' ability to identify letter names and letter sounds was significantly correlated to their writing skills (i.e., alphabet and name writing). In addition, the author found significant correlations among writing scores (i.e., letters and name writing), reading scores on the Dynamic Indicators of Basic Early Literacy

Skills (University of Oregon, Center on Teaching and Learning, 2018), and visual–motor scores on the Beery–Buktenica Developmental Test of Visual–Motor Integration.

The student with poor form constancy does not recognize errors in their own handwriting and may show poor recognition of letters or numbers in different environments, positions, or sizes. The student may be unable to recognize letters or words in different prints and therefore may have difficulty copying from a different type of print to handwriting.

If the student is unable to discriminate a letter, they may have difficulty forming it. A student with visual closure difficulty always needs to see the complete presentation of what they are to copy. A student with figure ground problems may have difficulty copying because they are unable to determine what is to be written; the student therefore may omit important segments or may be slower than peers in producing written products.

Visual–spatial problems can affect a student's handwriting in many ways. The student may reverse letters such as *m, w, b, d, s, c,* and *z* and numbers such as *2, 3, 5, 6, 7,* and *9.* However, letter reversals are developmentally appropriate until approximately the age of 7. If the student is unable to discriminate left from right, they may have difficulty with left-to-right progression in writing words and sentences. The student may overspace or underspace between words and letters and may have trouble keeping within the margins.

The most common spatial errors in handwriting involve incorrect and inconsistent spacing between writing units and variability in orientation of major letter features when the letter is written repeatedly. When a student has a spatial disability, they may be unable to relate one part of a letter to another part. They also may demonstrate poor shaping or closure of individual letters or a lack of uniformity in orientation and letter size. The student may have difficulty placing letters on a line and adapting letter sizes to the space provided on the paper or worksheet. Studies have explored the relationship between visual cognitive skills and handwriting and have found visual–motor integration to be the best predictor of handwriting.

Mathematics. Carlson et al.'s (2013) findings suggest that students with higher visual–spatial integration have superior math performance. Students with visual–perceptual problems can have difficulty aligning columns for calculation; their answers therefore are incorrect because of alignment problems, not calculation skills. Worksheets with many rows and columns of math problems may be disorienting to students with figure ground problems.

Students with poor visual memory may have difficulty using a calculator. Visual memory disabilities also may present difficulties when addition and subtraction problems require multiple steps. Geometry, because of its spatial characteristics, is very difficult for the student with visual-spatial perception problems. Recognition, discrimination, and comparison of object form and space are part of the foundation of higher level mathematical skills. The visual imagery required to match and compare forms and shapes is difficult for students with visual–perceptual problems, which interferes with their ability to learn these underlying skills.

BEST PRACTICES

Occupational therapists are often responsible for the evaluation of and intervention planning with students when visual–perceptual and visual–motor challenges are interfering with their academic learning.

Evaluate the Student

Occupational therapists identify and analyze possible causes and types of visual–perceptual and visual–motor dysfunction. The therapist initiates the evaluation by gathering an occupational profile, including the student's needs, problems, strengths, and concerns regarding valued occupations in the school setting. To identify visual–perceptual factors that limit occupational performance and participation, occupational therapists ask about and observe how visual–perceptual difficulties affect daily occupations. For example, the prerequisite skills of letter naming and phonemic awareness should be assessed early in kindergarten.

It is important to use multiple methods in the evaluation process (e.g., observation, interview, review of written medical and educational history, formal and informal tools). During the interview, the occupational therapist should ask the parents whether their child had an eye examination within the past year. Ruling out an acuity issue is critical. (Vision screening at school is often distance vision—far-point but not near-point, close-up objects).

The therapist can conduct observations by watching the student engage in daily activities during school routines (e.g., classroom activities—drawing and writing, dressing, playing computer games, playing ball, and moving around the classroom). Coté (2011) proposed that 4 general areas of cognitive processes that are related to visual analysis—imitation, analysis, imagery, and flexibility—be assessed in all visual perception tasks.

Cultural influences should always be considered in the evaluation process. For example, some cultures read and write from right to left or vertically on the page. Nonverbal communication, which is often based on facial cues and may vary with different cultures, can be a challenge for persons with perceptual deficits.

During the evaluation process, the occupational therapist generates and tests hypotheses to determine those factors that support or hinder the student's ability to engage successfully in valued occupations (AOTA, 2014b). Performance on visual–motor tests may indicate an underlying visual cognitive deficit, including

- Challenges with visual acuity,
- Difficulty with visual discrimination,
- Poor fine motor ability,
- Inability to integrate visual cognitive and motor processes, or
- A combination of these factors.

Therefore, careful analysis is necessary to determine the underlying problem. If visual deficits have been diagnosed by a vision professional, then the therapist could recommend instructional strategies to improve the student's performance within their visual capacities (Scheiman, 2011).

The occupational therapy evaluation should address relevant tasks and assess what may be affecting the student's performance. Normative assessments provide a standard measure of performance yet do not have ecological validity and do not consider the student's performance in natural contexts.

Formal evaluation tools commonly used in school practice include the following:

- Beery–Buktenica Developmental Test of Visual–Motor Integration (Beery et al., 2010),
- Developmental Test of Visual Perception (Hammill et al., 2014),
- Test of Visual–Motor Skills (Martin, 2010),
- Test of Visual Perceptual Skills (Martin, 2017), and
- Motor-Free Visual Perception Test (Colarusso & Hammill, 2015).

The therapist should use the information obtained with other information they have gathered to analyze the student's performance and determine the need for environmental or academic modifications or accommodations, assistive technology (Watson et al., 2010), and occupational therapy services.

Plan and Provide Effective Interventions

Intervention planning requires an understanding of the underlying reasons for difficulty as well as a delineation of the conditions that influence performance. Providing integrated services allows the occupational therapy practitioner to contribute discipline-specific information and strategies to enhance a student's abilities that are not typically within a teacher's expertise (Asher & Nichols, 2016). Intervention approaches may adapt the environment, promote strategy use, or address performance skills to optimize student participation.

Environmental adaptations

The occupational therapy practitioner can modify, adapt, or compensate by revising the context or activity demands to support performance in daily routines (Fox & Lincoln, 2008). When the task–environment demands are greater than the student's abilities, the therapist, in collaboration with the teacher, must adapt the environment or task to foster successful participation. The school environment includes the classrooms, cafeteria, playgrounds, restrooms, gymnasium, art room, and other areas, and all should be considered. For example, the student may have difficulty with "way finding," such as knowing how to get from the cafeteria to the classroom.

The occupational therapy practitioner can also foster performance through universal design for learning in the classroom, with environmental modifications. For example, when visually stimulating classrooms adversely affect a student's participation, the occupational therapy practitioner and the teacher can collaborate on how to lessen competing stimuli. Auditory books with text readers could help refocus visual attention to the reading process, for instance.

Strategy use

The occupational therapy practitioner can
- Foster self-generation of strategies (Grajo & Candler, 2014);

- Promote explicit instruction and feedback, model using clear explanations and pictures, break tasks into smaller units, and decrease support as the student becomes more independent (Vaughn et al., 2012); and
- Provide visual cues for letter formation, then ask the student to study the letter to form a visual image and then write the letter by memory.

Address performance skills

The occupational therapy practitioner can use several strategies to address students' performance skills:
- Create or promote skills through enriched contextual and activity experiences, thereby facilitating mastery and competence in context. Performing visual–perceptual skills embedded in natural contexts reinforces advanced skill development (Coté, 2015).
- Increase the student's engagement in reading and writing so they can use the skills they have learned more effectively and efficiently. Motivation toward achieving the goal is the driving force as the student self-organizes the many components (Case-Smith et al., 2010; Coté, 2015). These therapeutic activities should incorporate as many of the components of the visual process as possible (Coté, 2015).
- Direct students toward print when they are reading books, pairing verbal and nonverbal cues (e.g., say, "This is the front of the book," then sweep your hand across the cover; Frank, 2012). Other print concepts include where to start, which way to go, return sweep left, first and last, and the concept of letters.
- Provide structured activities to improve performance skills and measure progress toward targeted outcomes (Ratzon et al., 2007).
- Encourage students to use writing as a communication tool. During classroom activities, students can learn about letters and sound as a precursor to letter formation.
- Develop the skills students need for alphabet knowledge; rapid naming of letters, digits, colors, and objects; and name writing (Frolek Clark, 2016; National Early Literacy Panel, 2008) through sensory processing, attention and engagement, fine motor skills, and play (Coleman et al., 2016).
- Develop visual–spatial skills as potential avenues for targeted math and writing interventions (Carlson et al., 2013; Kaiser et al., 2009).
- Use strategies involving self-directed movement through space, such as the use of obstacle courses with word games to assist in higher ordered visual sight recognition and to foster movement through space.
- Haptic perception (e.g., exploring objects by feel to determine size, texture, and shape) can enhance visual perception (Gori et al., 2008).
- Increase the student's participation in self-chosen and structured reading occupations using self-generated strategies for the student to draw on when they face challenges in reading activities (Grajo & Candler, 2014, 2016).
- Engage in interprofessional collaboration (Asher & Nichols, 2016).

Education of the student and their parents, teachers, and caregivers can at times be the most helpful intervention for the student. This assists in increasing the stakeholders' awareness of the student's limitations and the functional implications of the visual–perceptual problems. Education helps others to view the student in a different way. For example, they understand the problem and can provide cues or environmental adaptations to support learning.

SUMMARY

Occupational therapists have much to contribute in the identification and intervention of visual–perceptual and visual–motor problems among students, an area that is often overlooked. During intervention, occupational therapy practitioners should document and empirically measure the real-life changes in occupational performance that come from changes in visual perception skills (Bendixen & Kreider, 2011). Efficacy studies on which intervention approaches are most successful are needed.

REFERENCES

American Occupational Therapy Association. (2014a). Guidelines for supervision, roles, and responsibilities during the delivery of occupational therapy services. *American Journal of Occupational Therapy, 68*(Suppl. 3), S16–S22. https://doi.org/10.5014/ajot.2014.686S03

American Occupational Therapy Association. (2014b). Occupational therapy practice framework: Domain and process (3rd ed.). *American Journal of Occupational Therapy, 68*(Suppl. 1), S1–S48. https://doi.org/10.5014/ajot.2014.682006

Asher, A., & Nichols, J. (2016). Collaboration around facilitating emergent literacy: Role of occupational therapy. *Journal of Occupational Therapy, Schools, and Early Intervention, 9*, 51–73. https://doi.org/10.1080/19411243.2016.1156415

Beery, K. E., Buktenica, N. A., & Beery, N. A. (2010). *Beery–Buktenica Developmental Test of Visual–Motor Integration* (6th ed.). San Antonio: Pearson.

Bendixen, R., & Kreider, C. M. (2011). *Centennial Vision*—Review of occupational therapy research in the practice area of children and youth. *American Journal of Occupational Therapy, 65*, 351–359. https://doi.org/10.5014/ajot.2011.000976

Carlson, A., Rowe, E., & Curby, T. (2013). Disentangling fine motor skills' relations to academic achievement: The relative contributions of visual–spatial integration and visual–motor coordination. *Journal of Genetic Psychology, 174*, 514–533. https://doi.org/10.1080/00221325.2012.717122

Case-Smith, J., Law, M., Missiuna, C., Pollock, N., & Stewart, D. (2010). Foundations for occupational therapy practice with children. In J. Case-Smith & J. C. O'Brien (Eds.), *Occupational therapy for children* (6th ed., pp. 22–55). St. Louis: Mosby.

Clark, G. J. (2010). *The relationship between handwriting, reading, fine motor and visual–motor skills in kindergarteners* (Unpublished doctoral dissertation). Iowa State University, Ames. Retrieved from http://lib.dr.iastate.edu/etd/11399

Colarusso, R. P., & Hammill, D. D. (2015). *Motor-Free Visual Perception Test* (4th ed.). Novato, CA: Academic Therapy.

Coleman, B., Corl, C., Davis, H., Perucco, A., & Tanta, K. (2016). Occupational therapy and preliteracy skills: An integrated approach to treatment. *Journal of Occupational Therapy, Schools, and Early Intervention, 9*, 6–11. https://doi.org/10.1080/19411243.2016.1141585

Coté, C. A. (2011). Levels of processing in visual perception tasks. *Early Intervention and School Special Interest Section Quarterly, 18*, 1–4.

Coté, C. A. (2015). A dynamic systems theory model of visual perception development. *Journal of Occupational Therapy, Schools, and Early Intervention, 8*, 157–169. https://doi.org/10.1080/19411243.2015.1034304

Every Student Succeeds Act, Pub. L. 114–195, 129 Stat. 1802 (2015).

Fox, T., & Lincoln, N. (2008). Verbal mediation as a treatment strategy for children with non-verbal learning difficulties. *International Journal of Therapy and Rehabilitation, 15*, 315–320. https://doi.org/10.12968/ijtr.2008.15.7.30455

Frank, S. (2012). *The use of explicit, non-evocative print referencing with at-risk preschool children: Implications for increasing print knowledge* (Unpublished doctoral dissertation). University of Kentucky, Lexington.

Frolek Clark, G. (2016). The occupations of literacy: Occupational therapy's role. *Journal of Occupational Therapy, Schools, and Early Intervention, 9*, 27–37. https://doi.org/10.1080/19411243.2016.1152835

Gilbert, C. D., & Li, W. (2013). Top-down influences on visual processing. *Nature Reviews Neuroscience, 14*, 350–363. https://doi.org/10.1038/nrn3476

Goldstand, S., Koslowe, K., & Parush, S. (2005). Vision, visual-information processing, and academic performance among seventh-grade school children: A more significant relationship than we thought? *American Journal of Occupational Therapy, 59*, 377–389. https://doi.org/10.5014/ajot.59.4.377

Gori, M., Del Viva, M., Sandini, G., & Burr, D. (2008). Young children do not integrate visual and haptic form information. *Current Biology, 18*, 694–698. https://doi.org/10.1016/j.cub.2008.04.036

Grajo, L. C., & Candler, C. (2014). Children with reading difficulties: How occupational therapy can help. *OT Practice, 19*(13), 16–17. Retrieved from https://www.aota.org/-/media/Corporate/Files/Practice/Children/classroom-trouble-learning-to-read.pdf

Grajo, L. C., & Candler, C. (2016). An Occupation and Participation Approach to Reading Intervention (OPARI) Part II: Pilot clinical application. *Journal of Occupational Therapy, Schools, and Early Intervention, 9*, 86–98. https://doi.org/10.1080/19411243.2016.1141083

Hammill, D., Pearson, N. A., & Voress, J. K. (2014). *Developmental Test of Visual Perception* (3rd ed.). Austin, TX: Pro-Ed.

Kaiser, M., Albaret, J., & Doudin, P. (2009). Relationship between visual–motor integration, eye–hand coordination, and quality of handwriting. *Journal of Occupational Therapy, Schools, and Early Intervention, 2*, 87–95. https://doi.org/10.1080/19411240903146228

Kavale, K. A., & Forness, S. R. (2000). Auditory and visual perception processes and reading ability: A quantitative reanalysis and historical reinterpretation. *Learning Disability Quarterly, 23*, 253–270. https://doi.org/10.2307/1511348

Lauwereyns, J. (2012). *Brain and the gaze: On the active boundaries of vision.* Cambridge, MA: MIT Press.

Magi, K., Kikas, E., & Soodla, P. (2018). Effortful control, task persistence, and reading skills. *Journal of Applied Developmental Psychology, 54*, 42–52. https://doi.org/10.1016/j.appdev.2017.11.005

Martin, N. A. (2010). *Test of Visual–Motor Skills* (3rd ed.). Novato, CA: Academic Therapy.

Martin, N. A. (2017). *Test of Visual Perceptual Skills* (4th ed.). Los Angeles: Western Psychological Services.

Matthews, A. J., & Martin, F. H. (2009). Electrophysiological indices of spatial attention during global/local processing in good and poor phonological decoders. *Brain and Language, 111,* 152–160. https://doi.org/10.1016/j.bandl.2009.09.002

Menghini, D., Finzi, A., Carlesimo, G. A., & Vicari, S. (2011). Working memory impairment in children with developmental dyslexia: Is it just a phonological deficit? *Developmental Neuropsychology, 36,* 199–213. https://doi.org/10.1080/87565641.2010.549868.

National Early Literacy Panel. (2008). *Developing early literacy: A scientific synthesis of early literacy development and implications for intervention.* Jessup, MD: National Institute for Literacy.

Ram-Tsur, R., Faust, M., & Zivotofsky, A. Z. (2008). Poor performance on serial visual tasks in persons with reading disabilities: Impaired working memory? *Journal of Learning Disabilities, 41,* 437–450. https://doi.org/10.1177/0022219408321141

Ratzon, N. Z., Efraim, D., & Bart, O. (2007). A short-term graphomotor program for improving writing readiness skills of first-grade students. *American Journal of Occupational Therapy, 61,* 399–405. https://doi.org/10.5014/ajot.61.4.399

Scheiman, M. (2011). *Understanding and managing vision deficits: A guide for occupational therapists* (3rd ed.). Thorofare, NJ: Slack.

Schneck, C. M. (2010). Visual perception. In J. Case-Smith & J. C. O'Brien (Eds.), *Occupational therapy for children* (6th ed., pp. 382–412). St. Louis: Mosby/Elsevier.

Schotter, E. R., Angele, B., & Rayner, K. (2012). Parafoveal processing in reading. *Attention, Perception, and Psychophysics, 74,* 5–35. https://doi.org/10.3758/s13414-011-0219-2

Solan, H. A., Shelley-Tremblay, J. F., Hansen, P. C., & Larson, S. (2007). Is there a common linkage among reading comprehension, visual attention, and manocellular processing? *Journal of Learning Disabilities, 40,* 270–278. https://doi.org/10.1177/00222194070400030701

University of Oregon, Center on Teaching and Learning. (2018). *Dynamic Indicators of Basic Early Literacy Skills* (DIBELS®, 8th ed.). Eugene: Author. Retrieved from https://dibels.uoregon.edu

Vaughn, S., Wanzek, J., Murray, C., & Roberts, G. (2012). *Intensive interventions for students struggling in reading and mathematics: A practice guide.* Portsmouth, NH: Center on Instruction.

Watson, A. H., Ito, M., Smith, R. O., & Andersen, L. (2010). Effect of assistive technology in a public school setting. *American Journal of Occupational Therapy, 64,* 18–29. https://doi.org/10.5014/ajot.64.1.18

Woodrome, S. E., & Johnson, K. E. (2007). The role of visual discrimination in the learning-to-read process. *Reading and Writing, 22,* 117–131. https://doi.org/10.1007/s11145-007-9104-8

APPENDIXES

Appendix A. The Future of School Occupational Therapy Practice

Joyce E. Rioux, EdD, OTR/L, SCSS; Pam Stephenson, OTD, OTR/L; and Gloria Frolek Clark, PhD, OTR/L, BCP, SCSS, FAOTA

The background of occupational therapy practice from the past through the present can be found in Chapter 1, "History of Occupational Therapy in Schools." This appendix focuses on the future vision of occupational therapy in schools—a vision that upholds school occupational therapy as an educationally necessary and relevant service linked to education and health that has evolved and gained support as administrators, team members, and parents understand occupational therapy practitioners'[1] roles and contributions.

So where is practice going over the next 10 years? What does school occupational therapy's future hold? How do practitioners meet these needs? In response to our questions, which we relayed using several sources (e.g., AOTA online forum, a town hall meeting at the 2018 Children and Youth Specialty conference, AOTA's communities of practice, occupational therapy practitioners with a specialty certification in school systems [SCSS] credential), occupational therapy practitioners and students identified their future visions. The 3 common themes that emerged—leadership, expanded roles, and recognition of occupational therapy as an inclusive profession—indicate that the future is in good hands.

2029: OCCUPATIONAL THERAPY PRACTITIONERS HOLD LEADERSHIP ROLES IN SCHOOL PRACTICE

The distinct value of school occupational therapy practitioners in practice, policy, advocacy, research, and leadership is now understood and recognized by local, state, and national stakeholders. Practitioners have expanded their knowledge and skills to achieve their SCSS, which is highly valued by practitioners and by local, state, and national educators. AOTA has increased support for school occupational therapy practitioners through annual specialty conferences, ongoing community of practice groups, and resources specific to practice in this area. Special committees have been funded to study areas of need (e.g., service gaps between what is happening in practice and what is best practice, service delivery models, evidence-based practices) and have strengthened school practitioners' role in practice, policy, research, and leadership.

Occupational therapy practitioners continue to work with the system (at local, state, and national levels) to enhance outcomes for all students. Their expertise in enhancing students' access, academic participation, functional life skills, and mental health (i.e., through promotion, prevention, and intervention) in the educational setting is highly valued.

The inclusion of management and administration continuing education and coursework at the college and university levels has prepared occupational therapy practitioners and students to gain leadership positions. Advanced or dual degrees in complementary fields of study (e.g., education, public health, business administration, jurisprudence) have been encouraged. Fieldwork sites in school administration are now available across the nation.

School occupational therapy practitioners are involved in local, state, and national committees (e.g., vocational assessment, literacy committees, multi-tiered systems of support, transition committees) and are using their knowledge and skills to have an impact on systems of change. Advocacy work at the systems level affects students across all age groups and has led to powerful outcomes. In addition, advocacy work at the state and national levels has positively affected education policy and research to enhance outcomes for students with disabilities. This advocacy work has brought awareness to this population along with a growing pool of resources to optimize students' capacity, strengths, and preparation for adulthood.

In the future, barriers in state policy that prevented advancement will have been removed. Occupational therapists have obtained the necessary credentialing and hold various leadership positions in local, state, and national educational agencies. Local roles include lead therapist, manager (e.g., assistant director or director of therapy services), administrator, and researcher. State roles include member of various statewide task forces or committees, consultant at the Department of Education, and state director of special

---

[1] *Occupational therapy practitioner* refers to both the occupational therapist and the occupational therapy assistant. The American Occupational Therapy Association (AOTA; 2014a, p. S18) states, "The occupational therapist is responsible for all aspects of occupational therapy service delivery and is accountable for the safety and effectiveness of the occupational therapy service delivery process" and "must be directly involved in the delivery of services during the initial evaluation and regularly throughout the course of intervention. . . . The occupational therapy assistant delivers safe and effective occupational therapy services under the supervision of and in partnership with the occupational therapist."

Copyright © 2019 by the American Occupational Therapy Association. All rights reserved. To reuse this content, contact www.copyright.com.
https://doi.org/10.7139/2019.978-1-56900-591-0.AppA

education, and national roles include member of national task forces or committees, staff at regional technical centers, and pediatric consultant at AOTA. People in these roles have knowledge of program evaluation and development, supervision and appraisal of personnel, management of fiscal and material resources, and implementation of educational services and programs. Their knowledge of educational laws and procedures, skills in critical thinking and ethical reasoning, ability to apply a holistic perspective, and strength in building interpersonal relationships support them in their roles.

Occupational therapy assistants who have obtained additional management training or advanced degrees have stepped into leadership positions on various committees and teams (e.g., assistive technology team, transition task force, state guidelines committee).

2029: THE SCHOOL OCCUPATIONAL THERAPY PRACTITIONER HAS AN EXPANDED ROLE

In the future, occupational therapy practitioners' active involvement in schoolwide initiatives, support of effective services through research, work with all students, and proactive versus reactive role in student programming will have led to 1 or more occupational therapy practitioners being assigned to a school building. The proximity and availability of practitioners to educators result in greater collaboration, opportunities for coaching, and a shared responsibility for targeting improved student outcomes.

Occupational therapy practitioners are integrated as core members of the educational team. This integration includes collaborative practices with other professionals across the team to serve the needs of the school population as a whole. Occupational therapy practitioners collaborate with colleagues to design interventions that support students' participation in school life. They use coaching to teach and empower others on the team and to ensure that students attain successful outcomes. Occupational therapists co-teach in classrooms and across school environments (e.g., academic, social, work preparation, extracurricular).

Occupational therapy practitioners embrace their full scope of practice and support the occupational needs of students, families, and school staff. They work beyond a primary lens of performance skills deficits and embrace a practice that is focused on student participation in and performance of meaningful and necessary activities. They collaborate with colleagues to support social participation and to design initiatives that promote resilience and positive mental health. They use their expertise to support the development of behavior management plans that maximize students' participation and occupational engagement at school.

Administrators and school personnel now recognize the distinct knowledge and skill set of occupational therapy practitioners as an essential component of the team. Practitioners are identified as valuable contributors, and they use their skills to develop and implement systemwide supports, including using their knowledge of universal design for learning (UDL), environmental modifications, and assistive technology to build supports for students' participation at school and transition to adulthood. Practitioners are valued for what they bring to the interprofessional team,

and this value is reflected in fair compensation, manageable workloads or caseloads, and full participation and inclusion in team meetings.

2029: SCHOOL OCCUPATIONAL THERAPY RECOGNIZED AS AN INCLUSIVE PROFESSION

With the growing trend toward diverse and culturally responsive education (e.g., UDL, differentiated instruction, school choice options), school occupational therapy practitioners are capitalizing on their holistic approach. Their distinct value is in adapting the environment to fit the learner; working with students to find balance and self-direction for their education; and supporting the health, well-being, and occupational needs of the school community (e.g., students, teachers, parents). Individual services are episodic (e.g., short-term intensive, transitional periods) and are based on evidence for interventions in school contexts that have the greatest effect on students' immediate and critical needs. Continuous services address the needs of all learners through co-teaching, life-centered planning, and coaching.

Technology is embedded in people's daily lives, and occupational therapy practitioners contribute their expertise on healthy developmental choices and intentional selection of technology, including services delivered through telehealth. Occupational therapists are actively involved in curriculum development and technology integration to promote responsible, ethical, and relevant use of technology as a tool and to collaborate on projects, solve problems, share information, critically analyze content, and serve as media mentors.

Technology is not a replacement for rigorous instruction or other means of learning content. Technology use is balanced with creative hands-on workstations and opportunities to conceptualize, make, collaborate, and interact with actual materials and tools. For students preparing for transition to adulthood, occupational therapy practitioners are capitalizing on their knowledge of mainstream technology and educating students in responsibly accessing telehealth, online education, electronic job application submissions, and social networking communities.

As education is preparing students for future jobs and careers, occupational therapy practitioners are supporting this education by contributing to discussions on, planning of, and collaboration on curriculum development. Practitioners are applying their knowledge of "the therapeutic use of everyday activities with individuals or groups for the purpose of enhancing or enabling participation in roles, habits, and routines in home, school, workplace, community, and other settings" (AOTA, 2014b, p. S1). They are instructional facilitators and strategists who help all students uncover their strengths, persist through challenges, and prepare for the future (e.g., postsecondary options, entrepreneurship, community living).

REALIZING THE FUTURE

The future of occupational therapy in schools parallels AOTA's *Vision 2025:* "As an inclusive profession, occupational therapy maximizes health, well-being, and quality of life for all people, populations, and communities through effective solutions

TABLE A.1. 2029: School Occupational Therapy Practitioners in Action

PILLAR	SAMPLES
Effective	▪ Conducting research and implementing interventions that meet Every Student Succeeds Act (2015; Pub. L. 114–95) criteria (U.S. Department of Education, 2016) for strong, moderate, and promising evidence. (E.g., strong evidence: well-designed experimental study, statistically significant effect of the intervention, large sample, multisite sample that overlaps with populations and settings proposed to receive the intervention). ▪ Completing program evaluations to streamline processes and improve client outcomes.
Leaders	▪ Directing energies to the systems level of education and the interconnections within. ▪ Seamlessly supporting all students, having a seat at the table in state educational agencies, and having a wealth of resources and supports at the national level (e.g., AOTA). ▪ Influencing educational policies, learning environments, and the complex system of education.
Collaborative	▪ Preparing occupational therapy students for school practice to ensure they are well versed in educational laws; possess skills to effectively collaborate with educators, other professionals, families, and students; and articulate the distinct value and contributions of occupational therapy in educational settings. ▪ Working collaboratively and respectfully on a school team to optimize the role of all professionals on the team.
Accessible	▪ Promoting healthy learning environments that are safe, positive, and supportive of all students' success in school, home, and the community. ▪ Applying a co-teaching model to implement evidence-based interventions and improve outcomes for entire classrooms.
Diversity	▪ Realizing equality in schools and opportunities for occupational therapists to assume formal administrative roles in education, accomplished through the partnership and advocacy efforts of academics, practitioners, and AOTA. ▪ Promoting and implementing programs throughout the grades to build community participation, engagement, and acceptance; emphasizing inclusive classroom communities, school communities, local communities, and global communities.

Note. AOTA = American Occupational Therapy Association.

that facilitate participation in everyday living" (AOTA, 2018). Embracing this vision to set a course, school practitioners have furthered their specialized knowledge, skills, and capacity in the 5 pillars of *Vision 2025* to progress into the future and beyond, as demonstrated in Table A.1.

REFERENCES

American Occupational Therapy Association. (2014a). Guidelines for supervision, roles, and responsibilities during the delivery of occupational therapy services. *American Journal of Occupational Therapy, 68*(Suppl. 3), S16–S22. https://doi.org/10.5014/ajot.2014.686S03

American Occupational Therapy Association. (2014b). Occupational therapy practice framework: Domain and process (3rd ed.). *American Journal of Occupational Therapy, 68*(Suppl. 1), S1–48. https://doi.org/10.5014/ajot.2014.682006

American Occupational Therapy Association. (2018). *Vision 2025. American Journal of Occupational Therapy, 71,* 7103420010. https://doi.org/10.5014/ajot.2017.713002

Every Student Succeeds Act, Pub. L. 114–95, 129 Stat. 1802 (2015).

U.S. Department of Education. (2016). *Non-regulatory guidance: Using evidence to strengthen education investments.* Retrieved from https://ed.gov/policy/elsec/leg/essa/guidanceuseseinvestment.pdf

Appendix B. AOTA Occupational Profile Template

OCCUPATIONAL PROFILE: EXAMPLE

Background Information: James is a student in 2nd grade. His physician recently diagnosed him with dyspraxia. In response, James' parents pursued a 504 referral. The building intervention team referred James for an occupational therapy evaluation on the basis of underlying motor concerns (e.g., using school materials, moving around the school, participating in recess). The occupational therapy evaluation starts with the completion of an occupational profile.

Copyright © 2017 by the American Occupational Therapy Association. All rights reserved. To reuse this content, contact www.copyright.com. Originally published in *American Journal of Occupational Therapy, 71*(Suppl. 2), 7112420030. https://doi.org/10.5014/ajot.2017.716S12

AOTA OCCUPATIONAL PROFILE TEMPLATE

"The occupational profile is a summary of a client's occupational history and experiences, patterns of daily living, interests, values, and needs" (AOTA, 2014, p. S13). The information is obtained from the client's perspective through both formal interview techniques and casual conversation and leads to an individualized, client-centered approach to intervention.

Each item below should be addressed to complete the occupational profile. Page numbers are provided to reference a description in the *Occupational Therapy Practice Framework: Domain and Process, 3rd Edition* (AOTA, 2014).

Client/Date: James LastName/09-20XX

<table>
<tr><td rowspan="5" style="writing-mode: vertical-rl">Client Report</td><td>Reason the client is seeking service and concerns related to engagement in occupations</td><td colspan="2">Why is the client seeking service, and what are the client's current concerns relative to engaging in occupations and in daily life activities? (This may include the client's general health status.)

504 referral. Recent diagnosis of dyspraxia. Does James have equal access to education in comparison with his grade peers? Physical barriers (e.g., using school materials, moving around school, participating in recess)?</td></tr>
<tr><td>Occupations in which the client is successful (p. S5)</td><td colspan="2">In what occupations does the client feel successful, and what barriers are affecting his or her success?

Loves math, counting up on his fingers, "math work makes you smarter." Likes to run at recess and think about how far away the planets are.</td></tr>
<tr><td>Personal interests and values (p. S7)</td><td colspan="2">What are the client's values and interests?

Interests: Learning about planets and space. Math, reading, being a "good" student.</td></tr>
<tr><td>Occupational history (i.e., life experiences)</td><td colspan="2">What is the client's occupational history (i.e., life experiences)?

Lives with mom, dad, younger brother. One fish and two dogs. Did not go to preschool. Family academically focused versus sports-, nature-, or physical-focused activities.</td></tr>
<tr><td>Performance patterns (routines, roles, habits, & rituals) (p. S8)</td><td colspan="2">What are the client's patterns of engagement in occupations, and how have they changed over time? What are the client's daily life roles? (Patterns can support or hinder occupational performance.)

Self-advocates for academic needs. Asks for clarification. Few peer interactions during unstructured activities. Runs along perimeter at recess versus joining games or using equipment. Left handed.</td></tr>
<tr><td colspan="2"></td><td colspan="2">What aspects of the client's environments or contexts does he or she see as:</td></tr>
<tr><td rowspan="2" style="writing-mode: vertical-rl">Environment</td><td></td><td>Supports to Occupational Engagement</td><td>Barriers to Occupational Engagement</td></tr>
<tr><td>Physical (p. S28) (e.g., buildings, furniture, pets)</td><td>Benefits from preparation for loud sounds. Preferred seating</td><td>Stairs, heavy cafeteria door, scissors</td></tr>
<tr><td>Social (p. S28) (e.g., spouse, friends, caregivers)</td><td>Supporting teacher (provided reading support last year). One friend who is good role model. Ignores classmates who say unkind things.</td><td>Seeks out adults versus children</td></tr>
<tr><td rowspan="4" style="writing-mode: vertical-rl">Context</td><td>Cultural (p. S28) (e.g., customs, beliefs)</td><td>Family values academics</td><td>None identified</td></tr>
<tr><td>Personal (p. S28) (e.g., age, gender, SES, education)</td><td>2nd grader. Feels successful at school. Advocates for self. Asks for clarification.</td><td>None identified</td></tr>
<tr><td>Temporal (p. S28) (e.g., stage of life, time, year)</td><td>None identified</td><td>Family identified that his play is not typical of peers. Does play with a cousin (girl).</td></tr>
<tr><td>Virtual (p. S28) (e.g., chat, email, remote monitoring)</td><td>Likes to look up space topics on computer</td><td>Holds the iPad close, computer close.</td></tr>
<tr><td rowspan="2" style="writing-mode: vertical-rl">Client Goals</td><td>Client's priorities and desired targeted outcomes: (p. S34)</td><td colspan="2">Consider: occupational performance—improvement and enhancement, prevention, participation, role competence, health and wellness, quality of life, well-being, and/or occupational justice.</td></tr>
<tr><td colspan="2">James does not identify any concerns or struggles at school. He reports that he likes school and likes his teacher. Likes to run and does not like to get distracted when running. Identifies one classmate who he sees as a friend. Enjoys quiet buses. Last year, seats were assigned on the bus. Likes to look out the window. Likes hugs from his family at the end of the day.</td></tr>
</table>

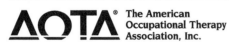

AOTA® **The American Occupational Therapy Association, Inc.**

Copyright © 2017, by the American Occupational Therapy Association.
This document is designed to be used in occupational therapy practice and education.
For all other uses, such as republishing or digital hosting and delivery, contact www.copyright.com or copyright@aota.org.

ADDITIONAL RESOURCES

For a complete description of each component and examples of each, refer to the *Occupational Therapy Practice Framework: Domain and Process, 3ʳᵈ Edition.*

American Occupational Therapy Association. (2014). Occupational therapy practice framework: Domain and process (3rd ed.). *American Journal of Occupational Therapy, 68*(Suppl. 1), S1–S48. https://doi.org/10.5014/ajot.2014.682006

The occupational profile is a requirement of the *CPT®* occupational therapy evaluation codes as of January 1, 2017. For more information visit www.aota.org/coding.

Appendix C. Occupational Therapy Intervention Plan

Client Information		
Name:	DOB:	School/Grade:
Parents:	Phone:	
Diagnosis or Conditions:		
Precautions:		

Intervention Goals: *Areas of Occupation to be Addressed:*
☐ ADLs   ☐ IADLs ☐ Education   ☐ Leisure   ☐ Play ☐ Rest/Sleep   ☐ Social Participation   ☐ Work

Intervention Approaches: Check/Describe
☐ Create/Promote   ☐ Establish/Restore   ☐ Maintain   ☐ Modify   ☐ Prevent

Types of Interventions: Check/Describe
☐ Advocacy   ☐ Education & Training ☐ Group ☐ Occupations & Activities   ☐ Preparatory Methods & Tasks

Service Delivery Mechanisms	
Frequency:	Duration:
Location of services:	Provider(s):

Discontinuation Plan (list criteria)

Outcome Measures (check)

☐ Health & Wellness   ☐ Occupational Justice   ☐ Occupational Performance   ☐ Participation
☐ Prevention   ☐ Quality of Life   ☐ Role Competence   ☐ Well-Being

Developed by:

Date Developed: **Date Revised:**

Source. Copyright © 2015 by Gloria Frolek Clark. Used with permission.

Copyright © 2015 by Gloria Frolek Clark.
https://doi.org/10.7139/2019.978-1-56900-591-0.AppC

Appendix D. Brief Audit of Occupational Therapy Documentation

Date of Review: _____				
Purpose: To identify documentation strengths and needs as part of employee appraisal				
Directions: Place a checkmark (√) in the box that best describes practitioner documentation.				
Coding Key: C = *complete*; IC = *incomplete*; M = *missing*.				
File Reviewed (file ID: _____)	**C**	**IC**	**M**	**Comments**
Recent evaluation or reevaluation report				
Current IEP				
Educationally relevant goals and objectives				
Recent intervention plan				
Contact report current				
Recent progress report				
Additional Documentation (if applicable)	**C**	**IC**	**M**	**Comments**
Medicaid documentation current				
Weekly schedule				
OTA supervision log current				
Mileage forms				
Timesheets				
Timely documentation submission				
Workspace organized				
Adhere to confidential practices				
General Comments:				

Reviewed Practitioner Signature _____ Supervisor/Auditor Signature _____

Date of Signature: _____

Note. IEP = individualized education program; OTA = occupational therapy assistant.
Source. Developed by Joyce E. Rioux. Used with permission.

Copyright © 2018 by Joyce E. Rioux.
https://doi.org/10.7139/2019.978-1-56900-591-0.AppD

Appendix E. Full or Partial Audit of Occupational Therapy Documentation

Date of Review: _____

Purpose: To align documentation with the official guidelines from the American Occupational Therapy Association (2018). The data collected should be analyzed to identify areas of strengths and needs

Directions: Identify the documentation reports that will be reviewed. Assess the documentation against the criteria listed. Place a checkmark (√) in the box that best describes practitioner documentation

Client: May include a person, group (e.g., classroom), and population (e.g., district)

Coding Key: C = *complete*; IC = *incomplete*; M = *missing*.

SCREENING REPORT	C	IC	M
Fundamentals • Each page of documentation includes: client's full name, date of birth, gender, file ID (if applicable). • Includes the type of documentation and date of services. • Professional signature (first name or initial, last name) and credential; cosignature and credential when required for documentation of supervision. • All errors are noted and initialed or signed.			
Client information Includes: Name, date of birth, gender, description of occupational history, experiences, and performance; health status; applicable medical, educational, and developmental diagnoses; and precautions and contraindications.			
Screening (request) information Includes: Date and source of request, reason for request.			
Brief occupational profile Includes: Client's reason for seeking occupational therapy services, areas of occupation in which the client is successful and challenged; contexts and environments that support and hinder occupational performance (e.g., patterns of living, interest, values); medical, educational, and work history; and client's priorities and targeted goals.			
Sources of information and results Includes: Types of assessment used (e.g., interviews, record reviews, observations) and description of results.			
Recommendations Includes: Professional judgments regarding strategies and instruction to be used to assist client in general education performance; need for complete occupational therapy evaluation.			
EVALUATION REPORT	C	IC	M
Fundamentals • Each page of documentation includes: Client's full name, date of birth, gender, file ID (if applicable). • Includes the type of documentation and date of services. • Professional signature (first name or initial, last name) and credential; cosignature and credential when required for documentation of supervision. • All errors are noted and initialed or signed.			

(Continued)

Copyright © 2019 by the American Occupational Therapy Association. All rights reserved. To reuse this content, contact www.copyright.com.
https://doi.org/10.7139/2019.978-1-56900-591-0.AppE

Client information Includes: Name, date of birth, gender, description of occupational history, experiences, and performance; health status and previous services required and accessed; applicable medical, educational, and developmental diagnoses; and precautions and contraindications.			
Referral information Includes: Date and source of referral, services requested, and reason for referral.			
Occupational profile Includes: Client's reason for seeking occupational therapy services; areas of occupation in which the client is successful and challenged; contexts and environments that support and hinder occupational performance; medical, educational, and work history; occupational and psychosocial history (e.g., patterns of living, interest, values); and client's priorities and targeted goals.			
Sources of information and results Includes: Types of assessment used (e.g., interviews, record reviews, observations, standardized or nonstandardized assessments) and description of results.			
Analysis of occupational performance Includes: Analysis of occupational performance and identification of factors that support and hinder performance and participation (objective and measurable identification of performance skills, performance patterns, contexts and environments, activity demands, outcomes of standardized or nonstandardized assessments, and client factors).			
Summary and analysis Includes: Interpretation and summary of the occupational profile and occupational performance issues, identification of targeted areas of occupation and occupational performance to be addressed, and expected outcomes.			
Recommendations Includes: Professional judgment regarding necessity for skilled occupational therapy services or other services.			
REEVALUATION REPORT	**C**	**IC**	**M**
Fundamentals • Each page of documentation includes: Client's full name, date of birth, gender, file ID (if applicable). • Includes the type of documentation and date of services. • Professional signature (first name or initial, last name) and credential; cosignature and credential when required for documentation of supervision. • All errors are noted and initialed or signed.			
Client information Includes: Name, date of birth, gender, description of occupational history, experiences, and performance; health status; applicable medical, educational, and developmental diagnoses; and precautions and contraindications.			
Occupational profile Includes: Updates on current areas of occupation that are successful and problematic; contexts and environments that support and hinder occupational engagement, summary of any new medical, educational, and work information; updates on or changes to client's priorities and targeted outcomes.			
Reevaluation results Includes: Focus of reevaluation; specific types of outcome measures from standardized or nonstandardized assessments used; and results.			
Analysis of occupational performance Includes: Analysis of occupational performance and identification of factors that support and hinder performance and participation (objective and measurable identification of performance skills, performance patterns, contexts and environments, activity demands, outcomes from standardized or nonstandardized assessments, and client factors).			
Summary and analysis Includes: Interpretation and summary of the occupational profile and analysis of occupational performance, identification of targeted areas of occupation and occupational performance to be addressed, and expected outcomes.			
Recommendations Includes: Changes to occupational therapy services; revision or continuation of interventions, goals, and objectives; frequency of occupational therapy services; and recommendation for referral to other professionals or agencies, as applicable.			

(Continued)

INTERVENTION PLAN	C	IC	M
Fundamentals ▪ Each page of documentation includes: Client's full name, date of birth, gender, file ID (if applicable). ▪ Includes the type of documentation and date of services. ▪ Professional signature (first name or initial, last name) and credential; cosignature and credential when required for documentation of supervision. ▪ All errors are noted and initialed or signed.			
Client information Includes: Name, date of birth, gender, and precautions and contraindications.			
Intervention goals Includes: Measurable and meaningful occupation-based long-term and short-term goals directly related to client's ability to engage in desired occupations and to justification of the need for skilled occupational therapy intervention to meet the goals. Goals are based on the evaluation or reevaluation in adherence to each payer source's documentation requirements.			
Intervention approaches and types of interventions to be used Includes: Intervention approaches (e.g., create or promote, establish or restore, maintain, modify, prevent); types of interventions (e.g., consultation, education process, advocacy, and therapeutic use of occupations or activities) used in individual or group sessions.			
Service delivery mechanisms Includes: Service provider; service location; and frequency, intensity, and duration of services for the individual needs of the client.			
Plan for discontinuation Includes: Discontinuation criteria, discharge setting, and anticipated follow-up care.			
Outcome measures Includes: Tools that assess occupational performance, adaptation, role competence, improved health and wellness, improved quality of life, self-advocacy, and occupational justice. Standardized and nonstandardized assessment methods used at evaluation should be readministered periodically to monitor measurable progress and report functional outcomes as required by payer source and facility requirements.			
CONTACT REPORT (THERAPY NOTES)	C	IC	M
Fundamentals ▪ Each page of documentation includes: Client's full name, date of birth, gender, file ID (if applicable). ▪ Includes the type of documentation and date of services. ▪ Professional signature (first name or initial, last name) and credential; cosignature and credential when required for documentation of supervision. ▪ All errors are noted and initialed or signed.			
Client information Includes: Name, date of birth, gender, diagnosis, precautions, contraindications, and variables that influence the client's condition.			
Therapy log Includes: Reflects the complexity of the client and the professional clinical reasoning and expertise of an occupational therapy practitioner required to provide safe and effective outcomes in occupational engagement and performance. Content includes date; length of service contact; type of contact; names and positions of persons involved; summary of significant information communicated during contact; client attendance and participation in intervention or reason service was missed; types and approaches of interventions used; client's self-report and response to intervention; adverse reaction or response to treatment; environmental or task modification; assistive or adaptive devices used or fabricated; statement of any training, education, or consultation provided; and client's present level of performance. Significant, unusual, or unexpected changes in clinical or functional status are reported. Objective measures used to assess outcomes should be repeated in accordance with payer and facility requirements and clearly documented to demonstrate measurable functional progress toward the client's goals.			

(Continued)

PROGRESS REPORT	C	IC	M
Fundamentals ▪ Each page of documentation includes: Client's full name, date of birth, gender, file ID (if applicable). ▪ Includes the type of documentation and date of services. ▪ Professional signature (first name or initial, last name) and credential; cosignature and credential when required for documentation of supervision. ▪ All errors are noted and initialed or signed.			
Client information Includes: Name, date of birth, gender, precautions, and contraindications.			
Goals Includes: Goals addressed during the provision of therapy services (IEP goals; goals on occupational therapy intervention plan).			
Summary of services provided Includes: Brief statement of frequency and duration of services; types and approaches of interventions provided; data collection procedures (age-appropriate standardized and nonstandardized assessments, tests, and measures) and results; measurable progress (or lack thereof); environmental or task modifications provided; adaptive equipment or orthotics provided; medical, educational, or other pertinent client updates; client's response to occupational therapy services; and programs or training provided to the client or caregivers.			
Current client performance Includes: Goal achievement and current performance in areas of occupation.			
Plan or recommendations Includes: Recommendations and rationale as well as client's input for changes or continuation of plan to include goals, frequency, intensity, or duration.			
TRANSITION PLAN	C	IC	M
Fundamentals ▪ Each page of documentation includes: Client's full name, date of birth, gender, file ID (if applicable). ▪ Includes the type of documentation and date of services. ▪ Professional signature (first name or initial, last name) and credential; cosignature and credential when required for documentation of supervision. ▪ All errors are noted and initialed or signed.			
Client information Includes: Name, date of birth, gender, diagnosis, precautions, and contraindications.			
Client's current status Includes: Current occupational engagement and performance skills.			
Transition plan Includes: Name of current service setting and setting to which client will transition, reason for transition, time frame in which transition will occur, and outline of activities to be carried out during the transition plan.			
Recommendations Includes: Recommendations and rationale for occupational therapy services, modifications, or accommodations needed, and assistive technology and environmental modifications needed.			
DISCONTINUATION REPORT	C	IC	M
Fundamentals ▪ Each page of documentation includes: Client's full name, date of birth, gender, file ID (if applicable). ▪ Includes the type of documentation and date of services. ▪ Professional signature (first name or initial, last name) and credential; cosignature and credential when required for documentation of supervision. ▪ All errors are noted and initialed or signed.			
Client information Includes: Name, date of birth, gender, diagnosis, precautions, and contraindications.			

(Continued)

Summary of intervention process Includes: Dates of initial and final service; frequency, number of sessions, and summary of interventions used; summary of progress toward goals; and occupational therapy outcomes (including initial and ending client status regarding engagement in occupations and client's assessment of efficacy of occupational therapy services).			
Recommendations Includes: Recommendations pertaining to the client's future needs; specific follow-up plans, if applicable; referrals to other professionals and agencies, if applicable.			

Note. IEP = individualized education program.
Source. Adapted from American Occupational Therapy Association (2018).

REFERENCE

American Occupational Therapy Association. (2018). Guidelines for documentation of occupational therapy. *American Journal of Occupational Therapy, 72*(Suppl. 2), 721241010. https://doi.org/10.5014/ajot.2018.72S203

Appendix F. Selected Assessment Tools for Analysis of Students' Occupational Performance

Disclaimer: This table catalogs the many tools cited in the chapters. This list should not be considered exhaustive but rather as a sampling of available tools.

DOMAIN OF OCCUPATIONAL THERAPY	SAMPLE ASSESSMENTS USED IN OCCUPATIONAL THERAPY PRACTICE IN SCHOOLS
Occupations ▪ ADLs ▪ IADLs ▪ Education ▪ Play ▪ Leisure ▪ Rest and sleep ▪ Social participation ▪ Work	**Everyday Activities** ▪ Adaptive Behavior Assessment System: School Kit (Harrison & Oakland, 2015) ▪ Canadian Occupational Performance Measure (Law et al., 2014) ▪ Child and Adolescent Scale of Participation (Bedell, 2009) ▪ Child and Family Follow-up Survey (TBI specific; Bedell, 2004) ▪ Child Occupational Self-Assessment (Keller et al., 2005) ▪ Children's Assessment of Participation and Enjoyment (King et al., 2004) ▪ Choosing Outcomes and Accommodations for Children (Giangreco et al., 2011) ▪ Goal-Oriented Assessment of Lifeskills (Miller et al., 2013) ▪ Making Action Plans (O'Brien et al., 2010) ▪ Participation and Environment Measure for Children and Youth (Coster et al., 2011) ▪ Pediatric Evaluation of Disability Inventory (Haley et al., 2012) ▪ Pediatric Evaluation of Disability Inventory Computer Adaptive Test (Haley et al., 2012) ▪ Perceived Efficacy and Goal Setting system (Missiuna et al., 2004) ▪ TEACCH Transition Assessment Profile (Mesibov et al., 2007) ▪ Transition Planning Inventory (Patton & Clark, 2014) ▪ Vineland Adaptive Behavior Scales (Sparrow et al., 2005) **ADLs** ▪ Brief Autism Mealtime Behavior Inventory (Lukens & Linscheid, 2008) ▪ Brief Assessment of Mealtime Behavior in Children (Hendy et al., 2013) ▪ Eating Profile (Nadon et al., 2011) ▪ Roll Evaluation of Activities of Life (Roll & Roll, 2013) ▪ Screening Tool of Feeding Problems (Matson & Kuhn, 2001) ▪ Screening Tool of Feeding Problems applied to children (Seiverling et al., 2011) **IADLs** ▪ Kohlman Evaluation of Living Skills (Kohlman Thomson & Robnett, 2016) ▪ Roll Evaluation of Activities of Life (Roll & Roll, 2013) **Education** ▪ DeCoste Writing Protocol–Revised (DeCoste, 2014) ▪ Functional Assessment and Curriculum for Teaching Students With Disabilities (Valletutti et al., 2008) ▪ Here's How I Write (Goldstand et al., 2013) ▪ Miller Function and Participation Scales (Miller, 2006) ▪ Perceived Efficacy and Goal Setting System (Missiuna et al., 2004) ▪ Personal Futures Planning (Mount, 2000) ▪ Preferences for Activities of Children (King et al., 2004) ▪ Promoting Alternative Tomorrows with Hope (O'Brien et al., 2010) ▪ Protocol for Accommodations in Reading (DeCoste & Wilson, 2012) ▪ Questionnaire of Young People's Participation (cerebral palsy specific; Tuffrey et al., 2013) ▪ School Assessment of Motor and Process Skills (Fisher et al., 2005) ▪ School Function Assessment (Coster et al., 1998) ▪ Test of Handwriting Skills (Milone, 2007)

(Continued)

Copyright © 2019 by the American Occupational Therapy Association. All rights reserved. To reuse this content, contact www.copyright.com.
https://doi.org/10.7139/2019.978-1-56900-591-0.AppF

	- The Print Tool (Olsen & Knapton, 2006) - Weekly Calendar Planning Activity: A Performance Test of Executive Function (Toglia, 2015) - Wisconsin Assistive Technology Initiative: Assessing Students' Needs for Assistive Technology (Wisconsin Assistive Technology Initiative Development Team, 2017) **Play and Leisure** - Assistance to Participate Scale (Bourke-Taylor & Pallant, 2013) - Paediatric Activity Card Sort (Mandich et al., 2004) - Pediatric Interest Profiles (Henry, 2000) - Test of Playfulness (Skard & Bundy, 2008) **Social Participation** - Evaluation of Social Interaction (Fisher & Griswold, 2010) **Work** - Assessment of Work Performance (Sandqvist et al., 2010) - Vocational Fit Assessment (Persch et al., 2015)
Client Factors - Body functions - Body structures - Values, beliefs, and spirituality	- Assisting Hand Assessment (Krumlinde-Sundholm et al., 2007) - Paediatric Pain Profile (Institute of Child Health et al., 2003) - Quality of Upper Extremity Skills Test (cerebral palsy and traumatic brain injury specific; DeMatteo et al., 1992)
Performance Skills - Motor skills - Process skills - Social interaction skills	**Motor Skills** - Beery–Buktenica Developmental Test of Visual–Motor Integration (Beery et al., 2010) - Bruininks–Oseretsky Test of Motor Proficiency (Bruininks, 2005) - Developmental Pre-Feeding Checklist (Morris & Klein, 2001) - Gross Motor Function Classification System (Palisano et al., 2007) - Gross Motor Performance Measure (Boyce et al., 1998) - Manual Ability Classification System (CP specific; Eliasson et al., 2006) - Movement Assessment Battery for Children–2 (Henderson et al., 2007) - Peabody Developmental Motor Scales (Folio & Fewell, 2000) - School Assessment of Motor and Process Skills (Fisher et al., 2005) **Process Skills** - The Adult/Adolescent Sensory History (May-Benson, 2015) - Beery–Buktenica Developmental Test of Visual–Motor Integration (Beery et al., 2010) - Behavior Rating Inventory of Executive Functioning (Gioia et al., 2015) - Developmental Test of Visual Perception (Hammill et al., 2013) - Developmental Test of Visual Perception: Adolescent and Adult (Reynolds et al., 2002) - Motor-Free Visual Perception Test (Colarusso & Hammill, 2015) - Sensory Processing Measure: School Form (Miller-Kuhaneck et al., 2007) - Sensory Profile™ (Dunn, 2014); Adolescent/Adult Sensory Profile (Brown & Dunn, 2002) - School Assessment of Motor and Processing Skills (Fisher et al., 2005) - Test of Visual–Motor Skills (Martin, 2010) - Test of Visual Perceptual (Martin, 2017) **Social Interaction Skills** - Every Move Counts (Korsten et al., 1993) - Social Responsiveness Scale (Constantino & Gruber, 2012) - Social Skills Improvement System: Rating Scales (Gresham & Elliott, 2008)
Performance Patterns - Habits - Rituals - Roles - Routines	- Canadian Occupational Performance Measure (Law et al., 2014) - Child Occupational Self-Assessment (Keller et al., 2005) - Children's Assessment of Participation and Enjoyment (King et al., 2004) - Short Child Occupational Profile (Bowyer et al., 2008)
Context - Cultural - Personal - Physical - Social - Temporal - Virtual	- Canadian Occupational Performance Measure (Law et al., 2014) - Child Occupational Self-Assessment (Keller et al., 2005) - Children's Assessment of Participation and Enjoyment (King et al., 2004) - Choosing Outcomes and Accommodations for Children (Giangreco et al., 2011) - Classroom Sensory Environment Assessment (Kuhaneck & Kelleher, 2015) - Making Action Plans (O'Brien et al., 2010) - Perceived Efficacy and Goal Setting system (Missiuna et al., 2004) - Personal Futures Planning (Mount, 2000) - School Setting Interview (Hemmingsson et al., 2005) - Short Child Occupational Profile (Bowyer et al., 2008) - Test of Environmental Supportiveness (Skard & Bundy, 2008)

Note. ADLs = activities of daily living; CP = cerebral palsy; IADLs = instrumental activities of daily living; TBI = traumatic brain injury.

REFERENCES

Bedell, G. M. (2004). Developing a follow-up survey focused on participation of children and youth with acquired brain injuries after discharge from inpatient rehabilitation. *NeuroRehabilitation, 19,* 191–205.

Bedell, G. (2009). Further validation of the Child and Adolescent Scale of Participation (CASP). *Developmental Neurorehabilitation, 12,* 342–351. https://doi.org/10.3109/17518420903087277

Beery, K. E., Buktenica, N. A., & Beery, N. A. (2010). *Beery–Buktenica Developmental Test of Visual–Motor Integration: Administration, scoring, and teaching manual* (6th ed.). Minneapolis: Pearson.

Bourke-Taylor, H., & Pallant, J. (2013). The Assistance to Participate Scale to measure play and leisure support for children with developmental disability: Update following Rasch analysis. *Child Care, Health and Development, 39,* 544–551. https://doi.org/10.111/cch.12047

Bowyer, P. L., Kramer, J., Ploszaj, A., Ross, M., Schwartz, O., Kielhofner, G., & Kramer, K. (2008). *The Short Child Occupational Profile (SCOPE), Version 2.2.* Chicago: University of Illinois at Chicago.

Boyce, W., Gowland, C., Rosenbaum, P., Hardy, S., Lane, C., Plews, N., & Harding, D. (1998). *Gross Motor Performance Measure manual.* Kingston, Ontario: Queen's University, School of Rehabilitation Therapy.

Brown, C., & Dunn, W. (2002). *Adolescent/Adult Sensory Profile: User's manual.* San Antonio: Psychological Corporation.

Bruininks, R. H. (2005). *Bruininks–Oseretsky Test of Motor Proficiency.* Circle Pines, MN: AGS.

Colarusso, R., & Hammill, D. D. (2015). *MVPT–4: Motor-Free Visual Perception Test.* Novato, CA: Academic Therapy.

Constantino, J. N., & Gruber, C. P. (2012). *Social Responsiveness Scale (SRS).* Torrance, CA: Western Psychological Services.

Coster, W., Bedell, G., Law, M., Khetani, M., Teplicky, R., Liljenquist, K., . . . Kao, Y. (2011). Psychometric evaluation of the Participation and Environment Measure for Children and Youth. *Developmental Medicine and Child Neurology, 53,* 1030–1037. https://doi.org/10.1111/j.1469-8749.2011.04094.x

Coster, W. J., Deeney, T., Haltiwanger, J., & Haley, S. (1998). *School Function Assessment.* San Antonio: Psychological Corporation.

DeCoste, D. (2014). *The DeCoste Writing Protocol: Evidence-based research to make instructional and accommodation decisions.* Volo, IL: Don Johnston.

DeCoste, D., & Wilson, L. B. (2012). *Protocol for Accommodations in Reading.* Volo, IL: Don Johnston.

DeMatteo, C., Law, M., Russell, D., Pollock, N., Rosenbaum, P., & Walter, S. (1992). *QUEST: Quality of Upper Extremity Skills Test.* Hamilton, Ontario: McMaster University, Neurodevelopmental Clinical Research Unit.

Dunn, W. (2014). *Sensory Profile™ 2.* San Antonio: Pearson.

Eliasson, A. C., Krumlinde-Sundholm, L., Rosblad, B., Beckung, E., Arner, M., Ohrvall, A. M., & Rosenbaum, P. (2006). The Manual Ability Classification System (MACS) for children with cerebral palsy: Scale development and evidence of validity and reliability. *Developmental Medicine and Child Neurology, 46,* 549–554. https://doi.org/10.1111/j.1469-8749.2006.tb01313.x

Fisher, A., Bryze, K., Hume, V., & Griswold, L. (2005). *School AMPS: School version of the Assessment of Motor and Process Skills* (2nd ed.). Fort Collins, CO: Three Star Press.

Fisher, A. G., & Griswold, L. A. (2010). *Evaluation of Social Interaction.* Fort Collins, CO: Three Star Press.

Folio, M. R., & Fewell, R. R. (2000). *Peabody Developmental Motor Scales: Examiner's manual.* Austin, TX: Pro-Ed.

Giangreco, M. F., Cloninger, C. J., & Iverson, V. S. (2011). *Choosing Outcomes and Accommodations for Children* (3rd ed.). Baltimore: Brookes.

Gioia, G. A., Esquith, P. K., Guy, S. C., & Kenworthy, L. (2015). *Behavior Rating Inventory of Executive Functioning* (2nd ed.). Lutz, FL: Psychological Assessment Resources.

Goldstand, S., Gevir, D., Cermak, S., & Bissell, J. (2013). *Here's How I Write: A child's self-assessment of handwriting and goal setting tool.* Framingham, MA: Therapro.

Gresham, F. M., & Elliott, S. N. (2008). *Social Skills Improvement System: Rating Scales manual.* Bloomington, MN: NCS Pearson.

Haley, S. M., Coster, W. J., Dumas, H. M., Fragala-Pinkam, M. A., & Moed, R. (2012). *Pediatric Evaluation of Disability Inventory Computer Adaptive Test.* Retrieved from http://www.pedicat.com

Hammill, D., Pearson, N., & Voress, J. (2013). *Developmental Test of Visual Perception* (3rd ed.). Austin, TX: Pro-Ed.

Harrison, P., & Oakland, T. (2015). *Adaptive Behavior Assessment System* (3rd ed.). San Antonio: Psychological Corporation.

Hemmingsson, H., Snaefridur, E., Hoffman, O., & Kielhofner, G. (2005). *The School Setting Interview.* Chicago: University of Illinois at Chicago.

Henderson, S. E., Sugden, D. A., & Barnett, A. L. (2007). *Movement Assessment Battery for Children–2.* San Antonio: Harcourt Assessment.

Hendy, H. M., Seiverling, L., Lukens, C. T., & Williams, K. E. (2013). Brief Assessment of Mealtime Behavior in Children: Psychometrics and association with child characteristics and parent responses. *Children's Health Care, 42*(1), 1–14. https://doi.org/10.1080/02739615.2013.753799

Henry, A. D. (2000). *Pediatric Interest Profiles: Surveys of play for children and adolescents, Kid Play Profile, Preteen Play Profile, Adolescent Leisure Interest Profile.* San Antonio: Psychological Corporation.

Institute of Child Health, University College, & Royal College of Nursing Institute. (2003). *Paediatric Pain Profile.* London: Authors.

Keller, J., Kafkes, A., Basu, S., Federico, J., & Kielhofner, G. (2005). *Child Occupational Self-Assessment.* Chicago: University of Illinois at Chicago.

King, G., Law, M., King, S., Hurley, P., Hanna, S., Kertoy, M., . . . Young, N. (2004). *Children's Assessment of Participation and Enjoyment and Preferences for Activities of Children.* San Antonio: Harcourt Assessment.

Kohlman Thomson, L., & Robnett, R. (2016). *Kohlman Evaluation of Living Skills* (4th ed.). Bethesda, MD: AOTA Press.

Korsten, J. E., Dunn, D. K., Foss, T. V., & Francke, M. K. (1993). *Every Move Counts: Sensory-based communication techniques.* Austin, TX: Pro-Ed.

Krumlinde-Sundholm, L., Holmefur, M., Kottorp, A., & Eliasson, A. C. (2007). The Assisting Hand Assessment: Current evidence of validity, reliability, and responsiveness to change. *Developmental Medicine and Child Neurology, 49,* 259–264. https://doi.org/10.1111/j.1469-8749.2007.00259.x

Kuhaneck, H. M., & Kelleher, J. P. (2015). Development of the Classroom Sensory Environment Assessment. *American Journal of Occupational Therapy, 69,* 6906180040. https://doi.org/10.5014/ajot.2015.019430

Law, M., Baptiste, S., Carswell, A., McColl, M., Polatajko, H., & Pollock, N. (2014). *Canadian Occupational Performance Measure* (5th ed.). Ottawa: CAOT Publications.

Lukens, C. T., & Linscheid, T. R. (2008). Development and validation of an inventory to assess mealtime behavior in children with autism. *Journal of Autism and Developmental Disorders, 38,* 342–352. https://doi.org/10.1007/s10803-007-0401-5

Mandich, A., Polatajko, H. J., Miller, L., & Baum, C. (2004). *The Paediatric Activity Card Sort (PACS)*. Ottawa: Canadian Association of Occupational Therapists.

Martin, N. A. (2010). *Test of Visual–Motor Skills* (3rd ed.). Novato, CA: Academic Therapy.

Martin, N. A. (2017). *Test of Visual Perceptual Skills* (4th ed.). Los Angeles: Western Psychological Services.

Matson, J. L., & Kuhn, E. D. (2001). Identifying feeding problems in mentally retarded persons: Development and reliability of the Screening Tool of Feeding Problems (STEP). *Research in Developmental Disabilities, 21,* 165–172.

May-Benson, T. (2015). *The Adult/Adolescent Sensory History.* Newton, MA: Spiral Foundation at OTA.

Mesibov, G., Thomas, J. B., Chapman, S. M., & Schopler, E. (2007). *TEACCH Transition Assessment Profile* (2nd ed.). Austin, TX: Pro-Ed.

Miller, L. J. (2006). *Miller Function and Participation Scales manual.* San Antonio: Harcourt Assessment.

Miller, L. J., Oakland, T., & Herzberg, D. S. (2013). *Goal-Oriented Assessment of Lifeskills.* Torrance, CA: Western Psychological Services.

Miller-Kuhaneck, H., Henry, D., & Glennon, T. (2007). *Sensory Processing Measure: Main classroom and school environments forms.* Los Angeles: Western Psychological Services.

Milone, M. (2007). *Test of Handwriting Skills–Revised.* Novato, CA: Academic Therapy.

Missiuna, C., Pollock, N., & Law, M. (2004). *Perceived Efficacy and Goal Setting system.* Oxford, England: Harcourt Assessment.

Morris, S. E., & Klein, M. D. (2001). *Pre-feeding skills: A comprehensive resource for mealtime development* (2nd ed.). Cambridge, MA: Academic Press.

Mount, B. (2000). *Person-centered planning: Finding directions for change using personal futures planning.* New York: Graphic Futures.

Nadon, G., Feldman, D. E., Dunn, W., & Gisel, E. (2011). Association of sensory processing and eating problems in children with autism spectrum disorders. *Autism Research and Treatment, 2011,* 541926. https://doi.org/10.1155/2011/541926

O'Brien, J., Pearpoint, J., & Kahn, L. (2010). *The PATH and MAPS handbook: Person-centered ways to build community.* Toronto: Inclusion Press.

Olsen, J., & Knapton, E. (2006). *The Print Tool.* Cabin John, MD: Handwriting Without Tears.

Palisano, R., Rosenbaum, P., Bartlett, D., & Livingston, M. (2007). *Gross Motor Function Classification System: Expanded and revised.* Hamilton, Ontario: McMaster University.

Patton, J. R., & Clark, G. M. (2014). *Transition Planning Inventory* (2nd ed.). Austin, TX: Pro-Ed.

Persch, A. C., Gugiu, P. C., Onate, J. A., & Cleary, D. S. (2015). Development and psychometric evaluation of the Vocational Fit Assessment. *American Journal of Occupational Therapy, 69,* 6906180080. https://doi.org/10.5014/ajot.2015.019455

Reynolds, C. R., Pearson, N. A., & Voress, J. K. (2002). *Developmental Test of Visual Perception: Adolescent and Adult.* Austin, TX: Pro-Ed.

Roll, K., & Roll, W. (2013). *The REAL: The Roll Evaluation of Activities of Life.* Minneapolis: Pearson.

Sandqvist, J., Lee, J., & Kielhofner, G. (2010). *Assessment of Work Performance (AWP) Version 1.0.* Chicago: University of Illinois at Chicago.

Seiverling, L., Hendy, H. M., & Williams, K. (2011). The Screening Tool of Feeding Problems applied to children (STEP–CHILD): Psychometric characteristics and associations with child and parent variables. *Research in Developmental Disabilities, 32,* 1122–1129. https://doi.org/10.1016/j.ridd.2011.01.012

Skard, G., & Bundy, A. C. (2008). Test of Playfulness. In L. D. Parham & L. S. Fazio (Eds.), *Play in occupational therapy for children* (2nd ed., pp. 71–93). Maryland Heights, MO: Mosby.

Sparrow, S., Cicchetti, D., & Balla, D. (2005). *Vineland Adaptive Behavior Scales* (2nd ed.). Circle Pines, MN: AGS.

Toglia, J. (2015). *Weekly Calendar Planning Activity: A performance test of executive function.* Bethesda, MD: AOTA Press.

Tuffrey, C., Bateman, B. J., & Colver, A. C. (2013). The Questionnaire of Young People's Participation (QYPP): A new measure of participation frequency for disabled young people. *Child Care Health Development, 39,* 500–511. https://doi.org/10.111/cch.12060

Valletutti, P. J., Bender, M., Smith Hoffnung, A., & Balin, U. C. A. (2008). *A Functional Assessment and Curriculum for Teaching Students With Disabilities—Volumes I–IV: Complete set.* Austin, TX: Pro-Ed.

Wisconsin Assistive Technology Initiative Development Team. (2017). *Wisconsin Assistive Technology Initiative: Assessing students' needs for assistive technology.* Retrieved from http://www.wati.org/free-publications/assistive-technology-consideration-to-assessment/

Appendix G. How to Incorporate *Best Practices for Occupational Therapy in Schools, 2nd Edition,* Into a 16-Week Occupational Therapy Curriculum

Directions: Instructors are encouraged to select or adapt this template for their class.

WEEK	TOPICS OR LABS INCLUDED, AS APPROPRIATE	SUGGESTED MATERIALS FROM *BEST PRACTICES*
Systems Based		
1	Influences on practice (e.g., history, laws, licensure, payment sources)	Chapters 1 (history), 3 (laws), 16 (Medicaid), and 27 (Section 504)
2	Applying the *OTPF–3* in schools	Chapters 2 *(OTPF–3)* and 4 (ethical reasoning); Appendix B (occupational profile)
3	Working on educational teams	Chapters 11 (family engagement), 12 (teams), and 13 (conflict)
4	Continuum of services (e.g.,workload, OTA partnership, MTSS)	Chapters 7 (OTAs), 14 (workload), and 26 (MTSS); AOTA (2014b; workload)
5	Additional roles of OTs and OTAs in schools	Chapters 8 (administrators), 9 (leadership), 10 (access), 21 (AT), and 22 (transportation); Appendix J ("Guidelines for OT Services in Early Intervention and Schools"; AOTA, 2017)
Individual Based		
6	Evaluation process: Determining strengths and needs	Chapter 40 (evaluation); Appendix F (assessments)
7	Documentation and setting student goals; evidence-based interventions	Chapter 45 (data collection); Appendixes C (intervention plan), D (brief audit of documentation), E (full or partial audit of documentation), and H (evidence)
8	Data-based decision making (e.g., progress monitoring)	Chapters 15 (program evaluation) and 45 (data collection)
9	Services with student and on behalf of the student (accommodations, modifications, support to school personnel)	Chapters 41 (interventions), 42 (group interventions), and 43 (telehealth)
Interventions		
10	Evidence-based interventions for all occupations in schools (e.g., self-care, play and leisure)	Chapters 46 (ADLs), 47 (mealtimes), 51 (play and leisure), and 53 (social participation)
11	Evidence-based interventions for all occupations in schools (e.g., literacy)	Chapters 17 (literacy and STEM), 49 (handwriting), and 50 (reading)
12	Performance-based interventions (as applied to school environment)	Chapters 54 (EF), 55 (fine motor skills), 56 (motor skills), 57 (sensory), and 58 (visual–motor)
13	School mental health and positive behavioral supports	Chapters 19 (school mental health), 30 (childhood trauma), and 31 (emotional disturbance)
14	Transition planning and adolescent topics	Chapters 23 (preschool transition), 24 (transition to work), 25 (transition to college), 48 (IADLs), and 52 (driving)
Education Disability Categories		
15	Student group presentation on disabilities	Chapters 28–39 (topics including ADHD through visual impairments)
Schoolwide		
16	Professional development in schools (plus any of the topics listed earlier)	Chapters 18 (health and wellness) and 20 (UDL); Appendixes A (future) and I (liability)

Note. ADHD = attention deficit hyperactivity disorder; AT = assistive technology; EF = executive functioning; MTSS = multi-tiered systems of support; OT = occupational therapist; OTA = occupational therapy assistant; *OTPF–3 = Occupational Therapy Practice Framework* (3rd ed.; AOTA, 2014a); STEM = science, technology, engineering, and mathematics; UDL = universal design for learning.

Copyright © 2019 by the American Occupational Therapy Association. All rights reserved. To reuse this content, contact www.copyright.com.
https://doi.org/10.7139/2019.978-1-56900-591-0.AppG

REFERENCES

American Occupational Therapy Association. (2014a). Occupational therapy practice framework: Domain and process (3rd ed.). *American Journal of Occupational Therapy, 68*(Suppl. 1), S1–S48. https://doi.org/10.5014/ajot.2014.682006

American Occupational Therapy Association. (2014b). *Transforming caseload to workload in school-based occupational therapy services.* Retrieved from https://www.aota.org/~/media/corporate/files/secure/practice/children/workload-fact.pdf

American Occupational Therapy Association. (2017). Guidelines for occupational therapy services in early intervention and schools. *American Journal of Occupational Therapy, 71*(Suppl. 2), 7112410010. https://doi.org/10.5014/ajot.2017.716S01

Appendix H. Evidence-Based Practice and Occupational Therapy in Schools

Elizabeth G. Hunter, PhD, OTR/L, and Deborah Lieberman, MHSA, OTR/L, FAOTA

Evidence-based practice (EBP) is an important component of occupational therapy practice. It is crucial for occupational therapy practitioners[1] to stay current on research in the field, particularly in their practice area. EBP is tripartite in that it relies on (1) research evidence, (2) practitioner expertise, and (3) client needs and preferences (see Figure H.1). All 3 components need to be included to provide best practice with a goal of efficiency and effectiveness. In schools, instruction is individualized and changes regularly; therefore, a strong foundation in which interventions are effective and supported by research is critical.

TYPES OF EVIDENCE

The best research evidence is usually found in peer-reviewed published research studies that have been conducted using sound methodology (Sackett et al., 2000). To provide EBP, practitioners need to recognize different types of evidence and understand that they provide stronger or weaker evidence. A magazine article (e.g., *OT Practice, SIS Quarterly Practice Connections*) reporting on a certain intervention is not the strongest evidence if it is based solely on opinion. Findings from a group or program trying to sell a product may not be unbiased because they may really be marketing a product rather than conducting rigorous research. Findings from research funded by a group that will benefit from the outcomes may not be considered strong evidence and may have a high risk of bias.

The goal is to find unbiased, well-designed, well-conducted research that is published in a peer-reviewed journal. Peer-reviewed journals, such as the *American Journal of Occupational Therapy (AJOT),* rely on outside, unbiased peer reviewers who do not stand to benefit from the findings of the research. This is the gold standard in research in terms of reporting research findings. Only studies that pass peer review will be published in a peer-reviewed journal. These are the data needed when conducting EBP.

There are many types and methods of research. All well-designed, peer-reviewed research publications are useful and informative for one reason or another. For decision making, it is important to feel certain that the study's outcomes are the result of the intervention being tested. The gold standard in assessing an intervention's efficacy is the randomized controlled trial (RCT), a study design in which participants are randomized into 2 or more groups. The groups receive different interventions, often standard of care (e.g., methods accepted by qualified practitioners) in 1 group and the intervention being tested in the other.

When the study has the appropriate number of participants, randomizing minimizes the risk of selection bias. In a perfect world, the participants and the people doing the assessments would not know which participants were in which group (double-blind study). Such a study is not always feasible in all settings or with all interventions; regardless, the RCT is considered the highest level of scientific evidence. Having said that, practitioners should not hesitate to consider lower level evidence to answer their specific focus questions, recognizing that lower level evidence is at risk for various biases and limitations, including the research design, and the findings need to be looked at with that in mind.

Qualitative research is often not included in analyses of scientific evidence and systematic reviews of interventions, but the findings from qualitative studies can provide important foundational understanding of factors such as client experiences and understanding events, among other issues. This knowledge can improve how a practitioner provides services and care. When looking for evidence to support an intervention, however, the experimental design is the first line of information.

ANALYZING EVIDENCE

Once a practitioner locates evidence, they have some work to do in terms of analyzing, appraising, and understanding the findings of a study. Three major factors—level of evidence, risk of bias, and findings and outcomes—need to be assessed and are described next.

---

[1]*Occupational therapy practitioner* refers to both the occupational therapist and the occupational therapy assistant. The American Occupational Therapy Association (AOTA; 2014, p. S18) states, "The occupational therapist is responsible for all aspects of occupational therapy service delivery and is accountable for the safety and effectiveness of the occupational therapy service delivery process" and "must be directly involved in the delivery of services during the initial evaluation and regularly throughout the course of intervention. . . . The occupational therapy assistant delivers safe and effective occupational therapy services under the supervision of and in partnership with the occupational therapist."

Copyright © 2019 by the American Occupational Therapy Association. All rights reserved. To reuse this content, contact www.copyright.com.
https://doi.org/10.7139/2019.978-1-56900-591-0.AppH

FIGURE H.1.	*Evidence-based practice* is the use of the best available research evidence combined with the practitioner's expertise and the client's needs and preferences.

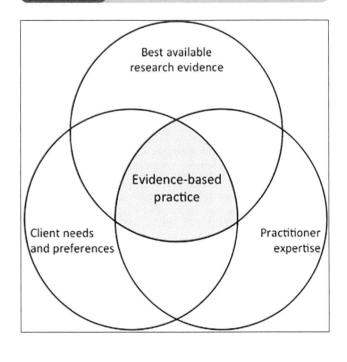

Level of Evidence

As we have discussed, different research designs have different levels of evidence. Level I studies, such as RCTs, are the gold standard. As one considers the lower levels of evidence in the hierarchy, the innate risk of bias increases. Therefore, identifying the study design is the first step in analyzing the evidence and beginning the process of assessing the trustworthiness of the findings and the application to practice. The levels of evidence are as follows:

- **Level 1A:** Systematic review of homogeneous RCTs (e.g., similar population, intervention), with or without meta-analysis
- **Level 1B:** Well-designed individual RCT (not a pilot or feasibility study with a small sample size)
- **Level 2A:** Systematic review of cohort studies
- **Level 2B:** Individual prospective cohort study, low-quality RCT (e.g., less than 80% follow-up or low number of participants, pilot and feasibility studies), ecological studies, and 2-group nonrandomized studies
- **Level 3A:** Systematic review of case-control studies
- **Level 3B:** Individual retrospective case-control study, 1-group nonrandomized pretest–posttest study, cohort studies
- **Level 4:** Case series (and low-quality cohort and case-control study)
- **Level 5:** Expert opinion without explicit critical appraisal (Howick et al., 2016).

Risk of Bias

Bias in research is a systematic error or deviation from true results, often resulting from limitations in study methods and procedures. Bias can cause something to be overestimated or underestimated. Either way, bias makes it very hard to trust research results. Better designed and conducted studies are more likely to end up with results that are unlikely to be false or misleading.

Bias can come from selection (characteristics of the participant group), performance (whether study participants and personnel know who is receiving which intervention), and detection (whether the assessor knows which participant is assigned to which group), as well as from how results are reported, whether all participants remained in the study from beginning to end, and others. It is important for practitioners to read research articles critically, assess the study design, and look for a very detailed description of the study procedures and outcomes.

Findings and Outcomes

When evaluating the evidence, assess the study for the significance of the findings. It is necessary to understand whether the findings were in fact statistically significant (e.g., were the outcomes significantly different between groups?). If the findings were not significantly different, occupational therapy practitioners should question implementing the intervention. Descriptions such as "the intervention resulted in a small improvement" and other vague statements such as "the intervention improved" are not very useful in evaluating the difference between the efficacy of interventions and determining whether to use the intervention in practice.

SYNTHESIZING EVIDENCE

The final step for a practitioner in terms of deciding which research to incorporate into practice is synthesizing all of the evidence. *Synthesizing the evidence* means looking at the level of evidence (study design), the risk of bias (study limitations), and the study results and merging the information. A practitioner may review 1 study or, even better, more than 1 study testing the intervention of interest. For example, 2 or more RCTs increases the strength and level of certainty of a given intervention. Having multiple studies to evaluate assists the occupational therapy practitioner in deciding whether the level of evidence is strong enough to implement the intervention in practice. Table H.1 provides information to evaluate the strength of the evidence for the intervention being reviewed.

Thankfully, practitioners can consider numerous systematic reviews related to different interventions, practice conditions, or populations. The benefit of finding a good-quality systematic review is that the authors have already reviewed, appraised, and synthesized specific studies and provided guidance on critical practice questions. Practitioners can evaluate single studies or multiple studies, or they can use existing systematic reviews to evaluate to what degree they can trust the findings and how sure they are that an intervention has the best available evidence to incorporate it into school practice.

TABLE H.1.   Strength of Evidence (Level of Certainty)

STRENGTH OF EVIDENCE	DESCRIPTION
Strong	▪ Two or more Level I studies ▪ The available evidence usually includes consistent results from well-designed, well-conducted studies. The findings are strong, and they are unlikely to be called into question by the results of future studies. ▪ All studies have moderate to low risk of bias.

Moderate	▪ At least 1 Level I high-quality study or multiple moderate-quality studies (e.g., Level II, Level III)
	▪ The available evidence is sufficient to determine the effects on health outcomes, but confidence in the estimate is constrained by such factors as
	  • The number, size, or quality of individual studies.
	  • Inconsistency of findings across individual studies.
	▪ The studies have moderate to low risk of bias.
	As more information (other research findings) becomes available, the magnitude or direction of the observed effect could change, and this change may be large enough to alter the conclusion related to the usefulness of the intervention.

Low	▪ Small number of low-level studies, flaws in the studies, etc.
	▪ The available evidence is insufficient to assess effects on health and other outcomes of relevance to occupational therapy. Evidence is insufficient because of
	  • The limited number or size of studies
	  • Important flaws in study design or methods
	  • Inconsistency of findings across individual studies
	  • Lack of information on important health outcomes.
	Many of these studies will have high risk of bias.
	
	More information may allow estimation of effects on health and other outcomes of relevance to occupational therapy.

Source. U.S. Preventive Services Task Force (2016).

EDUCATION PRACTICE: EVIDENCE-BASED INTERVENTIONS

Occupational therapy practitioners working in schools must also be knowledgeable about how *evidence-based interventions* are defined in education law. The Every Student Succeeds Act (ESSA; 2015; Pub. L. 114–95) defines the term *evidence based,* when used with respect to a state, local educational agency, or school activity, as an activity, strategy, or intervention that

  (i) demonstrates a statistically significant effect on improving student outcomes or other *relevant outcomes* based on—
    (I) strong evidence from at least one well-designed and well-implemented experimental study;
    (II) moderate evidence from at least one well-designed and well-implemented *quasi-experimental* study; or
    (III) promising evidence from at least one well-designed and well-implemented correlational study with statistical controls for selection bias; or
  (ii) (I) *demonstrates a rationale* based on high-quality research findings or positive evaluation that such activity, strategy, or intervention is likely to improve student outcomes or other *relevant outcomes*; and
  (ii) (II) includes ongoing efforts to examine the effects of such activity, strategy, or intervention. (§ 8101[21])

Table H.2 outlines the U.S. Department of Education's (2016) recommendations for identifying evidence across 4 different levels.

The Individuals With Disabilities Education Improvement Act of 2004 (Pub. L. 108–446) uses the term *scientifically based research* but does not define it. According to the No Child Left Behind Act of 2001 (Pub. L. 107–110), which was later replaced by ESSA, *scientifically based research*

(A) Means research that involves the application of rigorous, systematic, and objective procedures to obtain reliable and valid knowledge relevant to education activities and programs; and
(B) (i) Employs systematic, empirical methods that draw on observation or experiment;
(ii) Involves rigorous data analyses that are adequate to test the stated hypotheses and justify the general conclusions drawn;
(iii) Relies on measurements or observational methods that provide reliable and valid data across evaluators and observers, across multiple measurements and observations, and across studies by the same or different investigators;
(iv) Is evaluated using experimental or quasi-experimental designs in which individuals, entities, programs, or activities are assigned to different conditions and with appropriate controls to evaluate the effects of the condition of interest, with a preference for random-assignment

TABLE H.2.   U.S. Department of Education (2016) Criteria Recommended in ESSA for the Identification of Evidence

LEVEL	DESCRIPTION
Strong	▪ One well-designed and well-implemented experimental study (e.g., RCT) ▪ Statistically significant and positive effect of the intervention on student outcome or other relevant outcome ▪ Not overridden by statistically significant and negative evidence for the same intervention in other studies ▪ Has a large, multisite sample ▪ Has a sample that overlaps with the populations (i.e., the types of students served) and settings (e.g., rural, urban) proposed to receive the intervention
Moderate	▪ Must have at least 1 well-designed and well-implemented quasi-experimental study of the intervention ▪ Shows a statistically significant and positive effect of the intervention on student outcome or other relevant outcome ▪ Not overridden by statistically significant and negative evidence for the same intervention in other studies ▪ Has a large, multisite sample ▪ Has a sample that overlaps with the populations (i.e., the types of students served) and settings (e.g., rural, urban) proposed to receive the intervention
Promising evidence	▪ At least 1 well-designed and well-implemented correlational study with statistical controls for selection bias on the intervention ▪ Shows a statistically significant and positive (i.e., favorable) effect of the intervention on student outcome or other relevant outcome ▪ Not overridden by statistically significant and negative (i.e., unfavorable) evidence for that intervention from findings
Demonstrates a rationale	▪ Includes a well-specified logic model that is informed by research or an evaluation that suggests how the intervention is likely to improve relevant outcomes ▪ An effort to study the effects of the intervention, ideally producing promising evidence or higher, that will happen as part of the intervention or is underway elsewhere (e.g., another SEA, LEA, or research organization) to inform stakeholders about the success of that intervention

Note. ESSA = Every Student Succeeds Act (2015); LEA = local educational agency; RCT = randomized controlled trial; SEA = state educational agency.

experiments, or other designs to the extent that those designs contain within-condition or across-condition controls;

(v) Ensures that experimental studies are presented in sufficient detail and clarity to allow for replication or, at a minimum, offer the opportunity to build systematically on their findings; and

(vi) Has been accepted by a peer-reviewed journal or approved by a panel of independent experts through a comparably rigorous, objective, and scientific review. (No Child Left Behind Act of 2001, 20 U.S.C. § 1411[e][2][C][xi])

Taking this a step further, the Council for Exceptional Children (CEC; 2014) has developed explicit standards for categorizing the evidence base of practices in special education. These indicators and criteria apply to studies that examine practice or programs on student outcomes. Eight quality indicators are used to assess the evidence for various intervention and program practices:

1. **Context and setting.** The study provides sufficient information regarding the critical features of the context or setting.
2. **Participants.** The study provides sufficient information to identify the population of participants to which results may be generalized and to determine or confirm whether the participants demonstrated the disability or difficulty of focus.
3. **Intervention agent.** The study provides sufficient information regarding the critical features of the intervention agent.
4. **Description of practice.** The study provides sufficient information regarding the critical features of the practice (intervention), such that the practice is clearly understood and can be reasonably replicated.
5. **Implementation fidelity.** The practice is implemented with fidelity.
6. **Internal validity.** The independent variable is under the control of experimenter. The study describes the services provided in control and comparison conditions and phases. The research design provides sufficient evidence that the independent variable causes change in the dependent variable or variables. Participants stayed with the study, so attrition is not a significant threat to internal validity.
7. **Outcome measures/dependent variables.** Outcome measures are applied appropriately to gauge the effect of the practice on study outcomes. Outcome measures demonstrate adequate psychometrics.
8. **Data analysis.** Data analysis is conducted appropriately. The study reports information on effect size. (CEC, 2014, pp. 3–6)

Several research groups have published EBP documents that identify specific practices that have met the evidence threshold (e.g., National Professional Development Center on Autism Spectrum Disorder, What Works Clearinghouse).

Many of the models place stronger emphasis on research that has replicated studies of manualized or operationalized interventions (Cook & Cothren Cook, 2011). Occupational therapy practitioners working in schools must be familiar with evidence within the occupational therapy profession and the education–special education profession.

USE IN PRACTICE

Differences in the interpretation of EBP among occupational therapy practitioners and other members of the service delivery team may cause misunderstandings, because each team member is expected to adhere to the EBP standards set forth by their practice setting (Scheibel & Watling, 2016). Occupational therapy practitioners cannot continue to use interventions that they learned 15 years ago or that were presented at a conference but have no evidence base. They must implement current EBP into their daily practice, gather data, and use the data to make decisions about the effectiveness of the decisions (AOTA, 2017; Hanft & Shephard, 2016). Some practitioners are unsure how to incorporate research into their practice. Torres et al. (2012) authored a guide for special educators on implementing EBP that can be used by school occupational therapy practitioners. Their step-by-step process is as follows:

1. Determine the student's, environment's, and instructor's characteristics.
2. Search sources of EBPs.
3. Select applicable EBP.
4. Identify essential components of the EBP.
5. Implement the EBP in the cycle of effective instruction.
6. Monitor implementation fidelity.
7. Progress monitor student outcomes.
8. Adapt the EBP, if necessary.
9. Make data-driven decisions and return to previous steps as needed.

OCCUPATIONAL THERAPY RESOURCES

AOTA has developed a repository of EBP resources for practitioners, educators, researchers, and students. AOTA collaborates with teams of researchers to conduct systematic reviews and develop Practice Guidelines. The systematic reviews are published in *AJOT* and as Practice Guidelines. Also, critically appraised summaries are published on AOTA's website. The "Evidence-Based Practice" section of AOTA's website (https://bit.ly/2AQcbbQ) provides many different resources and tools to remain current and provide services that are informed and guided by evidence.

A journal club may be an efficient and effective way for a group of occupational therapy practitioners to explore and evaluate evidence. The Journal Club Tool Kit provides step-by-step instructions and templates that can help practitioners set up and run different types of journal clubs. For additional sources for EBP, see Table 41.3 in Chapter 41, "Best Practices in School Occupational Therapy Interventions to Support Participation."

SUMMARY

All occupational therapy practitioners have a professional responsibility to use evidence-based interventions. Gaining experience in EBP is a process and skill that are developed with time, perseverance, and experience. Many resources are available that can enhance practitioners' familiarity and experience with accessing and evaluating research to support the provision of EBP in the school setting.

REFERENCES

American Occupational Therapy Association. (2014). Guidelines for supervision, roles, and responsibilities during the delivery of occupational therapy services. *American Journal of Occupational Therapy, 68*(Suppl. 3), S16–S22. https://doi.org/10.5014/ajot.2014.686S03

American Occupational Therapy Association. (2017). Guidelines for occupational therapy services in early childhood and schools. *American Journal of Occupational Therapy, 71*(Suppl. 2), 7112410010. https://doi.org/10.5014/ajot.2017.716S01

Cook, B., & Cothren Cook, S. (2011). Unraveling evidence-based practices in special education. *Journal of Special Education, 47,* 71–82. https://doi.org/10.1177/002246691142087.

Council for Exceptional Children. (2014). *Standards for evidence-based practice in special education.* Retrieved from https://www.cec.sped.org/~/media/Files/Standards/Evidence%20based%20Practices%20and%20Practice/EBP%20FINAL.pdf

Every Student Succeeds Act, Pub. L. No. 114–95, 129 Stat. 1802 (2015).

Hanft, B., & Shepherd, J. (2016). *Collaborating for student success* (2nd ed.). Bethesda, MD: AOTA Press.

Howick, J., Chalmers, I., Glasziou, P., Greenhalgh, T., Heneghan, C., Liberati, A., . . . Hodgkinson, M.; OCEBM Levels of Evidence Working Group. (2016). *The Oxford levels of evidence 2.* Oxford, England: Oxford Centre for Evidence-Based Medicine. Retrieved from https://www.cebm.net/index.aspx?o=5653

Individuals With Disabilities Education Improvement Act of 2004, Pub. L. 108–446, 20 U.S.C. §§ 1400–1482.

No Child Left Behind Act of 2001, Pub. L. 107–110, 20 U.S.C. §§ 6301–8962. (2002).

Sackett, D. L., Straus, S. E., Richardson, W. S., Rosenberg, W., & Haynes, R. B. (2000). *Evidence-based medicine: How to practice and teach EBM* (2nd ed.). New York: Churchill Livingstone.

Scheibel, G., & Watling, R. (2016). Collaborating with behavior analysts on the autism service delivery team. *OT Practice, 21*(7), 15–19.

Torres, C., Farley, C. A., & Cook, B. G. (2012). A special educator's guide to successfully implementing evidence-based practices. *TEACHING Exceptional Children, 47,* 85–93. https://doi.org/10.1177/0040059914553209

U.S. Department of Education. (2016). *Non-regulatory guidance: Using evidence to strengthen education investments.* Retrieved from https://ed.gov/policy/elsec/leg/essa/guidanceuseseinvestment.pdf

U.S. Preventive Services Task Force. (2016). *Grade definitions.* Retrieved from https://www.uspreventiveservicestaskforce.org/Page/Name/grade-definitions

Appendix I. Importance of Professional Liability Insurance

Christopher M. Bluhm, CAE, CMA, CPA

During your career as an occupational therapy practitioner,[1] you may be subjected to the unfortunate experience of being accused of errors or wrongdoing. Students, their families, and even your employer could make accusations of improper conduct or treatment, unethical practices, or an intervention provided in unsafe conditions or manner. Complaints can be made immediately or they can be filed weeks or years later. Complaints can be filed with state licensing boards, employers, and the National Board for Certification in Occupational Therapy® or as civil court actions.

Defending yourself against even meritless charges can be expensive, exposing you to personal financial risk. Professional liability insurance should be part of your personal legal and financial planning, and the decision to purchase your own professional liability insurance is critical. The most common reason given for not carrying private liability insurance is "My company has insurance that covers my work." Unfortunately, there are instances in which employer coverage may not protect you. Consider the following:

- Will your company step forward when a claim is brought against you but not the company? According to published reports, about 40% of occupational therapy insurance claims are levied against employees and their personal insurance policy.
- If your company holds a "claims-made" policy rather than an "occurrence" policy (discussed later), your protection could expire when you leave their employ, but you could still be held liable for claims on services that occurred while you worked at that facility, which could come months or years after you have left.
- Claims could be made against you by your employer. These claims could include deviation from company policy in intervention or alleged improper conduct. One example is an occupational therapist who was sued by

a former employer; although the therapist's defense was successful, the case lasted years and produced legal expenses exceeding $120,000.
- You could be compelled to testify in a case involving a current or former employer and client (e.g., student) without any personal legal advisory support. In one instance, even though a practitioner was never charged with any wrongdoing, the practitioner was brought in to testify on a case in which the employer was the defendant; the practitioner's personal legal expenses totaled $1,800.
- Your work status as an employee or independent contractor or even providing services for free all create potential liability. Persons do not need to be paid to be held liable.

MANAGING YOUR RISK

Occupational therapy practitioners should take several vital steps to limit the possibility of claims and reduce their liability if a claim is filed:[2]

- Understand the scope of practice regulations in any state in which you provide services (see AOTA, 2014b). If employed by a school system or a contracting agency, then be sure all policies and procedures are within the scope of occupational therapy practice. You should feel comfortable asking about any discrepancies.
- Complete detailed, accurate, and timely documentation of student services, observations, and all communications with peers and family (AOTA, 2018). Incorrect or late documentation has been an important factor in past claims both for and against practitioners.
- Maintain a professional portfolio that includes artifacts and documents that support your professional development and continued competence in your area of practice. Make sure to keep your state license current. Having a portfolio before it is requested can more easily help in challenging claims made.
- Be familiar with and understand privacy requirements under the Family Educational Rights and Privacy Act of 1974 (Pub. L. 93–380), Health Insurance Portability and Accountability Act of 1996 (Pub. L. 104–191), Individuals With Disabilities Education Improvement Act of 2004 (Pub. L. 108–446), and Section 504 of the

---

[1]*Occupational therapy practitioner* refers to both the occupational therapist and the occupational therapy assistant. The American Occupational Therapy Association (AOTA; 2014a, p. S18) states, "The occupational therapist is responsible for all aspects of occupational therapy service delivery and is accountable for the safety and effectiveness of the occupational therapy service delivery process" and "must be directly involved in the delivery of services during the initial evaluation and regularly throughout the course of intervention. . . . The occupational therapy assistant delivers safe and effective occupational therapy services under the supervision of and in partnership with the occupational therapist."

[2]Much of the information in the document can be found in CNA and Healthcare Providers Service Organization (2017).

Copyright © 2019 by the American Occupational Therapy Association. All rights reserved. To reuse this content, contact www.copyright.com. https://doi.org/10.7139/2019.978-1-56900-591-0.AppI

Rehabilitation Act of 1973, as amended (2008; Pub. L. 93–112), as amended. Occupational therapy practitioners working in schools have a special obligation that all communication regarding a student, including that with teachers, peers, and families, be professional, courteous, and precise. Be careful that discussions of student progress and personally identifiable information cannot be overheard and that texts and emails protect students' privacy. Do not store personally identifiable information on your personal devices (e.g., iPad, storage drives). Avoid storing personally identifiable information on your computer. When providing itinerant services, any personally identifiable information (e.g., folders, reports) must be transported in a locked case. Avoid taking pictures of students with your cell phone, which could create a privacy risk (R. Argabrite-Grove, MS, OTR/L, FAOTA, AOTA Governance, Leadership Development and International Liaison, personal communication, January 7, 2019).

- Maintain appropriate diligence and supervision when working with students, and maintain a safe workspace. Claims have occurred from falls when occupational therapy practitioners were only momentarily distracted.

BASICS FOR SELECTING THE RIGHT INSURANCE POLICY

- When purchasing a policy, be sure to ask whether it is an occurrence-based or claims-made policy. *Occurrence policies* protect any covered incident during the policy period, even after the policy has expired or been canceled. *Claims-made policies* cover only claims made while the policy is in effect. An occurrence policy is most desirable but may not be available in all states.
- Most basic policies currently have a $1 million per occurrence and $3 million total liability coverage limits. Policies can also commonly be purchased with higher (e.g., $2 million, $4 million) limits, when appropriate. These standard employee policies should cost around $100 per year. Private-practice professionals and clinic owners will pay higher rates.
- A basic insurance policy may not cover everything. Some interventions, such as hippotherapy, may be deemed experimental and thus outside the scope of practice. If that is the case, these interventions may not be covered without a separate policy endorsement.
- With the expansion of online purchasing, several newer, smaller, online-only insurance companies are offering policies to occupational therapy practitioners. If you are considering an online-only company, be sure to ask

about their *A. M. Best rating,* a financial rating that compares companies' ability to pay out claims.

SUMMARY

Professional liability insurance plans are designed to protect personal assets by covering defense costs and civil claims, including compensatory damages, up to the policy limits. An employer's liability plan does not cover everything and may not cover you at all in some instances. Practitioners should carry their own liability coverage.

RESOURCE

- **CNA and Healthcare Providers Service Organization:** *Occupational Therapy Claim Report: A Guide to Identifying and Addressing Professional Liability Exposures* (http://www.hpso.com/Documents/pdfs/CNA_CLS _OT_032917_CF_PROD_ONLINE_040417_SEC.pdf). This guide has great information that extends the learning content of this appendix.

REFERENCES

American Occupational Therapy Association. (2014a). Guidelines for supervision, roles, and responsibilities during the delivery of occupational therapy services. *American Journal of Occupational Therapy, 68*(Suppl. 3), S16–S22. https://doi.org/10.5014 /ajot.2014.686S03

American Occupational Therapy Association. (2014b). Scope of practice. *American Journal of Occupational Therapy, 68*(Suppl. 3), S34–S40. https://doi.org/10.5014/ajot.2014.686S04

American Occupational Therapy Association. (2018). Guidelines for documentation of occupational therapy services. *American Journal of Occupational Therapy, 72*(Suppl. 2), 7212410010. https://doi.org/10.5014/ajot.2018.72S203

CNA & Healthcare Providers Service Organization. (2017). *Occupational therapy claim report: A guide to identifying and addressing professional liability exposures.* Retrieved from http://www.hpso .com/Documents/pdfs/CNA_CLS_OT_032917_CF_PROD _ONLINE_040417_SEC.pdf

Family Educational Rights and Privacy Act of 1974, Pub. L. 93–380, 20 U.S.C. § 1232g; 34 C.F.R. Part 99.

Health Insurance Portability and Accountability Act of 1996 (HIPAA), Pub. L. 104–191 42 U.S.C. § 300gg, 29 U.S.C. §§ 1181–1183, and 42 U.S.C. 1320d–1320d9.

Individuals With Disabilities Education Improvement Act of 2004, Pub. L. 108–446, 20 U.S.C. §§ 1400–1482.

Rehabilitation Act of 1973, Pub. L. 93–112, 29 U.S.C. §§ 701–796l.

Section 504 of the Rehabilitation Act of 1973, as amended, 29 U.S.C. § 794 (2008).

Appendix J. Guidelines for Occupational Therapy Services in Early Intervention and Schools

The primary purpose of this document is to provide guidelines for the provision of occupational therapy services in early intervention (EI) and school settings. This document is intended for an internal audience (e.g., occupational therapists, occupational therapy assistants, students in occupational therapy programs) as well as external audiences (e.g., school staff and administrators, regulatory and policymaking bodies, accreditation agencies) who seek clarification of occupational therapy's role related to these settings. Occupational therapy practitioners[1] often are supervised by people unfamiliar with occupational therapy practices; the principles (e.g., level of expected performance) included in these guidelines and other American Occupational Therapy Association (AOTA) documents can be used to enhance their knowledge about the profession.

Approximately 25% of occupational therapists and 18% of occupational therapy assistants work in EI and school settings (AOTA, 2015a). Occupational therapy practitioners work with children and youth, parents, caregivers, educators, team members, and district and agency staff to facilitate children's and youth's ability to participate in their *occupations,* which are daily life activities that are purposeful and meaningful to the person (AOTA, 2014b). Occupations are based on meaningful social or cultural expectations or peer performance. Examples include social interactions with peers on the playground, literacy activities (e.g., writing, reading, communicating, listening), eating school lunch, opening locker combination to access books and coat, ability to drive car to school. Occupational therapy practitioners apply their knowledge of biological, physical, social, and behavioral sciences to evaluate and intervene with people across the life span when physical, adaptive, cognitive, behavioral, social, and mental health concerns compromise occupational engagement.

Occupational therapy practitioners provide services to young children and families in EI and to students, families, and educational staff in preschool and school settings to support engagement and participation in daily living activities (e.g., activities of daily living, instrumental activities of daily living, education, work, play, leisure, rest and sleep, and social participation; AOTA, 2014b). These guidelines provide information about occupational therapy practice in schools, including the influences (e.g., legislative, professional, environmental, contextual) and roles that occupational therapy practitioners may assume. Each section outlines guidelines related to these factors for occupational therapy practitioners. The variability in policy and practices across states and school districts results indifferences in how occupational therapy service delivery is implemented in each state.

Influences on Early Intervention and School Practice

Legislation and Regulatory Influences

Occupational therapy practitioners working in EI and schools must adhere to federal, state, and local education policies unless they conflict with occupational therapy state regulations (e.g., licensure). If

---

[1]*Occupational therapy practitioners* refers to both occupational therapists and occupational therapy assistants. The *occupational therapist* is responsible for all aspects of occupational therapy service delivery and is accountable for the safety and effectiveness of the occupational therapy service delivery process. *Occupational therapy assistants* deliver occupational therapy services under the supervision of and in partnership with an occupational therapist (AOTA, 2014a).

Copyright © 2017 by the American Occupational Therapy Association. All rights reserved. To reuse this content, contact www.copyright.com.
Originally published in the *American Journal of Occupational Therapy, 71*(Suppl. 2), 7112410010. https://doi.org/10.5014/ajot.2017.716S01

inconsistencies occur, practitioners must work with employment agencies or district administrators to align policies to eliminate conflict. To ensure adherence to legislation and regulatory requirements in providing occupational therapy services, practitioners in EI and schools have a responsibility to

- Make recommendations for services in accordance with federal, state, and local policies and procedures related to EI and school practice, in both general and special education (see Table 1 for examples of relevant legislation);

- Apply information from state occupational therapy practice acts and rules (licensure) to service delivery in EI and schools; and

- Understand state regulations for Medicaid cost recovery and other payment sources and adhere to professional codes of ethics and billing requirements.

Table 1. Legislative Influences on Occupational Therapy Practice in EI and Schools

Law	Influence on Occupational Therapy Services
Individuals With Disabilities Education Improvement Act of 2004 (IDEA), Parts B and C	Part B mandates access to occupational therapy as a related service for eligible students with disabilities ages 3–21 years if services are needed for a student to benefit from special education. Part B is administered through state education agencies. Part C is voluntary at the state level and lists occupational therapy as a primary service for infants and toddlers ages 0–3 years who are experiencing developmental delays or have identified disabilities. Part C services may be administered through state education agencies, state health and human services agencies, or a combination.
Every Student Succeeds Act of 2015 (ESSA), a reauthorization of the Elementary and Secondary Education Act of 1965	ESSA ensures equal opportunity for all students in Grades K–12 and builds on previous legislation focusing on educational achievement. Bill includes occupational therapy as "specialized instructional support personnel" (SISP). SISPs should be included in state, local, and schoolwide planning activities as well as certain school-wide interventions and supports. ESSA is administered through state and local education agencies.
Section 504 of the Rehabilitation Act Amendments of 2004; Americans With Disabilities Act Amendments Act of 2008 (ADAA)	These civil rights statutes prohibit discrimination on the basis of disability for places that are open to the general public (ADAA) or programs receiving federal funds (504). Disability is defined more broadly than in IDEA. Children who are not eligible for special instruction under IDEA may be eligible under Section 504 or the ADAA for services including environmental adaptations and other reasonable accommodations.
Medicaid (Title XIX of the Social Security Act of 1965)	Medicaid is a federal–state matching program that provides medical and health services for low-income children and adults. Occupational therapy is an optional service under state Medicaid plans but is mandatory for children and youth under the federal Early Periodic Screening, Diagnosis, and Treatment (EPSDT) program. Although state Medicaid programs do not cover the costs of providing all services under IDEA in schools (e.g., services on behalf of the child), costs associated with providing medically necessary occupational therapy services provided directly to the child in EI and school settings can be reimbursed by Medicaid for students who are enrolled in the Medicaid program.
Family Educational Rights and Privacy Act of 1974 (FERPA) and Health Insurance Portability and Accountability Act of 1996 (HIPAA)	FERPA is a federal law that protects the privacy of education records, including health records, for children with disabilities in programs under IDEA Parts B and C. The law applies to all EI programs and schools that receive funds under an applicable program of the U.S. Department of Education. Service providers, school districts, and educational agencies billing Medicaid are also subject to HIPAA rules under protected health information provisions.
Improving Head Start for School Readiness Act of 2009	Head Start and Early Head Start are federal programs that provide comprehensive child development services to economically disadvantaged children ages 0–5 years, including children with disabilities, and their families. Early Head Start serves children up to age 3; Head Start serves children ages 3 and 4. Occupational therapy may be provided in these settings under the Head Start requirements or under IDEA.

(Continued)

Table 1. Legislative Influences on Occupational Therapy Practice in EI and Schools *(cont.)*

Law	Influence on Occupational Therapy Services
Assistive Technology Act of 2004 (Tech Act)	The Tech Act promotes access to assistive technology to enable people with disabilities to more fully participate in education, employment, and daily activities.
Healthy, Hunger-Free Kids Act of 2010	The National School Breakfast and Lunch Programs are required to provide food substitutions and modifications of school meals for students whose disabilities restrict their diets, as determined by their health care provider.
State education codes and rules	In compliance with IDEA Part B, state education codes and rules must include policies and procedures for administration of instruction and for special education. Local education agencies further define these policies for their specific school communities.
State Part C EI	If state chooses to use federal funds for EI services (Part C), it must provide statewide, comprehensive, coordinated, multidisciplinary, interagency EI systems with a designated lead agency. The lead agency determines policies and procedures for implementation and monitoring within the state.
State practice acts and rules (licensure)	Practice acts and rules provide stipulations for occupational therapy service delivery, including evaluation, intervention, documentation, and supervision of occupational therapy assistants. Ethical and behavioral expectations for professional conduct are often included.

Note. EI = early intervention.

Navigating the nuances of the vast regulatory landscape and keeping up with changes to each law can be a daunting challenge, especially for practitioners new to EI or school practice settings. Practitioners must make educating themselves and keeping up with regulatory changes a priority. AOTA provides leadership and resources that can assist practitioners with staying current on legislation that affects practice.

Individuals With Disabilities Education Improvement Act (IDEA; Pub. L. 108–446) Part C programs, which serve infants and toddlers and their families, may seek reimbursement for occupational therapy services from Medicaid or Medicaid managed care programs available in their state and from the family's private insurance. States vary in their agreements with third-party payers for reimbursement of EI services. Some states require the family to pay a portion of the cost of Part C services, typically determined according to a sliding scale based on family income, whereas others (known as "birth mandate states") cover all costs except those that can be billed to Medicaid. In all cases, compliance with documentation requirements is critical for facilitating optimum reimbursement for Part C programs.

States provide public schools the opportunity to receive Medicaid reimbursement for the costs of providing occupational therapy services to eligible school-age children under Part B of IDEA. Reimbursable services typically include occupational therapy evaluations and services provided directly to the child. As in IDEA Part C programs, documenting services so that Medicaid requirements are met is essential to ensure that public schools realize available Medicaid revenue under state laws.

Professional Influences

In addition to adhering to state regulatory requirements (licensure), occupational therapy practitioners are guided by several professional documents (e.g., AOTA, 2013, 2014a, 2014b, 2015b, 2015c). The *Occupational Therapy Practice Framework: Domain and Process* (3rd ed.; AOTA, 2014b) articulates occupational therapy's distinct role and contributions to participation through engagement in occupation. Occupational therapy practitioners use the *Framework* to guide them in their practice, including service delivery (e.g., approaches to intervention may include creating skills, restoring movement, maintaining safe access, modification of the environment, prevention of back injury through backpack awareness). Providing client-centered delivery of services using evidence-based practices (EBP) is inherent to occupational therapy practice. In addition to providing individual services to the child or youth, the occupational therapy practitioner may focus on family structure and resources; specific groups or populations (e.g., co-teaching in general education classroom), the school system or district (e.g., serving on curriculum or playground committees), and the community (e.g., school health and wellness initiatives). Early intervention programs through

Part B of the IDEA and the school programs through Part C of the IDEA provide a structure to these effective practice guidelines.

Guidelines for ensuring consistency with professional practice are as follows:

- The occupational therapist and occupational therapy assistant must demonstrate professional role performance and conduct aligned with AOTA official documents, state occupational therapy regulations, and best available evidence.

- The occupational therapist conducts evaluations aligned with current evidence and best practices across the home, preschool, school, and community environments (e.g., evaluate child in natural environment using observation and input from parents and others; identify priorities, concerns, and resources from the family [Part C] or from the day care, education, or transition team [Part B].

- During the evaluation, the occupational therapist must identify the child's performance in his or her occupations, the affordances and barriers to successful engagement, and expectations for the child's development and participation and synthesize information to develop a working hypothesis.

- In collaboration with the team, the occupational therapist identifies the young child's current performance and identifies priorities and concerns of the parent or caregiver to develop family or child outcomes (Part C) or identify the priorities and concerns of parents and school staff to develop goals for the school-age child (Part B).

- The occupational therapist must determine service recommendations on the basis of individual need, as indicated by the occupational therapy evaluation and data shared during the team process.

- The occupational therapist, with input from the occupational therapy assistant, develops an occupational therapy intervention plan (e.g., occupation-based goals, intervention approach, methods of service delivery) that provides a framework for the implementation of the individualized education program (IEP) and individualized family service plan (IFSP).

- The occupational therapist and occupational therapy assistant demonstrate service delivery aligned with current evidence and best practices across the home, preschool, school, and community environments (e.g., provide intervention in the natural environment to facilitate child development and skill building [Part C] and in the least restrictive environment (LRE) to enhance the child's benefit from education [Part B]; provide assistance to teachers to enhance the participation of children in school activities and routines, including provision of strategies for improving performance in these activities; use assistive technologies (AT), universal design for learning (UDL) principles, and environmental modifications).

- The occupational therapist and occupational therapy assistant apply knowledge of risk factors affecting growth, development, learning, and engagement in meaningful occupations during interventions to support health and participation.

- The occupational therapist and occupational therapy assistant monitor and document progress toward annual goals in accordance with organizational and professional (e.g., state licensure regulations, AOTA) requirements and measure outcomes.

- The occupational therapist determines the need for ongoing or discontinuation of services or for referral to other professional.

Environmental and Contextual Influences

Services under the Every Student Succeeds Act of 2015 (ESSA; Pub. L. 114–195) are provided to educational staff and children in general education, whereas IDEA requires services to be provided in the natural environment for infants and toddlers (Part C) or in the LRE for children and youth (Part B). When providing services, occupational therapy practitioners must understand the climate, culture, beliefs, and values of the family or school (Frolek Clark, 2013). Occupational therapy service delivery is influenced by the environment (e.g., social and physical) and context (e.g., cultural, personal, temporal, virtual), including where children and youth live (e.g., homes), learn (e.g., community, day care, classroom, music room), play (e.g., playgrounds, gymnasium), socialize (e.g., hallways, cafeteria), take care of needs (e.g., bathroom), and work (e.g., locations in the community). Exploring the dynamic connections among the student, occupations or activities, and the environment are critical during service delivery. Guidelines for addressing environment and context include the following elements:

- The occupational therapy practitioner must be knowledgeable about the systems that influence practice (e.g., state lead agency, education agencies, community organizations, medical providers) and establish access to community resources.

- The occupational therapy practitioner must understand the procedures and practices of the EI system, including those of the lead agency; the model of service delivery in the home; the definition of developmental delay; and the source of reimbursement (e.g., birth mandate state, third-party payer, payer of last resort; Part C).

- The occupational therapy practitioner must understand and apply principles of family-centered practice (e.g., empowering parents; building relationships; encouraging involvement in decision making; building on informal community support systems; being respectful of the family's culture, beliefs, and attitudes; Part C).

- The occupational therapy practitioner must understand the procedures and practices of the local education agency (e.g., multitier systems of support, UDL, bullying prevention), curriculum standards (e.g., developmental sequences, program of studies, standards of learning, adapted curricula, and high-stakes testing), and special education process (Part B).

- The occupational therapy practitioner must form effective partnerships with team members (e.g., parents, teachers) and the medical community to effectively identify children who may be at risk for a substantial developmental delay (Part C) or a child with a disability (Part B).

- The occupational therapy practitioner must provide interventions based on EBP for early intervention, school, and community settings (e.g., coaching families, social emotional development, safe transportation, driving).

- The occupational therapy practitioner must understand expectations at the district, classroom, and agency level (e.g., classroom routines, curriculum, literacy practices, AT, building rules; Part B).

- The occupational therapy practitioner must understand opportunities for students' postsecondary transition goals of function in education and employment, independent living, and social inclusion in communities.

Roles of Occupational Therapy Practitioners

Occupational therapy practitioners assume many roles during service delivery in EI and school settings. As described in the Professional Influence section, occupational therapy practitioners provide services to groups (e.g., students at risk for academic or behavior problems) and populations (e.g., general education classes in school; school district staff) as well as individuals.

With the passage of the ESSA, the role of specialized instructional support personnel (SISP), including occupational therapy practitioners, includes schoolwide interventions and supports. Additionally, IDEA's inclusion of early intervening services (EIS) allows SISPs to support general education children (kindergarten through grade 12) who are at risk in academic and behavioral areas and offer professional development and training to teaching staff. Contributions by occupational therapy practitioners to response to intervention (RTI) frameworks and multitiered systems of support (MTSS) demonstrate occupational therapy practitioners' role in working at the system level (e.g., school district, building, classroom levels). Table 2 provides examples of the roles for occupational therapy practitioners.

As service providers in EI and school settings under IDEA, occupational therapy practitioners fulfill role responsibilities including service provision to children and youth, families, teams, organizations, and communities. Table 3 lists the core responsibilities of all practitioners working in these practice settings;

Table 2. Examples of Occupational Therapy Practitioner Roles Under ESSA (General Education)

Role and Description	General
Consultation	• Stakeholders to be consulted regarding the development of State Accountability Plans, which are replacing the annual yearly progress (AYP). • Assist with information about assessment of schools and development of alternative academic achievement standards for students with the most severe cognitive disabilities.
Schoolwide systems of support	• Provide services to support at-risk students. • Improve student performance through schoolwide programs (e.g., positive behavioral interventions and supports, RTI, MTSS, antibullying strategies). • Implement schoolwide positive behavioral interventions and supports, including coordination with similar activities carried out under IDEA, in order to improve academic outcomes and school conditions for student learning.
Professional development and training	• Provide professional development, preparation, and training programs with teachers and other staff.

Note. ESSA = Every Student Succeeds Act of 2015; IDEA = Individuals With Disabilities Education Improvement Act; MTSS = multi-tiered systems of support; RTI = response to intervention.

Table 3. Examples of Occupational Therapy Practitioner Roles in Part C and Part B of IDEA

Role and Description	For Both Part C and Part B unless specified
Evaluator (primarily the occupational therapist role; under the supervision of the occupational therapist, an occupational therapy assistant may assist in data collection).	• Under IDEA Child Find, identify children who are suspected of having a disability. • Serve as an evaluator for the team to determine each child's eligibility under IDEA Part C or Part B (special education). • Serve as an evaluator under IDEA to determine each child's strengths and needs, including need for occupational therapy (Part C, as an EI service; Part B, as a related service). • Document referral source, reason for services, dates of services for data gathering and planning, and results of evaluation (report). • Serve as an evaluator for children's assistive technology needs • Conduct reevaluations to determine child's strengths and ongoing needs. **Part C: Early Intervention** • Identify the family's concerns, priorities, and resources during the evaluation of the child. • Gather relevant data to address the functional needs of the child related to adaptive development, adaptive behavior, and play and sensory, motor, and postural development. • Synthesize information and collaborate with family to identify possible outcomes and need for services. **Part B: Preschool and School** • Provide educational and behavioral evaluations, services, and supports to enhance general education instruction for students at risk (K–12). • Solicit input from child, family, school personnel, and others. • Gather relevant functional, developmental, and academic information (e.g., conduct interviews, review existing evaluation information; use assessment tools and strategies; observe child across relevant contexts) to obtain reliable information about what the child knows and can perform academically, developmentally, and functionally. • Synthesize information and collaborate with family and educational staff to identify goals and need for services.

(Continued)

Table 3. Examples of Occupational Therapy Practitioner Roles in Part C and Part B of IDEA *(cont.)*

Role and Description	For Both Part C and Part B unless specified
Service coordinator for children and family (Part C) (only occupational therapist role)	• Demonstrate leadership by serving as service coordinator. • Collaborate with families to enable them to receive the services and rights under Part C. • Accurately interpret and communicate evaluation findings collaboratively with family members. • Coordinate all evaluations, the development and review of the IFSP, all services on the IFSP, any funding sources, and development of a transition plan within the established timelines and procedures. • Engage in collaborative decision making and problem solving with IFSP team.
Case manager for students (Part B) (only occupational therapist role)	• Demonstrate leadership by serving as case manager. • Synthesize evaluation findings and, in collaboration with the IEP team, identify and prioritize meaningful educational goals. • Engage in collaborative decision making and problem solving with IEP team. • Collaborate to develop and implement comprehensive transition plans.
Service provider	• Design and implement interventions that are congruent with expectations in the setting and culture. • Embed therapy interventions into the context of child's environments and routines. • Gather data to determine the effectiveness of the intervention and guide changes to the intervention. • Document performance changes and service provision (e.g., daily logs, progress notes, intervention plans, reports) in commonly understood and meaningful terms. • Use modifications, adaptations, and assistive technology, as needed, to enhance developmental, functional, or academic skills. • Document services ethically and accurately for third-party payers. • Provide mental health promotion, prevention, and intervention services to children and youth. • Demonstrate knowledge of evidence-based research in this area. • Use knowledge of current research when planning intervention approaches and strategies. **Part C: Early Intervention** • Actively participate with the team in the development of the IFSP in accordance with the priorities and preferences of the family and child (the occupational therapy assistant provides input under the supervision of the occupational therapist). • Occupational therapist designs the intervention to meet the stated IFSP outcomes; the occupational therapist or the occupational therapy assistant implements intervention and strategies. • Assist in the transition of child to community or Part B programs. **Part B: Preschool and School** • Actively participate with the team in the development of the IEP to document the child's strengths and needs, prioritize goals, and determine services (occupational therapy assistant provides input under the supervision of the occupational therapist). • Occupational therapist designs the intervention to meet the child's IEP goals; the occupational therapist or the occupational therapy assistant implements intervention and strategies. • Support student's achievement of postsecondary transition goals of function, education and employment, independent living, and social inclusion in communities.
Collaborative team member	• Form partnerships and work collaboratively with others to contribute to the understanding of the nature and extent of the child's strengths and needs. • Demonstrate effective communication and interpersonal skills (e.g., active listening, collaboration, coaching). • Actively participate in team decisions (e.g., eligibility, transition, behavior needs) using clinical reasoning (the occupational therapy assistant provides input under the supervision of the occupational therapist). • Promote inclusion of the child within the home, school and community settings.

(Continued)

Table 3. Examples of Occupational Therapy Practitioner Roles in Part C and Part B of IDEA *(cont.)*

Role and Description	For Both Part C and Part B unless specified
Educator and trainer	• Build the capacity of relevant stakeholders and teams through instruction, technical assistance, and training. • Educate family, children, school staff, and administration (e.g., resources, inservice, presentations, serving on committee). • Conduct trainings addressing strategies to best support children in natural environments and to empower families. • Educate EI teams on family-centered principles that empower families and respect families' culture, beliefs, and attitudes. • Educate school personnel on schoolwide programs (e.g., UDL, mental health, self-regulation).
Resource (Consultant)	• Provide technical assistance to teams, family, and community as necessary. • Assist the EI team in identifying resources for families (e.g., transportation options, child development). • Promote the child's access to school environments, instruction, and social communities. • Promote national, state, and local priorities for the participation and education of all children and school improvement. • Serve on committees and teams to address school and community challenges (e.g., evidence-based curriculum, accessible community participation, social community engagement, mental health and fitness). • Assist administrators and policy makers with the development of systemwide educational supports and programs.
Advocate	• Advocate for schoolwide initiatives that promote learning, health, wellness, and engagement (e.g., multitiered systems of support, also known as RTI; playground safety; mental health; ergonomics; fitness). • Promote understanding of diversity. • Advocate for access to occupational therapy services, when appropriate, for children and families in EI; teachers and children in general education; and children in special education programs and educational staff. • Provide guidance on the developments in educational, social, and health care policy and research that affect EI and school therapy services.
Leader	• Supervise occupational therapy assistants (only an occupational therapist role). • Supervise professional students and school personnel who implement occupational therapy recommendations. • Participate in the mentorship process to build knowledge and skills in the practice area. • Address trends in occupational therapy service provision by gathering, synthesizing, and evaluating data (only an occupational therapist role). • Educate others on the role of occupational therapy in this setting. • Assume personal responsibility for professional development. • Promote development of job descriptions, recruitment, orientation, and professional development for occupational therapy practitioners. • Manage workload and needs related to the job description.
Researcher	• Conduct program evaluation to determine effectiveness. • Design or assist in research studies in this setting.

Note. EI = early intervention; IEP = individualized education program; IFSP = individualized family service plan; RTI = response to intervention; UDL = universal design for learning.

however, because of the difference in procedures and practices, the roles and responsibilities vary by state and school district. Because of the level of analysis and decision making required, only an occupational therapist may fill the evaluator, service coordinator, and case coordinator roles. Although agencies may create service coordinator or case coordinator positions and hire occupational therapy assistants in those capacities, such employees are not typically working as occupational therapy practitioners. The other roles may be filled by an occupational therapist or occupational therapy assistant in accordance with agency and state policy.

Summary

In EI and school settings, occupational therapy practitioners use their expertise to enhance participation in activities and occupations for children and youth. Occupational therapy practitioners also provide resources for and build the capacity of families, caregivers, and education staff. The guidelines presented in this document serve to empower occupational therapy practitioners working in EI and school settings with the resources to achieve positive outcomes and demonstrate the distinct value of their practice in these settings.

References

American Occupational Therapy Association. (2013). Guidelines for documentation of occupational therapy. *American Journal of Occupational Therapy, 67*(Suppl.), S32–S38. https://doi.org/10.5014/ajot.2013.67S32

American Occupational Therapy Association. (2014a). Guidelines for supervision, roles, and responsibilities during the delivery of occupational therapy services. *American Journal of Occupational Therapy, 68*(Suppl. 3), S16–S22. PubMed https://doi.org/10.5014/ajot.2014.686S03

American Occupational Therapy Association. (2014b). Occupational therapy practice framework: Domain and process (3rd ed.). *American Journal of Occupational Therapy, 68*(Suppl. 1), S1–S48. https://doi.org/10.5014/ajot.2014.682006

American Occupational Therapy Association. (2015a). *2015 salary and workforce survey: Executive summary.* Retrieved from http://www.aota.org/Education-Careers/Advance-Career/Salary-Workforce-Survey.aspx

American Occupational Therapy Association. (2015b). Occupational therapy code of ethics (2015). *American Journal of Occupational Therapy, 69*(Suppl. 3), 6913410030. https://doi.org/10.5014/ajot.2015.696S03

American Occupational Therapy Association. (2015c). Standards of practice for occupational therapy. *American Journal of Occupational Therapy, 69*(Suppl. 3), 6913410057. https://doi.org/10.5014/ajot.2015.696S06

Americans With Disabilities Act Amendments Act of 2008, Pub. L. 110–325, 122 Stat. 3553.

Assistive Technology Act of 2004, Pub. L. 108–364, 118 Stat. 1707.

Elementary and Secondary Education Act of 1965, Pub. L. 89–10, 20 U.S.C. § 6301 et seq.

Every Student Succeeds Act of 2015, Pub. L. 114–195, 114 Stat. 1177.

Family Educational Rights and Privacy Act of 1974, 20 U.S.C. § 1232g, 34 CFR Part 99.

Frolek Clark, G. (2013). Best practices in school occupational therapy interventions to support participation. In G. Frolek Clark & B. E. Chandler (Eds.), *Best practices for occupational therapists in schools* (pp. 95–106). Bethesda, MD: AOTA Press.

Health Insurance Portability and Accountability Act of 1996, Pub. L. 104–191, 110 Stat. 1936.

Healthy, Hunger-Free Kids Act of 2010, Pub. L. 111–296, 124 Stat. 3183.

Improving Head Start for School Readiness Act of 2007, Pub. L. 110–134, 121 Stat. 1363, 42 USC 9801 et seq.

Individuals With Disabilities Education Improvement Act of 2004, Pub. L. 108–446, 20 U.S.C. § 1400 et seq.

Rehabilitation Act Amendments of 2004, 29 U.S.C. §794.

Social Security Act of 1965, Pub. L. 89–97, 79 Stat. 286, Title XIX.

Resources

For information on rights and privacy rules related to IDEA, refer to the following sites:

- DaSy Center. http://dasycenter.org/category/privacyguidance/
- United States Department of Education. http://www2.ed.gov/policy/gen/guid/fpco/ferpa/index. html
- United States Department of Health and Human Services. http://www.hhs.gov/hipaa/for-professionals/ faq/513/does-hipaa-apply-to-an-elementary-school/index.html
- For EBP, refer to the following documents, which were designed to share current research:
- Bazyk, S. (2013). *Mental health promotion, prevention, and intervention with children and youth.* Bethesda, MD: AOTA Press.
- Bazyk, S., & Arbesman, M. (2013). *Occupational therapy practice guidelines for mental health promotion, prevention, and intervention for children and youth.* Bethesda, MD: AOTA Press.
- Chandler, B. (2010). *Early childhood: Occupational therapy services for children birth to three.* Bethesda, MD: AOTA Press.
- Frolek Clark, G. & Chandler, B. (2013). *Best practices for occupational therapy services in schools.* Bethesda, MD: AOTA Press.
- Frolek Clark, G., & Kingsley, K. (2013). *Occupational therapy practice guidelines for early childhood: Birth through 5 years.* Bethesda, MD: AOTA Press.
- Frolek Clark, G. & Handley-More, D. (2017). *Best practices for documenting occupational therapy services in schools.* Bethesda, MD: AOTA Press.
- Jackson, L. (2007). *Occupational therapy services for children and youth under IDEA.* Bethesda, MD: AOTA Press.
- Hanft, B., & Shepherd, J. (2016). *Collaborating for student success* (2nd ed.). Bethesda, MD: AOTA Press.
- Tomchek, S., & Koenig, K. P. (2016). *Occupational therapy practice guidelines for individuals with autism spectrum disorder.* Bethesda, MD: AOTA Press.

Authors
Gloria Frolek Clark, PhD, OTR/L, BCP, SCSS, FAOTA
Patricia Laverdure, OTD, OTR/L, BCP
Jean Polichino, OTR, MS, FAOTA

for

The Commission on Practice
Kathleen Kannenberg, MA, OTR/L, CCM, *Chairperson*

Adopted by the Representative Assembly Coordinating Council (RACC) for the Representative Assembly, 2017

Revised by the Commission on Practice 2017

Note. This revision replaces the 2011 document *Occupational Therapy Services in Early Childhood and School-Based Settings,* previously published and copyrighted in 2011 by the American Occupational Therapy Association in the *American Journal of Occupational Therapy, 65,* S46–S54. https://doi.org/10.5014/ajot.2011.65S46

Copyright © 2017 by the American Occupational Therapy Association.

Citation. American Occupational Therapy Association. (in press). Guidelines for occupational therapy services in early intervention and schools. *American Journal of Occupational Therapy, 71*(Suppl. 2), 7112410010. https://doi. org/10.5014/ajot.2017.716S01

INDEXES

Subject Index

Note: Page numbers in italics indicate figures, tables, and exhibits.

A

academic calendar, and fieldwork, 44
academic degree programs, 202
academic fieldwork coordinator (AFWC), 43, 47–48
  collaboration with institution, 47
  designation of program contact, 47
  familiarity with curriculum, 47
  legal responsibilities, 47–48
  preparation monitoring, 47
academic performance
  ADHD and, 229
  autism spectrum disorder and, 236
  childhood trauma and, 244, 245
  emotional disturbance and, 259–260
  literacy and, 136–137
  low-incidence disability and, 284
  traumatic brain injury and, 315–316
  see also mathematics; reading
academic persistence, 201
access, 77–84
  assistive technology for, 173
  barriers to, identifying, 81–82
  best practices for, 81–83
  changing environment or activity to promote, 82
  to cultural context, 78
  to educational programs with peers, 79–80
  to effective instruction and curriculum, 80
  essential considerations for, 78–81
  to extended school year services, 80
  to homebound services, 80
  legal right to, 24, 77
  to occupational therapy, 81
  occupational therapy education about, 38
  to personal context, 78
  to physical environment, 24, 79, 161–162, 299

to programs, 24
providing services on behalf or with student for, 82–83
reasonable modifications for, 77, 80–81
to school meals, 77, 80–81, 395
to social environment, 79
to temporal context, 78–79
to virtual context, 79
to vocational education, 77
see also universal design; universal design for learning
accommodation, 79, 342–345
  definition of, 343
  for emotional disturbance, 258
  for hearing impairment, 268–269
  for physical disability, 299
  Section 504, 223–225
    selection of, questions guiding, 223, *223*
  for specific learning disabilities, 310
  for visual perception, 494
accountability, 119
  see also program evaluation
Accreditation Council of Occupational Therapy Education (ACOTE), 36, 43, 48, 358
accreditation of private schools, 368
ACEs (adverse childhood experiences), 243
  see also trauma, childhood
acoustics, classroom, 268
activities
  changing, to promote access, 82
  definition of, 344
  enriched, 345
  intervention, 344–345
  as intervention, *16*
activities of daily living. *See* ADLs
activity analysis, 82, 389
activity-level evaluations, 476
activity modification, 82

actual work, 115
acute condition, 291
ADA (Americans With Disabilities Act of 1990), 24
ADA Amendments Act of 2008 (ADAAA), 24, 219
  access under, 77
  collaboration for access under, 93
  comparison with Section 504 and IDEA, 220–222, *221*
  definition of disability, 222
  postsecondary education under, 202, *203*
  transition under, 194
  transportation under, 177
ADA Information Line, 24
adaptive behavior, 272
Adaptive Behavior Assessment System, 391, 408
ADAS (advanced driver-assistance systems), 438
ADHD. *See* attention deficit hyperactivity disorder
ADHD Rating Scales, 230
adjustment to school, 187, 190
ADLs, 387–394
  activity or task analysis, 389
  assessing environment and context, 388–389
  assessment tools for, 517
  best practices for, 388–391
  coaching, 391
  collaborative goals for, 387–388
  context-focused therapy for, 389
  educating students, parents, and educational personnel on, 390–391
  essential considerations for, 387–388
  evaluation of, 388–389
  health conditions and, 388
  interventions for, 389–390
    altering environment, 390

Copyright © 2019 by the American Occupational Therapy Association. All rights reserved. To reuse this content, contact www.copyright.com.
https://doi.org/10.7139/2019.978-1-56900-591-0.Subject Index

Citation Index

Note: Page numbers in italics indicate figures, tables, and exhibits.

Copyright © 2019 by the American Occupational Therapy Association. All rights reserved. To reuse this content, contact www.copyright.com.
https://doi.org/10.7139/2019.978-1-56900-591-0.Citation Index